HOSPITALS
&
NURSING HOMES
Planning, Organisations & Management

The hospital is an integral part of social and medical organization. The function of which is to provide for the population complete healthcare, both curative and preventive, and whose outpatient services reach out to the family and its home environment; the hospital is also a centre for training of health workers and for biosocial research.

HOSPITALS
&
NURSING HOMES
Planning, Organisations & Management

Syed Amin Tabish

JAYPEE BROTHERS
MEDICAL PUBLISHERS (P) LTD.
New Delhi

Published by

Jitendar P Vij
Jaypee Brothers Medical Publishers (P) Ltd
EMCA House, 23/23B Ansari Road, Daryaganj
New Delhi 110 002, India
Phones: 23272143, 23272703, 23282021, 23245672, 23245683 Fax: 011-23276490
E-Mail: jpmedpub@del2.vsnl.net.in
Visit our website: http://www.jpbros.20m.com

Branches

- 202 Batavia Chambers, 8 Kumara Kruppa Road
  Kumara Park East, **Bangalore** 560 001, Phones: 2285971, 2382956
  Tele Fax: 2281761, e-mail: jaypeebc@bgl.vsnl.net.in
- 282 IIIrd Floor, Khaleel Shirazi Estate, Fountain Plaza
  Pantheon Road, **Chennai** 600 008, Phone: 28262665 Fax: 28262331
  e-mail: jpmedpub@md3.vsnl.net.in
- 4-2-1067/1-3, Ist Floor, Balaji Building, Ramkote Cross Road
  Hyderabad 500 095, Phones: 55610020, 24758498 Fax: 24758499
  e-mail: jpmedpub@rediffmail.com
- 1A Indian Mirror Street, Wellington Square
  Kolkata 700 013, Phone: 22451926 Fax: 22456075
  e-mail: jpbcal@cal.vsnl.net.in
- 106 Amit Industrial Estate, 61 Dr SS Rao Road
  Near MGM Hospital, Parel, **Mumbai** 400 012
  Phones: 24124863, 24104532 Fax: 24160828
  e-Mail: jpmedpub@bom7.vsnl.net.in

Hospitals and Nursing Homes: Planning, Organisations & Management

First Edition: **2003**

Reprinted 2005

ISBN 81-8061-154-X

Typeset at JPBMP typesetting unit
Printed at Gopsons Papers Ltd., A-14, Sector 60, Noida

To
my parents
(Syed Ghulamuddin and Syeda Zainab)
my wife (Farhat)
and my children
(Syed Abeer and Syed Nabil)
without whose inspiration and sacrifice
this work could not have materialised

Preface

This book has been developed so that those involved in planning, designing, building, and operating healthcare facilities can understand and appreciate all the work required to produce a facility that will be as reasonably safe and efficient as possible for staff to work in and for patients to be treated and housed in. This book provides the step-by-step process of planning and state-of-the-art design to achieve a viable facility to meet this objective. It covers the planning and design problems of hospitals with a deep insight.

A hospital is a community in which the interaction of individuals is fundamental to the successful working of the whole. The great depth of technical knowledge required for the design, enables the complexities to be brought together into a whole concept which respects the fundamental requirement, to build a community.

The process of planning, design and construction of hospitals involves the coordination of many groups and agencies on many levels. A endeavour has been made to sort out the many ingredients necessary to construct a hospital and presenting them in such a way that the whole process can be comprehended and showing how the multitude of requirements necessary in building a hospital can be satisfied (the order of topics).

Materials have been organised as much as possible in the order in which events occur.

Healthcare facility planning and construction could be the result of a growing population; an aged building becoming too aged; or a desire of benefactors to help others by contributing to the building of a hospital in memory of someone. The result is a decision by some group, administration, or agency to build a particular type of hospital in a certain location.

Even after construction, the operation of a hospital requires more surveillance because of the nature of its activities and its special occupants. Any modification, therefore, must be viewed with more than normal concern.

The process of planning, design and construction of a hospital has become a complicated one. These are building codes, fire codes, health codes, inspection agencies, certificates of need, certifications, licensure, accreditation—all in order to build a healthcare facility.

Balancing needs, desires, costs, and regulations, in the planning, design and construction of a hospital requires knowledge of a host of complicated and hospital care is a dynamic process. Architecture for health has to strive for shells for living, continuously changing organisms. Health facilities have, after being designed, built and commissioned, to be maintained, adapted to changing requirements and have also been modernised. This means architecture for health leads into planning which is continuously escorting the life and the operation of the facility.

Planning, organisation and management of healthcare facilities are more and more influenced by the rapid developments of information and computerisation. Modern informatics open up for us, new different possibilities in the functional and architectural composition of healthcare facilities, respectively.

Dealing with hi-tech medicine on the one hand, and with conditions of limited resources on the other, one has to become more conscious of the time factor. In planning under limited resources, adaptability to changing (and usually increasing) demands is indispensable if misinvestments are to be avoided.

We have to learn to think of setting limits and to design and organise for efficiency, economy and humanity.

This book presents new planning concepts and recent trends in the hospital architecture that ought to be thoroughly considered by hospital administrators and trustees in anticipation of their arduous work with architects, consultants, and responsible staff members over the problems involved in trying to make their buildings, as up-to-date as possible to accommodate the current technology and as adjustable as possible for the new, revised, or expanded functions that they will be expected to house in the future.

The aim of this book is to introduce the reader to some of the basic ideas and research in hospital planning, design, construction, organisation and management. Each chapter of the book deals with a particular topic beginning with a theoretical framework from which the subject could be approached. I hope that the book will be particularly relevant for administrators or chief executive officers of a facility and their staff; healthcare facility board members; building committees; medical facility plant engineers; healthcare architects, designers; and engineers; contractors; financial advisors; business, economics, architecture, hospital administration students who plan to enter the healthcare field; and medical and nursing personnel who are responsible for the planning, organising and management of a healthcare facility.

This book is useful particularly for clinical directors/head of the clinical and paraclinical departments; unit managers; in-charge of service departments, laboratories and patient care areas. All therapeutic and diagnostic facilities have been discussed in detail with extraordinary emphasis on nursing zone, clinical zone, support zone and utility services.

An endeavour has been made to place under one cover a lot of material that heretofore was scattered throughout various books, articles, and documents to make it the most comprehensive treatment of this subject to date.

I am extremely grateful to Mr RK Yadav, Director Publishing, M/s Jaypee Brothers Medical Publishers, for his unswerving dedication, commitment and conviction of courage to advance medical knowledge by encouraging promising authors to put their ideas into action.

Syed Amin Tabish

Contents

Part-one
Healthcare Facility Planning: Past, Present and Future

Part-two

Hospital: Design and Development

From "An" Idea to "The " Idea

Design and Construction

Part-three
Hospital Administration

Health is a social value. This is reflected in provision of services, which need to consider ethical and philosophical issues as well as medical-scientific and medical-behavioral issues. Concern for the care of the human being as a whole in the hospital needs contribution of all the human services.

The Hospital should reflect the rhythm of the local culture, civilization and historical heritage and simultaneously be flexible enough to accommodate modern methods of health-care facilities.

The planning of any segment of the health service system should be determined by and shaped around the life patterns and value systems of the population to be served.

Part One

Healthcare Facility Planning: Past, Present and Future

✍ Growth

✍ Planning

✍ Emerging Approaches

✍ Recent Trends

1 The Art and Science of Medicine

Health is a social value. This is reflected in provision of services, which need to consider ethical and philosophical issues as well as medical-scientific and medical-behavioral issues.

Medicine and other subjects associated with health have a fascinating story, reaching far into the past, and progressing with increasing speed after innumberable false starts and tragic disappointments.

Medicine deals with health and disease. Four phases are discernible in its history: (1) primitive ignorance and superstition with resulting fear of disease; (2) accumulation of experience in managing disease, culminating in a professional group specially trained in ministering to the sick; (3) gradual growth of verifiable knowledge of the causes of illness, with recent application to the prevention of disease; and now (4), with knowledge applied to the control of disease, the effort to promote optimum health places emphasis on preventive rather than curative medicine.

There have been more advances in medicine in the past 100 years (twenty-first century) than in the 500 years before that, and that there were more advances in that 500 years than in the previous 5000 years. The twenty-first century may prove to be the golden age of medicine. The result of all this progress has been added years to the life and life to the years of the individual. The twentieth century has been a period of revolutionary change in medical therapy. Before 1900, there were few drugs which were specific treatment for specific diseases. However, the drug industry has become one of the largest industries. Today, the strength and purity of drugs are rigidly standardized. Much of the research that goes into discovery of new drugs is carried on by the drug industry. After a new substance has proved useful in treatment, the drug companies use their individual skills to make the drug available at a practical price.

Development of a strong public health system involving immunization, early warnings of epidemics and quarantine has greatly reduced the threat of worldwide pandemics. The prime weapon in prevention is vaccine for children. Viral vaccine development has progressed most since 1930's after a yellow fever vaccine, which was produced by Max Theiler.

With the development of measures to prevent and treat surgical shock, and measures to prevent infection made possible by the antimicrobial, many surgical operations that were not attempted in the previous century, are being performed routinely now-a-days.

Open heart surgery, surgery of brain, organ transplantation (kidney, liver, cornea, heart, pancreas, etc) hip and joint replacement, advances in plastic surgery, fetal surgery, minimal access (keyhole) surgery, bone marrow transplantation, prosthetics (Artificial limbs), telemedicine, molecular genetic interventions in vitro fertilization, etc.have also been introduced in the twenty-first century.

Advances in radiodiagnosis, imaging and nuclear medicine ultrasonography, CT Scan, magnetic resonance imaging, digital subtraction angiography, positron emission tomography, C-arm fluoroscope, color doppler, tread mill, cardiac catheterization, angiography, laparoscopy, fibrotic endoscopy, lithotriopsy, ERCP, linear accelerator, the cobalt therapy machine, gamma camera, computerized treatment planning system, brachytherapy, gamma knife,etc. have revolutionized diagnostic facilities. Laboratory medicine has also flourished. The advent of electron microscopy, multichannel auto-analyzers, spectrophotometers, etc. are of a great help to the clinician.

Advance in anesthesia (like ventilators, potent and safe anesthetic agents), psychiatry, pharmaceuticals, nephrology (dialysis), hematology, telemedicine, medical laser immunology, monoclonal antibodies, immunology the mapping of the human genome, cloning and preparation of various parts of human body, etc. have substantially reduced the mortality.

Medicine of the recent decades has been faced with rapid experience of biophysics, bioengineering, biomathematics, molecular biology and the integration of skills of the biologist and the engineer. The application of energy sources such as ultrasonic laser light beam, radioactive energy and heat-sensitive crystals, is reflected in the automatic sampling and analysis of body fluids, monitoring for critical care, artificial organs, prosthetic devices, physical therapies and computer technology. When properly performed, for the right reasons and at the right time, surgery ranks as the uppermost echelon of effectiveness in medicine.

A hospital is an integral part of a social and medical organization. The function of which is to provide for the population complete health care both preventive and curative and whose outpatient services reach out to the family and its home environment; the hospital is also a center for biosocial research (WHO).

Hospitals arouse strong emotions. Doctors, nurses, paramedics remembering the excitement of their early training years, associate hospitals with youth, vigor and the possibilities presented by a new career. The heady mixture of large numbers of young men and women exploring new ideas together remains as an affectionate memory with most medical professionals for the rest of their working lives.

For the general public the perception is different. Most people fear the prospect of entering a hospital, even as a visitor. This is ultimately, because numbers of people who enter hospitals die there. Hospitals have an alien feel for most members of the general public, which is not understood by people who work in them.

Health is a fundamental human right, the essence of productive life, an integral part of development and central to the concept of quality of life.

Culture, Health and Illness

To the members of all societies, the human body is more than just a physical organism, fluctuating between health and illness. It is also the focus of a set of beliefs about its social and psychological significance, its structure and function. The body image (used to describe all the ways that an individual conceptualises, and experience, his or her body), then, is something acquired by every individual as part of growing up in a particular family or society. The body image is influenced by social and cultural background and can have important effects on the health of the individual.

In most societies people suffering from physical discomfort or emotional distress have a number of ways of helping themselves or of seeking help from other people. Within these societies there are many groups or individuals, each offering the patient their own particular way of explaining, diagnosing and treating ill health. To the ill person the efficacy of the health care system in relieving suffering is important.

In most countries, scientific medicine is the basic of the professional sector, which comprises the organised, legally sanctioned healing professions such as allopathy.

The dominant system of health care of any society cannot be studied in isolation from other aspects of that society, because the medical system or professional sector of health care does not exist in a social or cultural vacuum. Rather, it is an expression of and to some extent a miniature model of the values and social structure of the society from which it arises. Different types of societies therefore, depending on their dominant ideology, produce different types of medical system, and different attitudes to health and illness. One society may see free (or relatively inexpensive) health care as a basic right of citizenship, or the basic right only of the very poor or the very old, while another may see medical care as a commodity to be bought only by those who can afford it. In the latter case, the pursuit of profits in health care will exclude many of the poorer members of society who do not have the resources to pay for it. Whatever the type of society, the medical system not only reflects these basic values and ideologies, but in turn helps also to shape and maintain them.

In most countries, the main institutional structure of scientific medicine is the hospital. The ill person is removed from family, friends and community at a time of personal crisis. In hospital they undergo a standardized ritual of depersonalization' becoming converted into a numbered 'case' in a ward full of strangers. The emphasis is on their physical disease, with little reference to their home environment, religion, social relationships, moral status, or the meaning they give to their ill health. Hospital specialization ensures that they are classified, and allocated to different wards, on the basis of age (adults, pediatrics, geriatrics), gender (male, female), condition (medical, surgical or other), organ or system involved (neurosurgery cardiology), or severity (intensive care units, accident and emergency departments). Patients of the same sex, similar age range and similar illness often share a ward. All of them have been stripped of the props of social identity and individuality, and clothed in a uniform of pajamas, nightdress or bathrobe. There is a loss of control over one's body, and over personal space, privacy, behavior, diet and use of time. Patients are removed from the continuous emotional support of 'family and community, and cared for by healers whom they may never have seen before. In hospitals, the relationship of health professionals, doctors, nurses, technicians with their patients is largely characterized by distance, formality, brief conversations and often the use of professional jargon. Hospitals have been seen as 'small societies'; with their own implicit and explicit rules of behavior. Patients in a ward form a 'temporary community of suffering' linked together by commiseration, ward gossip, and discussions of one another's condition. The health involves individual, state, and international responsibilities and is worldwide social goal. Health care refers to a multitude of services rendered to individuals, families or communities by the agents of health services or professions, for the purpose of promoting, maintaining, monitoring or restoring health.

Medical care refers chiefly to those personal services that are provided directly by the physician or rendered as a measure of physician's instructions.

The hospital should reflect the rhythm of the local culture, civilization and historical heritage and simultaneously be flexible enough to accommodate modern methods of health care facilities.

A hospital building, being an embodiment of life, should be conceived as a living entity where from follows function. A building without comfort, safety, and inviting quality, peace, silence, beauty and proper atmosphere has no significance as architecture.

The art and science of medicine, concerned with man as man, requires pleasant and peaceful environment that will restore the dignity of a man who has lost his own in the operation theatre or other patient care area.

Medical Care

Medical Care cannot be separated from the buildings in which it is delivered. The quality of space in such buildings affects the outcome of medical care, and architectural design is thus an important part of the healing process.

Hospitals are spaces for healing. Their functional and spatial requirements differ from those of other public buildings. Yet, because of the technical complexity of hospitals and their immense cost, optimal orientation, scale, and symbolic meaning are often not achieved. It is possible to provide both successful function and good architecture by listening to patients (suggestions from patients are critical to designing spaces that enable patients to heal). This patient-centered approach is part of a larger movement towards involving patients in the healing process. Hospitals also improve by learning from their experience. Good architecture can be created in expansion or renovation projects, as well as in new facilities.

Many of the qualities of space that are pleasing in hospitals are fundamental to good design in all types of buildings. In this regard a well-designed hospital reflects the art and skill of architects in the practice of their craft. A balance between function and anesthetics is essential.

It is of increasing importance for hospital buildings and facilities to be available in such quality and quantity as these will permit and indeed promote all reasonable economies without denying any applicant the immediate benefit of the multiplying improvements in patient care.

The language of medical care can influence legislation, philanthropy, trusteeship, medical practice, and all else that makes up the hospital effort on the planning or operational level. The word hospital must be defined workably before the job of functional planning is begun.

The hospital is an indispensable communal institution, brought into existence in response to an environmental need. The hospital is maintained for the centralized, collective, sheltered, expert care of the sick who cannot, or should not be cared for anywhere else.

There must be an understanding of the methods by which the variables in a programme can be isolated, evaluated, and reflected in the final building plan, all in proportion to their relative importance. This calls for full knowledge of the functional programme and of the whole planning process. A competent architect can design any space if he knows what is to be done in the space, what persons are expected to do it and what special equipment and physical conditions are required. The architect has to meet the challenge of satisfying the highly demanding functional requirements and still to create a beautiful building.

Challenges

In addition to the share size and complexity of its technical planning problems, hospital design presents a challenge to administrator, hospital consultant and architects. The design has to have sufficient clarity of form to be understood by all who use it.

No matter how complex a hospital may be, its map must be easy to understand by all its users. Each separate department needs its own identity and within it, its own map, its own public and private spaces as well as its own front door. The hospital must be designed so as to allow the identity of the many 'families ' which form its work force to be identifiable, physically, from inside the complex. Hospital should be designed as a complex with separate parts, just as a village is constructed of separate, identifiable buildings. A hospital needs to absorb change, as a continuous process of change occurs throughout its life, which causes modification to be made to each of the individual departments.

The physical form of the hospital will change over a period of time as it responds to internal and external forces and will acquire complexity as it ages. The architect must bring order to the process of change by designing the building round a binding center. The architect must design a street system, locate the front doors and allow the inhabitants of each of the departments to effect the changes required to serve changing functions without distorting the image of the whole.

Different patients have different needs, and different clinicians have different methods of treating their patients. This freedom of method of choice must be preserved.

Complexity and a high degree of technical mechanization have often been mistaken for qualitative superiority. Modern medicine, with its emphasis on technology and specialization, is threatening to dehumanize hospital care. Increased specialisation in hospitals has led to a form of alienation from the border aims of the health service. Hospital care must be rehumanised. Concern for the care of the human beings in a whole as the hospital needs contribution of all the human sciences.

The medical need is a matter of judgment and not an absolute state. Patients generally desire convenient access to immediate, considerate, and knowledgeable medical care, which should also be comprehensive, co-ordinated and continuous. The planning of any segment of the health service system should be determined by and shaped around the life patterns and value systems of the population to be served.

The availability of medical personnel and economic resources have to be analyzed to make an efficient medical and social service possible. Trained personnel, material resources, and all other forms and measures of help to the patient should be coordinated, so that the assistance could be delivered rapidly and competently. Objective criteria are needed for establishing each patients diagnosis and the status of his condition when he enters the health care system.

Every citizen should be able to enter the healthcare system within reasonable time at any time and, with the certainty that the appropriate level of care for him is available.

The hospitals should invariably be designed in support of the needs of the health centers and other healthcare units rendering primary care at the peripheral level.

The hospital with its specialized facilities and staff has to limit itself to the functions that cannot be performed elsewhere, channeling a number of functions to a closely associated, carefully planned, less expensive satellite facility network and not to divert scarce resources to uses for which they are not needed.

Hospitalization ought to be reserved to the greatest extent for patients whose conditions require highly qualified staff and complicated apparatus, whereby the quality levels of hospitals and other healthcare facilities have to be made distinct.

In the effort to assign the patient to a service area according to the extent of care required, six elements have been introduced: critical care, intermediate care, self-care, long-term care, home care, and ambulatory (outpatient)care. The inpatient care has three broad levels: critical or intensive, intermediate and minimal.

Specialist hospitals promote high standards. The fact that the staff deal only with a small range of disease, leads to their developing special skills.

The categorization and differentiation of hospitals on the availability of medical expertise and proper use of facilities will most likely become a major healthcare planning feature.

Hospital Planning

An efficient hospital requires a well-balanced organization for compassionate care within an adequate technical and environmental framework.

In the field of hospital planning three quite distinct worlds—the ordinary physical world; the mental world; and the world of actual or possible objects of thought, the world of concepts, ideas, theories, arguments and explanation are clearly felt.

The hospital works under the control of two distinct boundary systems; the higher one is the hospital organization, which harnesses the lower one, which in itself consists in several levels of functions and functional procedures on which the success of the hospital depends. Each level is relying for its working on the level above it.

Planning involves and requires understanding and evaluation of the current cultural mainstreams, the economic and technological conditions, and the goals of the community.

Total project cost considerations are planning, financing, construction, and equipment. The equipment costs alone account for about 30 percent of the total.

The hospital planning process concentrates on the designing of buildings and their architectural appearance and devotes inadequate attention to the planning of organizations and equipment as well as accommodating them and generating spaces to meet policies. The long-term cost of operating a hospital can be greatly increased by the initial failure to plan proper systems and equipment.

The objectives of hospital planning should be fully understood. The implications of planning ideas, data and designs, when they progress from the idea to a staffed and maintained hospital should be predictable.

A hospital emerges in three interdependent processes: analysis-planning-programming, designing and construction. Maximum efficiency should be sought for every precise function. The known depths of all involved factors have to be viewed at from a proper angle simultaneously and synthetically. The concurrent requirements of complex systems have to be assembled and balanced.

To secure a good facility, during the initial period of planning the main medical, ecologic, managerial, economic, social demographic, and technological factors and possibilities have to be identified.

Planners and architects must also take into account existing and emerging trends (that shape the health facilities) for the provision of health care. Technologies can be created to satisfy recognized demands. The basic decisions to be taken concern the character, the size and the siting of the hospital as well as the degree of the hospital's adaptability to future developments.

The programme should include the facts, intentions, and assumptions about the organization stated so early that a facility can be drawn from it. It is important to dress the hierarchy of the requirements, necessities and solutions. A functional programme can be used to clarify terminology, common understanding, and agreement among the parties involved. The programme is a reference to original intent for years to come, and is also an instrument to determine the staffing levels for selection of equipment and thus may serve as a means for organization of capital and labour.

The value of a brief should be measured by how well the strategic lines along which the hospital can be designed, are specified.

In a dynamic programme, the criteria for the physical design and the qualitative requirements on the medical standard and other standards should represent a range of realistic variables, the assignment of priorities, and the phase mode if such is a value.

The final phase consists of an explicit description of the hospital at a chosen point in time. The care needs of patients should directly dictate the character of every care function throughout the hospital.

FURTHER READING

1. Helman, Cecil: Culture, Health and Illness: An introduction for Health professionals, 2nd edn. Butterworth & Co. London 1990.
2. Norman Vetter: The Hospital: from the centre of excellence to community support. Chapman & Hall. London 1995.

2 The Hospital

Since many health problems require a level of medical treatment and personal care that extends beyond the range of services normally available in the patient's home or in the physician's office, modern society has developed formal institutions for patient care intended to help meet the more complex health needs of its members. The hospital, the major social institution for the delivery of health care in the modern world, offers considerable advantages to both patient and society. From the standpoint of the individual, the sick or injured person has access to centralized medical knowledge and technology that will render treatment which is thorough and efficient from the standpoint of society, hospitalization both protects the family from many of the disruptive and injured into medically supervised institutions where their problems are less disruptive for society as a whole.

The Hospital as a Social Institution

The development of hospitals as institutions providing medical services for the general public proceeded in pace with the prevailing needs, beliefs, values and attitudes of the societies they served. Historically, hospitals had passed through four distinct phases of development (1) as centers of religious practice; (2) as poor houses; (3) as death-houses; and (4) as centers of medical technology.

Hospitals as Centers of Religious Practice

Although the Romans were the first to establish separate medical facilities (for economic and military reasons) which had been described as hospitals, the origin of the institution we know today as the hospital has usually been associated with the rise of Christianity. Christian theology emphasized that human beings were duty-bound to provide assistance to the sick and needy; this belief was reinforced by the notion that spiritual salvation could be obtained by whoever provided such a service. Consequently, the Roman Catholic Church encouraged its Clergy to found hospitals and to localate these hospitals near churches as an intergral feature of Christian religious endeavour. Further more, during the period of the Crusades between 1096 and 1291, many hospitals were established along the routes taken to the Holy Land by the Christian armies. Secular benefactors such as kings, queens and other members of the nobility, wealthy merchants, artisan and craftsmen's guilds, and municipalities also founded hospitals. By the end of the fifteenth century, an extensive network of hospitals was known to have existed throughout Western Europe.

The medieval Hospital, however, was not a hospital by any modern standard. True, these hospitals were community centers for the care of the lower-class sick; yet the medical care, supervised and largely performed by clergy and nuns, consisted primarily of a rudimentary form of nursing. The primary functions of the medieval hospital were the exercise of religious practices and the extension of charity and welfare services to the poor, including both the able-bodied and the sick. These early hospitals, therefore, provided a wide spectrum of social tasks for the benefit of the lower classes, especially the provision of food, shelter, sanctuary and prayer as well as nursing.

During the Renaissance and the Reformation, the religious character of the hospital began to disappear as increasing numbers of hospitals were placed under the jurisdiction of secular authorities. Nevertheless, three basic features of the modern hospital are derived from the influence of the Church. First, the concept of a service oriented toward helping others has become a guiding principle for the manner in which hospital personnel are required to approach their work. Second, hospitals are supposed to have a "universallistic" approach. That is, to accept for treatment of all people who may be sick or injured, And third, the custodial nature of hospital care has been facilitated by housing patients within the confines of a single location.

Hospitals as Poorhouses

The secular control of hospitals marked a period of decline for the development of Europe's hospital system. Even though monks and nuns continued to work in hospitals, the removal of the centralized authority of the Church left hospitals under many separate administrations, usually those of municipal governments. Without general regulations pertaining to hospital administration, individual hospitals were free to pursue any course of action they desired. This situation encouraged abuse, particularly in regard to neglect of facilities, misappropriation of funds, and the lowering of prevailing standards of patient care. In England the suppression of the monastery system in the mid-1500 led to the collapse of the English hospital system as many hospitals, left without personnel or money, were forced to close down. The few remaining hospitals limited their services to people who were actually sick and who could be cured. While this policy relegated the poor, both the incurably ill and the able-bodies, to poorhouses or to the streets for their support, it marked the beginning of a new definition of hospitals as institutions active in curing the sick and injured so that they could return to society.

However, by the end of the sixteenth century, the economic and social conditions of the poor worsened to a considerable degree. Unemployment, higher prices, and the loss of land created a serious problem of vagrancy throughout Europe. Many vagrants claimed to be sick or crippled, and they crowded wherever hospital facilities were available. In accordance with the new definition of social welfare as a community rather that a church responsibility, measures were eventually taken by city and national authorities to provide public assistance. Many hospitals were reopened, but they soon acquired the characteristics of boarding houses because they offered food and shelter to the poor, regardless of whether they were sick or healthy. Those persons living in hospitals who could work were required to pay for their lodging, while hospitals became little more than social "warehouses" where invalids, the aged, orphans, and the mental ly defective could be sent and thus removed from the mainstream of society. Even today in the United States, people with chronic health problems requiring long-term hospitalization—the insane, the incurable, and individuals suffering from highly infectious diseases tend to be sent to public institutions, while private hospitals tend to accept patients with acute disorders.

Hospitals as Death Houses

Following the Renaissance and the Reformation, the outward character of hospitals appeared to change very little from that of a public institution whose purpose was to provide welfare services for the lower social classes on behalf of the communi ties in which they were located. Nonetheless, changes were taking place as physicians discovered that hospitals contained large numbers of sick and injured (and also generally powerless) people whose health problems could be studied and upon whom the various evolving techniques of medical treatment could be practiced.

Physicians had first begun to associate themselves with hospitals during the fourteenth century; initially they had little influence because they were not members of the hospital staff and provided their services on a purely voluntary basis. By the seventeenth century, however, physicians acquired a virtual monopoly over the existing body of medical knowledge that placed them in the position of first advising and eventually directing all patient care within the hospital. As physicians became increasingly influential, non-medical hospital tasks gradually disappeared. By the early nineteenth century, hospitals had clearly assumed their present-day role as institutions for medical care, for medical research, and for the education of medical students.

Although medical treatment was recognized as the primary function of the hospital in the eighteenth century, the primitive level of that treatment produced few cures. Trained physicians were unable to achieve consistent results with their techniques and accordingly, neither they nor hospitals were held in high esteem in the general population. Because very few patients survived treatment despite occasional heroic efforts, hospitals acquired an image as places where the poor went to die.

The high death rate in hospitals was also related to appalling living conditions provided to the patients. Typically, hospitals were dirty, poorly ventilated, and filled to capacity. Often more than one patient was placed in a single bed regardless of the patient's disorder, and treatment was usually carried out publicly in the ward itself. Surgery was limited at that time mostly to amputations and childbirth, plus the purging of fevers with various options bloodletting to eliminate "excess" blood, and the removal of the dead all occurred in the same general area where patients ate and slept. Nor did the attending physicians and surgeons practice even the most rudimentary standards of sanitation, moving from bed to bed and treating great variety of disorders, including those who were infectious, without washing their hands or changing their clothes. Thus, it is not surprising that hospitals were regarded by most people as place where only the lower social classes went to die.

Hospitals as Centers of Medical Technology

Since the end of the nineteenth century, a new image of hospitals evolved as institutions where patients of all social classes could generally expect to find the highest quality medical care and could reasonably expect to be cured of their disorders. Three major factors were responsible for this change. First was the fact that medicine had indeed become a science in terms of employing the scientific method to seek out accurate medical knowledge. and to develop successful techniques that could be employed in a consistent manner. Of particular importance was increased knowledge about human physiology and the development of the science of bacteriology; also important was the perfection of either as an anesthetic, which allowed surgery to be performed in a relatively painless fashion. Since the new medical technology required extensive and often expensive facilities, these facilities were centralized in hospitals so that they could be available to most physicians. Hospitals eventually became places where physician also referred their upper- and middle-class patients, since the most advanced medical technology was located there. While the poor generally remained in charity status as hospital patients, a new type of patient came into being—private patient—who required private accommodations, usually had a private physician, and who paid for hospital services.

A second important factor, concomitant with the development of medical technology, was the discovery and use of antiseptic measures in the hospital to help curtail infection. Hospitals were not only properly cleaned and ventilated, but patients with infectious diseases were isolated in special areas of the hospital, and hospital staff members were required to wash their hands and change their clothing after working with these patients. The use of such items as surgical masks, rubber gloves, and sterilized surgical instruments became common place. These procedures not only reduced the number of deaths among hospital patients, but also reduced the amount of time required for patient's recovery.

Third, there was a significant improvement in the quality of hospital personnel. Especially important was the entry on the scene of the trained nurse and the laboratory technician, whose specialized skills were able to support the physician in his or her primary role of diagnostician and practitioner. In the twentieth century, the hospital became the major institutional resource available to society for coping with problem of health and illness.

Modern Hospital

The hospital is an integral part of a social and medical organisation, the function of which is to provide for the population complete health care, both curative and preventive, and whose outpatient services reach out to the family and its home environment; the hospital is also a centre for the training of health workers and for biosocial research.

The hospital can be defined as an institution whose primary function is the provision of a variety of diagnostic and therapeutic services to patients, both in the hospital and in outpatient clinics. It is the umbrella organization under which many individual health care professionals provide some or all of their services. More than 30 disciplines are represented in most hospitals, each having its own professional structure, body of knowledge, code of ethics, and technical procedures. A hospital is also a social institution, dealing daily with a broad panorama of human hopes, fears, and concerns, Finally, a hospital is a business, responsible for the efficient, cost-effective provision of a wide range of services.

Functions

The universal function of the hospital is patient care. In addition, many hospitals also have a commitment to the education of health professionals, biomedical research, and community outreach services.

Patient Care

A hospital's primary concern is the patient in need of health care services. These may include diagnosis, treatment, rehabilitation, and preventive care. In the past, care was often centered primarily on the hospitalized patient. Today, hospitals provide many services for the outpatient or ambulatory patient who receives services without spending the night in the hospital. Patient care is usually directed by physicians. Physicians are assisted by hospital staff consisting of a wide variety of health care professionals. Because of this unique arrangement for delivering a service, hospitals, and physicians are truly partners in the provision of health care.

Education

The medical and nursing professions have historically depended on hospitals for clinical training and education. Today, ancillary and paramedical personnel also receive much of their education in hospitals. Written affiliation agreements with teaching institutions commit hospitals to support the education programmes and are usually very specific with regard to these sources and opportunities to be provided for continuing education opportunities for their own personnel.

Research

Some hospitals, particularly those with educational affiliations, regard research as an important function of the institution. These hospitals coordinate the work of the scientist and clinician to promote the development of research that may be applied to the practice of medicine.

Community Outreach Services

In the largest sense, hospitals are community servants, responding to the health care needs and desires of the surrounding community. Recently, hospitals have taken a more active role in community service through outreach programmes, promotion of good health habits, and emphasis on preventive medicine.

Classification of Hospitals

Hospitals can be classified according to various criteria, including length of stay, types of services offered, control or ownership, levels of care and the institution's teaching or non-teaching role.

Short-term, or acute care, hospitals are those in which the average stay is relatively short. Institutions such as nursing homes and rehabilitation hospitals are defined as long-term. Psychiatric hospitals often fall into this category as well.

Types of services offered include general, psychiatric, raehabilitation, pediatric, tuberculosis, maternity, and other specialized care, some hospitals specialize in only one type of service. Others offer a variety of services.

Type of control or ownership is another criterion for classifying hospitals: voluntary, non-profit institutions, including community hospitals and those affiliated with church groups, religious orders and fraternal orders; proprietary, which means they are operated for profit and privately owned, either by a small group or by corporations with stockholders, those owned by state or local governments and operated by the federal government (Table 2.1).

"Levels of care" refers to a relatively new concept that involves the type of disease treated, the level of training of the physician treating the disease, and the facilities and services necessary to support the physician. Levels of care include primary (basic), secondary (specialized), and tertiary (highly specialized) care.

Table 2.1: Hospital classifications

Clinical	Ownership and control
General medical and surgical	Governmental
Speciality	Army, Navy, Vetrans
Internal medicine	Administration public health service
Psyehiatric and nervous disease	State
Tuberculosis	County
Communicable disease	City
Pediatrics	Non-government
Surgery	Private for profit
Orthopaedic	Non Profit
Gynaecologic	Church
Otolaryngologic	Fraternal order
Maternity	Community
Length of stay	Non-profit private
Short-term	By accreditation*
Long-term (Chronic)	Accredited
Custodial (Long-term)	Non-accredited

* Joint commission on accrediation of hospitals

What are teaching hospitals. A major teaching hospital is one which is used extensively for the clinical instruction of medical school students. A minor teaching hospital is used only for a limited number of student instruction, such as occasional demonstrations or clinics.

Traditionally teaching hospitals are places where the new medical graduates seek postgraduate training. They almost always undergo 1 year of hospital training as an intern. They may frequently spend 2 or more additional years in a hospital as a resident in some speciality, such as internal medicine, surgery, pediatrics or radiology.

Industry also recognizes the importance of the teaching hospital by virtue of the special coverage it receives from the company's medical service representatives as well as its desire to financially support both educational and research programmes.

Because teaching hospitals act as referral centres for the more seriously ill patient, third party payers have been, in recent years, reimbursing these hospitals at a higher rate than small suburban institutions with no special programmes for the care of these cases.

Mostly young physicians entering practices look for locations in a teaching hospital because such institutions assure them of the most contemporary educational opportunities coupled with broad experiences in the clinical care of patients, teaching and research.

Statistical Indicators

Hospital size or activity is commonly described by using a variety of statistical indicators. Each hospital calculates its individual statistics. Monthly and annual averages are published in various statistical sources.

Number of Beds

The number of beds is often used as an overall indicator of size, services, and occupancy, A hospital bed" is defined as one that is available for 24-hour occupancy by inpatients during their period of hospitalization.

Inpatient Admissions

These statistics include number of admissions, average length of stay, and number of patient days. Inpatient statistics are a key indicator of hospital use.

Outpatient Visits

The number of outpatient visits have recently assumed increased importance. It points to a national trend towards greater use of clinics for certain conditions and procedures, primarily as a less-expensive alternative to inpatient care.

Procedures

The number of procedures, such as tests, X-rays or treatments, of clinical services is a standard gross indicator of volume in these areas.

Hospital Requirements and Standards

Hospitals standards are the basic minimum requirements for health care institutions some standards are mandatory, such as those established by federal and state agencies. Others are voluntary, such as those developed by associations or voluntary review bodies.

Licensure

In most states, the law requires hospitals to be licensed, usually by the state's health department. The purpose of a state's licensing law is to "further protect the public health through the development and enforcement of standards for the care of individuals in hospitals, and for the construction, maintenance, and operating of hospitals". Such a licensing law is usually accompanied by state hospital regulations, which may detail such requirements as sanitary and safety regulations. Hospitals may also be bound by local municipal ordinance that provide another check on the quality of care and facilities.

Accreditation

The Joint Commission on Accreditation of Hospitals (JCAH) is an independent, volunteer, not-for-profit organization formed in 1951 in the USA to develop quality standards for hospitals. Any hospital may request evaluation by the JCAH. The evaluation is done for a fee by a survey team that "measure" the hospital's services organization, and governance against a set of published standards.

These standards are periodically reviewed and revised by the JCAH.

Accreditations awarded for a period of three years to hospitals that comply with the JCAH standards. While JCAH accreditation is voluntary, it is widely recognized and highly desirable.

Other Standards

To be eligible to receive reimbursement for medicare and medicaid patients in the USA, a hospital must meet minimum standards of care as spelled out in the Medicare regulations. Also, most professional associations have developed standards for hospitals that provide clinical facilities for use in teaching programmes. These standards spell out the minimum requirements that must be met for the hospital to affiliate with the teaching programme.

The Hospital-Patient Role

While hospital services are oriented towards a supportive notion of patient welfare, hospital rules and regulations are generally designed for the benefit of hospital personnel so that the work of treating large numbers of patients can be more efficient and easier to perform. Consequently, the sick and the injured are organized into various patient categories (maternity-obstetrics, neurology, cardiology, orthopedics, urology, pediatrics, psychiatry) that reflect the medical staff's definition of their disorder and are then usually subject to standardized, staff-approved medical treatment and administrative procedures.

While it can be argued that standardizing patient care results in increased organizational efficiency and ultimately serves in the best interest of the patient—a prominent theme of the hospitalization experience noted by medical sociologists has been that of depersonalization. Patients in general tend to be devalued by hospital personnel even before they are admitted to the hospital because they are old, sick, or defective in some way. In other words, hospital patients are more than just dependent upon other people, but they are also less than "ideal".

Personnel in hospitals do not necessarily have the express goal of making their patients feel depersonalized, but the organization of the hospital's work does favour rules and regulations that reduce patient autonomy and encourage patient receptivity of the hospital routine. Another important factor is the work situation itself. Nurses who had difficulty tolerating the work in intensive or coronary care hospital units felt oppressed by "repetitive exposure to death and dying, daily contact with mutilated and unsightly patients, formidable and demanding work loads, limited work space, intricate machinery, and communication problems involving physicians, staff, and families". The intensive care ward is thus an example of a work situation that generates pressures of a dehumanizing nature as a result of staff attempts to cope with inherently intense psychological stress. Furthermore, on the surgical wards patients are so concerned about themselves that if the nurses do take a personal interest in them, they demand increasing amounts of the nurses' time and energy.

Yet it should be noted that the process of depersonalization is not just a result of the manner in which large numbers of patients are managed or the work conditions, but it is also related to the patient's subjective experience of feeling sick. Most reports of depersonalization commonly cite the experience of one's self as a physical object or thing. A second common experience is the feeling that one's own psychological self is isolated from other psychological selves (other people). Further more, bodily symptoms such as pain can create a sense of separation within the individual of the physical self from the conscious psychological self. This inner alienation, in addition to the feeling of isolation from others, compounded by the doubt, uncertainty, and confusion that often accompany feelings of illness, can create for patients a sense of inadequacy and inability to control their lives. This attitude of incompetence is further intensified by the patient's having to assume an institutional role like the sick role, in which he or she is officially depended and excluded from decision making. The process of depersonalization is undoubtedly enhanced by the need of the physician or nurse to have access to the patient's body. No matter how legitimate this may be, the exposure and giving over of one's body to strangers can be degrading and humiliating experience, though it is intended to be therapeutic.

Patients are alienated from their usual lives and reduced to a largely impersonal status in the hospital through three basic mechanisms of hospital processing: (1) stripping, (2) control of resources, and (3) restriction of mobility. When patients present themselves for treatment in a hospital, they bring with them a particular social identity, this represents their attitudes, beliefs, values, concept of self, and social status, all of which form the basis for their manner of presenting themselves to the world. Stripping occurs when the hospital systematically divests the person of these past representations of self. The patient's clothes are taken away and replaced with a set of pajamas; regardless of whether the pajamas are the property of the hospital or the patient. The simple fact of wearing pajamas serves as a uniform that identifies that person as sick and restricts movements to those areas of the hospital in which pajamas (patient dress) are authorized. Personal belongings of value are taken away and locked up for safekeeping by the staff. Visiting regulations control not only when patients are allowed to have visitors, but also who is allowed to visit. In addition, the staff supervises the patient's diet, decides when the patient should be asleep or awake, and in essence controls the general conduct of the patient's social life in the hospital. The hospital routine for one patient is very similar to the routine of others having the same or similar health problems.

Another important feature of hospitalization is the control of resources by the staff. Code includes under the control of resources not only physical items, like bedclothes and toilet paper, but also the control of information about the patient's medical condition. For example, patients are normally not aware of their prognosis or the results of laboratory tests and X-rays unless the physician decides to inform them. On such occasions doctors and nurses will even deliberately limit communication with patients discovering their mistakes and shortcomings. A major complaint of patients including patients who were dying is the difficulty they have in obtaining information about themselves from their doctors.

In general, all patients are entitled to full knowledge about their medical condition, and it is incumbent upon the doctor to help them cope with this information. The denial of this information contributes to a sense of uncertainty among patients and lessens their perceived ability to control their own lives.

The third aspect of depersonalization is the restriction of mobility. In most hospitals, patients are not allowed to leave their wards without the permission of the head nurse, who is usually required to know the location of all patients at all times, when patients do leave the ward to travel to another area of the hospital, they are generally accompanied by a nurse, nurse's aide, or orderly, when patients are admitted to the hospital and also when discharged, they are taken in a wheelchair between the ward and the hospital entrance regardless of their ability to walk because the hospital is 'responsible' for them whenever they are inside its walls. The result is that even the ability of patients to move about is supervised and controlled.

JOINT COMMISSION ON ACCREDITATION OF HEALTHCARE ORGANIZATIONS

The Joint Commission on the Accrediation of Healthcare Organizations (JCAHO) can trace its root as far back as 1917, when the Americian College of Surgeons sought improvement in hospital surgery. Today's commission actually began operation in 1951 with commissioners appointed from the American College of Physicians, the

American College of Surgeons, the American Hospital Association, and the American Medical Association. These four corporate members appointed a total of twenty commissioners. This model remained intact until December 1979, when the corporate membership was expanded to include the American Dental Association, which provided one more voting seat and increased board membership to twenty-one. The commission was known as the Joint Commission on Accreditation of Hospitals (JCAH) until 1987, when it adopted its current name.

JACHO's purpose is to promote high-quality patient care through a process in which hospitals voluntarily seek accreditation. The word "voluntarily" is important to note. The JCAHO survey team is invited by healthcare organizations to conduct an evaluation of hospital services. JCAHO should be viewed as a self-policing programme because the Commission's activities are paid for by the healthcare organizations that use its programme.

Standards and Inspections

The Commission produces and revises its standards each year through the publication of the Accreditation Manual for Hospitals (AMH). The AMH is generally published several months before the beginning of the calendar year in which the standards will go into effect to give organization's time to review and implement standards compliance before the effective date. The AMH, which is designed for use in facility self-assessment, is the basis for the Commission surveyors' report.

The JCAHO survey (inspection) team generally consists of a physician, a hospital administrator, a registered nurse, and an ambulatory care surveyor. The full team is not always used in small facilities.

On completion of all on-site inspections, the surveyors hold an exit conference with the hospital's top administrators. The Commission requests that this conference be limited to six people. At the request of the hospital the surveyors will conduct a summation conference for all hospital staff.

Type of Accreditation

On completion of the on-site JCAHO survey, the commission staff evaluates the results of the survey, along with any other relevant data to determine the type of accreditation status to be granted. There are three types of accreditation.

Conditional accrediation is granted to facilities that are not in substantial compliance with JCAHO standards but are judged to be capable of expeditious resolution of performance deficiencies. A resurvey is scheduled for six months after the commission's acceptance of the hospital's plan for correcting deficiencies.

Accreditation with Type I recommendations accredits the hospital for three years. The commissions monitors the hospital's efforts to improve in the areas of concern and to achieve significant compliance with a specified period of time.

Full accreditation, which lasts for three years, also generally contains some Type II recommendations, which indicate areas that need improvement. These areas are reviewed carefully in subsequent inspections.

Once a hospital has received accrediation it is subject to reinspection at any time during the accreditation period.

Quality Assurance and Agenda for Change

The Commission continues to place a great emphasis on its quality assurance (QA) standard. In short, this standard requires hospitals to monitor and evaluate the appropriateness of patient care, to pursue opportunities to improve care, and to resolve identified problems. Ongoing measurement, analysis of measurement findings, corrective or improved actions, and documentation are all facets of the QA function.

In 1986 the Commission introduced a new concept, "Agenda for Change", (further developed

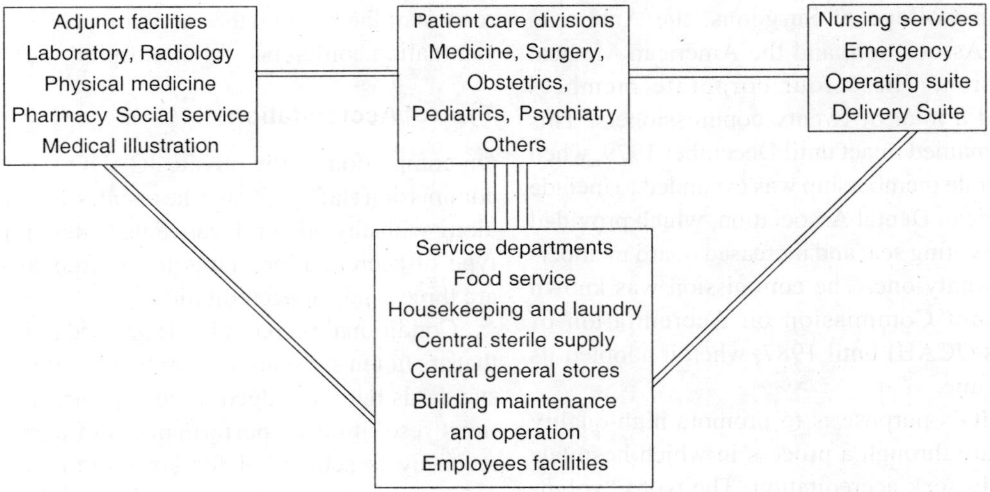

Fig. 2.1: Functional relationships, hospital divisions

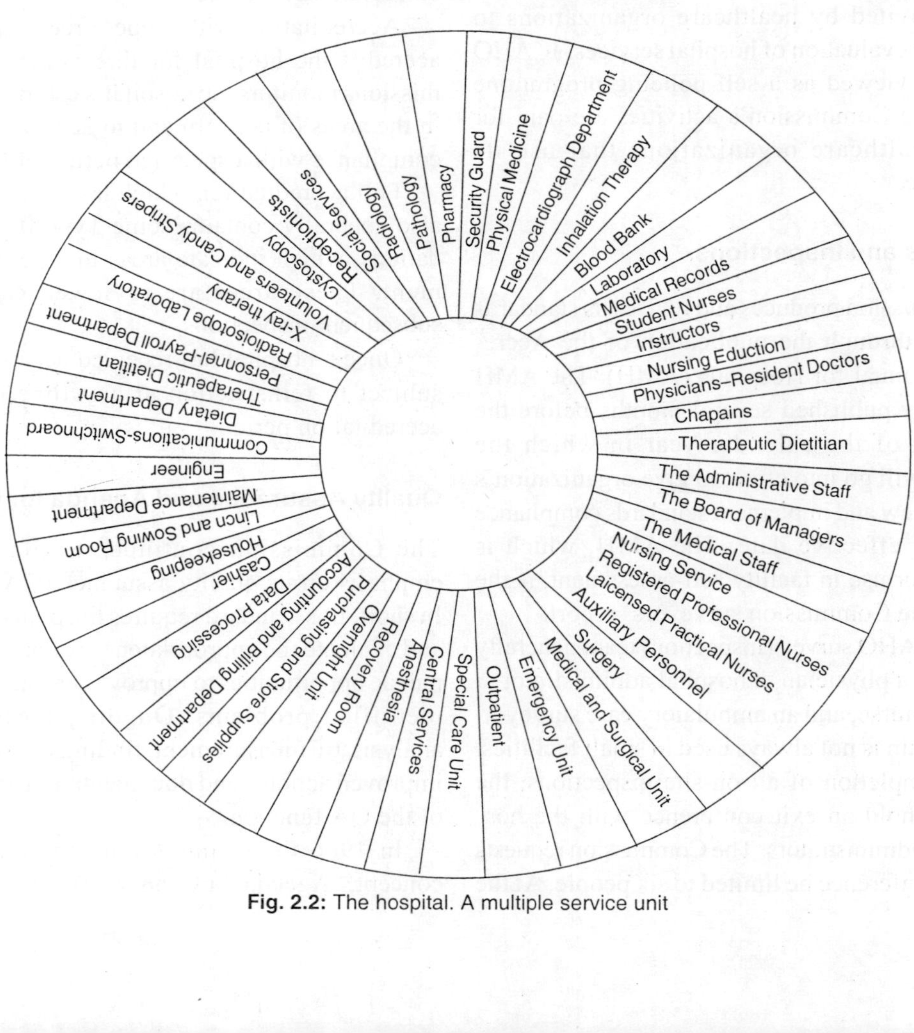

Fig. 2.2: The hospital. A multiple service unit

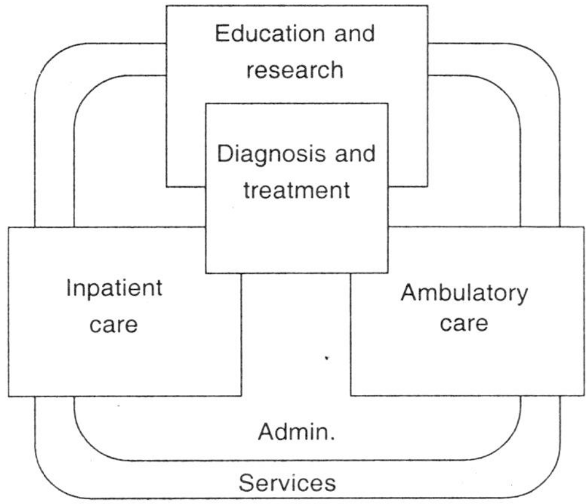

Fig. 2.3: Hospital sectors diagram of relationships

in 1991). The two basic elements of this concept are the processes and the outcomes of patient care, with a goal of continuous improvement of patient care services.

The "Plant, Technology, and Safety Management" section of the JCAHO 1990 Accreditation Manual for Hospitals alludes to the provision of a safe environment. Standard PL. 1 requires "a safety management programme that is designed to provide a physical environment free of hazards and to manage staff activities to reduce the risk of human injury."

Requirements PL 1.1 refer to traditional safety areas—not security. PL 2 deals with the area of fire safety. Both of these standards, however, directly involve security department operations.

The Hospital's Changing Role

Health delivery systems are changing at an increasingly faster pace. England is experiencing some shifting from socialised medicine to private care. In the United States the change is toward more government control. Under Candadas changing system, everyone receives government-mandated healthcare.

Hospital care constitutes as major part of the delivery of healthcare. However, there is more emphasis on ambulatory care.

With diversification, hospitals acquired a keen sense of the need to compete for patients.

The hospitals of the future will provide a core of high-level inpatient services for chronic and critical-care units of today.

FURTHER READING

1. Colling, Russel L: Hospital Security (3rd edn) Bulterworth-Heinemann, Stoneham, MA 02180.
2. Generald McManis,"Challenges of New Decade Demand Break with Tradition," Modern Healthcare. January 1990.
3. Llewelyn-Davies anc Macanlay HMC: Hospital Planning and Administration. World Health Organisation, Geneva, 1966. Closure by 1993.

3 Hospital Organization and Structure

People generally view a hospital as a place in which the sick and injured receive medical care. Throughout its evolution, this has been the hospital's primary mission. However, the hospital has important secondary functions, including the education of physicians and paramedical personnel. The prevention of disease and promotion of health standards and the perpetuation of medical research.

A hospital is a corporate entity like any other business and should be viewed as a business within the framework of a patient care system. The hospital includes such supporting elements as income, operating expenses, politics, reporting levels, and vast interactions with the public, patients, employees, and physicians. Differences between hospitals and other business do exist. The chief difference is the power structure that operates in the medical facility.

Within the organization, those with certain levels of status possess the right to control the actions of those with lesser status. This right may be formal in that it has been legitimized in the system's organization or it may be informal. In that an individual develop's some degree of influence in the decision-making operations of the system. Although the hospital administrator holds the institutionalized right to control the actions of others in the system, he or she is not a free agent in the decision-making process because in the final analysis, the administrator is subordinate to the board of trustees. The final rights of power are ultimately vested in an authoritative board that is not involved in the day-to-day direction of the organization.

Few other organizations have as complex an organizational structure or bring together as many kinds of people, with all kinds of attitudes and dispositions, to carry out as great a variety of work as hospitals do. The fusion of these diverse talents into exactness of action, with human lives at stake, requires administrative concepts found only in the healthcare setting (Figs 3.1, 3.2 and 3.3).

Patients and Visitors

Each year millions of patients are cared for in the hospitals, nursing homes, and thousands of outpatient clinics and physician's offices. In addition, more than one million patient's are treated daily in hospital outpatient facilities, including emergency rooms.

The number of visitors per patient varies according to the type of patient. For example, visitors to pediatric patients greatly exceed the number of

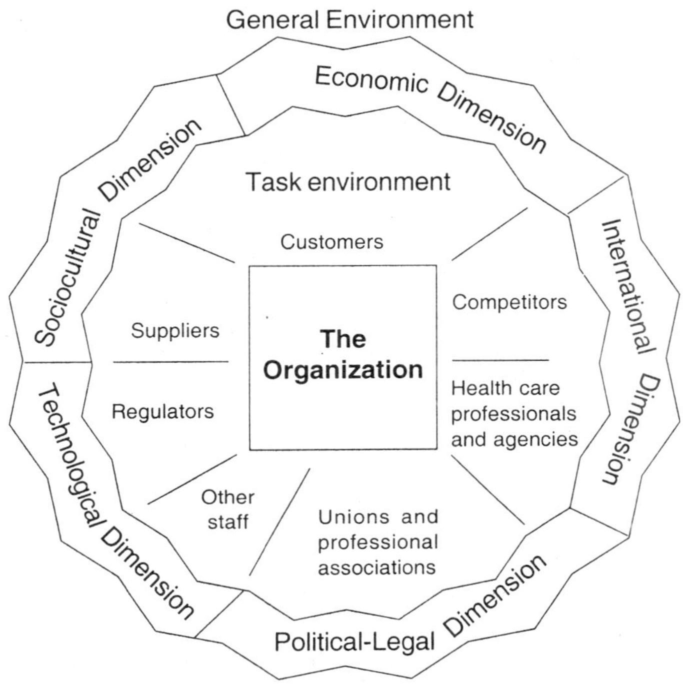

Fig. 3.1: The organisation and environment-I

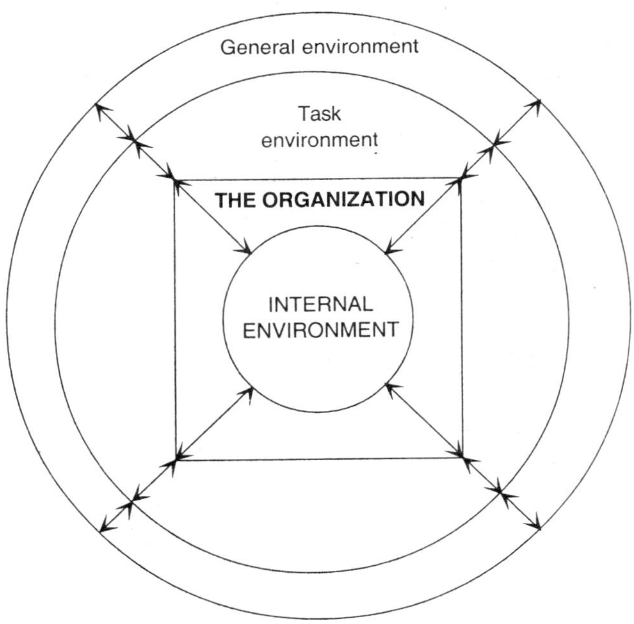

Fig. 3.2: The organisation and its environment-II

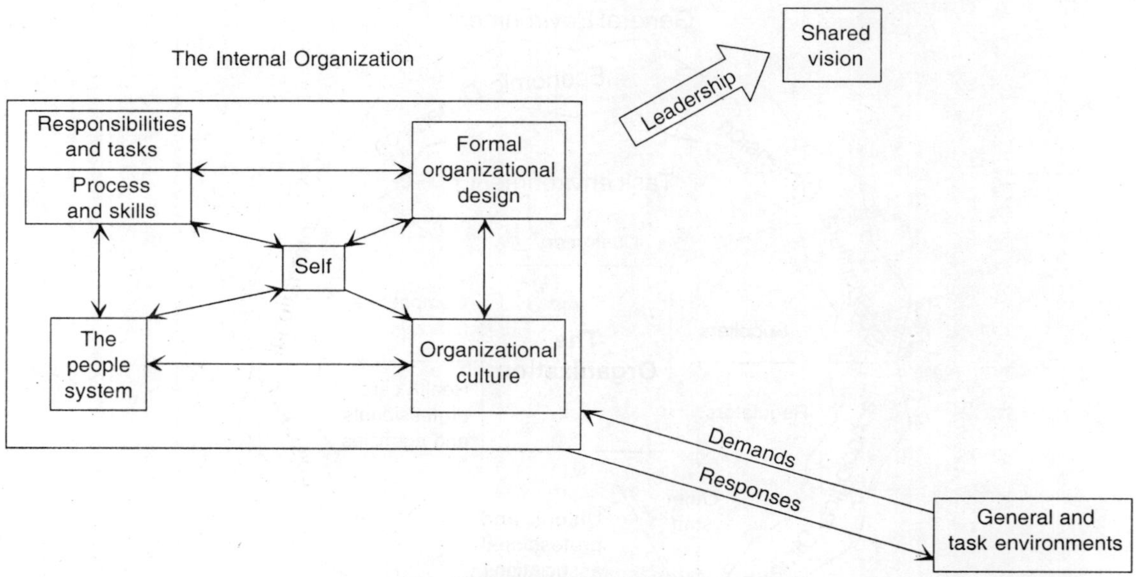

Fig. 3.3: The Internal organisation

visitors to long-term, upper-respiratory-disease patients. As a rule of thumb, each patient receives approximately three to four visitors per day. Hospital public relations and marketing efforts have encouraged an increasing number of people to come to the hospital to visit. A good example of increased visiting can be found in maternity patient care. Birthing rooms and the once tightly controlled newborn nurseries are often full of friends and relatives.

Friends and relatives of inpatients are not the only visitors who arrive daily at hospitals in large numbers, people who go to the hospital for clinic/outpatient services often are accompanied by others. These visitors are not only supporting people but also often are young children for whom no other care is available. These visitors can present unique situations for hospital security. Another group of visitors are those who accompany an injured or a sick person to the hospital emergency department.

Hospital Employees

Hospital employees are a major component of the healthcare delivery system. As shown in Figure 3.4, the largest single cost in operating a hospital is the labour—the employees required directly or indirectly to render patient care. The typical hospital has approximately four employees per patient. This number, of course, varies with the mix of specialities and types of patients in the each hospital. In the years ahead, continued growth and occupational diversification are expected.

Various studies reveal that some of the most stressful occupations are in the healthcare field. It is generally well accepted that responsibility for people causes a higher level of stress than responsibility for things. The hospital employee is not only responsible for patients but also must ensure the satisfaction of other groups, including families, physicians, accrediting bodies, and licensing authorities.

The percentage of employees in any given position or work group caries among healthcare facilities, depending on size and primary mission. In this frame of reference, primary mission refers to whether the hospital's emphasis is on teaching, research, rehabilitation, clinical care, or medical speciality. Today a hospital may employ people in as many as 175 different job skills or classifications.

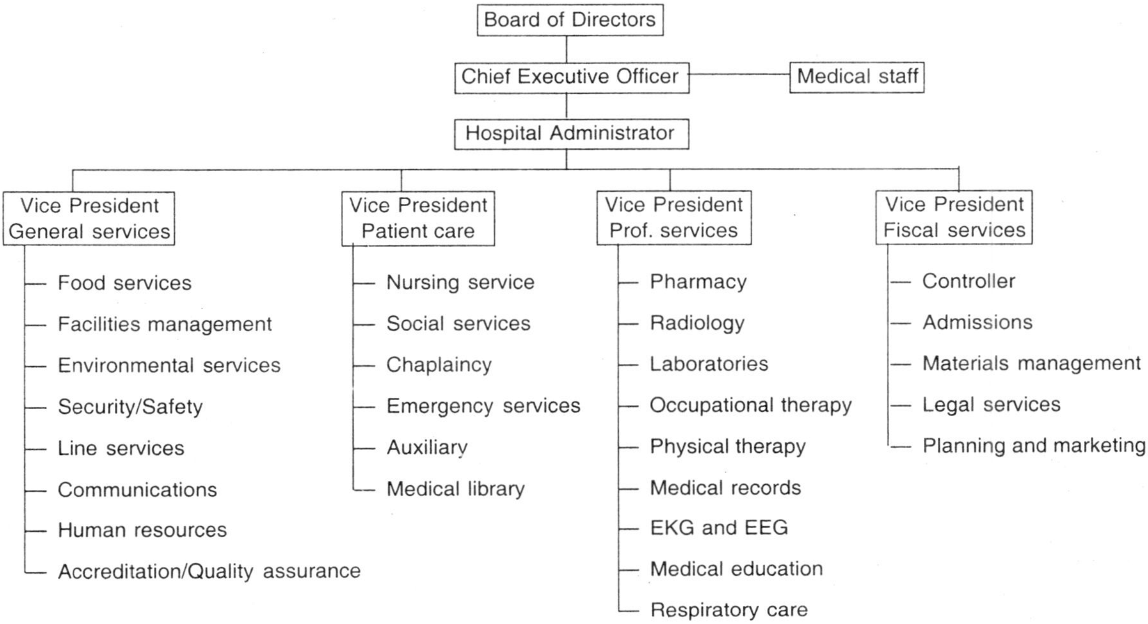

Fig. 3.4: A representative example of hospital organizational structure

In some job categories, as many as half of the employees are replaced each year. This places a heavy burden on management in recruiting, screening, testing, checking reference, orienting, training, and supervising. The days of the dedicated, religiously motivated worker are almost over. Today health proffessional can essentially be classified as a transient worker.

A large number of professionals work in hospitals. In general, more than 65 percent of the personnel in a healthcare organization have professional status. This is a handicap in terms of administrative control because a professional, and a highly specialized group is inherently more autonomous than non-professional group. It is often said that the administrator of a modern healthcare facility is merely a coordinator who makes certain that all the resources come together at the right time and the right place to produce excellence in patient care.

Medical Staff

Medical staff are effectively organized and usually have exceptionally good channels of communication with the board of trustees. The medical staff can be the main support of the administrator and conversely when the medical staff withdraws their support, the administrator almost inevitably is the loser.

The physician and the nurse are two primary caregivers, and they interact to a great degree. Physicians regard nurses as subordinates who take their orders and translate them into action for the benefit of the patient. Modern nurses view the relationship in an entirely different light. As some leaders in the nursing profession have expressed it, the nurse works with-not for-the doctor.

Not all physicians who interact in the hospital have the same responsibilities and privileges. Medical staff are typically broken down into the following general categories:

The accredited medical staff is composed of those physicians and dentists who have recently been appointed to the medical staff. Like the active staff, they have full admitting privileges.

The honorary medical staff comprises members of the staff who have rendered meritorious service to the hospital or who are properly qualified physicians of national repute and standing. They have no administrating privileges.

The consulting medical staff consists of physicians and dentists promoted from the active or courtesy staff for meritorious service rendered to the hospital, Physicians who have attained-national recognition in their specialty, and certain other physicians. They generally have full admitting privileges.

The courtesy medical staff is composed of physicians and dentists who are qualified to practice at a particular hospital but do not wish to participate in medical staff affairs.

Today, physicians successfully compete with hospitals for a significant share of the ambulatory-care market. They are able to use an increasing number of diagnostic and therapeutic technologies in their office. On the other hand, like hospitals, physicians must face new reimbursement systems, the high cost of operating a practice, new high-cost technologies, greater liability, and the administration of complex managed-care arrangements. The need for a working partnership between hospitals and physicians still exists, and thus, only the structure and philosophies will change. Hospitals must foster new and better relationships with physicians as they have to compete with other hospitals for physician-generated inpatient revenues.

Committees

A committee is a group of people to whom some matter is committed. This group may be called a task force, commission, or team. Committees are assembled for many reasons, one of which is the advantage of group deliberation and judgment.

Few organizations exist with more committees functioning on a routine basis than the hospital. Committees are quite beneficial in the hospital setting and serve to coordinate plans and the execution of programmes. The dynamics of patient care involve so many different and varied disciplines that administrative decisions must be as fully integrated as possible. Figure 3.5 lists typical hospital committees and given an overview of the number and diversity of committees commonly found in today's healthcare facilities.

Typical Hospital Committees

Executive committee	Graduate medical education
Cancer	Continuing medical education
Infection	Emergency room
Credentials	Medical records
Utilization review	Risk management
Hospital safety	Tissue and transfusion
Product education	Medical audit
Surgical audit	Obstetrics and Gynaecology audit
Anesthesia audit	Ophthalmology unit
Emergency room audit	Senior citizen's health center
Medical governing council	Surgical governing council
Alcohol rehab. advisory	Procedural
Disaster	Psychiatric advisory
Psychiatric	Council on education
Council on patient care	Council on quality control
Library	Rehabilitation advisory
Joint conference and Long range planning	Accreditation/Quality assurance research
Computer utlization	
Maternal and prenatal mortality	
Morbidity	IUC
	Therapeutic abortion
Prenatal advisory bylaws	Nominating
Social services	Nuclear medicine
Staffing	Staff nurse council

Fig. 3.5: Example of hospital medical staff committees

Beyond doubt, committees are both time consuming and costly. If a committee is supposed to reach a unanimous or near-unanimous decision, the discussion is likely to be lengthy. On the other hand, if a decision is reached rather quickly, the meeting might have been unnecessary in the first place.

Committees tend to seek conclusions on which all can agree—whether from feelings of politeness, mutual respect, or humility, especially in small group situations. It is generally agreed that all decisions directly or indirectly affecting patient care must receive maximum input and necessary deliberations. Regardless of its shortcomings, a primary mechanism used to reach such decisions in hospitals is the committee. For this reason, the magnitude of committee action in healthcare facilities is not likely to decrease in the future. There is a trend, however, to reduce standing committees in favor of ad hoc committees. An ad hoc committee is assembled for a specific purpose and disbanded once the work has been completed.

Clinical Departments

The degree of departmentalization of the clinical divisions of the hospital depends almost entirely upon the degree of specialization of the medical staff. In small communities, one would expect to find two major departments in a hospital, medicine and surgery. Supportive services such radiology and pathology are also offered but are generally limited in their capability to provide service. In those areas where there are two or more small hospitals, it is common to have a single departments of pathology or radiology servicing both institutions. However, in the large metropolitan areas, the hospital staff is highly specialized and therefore greater subdivisions with a particular department.

Generally, the department of medicine includes the following subdivision.

Internal medicine
Allergy
Cardiology
Infectious diseases
Dermatology
Endocrinology
Geriatrics
Immunology.
Pediatrics
Gasteroenterology
Nephrology
Neurology
Psychiatry
Respiratory medicine
Rheumatology

The department of surgery is generally divided into the following:

General Surgery
Orthopedic surgery
Neurologic surgery
Obstetrics and Gynecology
Ophthalmology
Dental and oral surgery
Pediatric surgery
Otolaryngology
Plastic surgery
Gasterointestinal
Thoracic surgery
Urology
Cardiovascular surgery

In addition, there may be a division of general practice as well as a division of physical medicine and rehabilitation within the hospital.

Each of these sub-divisions usually has a chief-of-service who in turn is responsible to the department chief. In addition, the medical staff is organized in such a manner so as to provide fair representation of each individual on the staff through so the administration and the governing body.

The larger and more specialized medical staff is indicative of the fact that the institution is a teaching hospital. Because the description "teaching hospital" has been misused, the American Hospital Association describes such an institution in the following manner.

A hospital that allocates a substantial part of its resources to conduct in its own name or in formal association with a college or courses of institution in the health disciplines that lead to the granting of recognized certificates, diplomas or degrees, or that are required for professional certification or licensure is a teaching hospital.

The association also placed the following interpretation on the definition.

The allocation of resources and facilities, personnel, and funds must be adequate to demonstrate the discharge of teaching programmes.

Educational programmes or courses of instruction are "formal" when based upon published or recorded curricula covering specified periods of study and have faculty qualification and student admission requirements established or agreed to by the hospital. They are "not work and learn" or "on the job training" assignments that primarily augment the hospital's capability to provide service. Further, the hospital controls or agrees to the appointment of faculty and selection of students except during the term of agreement that gives a college or medical school exclusive authority therefore.

Certificates, degrees or diplomas must be recognized and accepted by national educational agencies, (Medical Council) professional qualifying bodies or state approving authorities. This implies that the courses of educational programmes meet standards generally recognized in the health field.

Support Services

To those unfamiliar with the hospital environment, it would seem as though the hospital consisted of the clinical departments only. Actually the clinical departments would not be able to function without the supporting services. Amongst the supporting services are the nursing departments, the dietary service, laboratory service, the medical records department, the blood bank, radiodiagnosis, the central sterile supply and the social service department.

There are other services clinically essential to the operation of the hospital such as the maintenance and engineering divisions.

Nursing Service

The revolution in medical care has had its effect on the other health professions. For nursing, keeping pace with medicine has meant many changes in practice. The nursing team, made upon workers with varying degrees of nursing skill and directed by a professional nurse, now replaces the single nurse who once did everything for the patient, Today's nursing practitioner recognizes social, psychological, or religious problems with the patient that might influence his physical well-being and refer those that lie outside the province of nursing to the person most competent to deal with them. Helping the patients to help themselves is another new element of nursing practice added because of increased emphasis on self care by the patient as an aid to early recovery.

Nursing care encompasses health promotion, the care and prevention of disease or disability, rehabilitation, teaching, counselling, and emotional support as well as to take care of the ill.

Nursing care is an integral part of total health care and is planned and administered in combination with related medical, educational and welfare service.

The nursing service is organized similarly to any other large service of the hospital. There is at its head a Chief Nursing Officer who is generally an experienced nurse with administrative talent. The administrative nursing service carries ultimate administrative authority and responsibility in one or more health facilities for the nursing services provided to individuals and families. As a member of the administrative staff, the administrative nursing service participates in formulating policy, and devising procedures essential for the achievement of objectives and in developing and evaluating programmes and services. In those institutions where the school of nursing has been separated from the nursing service, the individual heading the school assumes a position of responsibility similar to that of the Chief Nursing Officer and may be responsible directly to the Chief Executive officer of the hospital.

Dietetic Services

An essential service of each institution is that of the dietary department. The JCAH requires that the dietetic service be organized in such a manner that it shall effectively apply the principles of the science of nutrition to the preparation of palatable and appropriate food. The services are generally directed by a qualified person and staffed by adequate numbers of dietitians and technical and clerical personnel.

In addition to the purchasing, planning and preparation of menus, both for patients and employees, the dietitian is generally responsible for recording dietary histories of patients such as those with food allrgies and those unable to accept a limited diet regimen: interviewing patients regarding their food habits; counselling, patients and their families concerning normal or modified regimens, and encouraging patients to participate in planning their own normal or modified regimens; and participating in appropriate ward rounds and conferences.

Medical Records Department

Every hospital is required by law to maintain adequate medical records on their patients. These must be accurately documented, readily accessible and can be easily used for retrieving and compiling information.

The purposes of the medical record are:

- To serve as a basis for planning and for continuity of patient care.
- To provide means of communication among the physician and any professionals contributing to the patient's care.
- To furnish documentary evidence for the course of the patient's illness and treatment during each hospital stay.
- To serve as a basis for review, study and evaluation of the care rendered to the patient.
- To assist in protecting the legal interest of the patient, hospital and responsible practitioner.
- To provide data for use in research and education.

The medical record must contain all significant clinical informations and should be sufficiently detailed to enable another practitioner to assume the care of the patient at any time. A consultant should give an opinion after his examination of the patient and the practitioner should give affective continuing care to the patient.

A complete medical record is one which includes identification and sociological data, personal family history, history of present illness, physical examination. Special examinations are such as consultation, clinical laboratory data, X-ray and other examinations, provisional or working diagnosis, medical or surgical treatment, gross and microscopic pathologic findings, progress notes, final diagnosis, conditions on discharge follow-up, and autopsy findings.

Identification data in the medical record are generally provided on what is known as the admission sheet. This sheet generally contains such pertinent information as the unit record number, the patient's name, address, name of the patient's spouse, sex, date of birth, birth place, marital status, occupation, referring, family physicians name and address, admission diagnosis, date and time of admission, and destination within the hospital. Attached to the admission sheet, one may generally find consent forms for the authorization for medical or surgical treatment, authorization for the release of information to insurance companies, and general authorization for the release of information to other physicians or attorneys.

The admission history sheet usually provides space for recording the name of the information as well as the name of the individual taking the history. The purpose of the admission history is to record the patient's chief complaint and a description of his present illness. In addition, it provides the opportunity of protecting the provisional or admitting diagnosis which is usually made on every patient at the time of admission.

The history and physical examination sheet provides the physician with such information as hospital admissions that have taken place in the past with their subsequent diagnosis, operations and major injuries that have been experienced by the patient, the history of childhood and adult infectious diseases, if applicable, pregnancies with dates, out come and complications, immunization data, a history of transfusion with dates, reactions and complications, current medications, sociological data covering habits with alcohol or tobacco, diets, height, weight, date of birth, place of birth, education, military history, occupational history, marital status, health of spouse, family history.

The physical examination sheet consists of a routine systematic review of skin, head and neck, cardiorespiratory, breast, gastrointestinal, urinary, genitalia, endocrine-metabolic, lymph nodes and hematological, muscular skeletal and extremities, urologic, psychiatric, and allergy.

Once the physician has obtained all of this information, he then proceeds to record in the medical record a suggested programme to be followed during the hospitalization of the patient.

Signed laboratory sheets are entered into the patients medical record. The laboratory reports include those obtained from chemistry, hematology, microbiology, serology, pathology as well as radiology. For this purpose, hospitals have a preprinted from which permits for the recording of data under each of the specific sections. However, some hospitals find it practical to paste the original laboratory reports into the medical record.

All treatment procedures performed upon the patient are recorded in the medical record. Operative notes are also included in the record and contain both a description of the findings as well as a detailed account of the techniques used and the tissues removed.

Progress notes are made in the medical record for the purpose of providing the physician with a chronology picture and analysis of the clinical course of the patient.

Upon the completion of all the diagnostic procedures to be performed, it is mandatory that the physician enters into the medical record a definitive final diagnosis which is based on the terms specified in the standard nomenclature of diseases and operations.

Upon discharge from the hospital, the patient's record will have entered into it a discharge summary. The purpose of this is to provide a recapitulation of the patient's hospitalization. In some hospitals, a copy of this discharge summary is forwarded with the patient whenever, he is transferred either to another hospital or to an extended care facility or nursing home. Some of the items contained within the discharge summary include a brief history, results of the physical examination, laboratory data, a description of the patient's hospital course, the diagnosis, the present condition, medications that have been sent with the patient, a listing of the operations performed.

If the patient has died while in the hospital, and an autopsy has been performed, the medical record will contain a complete protocol of the findings that have resulted from the autopsy.

Pathology Services

The chief of the Pathology Service is a member of the medical staff and has undertaken special training in pathology. In addition to the cytologic and gross anatomic analysis performed within the department of pathology, most hospital's group clinical laboratories within this division laboratories such as clinical chemistry, microbiology, clinical microscopy, hematology, and serology are but a few examples.

Blood Bank

Because of the essential nature of blood as a therapeutic agent, most hospitals operate a blood bank. This service is generally under the supervision of a licensed physician who has a basic interest in hematology. However, some hospitals assign the blood bank to the department of pathology because of its laboratory-like operation.

Radiology

One of the most important of the scientific and therapeutic facilities of the hospital is the department of radiology. Radiology is that branch of medicine which deals with the agnostic and therapeutic application of radium energy, chiefly in the form of roentgen rays and radium. The department is under the supervision of a qualified radiologist.

Radiology services are performed only upon the written order of a member of the medical staff who has been granted clinical privileges in the hospital. The therapeutic use of radium or sealed radioactive sources in the hospital is limited to physicians who have been granted this privilege, after consultation with and consideration of the recommendations of the radiologist and/or a radiation safety committee. Only persons who have suitable training and experience are permitted to handle radioactive materials.

The department of radiology generally consists of physicians who are trained as radiologists, physicists, technicians, radiotherapists, isotopepharmacists, nurses, orderlies and secretarial personnel.

Medical Social Service Department

The Medical Social Service Department is an important liaison between the hospital and the patient and his community. The qualified social worker represents a discipline whose professional focus is on the social aspects of the patient and his family, social service personnel generally provide information relating to medical social study of appropriate patients: social therapy and rehabilitation of patients home environmental investigations for attending physician: cooperative activities with community agencies; social service summaries: and follow-up reports of discharged patients, confirming disposition, when obtained.

Anesthesia Service

The Anesthesia Service of a hospital is generally directed by an anesthetist who has had special training and is responsible for the following: Quality of anesthesia care rendered by anesthetist in the surgical and obstetrical area; availability of equipment necessary for administrating anesthesia and for related resuscitative effect; development of regulations concerning anesthetic safety; and retrospective evaluation of all anesthesia care.

Anesthesia care is usually provided by anesthesiologists, qualified nurse anesthetist, or appropriately supervised trainees in an approved educational programme.

Central Service Department

The Central Service Department furnishes all supplies required for the nursing units. These supplies include sterile linen, sterile kits, operating room packs, needles, syringes, and other medial surgical supplies. In addition the personnel in this department clean, inspect, repair, assemble, wrap, and sterilize special treatment trays for the various nursing units.

Pharmacy

A hospital is truly a "city within a city"—within its four walls there is an operation: a hotel which manifests itself by the patient's room accommodations; a dormitory for the student nurses, residents and interns; a school for the training of nurses, technicians, dietitians; laboratories; a pharmacy; food vending operations a laundry and linen service; housekeeping services; engineering power generating services; delivery services; a post office: a massive internal and external communications system; blood bank: accounting and credit services; a public relations department; a motor service and security patrols.

Although the pharmacy department is only one of the many divisions of a hospital. It exerts a great deal of influence on the professional stature of the hospital as well as upon the economics of the total operational costs of the institution because of its inter-relation with and the inter-dependency of these other services upon it.

This is not true in the hospital or in an extended care facility. In this setting, we find interjected into the doctor-pharmacist-patient triad, the professional nurse who assumes the major responsibility of administering all medications to the patient (unless the patient is on a self-medication regimen).

Hospital Contractual Relations

Because of the high cost of delivering health care, governing boards of hospitals have resorted to various means of reducing operating costs. In some institutes, this has been achieved via shared services agreement. Contract management and institutional management contracts. Yet others have gone the corporate reorganization route.

Shared Services

Sharing of services offers a viable option to health care institution in providing extensive and high-quality services in a cost-effective manner. Such services include both administrative and clinical activities. Shared services of an administrative nature can be defined as those support services that are not normally involved in the delivery of direct patient care and are not normally revenue producing. These services are easier to develop than clinical shared services programmes because they do not directly involve the medical staff had fewer external elements, and often can be implemented by the hospital's chief executive officer.

Clinical shared services can be defined as those services that are normally involved with the delivery of direct patient care, are usually revenue producing, and may have a significant impact on the financial resources of the participating institutions.

Hospitals may develop and participate in various types of arrangements to recognize and operate shared services programmes, including.

a. *Referral service* a service maintained by one member of a group of health care institutions.
b. *Purchased service* any service for which an institution pays directly.
c. *Multisponsored service* a service jointly controlled and operated by a group of institutions generally involving a legal agreement among the sponsoring hospitals.
d. *Regional service* a service sponsored by an association of institutions through a community hospital council, a state hospital association or special association or organization formed for a specific purposes.

Contract Management

A departmental management contract (DMC) is arranged agreement between a health care institution and a contractor, under which the contractor provides to the institution various management functions and which may include other services in return for a fee.

A DMC differs from consultative services in several respects. Consultative services are most frequently specific in nature, limited in scope and used only periodically. On the other hand, DMCs are ongoing and comprehensive, and relate to, day-to-day operation of a department, and combine consultation with the authority and responsibility for action and implementation.

Once a contract has been agreed upon, the hospital and contractor must develop plans to ensure a close day-to-day working relationship. The initiator's management should commit itself to regular monitoring of the contractor's performance under the contract, just as it would evaluate the performance of any of its internally provided services.

With proper organization and supervision, the well-qualified department head who is provided with adequate resources should be able to equal or exceed and advantages of maintaining in-hospital services include-greater employee loyalty; scheduling flexibility; better interdepartment cooperation and teamwork and lower overhead costs. Advantages of contracting for services include—reduced costs, provides skills not readily available to the hospital: improves efficiency of the department served and reduces the number on the payroll, thus lowering the cost of fringe benefits. Contractors claim that their services offer the following advantages, higher productivity, better supervision custom-designed services, familiarity with labor demands, research capability and provides equipment and supplies at a lower cost because he has the price advantage of a quantity discount.

Institutional Management Contracts

With tight fiscal constraints being placed on hospitals coupled with a shortage of highly trained business-type executives to manage them, trustees have entered into institutional management contracts (IMCs).

The American Hospital Association defines an institutional management contract as one of the many types of arrangements through which health care institutions can obtain the services of other organizations or provide services to other organizations. An IMC is a formal agreement in which a hospital or other organization contracts with the governing board of a hospital to assume the responsibility for general management of the hospital. This managing organization appoints the administrator and has overall day-to-day management authority and responsibility for the man aged hospital, subject only to the direction of the governing body. Subject to the terms of the contract and local law, the managed hospital may retain total legal responsibility and ownership of the facility and its assets and liabilities.

Potential contractors for this service include autonomous hospitals, tax-exempt multihospital systems, shared service organisations, investor-owned multihospital systems, hospital association and firms specializing in management contracts.

Among the reasons hospitals enter into management contracts are economies of scale: access to specialized consultants in finance, reimbursement, and management systems; procurement of qualified management personnel; resolution of financial difficulties and assistance in dealing with *liceing*, planning and related regulatory requirements.

Hospital Reorganization

Regulatory and competitive pressures are requiring hospitals and other healthcare providers to examine their organizational structures, and to realign those structures to place themselves in a more flexible posture to compete on an as nearly equal basis as possible in a healthcare delivery system undergoing revolutionary changes.

Organizational and entity structure has come to be recognized as an important weapon in a healthcare facility's aresenal for confronting these regulatory and competitive pressure that will only intensify in the future.

As a result, institutions are now reassessing their modes of operations, and are restricting or have restructured to protect present and future assets, develop and safeguard a wide variety of new sources of revenue, attract additional funds through philanthrophy, and to raise venture and equity capital through cooperative ventures.

The response of the industry has been a realignment of corporate structure.

Essentially, this has involved (a) the transformation of the existing hospital corporation into a parent corporation, deprived of its authority to operate a hospital: (b) the creation of a new subsidiary corporation to operate the hospital: and (c) the creation of other subsidiary corporations to operate various business enterprises.

DESIGN STRATEGIES TO ASSIST HEALING

The health care delivery systems in many countries are changing rapidly to meet the challenge of providing universal health care to expanding and ageing populations with continuously developing new health threats and limited resources. USA is struggling to increase access and reduce costs at the same time. Newly industrialised nations such as Korea, Taiwan and Malaysia are extending more health services to a broader segment of population, China is adding more aspects of Western medicine and service to its health system, and Japan is facing the largest wave of ageing population as it works at reducing acute care length of stay. The basic principle which must direct changes in all of these countries is to increase the effectiveness of health care services—that is, to produce the highest possible value for the expenditure. Ultimately to achieve the highest value and effectiveness, the physical environment for delivery of health services must join the medical services and organisations, and social environments in contributing to the patients, health and healing.

A physical environment for healing must satisfy two conditions:

1. It should do no harm. It should be safe in configuration and material usage in providing adequate temperate and clean air and providing adequate and safe noise and light levels.
2. It should facilitate medical service. It should balance adequate stimulation with over stimulation, induce positive physiological responses, and enhance patient control and participation in the environment.

There is a growing body of evidence that certain physical environment issues directly influence a facilities. Health facility designers who pursue this body of research can find a number of well-documented studies which provide substantial evidence of the probable positive effect of certain environmental conditions.

The following are some of the key environmental issues essential to a health environment. While the list is by no means exhaustive, and there needs to be continuing empirical research into these and other environmental influences, the potential for improving the effectiveness of the environment through careful design of these issues alone is very high.

Sound

Sound generated by the environment with no specific human purpose is noise, which can be positive for example sounds from nature, such as birds or breezes, or negative, as it often is with man-made sounds such as machine or intrusive activity noise.

Loudness and control are two key variables in noise. Studies of nursing units have shown that average sound levels range from 50 to 60 dB (A) (decibels adjusted for human hearing range) at different times of the day, with frequent peaks up to 120 dB (A) (dropped utensils, slammed doors, and so on). The United States Environmental Protection Agency (EPA) recommends 45 during day time and 35 dB at night in nursing units. Fifty-five dB has been shown to arouse infants from light sleep and 70 dB prevents sleep. Studies of nursing homes have shown that night time changes in noise levels greater than 60 dB happen more than 30 times a night and are a major source of sleep deprivation. One study showed higher use of pain medication in a recovery room during periods of high noise levels. Sound effects on patients can be compounded by ototoxic drugs. For the elderly and other hearing id, high noise levels add to confusion and disorientation by masking auditory signals and conversation. Studies have demonstrated the negative effects of noise on key physiological parameters such as neuroendocrine reactions.

Health facility design strategy should set goals for accept able noise levels (close to EPA's recommendations) and achieve them through:

- Source attenuation (location isolation, insulations, bumpels)
- Source elimination (phone bells, intercoms, audio-pagers printers)
  — General acoustic attenuation (adequate ceilings, walls,
  — Patient control (television, fans, doors).

Beyond control of noise a design strategy should incorporate positive use of sound as a contributor to wellness. Natural sounds, particularly water, has a calming and relaxing effect which is underused in health care.

Selective use of music, with adequate concern for patient control can also contribute positively. While we have found no significant empirical research supporting positive physiological responses to these controlled uses of sound, there are behavioural studies documenting modifications achieved by controlling loudness and tempo of music.

Light

Light is essential to vision, and affects health in other ways including synthesis of vitamin D and levels of plasma bilirubin. There is also significant evidence of light/dark cycle effects on biochemical and hormonal rhythms. Factors in human response to light include:

- Intansity (relative brigtness)
- Color rendering
- Temperature of light (distribution of wave-lengths)
- Temporal pattern of exposure and
- Source (direct).

There is a significant difference in the need for intensity of light between tasks and between groups, Elderly people require three times the light intensity required by young adults for the same activities. Excessive light levels in neonatal units have been shown to be harmful to infant development.

Colour rendering is particularly important in design (short wavelength) end of the color spectrum. Color rendering is important to everyone in terms of perception of healthy or sickly skin tone, and accurate perception of colour variety.

Light temperature is integral to color rendering. In candes cent light temperature is the 2850°K range area at 6400°K and render colors very cool or blue. The best color rendering balance is in the range of 3500°K which can be achieved by a number of sources including newer energy efficient types.

The temperal pattern of light acts as both inducer and timer of glandular and metabolic functions. Artifical light can either be ignored or used to reinforce the day/night cycle.

The source of light, whether direct or indirect, is a key actor in controlling glare. Glare directly interfaces with the ability to clearly see the environment. Peripheral glare causes eye fatigue and loss of concentration. Glare significantly compounds problems for the elderly,

Design strategies for a healing lighting environment should accomplish the following.

- Provide artifical light from sources that have high color rendering indices and are in the 3500°K temperature range
- Provide general illumination from indirect sources, at reasonable intensity for most uses (25-35fc) but increased for primarily elderly population uses
- Provide intensity variability in general illumination so that spaces may be adjusted for active outward activities (high levels of illumination) or for more passive, inwardly focused activity (lower levels of illumination)
- Add sparkle point and focal glow for variety and object rendering
- Relate general illumination temporal patterns closely to diurnal patterns.
- Ensure access to unfiltered daylight for long-term patients (that is, access to outdoors)
- Provide for patient control of light within their territorial space, and
- Provide non-glare visual access to outside wherever possible from spaces occupied continuously for any significant length of time.

Color

Color is an essential of visual stimulation in the environment, Lack of variety in color in the environment causes sensory deprivation, diminished concentration and attention lapses, and fading perceptual ability. The importance of color to perception is demonstrated by the fact that children will sort objects by color before shape.

Color attributes include:

- Hue (dominant wavelength)
- Brightness (luminance), and
- Saturation (purity of wavelength)

There is general agreement that warm colors (long wavelength such a redorange) induce outward oriented active behavior (particularly when combined with high illumination) and that cool colors (short-wavelengths such as blue and particularly at low illumination) induce inward oriented, passive behaviour.

Color is critical to distinguishing edges, shape or an object from its background, and there are number of color relationships which creat contrast essential to these perception. These include contrast in hue, or saturation, or light to dark, or warm to cool and a number of others.

Elderly people have reduced sensitivity to the short wavelength end of the color spectrum (blues and the like), reduced color differentiation, extended duration of figure aftereffects and other visual degeneration which affects their color perception.

Color can be used to signal pathways or use areas (cueing) or to identify a place or thing (coding). A study of elderly demented patients demonstrated successful use of negative cueing (cueing out areas to be avoided) but was not successful with coding for the patients own room.

Design strategies for a healing colour environment must include:

- Balance between understimulation of extreme unity and overstimulation of extreme complexity
- Use of cueing and coding to aid way-finding and understanding ability.

Other Design Issues

There are a number of other design issues which are equally important as sound, light and color in a healing environment. Because of limitations on the length of this article, I will describe them in summary form only.

Temperature, humidity and air change rate are all key issues. These issues are influenced by need for energy efficiency. The comfort and purity of the air provided are both critical to the healing process, as is also perceived control over the patients territory by the patient (and staff territory by staff). A balance in air change rates and energy consumption must be struck which heightens the importance of exhaust heat recovery. Odor and aroma are two sides of a coin that can be negative and positive. Uncontrolled smells (odors) must be eliminated. Some aromas can however be effectively used as stress reducers.

Vanilla is one that has been used effectively in the hospital environment to lift spirits and provide positive distraction from stressful events.

Nature

There is ample evidence that exposure to nature through interaction or access to views has a positive healing effect. Ulrich's now famous study of cholecystectomy patients which showed shorter length of recovery less use of potent analgesic, and fewer complaints from patients with a nature view is currently the strongest case made fire, water plants and fish tanks have all been used effectively as well as views of nature and access to garden courts.

Materials

Material selection is critical in a number of ways. First, it is essential to select non-toxic, non-allergenic and non-bacterial harbouring materials for patient safety. This is a difficult specification and must research is currently going on, particularly in relation to the toxicity issue, second, materials need to be selected and designed for safe use. This is particularly true for flooring and stair materials. In the USA, slip and fall injuries are the leading cause of claims against architects, and stairs are identified as the most dangerous consumer product by the US consumer product safety commission. The physical environmental actors contributing to these problems include confusing patterns and other visual miscues, glare, indequate or too highly contrasting coefficient of friction and poorly designed material intersections. Finally, materials can also contribute positively to healing through stimulating and engaging the tactile senses and through a connection to nature in nature materials.

Esthetic Form

The principal aspects of architectural design, building form, and detail are important factors in the healing environment, the building form must evoke positive, reassuring responses both from recall of reassuring forms but also from esthetic pleasure. That "God is in the detail" is true only if the details transmit a notion of caring thoughtfulness and appropriateness. Again, a balance between unity and complexity is essential to appropriate engaging stimulation of healing.

None of the design strategies described here is unique to a healing environment. Rather, they are universal hallmarks of thoughtful architectural design. The fact that there is a growing body of research on the positive physiological and psychological impact of these strategies is helpful in overcoming the purely functionalist tradition which undervalues this more holistic attitude toward the physical environment.

In order for a health facility to accomplish the mission of a healing environment: to do no harm, facilitate medical service and contribute to healing—its design must incorporate this holistic approach to all aspects of the physical environment.

FURTHER READING

1. Accrediation Manual for Hospitals 1991, Joint Commission on Accrediation of Hospitals, Chicago, ILL Page IX 1991.
2. American Hospital association Guidelines for Shared Services for Hospitals Catalog No G028. AHA. 840N. Lake Shore Drive. Chicago, 60611, 1977.
3. Definition of a Teaching Hospital. American Hospital Association Memorandum, November 1-15, 1967.
4. Diagnostic Related Groups. Their importance in Medicare Payments to Hospitals. Ernst and Whinney Document No.158341, 1980.
5. Hassan WME: Clinical Pharmacy-The Medical Record drug Topics, **114**:16, [April] 1970,
6. Huffman, DC.Jr and Kilgore, Susan, M: Changing Concepts in Hospitals Reimbursement. Curr. Concepts in Hosp. Pharm Mgt: **6**: 13-18, 1984.
7. In Pursuit of Quality-Hospital Nursing Service, National League for Nursing New York. 1964.
8. Job Descriptions and organizational Analysis for Hospitals and Related Health Services, U.S. Government printing office, Washington, 1952.
9. Jonaseen JO: Design Strategies to Assist Healing Hospital management international 1995.
10. The Revised DRGs: Their importance in Medicare Payments to Hospitals, Ernst and Whinney Document N0.158-442, 1983.

4 Growth of the Modern Hospital

A Hospital is a human invention, and as such can be reinvented at any time. Hospitals are connected with matters that affect life and death. Once these absolutes are mentioned, normal methods of evaluating results become difficult to apply; when life is at a stake, people naturally feel that only the best is acceptable

Any form of financial limitation is apt to be seen as an inhuman restraint. Escalating costs are accepted as a matter of course. It is assumed that more sophisticated modern procedures automatically justify a correspondingly heavier investment in building and engineering.

Historical records show that efficient hospitals were constructed in India by 600 BC. During the splendid rule of Empire Ashoka (273-232 BC), Indian Hospitals looked like modern hospitals. They followed principles of sanitation, and ceserian section's were performed with close attention to technique in order to save both mother and infant. Physicians were appointed one for every ten villages to serve the health care needs of the population, and regional hospitals for the infirm and destitute were built by Buddha.

The development of efficient hospitals was an outstanding contribution of Islamic civilization. The Roman military hospitals and the few Christian hospitals were no match for the number, organization, and excellence of Arabic hospitals (6th-7th century).

During the time of prophet Mohammad (PBUHS), a real system of hospitals was developed. Asylums for the insanes were founded ten centuries before they first appeared in Europe. Islamic Physicians were responsible for the establishment of pharmacy and chemistry as science.

Some of the best known of the great hospitals in the Middle Ages were in Baghdad, Damascus and Cairo. The ideal modern hospital is a place where people seek and receive care and where clinical education is provided to health professionals at the same time. It provides continuing education for the practicing physicians as well as increasingly serves the function of an institution of higher learning for entire community. Besides, it conducts investigation studies and research in medical sciences.

The construction of modern hospital is influenced by central/state government laws and accreditation of Hospital policies of voluntary organization like Joint Commission of Accreditation of Hospitals.

Health problems are identified in relation to the population at risk in the planning area. Within each relevant population group the planner must identify, the nature and importance of individual health needs, as well as the extent to which these needs are currently translated into demands for health services. Assessment of problems should allow for both cause and effect.

Estimation of the demand and need for hospitals rests on several factors—population, economic level of the area planned for, and the availability of funds for hospitalization. The accessibility of facilities help to determine the effective demand. The age pattern also affects demand for health care facilities. Past utilization rates and trends are probably the best indicators for short-term chances in demand for the future.

After basic information is collected on the current parameters, changes should be predicated for the future; increase in population and increase in per capita utilization. Also migration patterns and changes in birth rates should be projected. Besides projections of objective needs and anticipated government policies and priorities should be realistically considered. Planners must build for the future, not the past, anticipating worldwide trends, such as urbanization, and plan for facilities to meet these major trends.

Key Issues

There are a number of change factors that will have a significant impact on the provision of health facilities for the feature:

- Health transition
- Medical technology
- Consumer expectations and quality of care
- Demographic and epidemiological pressures
- New inventions in basic, applied and medical sciences
- Incorporation of electronic and computer technology—information superhighway.

Other issues that should be considered now if the health care organization are to develop in a way that will respond to future needs

- Decentralization of some services into the community
- Shift from inpatient to day care facilities
- Organization of services around specialist equipment/expertise,
- Shift to high technology, short stay, high dependency inpatient care,
- Effect of information technology on hospital layout,
- Changing patterns of care,
- Reallocatin of space to meet changing needs,
- New objectives for ward design.

Trends that may have greatest impact on the future of the new hospital include:

- Aging (increase in average lifespan)
- Competition (on price)
- Conglomerates (multi-institutional system)
- Integrated health plans: Health insurance plans, government health programs, (Health maintenance organizations, preferred provided organization, insurance companies, etc.)
- Corporate practice (capitation and Prospective payment)
- The new consumer (quality conscious and price sensitive)
- Information and Telecommunication (providing information therapy to consumers, computer systems and video conferencing telemedicine).
- Shifting value of money

Change from inpatient to day-care, fee for service to capitation, from public to private, health promotion, etc).

- Revolution in technology: (computerization, artificial intelligence, office automation, genetic engineering, super drugs, bio-replacement technology, organ transplantations laser surgery, etc).
- Medical Ethics: (issues of life and death, *in utero* surgery, etc).

Progressive Patient Care

This is one of the innovative concepts of organization of hospital facilities, services and staff around the medical and nursing needs of the patient,

tool to increase the productivity, the effectiveness of patient care and efficiency in hospital services. It consists of grouping of patients according to their degree of illness and need for the care; planned and organized units are set upon which patients are admitted in ward in accordance with their degree of illness and need for care.

Elements of progressive patient care include:
- Intensive care,
- intermediate care,
- self-care,
- long-term care,
- outpatient care.

Intensive Care

- 2 to 5 percent of total beds
- space: 140 SFT/bed.

Intermediate Care

- For moderately ill patients
- 30-35 bedded wards
- Rigg's pattern of ward of one, two, or four bedded rooms may be provided.

Self Care

- For patients convalescing or requiring diagnosis or some preoperative cases,
- Patient permitted to follow home-life routine,
- Ward should be located nearer to diagnostic facilities.

Long-term Care

- Geriatic, rehabilitation and amputation cases,
- 40-55 bedded ward, located on ground floor,
- 125 SFT in single room, 100 SFT in multiple bed rooms.

Integrated System of Services

Each department needs to be freely sited with space around for outward expansion and planned internally to allow for change and future expansion at minimum cost and without disruption to its everyday functioning. The aim for expansion in small manageable increments can be reached by providing free-ended buildings with extendible corridors. To adapt itself to organizational change during different stages of growth, a hospital most do so while maintaining the central communication routes (circulation) viable and while retaining adequate access to the communications network at all times.

To cater for internal flexibility there is a need to consider the concept of "long life, loose-fit buildings"-buildings that bride the gap between the long life expectancy of the building itself and the short life of functions it houses.

To achieve maximum flexibility, there is a need to provide a system of vertical ducts and penetrable flooring at regular intervals, as integral part of the structure, to cater for present and future use.

A standard space module used throughout the building will ensure compatibility between structure, room dimensions, service facilities and fittings.

Landscaping

The landscape provides a picture and an apt setting for the building by highlighting its scale, its color scheme, by focussing the eye on important views and by screening out the negative views of the structure. A carefully landscaped environment can be of immense therapeutic value as it evokes interest and cheerfulness and brings one closer to the nature.

PLANNING THE WHOLE HOSPITAL

Peoples' expectations from hospitals have changed over the centuries.

Key Dates

Gradually, the idea that hospitals were about life rather than death began to dawn. They key dates may be said to be:
- 1846-discovery of anesthetics,
- 1866-Lister's use of carbolic sprays for antiseptic surgery.

- 1886-Van Bergman's introduction of aseptic techniques, the sterilising of instruments and the use of autoclaves.

  These successes gradually extended the range of surgery and the area of ancillary accommodation associated with it.
- 1895-Roentgen used X-rays as an aid to diagnosis. Laboratories similarly added a new dimension to medicine and enormously extended the use of pharmaceuticals. With active interventions as their primary function, hospitals became places where life could not only be saved, but the quality of life also be improved.

Ownership

After second World War, the ownership and control of hospitals assumed a different pattern in each country.

- Voluntary and charitable organizations
- Municipal authorities
- State.

Rationalization

- Reorganizing health care facilities on nationwide scale in Britain.
- Emergence of District General Hospital as the cornerstone of the service
- Hospital plan; to give the hospital service both the physical equipment and the pattern and setting which will everywhere place the most modern treatment at the service of patients and enable the staff who care for them to exercise their skill and devotion under the best possible conditions.

District General Hospital

In the UK professor Thomas Mckeown believed that the District General Hospital should mirror the pattern of morbidity of community it serves, should have not less than two consultants in each speciality and training facilities should be incorporated for all medical, nursing and paramedical personnel.

Unprecedented Expansion on all Fronts

- The rate of increase both in the complexity and the size of the hospitals.
- A typical 19th century hospital had a gross area of about 20 m^2/bed, wards accounted for more than half of this space.

Zoning Concept

- The nursing zone: here patients are fostered throughout their stay in hospital. It deals with people.
- The clinical zone: Consisting of diagnostic and treatment facilities primarily associated with technical equipment required for procedures on patients.
- Support zone: comprises kitchen boiler house, stores, laundry, cafeteria, etc. accommodated all the supporting services.

The key to hospital planning is the manipulation of these zones and their relationship to produce a fully functional, integrated hospital.

Changing Rates of Growth

- The zones increased due to expanding brief.

Indeterminancy and Obsolescence

Indeterminancy is an architectural principle enabling building to grow with order and change with calm.

Functions change so rapidly that designers should no longer aim for an optimum fit between a building and function. The real requirement is to design a building that will inhibit change of function least, and not one that will fit specific function best.

Universal Space

Universal space is a series structurally uninterrupted floors, to which any services such as electricity, gas, water, could be brought from above, and from which all wastes could be taken from below.

- The building is permanent, but its uses are constantly changing.

- Hospitals designed on the engineering floor sandwich principle (complete engineering subfloors nearly 2 m high are provided, instead of treating services as additions and concealing them in ducts and false ceilings).

Combating Obsolesence

Construction should proceed in parallel with decision making and the choice of equipment could be postponed until the last possible moment, for which rapid advances in technology the latest piece of equipment is often the most cost-effective. The possibility of obtaining the latest model and plugging it in without incurring the penalty of contract variation orders is an important consideration.

Plug-in departments and systems development programme, an array of standard building envelops, housing different departments which could be selected and assembled into a whole hospital to meet varying demands and site conditions.

- Designed on modular basic with 15 m clear spans, so that they could be plugged into the mainly, horizontal network of corridors and ducts serving the hospital.
- It provides a flexible link between interchangeable components which can be installed or replaced, to keep pace with technological progress.

A Brave new World

The enormous growth of population, the increase in GNP and the rise in the standard of living encouraged every one to think big.

Changing Need for Beds

The most expensive element in health care is the hospital bed. The most obvious way to economise is not to have build any beds at all:

- Home care and self care (if the patient can be treated at home in his own bed, then there is no need to provide a second bed in a hospital).
- Preventive medicine and early diagnosis have almost eliminated the need for beds for TB, Polio and venerial disease.

The demand for hospital care will depend on:

- accessibility
- availability of beds
- prevalence of disease
- the reputation of the hospital
- the attitude of doctors
- the cost of utilization.

This in turn will depend on whether the cost is borne by individual or the community, either directly or through financing agency.

The number of beds available varies in different countries.

Six beds/1000 pop. (Spain), 8/1000 (Britain), 11/1000 (France), 15/1000 (Sweden) and 0.9/1000 (India).

Throughput of Patients

- The number of beds needed depends on the throughput of patients.
- The shorter the length of stay and the quicker the arrival of the next patient, the fewer the beds required.

Alternative Strategies

One of the most promising alternative strategies may be to think of planning health services from the base upwards rather than planning from the district hospital downwards and shift some of the functions performed in the large hospitals into less sophisticated but adequately equipped places nearer to the community served.

Better Value for Money

- Day-care services (flexible use of space is extended to whole hospital)
- Cottage hospitals (less sophisticated surroundings)
- Reduction in on costs (percentage addition which has to be made to take account of

peculiarities of site, additional foundations, height allowance, airconditioning ,etc.). Careful choice of site meant that the building could be contained in two storeys. Courtyards provide natural light and ventilation. Communications-the corridors and ducts linking the departments together-are reduced. Instead of conventional boiler house with its factory chimney, distributing steam to all parties of the hospital, small interconnected roof top boiler houses are located near the centers of demand. Artificial ventilation is restricted to the clinical zone at the core of the hospital.

Nucleus Concept

In the nucleus concept the aim is to build a hospital in phases: the first phase 300 bedded nucleus, capable of expansion by further self-contained phases to 600 beds.

It is a highly versatile and economic answer to the problem of growth and change. Gross area per bed has been brought down from 75-80 m^2 to 50-60 m^2 in the UK.

Need for Business-like Approach

There can be no such thing as an "ideal hospital" to which all must conform. The secret of success lies in controlling demand and allocating resources to achieve the best balance between the two.

The recognition that local needs are best satisfied by making the most of what can be found on the spot, holds promise of much greater variety in the future.

The Planner's Response

In recent years, considerable research and development work have been undertaken with the aim of reducing both the cost and time-scale of hospital building. Space, previously visualised as a series of self-contained department units, is now viewed as a resource which can be programmed overtime and shared between adjoining or associated functions. In addition, more flexible design solutions have opened up the possibilities of reduced functional content, and of construction and commissioning in stages. Today general hospitals and teaching hospitals are being planned to accommodate upto 1000 beds within average area per bed of 60 m^2 and 110 m^2 respectively.

In an attempt to contain the high costs of building hospitals in multi-storey, and deep-span, forms, a horizontal courtyard strategy was developed in the UK during the 1960s. Instead of the vertical arrangement in the tower-on-podium the zones are related horizontally, in the form of simple two-storey structures tailored in plan and section to the particular functional and environmental needs of each zone. Two basic layouts have been developed; extended courtyard and compact courtyard.

Hospital planning is primarily concerned with putting together the 30 or more separate departments to form a functional and viable whole. Functional zoning can facilitate this process. It will permit the tailoring of plan shape, volume, structure and environmental services to suit the needs of groups of departments with similar characteritics. The clinical zone requires deep planned, high volume, uncluttered and hygienically finished spaces suitable for sophisticated equipment and support systems. The nursing zone needs an appropriate environment for fostering sick people during their brief stay in hospital. Storage and processing areas can be housed in separate structures with industrial-standard finishes, to form the support zone. Fire safety may require the separation of such high life-risk areas as the nursing zone from other high fire-risk areas suh as the support zone. Each zone should be free to grow and change without affecting the integrity of other zones.

Since the beginning of the twentieth century, various planning strategies had been devised to meet the requirements of differing health needs, cultures, climates, sites and budgets. Most of these can be classified into two main groups—vertical and horizontal.

In vertical strategies, the zones are arranged one above the other so that the movement is mainly horizontal.

In the UK, the "one-shot" compact tower-on-podium was abandoned in favour of horizontal strategies, like the the spine and pavilion, which envisaged future expansion of all zones, limited only by the 30-40 acre sites. Extended courtyard is similar to the spine and pavilion layout but the accommodation is planned around open courtyards instead of separate pavilions. The height is normally limited to 4-storeys. The zones are linked horizontally at upper levels as well as at ground floor level, via a central spine corridor system which affords easy access for patients visitors and goods to all departments. Dependence on lifts is much reduced.

The nucleus programme was developed in response to the demand for containment of the scale and cost of acute care hospitals. It provided nationally for a large pre-planned initial phase, or nucleus, of general hospital, which could subsequently be extended if required. The size of the nucleus is limited to around 300 beds (18,000 m^2) and it is designed to be fully operational in its own right.

Universal space strategies incorporating interstitial floors usually involves high capital costs. Overall floor areas (including sub-floors) are in the range 130 to 300 m^2 per bed.

However, it is claimed that subfloor eliminates the need for definitive programmes and permits an easy installation of engineering services and equipment. These systems (Horizontal monolith) were popular during the growth period (1965-75) and various examples were build in the USA and UK.

THE NURSING ZONE

The nursing zone has come a long way from the old barrack-like basic ward packed with bedridden patients. Each new development has in Europe been accommodated by adding more and more rooms or more square meters while in the USA, planners tried to get back to the old nineteenth-century ideal of nursing a patient in his/her own home, giving him/her all the home comforts in a clinical setting. The problem was seen, in over simplified terms, as "How to make a hospital more like a hotel"—home away from home—the plaza suite with nursing care instead of room service.

The nursing zone includes all those areas used for fostering patients during their stay in hospitals. It is in full occupation 24 hours per day. It makes the heaviest demands on numbers of staff employed, materials and energy. Although it now constitutes less than half the total area of the hospital, its sizes and shape will often dictate the overall design of the whole complex.

There is a wide disparity in the gross area per bed in nursing zones currently being planned in different countries. The figures stretch from 18 m^2 in the UK to 43 m^2 in Sweden. In Scandinavia the preference for single bedrooms, and in USA for two bed rooms and in UK for 4-6 bed bays in open wards, partly accounts for this difference. But as with the numbers of beds provided by each country per 1000 population the differences go deeper than variations in climate or standard of living. Cultural factors and nursing traditions are equally important.

The nursing zone comprises one or more nursing units. A nursing unit consists of three elements: patient space (beds, toilets and day space); nursing space (staff base, utility rooms, offices) and corridors.

The different ways in which these elements are arranged can be classified into a number of different types. Starting with the simple open Nightingale form, changes have been introduced in the pursuit of more privacy (corridor or continent) greater amenity for patients and staff (duplex or Nuffield) compactness (racetrack or double corridor); economy (courtyard, a naturally ventilated version of the above); better observation of all patients (cruciform or cluster); shorter distance between patient and nurse (radial).

Each type represents some compromise between privacy for the patient and good nursing supervision (Fig. 4.1). Some like the single room plans, score high marks on one count, others like the open ward on another. But each new development seeks to capitalise on what has gone before. Collectively, they represent a movement to the dedication of the nurses, who stated the requirements and the inventiveness of the architects, who arrived at the solutions.

Although different countries attach importance to different factors in ward design, some objective yardsticks are useful. One of these is staff-patient contact. A crude measure of this is the average distance in a ward between the bed and the nurses base. The closer the nurse is to the patient, the better (Fig. 4.2).

Economy is another factor which cannot be ignored. An efficient plan is one in which every square meter of space is in use for the maximum of hours per day. A corridor is of course necessary, but it is only used intermittently. If doors are kept closed, a nurse in a corridor is out of sight and out of touch. The number of beds per 3 m run of corridor is therefore a useful indicator. The higher the number, the more efficient the arrangement (Table 4.1).

The amount of space in a nursing unit which is allocated to accomodate the patient varies widely from country to country (Fig. 4.3). Space allocations are influenced by several factors: open or corridor layouts, number of beds in a room, bed spacing, ratio of toilet accomodation, provision of sitting up space, etc.

In England larger rooms, each with 5-6 beds and integral day space are preferred. Generous bed spacing (2.4 m) permits the use of curtains, giving a degree of privacy to each patient. The spacing of beds is governed by nursing procedures requiring the circulation of treatment trolleys, drip-stands, wheel-chairs, etc; 2.5 m also allow room for a locker and a chair.

The location of space for nursing ancillaries staff base, utility rooms, stores, treatment rooms, etc. will depend on the central system and Decentralized system.

The most important decisions in planning the nursing zone are the number of beds per nursing unit and the way these beds are arranged; whether in open wards or multi-bed bays or room, or in single rooms. Such decision will influence the amount of space required for corridors

There are four alternative ways of arranging 24 beds in a ward and the effect on the length of corridor needed to gain access to these beds. Because ward corridors need to be wide enough to allow movement and turning of beds, the width has to be constant 2.1 m (Fig. 4.4).

The final stage in the planning of the nursing zone is evaluation and feedback. When the enormous differences in capital, maintains and staffing costs of different ward types is taken into consideration, and the wide variety of ways of satisfying staff and patients needs, the importance of evaluation can hardly be overemphasized. There is a need for fresh experiments in producing more efficient and more cost-effective ward designs in the future.

THE CLINICAL ZONE

The clinical zone is of course the most expensive area to build and equip. Because of its centralization, its expansion and contraction has a vital effect on the size of the rest of the hospital. The strategies for containment include: concentration and consolidation of resources; versatility of accommodation; mechanization and miniaturization and finally more consideration for the patient's convenience by relocating some services nearer his/her own home and so freeing more space for procedures that can only be carried out in hospital.

In temperature climates the cost of engineering services can be reduced if rooms requiring air-conditioning are concentrated in one zone. A central treatment area can take the place of dispersed treatment rooms previously attached to each nursing unit, surgery, emergency and obstetrics, can also

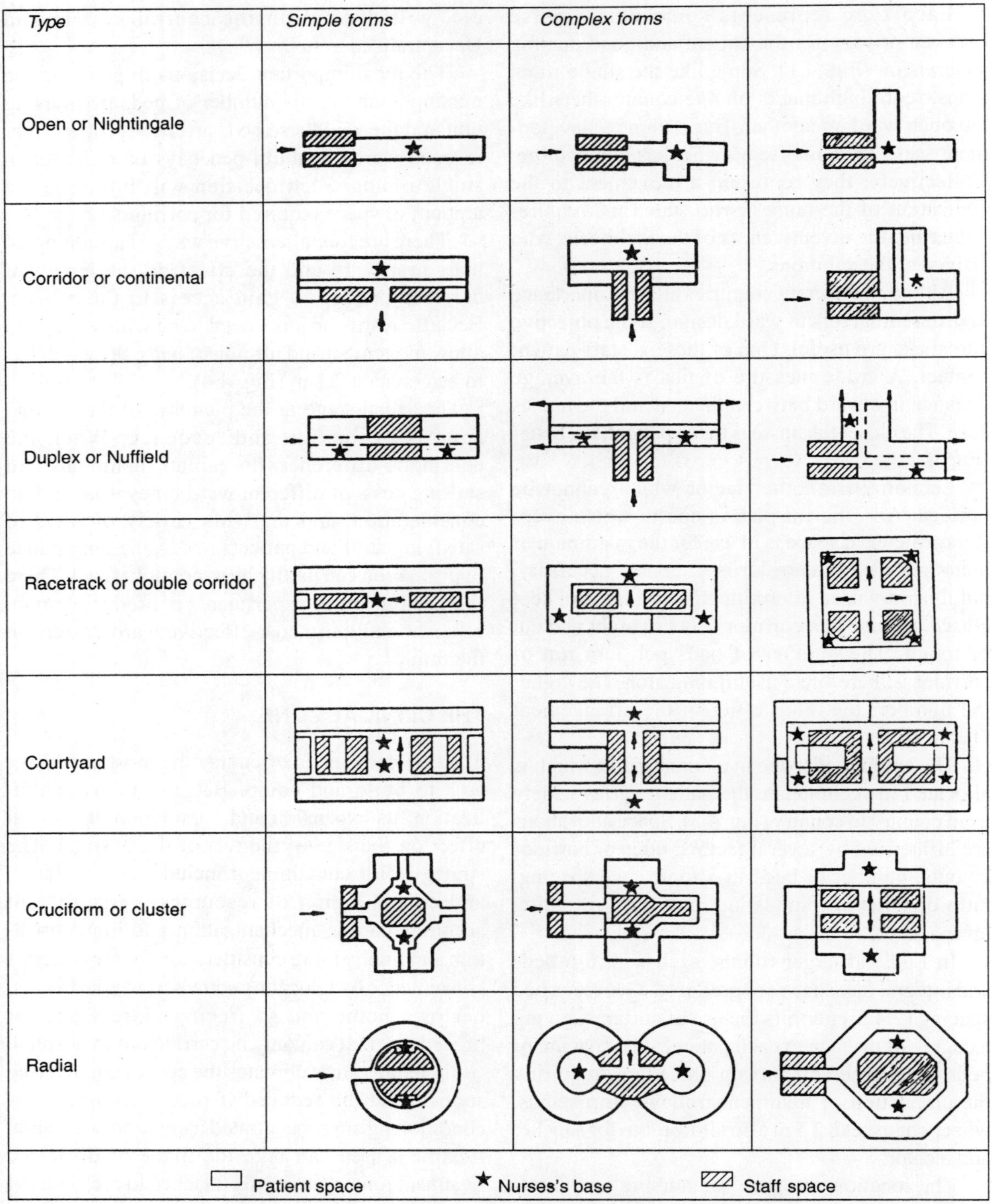

Fig. 4.1: Comparative ward layouts

Table 4.1: *General hospitals 100-400 beds.*
(Based on recent examples in UK, W Germany, Switzerland and Middle East)

	100 beds	*Net space m^2*	*200 beds*	*Net space m^2*	*300 beds*	*Net space m^2*	*400 beds*	*Net space m^2*
A. *In-patients wards*								
Medical/surgical	84 beds	1210	140 beds	180	196 beds	2825	252 beds	3630
Pediatric	—		46 beds	730	69 beds	1100	69 beds	1100
Obstetrics	20 beds	290	25 beds	365	25 beds	363	50 beds	730
Psychiatric	—	—	—	—	—	—	30 beds	480
		1500		2965		4290		5940
B. *Out-patients*								
Consulting clinics	12 C/E rms	350	18 C/E rms	505	24 C/E rms	670	30 C/E rms	840
Emergency	1 dept		1 dept	590	1 dept	590	1 dept	590
		350		1095		1260		1430
C. *Diagnostic/treatment*								
Radiodiagnostic	2 rooms	220	3 rooms	310	4 rooms	415	5 rooms	520
Radiotherapy/ nuclear medicine	—	—	—	—	—	—	—	—
Operating/endoscopy	2 tables	290	3 tables	580	4 tables	620	5 tables	790
Intensive treatment unit/ Coronary care	4 beds	140	6 beds	210	8 beds	280	8 beds	280
Laboratories incl-post-mortem	1 dept	110	1 dept	260	1 dept	390	1 dept	390
Functional diagnosis	included	—	included	270	included	—	1 dept	160
Rehabilitation	1 dept	135	1 dept	270	1 dept	405	1 dept	540
Obstetric delivery	1 dept	180	1 dept	365	1 dept	365	1 dept	480
Day care	1 dept	120	1 dept	235	1 dept	335	1 dept	450
		1195		2230		2830		3610
D. *Administration*								
Central administration	100 beds	290	200 beds	320	300 beds	345	400 beds	460
Medical administration	100 beds		200 beds		300 beds	60	400 beds	80
Admission. reception, etc.	100 beds		200 beds	225	300 beds	340	400 beds	450
Staff facilities	100 beds	140	200 beds	280	300 beds	425	400 beds	560
		540		825		1170		1550
E. *Industrial*								
Kitchen	100 beds	260	200 beds	410	300 beds	445	400 beds	480
Laundry	100 beds	260	200 beds	—	300 beds	—	400 beds	480
Stores	100 beds	150	200 beds	170	300 beds	225	400 beds	340
Sterile:/disinfect:	100 beds	100	200 beds	160	300 beds	280	400 beds	280
Pharmacy	100 beds	80	200 beds	160	300 beds	240	100 beds	420
Workshops	100 beds	120	200 beds	200	300 beds	300	400 beds	420
Plantrooms	100 beds	230	200 beds	250	300 beds	280	400 beds	370
		940		1350		1800		2790
H. *Circulation* (percentages are of net space)	(60%)	2715	(60%)	508	(60%)	6810	(60%)	9190
Total gross space	108 beds	7240	217 beds	13545	298 beds	18160	409 beds	24510
Space per bed		67 m^2		63 m^2		61 m^2		60 m^2

Example	*Type*	*Form*	*Average distance nurse-bed (m)* 0 5 10 15 20 25 30m
St Thomas' UK 1870	Open	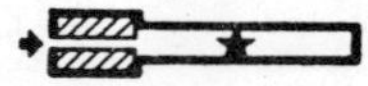	9.3
Grantham UK 1982	Open	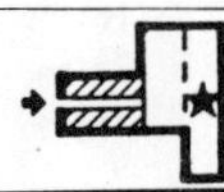	9.8
Varburg Sweden 1978	Corridor		22.4
Airedale UK 1963	Corridor		18.4
Holy cross USA 1963	Racetrack	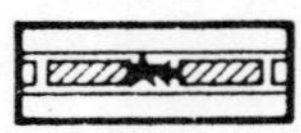	16.5
Gelsenkirchen W Germany 1977	Recetrack		15.3
Hvidovre Denmark 1978	Courtyard		26.5
West Suffolk UK 1972	Courtyard	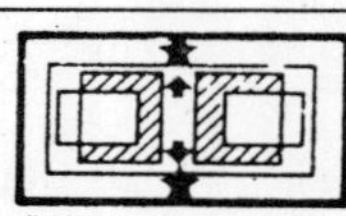	19.3
Newham UK 1982	Cruciform	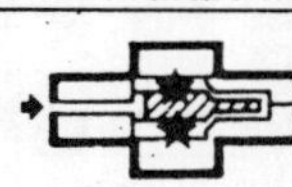	11.5
S. Western RHA UK 1983	Cruciform		9.8
Jegensdorf Switzerland 1978	Radial		10.4
Nordenham W. Germany 1974	Radial		9.3

Fig. 4.2: Staff-patient contact

Table 4.1a: Number of beds to corridor length

Example	*Room type*	*Built form and corridor type*	*Total length of corridor (m)*	*Number of beds in unit*	*Number of beds 3 m run of corridor*
Newham, UK 1981 (Nucleus)	Mainly 6-bed rooms	Cruciform Part double part single corridor	72.0	56	2.33
Frimley Park, UK 1974 (Best buy)	Mainly 6-bed rooms	Courtyard Single corridor	99.0	68	2.06
Nordenham, West Germany, 1974	Mainly 2-bed rooms	Radial Part circular corridor	99.0	60	1.82
Gelsenkirchen, West Germany, 1977	Mainly 3-bed rooms	Racetrack Double corridor	134.0	78	1.74
High Wycombe, UK 1966	Mainly 4-bed and 6-bed rooms	Racetrack Double corridor	78.0	40	1.54
Centinela valley USA, 1969	All single rooms, beds at right angles	Racetrack Double corridor	70.0	34	1.47
Valley Presbyterian USA, 1974	All single rooms, beds at right angles	Radial Circular corridor	66.0	32	1.45
St Marks USA, 1974	All single rooms, beds at right angles to corridor	Radial Triangular corridor	87.0	35	1.21

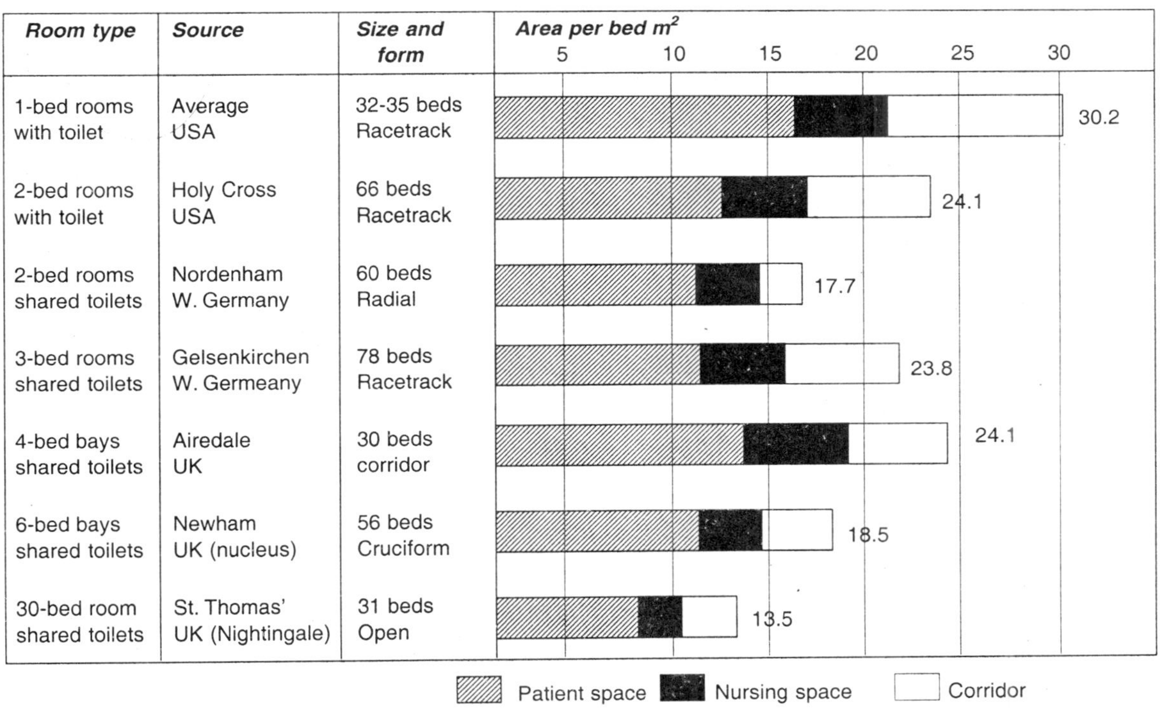

Fig. 4.3: Comparing different standards of patient accommodation and illustrating the effect on the allocation of patient space, nursing space and corridor space

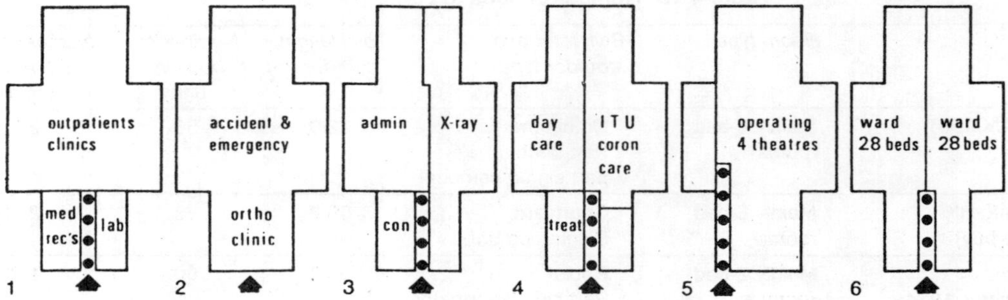

Fig. 4.3a: Cruciform templates contain standard departments; each template is approximately 1000m^2 in area and is based on a 16.2m module

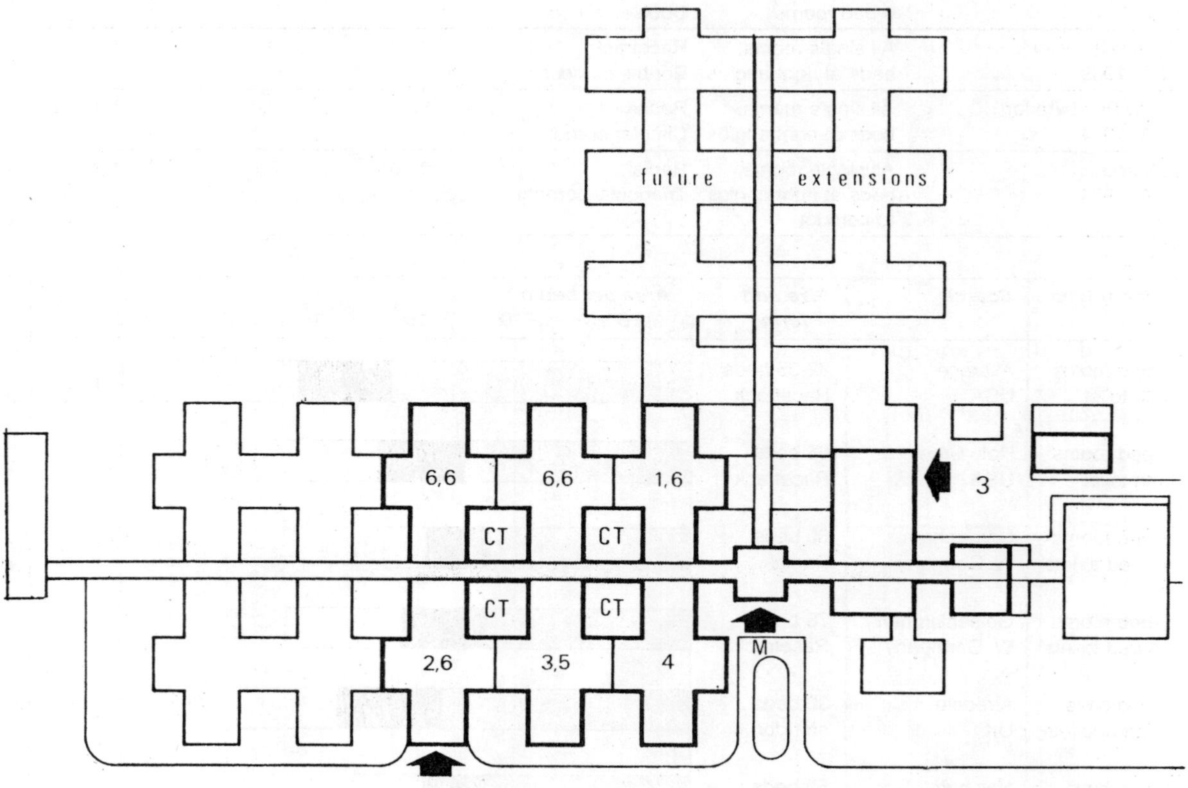

Fig. 4.3b: Block schematic plan of illustrating how the templates, numbered 1-6, are assembled into a two-storey courtyard development arranged on either side of a central spine corridor system which also carries the main services distribution and plant rooms. Unnumbered templates indicate how the hospital can be extended up to 800 beds

be placed side by side. As acceptable appointment system could be devised to reduce the area of waiting space required, while at the same time of course increasing the convenience of patients and

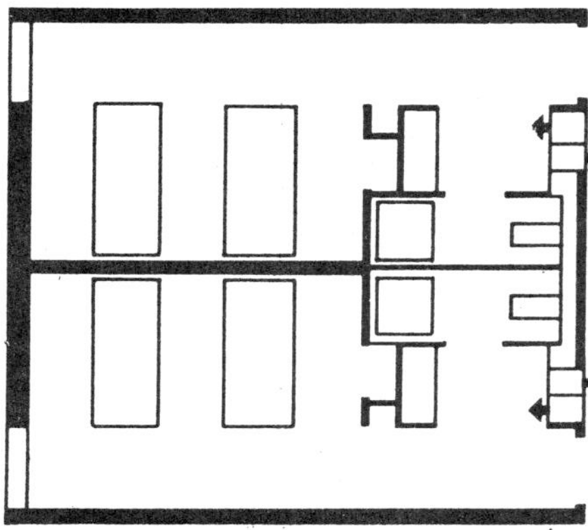

Fig. 4.3c: Holy cross hospital, Maryland, USA: typical patient suite comprising a bedroom sized to accommodate one or two beds together with shower, wc, basin and wardrobe. Note 'nurse server' on corridor wall. The total floor area is substantially in excess of European standards

their escorts. Zeidler has developed the sub-zero lab system for the McMaster Health Science centre in Canada. Here, completely serviced prefabricated standard demountable units can be assembled and atteached to the energy harness of the building at strategic points in the clinical zone. Each one is a kind of mini-lab on wheels.

Progress towards the better use of operating theaters can only be made if and when those directly

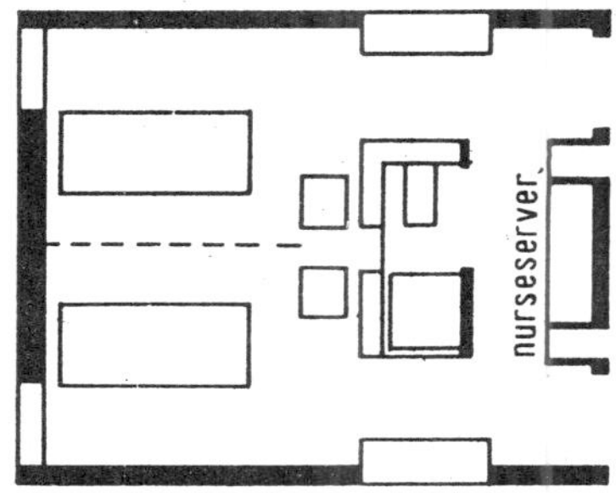

Fig. 4.3d: Mercy Hospital, San Juan, USA: alternate layout with beds placed at right angles to external wall. This arrangement gives improved privacy when the room is occupied by two patients

concerned in running these units are prepared to analyze and discuss the problem. The important factors that affect the utilization include: extending the use of theaters outside prime time (daytime week day periods), the effect of bed allocation, admission policies and length of stay, treatment facilities (anesthetic rooms, recovery rooms), the efficiency of schedules, etc.

Ultra Clean Air System (UCA) is a development of the laminar flow principle. Air is blown from the ceiling downwards at 20 m a minute in a unidirectional manner over an area 3 m square. An ultra-clean area is formed immediately around the operating table. This effectively isolates the table

National examples	Beds in room	Bed spacing	Ratio of fittings to beds					Net area of bedroom (m^2/bed)
UK St Thomas	30	2.40	1:15	1:15	1:15	1:6	✓	7.00
UK Newham	6	2.50	1:14	1:28	1:6	1:6	✓	10.20
USA Holy Cross	2	1.98	1:28	1:2	1:2	1:2	✓	8.25
Sweden	4	1.85	1:30	1:4	1:4	1:4	✓	9.72
Denmark	4	1.83	1:28	1:4	1:2	1:2	✓	8.89
West Germany Gelsenkirchen	3	1.68	1:39	1:3	1:3	1:3	✓	7.85
West Germany Nordenham	2	1.68	1:30	1:30	1:2	1:2	✓	8.75
Switzerland	2	1.68	1:26	1:26	1:5	1:2	✓	11.79

Fig. 4.3e: Patient room: comparative standards in various countries

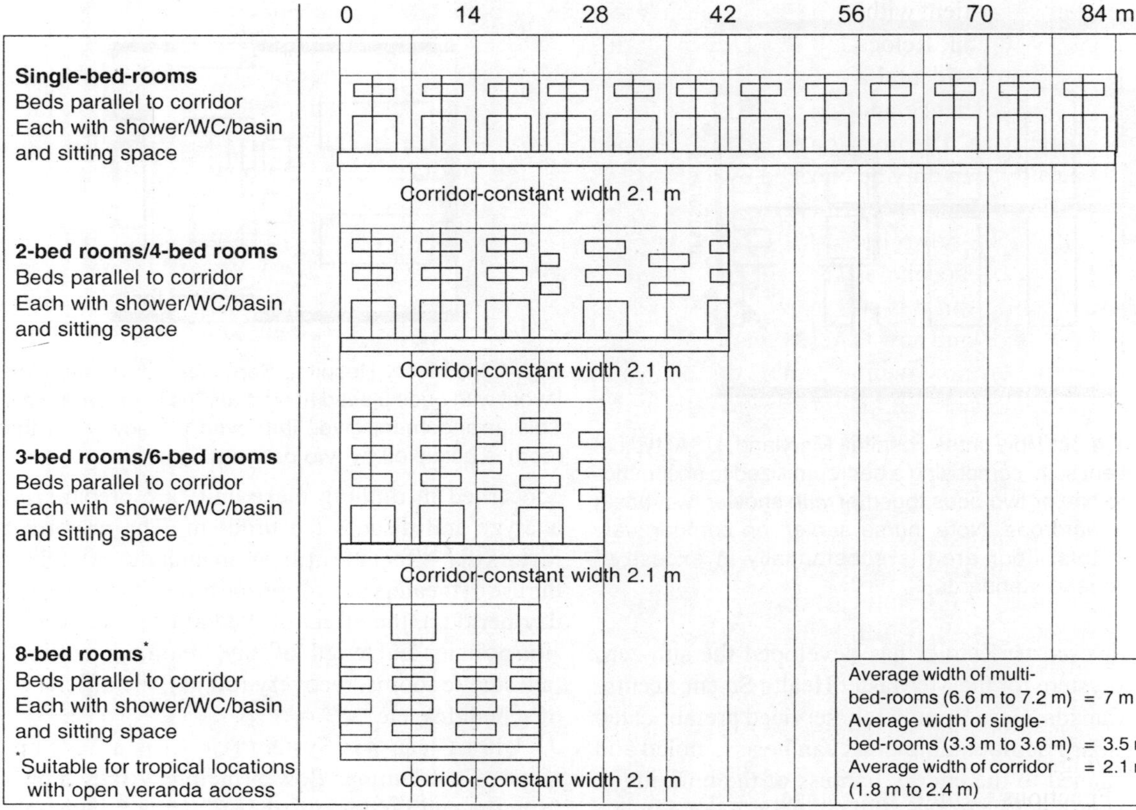

Fig. 4.4: Alternative arrangements for 24-bed ward

and the instruments from the rest of the theater suite. The surgical team can be equipped with special growth and mask fitted to the suction outlet. The rest of the theater staff are therefore outside the ultraclean "enclosure", and their cleanliness is of comparatively of little importance.

The use of UCA systems and their development may well have a profound effect on theater planning and design, leading to a reduction in compartmentalisation. Already open plan multi-table operating theaters using laminar-flow enclosures have been built in Switzerland and South Africa.

The use of UCA enclosures will result in better space utilization and more efficient development of staff. It may well be that such a department will offer more patients more surgery in safer surroundings built in a smaller space, for less money.

The enormous increase in X-ray examinations and laboratory tests has led to the mechanization of some processes previously carried out by hand. File processors eliminate the need for darkrooms. Auto-analyzers process 3 man-weeks worth of tests in 8 hours. The unit dose system, enabling the pharmacy to supply a nurse with a specific dosage of a particularly drugs, to be taken at a particular time by a particular patient means that all the work of preparation and measurement can be done more accurately in advance. These developments ease the pressure on the clinical zone.

X-ray images can be transmitted by wire, so that hospitals can have the benefit of an interpretation by a radiologist sitting at a central point. His diagnosis can be given immediately without waiting for films to be developed and despatched; and, more important for patient without a special journey to a specialist hospital. Relocation of as many service as possible in residental areas will greatly add to patient's convenience and reduce the pressure on the clinical zone. The invasion of the clinical zone by the healthy can only be checked by a change in attitude. People must accept more responsibility for the health of their own bodies.

The modern hospital is very young institution. As an organization it is still learning how to cope with its mission and how to behave rationally. This is where the task of hospital administration lies. It asks for much specific knowledge and skills, for perseverance and patience and above all for courage.

The growth of the clinical zone effects the advances in diagnostic and treatment techniques that have taken place in twentieth century. A general hospital today will require about three times the area to house its clinical zone that it did at the turn of the twentieth-century.

This is the most highly serviced and most expensive part of the hospital. It is also the fastest-growing.

Functions forming the clinical zone include:

- Operating theater
- Radiodiagnosis
- Rehabilitation
- Laboratories.

In recent years, planners have sought to break down departmental boundaries, so that one department can flow into another open-ended sections permit future expansion.

THE SUPPORT ZONE

The support zone is the third main section of the hospital: it includes those areas not already allocated to the nursing or clinical zones. Its purpose is to satisfy all their physical and material needs: food, energy, goods and services. It has to provide for the reception, handling, distribution, storage, and disposal of everything that comes into or goes out of the hospital.

The growth of the support zone is comparatively recent. As new developments took place extra buildings were added: workshop to maintain furniture and equipment, garages for ambulances, a transformer station, a telephone exchange, changing rooms, cafeteria, educational and recreational facilities, shops and a bank.

Dominating the whole complex might be a huge factory chimney, a water tower, and boiler house supplying central heating and steam for the laundry, CSSD and kitchens. All buildings on the site would be linked by the complex infrastructure of walkway ducts housing engineering services requiring constant maintenance and attention, while above ground, more and more of the landscape was taken over by an ever-growing care park.

The enormous area required to house these activities prompted planners to take a fresh look at what was going on instead of providing for them on an additive basis, could they not be grouped together into one zone with a more orderly system of distribution and disposal (concentration)—the whole process of supply, processing and distribution. The whole process of supply, processing and distribution in some hospitals is fully automated.

The next development to hit hospitals was air conditioning. The heating, cooling and humidification of the air is carried out at each air-handling unit. A hot and cold dual duct system provides air at high velocity to air mixing boxes, from which it is distributed at low velocity to the rooms below. Refrigeration for the air-conditioning is by absorption type units situated centrally on the roof with cooling towers above.

A Canadian research team recorded its conviction of the potential advantages of the adoption of interstitial space for all future hospitals of over 400 beds. Some hospitals have provided complete floors entirely dedicated to the maintenance and distribution of engineering services. Interestial space not only enables routine maintenance to be carried out with less disturbance, it accommodates change of use on the clinical or nursing floor above or below. It postpones obsolescence and makes possible plant replacement with less disruption when the time comes to introduce more up-to-date equipment. It opens up a new dimension for the supply zone. Planners began to see interstitial space (in some hospitals occupying some 40 percent of the total volume) as a new way to accomodate unknown future requirements.

All these extensions of the supply function led to higher and higher energy consumption. This in turn stimulated the concept of total energy: the idea that the hospital should generate its own electricity. Fuelled partly by burning waste products, it would make use of surplus energy to boost the grid.

It is a question of choosing, in each particular situation, methods which are most appropriate to the climate, customs and economy of the community to be served.

The support zone comprises several departments including hospital kitchens, laundries, bulk stores and energy centers. There are only two areas which are unique to hospitals: central sterilizing and disinfecting departments and manufacturing pharmacies.

The main difference between hospital support functions and those in other building types is centered on the need for most materials to be moved to a static consumer, mainly on a routine basis but sometimes in a hurry. It is this problem of materials handling with the logistics of supply and disposal, which has produced solutions which are unique to hospitals.

Until recently, most hospitals have been planned with comprehensive support zones within the building, either in the basement (vertical schemes) or in a separate but linked block (horizontal schemes). Today, due mainly to technological developments in catering, sterilizing and laundry equipment, it is more efficient to provide those services on area or regional basis.

This, with the increasing use of commercially supplied disposable, has resulted in the reduction of the support zone within the hospital.

The method of distributing supplies requires careful integration with the overall design of the building. More recently, various systems have been developed, offering more flexibility in use and taking account of future growth and charge in addition to manually operated trolleys or carts, these include automated costs and locomotive train systems.

Early consideration of the location and type of energy source and of the method of distributing energy throughout the building area of vital importance in whole hospital design. They can substantially influence both capital and revenue costs.

PROCEDURES FOR THE PLANNING OF HOSPITALS

There are two approaches to the business of organizing the design process.

Medical Approach

It starts from the premise that hundreds of hospitals have already been built. They are working acceptably in terms of function and cost.

Eighty percent of effort will go into twenty percent of product. Typically, many of the finest European hospitals were designed on this basis.

The Lay Approach

It starts from the assumption that a hospital, like any other building exists to house an organization. It is an inside-out approach. Design is achieved after a process of logical rational, sequential thought, starting from a statement of need, a description of work to be done and the objectives to be achieved. Typically, it flourished in America. It has the merit of economy of effort.

Objective Criteria

Teams comprisiing of a doctor, a nurse, an administrator, an architect, a mechanical engineer, a quantity surveyor are set up for planning of a hospital. The project of course benefits from a team approach.

Project Teams Working Methods

The object is to define what activities will be carried out in every part of a hospital, and how they will be accommodated. This is proceeded by a detailed investigation of existing practice. The various specialists incharge of each department are visited in turn and interrogated by the team. They are questioned on a room-by-room basis and notes are taken of the estimated space requirements, and on environmental conditions, sound insulation, sound absorption, day lighting, view out and view in, the type and number of people using each space, the duration, frequency, and times of occupation, the size and weight of equipment used or stored, etc. The standard work-study questions are put; who does it? Where is it done? Who else could do it? How is it done? What other ways of doing it? Where else could it be done?

The collection of information has become a highly sophisticated art. Elaborate checklists are prepared to ensure that nothing is missing. As soon as the written collection of data is complete, it is followed by room loading sheet giving engineering requirement's socket outlets, lighting points, etc and 1:50 scale plans and elevations are drawn and returned to the user specialists for checking and initiating. All this often takes a year or more to produce, but it is thought to be necessary if the room provided is to be used effectively without some costly last-minute alterations.

Step-by-Step Procedure

This describes a logical sequence to be followed by project teams from feasibility studies though operational policies, sketch design (Schematics), detail design, contract documents, construction, commissioning and occupation, to evaluation and feedback.

Plans are achieved by the process of logical, rational, sequential thought rather than by inspiration. The step-by-step advance reduces risk of failure though incompetence or inexperience. Safe and slow it is ideally suited to a governmental machine of financial orthodoxy, regional quality, and public accountability.

It imposes a delay on the production of hospitals.

Standardization

The classic aim of standardization are economy of professional staff, and concentration of design effort leading to a better product, which in turn increases demand and makes possible mass production and higher output for less cost.

There are two approaches to standardization. The first is to produce standard plans (whole buildings). The second is to produce standard components (the bits and pieces).

CONTAINMENT

The first question to be asked is why most hospitals always take so long to build and cost so much? And the second is: is there anything to choose between the medical and lay approach? The best way to answer these questions is to look very closely at the various procedures being advocated today and observe what happens in practice, as opposed to what is supposed or desired to happen operational research.

Someone Incharge

Hospitals need take on longer to design and build than other complex buildings. There must be a client, to manage the briefing and design evaluation process and ensure that all the pressures are balanced by an objective authority. The cost of hiring an incharge will be repaid many times over by the savings on the capital cost of building, and what is far more important, the functional efficiency and therefore the running costs of the future hospital.

The Probject Director

The team leader may be an outside consultant or an in-house appointment. He should have demonstrated marked skills as an entrepreneur.

He must be able to command the respect of all parties concerned. The project director is coldly rational, processing raw data into rational information, stimulating the clients to make decisions.

Table 4.2: Teaching hospitals 500-900 beds.
(Based on examples in UK, Belgium, W. Africa, USA and Far East)

	500 beds	*Net space m^2*	*600 beds*	*Net space m^2*	*700 beds*	*Net space m^2*	*800 beds*	*Net space m^2*	*900 beds*	*Net space m^2*
A. In-patients wards										
Medical/surgical	364 beds	6190	420 beds	7140	504 beds	8570	580 beds	9860	644 beds	10950
Pediatric	69 beds	1360	92 beds	1810	92 beds	1810	115 beds	2265	115 beds	2265
Obstetric	50 beds	815	75 beds	1185	75 beds	1185	75 beds	1185	100 beds	1550
		8365		10135		11565		13310		14765
B. Out-patients										
Consulting clinics	All depts	3190	All depts	3825	All depts	4460	All depts	5100	All depts	5740
Emergency department	1 dept	1125	1 dept	1125	1 dept	1500	1 dept	1500	1 dept	1500
		4315		4950		5960		6600		7240
C. Diagnostic/treatment										
Regional specialities*	—	—	—	—	1 dept	500	1 dept	500	2 dept	1000
Radiodiagnostic	7 r/d rms	825	9 r/d rms	1060	11 r/d rms	1300	13 r/d rms	1535	15 r/d rms	1770
Operating/endoscopy	6 tables	990	8 tables	1320	10 tables	1650	12 tables	1980	14 tables	2310
Intensive treatment unit/recovery	25 beds	415	30 beds	495	40 beds	660	45 beds	745	50 beds	830
Clinical service beds	All depts		All depts		All depts		All depts		All depts	
Mortuary and post-mortem	1 dept	3080	1 dept	3700	1 dept	3850	1 dept	4110	1 dept	4625
Functional diagnosis	1 dept	1000	1 dept	1200	1 dept	1310	1 dept	1500	1 dept	1600
Rehabilitation	1 dept	1000	1 dept	1280	1 dept	1400	1 dept	1600	1 dept	1600
Obstetric delivery	1 dept	750	1 dept	800	1 dept	1050	1 dept	1200	1 dept	1600
Day care (endoscopy)	2 tables	110	3 tables	165	4 tables	220	5 tables	275	5 tables	275
		8170		10020		11940		13445		15610
D. Administration										
Central administration	500 beds	750	600 beds	960	700 beds	1050	800 beds	1200	900 beds	1350
Administrative units	500 beds	940	600 beds	1200	700 beds	1310	800 beds	1500	900 beds	1690
Social medicine	1 dept	1000	1 dept	1200	1 dept	1200	1 dept	1200	1 dept	1200
Social services	500 beds	1810	600 beds	2320	700 beds	2540	800 beds	2900	800 beds	3260
		4500		5680		6100		6800		7500

Contd....

Contd....

	500 beds	Net space m^2	Net 600 beds	space m^2	Net 700 beds	Net space m^2	Net 800 beds	space m^2	900 beds	space m^2
E. Industrial										
Kitchen	500 beds	700	600 beds	760	700 beds	885	800 beds	1010	900 beds	1135
Laundry	500 beds	560	600 beds	560	700 beds	655	800 beds	750	900 beds	840
Stores	500 beds	750	600 beds	900	700 beds	1050	800 beds	1200	900 beds	1350
Sterilising	500 beds	340	600 beds	340	700 beds	340	800 beds	450	900 beds	450
Pharmacy	500 beds	450	600 beds	450	700 beds	525	800 beds	600	900 beds	675
Workshops	500 beds	480	600 beds	525	700 beds	615	800 beds	700	900 beds	700
Plantrooms	500 beds	500	600 beds	600	700 beds	700	800 beds	800	900 beds	900
		3780		4135		4770		5510		6050
F. Teaching/research										
Teaching units	150 student	1250	180 student	1500	210 student	1750	240 student	2000	270 student	2330
Teach/research labs	150 student	1500	180 student	1800	210 student	2100	240 student	2400	270 student	2700
Lecture/classrooms	150 student	690	180 student	825	210 student	960	240 student	1100	270 student	1285
Library/TV/cloaks	150 student	1810	180 student	2175	210 student	2535	240 student	2900	270 student	3260
		5250		6300		7345		8400		9575
G. Dental										
Hospital and school	N/A		N/A		N/A		100 student 2120	2120	100 student 2120	2120
H. *Circulation* (percentages are of net space)	(60%)	20495	(60%)	24555	(60%)	28430	(60%)	33535	(60%)	37500
Total gross space		54875		65775		76110		89720		100360
Space per bed	508 beds	108	617 beds	107	711 beds	107	815 beds	110	909 beds	110

*Regional specialities: radiotherapy, nuclear medicine, haemodialysis, burns

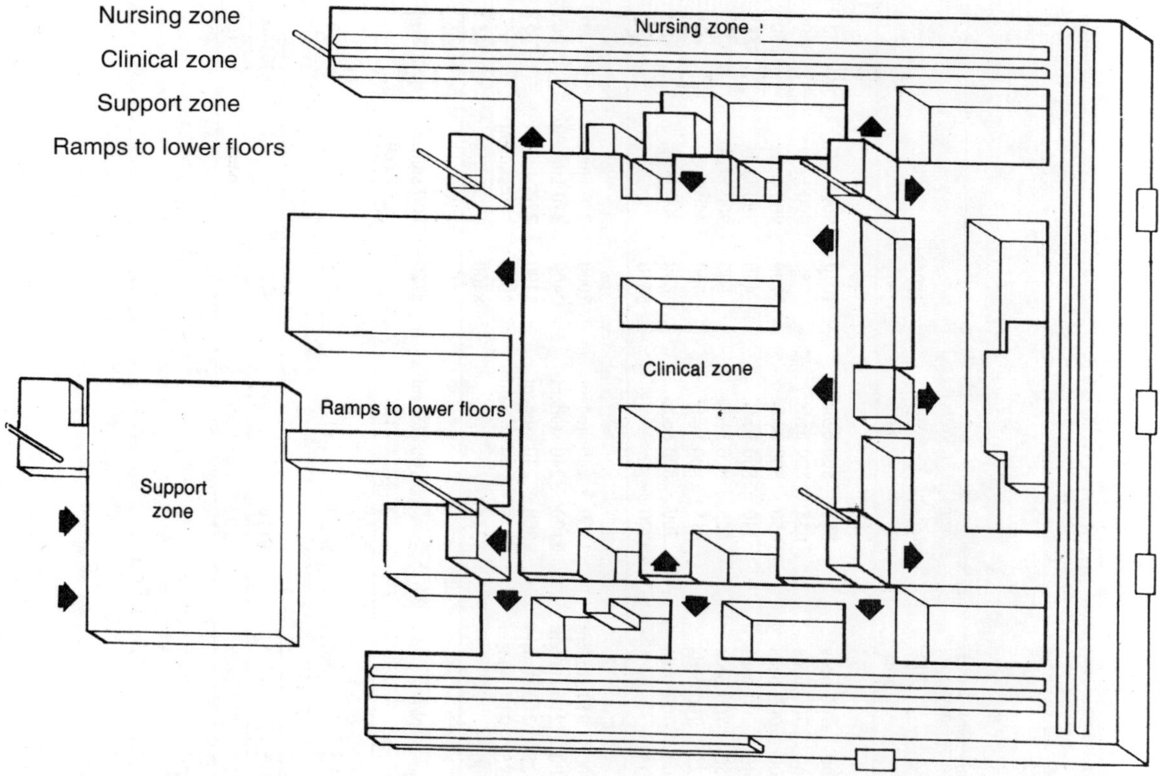

Fig. 4.5: King's Lynn Hospital, UK: a Best Buy hospital. Axonometric showing position of support zone and its relationship to the user zones. A locomotive train system was developed for the Best Buy hospital similar to that used at Baltimore. The support zone, conceived as a separate single-storey industrial type building, is placed at a level midway between the two floors of the main complex. Single flight ramps, one up and one down, link the support zone to the ring main corridors at each level. The trains move in a clockwise direction, dropping off and collecting trolleys in the turn-around spaces outside the user department entrances

He works with his head. The design architect works with his heart instinctively translating his brief into form and content.

The first job of project director is the preparation of a certificate of need. This sets out the short- and long-term aims, service, costs benefits and anticipated use of facilities. Once approved by the government, the promoter can claim the financial benefits to which he is entitled.

Obtaining Consensus

After carrying out the usual collection of data and interviews, the project director and his team conduct a series of work session. These take place in the clients' backyard. They consist of intensive day and night session, lasting perhaps a week. Conflicts between different groups are brought out into the open and their effect on space allocations and cost illustrated by graphic display.

The probject director has 4 fields of manoeurvre form, function, economy and time. In order to achieve best value for money he should be free to operate in at least one, and preferably in all four.

Hospitals come in many shapes and size (high rise, low rise, monoblock, etc). Similar functions can be achieved by many different operational policies (e.g. linen exchange or laundary annexe).

Cost consequences and methods of circulation are almost equally variable (e.g. ramps or elevators). He should also be free to decide as and when to let a contract (whether to go ahead immediately or bank his money and wait for a more favorable tendering climate).

As soon as the week of intensive work sessions is over, there is an interval of 2-4 weeks. During this period, the project director and his team check the evidence they have received to make sure that it includes all the hopes and aspirations of the client groups. He then completes his brief, his statement of the problem to be solved, expressed in terms of form, function, money and time.

During the work sessions, the architect and his team of consultants are present. But they play a passive role, answering questions if asked. Their job is to listen and observe, so that they are aware of the problems to be solved and they reason behind the project director's decisions. An explicit and open process conducted in this way at the work sessions, leads to a clear understanding of the project first by the client and later by the designer.

On receipt of this brief, the architect prepares his sketch designs or schematics exactly as he would if entering a two-stage competition. The project director calls for alternative solutions from the architect, if necessary, adjudicates. The selected scheme is then developed into detailed designs and once approved, translated into contract documents.

FAST TRACK

Every means of shortening the production process is worth pursuing: word processors, computer-assisted drafting methods and all mechanical aids at the disposal of the design team.

One of the most impressive strategies for saving time is known as fast-track. The aim is to telescope operations that are normally sequential, so that they can be stated in quick succession and completed almost simultaneously.

Fast track depends on the use of predetermined envelopes such as nucleus. The number and configuration of these envelopes can be quickly determined at sketch design. Approximate bills of quantities can be prepared in advance and priced, directly or by reference to previous contracts. Tenders can therefore be obtained at a much earlier stage and a contractor appointed immediately. While foundations are being dug, detailed design development is completed and orders placed for equipment. As soon as it arrives on the job, the contractor is ready to install it.

TURNKEY

Turnkey is a time-saving procedure. It has been especially successful in developing countries. Modern turnkeys combine competitive tendering and design competition in one package. The normal turnkey is contractor led. The client—government department, public authority or private developer—prepares (or has prepared by his project director) a detailed program and specification, including in some cases draft schematics. Meanwhile contractor-led consortia are invited to prequalify with the client-authority. The client then selects a short list of turnkey consortia (which normally include, in addition to the contractor, the medical equipment supplier, architect, mechanical and electrical consultants and cost consultants, all appointed by contractor). The project director will advise the client on the selection of the short list.

The tender documents (program and specifications) are given to the selected consortia, who will then bid for the design, construction and equipping of the hospital (often this will include a two-year training and maintenance programme on completion of work).

Turnkey contractors are usually given a period of two to four months to complete their bids for a hospital of 300-500 beds. This very tight period makes great demands on the contractors, design consultants, who normally have to produce final design documents to satisfy the contractors need for a form price-base and the demands of the project director who, being responsible to the client both for design and supervision, needs to be satisfied that he is getting a sound design.

The successful tenderer is usually given a start-up period of 3 months before work must commence on site, and it is during this period that his design consultants have to produce working drawings.

The whole design period is thus telescoped into between 5-7 months for a hospital of 300-500 beds.

It has been observed that keen competition makes this a very attractive method for a founding authorities.

Not only will there be a low bid from the contractor but also the design, which is included in the bid price, is being done for an all-in fee of between 2-3 percent of all disciplines. All the clients pay in fees is for the project director to check the tenderer work and carry out the supervision on site.

The Need for Further Experiment

Quick decisions are best obtained from a knowledgeable client who has discretion, with carefully defined limits, to spend money as if it were his own. Those most likely to be capable of exercising the function of client are those working closest to the patient, or those in a portion to get an immediate reaction from users so that they can revise plans or incorporate improvements quickly in subsequent designs. This kind of flexibility is likely to be inhabited by remote control. A better service could almost certainly be provided if the people responsible for managing hospital construction or reconstruction could be more clearly identified and rewarded.

STEPS IN PLANNING

It is necessary to:

- Proceed in an orderly manner through a series of stages in the planning and building of hospital.
- Appropriately qualified planning staff must be available at each stage and must be given sufficient time to do the necessary work in a careful and accurate manner.
- Sufficient time be allowed in the early stages of planning.
- Time spent thinking out clearly what the requirements of the hospital are will save both money and time in the long run.

Stage I

Planning team should be assembled and given the task of preparing the architect's brief.

Project team comprises:

- Hospital consultant
- Administrator
- Architect
- Sociologist.

Tasks of the Project Team

i. To establish the need for the particular hospital under construction in relation to the regional plan, based on population and morbidity data of the region; projections of changes in population, and economic conditions in the area; and projections of the future development of the medical service.

ii. Determine the site
   - Survey existing health facilities in the area and projections of the future development of transport, economic development, and the general building programme in the area.
   - Planning team will need to collaborate closely with the authorities concerned with the economic development of the area and with the town and the country planning authorities.
   - Approximate estimates of the capital and running costs can be made and a master plan prepared.

Stage II

Preparation of the Architect's Brief

- Determine (in quantitative terms) the services to be provided in the hospital.

- The preparation of schedules of accommodation based on the requirements of services.
- Team should be enlarged to include:
  - One architect and
  - Nursing administrator
- In determining the services to be provided, it will be necessary to consult, on an ad hoc basis, medical specialists as particular problems arise.
- The architect's brief should be complete at the end of this stage, comprising of: general descriptions of the scope and functioning of each service, together with approximate floor areas, and notes on any special requirements or special equipment.

Stage III

- Design of the hospital from the brief by the architect.
- Mainly the work of architect. The team should include architects, mechanical engineer and civil engineer.
- The design costs are likely to amount to 10-12 percent of the building cost.

During the process of design, the medical and the administrative members of the planning team will operate as consultants to the architects and engineers, answering their questions and defending the requirements of the hospital in detail.

1. Preliminary designs will be produced and submitted to the planning team for any modifications.
2. The architects and engineers can proceed to prepare working drawings—a complete set of instructions to the contractor for the building of the hospital, they will show the whole of the construction process in minute details, and will be accompanied by specifications and bills of quantities.

Close and continuous collaboration is needed at this stage among architects and medical and nursing members of the planning team.

As the drawings proceed to greater, detail the advice of medical members of the planning team will be needed on a day-to-day basis by the architects.

Extra costs and severe delays will be involved if there are any important modifications in the design of the hospital during the working drawing stage.

Final Stage

Actual Building of the Hospital

- Carried out by contractor, who may be selected by competitive tender, his work will be controlled and supervised by the architects and consulting engineers. Modifications at this stage should be avoided as far as possible. It is important, when selecting a contractor to investigate the capacity of his firm is terms of managerial personnel and plant capacity.

During the construction, it will be necessary to set up a second team in addition to the planning team to prepare for the commissioning of the new hospital. This team should include experienced administrator and certain key members of the staff of the hospital. If possible the Hospital Administrator, Nursing Administrator, Chief of Medical and Surgical Services should be appointed a year or two before the hospital is likely to be finished so that they can take part in the work of the commissioning team. The functions of the team include:

- To decide in detail, the staffing required, and to arrange for the engagement of all staff.
- To schedule the acquisition of items of furniture and equipment down to the last tea spoon, and to arrange for their purchase and delivery at the appropriate time.
- To plan and carry out special staff training courses to give the staff the experience and the confidence to enable them to function under new conditions. The key members of the new staff may be sent for training to modern hospitals in other parts of the country or, perhaps, abroad, where the methods and the equipment proposed for the new hospital may have been recently put into operation. This orientation is vital.

ESTIMATION OF REQUIREMENTS

- Determine the broad requirements for the new hospital.
- Establish the area and population likely to be served by the new hospital.
- Estimate the demand for medical care (personal experience supported by morbidity pattern will determine the need).
- Predict broadly the demand for care in each speciality.
- Both the staffing and the planning of the building must start from such predictions.
- Once the assumed number of patients presenting for care in the various departments of the hospital has been established, the requirement for the hospital can be estimated.
- Assuming that a certain number of out-patients will present themselves at surgical clinics in a month, then the staffing of the clinic and the number of consulting rooms can be determined by making an estimate of the average length of time each consultation will require. Similarly, in determining the number of beds that may be needed for medical cases, surgery, obstetrics, and other departments, it will be necessary to make estimates not only of the number of patients who will present themselves for admission, but also of their length of stay in the hospital.
- From the number of beds and from the predicted number of out-patient attendance, it is possible to proceed to an approximate definition of the requirements for the medical; services departments (Radiodiagnosis, Laboratory etc.).
- Draw up rough figures for the population at the hospital site, including the patients and the staff of various categories (required for requirements for catering, laundry, stores, boiler house, etc.).

Also keep a provision for staff housing to be estimated.

Establish in broad terms:

- The volume of building required for the various departments of the hospital.
- Estimte the demand that the hospital will make on the public services, such as water, electricity, gas, and sewage disposal.

An architect should be able to give the hospital authority some idea of the cost of the project in round figures at this time. Operational costs of the hospital and the staff salary can be approximated.

Architect can make a master plan for the hospital development once a site has been chosen.

Proper understanding of the community, facility planning which is relevant, appropriate, and cost-effective to local conditions, through intersectoral coordination and cooperation, technology evaluation of equipment and dedicated team of professionals in the project team and community participation are some vital pillars of hospital planning.

Proper thought needs to be given during construction, for minimizing operating cost. By providing durable internal and external finishes, hygiene flooring and sanitary fittings, alongwith ducts and pipes of appropriate size, operating cost should be minimized.

Use of locally available building materials and skills are a valuable means of providing appropriate facilities. Imported equipment and materials are very expensive.

If there is an approach to design which will permit the designer to fully educate himself with what has gone before him in a given area of design, and at the same time keep the spark of creativity alive, this would be the ideal approach to hospital design.

At the time of planning, thought is to be given how best to plan the building where better maintenance is not only possible but also need for it minimal.

The functional aspect of the hospital should get precedence (design follows function) over the architectural and anesthetic aspect at the hands of the architect.

There should be flexibility in the design and provision for future expansion. A hospital must have an inbuilt capacity for natural expansion with minimum disruption.

There is enough scope for use of value engineering techniques to reduce the costs without affecting the performance. Economy in construction is of paramount importance and all out efforts should be made to achieve this.

Thought should be given to energy conservation and saving. If energy systems are designed to satisfy peak energy uses during extreme whether conditions, then the system operates at this peak design, resulting in avoidable excess consumption of energy. Similarly, design criteria regarding comfort levels and air and air changes influence the energy consumption. Bifurcation of areas according to their requirement will result in energy saving. Sophisticated control systems. Control supply to energy at the rate required to satisfy the energy needs. The type of control, energy distribution, hours of operation and thermal quality need special consideration. The hospital can use natural light throughout the year.

Hospitals must be capable of offering a care of a high priority health services and a corollary of secondary health services and funds must be provided accordingly. The aim should be to provide a minimum amount of permanent structure and an optimal amount of infrastructure in order to achieve maximum.

FURTHER READING

1. James, W Pau, Tatton-Brown, William: Hospitals—design and development. Architectural press Ltd. London 1986.
2. Putsep E: The Modern Hospital: International Planning Practice, Lloyd-luke, London 1979.

5 Changing System of Health Services Concepts

Hospitals have undergone a remarkable change both in the industrialised nations and developing countries. They are, or should be, dynamic institutions and in any society the only thing constant is change. The hospitals have to adopt a concept of providing Primary Health Care (from the centre of excellence to community support). Directly or indirectly, every person from birth to death, at one time or another, pins hope on the positive outcome of the health services, these institution provide. There has been very rapid change in last three decades in functioning of hospitals due to technological advances and knowledge explosion which had direct bearing on patient care.

- Emergence of corporate hospitals.
- Hospital-based approach to group practice and
- Role of hospital in primary health care.

Creative ideas such as day care facilities, transferring clinical activities that once were undertaken only in the very heart of the institution, in ward, operating suites and special units" to outpatient department, outreach programme and home and community care services. In recent years, hospital practice in all countries have been made effective by changing socio-demography and financial circumstances.

Now-a-days lot of importance is given to quick turnover of patients to reduce cost and thus to save many. To supplement the hospital cost, various types of insurance programmes are also offered. Above facts have major influence in the planing of new hospitals.

The other factors which have direct bearing on hospital planning are:

a. Costly diagnostic services cannot be provided in all hospitals. Thus, there should be proper choice of place and services to be rendered.
b. Tertiary care cannot be provided in all places due to high cost and lack of availability of trained manpower.
c. Design should follow function. However, the proper use of esthetic quality and humanized surroundings must be kept in mind so that it looks attractive and patient should feel homely.

Health Care System

Health care system comprises of different institutions which are graded according to the rank they have to fulfil. In many developing countries it is classified as different level of care.

A study of activities in health centres of different level is a prerequisite to planning as it answers several crucial questions.

For health centres of different sizes and with different functions, what is the proportion of

Level of care	Medical facility	Level of decision
Village	Health station	Village health guide
Primary	• Dispensary, Health centre	Medical officer
Secondary	• District hospital or similar	General duty medical officer/Specialist
Tertiary or provincial hospital	• National or Teaching	Specialist/Super specialist

working hours devoted to various broad activities of or definite tasks.

Which different categories of staff are needed and in what proportion?

What are the space requirements to discharge these functions?

What is the inter-relationship between these functions and consequently, what layout will be more convenient?

As conditions vary from place to place, it is necessary to undertake such a study for each project.

Design and Architecture of Health Centres

Grouping of closely related activities should be put together in one area. All areas should be located in relation to one another to allow direct communication and easy flow of patients, staff and services. The design and the structural system should allow maximum flexibility and expendibility.

All activities in the health centre may be grouped in four general areas:

- Clinical area

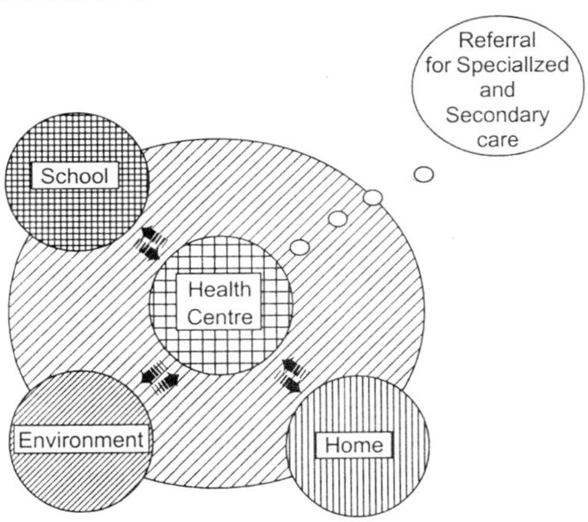

Fig. 5.1: Relationship between health centre, community and higher-level

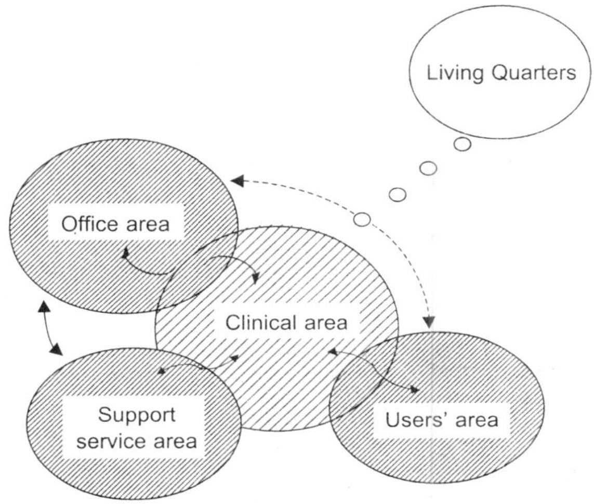

Fig. 5.2: Relationship between activities and space in a health centre

- Users area
- Office area
- Support service area

Users area, (layout and size) will depend on local tradition, size of the health centre and patient flow as determined by the working system of the health centre. The waiting area may consist of single waiting area for both sexes, there may be an additional special waiting area for maternal and child care; and, in the case of large health centres with a great variety of services, more waiting areas may be warranted. Toilets for each sex should always be provided separately.

Clinical area, consists of examination and treatment rooms, the bigger the health centre, the more specialized facilities (such as maternal and child-care room, dental treatment room, labour room, etc.) may be needed.

Supporting services area, which consists of laboratory space, will vary from a small counter for microscopy to a laboratory (about $18m^2$ per 1000 tests per month); pharmacy and integrated or separate storage area for supplies: pantry or kitchen, which may even be used for training purposes if big enough (about 20 m^2); and cleaner's room (or at least a cupboard).

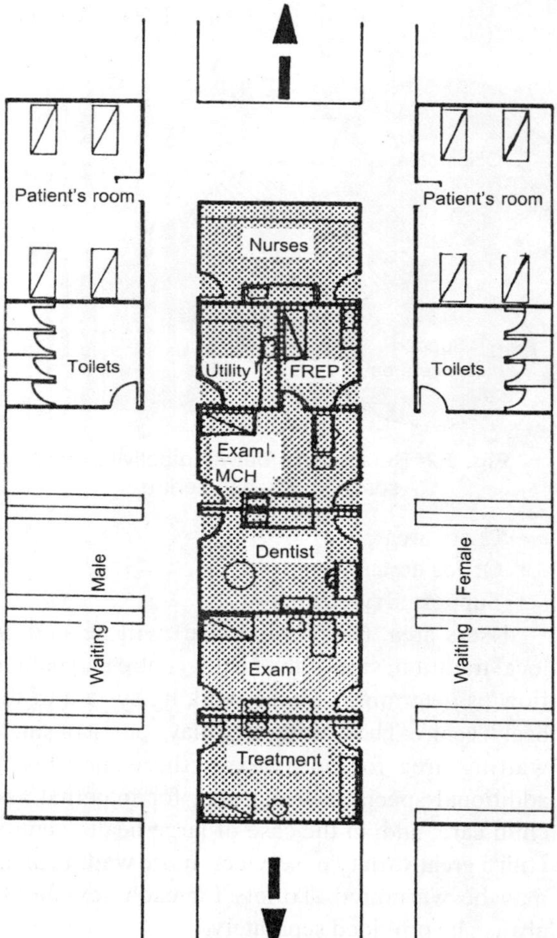

Fig. 5.3: Clinical area and user area

Office area for clerks, sanitary attendants, health visitors and other (minimum of 4 m^2 persons).

In larger health centres there may, in addition, be an area for the in patient care of emergency cases awaiting transfer or for deliveries; in that case, there should also be at least two rooms with toilet and shower facilities, as well as a clean working area for the nursing service and an area for disposal of dirty linen, etc.

The relationship between these areas is illustrated in Figure 5.4.

The spatial relationship diagram may be translated into various architectural schemes for small health centre layout as depicted in Figures 5.5, 5.6 and 5.7.

Norms

Inpatient is not only a place for admitting a patient who cannot be treated outside hospital, but also a place of training for doctors and paramedical staff. In developed countries, inpatients are likely to fall into one of five broad care groupings, in them proportions are shown.

1. *Intensive Medical Care* Where continuous medical and nursing observation and mechanical assistance is necessary to maintain life
2. *Intensive Nursing Care* Where patients are unable to leave their beds, and where they are in need to continuous nursing, observation and physical assistance.
3. *Medium Nursing Care* Where patients are also to leave their beds for short periods (upto four hours) each day with assistance which ambulant.
4. *Low Nursing Care* Where patients are able to leave their beds for more than four hours per day, requiring minimal assist ance.
5. *Self Care* Patients leading apparently a normal life, who are in hospital for observation.

Using a similar classification, the proportions of patients in a developing country are likely to be considerably higher in the intensive and medium care categories. perhaps upto 75-80 percent of total patients being within these two areas.

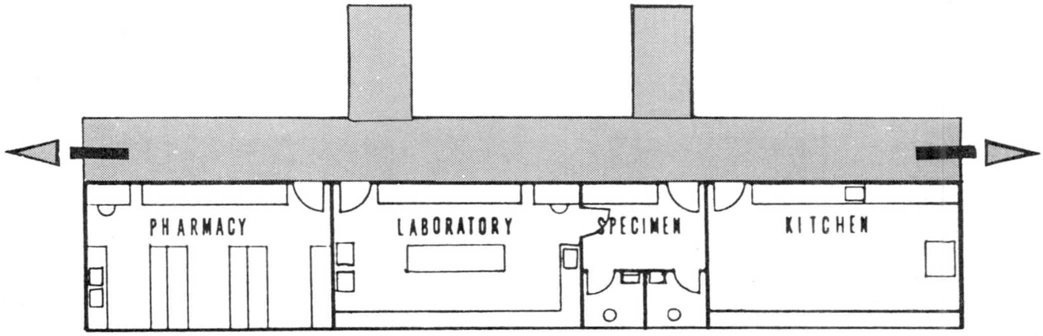

Fig. 5.4: Supporting services

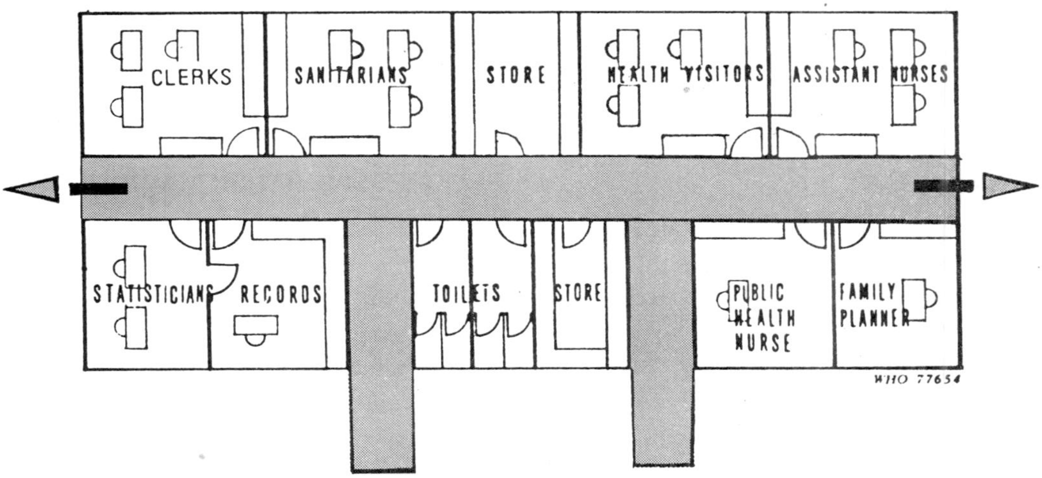

Fig. 5.5: Office area

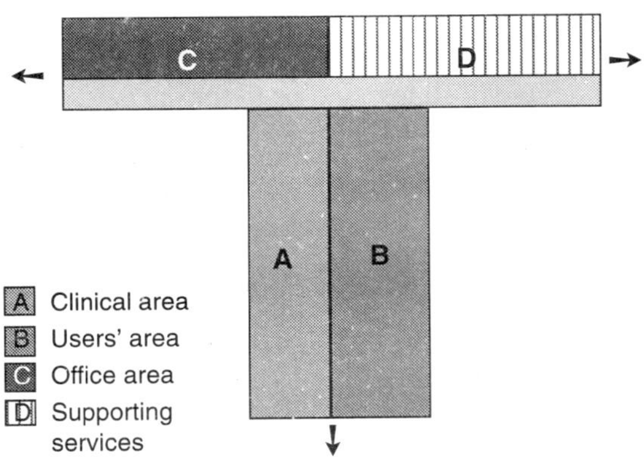

Fig. 5.6: Layout scheme for small health centre

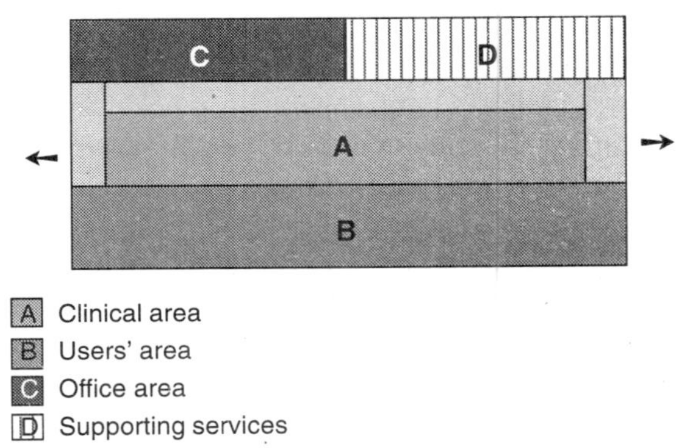

Fig. 5.7a: Layout scheme for small health centre

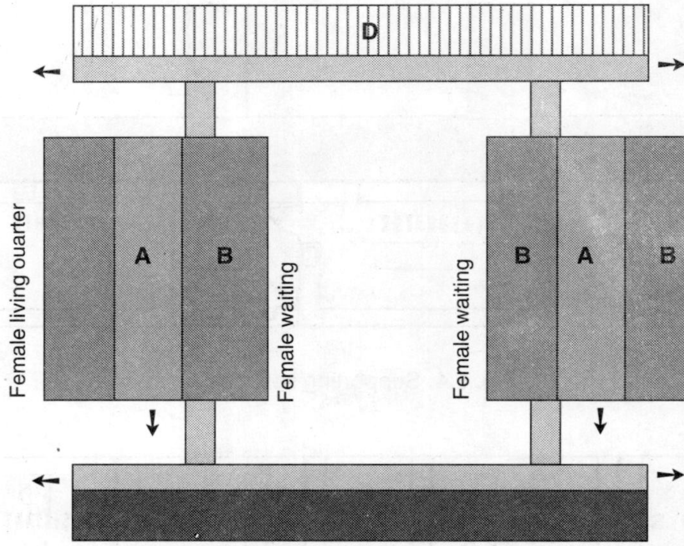

Fig. 5.7b: Layout scheme for large health centre

Size of Nursing Unit

The size of nursing unit depends on the most effective deployment of available staff. For every ward there is minimum need of one sweeper and one ward boy for all 24 hours. Keeping in view 8 hours shift, there will be need of 4 personnel, for every 10 beds one person will be provided (thus 40- bedded ward will be ideal.).

Outpatient Department

Ambulatory care is the medical care provided to patients who are not confined to bed. It can be provided at a general practitioner's or specialist's practice premises or at a health post, health centre or hospital. The function of out-patient services of a hospital is to provide diagnostic, curative, preventive, and rehabilitative service on ambulatory basis to the people of the community. The extent of these functions established by the individual hospital will vary, according to aim of hospital, expectation of community and political will, the scope and form will take a dramatic change. It can reduce pressure an inpatient care, which can be achieved by increasing diagnostic and treat ment service.

PROGRESSIVE PATIENT CARE

Progressive patient care is one of the innovative concept of application of modern management techniques to increase the following:

- The overall productivity in hospital
- The effectiveness of patient care
- Efficiency (reduction in cost)

Organization of hospital facilities, services and staff. It is also described as tailoring of hospital services to meet the patient needs or as the right patient on the right bed with the right services around him.

It consists of grouping of patients according to their degree of illness and need for the care rather than traditional grouping according to sex, age, type of illness, planned and organized with their degree of illness and need for care.

Elements of Progressive Patient Care Include

- Intensive Care
- Intermediate Care
- Self Care
- Long-term care
- Out-patient care

Intensive Care Unit (ICU)

Intensive care is meant for critically ill patient.
- Multiple injury or burn cases
- Acute coronary occlusion.

The ideal location is near operation theater but not very far from emergency department. Minimum 2 percent of total bed in large hospital should be earmarked for ICU:

for 200 beds = 2-3 beds
for 300 beds = 3-4 beds
for 400 beds = 4-5 beds
(*General guideline:* about five percent of total bed strength)
Space = 140 square ft. per bed.

Equipment and Drugs for ICU

- Life-saving drugs and equipment
- Cardiac arrest trays
- Tracheostomy trays
- Intermittent positive pressure equipment
- ECG monitor
- Pace-maker machine
- Portable X-rays
- Sterile supplies: treatment and procedure sets
- Blood bank facilities

  Staffing pattern for ICU
  - Anesthetist-overall incharge
  - One Medical Officer (with background of surgery or anesthesia) for round the clock coverage
  - One Nurse/Patient per shift

Intermediate Care

Moderately ill patients and patients who require palliative treatment:
- Pneumonia case (moderately ill)
- Acute cholecystitis.
- Uncomplicated abdominal surgery
- Partially recovered patients (from ICU)

Services

Intermediate care is similar to those given in general or surgical unit.

Staffing

- Similar to that of general ward
- Nursing staff vary with each shift
- Morning-1 for 6-7 patients
- Evening 1 for 8-10 patients
- Night 1 for 12-15 patients.

Number of Beds 30-35

Rigg's pattern of ward of one, two or four bed rooms.

Self Care

- *Patients* convalescing or requiring diagnosis.
- New diabetic patient who requires precise dietary management, frequent laboratory tests, insulin dose adjustment.
- Post-coronary patients,
- Patients requiring frequent radiation or physio-therapy,
- Some pre-operative cases

Services

- Educational and Supervisory.
- Patients permitted to follow home life routine.

Staffing

- One nurse for 10-15 patients.

Ward

- Located convenient to diagnostic facilities.

Long-term Care

- Diabetic amputee,
- Severe arthritis, etc.
- Geriatric and rehabilitation cases

Staffing

- Morning 1 nurse for 3 patients
- Evening 1 nurse for 4 patients
- Night 1 nurse for 5 patients

Design

LTC Unit : 40-55 beds
Location : Ground floor for outdoor recreation and rehabilitation therapy.

Area

- 125 sq. Ft. in single room
- 100 Sq.ft. in multiple bed rooms.

Home Care

It means that hospital services are extended to the homes of the patients.

Home-care team visits the patient in his/her home.

Advantages of progressive patient care concept include: effective and efficient use of hospital resources, better and uniform nursing facilities to the patient grouped, grouping of patients creates better environment in the wards, and home-care services help the hospital to coordinate its work with community health and social services.

LOOKING AHEAD

- Regional planning and programming of establishments constitute one phase in the overall process of sectoral planning and take their appropriate place within it.
- Sectoral planning is compatible with and follows logically from national planning and the relevant development plans.
- The regional investment plan is part of the sectoral investment plan, which in turn is part of the national investment plan.
- The regional plans give rise to local projects for facilities, which require a study and a special methodology for their planning and programming; they must be governed by and respond to the requirements of the plans and programmes for development and extension of services in the region.
- Multidisciplinary participation is essential in the preparation of the plans and studies at every level. The architect who specializes in health service buildings is an important member of the working team.
- The standardization of architectural designs and equipment, on an integrated basis, through "model units" for sectors, constitutes an extremely valuable procedure for shortening construction times, reducing costs, and facilitating operation and maintenance, especially in establishments of the primary, basic and intermediate levels.
- For the primary level, possibilities of rapid, economic and satisfactory mass construction of facilities must be explored by considering very simple solutions with intensive community participation.
- The optimum size of hospital facilities will depend mainly on the facilities for ambulatory and inpatient care and community protection required by the actions and activities planned to be developed by the whole service in the medical-architectural programme, at a level of capacity and complexity commensurate with the level of regionalization and the size of the population to be served.
- Standardization of accommodation units and equipment is highly necessary and useful and facilitates rationalization of architectural designs and staffing patterns, with great advantages in respect of installation, running and maintenance costs and of training and mobility of personnel.
- It is desirable to consolidate the isolated efforts being made at country level to obtain national standards for design and equipment of health facilities. This could be achieved by convening expert committees to study and harmonize them at the international level, thereby optimizing

the employment and use of resources, reducing installation, maintenance and running costs, promoting and encouraging multinational programme integration, and stimulating regional production of materials and equipment.

It is necessary to establish methodologies for the development of investments in health facilities, identifying the stages to be accomplished, the activities to be developed, the sequence for their implementation, those taking part and responsible for carrying them out, the requirement to be met in each case and the probable time needed for implementation, establishing the coordination mechanisms necessary in the process and facilitating technical decision-making.

FURTHER READING

1. Kleczkowski BM, Pibouleau R: Approaches to Planning and Design of Health Care Facilities in developing countries. World Health Organization, Geneva, 1976.

6 Changing Concepts in the Health Facility Planning

In evolving hospital concept, the architects and planners have to keep pace with the development in modern medicine, nursing technique and general community expectations. Medical technology is developing very fast so much so that often hospitals become outdated even before they are put to use. There has been very rapid change in last five decades in functioning of hospitals due to medical advances which have direct bearing on patient care.

Medicine is an everchanging subject. Discoveries and inventions keep on changing the paradigm of health care delivery. Recent trends in molecular biology, pharmaceuticals and surgical interventions have not only prolonged the life but also improved the quality of life. Information superhighway has turned the world into a 'Global Village'.

These factors have major influence in the planning of new hospitals. The other factors which have direct bearing on hospital planning are:

- Costly diagnostic services cannot be provided in all hospitals. Thus, there should be proper choice of place and services to be rendered.
- Tertiary care cannot be provided in all places due to high cost and lack of availability of trained man power.
- Design should follow function, however, the proper use of esthetic quality and humanized surrounding must be kept in mind so that it looks attractive
- A study of activities in health facilities at different levels is a perequisite of planning as it anweres several important question
- For health centres of different sizes and with different functions, what is the proportion of working hours devoted to various broad activities or definite tasks:
  a. Which different types of staff are needed and in what proportion?
  b. What are the space requirements to discharge these functions?
  c. What is the inter-relationship between these functions and consequently, what layout will be more convenient?

As conditions vary from place to place, it is necessary to undertake such a study for each project.

Health Centres

Grouping of closely related activities should be put together in one area. All areas should be located in relation to one another to allow direct communication and easy flow of patients, staff and services. The design and the structural system should allow maximum flexibility and expandability.

Developments in medical sciences and equipment technology have offered many new diagnostic and therapeutic modalities namely ultrasonography, computerized axial tomography, nuclear magnetic resonance imaging, non-invasive cardiac diagnosis, coronary angiography, invasive cardiophysiology, hemo-dynamic studies, pulmonary functions, endoscopic techniques and procedures, lasers, etc., which are now reliable, precise, easy to run and apply. Many of these have special physical requirements including controlled environment, energy and other engineering services. Since these are capital intensive, there has been an increasing concern to effect economy in their use.

Task before the architects therefore will be to determine the broad requirement for the hospital system. The system should be able to provide reasonably effective services to patients. Further, workloads and the required activities of any healthcare institution are never predictable in detail. Architects therefore, must recongnise the two main problems, expansion and flexibility to keep pace with the rapidly developing technology in medical sciences. Physical planning must allow for future expansions in all major functional areas of the hospital and for internal adjustments in the use of space to desired degree of changes must be feasible.

Functionally a hospital has six major facility zones:

1. Accident and emergency.
2. Ambulatory care (outpatients department).
3. Diagnostic and therpeutic facility.
4. In-patient (nursing care) units.
5. Administration department and business.
6. Hospital engineering services.

Each of the functional components need to be suitably placed depending on their inter-relationship but with shortest possible travel to achieve efficiency. These facilities do require their independent access and related parking lots. However, for reasons of overall control and security, entries and exits are to be kept to the minimum.

a. Emergency Department is an independent unit to function round the clock like a mini hospital. Entry to this department has to be prominant and self-guided so that a very minimum time is lost in giving immediate treatment to casualty and emergent cases arriving in the hospital.
b. Ambulatory care unit has to perform three main functions:
   - to diagnose and treat patients at an early stage.
   - follow up treatment after discharge from the hospital and
   - to institute health education programme to educate the public in environmental hygiene.

   The outpatient department in a hospital has very important role in health care delivery. A well organised and well equipped outpatient department can play key role in reducing the load on the inpatient beds and save a lot of time and expenditure. Emphasis is now more on outpatient facilities which are likely to increase substantially thereby reducing the load of inpatients and the cost the hospital projects as a whole. Facilities of this unit are termed as:

   - Clinics for various medical and surgical discipline.
   - Supporting facilities like laboratory, injection rooms, etc.
   - Pharmacy and Blood Bank.
c. Diagnostic and therapeutic facilities include: the radio-diagnostic and imaging department, clinical pathology as diagnostic facilities whereas radiotherapy, operation theaters, rehabilitation and physiotherapy as therapeutic areas are to serve in common to outpatient department and inpatient nursing care units. These facilities are to be suitably placed at different levels in consideration of their functional use and degree of necessity to dependent departments.

Diagnostic and imaging units generally deals with radiography and flouroscopy, ultrasound, nuclear medicine and CAT Scan, etc. This being a fast developing technique should be designed keeping in view the future scope of expansion.

Laboratories are concerned with the analysis of diseased tissue and fluids and other elements in the body. This department may comprise activities like Biochemistry, Microbiology, Clinical Pathology, Hematology, Histology, Cytology and Serology. Other activities connected with the department are mortuary and autopsy.

Radiography

Radiography includes treatment of various types of radiations, ranging from superficial therapy to megavoltage therapy. Size of department depends upon the load, scope of work and type of equipment employed. High degree of radiations, protective measures and air conditioning for the efficient functioning of the electronic equipments are the essential design requirements for the department.

Operation Theater

Hospital is technically a therapeutic aid in which a team of surgeons, anesthetic, nurses and sometime pathologists and radiologists operate upon or care for the patients. Location of the department should be decided on factors like quiet environment, noise-free atmosphere, conditions free from contamination and possible cross infection and convenient relationship to surgical wards, intensive care unit, radiology, pathology, blood bank and central sterile service department.

Understanding of medical and surgical needs of the patient during surgical procedures and the role of environment, sterilization and aseptic techniques in the control of nosocomial infections have led to the development of modern concept of zoning namely protective, clean, sterile and disposal zones in operation theratre design. Filtration and recirculation of conditioned air and scavanging of expired anesthetic gases have further enhanced safety and comfort of the patients and surgical team.

Rehabilitation and physiotherapy department provides treatment facilities to patients suffering from crippling diseases and disabilities. These facilities are classified as physical and electrotherapy, hydrotherapy, occupational therapy and exercises.

In-patient Nursing Care Units (Wards)

In-patient nursing care units (wards) occupy the maximum share of hospital space. Concept of providing this facility is fast changing due to policy of early ambulation and in fact only a few patients really need to be on bed. Nursing care is broadly classified into general wards, speciality-wise wards and intensive care units. Basic consideration in placing wards is to ensure sufficient nursing care, segregating patients according to three categories, locating them according to the needs of the treatment in respective medical discipline and controlling cross infection. Speciality-wise wards however, should be located closer to their respective outpatient clinics to act as self-contained centres.

In planning a ward, the aim should be to minimize the work of the nursing staff and provide basic amenities to the patients within the unit. Ward pattern has undergone a radical change from Nightingale ward to Rigg's ward. Many variations and modifications of the concept are meeting specific socio-medical requirements while attempting to enhance the efficiency of nurse-patients interaction, observability, lighting and other physical requirements, replenishment system for supply of diet medical and surgical supplies, linen and other materials at the doorstep of nursing activity have further relieved the nursing staff on non-nursing functions to attend patient centered activities.

Norms

In-patient Department

In-patient is not only a place for admitting a patient who cannot be treated outside hospital, but also a place of training for doctors and paramedical staff.

In-patients are likely to fall into one of five broad care grouping in the proportions shown.

1. *Intensive Medical Care* Where continuous medical and nursing observation and mechanical assistance is necessary to maintain life one percent.
2. *Intensive Nursing Care* Where patients are unable to leave their beds, and where their is need to continuous nursing, observation and physical assistance. 20-25 percent.
3. *Medium Nursing Care* Where patients are able to leave their beds for short periods (upto four hours) each day with assistance 20-25 percent.
4. *Low Nursing Care* Where patients are able to leave their beds for more than four hours per day, requiring minimal assistance 20-30 percent
5. *Self Care* Patients leading apparently a normal life, who are in hospital for observation 5-10 percent.

Using a similar classification, the proportions of patients in a developing country are likely to be considerably higher in the intensive and medium care categories, perhaps upto 75-80 percent of total patients being within these two areas.

Out-patient Department

"Ambulatory Care" is the medical care provided to patients who are not confined to bed. It can be provided at a general practitioner's or specialist's practice premises or at health post, health centre or hospital. The functions of outpatient services of a hospital are to provide diagnostic, curative, preventive, and rehabilitative service on ambulatory basis to the the community. The extent of these functions established by the individual hospital will vary, according to aim of hospital, expectation of community and political will. The scope and form is undergoing dramatic change. If it functions well, it can reduce pressure on inpatient care, which can be achieved by increasing diagnostic and treatment service.

Planning is a dynamic process and necessary for orderly development. It can be carried out at many levels of detail and in many timeframes. To assure a smooth, orderly project the first step in the planning process is to establish a schedule for the entire project:

- Preplanning schedule.
- Determination of community need for healthcare.
- Evolution of existing conditions.
- Demographic survey of the community.
- Statement of goals and objectives related to community needs.
- Capital financing plan
- Operational programme to meet goals and objectives.
- Master development plan as a framework, including gross departmental area allocation.
- Schematic plans,and construction staging.
- Cost analysis.
- Detailed space programme of first stage for construction.
- Equipment list.
- Design of first stage
- Construction of first stage.
- Evaluation of operation and feedback.

A hospital brings together the wide spectrum of knowledge, professional skill, and physical facilities so that the present and future generation will advance in health and well-being. If it can be designed in proper fashion it can combine science and wisdom to create holistic approach to health care. The architect has the task of designing a highly complex structure for a very complex organization, but his design has to have sufficient clarity of form to be understood by all who use it. In addition, he has to design individual territories—the departments for each of the groups whose successful interaction is the basis of the work of the hospital. Each separate department needs its own identity and within it, its own map, its own private and public space as well as own frontdoor. The design must allow the identity of many families which form its work force to be identifiable, physically, from inside the complex.

Hospital design must have flexibility, to adopt change and its concern should be the quality of medical care and the improvement of its standards.

It is accepted that planning and proper programming is essential to strengthen the health care facilities. Every country should accept it as its responsibility to design and implement changes that enhance the performance of the total health service delivery system in a balanced and integrated manner, because hospital is a complex organization.

The idea of planning is to prevent the haphazard mushrooming up of structure, to prevent fragmentation of function and to promote logical flow of patient, staff and equipment and to attain a fair degree of uniformity and standardization.

The implementation of a health care facility project could be regarded as a sequence of phases.

Formulation consists in establishing the need for a facility; in making sure that its erection would be in accordance with stated policies and priorities, in ascertaining that the resources (money and manpower) necessary for its realization and operation are available, or will be available when needed. At the end, formation of planning team should be made.

Site Selection

It is important for hospital building. It must have the following characteristics:

- Easy approach by people
- Enough land availability
- Sub-soil water must be deep
- Sufficient supply of water and electricity.

While selecting the site, one must keep in mind, any further expansion in future size of land required is as follows:

50 beds	10 acres	Single storey
100 beds	15-20 acres	Single Storey
200 beds	20-25 acres	Double storey
500 beds	55-70 acres	3-5 stories
700 beds	80-90 acres	4-6 stories
1000 beds	90-100 acres	6-9 stories.

Basement is possible if the sub-soil water is below 25 feet in mid monsoon time.

Preparation of architect brief After obtaining requirement of clinical and nursing departments supportive service, administrative and business and utility services, a general outline of requirement be prepared to provide the client with an appraisal and recommendation, so that it can be ensured that the project is functionally, technically and financially feasible.

The client's task is to establish a suitable project management organization which can develop the project brief by considering and analyzing all important factors.

Design Plan (Fig. 6.1)

While designing differnet zones, there is a need to establish relationship between activities and space in a health centre. Circulation area such as corridors, entrance halls, staircase, etc. in the hospital building should not be less than 30 percent of the total area of the building.

Basic circulation pattern depends upon land availability, and environmental circumstances, however, it may be any one of the following:

- radial-linear
- tree-shaped or dendritic-grid.

The other relevant details need to be kept in mind are as follows:

Water Supply

About 300-500 liters of water per bed per day (excluding water for gardening) is to be catered for. Water supply should be preferably from two sources. Reserve water for 7 days if from a single source and 2 days if from two sources.

Electricity

Electricity supply should be from 2 grid/3 grid (source). In addition, generator supply for certain essential areas should be catered for. Even for more essential equipment there should be provision for uninterrupted electric supply. Requirement for the hospital is One kv per bed per day.

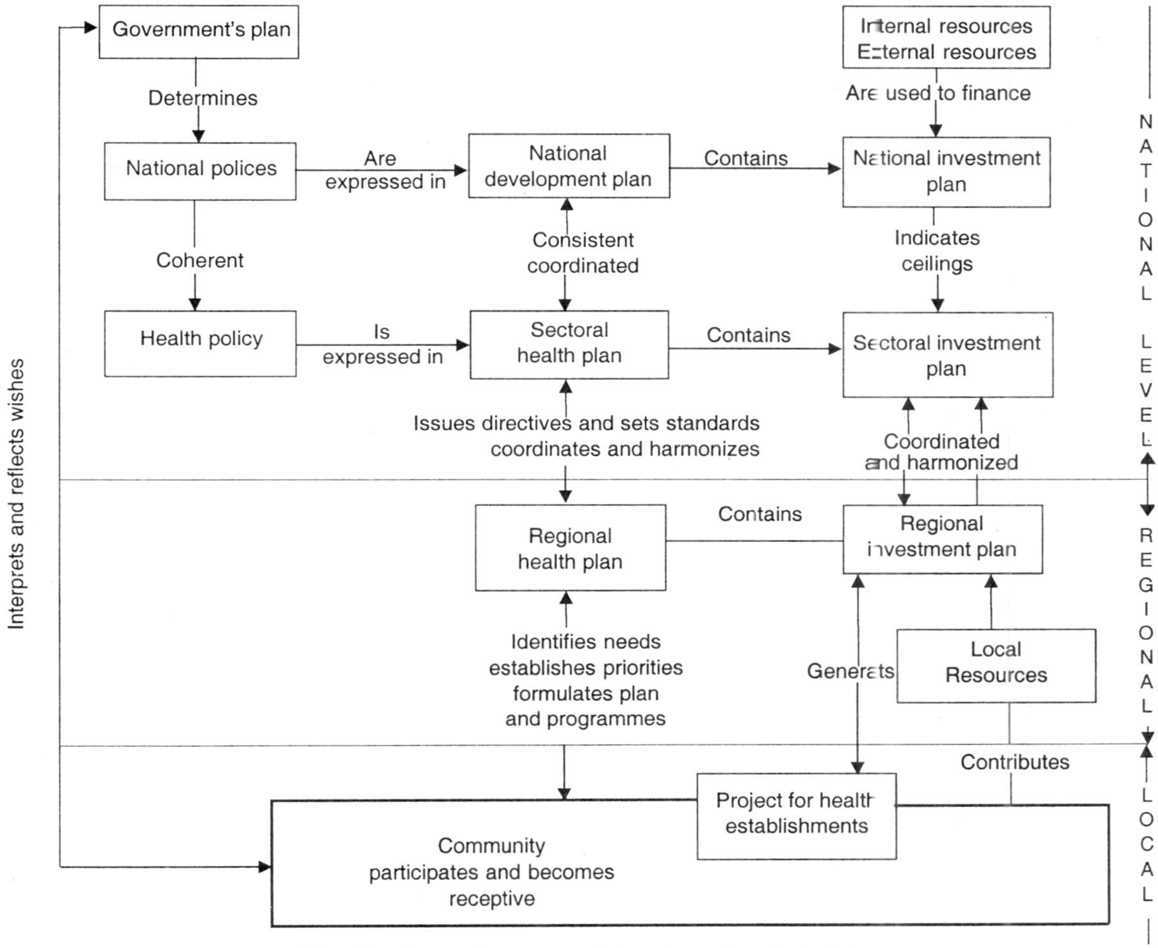

Fig. 6.1: General process of planning a health facility

Sanitary Requirements

Toilet for an individual room (single or two bed) in a ward unit shall be 3.5m^2 comprising a bath, a wash and WC. Toilet common to serve two such rooms shall be 5.25m to comprise a bath, a WC in a separate cubicle and a wash basin. For a multiple beded ward unit, requirement of fitments is given below:

Items	*Quantity*
Water closets	1 for every 8 beds (male)
	1 for every 6 beds (female)
Ablution taps	1 for each water closets plus 1 water tap with drainage arrangement in the vicinity of water closets
Urinals	1 for every 12 beds
Bath	1 bath with shower for every 12 beds
Bed pan washing sinks	1 for each ward in dirty utility and sluice room.
Sinks and dishwasher	1 for each ward in ward pantry.

Biomedical waste (soiled, semi-soiled and liquid) amounts to 2 kg per bed per day. The hospital drainage should be connected to the main town drainage system. A sewage treatment plant is desirable for a large teaching general hospital

Certain General Parameters

Hospital Space Module is taken as 3.5 sqm. This space is enough to accommodate a toilet comprising a WC, Wash basin and a shower. 7 Sqm. is enough for the routine hospital bed, and 14 sqm. will be required for each bed in the Intensive care unit.

a. *Hospital Engineering Grid* is taken as 1.6 m one and a half grid i.e. 2.4 m is the desired width of a corridor. Width of door, window etc. can also be expressed in the form of a grid.
b. *Plinth area* With all constraints the recommended area per bed is 75 sqm. whereas in developed countries it is 150 sqm.
c. *Floor height* The height of all the room in the hospital should not be less than 3 m and not more than 3.65m.
d. *Head room* The minimum height under the beams, fans,lights and other fixture on the ceiling should not be less than 2.6m. measured vertically from the floor.
e. *Dedoing* It should be generally upto a height of 1.2 m. In bathroom upto 2 m. and in operating and delivery room dedoing should be the complete floor height.
f. *Door* The minimum width of doors should not be less than 1.6 m. and height 2.1 m.
g. *Ventilation* There should be sufficient ventilation in hospital. As far as possible, there should be cross ventilation thus size of window should be 20 percent of the floor area.
h. Exhaust fans should be provided as per following scales.
   - Operation theatres and delivery suites—20 air changes per hour
   - Radiography room, Radiothapy room—08 air changes per hour.

i Traction—the traction system of the hospital may be divided into two parts extramural and intramural.

The extramural system is the ambulance service. The intramural system includes ramps, lifts, conveyor belts, and dumb waiters and trolleys etc.

j Lifts (automatic control) with speed of 0.36 m. and 0.75 per second for hospitals of two or more stories are to be provided at the following scale:

Two storeyed building lift	Stretcher-cum passenger	Service
Upto 199 beds	One	Nil
200 to 399 beds	Two	One
400 to 499 beds	Three	One
500 to 599 beds	Four	One
600 to 699 beds	Five	One
700 to 799 beds	Six	Two
800 to 1000 beds	Seven	Two

k. *Fire protection* In a high-rise building the following systems should be provided:
   - Fire safety system
   - Fire detection system
   - Fire alarm system
   - Fire fighting system

Design Competition

If the hospital is big, tender can be introduced to invite the architects for design competition and rate. A group of users and experts can choose best design and rates, etc.

Construction by Contractor

A project like hospital has to be contracted only at reasonable price with reputed contractor. A tender has to be issued by engineering department with full and complete specification stating type of work, excepted cost, period of completion,etc. The planning team should take a decision regarding allotment of work. Management must exercise proper control on construction.

Control

Control is an integral part of the project management process. It aims at regular measurement of achievement and monitoring by comparison with planned progress. When deviations from planned progress occur, plans may have to be changed. Time is very important and the control process should aim at early discovery of any departure from the planned course so that adjustment can be in time to be effective

Control information provides a basis for management decisions, and the following requirement should be satisfied by an effective control system.

It should draw immediate attention to significant deviations from what is expected. It should focus on the exception rather than the rule.

True and meaningful comparisons can be made possible.

The information should indicate in due time what corrective action is necessary and by whom, the action should be taken. It should also, as far as possible, indicate what consequences any deviation from the plan is likely to have on any other planned activities, especially the time-schedule, in order to help the project manager to modify his plans accordingly.

Control information should be expressed in a simple form so that it is readily understood by those who have to make use of it.

Key areas of control must be chosen with care so that the results of control are worth the time and effect expended.

Figure 6.2 outlines a generic schedule of the facility development process with an appropriate timeframe for each activity. The sequence and duration of each of these activities vary somewhat depending on project scope and implementation strategy.

Working with a qualified external planning team and following the guidelines of reasonable schedule, the institutions role in the process is to review, comment, and make timely decisions on the work or recommendations of the external team that is made up of health care consultants, architects/engineers, construction managers, and other consultants and advisors. This review-and response interaction among the various parties may require administrative and board decisions before the next phase of activity can begin.

Quality Leadership

For a project team to succeed in its task, it needs technical knowledge, expertise in the subject, know-how to work as a team, plan, conduct good meetings, manage logistics and details, gather useful data, analyse the data, communicate the results and implement changes.

With quality leadership, use of scientific approach becomes standard procedure. The focus is on improving products and services by improving how work gets done (the methods) instead of simply what is done (the results). Quality leadership emphasizes results by working on methods.

Principles of quality leadership include: customer focus, obsession with quality, recognising the structure in work, freedom through control, looking for faults in systems, teamwork, and continued education and training. Project teams are a crucial tool for quality improvement. The success or failure of projects will have great impact on the health facility.

Project team members learn how to work as a team and how to improve processes using scientific tools and techniques.

The basic statistical tools used most frequently in a scientific approach to quality improvement include: Flowcharts, Pareto chart, Cause-and-effect diagram, Operational definitions (what something is and how it is measured), Stratifications (to pinpoint a problem by exposing where it does and does not occur. It lets teams avoid wasteful effort, directing their energies to the most potentially fruitful areas), time plots (used to examine data for trends or patterns that occur. Overtime; the data points plotted in time order), Control chart (used to monitor a process to see whether it is in statistical contrtol. It also indicates the range of variations built into the system), Check sheets (used to record data), Scatter Diagrams (display the relationship between two process characteristics), etc.

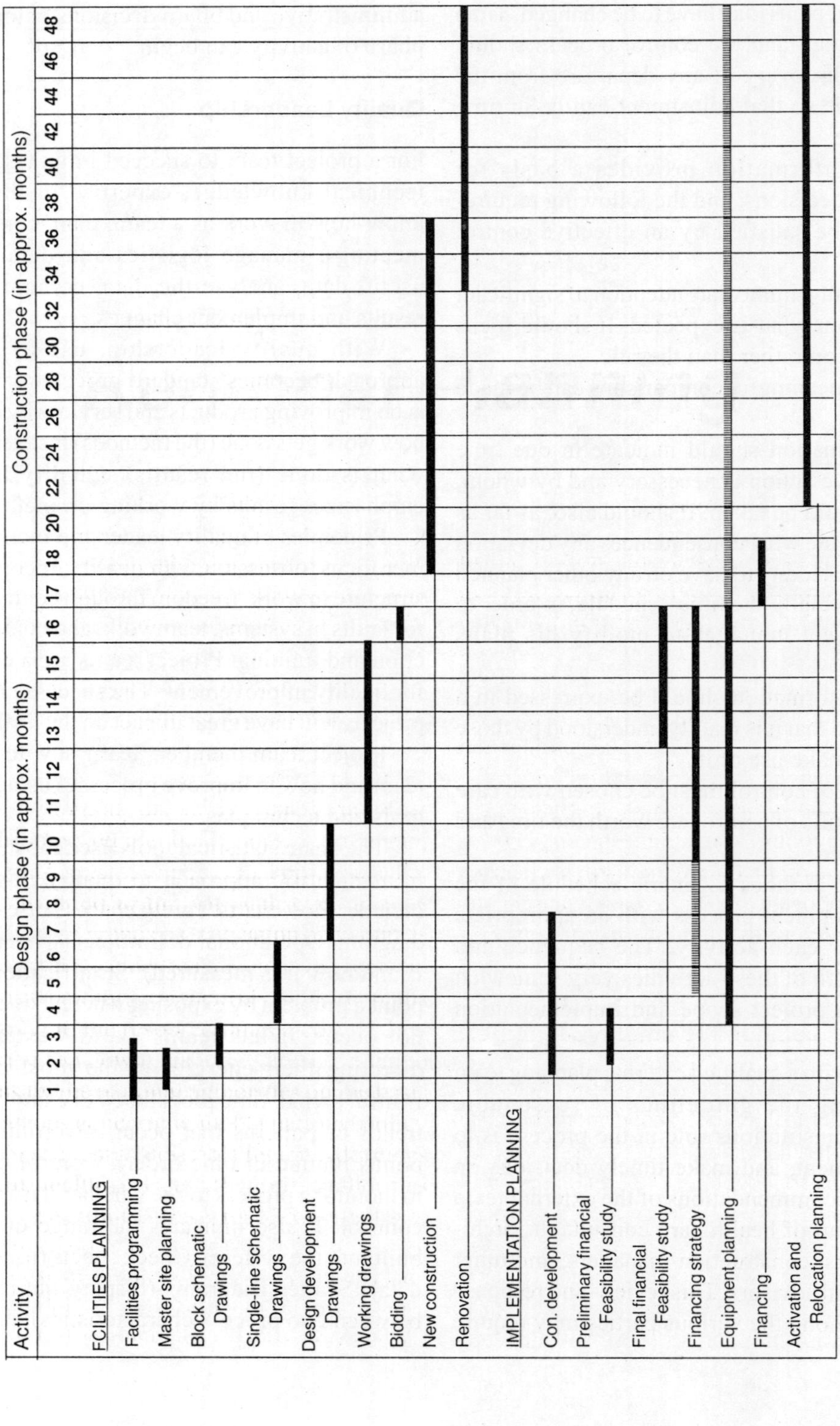

Fig. 6.2: Stages in facility development

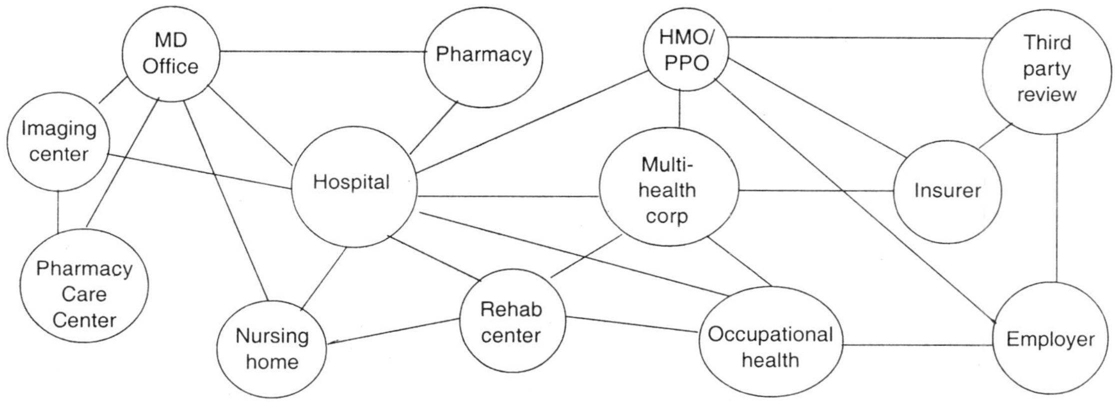

Fig. 6.3: The health care network

The success of a project depends largely on getting everything set up correctly: choosing an appropriate process, selecting appropriate team members, and doing the ground work, so a team will know what the project is all about.

The following activities must be incorporated into every step of project:

- Maintain communication
- Fix obvious problems
- Look upstream
- Document progress and problems
- Minitor changes.

Teams must spend time in the early stages of their project planning how the project will unfold. Planning is the heart of using a scientific approach to quality improvement. Ten ingredients for a successful team include:

- Clarity in team goals
- An improvement plan
- Clearly defined roles
- Clear communication
- Beneficial team behaviours
- Well-defined decision procedures
- Balanced participation
- Established ground rules
- Awareness of the group process
- Use of the scientific approach.

When quality is increased by improving processes, productivity improves. Better productivity lowers unit costs, which in turn lowers prices.

FURTHER READING

1. Putsep E: The Modern Hospital: international planning practice, Lloyd-Luke, 1979, London, 1979

7 Regional Planning

An essential precondition for drawing up the health plan is to have regional plans for the sector in which specific account is taken of the needs of the area in terms of facilities and the investments that must be made in order to carry out the plan (*See* Fig. 6.1).

Regional planning has great importance as the basis for the overall planning process of the sector. Two main planning systems have emerged:

- From the bottom up: local requests are examined, screened and consolidated at regional level, thus constituting regional proposals that are transmitted to the national level. On the basis of these proposals, allocation of resources to regions are decided at national level; regional and local authorities then revise their plans according to the resources allocated.
- From the top down: resources are allocated to regions by the national authorities on the basis of decisions concerning global national policy and, consequently, desirable regional development of health services. Regional authorities in turn distribute these resources to local authorities.

The phase of regional planning can be divided into two stages: a first stage of planning and programming of the network of facilities needed to carry out the health tasks and activities a signed to the region, and a second stage at which the general features of each facility are planned. Consideration is particularly given here to those aspects of the regional plan which relate to investments in physical construction and, specifically, those relating to the planning and programming of hospital facilities.

It is highly desirable that regional plans be implemented in the short-, medium- and long-term. It, thus becomes posible to gearup the planning of physical facilities to projections of the available economic and human resources necessary for operating these services and to educate the community in the optimum utilization of the services available.

Regional Systems of Facilities

The planning of the system of facilities for the area is based on the needs derived from the programme. The location, type and characteristics of the facilities are adapted to the levels of care adopted for the regionalization of services, considering that each facility does not constitute an independent or isolated service but an integral part of the system (Fig. 7.1). The existence or creation of each facility should be justified in so far as its functioning contributes rationality to meeting the health care needs of the locality concerned and of the region, its activities fitting into an ordered whole which delivers the right service at the right time, with the greatest efficiency and at the least possible cost to the system.

Once the main lines have been drawn showing the need to create or improve installed capacity and the main characteristics required of each facility have been determined, the general frame of reference for necessary future investments will have been established. The investment plan for the improvement and expansion of existing facilities or the creation of new ones should be a direct response to real health needs and the requirements of the area.

A study preparatory to planning the services for the region should comprise a meticulous general survey of the area concerned, convering the following points:

- Geographical, climatological, geological and other features;
- Distribution of the population, degrees of rural dispersion and urban concentration, demographic characteristics and projections, migration, etc;
- Physical integration of the region, communications systems, distance and time, accessibility, etc.
- Cultural and educational levels, habits, customs, literacy, schooling, etc.;
- Income levels, regional and local types of economy, sources of production, per capita income, family income;
- Public services available (both rural and urban), water supply and sewerage systems, energy, disposal of solid wastes, transport, town-planning activities;
- Health situation, mortality, morbidity and fertility rates, life expectancy, prevalent diseases, nutrition, housing, recreation, etc.;
- System of regionalization of health care in the area, participating bodies, systems of administration and operation of the services, sectoral and multisectoral programmes, degrees of integration of activities, co-ordination, etc.;

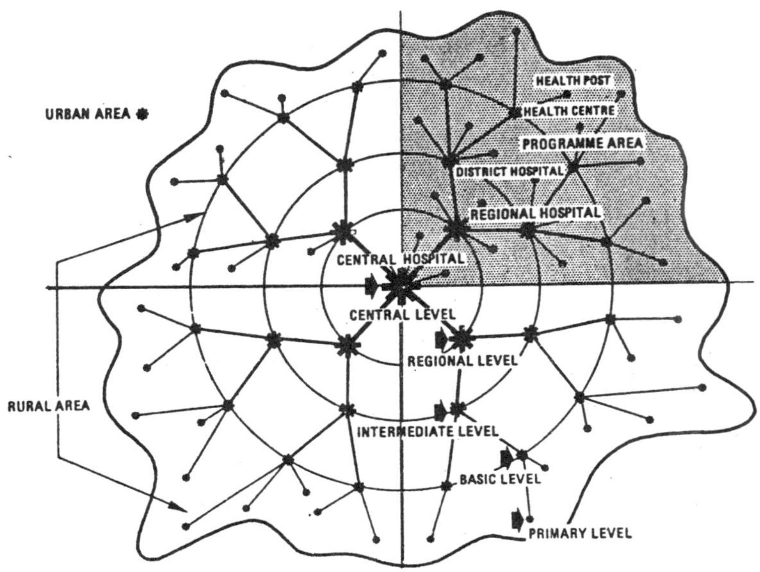

Fig. 7.1: Theoretical example of general pattern of regionalization showing programme area and type of facility

- Existing health resources (physical, human and economic), expenditure on health and its cost components, coordination of financing, degree of potentialization of the services, census and physical and functional inventory of establishments, maintenance, etc.;
- Coverages, size of population covered by types and sources of care, levels, etc.;
- Supply of and demand for services, demand met and unmet, distribution of demand by volume and type, etc.; and
- Local and regional prospects for development, foci of development, economic infrastructure projects affecting the region; landholding system, settlements, etc.

The investigation, study and analysis of all these aspects should be conducted with the aim of making a serious contribution to knowledge of the health situation in the atrea and especially of how these aspects affect the prevailing health level and conditions in the region. The important thing is to keep in mind the directives, guidelines, standards and, especially, priorities established in the health plan, the available resources and the programmes in course of implementation or due to be implemented. These data will provide an overall picture that will enable the needs in terms of facilities and the investment requirements for the zone to be determiend and their type and very broad characteristics to be fixed.

Specific Projects for Facilities

Normally, the facilities to be created form part of a classical type of health service, i.e., a regionalized medical care system comprising:

primary level,
basic level
intermediate level
regional level, and
central level.

Each of these levels possesses, from the physical point of view, highly specific design and equipment features; consequently, the needs at each level with respect to environment, equipment and installations must also be planned and programmed individually in the light of the functions which the facilities are expected to perform.

Primary and basic levels The primary and basic levels facilitate the rapid extension of coverage to the most unprotected part of the population by constituting the spearhead for the penetration of extension of the health activities of the system. They are therefore the facilities which make the greatest demand on resources in the developing countries.

The planning and programming study should be condcuted in two phases: firstly, an investigation of the localities which the regional plan indicates to be potentially suitable for coverage; and, secondly, classification and selection of facilities, taking into acount the available resources.

The purpose of the investigation phase is to produce fuller knowledge of the localities as regards the following aspects:

- Characteristics, level and type of the construction work to be undertaken, identifying the requirements for erection, extension or remodelling of buildings and provision of emergency and maternity beds;
- The time required for the work, taking into account local construction materials and facilities available, with an indication of the starting and finishing dates;
- The body responsible for the work and the participation of other sectors;
- The body immediately above to which the facility will be attached functionally and administratively, for purposes of supervision, provision of supplies and referral of patients;
- Geographical accessibility of the higher-level facility, with an indication of the type of link-up, distance and time;
- The building construction and equipment costs;
- The source of financing; and
- The manpower and economic resources that are available or will have to be provided for operation of the service.

Next, a study must be conducted to grade and select facilities according to the priorities indicated by the selection criteria, of which the most impor-tanmt are:

- Inclusion in and support to comprehensive development programmes in the area;
- Need for the service in order to conduct programmes of the sector and degree of participation and motivation of the community for its acceptance;
- Time required for execution of work and anticipated date of opening;
- Resources, particularly human, available for operation;
- Coverage to be provided;
- Degree of accessibility, considering how isolated the area is;
- Degree of integration into the regionalized system provided for in the plan; and
- Complementarity of contribuions to set up the facility.

Self-help and community participation constitute a valuable contribution which must be encouraged and turned to account; this will be reflected in a feeling of community participation in obtaining the service, to the great benefit of its acceptance, utilization and subsequent maintenance.

The great demand for facilities at these levels and their simplicity make it very useful to have model types of project, standardized as regards their architectural design and equipment, which can with very slight modifications be adapted to the specific conditions of the sites chosen for their erection. Primary level facilities are, for example, health posts, health points, health stations, dispensaries, etc.; at the basic level there are such facilities as health centres, polyclinics, etc. The function of both levels is to provide ambulatory care and sometimes, in the case of the health centres, inpatient care for emergency or maternity cases.

Health posts are facilities whose running is entrusted with community health promoters or nursing auxiliaries, with periodic supervision and support by professional staff from the higher levels. Their accommodation facilities are generally limited to two or three units: patients' waitingroom, workroom a small medicine stores that may or may not be included in the workroom, and toilet facilities for public and staff. Where there is no public water supply or sewerage service, the health post must be equipped with the simplest and most uncomplicated systems to replace them, thus providing a working example of basic rural sanitation measures such as latrine construction, water supply, waste disposal, protection from and elimination of vectors, etc.

Health centres usually have regular or permanent professional staff; their physical needs vary according to the range of their responsibility, the size of the population to be served, the primary services requiring supervision, the possibilities of access to the higher level and the human resources available. There exists two types: the health centre without beds, and the health centre with beds. Health centres with beds generally represent the second stage in the development of the original health centres, which is reached by successive extensions.

Health centres require greater facilities than health posts: they must have separate rooms for administration, consultations and treatment and, if possible, laboratory and X-ray installation. The beds, if they have, are generally earmarked for short-term hospitalization of patients in emergencies or for referral and for hospitalization of maternity cases; if maternity cases are accepted, the centre will be provided with the necessary delivery room and annexes.

Facilities at the intermediate level are usually general hospitals of between 100 and 200 beds which provide care in the four basic specialities (internal medicine, surgery, obstetrics and pediatrics) and have all the relevant facilities for these. It is usual for this type of facility to start with a smaller number of beds which is then progressively increased. It is not advisable, however, for the final capacity to exceed the initial capacity by more than 30%, since the general services have to be planned from the start to meet the final demand of the establishment. The architectural design should therefore be executed in full from the start so that the facility may be developed progressively by stages, without interfering with normal functioning and causing the least possible inconvenience to the users.

It is possible at this level for hospital design and equipment to be completely standaridzed, so as to obtain a "standard model"; but it is more practical and advisable to standardize basic sectors of the hospital, i.e., to construct "model units" for the various suites corresponding to the main departments such as non-medical services.

Regional level To this level belong hospital facilities located in urban centres of some importance, i.e., districts or medium-sized towns which generally corresponding to the poles of development of the area and are the centre of its government and administration. This level constitutes the hub around which the health system revolves: from it radiates the region's medical care programmes.

The regional level facility usually takes the form of a general hospital of 200 or more beds, its capacity depending on the size and requirements of the area and, in particular, at the degree of integration of the area under its responsibility and at the level of development and efficiency of the peripheral services under its jurisdiction.

These hospitals provide outpatient and inpatient care in the four basic specialities and in the sub-specialities required to meet the local and area needs. The capacity and level of organization of the hospitals is such as to permit the satisfactory solution of all the specialized care problems of the health care facilities within the system and to ensure the community as a whole a comprehensive, prompt and adequate service.

Central level The function of facilities at this level is to provide specialized medical services for selected patients who require particular conditions of care and treatment and, in addition, to perform specific tasks in high-level research and training of specialized staff. Because of their great complexity and the high concentration of resources required for their installation and operation, together with the fact that their field of activity is generally nation-wide or covers several regions, their planning lies in part outside the scope of the regional system and belongs more properly to the sectoral planning system; nevertheless, the programming studies can again be conducted according to the methodological guide which is given below as a model for intermediate and regional establishments.

Coordination

The most characteristic health establishments are hospitals, whether of the intermediate, regional or central level. Table 7.1 shows methodological guide for planning of hospital projects..

Determination of Size

Once the location and level of the hospital to be set up are specified in the regional health facilities plan, the determination of its size constitutes one of the most important aspects of its programming. The size is governed by the service capacity to be provided and, in general, it can be assumed that it will depend on the number of admissions and consultations; in turn, the admissions and consultations will be reflected in the number of beds and consulting rooms that will have to be provided. The volume and capacity of the other services will be proportionate to the figures for admissions per bed and consultations per consulting room obtained as a result of the basic calculation of the size of hospital required.

There exist various methods for calculating these two factors, ranging from the simple application of indices per head of population to

Table 7.1: Methodological guide for planning of hospital projects

Stage	*Action or Activities*	*Objectives*
Investigations	• Delimitation of area to be served • Study of community involved • Study of health situation	To define and get to know: • Universe of work • General frame of reference • Specific health framework
Analysis and Conclusions	• Establishment of health diagnosis • Presentation and evaluation of course of action	• To identify problems in respect of importance and magnitude • To define the problem field • To determine responsibilities • To indicate possible solution
Decision	• Selection of alternative • Inclusion of alternative in plans of action	• To determine responsibility *vis a vis* the problem and agree to contribute to its solution
Preliminary studies	• Medico-architectural programme • Preselection of site • Preliminary architectural project • Preliminary equipment project • Preliminary equipment project • Estimation of cost of building, equipment, training of personnel and operation • Feasibility study of execution and financing	• To prepare base for solution and harmonize them with: Available resources Fundable resources Mobilizable resources
Final studies	• Selection of site • Preparation of architectural, engineering and equipment project • Formulation of staff training plan • Definition of methods and systems of administration and operation • Final studies on financing of the installation and future operation	To have all the necessary studies ready for: • Commencing the installations • Training the personnel • Administering and operating, every thing • Establishing a complete programme for its financing
Execution of installations and preparation for operational phase	• Putting out to tender and award of contracts for construction, equipment and inspection of installations • Execution of installations • Preparation of personnel • Framing of administrative and operational regulations • Promotion of demand for the service • Appropriation of economic resources for operation	• To have the installations, personnel, systems and operational methods required for implementing the solution • To have informed and educated public demand • To have funding for operational phase
Acceptance dry run	• Drawing up of records and inventories of building and equipment • Testing of installations • Verification of capability of personnel and efficiency of operational methods	• To know the present installed
Opening	• Initiation of activities	• To solve the problem in the way provided for

complicated formulae involving a number of factors such as mortality among patients per 1000 persons who are in touch with a physician, morbidity requiring hospitalization, average length of stay in the hospital of the area, etc.; these methods require a considerable body of statistical data, which are usually not all available or reliable in the developing countries.

Calculation of bed requirements First, the following will have been determined or assumed: universe of work in terms of population, the establishment is responsible for serving, including both the direct population of the locality and the indirect population of the catchment area; number of admissions which it is aimed to be able to deliver to both population groups; the average length of stay that it is expected to be working with; and the occupancy rate desired for the hospital. The method is illustrated by the following example:

Data

Direct population	20,000
Indirect population	100,000
Admissions per year per 10 inhabitants, direct population	1
Admissions per year per 10 inhabitants, indirect population	0.3
Average length of stay	10
Hospital occupancy rate	80%

Procedure

Direct population × admissions/year/10 inhabitants = Admissions/year direct population

$$20{,}000 \times 1/10 = 2000 \text{ admissions}$$

Indirect population × admissions/year/10 inhabitants = Admissions/year indirect population

$$100{,}000 \times 0.3/10 = 3000 \text{ admissions}$$

Total admissions/year 5000

Total admissions/year × average stay = total bed-days/year

$$5000 \times 10 = 50{,}000 \text{ bed-days/year}$$

$$\frac{\text{Total bed-days/year}}{365} = \text{Total bed-days with 100\% occupancy}$$

$$\frac{50{,}000}{365} = 137 \text{ beds occupied 100\%}$$

$$\frac{\text{Total bed-days with 100\% occupancy}}{\text{Occupancy desired}} = \text{Beds with 80\% occupancy}$$

$$\frac{137}{0.8} = 172 \text{ beds}$$

Calculation of consulting-room requirement Indices are assumed for consultations to be delivered both to the direct population and to the area. Indications are also given of: the average number of first and of subsequent consultations given in the area; the estimated duration of each consultation; and the time during which the consulting rooms are in use.

Data

Direct population	20,000
Indirect population	1,00,000
Consultations per person per year, indirect population	2
Consultations per person per year, indirect population	0.5
Average first consultations in the zone	20%
Average subsequent consultations in the zone	80%
Time taken for first consultation	30 minutes
Time taken for subsequent consultations	15 minutes
Hours of work of consulting room	6 hours

Procedure

Direct population × consultations/person/year Consultations per year, indirect population	=	20,000 × = 40,000 consultations
Indirect population × consultations/persons/year	=	100,000 × 0.5 = 50.000 consultations
Consultations per year, indirect population		
Total consultations per year	=	90,000 consultations
$\frac{\text{Consultations/year}}{\text{Working days}}$ = Consultations/day	=	$\frac{90{,}000}{300}$ = 300 consultations/day
Consultations/day × % first consultation First consultation/day	=	300 × 0.2 = 60 first consultations/day
Consultations/day × % subsequent consultations Subsequent consultations/day	=	300 × = 240 subsequent consultations/day
First consultations/day × time = time first consultation	=	60 × 30 = 1800 minutes
Subsequent consultations/day × time = time subsequent consultations	=	240 × 15 = 3600 minutes
Total time	=	5400 minutes
$\frac{\text{Total time in minutes}}{60}$ = Hours consultation/day necessary	=	$\frac{5400}{60}$ = 90 consulting room hours/day
$\frac{\text{Consulting-room hours/day}}{\text{Consulting hours}}$ = Consulting rooms	=	90 = 15 consulting rooms

FURTHER READING

1. Jorge de los Rios Mazure: Regional Planning of Health Facilities, in Approaches to Planning and Design of Health Care Facilities in Developing Areas. Kleczkowski, Pibouleau (Eds): World Health Organisation, Geneva, 1976.

THE PLANNING ORGANIZATION MACHINERY

The planning teams' responsibilities include the compilation of the programme or brief which will spell out: the role of the hospital in the general health care delivery plan in relation to other services and buildings; the scope and range of functions and services to be included in the building; the policies for the operation and management of the organization within the building; a schedule of accommodation if possible; environmental design considerations; and a cost target. This brief or programme (statement of intent to create an organization and house it in a building), is usually produced by the central or regional authority to which the members of the planning team belong. Their responsibility does not end with the production of the brief; they are responsible for holding meetings with the design team during the development of the design, to ensure that aims and intentions are being met, to ensure that local or user needs are satisfied and see to it that the project is managed properly, that equipment of the required type is ordered in time, that key staff are trained in advance of the completion of the building, and that the cost and time limits are not being exceeded. Planning teams draw their data from official policy and guidance, research and development activities, general literature, and hospital users. The planning team would normally consist of specialist planning doctors, nurses, architects, engineers, quantity surveyors and administrators so as to ensure firstly, that the programme is a comprehensive statement of intent, and, secondly, that as the meetings develop there is a planning team member to answer questions on any aspect of the project. The specialists on planning teams ensure that links with fellow professionals on design teams are strong and that specialist questions are not only understood properly but answered adequately.

When they come together, the planning team and the design team merge into one project team, as their aims are identical.

The responsibility of the design team is to respond to the programme and develop the design through all stages, supervise the construction and hand over the completed building on time and within the scheduled cost. Members of the design team are building works professionals, architects, engineerings, quantity surveyors and soon in brief, the building designers.

The responsibility of the project manager is to ensure progress on the project and to construct programmes for the completion of the various parts of the work. The importance of a detailed time table for all stages of a project, including commissioning, cannot be overemphasized.

The multiprofessional team is thus made up of a range of professionals working together, planning and designing, and able to talk either collectively as a project team or professional. Each representative of both user and designer professions provides a focus of knowledge, the doctors and nurses being continually refreshed by close contacts with, but not involved in, day-to-day hospital practice.

The Multiprofessional Planning Team

A truly representative multiprofessional planning team combines both clients and those undertaking the work as a balanced whole, with responsibility for preparing project policies and programmes. Further, the multiprofessional planning team provides the focus for communication between hospital users on the one hand and the project design team on the other.

Doctors are key members of the client group on the planning team. It is obviously impossible for every medical speciality to be represented for the team and practising clinicians are only likely to be involved in a major building project once in their lifetime; furthermore, a practising clinicians would be prone to impress too strongly their own individuality on the design of their own department—a problem frequently encountered in teaching hospitals. Specialist advisors are, however, co-opted on to planning teams from time to time to give specialist advice.

Nurses and administrators on planning teams fulfil a role similar to that of the planning doctor. The hospital administrator brings to bear an overall view of hospital organization and management, which includes special interests such as logistics and catering.

The multiprofessional planning teams thus include people who may be regarded as proxy clients. The planning team is in an ideal position to communicate with three groups: those who use hospitals (the clients); those who pay for them (government or other corporate bodies); and those who design and building them (design firms, employed consultants).

From the planning team viewpoint, the combined knowledge and experience of doctors, nurses and administrators, together with the environmental concerns of their design—trained collaborators, is taken as representing the patient's total needs.

These work professionals will have made a special study of the problems of hospital design and, in addition to forging the technical links betwen planning and design teams, they will ensure that the brief is realistic and attainable in terms of the schedule of accommodation, engineering services, costs and the programme. They will also act as policy advisors, e.g., on standards of space and environmental conditions in the various hospital departments, and as technical advisors generally to their planning team colleagues.

The climatic, socioeconomic, political, education, manpower, commercial and maintenance conditions applying in developing countries, which can vary widely from region to region, make it essential that planning teams in such countries spell out their requirements clearly. This is particularly important when foreign design teams are employed. Planning teams can, of course, be modified to suit particular circumstances.

It is important to ensure that one only builds what one needs to build and then only in the most effective and economical manner.

All these professions have legitimate and constructive contributions to make to the planning and design processes. For the production of an optimum design solution, it is, however, the bridging of the gaps between the areas of purely professional responsibility that becomes more important than narrow professional knowledge itself. Bridging these gaps appears to be a question largely of establishing a common technical language as a vehicle for understanding and finally defining common objectives.

Doctors and nurses on planning teams are responsible for the quality of both patient care and the therapeutic environment. Architects and engineers are responsible for meeting these demands. As a result of their continuing responsibility, architects and engineers and to a lesser extent planning doctors and nurses have developed certain common fields of interest such as user satisfaction, ease and cost of maintenance and environmental quality. Professional pride also plays an important part. Doctors, nurses, architects and engineers conceive the design and the architects, engineers and constructors give birth to it. Their responsibility for the whole thing remains clear-cut.

The quantity surveyor sees his role as being to secure what he calls "value for money". For the most part, the task of the quantity surveyor has become cost "control" in the shallowest sense of the word. The fields he is expected to cover-i.e., building economics, cost planning, performance specifications, etc. require a width and depth of knowledge which can only be achieved fully when the rest of the planning team is very sympathetic.

The administrator is frequently cast in the role of manager for total design and building process.

Both health care planners and health facility planners should be trained at the earliest possible moment either to undertake the work themselves or to scrutinize critically the work of others commissioned to do it on their behalf.

The planning of health services should precede the planning of health buildings.

The planning team will consist of the professionals discussed earlier; it will normally be under the chairmanship of an administrator; and it will have a secretary who is again normally an administrator. The team occupies a position between the bodies providing the money and establishing policy on the one hand and hospital users and designers on the other; therefore, clearly defined communication lines are essential.

At the top level is a subcommittee of the higher authority (regional or national) charged specifically with responsibility for capital projects. This top-level group is known variously as the steering committee, development committee or central planning group. This is the highest level in the project planning system. In addition to coordinating information flow and standards, the central planning group has responsibility for determining planning and design policies, i.e., the nature, type and location of health care buildings, their content, servicing arrangements and building standards. This group also settles disputes which cannot be resolved at planning team level.

Below the central planning group comes the multiprofessional planning team or teams. It is essential therefore to establish various levels of importance in decision-making and to get these agreed before starting to plan a project, otherwise all decisions will have to be taken at the highest level. Coordination between the central planning group and the planning team is usually achieved by making someone a member of both bodies; often this is either the planning team chairman or secretary.

At the grassroots level, carying out detailed investigations into some aspect of function or design on behalf of a planning team, come the working parties or subgroups which often include hospital users. If planning is well organized, these subgroups can examine functional or design problems on behalf of more than one planning team. Indeed, such an arrangement has been found to be helpful where standard policies or design solutions are being sought.

Coordination between planning teams and subgroups is achieved by having representation from the planning team on the subgroup, according to the subject under discussion.

The complex primary task of briefing, designing and building hospitals and the complementary task of monitoring their progress, cost and general design and construction standards in such a way as to ensure that individual projects conform to the national and/or regional plan has prompted a number of countries to develop a capital project's management code. The purpose of such a code is to provide a "route-map" through the project for all parties involved and at all levels; a series of stages in the development of a project are established and their relationship to generally applicable data pointed out. The code serves as a reference point so that each planning team member can relate his tasks to those of his colleagues within the framework of a project as a whole. Indeed, some form of management code is essential where independent consulting design teams are employed so that both they and their employers know the process involved and at what point consultation cost checks and approvals to proceed are required.

Projects are made up of a large and complex set of substages which have to be completed in time and within cost limits if the whole project is to succeed. It is therefore, essential, firstly, to know what the stages are and, secondly, to know how long each should take; if this is known then targets for both the parts and the whole can be set. But there is a further point: projects can be compared and it can be established at which stages some are taking, or might take longer than the norm. The programme can then developed accordingly.

A capital projects management code can be refered to simply as a plan of work and in hospital design practice the projectcost is also checked as the design develops. This continuous checking of costs could be considered as obsessional and as adding to the gross cost largely because of delays at the various checking points. Those who take this view argue that the procedures should be kept simple, the number of check-points kept to a minimum, and a gross sum allocated to the project to be spent as the team consider reasonable, provided it is not exceed.

The Department of Health (UK) particularized a system for the processing of hospital schemes; this appeared under the codename "Capricode". The system has been brought upto date and the latest version calls for details (at Stage 1A) of the relationship of the project to area and regional strategy point referred to above. Capricode consists of six main stages:

Stage 1 Outline project intentions

Stage 2 Planning-project and first scheme

Stage 3 Design and cost planning

Statge 4 Contract and construction

Stage 5 Commissioning

State 6 Evaluation

Capricode has evolved over a number of years and has developed into a most comprehensive management tool but clearly, in order for it to work efficiently, it requires a great deal of expert knowledge and back-up data.

As in Capricode, approvals are required here also before proceeding to the next stage and again, in order for a sensible proposal to emerge, a great deal of data are required about hospital planning in general and about areas, capital costs, staffing, equipping and running costs in particular.

The study of such systems could greatly help developing countries in evolving their own capital projects management code but here again it must be emphasized that to adopt any system with only superficial modifications would be a mistake with far-reaching consequences. These systems should be considered as answers to definite problems. In each country, most data concerning the problem, especially those relating to manpower available for project management, are different; the answer will therefore be different, although the reasoning behind the problem-solving process will essentially be the same.

Rationalization, Standardization and Reuse of Planning Data

The Departmentof Health and Social Security of the United Kingdom has, over the years, developed what is known as its "Systems and Standards" approach wherein the various stages in the design and building process are formalized into a systems approach, with each stage served by a bank of generally applicable data. This technique maximizes the use of previously taken planning and design decisions and ensures that new decisions are taken into the system in such a way that they also can be reused wherever appropriate, and perhaps a previously taken decision droped from the system.

The main stages in the "Systems and Standards" approach are as follows:

- Briefing
- Designing
- Producing (the drawings and other design information)
- Constructing
- Commissioning (i.e., bringing the hospital into use)
- Evaluating

No matter how experienced the planning team, they can only do their job really efficiently if they have easy access to proven data at the correct stage of the project; the data bases have therefore been established bearing this point in mind. The activity data base contains agreed standard operational policies and schedules of acommodation for all the departments of a hospital together with a comprehensive range of activity data information. Basically, activity data are collected on two types of sheet known as A and B, the A sheet referring to the activity space and the B sheet to the activity units which are required within that space to make it function properly.

Sheets have been prepared for every room in the hospital so that a planning team no longer has to start from the beginning but may call for existing policies and activity data and need only validate the information for its own project. Standardization in this sense, therefore, does not preclude participation or unique project decisions where these are seen to be essential; rather, it provides data for validation, with all the benefits described above.

The planning of health buildings may be considered under three headings: planning personnel; planning procedures; and planning data.

Highly skilled health facility planners blend both training and experience.

Multiprofessional planning teams, together with their economic and administrative colleagues have responsibility for health care building at a regional or national level, who fasion the procedures through which the programme is processed and monitored.

A health building is an expensive tool. Not only is the initial investment important but the running costs are an ever-increasing burden that will have to be borne year after year. The planning teams and the planning organizations in each particular country therefore carry a tremendous responsibility. They must see to it that the buildings they bring into existence cover essential needs and are adapted to the cultural, technological and economic conditions of the country. Moreover, they must ensure that the ideas they have expressed in their programmes and designs can readily become a reality, answering the expectations of all and not creating problems in staffing and operation.

FURTHER READING

1. Raymond Moss: The Planning Team and Planning Organization Machinary in Approaches to Planning and Design of Helath Care Facilities in Developing Areas, Kleckzowski and Piboulean (Eds): World Health Organisation, Geneva, 1976.

8 Planning Health Facilities

Construction of health facilities on the basis of well-conceived plans is important, not only because of the large capital outlays involved but also because of the long-term recurrent cost implications associated with construction decisions. New health facilities in large developed countries can absorb billions of dollars worth of resources each year. Moreover, unneeded facilities can add upward of three hundred dollars per day per patient for cost of unnecessary hospitalizations that occur when the supply of hospital beds is not constrained. Avoidance of these costs can result in savings of as much as 10 percent of the annual health budget.

Savings of this magnitude are important in developing countries with far more critical resource constraints. Hospital operating costs account for the majority of the health budget in most developing countries. This underscores the need for objective appraisal of the need for additional hospital facilities balanced against the possibility of greater expansion of less sophisticated and expensive forms of care. Whatever the outcome of that appraisal, careful design of the needed facilities to maximize efficiency and productivity can limit operating costs substantially.

Needs Assessment

The construction of general hospitals utilizes the bulk of resources for construction of health facilities. The current trend is away from construction of special acute hospitals. Specialist hospitals occupied a vogue in the early part of the twentieth century but have grown increasingly less suitable in view of modern demands for shared services such as X-rays, laboratories and laundry, Also, special-purpose, acute-care hospitals require large populations with easy access for full utilization.

Similarly, special-purpose chronic disease facilities such as tuberculosis hospital see declining in importance. The increased use of psychotherapeutic agents has markedly reduced the demand for mental hospital, which were really more custodial institutions than health facilities anyhow.

As population age, there has been a marked increase in the demand for construction of another custodial type of institution—the nursing home, with increasing numbers of elderly people who cannot be cared for at home, the construction of new nursing homes, and the conversion of existing buildings into nursing homes have been major thrusts in the health facilities construction industry.

In addition rehabilitation hospital for the chronically disabled have taken an increasing part of the health facilities construction budget. As the population age in developing countries, and as the trend toward nuclear families increases, they will require more long-term care facilities.

Teaching hospitals are one special examples of hospital requiring special skills in planning to integrate the research and teaching functions of the facilities with the service function.

In addition to hospitals health facilities include health centers, satellite health posts, group practice buildings, individual patients' and dentists' office' special free standing out-patient clinic (such as health department clinic), and free-standing minor surgical, X-ray, diagnostic, and laboratory facilities. Planning effective, inexpensive health centers and health posts are particular challenges for planners in developing countries

Demand and Need

Estimation of the demand and need for hospitals rests on several factors. The first and most important is population. However, major difference in hospital beds to population ratio exist. Even within developed countries some are 50 percent higher than other (ranging from roughly four to six short-term per thousand population).

The second factor is the economic level of the area planned for. For example, there is a fifteen-fold (1500 percent) difference in the number of hospital beds per thousand persons in Nigeria and in Canada. Third, the availability of funds for hospitalization modifies the demand on these beds by the population at various economic levels. The general availability of public and private insured hospital care has greatly increased the demand for hospital care in many countries.

Fourth, the accessibility of facilities helps to determine the effective demand. If the facilities are readily available by normal means of transport, they are more heavily utilized. Fifth, the age pattern also affects demand for health care facilities, particularly hospitals. Older populations almost always have a higher use rate. Sixth, past utilization rates and trends are probably the best indicators for short-term change in demand for the future.

There will be demand for as many hospital beds as are built, applies to a large spectrum of ratios of hospital beds to population.

Facilities Surveys

The need for facilities must be judged against current availability. The most easily available sources of information on existing facilities are government records and those of licensing and accrediting agencies. In virtually all of the developed countries, health facilities require some process of licensing or accreditation or both. These procedures call for examination of the facilities and reports on their structure and services. In less-developed countries, detailed information is often not available and if one wishes to plan, it is essential to make special surveys of existing facilities to determine whether they are usable or not.

Surveys should include structural reviews of the condition of the building, and so on: and its fire resistance.

Mechanical devices should be surveyed to determine condition and safety. The services such as water, sewage, electricity, and gas should be reviewed to determine their adequacy and safety.

Access to the facility should be reviewed to determine any barriers to utilization of the structure by the public. Information should also be gathered on types of services, the health unit is prepared to offer, as well as the number of services actually performed in relation to capacity.

Cost Analysis

Estimation of Costs of Construction

Hospital costs vary greatly depending on locality, availability of capital, and interest rates charged.

There are two good sources of current information on hospital construction: the Dodge Building Cost Calculator and Evaluation Guide and Means Building Construction Costs Data. These manuals give costs of the different elements of construction for hospitals built in the past in different parts of the United States. They enable one to make comparisons' purposes. Less-developed countries have less information and a greater spread of construction costs.

Conversion of Capital Costs to an Annual Basis

In many developing countries, the government pays for the cost of all construction, which is budgeted as a one-time capital cost. However, there is an increasing trend towards use of non-governmental funds for hospital construction and for a realistic allocation of the governmental funds on an annual cost basis. This is particularly true as the use of government loans or bonds to finance construction of government hospitals increases.

To convert the cost of construction to an annual basis, one should use the concept of debt servicing charge: Such a charge includes the payback of principal, plus the interest on the remaining principal. For example, one may have a twenty-year loan in which one-twentieth of the principal is paid back each year, along with annually decreasing payments of interest. A more common method of allocation of debt servicing charges is to make equal payments each year for the twenty-year period of the loan. In this case the payments for the earlier years have a much higher component of interest and the overall interest charges over the twenty-year period are larger. However, in the real world, where inflation is a fact of life. It is probably advantageous to defer payback as long as possible, even if the overall interest charges are higher, as the payback in later years will be with deflated money. A practical tip for health facilities planners is to learn to use one of the inexpensive financial calculators to estimate the impact of different systems of allocation of the debt-servicing charges for hospital construction.

Comparison of New Facilities Cost with Old

In estimating the costs of operating new facilites, one starts with the debt servicing charges, unless one is operating in a system in which the capital costs are maintained in a completely separate budget. Even in this case an estimation of "shadow pricing" of debt servicing costs is important for reaching rational decisions on whether or not to construct a new facility.

In addition to the cost of debt servicing, one must estimate the cost of maintenance of the facility. Maintenance cost for a new facility may be substantially less than that for an existing one. Figures should be available from the hospital budgetary department on the costs of maintaining the old facility, through those should be judged according to whether the upkeep has been adequate. Estimates of future costs of maintaining the proposed facility should be appraised as realistically as possible, of course, rather than relying on optimistic hopes or contractor promises.

Sources of Funding for Construction

Essentially all funding is financed by loans which depend on current interest rates and the existing money market. In developing countries where the government finances hospital construction, the interest rates are often hidden as construction costs become a part of the national debt. International agencies provide funds on varying terms. For some purposes, for example, the World Bank can be a source of substantial funds at low interest. Numerous other possibilities include fund raising within the community; short-term debt financing; issuance of bonds, both tax-exempt and taxable; convertible mortgages; and other sources of private funding, Frequently funds gathered from the community or from individuals or through loans are matched by state and local authorities; often the local funds are augmented by central-level matching grants or loans. The terms of the financial arrange ments are sometimes dictated by the nature of the institution that will operate the health facility.

These complex elements come together to give rise to the debt servicing cost (interest plus payback of loan), which must be counted as part of the ongoing operating expenses of the health facility.

Operating Costs

The decreased cost of operating new facilities compared to old includes efficiencies that can be built into new facilities through such techniques as automation, spoke construction of facilities, and progressive patient care (intensive, intermediate, minimal). Hospital administrators and system analysts should be called on to make estimates of the saving in personnel and materials through the use of new systems in comparison to old systems before reaching decisions as to whether to continue with the old system, to renovate or to build anew.

Operating costs vary by size of hospital, by ownership, by type of hospital and, of course, by country. There is no consensus as to the most cost-efficient size of hospitals in the broad range of one hundred to one thousand beds. In developing countries operating costs may be as low as 10 percent of US costs because of their large, low-paid personnel component.

Focus on Implementation

The tug between elegance and economy is ever-present, and much of the pressure generated in society favors construction of expensive health facilities. Builders, insurers, as well as health providers exert pressure on governing bodies, boards of trustees of nonprofit organizations, and other decision-making groups to opt for new construction.

Another likely trade-off concerns is, site selection of the cheaper peripheral location which is less convenient to the bulk of potential users versus a more expensive central site. Efficiency in operation must be balanced against construction costs. Similarly, less flexibility in construction might lead to decreased construction costs, but must be balanced against the problem of early obsolescence. Furthermore, particularly in the developing countries, the cost of building hospitals must be balanced against the cost of building health centers and health posts This, in effect, is a decision on how to divide resources between urban and rural populations.

Planners should be familiar with the new techniques in hospital architecture such as: (1) the computer design for similar health facilities. (2) the "fast tract" system for initiating construction before design in complete (to prevent increased construction costs from inflation), (3) the use of interstitial floors to provide easier access for the various services such as water and electricity, (4) the use of traffic models for hospital design, and (5) the use of flexible designs with open options for expansion or change of facilities.

Master Planning

While it is essential for health planners to be knowledgeable of the basic elements of individual facility construction, it is also important for them to have a grasp of overall planning of facilities to serve regions, provinces, and entire nations. The starting place for master planning is the population, its distribution and its demographic attributes, such as aged distribution, birth rate (for calculating maternity services), economic levels, and current patterns of utilization of facilities.

After basic information is collected on the current parameters, changes should be predicted for the future: increase in population and increase in per capita utilization. The increased per capita

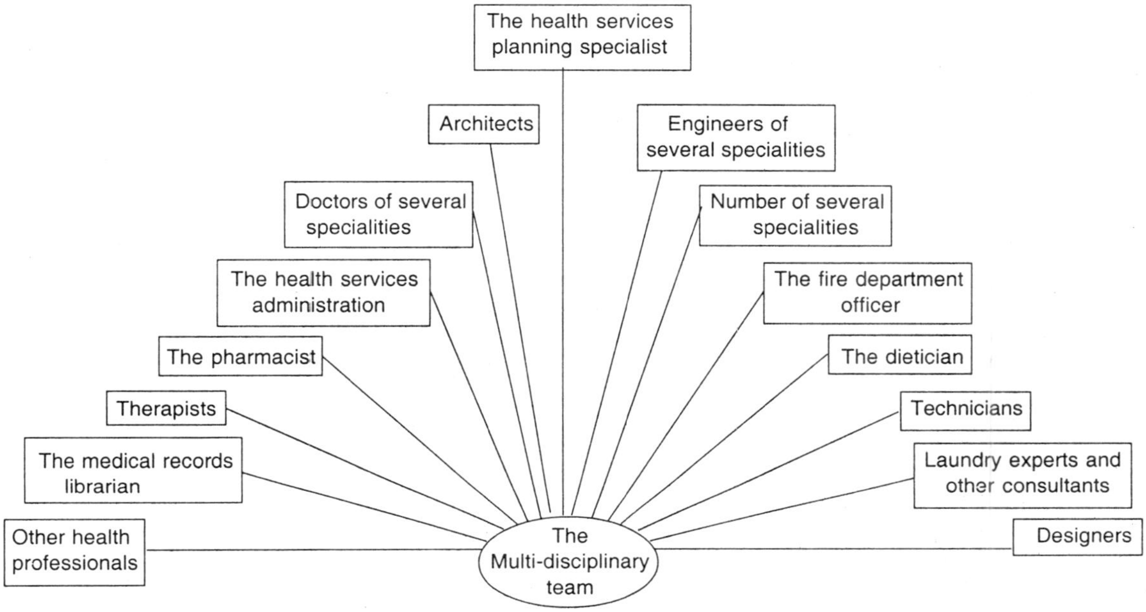

The setting of standards is probably the only occasion when such a team can be brought together to guide future planning efforts all over a developing country. An academic study by too narrow a group cannot improve health facility conditions, as those who use the standards in remote areas for their decision-making will not be able to adapt unrealistic, academic or biased regulations to local conditions. Such theoretical standards are immediately proved inadequate and, their credibility being lost, fail to produce the desired results.

Fig. 8.1: Specialists involved in setting standards for health care facilities

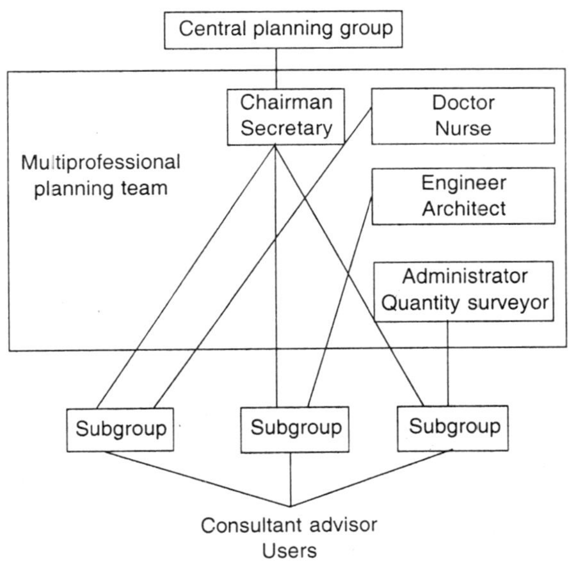

Fig. 8.2: Example of coordination between planning team and subgroups

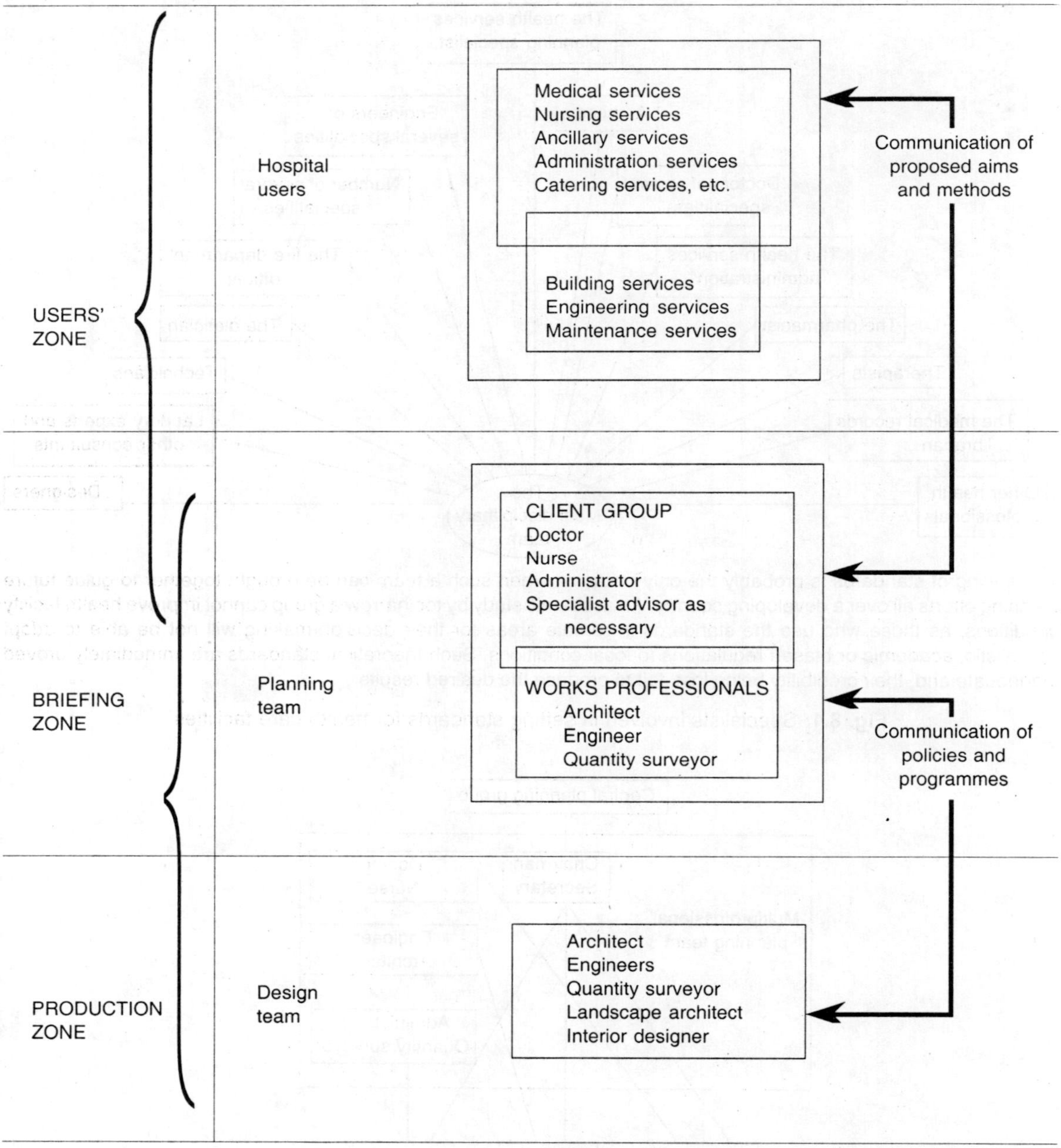

Fig. 8.3: The multiprofessional planning team

utilization will arise from increased economic levels and social changes such as preference for modern medical facilities instead of traditional medicine. Also migration patterns and changes in birth rates should be projected. In general, the same factors determining the need for additional health

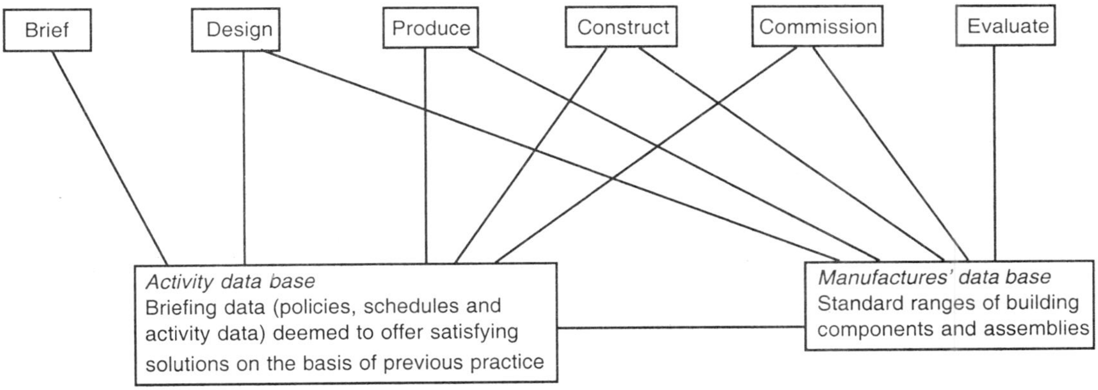

Fig. 8.4: The "systems and standards" approach

personnel dictate the need for facilities in which the additional personnel will work.

Besides projections of objective need, current and anticipated government policies and priorities should be realistically considered. Attitudes toward primary health care in comparison to high-technology specialized services should be appraised along with regional preferences and attempts to overcome existing inequities. One must always contend with the winds of political factors. However, should force any alterations on political grounds to be made in the best professional and technical master plan that can be developed.

Master planners must take a comprehensive view of the rapid changes that are occurring in most developing nations. They must build for the future and not the past, anticipating worldwide trends, such as urbanization, and plan for facilities to meet these major trends.

Use of Consultants

Once the decision to build a facility has been made, specialized architectural firms dealing primarily in health facilities should be consulted. Health facilities construction is a very special field in which many architectural firms have no competence at all.

In planning the actual design of a facility the basic team should include architects, engineers, hospital nursing supervisors, and informed representatives of the patient population. Frequently architectural firms have numerous planning sessions, involving community and health professionals, before any design is initiated.

FURTHER READING

1. *Appropriate Industrial Technology for Drugs and Pharmaceuticals,* Vienna: United Nations Industrial Development Organization. 1980.
2. Bridgman RF, MI Roemer: *Hospital Legislation and Hospital Systems*, Public Health Papers No. 50, Geneva: World Health Organization, 1973.
3. Cheesbrough M, J McArthur: *A Laboratory Manual for Rural Tropical Hospitals*, Edinburgh: Churchill Livingstone, 1976.
4. Dodge: *Building Cost Calculator and Evaluation Guide*, New York: McGraw-Hill Information System Co. revised annually.
5. Godfrey RS (Ed.): *Building Construction Costs Data*, Kingston MA: RS Means Co. Inc. revised annually.
6. Health: United States 1985, US Department of Health and Human Services, Public Health Service Publication No. PHS 86-1232, Hyattsville, MD: *National Center for Health Statistics*, December 1985.
7. Mein Philip, Thomas Jorgensen: Design for Medical Building: Manual for the planning and Building of Health Care Facilities Undér Conditions of Limited Resources, Housing Research and Development Unit. Nairobi: University of Nairobi, 1975.

8. Price DL: "Fast Tract and New Methodology in Hospi tal Planning and Construction" *Hospital Progress,* 53, **6**: 50-57, 1972.
9. Shastri JB: "Physical Planning and Primary Care: The problems of Developing Countries," *World Hospitals*, 14, **3**: 156, 1978.
10. Smythe CM: "New Resources for Medical Education: Start-up. Expenditures 22 New U.S. Medical School," *Journal of Medical Education*, **47**: 690-701, 1972.
11. Weeks J, G Best: "Design Strategy for Flexible Health Sciences Facilities," *Health Services Research*, 5, **3**: 263-84, 1970.

9 Renovation

Concurrently as hospital and healthcare services change to accommodate new services in response to a shift in healthcare emphasis and the increased demands of patients, the use of existing physical space also changes. An original approach is required to utilize available structures the best, and to avoid the need for constructing new spaces.

How to meet the ever-increasing demands for healthcare services within today's limited parameters in the question. Healthcare systems of the world have a significant amount of space available. To make affective use of that space presents a challenge to the planners, the architects, and the operators; one approach is the renovation of existing structures to provide new service in old, but remodeled, space.

The potential for a positive renovation programme is always present during the physical life of a building. But the scope of a renovation programme may vary quite widely, as may the advantages to be obtained. The possible benefits of such a programme may include some of the following, but there are also other possibilities that may result from the unique location or programme of an individual institution.

A number of hospitals, particularly older urban ones, are located on prime real estate in a strategic location in a city. As the physical structure ages, the question of possible replacement of the hospital with a new modern structure will inevitably rise. Unfortunately, because of the lack of availablility of land in the area of the existing hospital, a new hospital will, of necessity, have to be located a good distance away. A renovation programme will allow the hospital to remain at the same site.

The service area of a hospital will have been established over a period of any years. Remaining on the old site allows the hospital to continue to provide service to the local population. A renovated facility will allow it to do so at an improved quality level.

The medical staff of a hospital are an essential component and, over the years, will have developed a close relationship. A renovation programme undertaken in full co-operation with the staff, will cement these loyalties and allow the staff to offer quality care to their patients.

The operation of a hospital is a competitive business. A successful renovation programme will allow for an increased scope of services, both inpatient and ambulatory, and may lead to an increased market share and an improved balance sheet.

Although a hospital may be nearing a functional and operational obsolescence, the physical structure which houses the operation will still retain many positive aspects. A renovation programme will allow for continued use of these structures. Spaces will be converted to provide new and, perhaps, more complex services. Frequently this will require only cosmetic changes rather than a significant construction estimate.

A major renovation programme may change the image and the thrust of the hospital. Smaller and specific programmes can, however, produce positive results far beyond their cost. These indicate the upgrading of a service to enable it to offer new and improved factors of care, or the addition of a new service in space that was previously unused or under-utlised.

A cosmetic programme can create a patient-friendly hospital that attracts and retains both patients and staff by replacing the sterile and bleak appearance of the hospital with a comfortable and warm atmosphere, This may only require the use of-coordinated colour scheme, carpeting, effective use of natural light, or appropriate interior design. The result will induce the patient, the family and the visitors to return to this hospital when the need arises.

Many older hospitals will find that they have structure, which is no longer operational, such as School of Nursing or a nurses' residence. This space can often be effectively used for expanded healthcare service: possible functions could include an increased ambulatory care service, a women's health centre, a pain clinic, an AIDS resource, or any of a number of similar services that can operate reasonably independently. It must be cautioned that a need must be identified before a service is created or expanded. A renovation programme, done only for the sake of renovation, will be destined to fail.

Potential Renovation Programmes

A wide range of possibilities exists for potential renovation programmes. The range may vary from a small project undertaken in a small corner of the hospital to major addition, or partial replacement, on the existing site. If properly planned all will result in advantages.

Prior to major renovation programme it's often necessary to answer a basic question—should a new facility be built or should the old one be renovated?

There is no single, nor simple answer. There is however, a basic principle which should apply—this is the presence of an updated master plan of the future which clearly identifies the purposes and the goals of the institution. Within the context of the master plan, the administration must develop answers to a series of questions. These will include a full review of the project and its ramifications, both large and small.

If a new location is being considered, what is the size and social and economic profile of the new service area population versus the old? What is the competition in the new area? Who will be the medical staff at the new hospital? what are the capital cost implications? What can be done with, or realized from, the existing hospital? What are the comparisons of the operating costs? These answers, and a multitude of others, are required for an informed decision.

If renovation appears to be a reasonable option, the planning groups should consider how the programme will affect the hospital in total, as well as the individual departments. Will it be possible to complete the required construction and continue to operate at an acceptable level? What degree of construction is desired, and what is necessary? Is the programme financially feasible? Are the proposed physical areas adequate for the new services, even with intensive renovation? Will this compromise the long-term future of the hospital in any way?

Every renovation programme should be evaluated. The larger the programme proposed, the greater will be the impact. The process must therefore, be indepth extensive.

If a positive decision is made to undertake a renovation programme, then the planning for implementation can proceed. As previously mentioned,it is essential the hospital have a master plan.

The proposed renovation project should conform to this plan and the programme should be fully integrated into the plan.

The renovation programme is developed in detail within this master plan. A necessary element is the presence of a hospital planning consultant and an architectural firm with experience in renovation projects. The approach requires considerations, slightly different from new construction, which include a commitment to obtain the fullest potential possible; a consideration of the need for ongoing hospital operation including seasonal variations, and the effect on loss of income or increased operating costs; and the effect on loss of income or increased operating costs; and an increased need to cooperate closely with the operational personnel. The presence of this experienced planning element will assist in reaching a positive result.

The potential for renovation projects to improve effectiveness, scope of care offered, quality of care, and all other elements of the hospital is immense. In many countries, a full appreciation of this potential has not yet been reached. A greater understanding of this area of planning and construction, and an increased application of this concept to the healthcare system will result in positive benefits to all involved parties.

FURTHER READING

1. Flynn DF: Renovation: an integral potential. Hospital Management International. IHF, London, 1988.

10 The Process of Planning

Effective planning requires step-wise application of selected multidisciplinary methods and procedure to designated programmes and projects within specified timeframes. Planning is not simply a technical exercise. However, it is an ongoing process of learning, adapting to change, and educating.

Scope and Structure

Planning can be separated into comprehensive planning, programme planning, and project planning. Comprehensive planning normally provides a framework for the other types and is more closely associated with policy analysis than with details of implementation. Although concerned with practicability and feasibility, attention is on general considerations such as priorities and the relative contributions to be achieved by various types of health investment. A major interest is the balance between health services and the other important facets of socioeconomic development. With the increased specificity associated with programme and project planning, greater attention to implementation, especially in relation to time scale and target setting, is obviously needed.

Plans are also distinguished according to the planning horizon encompassed. Long-term perspective plans typically cover twenty years. Intermediate term plans most often look five years forward. Finally, there are annual plans closely tied to the yearly budgeting cycle. As in the case of comprehensiveness, the time dimension of planning bears on proximity to implementation. Perspective plans establish long-term policy directions. At the other extreme, annual plans are closely targeted plans of work for direct administrative action.

In practice, intermediate-term plans have been the most common. Often these have borne little resemblance to annual budgetary allocations which serve as the basis for action. Plan implementation has suffered as a consequence. Intermediate-term plans have also been constrained in their ability to innovate. Development of health personnel and facilities is a time-consuming endeavour that requires a perspective view extending beyond five years. More broadly, basic changes in the balance between sophisticated hospital care and community-based, primary health care are not accomplished quickly or easily. Increasingly, therefore, long-term perspective planning is employed to provide the basic framework within which rolling intermediate-term planning and annual plan implementation take place. The structural framework for planning must be adjusted to reflect this orientation.

In the interest of providing continuity between planning and implementation, an early decision must be made about the relative balance of planning responsibilities to be given to representative consultant groups and to a planning unit composed of full-time staff professionals. A spectrum of different arrangements may be necessary at various levels in the planning hierarchy.

The process of bringing together appropriate groups of health officials, members of professional societies, interested voluntary agencies, and general consumer representatives under whatever title or terminology will be called for present purposes "the part-time committee approach". Thus, the approach is exemplified by the pattern of health planning developed in India in the preparation of the health components of the successive five-year plans, the National Planning Commission (established in 1950) was composed of the Cabinet members and distinguished leaders representing many disciplines. The Prime Minister of India is the chairperson of the Planning Commission. The Planning Commission aims at providing total and comprehensive socio-economic development planning, with major emphasis on policy planning. The Health Panel of the Planning Commission similarly was composed of distinguished leaders interested in health services. Under this Health Panel, there were numerous committees which had the primary responsibility for decisions required in formulating the plan

In the other polar type of organization, planning has revolved around an elite fultime professional group of planners. The classic example is the Soviet System of Planning. A major burst of activity tends to occur during the preparation of a five-year plan; with a full-time professional group, however, planning tends to be done more on a continuing basis. The professional planners tend to work through their own hierarchy, which reaches out from the center.

Evidence is increasing that the best planning requires an appropriate mixture of the committee approach and a full-time professional planning unit. The planning unit can be compared with the executive branch, while the various commissions, councils, and committees have functions which more nearly resemble legislative responsibilities. In general, an approximately equal balance of the two components is probably desirable in the central, organization of planning, At the middle level, effective professional units are probably more important. At the local level the committee approach becomes particularly important.

The balance of the two organizational components also varies according to the type of planning activity. The committee approach is particularly necessary in comprehensive and perspective planning, while professional expertise is most needed in programme and project planning and in preparation of annual plans of work. Perhaps this is one of the reasons why the far project and programme-planning have been more effectively carried out than comprehensive planning.

The professional composition of the planning unit staff is determined by the local situation and traditions. Certainly, nothing causes planning to fall into disrepute among health personnel as quickly as a lack of health professionals in the planning groups. These health professionals should be respected for their practical experience and technical competence. Although a new speciality of health planning has developed, it seems desirable that professionals who take this special training should first have practical experience in general health programmes. Of great importance in organizing the information system and undertaking the necessary analyzer is strong representation of statistical skills. In view of the mounting evidence that the new techniques of systems analysis and operations research have much to contribute to health planning some representation from this area should be incorporated, especially at the higher levels in the planning hierarchy. The planning team should also include a member with competence in health economics. Additional specialities which can profitably be included, are public administration and the social sciences. Because of the tremendous importance of budgeting procedures in ensuring implementation, special expertise in budgeting and accounting is valuable. Finally, as planning focuses on particular substantive areas, such as the control of particular diseases or special subjects such as sanitation, the best technical experts in these areas must be available.

In setting up a smoothly functioning planning machinery, it is vital to define clearly the role of each member of the planning team. Assigning technical responsibilities usually appears fairly obvious. Clear statements of responsibility are needed. However, to define the relationships among the professional planners and the innumerable other groups and individuals who should be involved in the planning process, such liaison relationships may sometimes be shared among members of the planning team. For optimum implementation a direct linkage with all levels of the administrative hierarchy and with the institutions where health activities are carried out is also necessary.

Centralization/ Decentralization

On the spectrum ranging between complete centralization and decentralization, the appropriate balance point in any planning situation must be determined by complex local considerations. In general, the most important determinants are intangibles in the local political and social milieu. Popular participation is largely conditioned by tradition and culture.

The usual tendency is to have too much centralization initially. This may be partly because most early efforts in planning were in situation which provided maximum centralized control, such as the planning were in situations which provided maximum centralized control. This is certainly the most comfortable situation in which to plan. The planner works in a clear hierarchy, assuming that it is possible to convince the decision makers at the top about the appropriateness of the plan. The planner has the feeling that implementation will naturally follow.

Centralized Responsibilities

Early in the planning process, aims must be defined, and this requires a large measure of central direction. Local units, of course, should have some opportunity to contribute ideas and suggestions. The real work of defining plan goals and balancing their importance, however, requires the highest level of responsible policy-making representation. A broad range of understanding is necessary, especially in relation to other aspects of development such as roads, communications, education, and economic growth.

Planners must be told what the health services will have to work with and then judgments must be made at the central level concerning limitations to be placed upon the funds and personnel which are centrally controlled. The central unit must also make overall estimates of contributions expected from local participation, allowing for variation in what individual peripheral units actually decide to contribute to particular health activities.

A third responsibility which is primarily centrally controlled is adherence to basic plan priorities. This means that in the implementation process special central effort will have to be directed towards stimulating action in areas of deficiency.

Similarly, the establishment of the total organization and machinery of planning is primarily a central responsibility. The objective should be to have the planning machinery reach out as far as possible through the total range of public and private health services. Efficiency demands a certain degree of standardization in relationships.

A final planning activity has to be built into the routine of any good local administration; the principal responsibility for evolution as part of the planning process should, however, provide a considerable degree of external objectivity. An important part of such overall evaluation is comparison with other areas and projects, and this can clearly be done best at the central level.

Decentralized Responsibilities

The components of decentralized responsibility in planning are those residual functions not assumed by central authorities.

Effective data gathering is organized centrally, but the quality obviously depends on local involvement. If personnel at the periphery where the data originate know the purpose for which the data will be used, then there will be much more interest and precision in obtaining valid information. Any sort of feedback by which peripheral units can see the tangible contributions of their data will lead to an automatic improvement in validity.

Particularly important is that planning detailed programmes be done by peripheral units. Nothing promotes successful implementation as much as having communities feel that the planning hierarchy has been set up mainly to help them with their own planning. The most successful planners create a feeling of participation at peripheral levels so that credit for achievement is also decentralized.

At the local level, success in plan implementation depends on the participation of several diverse groups. Perhaps most important are the local professionals who are directly responsible for health services.

Efforts to include lay and consumer groups in the planning process also facilitate effective implementation. A major benefit is that such involvement can provide direct access to major gaps and areas of deficiency in services. Consumer participation is most essential in programmes which have a large component of personal services.

As a local planning unit undertakes implementation of plans, it is important to recognize that a major ingredient of success is the art of capturing the right moment. Since implementation requires the interaction of multiple forces, a high degree of opportunism is needed.

Planning as an Educational Process

Planning is largely an educational process. Planner's efforts will be proved effective not so much by what they do themselves as by what they persuade others to do. In spite of all that is said about the difficulty of educating the public, planners often need to concentrate even more educational effort on administrators and health personnel. The opinions of health workers are often harder to modify than public attitudes because of their greater personal investment in traditional ways of doing things.

A simple definition of organized planning is the use of systematic approaches to enable diverse individuals to agree on mutually satisfactory ways of carrying out complicated activities. Good planning should be realistically recognized to be a slow process.

Developmental change is primarily dependent on improved motivation. Public motivation starts with an interest in the immediate benefits of medical care. Professional guidance is needed in adjusting to a time scale of expected health improvements in which the public learns to think beyond immediate needs for curative services to the greater, through delayed, benefits of preventive and promotive activities.

Health personnel and administrators tend to be somewhat ambivalent in their approach to planning activities. Their investment in traditional activities and personal career goals makes them suspicious of planned change. A favorable motivation to change can be induced most readily by deliberate manipulation of incentives career and monetary rewards can be related directly to demonstrable improvements in services offered. An educational approach to plan implementation should be characterized by efforts to promote cooperation rather than to impose coordination.

Stages of the Planning Process

Planning explores the uncertainties of how the best use can be made of limited resources to meet priority needs. It has, therefore, much of the intellectual challenge of research.

Planning is a dynamic process; hence it is not in practice a single movement up a rigidly structured static stairway of steps. Rather it is an unending upward spiral of incremental efforts toward improvement. The purpose of the present categorization of the elements of the planning process is to provide a general framework or outline of functions to be performed to ensure a systematic approach.

In reality, many activities should be carried out concurrently, providing a mutually supportive flow back and forth among various stages of the process, depending on local conditions and requirements such variations lead at different times and places to great differences in the balance among the amounts of planning input required for various steps of the process. The structure and function of the planning machinery must also be adjusted to local conditions. Flexibility is desirable, especially at the start, when adaptations are more necessary and frequent.

Developing Planning Competence

In any planning structure the policy-making body must represent the political power structure, the general public, and health professionals. The balance among these three groups is determined largely by the type of planning to be undertaken. In comprehensive planning it is particularly important to ensure that the health activities fit general public desires. Hence, the proportionate representation of consumers should be great. In many types of programme planning and project planning, which should themselves fit in with a general comprehensive plan, the particular competence required is more technical in nature; thus, representation on the policy making group can be weighed more toward the health professional.

In general, the planning units should be closely associated with administrative structure but not directly involved in administration. Its success is often determined by its ability to make itself useful to administrators. Effective planning, however, requires the ability to move easily at all administrative and organizational levels and lines of communication.

Since planning is largely an educational enterprise, substantial effort must be devoted to teaching the planning methods to be used throughout the administrative structure. Once the members of the planning unit have themselves received the best training available, they should organize special training programmes for those with whom they work. Some of the most effective planning organizations have devoted a great deal of energy to organizing short courses in planning which are arranged by all levels of health personnel. In addition to teaching technical planning, data gathering skills, economic theory, and analytic methodology, such a systematic educational programme can have a unique impact by developing enthusiasm and a spirit of cooperative action.

Statements of Policy and Broad Goals

Planning policies and goals must be politically determined. Skill must be developed in gauging and mobilizing political opinions. In order to set the stage for effective implementation of the plan, it is essential to make sure at the start that planning goals fit the policies of the political group responsible for implementation

One of the best educational manoeuvres that a planning group can use in conditioning the political structure to which it is responsible is to require the policy-making group to go through the difficult exercise of explicitly starting plan aims. By taking the time at the beginning to induce policymakers to arrive at explicitly statements, much time is saved later when the details of planning and implementation are being worked out. An important step at this stage is to distinguish clearly between long-term goals and short-range objectives. Both should be stated with clear recognition of time and priority implications.

To ensure that planning is dynamic rather than static, they must recognize its cyclic nature. After following the steps of the planning process through a plan period, the time comes when policy makers are back to the first step again and must revise the plan objectives on the basis of experience gained. Continuity must be maintained by constantly looking ahead to the next plan period.

Information for Planning

A particular benefit of good planning is that it provides a basis for judgment in sharpening the selection of truly useful data.

In health planning, data customarily start with demographic information. The basic unit of health-care is obviously the number of people to be served and their distribution. Because of the rapid rate of population growth in most developing countries, it is particularly essential to have the most accurate population projections possible.

The Second category of information is epidemiologic, specifically information on the frequency and distribution of major health problems. In developing countries, this is often very spotty. Because of the chronic difficulty of collecting accurate mortality and morbidity information, an immediate need is often times to organize some sort of sample survey. Certainly, the patient selectivity factor makes hospital and other, institutional reports of disease only minimally useful.

In many places the most serious deficiencies of planning information are in economic data. Most health people have little idea of what sort of information might be useful for economic analyses. The simplest type of information is usually accurate cost accounting of specific health activities.

Another category of information which usually must be specially developed for planning purposes concerns the utilization of facilities and the functional patterns of work of various types of personnel. Planning can make its most dramatic contri butions in short time periods by increasing efficiency of utilization. This requires careful attention to the process of setting work standards and performance budgeting. Without an adequate data system, such rationalization of the services is obviously impossible.

Priority Statement of Health Problems

Setting priorities is considered by most health administrators to be the heart of the planning process. The steps leading up to this point can in a way be considered preparation for the crucial decisions involved in priority setting. Once priorities have been set, the subsequent steps can be considered progressive moves toward implementation. In priority setting judgment, wisdom is most needed, together with a uniquability to synthesize the numerous relevant details. It is the part of the planning process which is usually considered most intuitive. Priority setting, however, can perhaps benefit more than any of the other steps from being made an explicit and defined exercise.

The greatest skill required in priority setting is to balance variables which have very different quantitative relation ships and in fact lie in different dimensional scales.

The health planner must develop skills sufficient to provide a balanced approach to each. Particularly needed are valid specific indices for both the quantitative and qualitative types of information implied in these judgments. Despite all attempts at measurement and specific categorization, the planner will, in the end, have to rely on the indefinable elements of wisdom from experience or room evaluation of previous plans in making the final decisions.

Plan Outline

With the priority decisions in hand, it is necessary to begin to work out the alternative proposals which represent possible ways of coping with the health problems defined. A clear statement of alternative approaches provides a basis for deciding what should in fact be done. This involves actually specifying many of the underlying considerations which were gathered and balanced in the course of priority setting. The advantages at this stage of a clear outline for each alternative approach is that it provides a ready basis for comparison. Particular points to be included in the outline include: (1) a clear definition of the technical aspects of the programme, (2) the organization framework required, (3) the personnel and facilities needed, (4) costs in comparable financial terms, and (5) approximate benefits to be expected in relation to priority of concern.

Since decisions between alternatives must be based largely on a cost-benefit type of judgment, it seems that benefits should be greater in programmes that have multiple health contribution.

At this point, the distinctions among comprehensive planning, programme planning, and project planning should be recalled comprehensive planning provides the general framework for development; it is particularly concerned with the problem of priorities and the relative stress to be given to various programmes and projects. It provides the overall conceptual structure within which programme and project planning can be done. The most effective detailed planning, then, is at the programme and project level, programme planning is directed toward broad-impact health activities directed against single health problems.

Development of Detailed Plan

Construction of a detailed plan document is usually worked out in phases. Long-term goals are specifically stated, along with the proposed steps necessary to carry them out. Any programms requiring several years must be stated in flexible terms. Increasing detail and specificity can be introduced for more immediate periods, such as the next year.

The probability of achieving successful implementation of a detailed plan is proportionately increased with greater local involvement in the programming. If local units can be assigned responsibility for developing detailed programmes on the basis of general procedures set up by the central unit, more spontaneous enthusiasm and active participation will be brought to the task.

In shifting the planning balance toward decentralization and local involvement, two major controls should be built in by central planning units. The first is the development of appropriate standards for performance.

Similarly, target setting is an appropriate part of the central unit's responsibility. Targets should be specified according to quantitative indices of performance and within a clearly stated time framework. As with standard-setting, establishment of precise targets can be expected to improve with progressive implementation in successive plan periods. Both standard-setting and target-setting should be attempted from the beginning, however, in order to provide a rational basis for evaluation. Above all they should be realistic and based on the general human response that work effectiveness improves most if built on a reasonable experience of success.

Implementation

The concept of planning as a dynamic and continuing activity requires that implementation be an integral part of health planning.

Implementation can be considered an important part of the planning process from two quite distinct points of view. Traditionally, comprehensive planning has been considered a process in which the entire health service should be involved; planning has been viewed as only a normal step in good administration. In this inclusive view implementation is intimately associated with both planning and administration, so that the three aspects are not easily separated.

Clearly, the plan itself must incorporate detailed planning for implementation, but the health planner must set up the conditions which give the plan the greatest likelihood of being successfully carried out.

The first tactical step in plan implementation is to gain acceptance of the plan. A completely innocuous plan which merely confirms existing conditions, of course, has the best chance for acceptance. The more innovative the plan proposal, the more difficulty there will be in inducing political leaders, health personnel, and the public to agree if a plan is to do some good, it should contain the seeds of progressive change.

The probability of acceptance of plan proposals increases proportionately with the extent to which health personnel, political leaders, and the consumer public participate in the planning process.

Evaluation

Evaluation is such an important part of the total dynamic process of planning that many functioning units are called planning and evaluation units.

Two fundamentally different type of evaluation must be distinguished: Continuing evaluation for administrative purposes and periodic, more focused evaluation specifically for plan revision. Particularly important to the administrator is continuing self evaluation by local administrative health units. If the planning process can encourage local units to undertake systematic self-evaluation and provide them with appropriate know-how and mechanisms, this will be perhaps the best possible means of building in continuous improvement, In addition, a major role of the planning organization is to undertake continuing administrative evaluation to see that standards and targets are being met. One of the best ways for planners to establish their usefulness is to show that they can fulfill an important service role to the administrators. A natural service activity with great practical value to most senior administrators is a tough, frank approach to evaluation. In any centralized/decentralized balance, this naturally tends to continue as an important role of the central units.

The second major type of evaluation is more definitely related to the planning process. A centrally directed activity has to be set up with the primary purpose of quantifying achievement in particular planning periods. Such activity tends to be timed to precede the evolution of a new major plan or the modification of an existing one. This kind of exercise should extend considerably beyond mere measurement of achievement in terms of previous standards and targets. It should concentrate on assessment of such basic issues as whether the original goals and objectives were in fact appropriate; whether resource development is actually moving in the direction most suited to local conditions, in terms of both facilities and personnel; whether the priority setting was, in face, justified by further experience: and especially whether the data gathering system is producing useful information. It has to be worked out with as much ingenuity and innovative precision as any other part of the planning sequence.

At the heart of all health planning methodology is the desire to improve health system performance. We need a clear perception of that system and its component parts. Second, in line with concern for improvement, we examine the hierarchy of goals and objectives that drives the process of planned change. In addition to a conceptual understanding of the system and its purposes, planning in practice requires an analytical framework for concrete appraisal of the various functions of the system.

CONCEPTUALIZATION OF THE HEALTH SERVICES SYSTEM

Conceptually, (approach portrayed in Fig. 10.1) health services draw upon resources in response to certain health problems for the purpose of producing an outcome in the form of improved health status. Such a broad conceptualization is of course, of little practical value in coming to grips with real conditions, we must look more carefully therefore, at each system component in turn (Fig. 10.1).

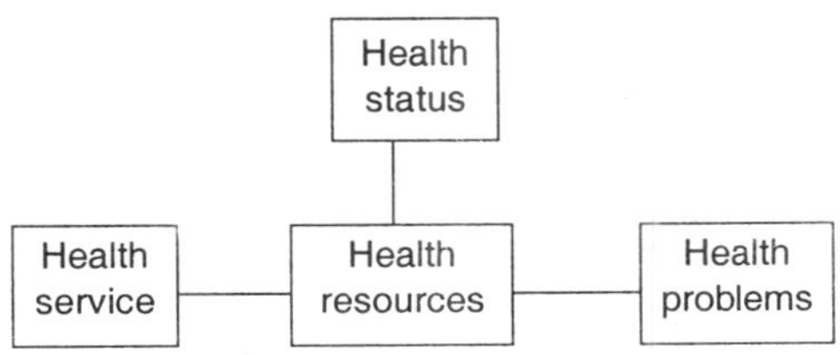

Fig. 10.1: Health care system overview

People and their Problems

Health problems (Fig. 10.2) are identified in relation to the population at risk in the planning area. Effectively, then, they have epidemiologic numerators, demographic demoninators, and geographic bounds. The last item depends upon the mandate of the planning body, the location of health resources, political jurisdiction, transportation and communication patterns, and population concentration.

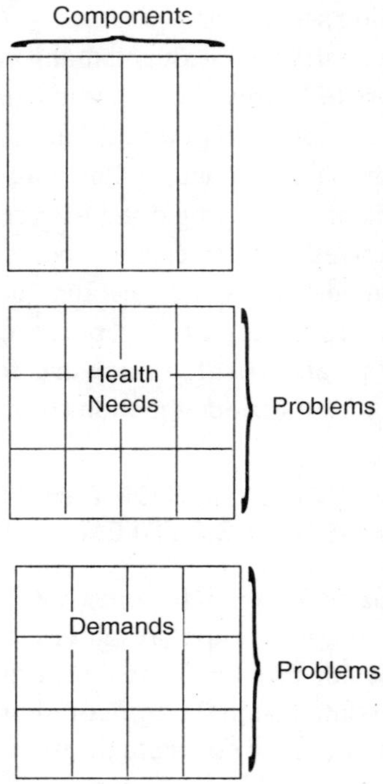

Fig. 10.2: Detailed view of health problems

Demographic considerations are based upon the fact that different segments of the population vary in the type and magnitude of their health needs as well as in their utilization of health services. A planner is especially interested in identifying important population characteristics that are likely to change in relative importance. As a minimum, the population breakdown should include age, sex, and place of residence. Frequently it is advisable to add social class and/or educational attainment, race and participation in health insurance programmes.

Within each relevant population group the planner must identify the nature and importance of individual health needs, as well as the extent to which these needs are currently translated into demands for health services. Assessment of problems should allow for both cause and effect. Identification of problems according to the International Classification of Disease may be useful. Furthermore, within this classification system a planner will probably be concerned with morbidity and disability or loss in productive capacity as well as mortality.

Classification of health problems by disease not only provides information on effects in terms of mortality and morbidity but also suggests specific disease agents as causal factors. In addition, more general hazards to health should be identified through reference to water supply sources, sewage and waste collection system, feeding practices, food protection mechanisms, housing conditions, and vector control. Table 10.1 summarizes the essential items of information needed under this and the other headings to be considered.

Health Resources

In considering health resources (Fig 10.3). planners must separate human, physical, and financial components. They must determine the available quantities and locations of different kinds of health

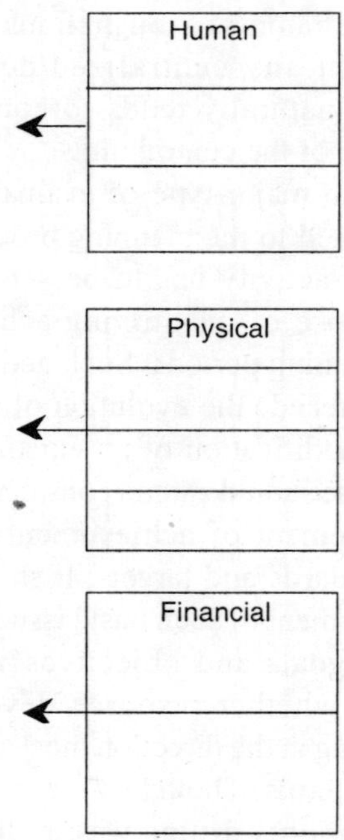

Fig. 10.3: Detailed view of health resources

Table 10.1

1. Population size and Characteristics:
   - Age-sex distribution
   - Geographical distribution
   - Transportation and communications patterns
   - Educational attainment
   - Socioeconomic status
   - Health insurance coverage.
2. Health Status and problems:
   - Disease-specific and age-specific mortality, isability, morbidity rates
   - Water supply sources
   - Sewerage and waste collection practices
   - Food protection mechanisms
   - Housing conditions
   - Vector control practices
   - Fertility rates.
3. Human Resources:
   - Mix of active personnel among major categories
   - Attrition rates
   - Age-sex distribution
   - Type of practice
   - Affiliation
   - Location of practice
   - Training limitations
   - Training capacity by :
     — Location and type of institution
     — Enrollment by location and type of institution.
     — Available teachers
     — Available funds for training
     — Size of pool of potential applications.
4. Physical Resources and Organization:
   - Geographical distribution
   - Diagnostic and treatment services provide
   - Sponsorship
   - Organizational relationships and referral patterns
   - Political factors influencing organizational authority responsibility.
5. Financial Resources:
   - Geographical variations in income
   - Sectoral distribution of GNP
   - Investment patterns contributing to development
   - Availability of foreign exchange
   - Health expenditures relative to GNP
   - Health budget relative to total public expenditures
   - Private *vs* public expenditure in health
   - Current budget *vs* development budget
6. Service Statistics
   - Utilization rates
     — Annual physician visits per person
     — Annual dentist visits per person
     — Hospital discharges
     — Hospital bed days
     — Pre-natal visits per live birth
     — Well-child visits per live birth
     — Attended deliveries by category of attention
   - Coverage
     — Demographic and epidemiologic characteristic of population served
     — Costs and charges for services
     — Sources of payment
     — Productivity standards

workers, inventory existing facilities of various. kinds (public and private), and identify various revenue sources.

Human resources must first be viewed with respect to existing supplies and then in terms of the training infrastructure as it could affect future levels. Enumeration of current providers should include community volunteers and indigenous practioners of local importance, as well as the main categories of professional, para-professional, and auxiliary workers employed in the formal health care system. In addition to numbers, the planner is interested in the age and sex distribution, affiliation, and type and location of practice.

Like human resources, physical facilities fit into a number of categories which must be separately identified and inventoried. These include hospitals, dispensaries, clinics, and private sources of personal care, as well as water, sewerage and other environmental systems.

The degree of detail embodied in the information depends upon the availability of data and the uniqueness of given resources. Apart from the detail with which records are maintained, the essential criterion of interest to planners is the degree to which facilities can be substituted for one another. Thus, they require a geographical beakdown in order to recognize differences in population groups served, distinctions are also made on the basis of differences in diagnostic and treatment facilities, consequently, information is assembled with respect to short-term general, long-term rehabilitation and mental institutions, along with the availability of various clinical and laboratory services within the institution. Frequently, distinctions must be made on the basis of the goals of individual health agencies which arise from different sources of sponsorship, and these distinctions may be reflected in the financial structure and organization of the agency. Hence, health planners are likely to distinguish among government, proprietary, religious, and other types of institutions.

Once the planners have appropriately classified a facility, they must place a value on it, usually in both physical and monetary terms. For example, a hospital might be identified as a two-hundred-bed institution with a certain replacement cost. In looking to the future, the age of existing installations is an important factor just as the age distribution of physicians is an important personal consideration.

Although categorization is necessary to the inventorying of resources, attention must also be given to coordination and interactions among categories. Existing referral patterns must be recognized along with the impact that such factors as increased dependence upon extended care facilities would have upon the need for beds in short-term general hospitals.

Health Services

Figure 10.4 depicts schematically the structure of health services that develop from the organization of resources to satisfy health demands. It also shows the impact of these services upon health status. Health services include diagnostic, treatment, and rehabilitative components. From the standpoint of planning and evaluation, these services should be viewed in functional rather than organizational terms. The planner must understand the present health service structure in terms of the performance of certain functions, each of which is a specific combination of human physical, and financial resources organized to satisfy to some extent one or more existing health demands.

In viewing the health services structure explicit recognition should be given to the preventive aspects. Primary disease prevention, such as immunization, has an impact extending beyond the health services box of Figure 10.2 secondary prevention as a category of service, such as early detection of cervical cancer, has its major effect at the diagnostic stage, whereas tertiary prevention occurs largely at the treatment stage, as in the case where stroke patients are treated in a manner that minimizes muscular deformities and subsequent problems of rehabilitation.

The health field is unique in the extent to which supply and demand interact. This is exemplified by contentions that physicians largely create a demand for their own services and that utilization of hospital beds is in large measure determined by their availability. A complete and realistic appraisal of the health services structure, therefore, must include factors that influence demand for services.

Actual measurement of services rendered should include, to begin with, a compilation of resource utilization data such as the annual number of physician visits and hospital discharges and durations of hospital stay. Recognition of the key role of financial mechanisms in determining the nature and volume of services actually provided is important, and planners, must know a good deal about the costs and sources of funding such services. In a broader sense they should be cognizant of the current magnitude of health expenditures in relation to the size of the total economy, along with future trends in both.

Besides recording the mere utilization of services, indices that relate services rendered both to the available resources and to the client population should be created. Examples of the former include hospital bed occupancy rates, average outpatient visits per health center per day, number of deliveries per midwife, and average cost per

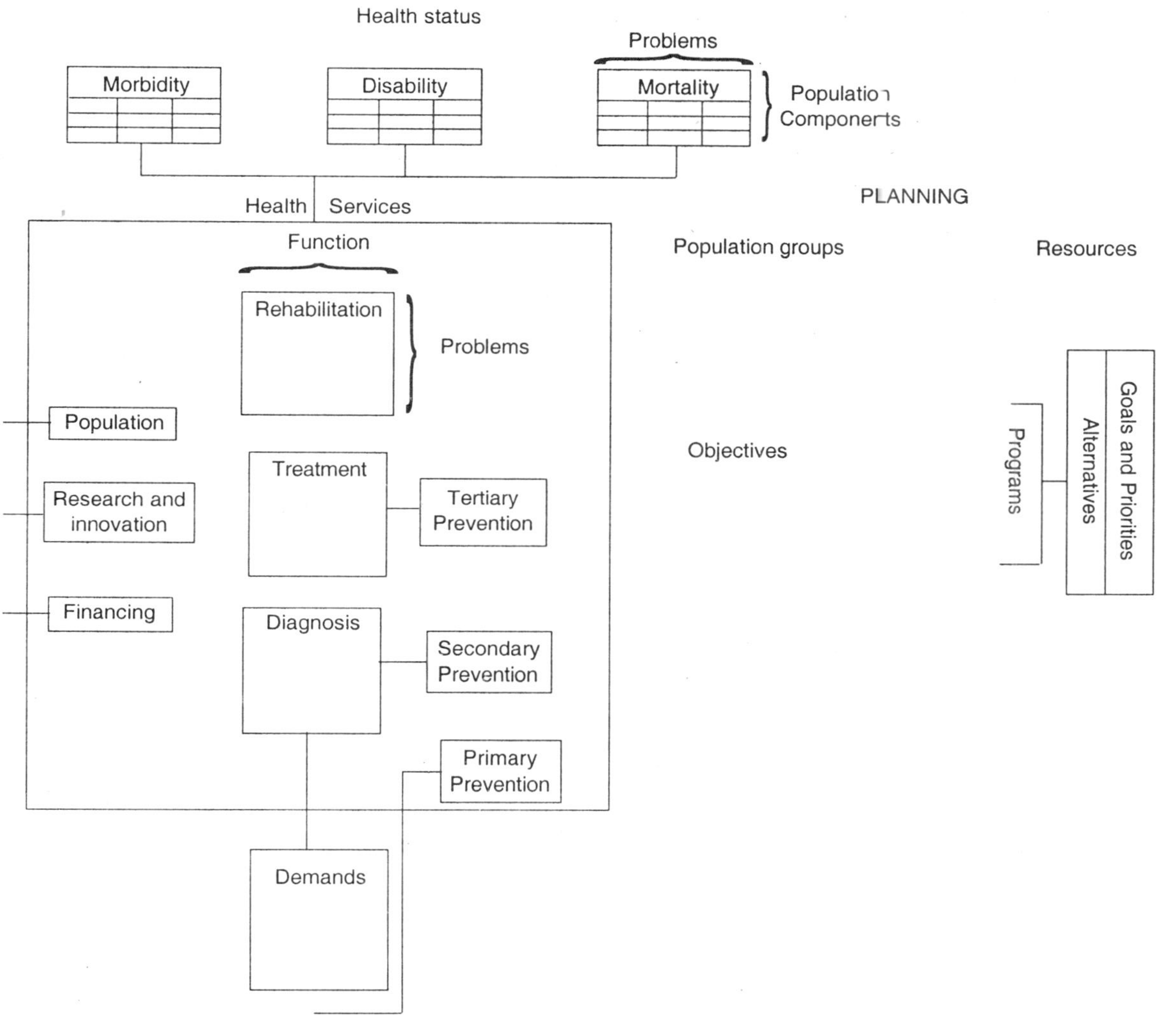

Fig. 10.4: Detailed view of health services and health status with planning

immunization. Indices related to the client population are illustrated by the proportion of deliveries attended by trained personnel and the proportion of underweight children served by feeding centers.

Health Status

For schematic purposes, health status can be considered in terms of mortality, disability, and morbidity. Morbidity is linked to population, indicating that the entire health system is dynamic. That is, we are interested in the ability of the health services to modify and improve health status and to return health individuals to the population. This suggests, furthermore, that each health status component (mortality, disability, and morbidity) should have the same subdivisions by population groups and health problems. As a result, a planner must identify not only the major causes of health needs but also areas in which these needs are not being met satisfactorily.

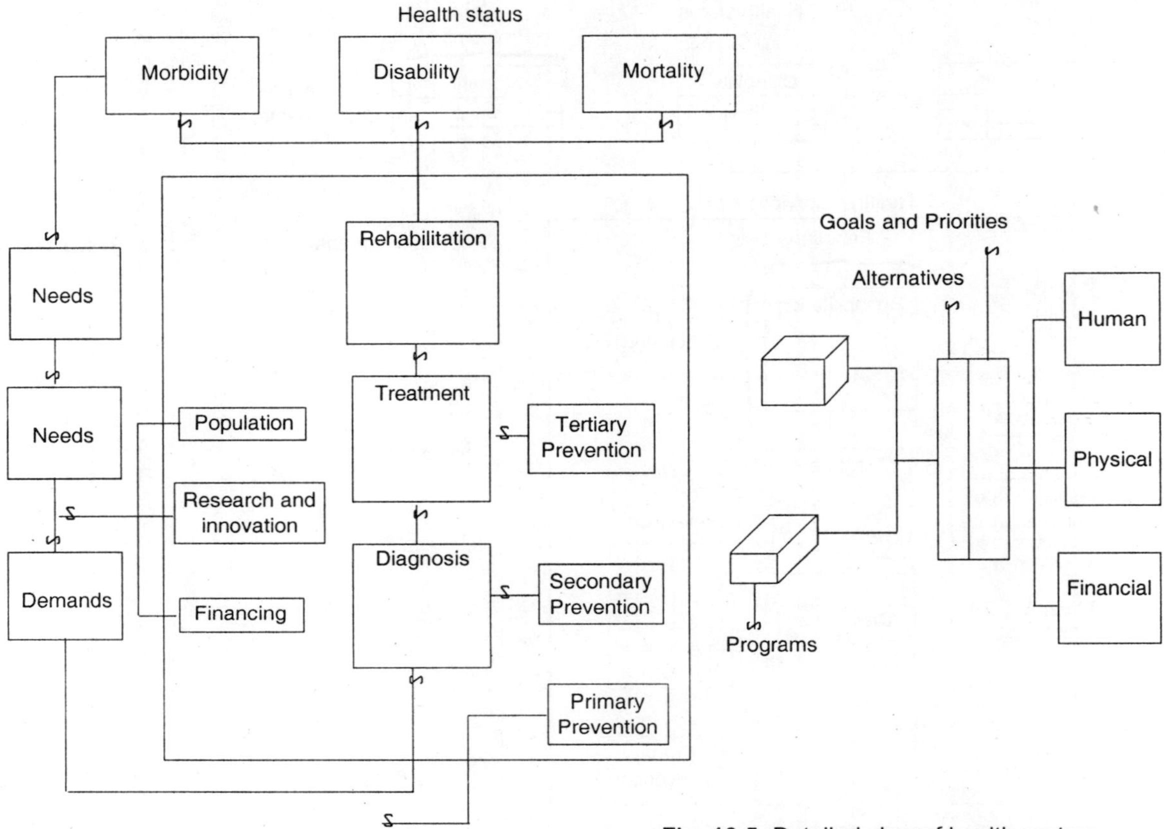

Fig. 10.5: Detailed view of health system

Impact of Planning

The health system components and linkages exist regardless of the role that health planning may play. Planning does, however, carry with it the potential for improving the performance of the system. Inherent in the notion of improvement is the specification of goals, or norms, towards which conscious effort is to be directed.

The core of planning, then, is the analysis of alternative means of moving toward identified health goals in the light of specified priorities and existing constraints. The selection process results in variety of programme packages. Each programme, which is directed at one or more health problems, is designed to achieve specific measurable objectives through a certain combination of resources oriented toward particular population groups.

All the health system components are brought together in Figure 10.5. It is considerably more detailed and expresselly incorporates the role of planning into the schematic representation.

THE ESSENCE OF PLANNING

The core of planning is analysis (in the face of con straints) of alternative means of achieving established goals ranked in some order of priority. The two factors—goals and analysis form the core of the practical process of planning.

Goals and Priorities

Mission describes an organization's reason for existence, the general functions of services it performs, and the limits of its jurisdiction and authority. The mission of a state or local health department might be the protection and advancement of the public health of the population of that state or community within certain legally specified limitations.

A goal is a long-range specified state of accomplishment towards which programmes are directed. It is not cast in terms of current availability of resources or a fixed time for achievement, but it must be consistent with the mission. In the health field, the goal is usually stated in terms of completely overcoming a health problem or reducing it to the extent the state of the art permits.

An objective is stated in terms of achieving a measured amount of progress toward a goal. It must include a specification of:

1. **What?** the nature of the situation or condition to be attained.
2. **How much?** the quantity or amount of the situation or condition to be attained.
3. **When?** the time at or by which desired situation or condition is intended to exist.
4. **Who?** the particular group of people or portion of the environment in which attainment is desired, and
5. **Where?** the geographic area to be included in the programme.

A target establishes a measured amount of output to be achieved in relation to a health objective through a specific programme activity, whereas objectives are set with respect to needs in the client population. Targets are set with respect to service providers. The targets should be based upon realistic performance standards.

Alternatives and Constraints

Targets can be established only after particular programme have been selected from set of alternatives. Moreover, reasonable objectives can only arise from a consideration of the costs and resources required to achieve the benefits that underlies contemplated objectives.

To be most effective, consideration of programme alternative should proceed within the framework of the health functions of particular concern. To illustrate, one agency has established the following nine study areas: reproduction, nutrition, dental and oral health, infectious and communicable diseases, trauma and safety, chronic diseases, handicapping conditions, mobility, and mental disorders. Other planners might prefer a breakdown in terms of personal preventive, curative, and rehabilitative activities; environmental sanitation, mass campaigns against communicable disease and so forth. These functions could be analyzed further with respect to such important dimensions as age or urgency of need (emergency, acute, and chronic conditions).

Broad goals consistent with the overall mission of the enterprise are established. The, specific quantified objectives are developed with the aim of effective functioning of the health services system. Progress towards the achievement of these objectives is made by means of health programmes. These programmes which organize activities for the efficient utilization of combinations of resources have certain targets. A meaningful comparison can be made between the activities per formed and the degree of attainment of targets and objectives. The functional analysis seeks to establish: (1) the level of activities and resources, currently devoted to each of the functions (2) the extent to which community needs remain unsatisfied in various areas, and (3) the potential for modifying or expanding services to meet these needs.

The key to meaningful analysis is to employ measures of need and resource availability that are mutually compatible. To measure need in strictly epidemiologic terms of disease prevalence and mortality rates, while resources are described in economic and financial terms of budgets and staffing patterns, is not very helpful analytically, rather, needs and resources must both be translated into service terms for the sake of comparability to enable judgments about reallocation of resources to be made rationally. Productivity standards are needed to translate the availability of human resources into services potential. Among the various means of assessing provider effort, work sampling techniques adapted from industry have proved to be especially useful. On the needs side, streamlined community sample surveys have been designed to transcend mere service utilization to measures of fundamental need. For evaluating provider-client interactions, patient flow studies have been developed. These determine the content, quality, and appropriateness of service rendered, as well as the time required, including patient waiting time. Finally, special techniques of cost analysis have been devised to transform cost information into meaningful functional terms.

As increased attention is directed to providing improved coverage with cost-effective services, such analyses make more visible possible impacts upon functional emphasis and demands for scarce resources.

THE INFORMATION BASE

The ability to engage in systematic analysis and to undertake rational planning obviously depends upon the availability of useful information. Four levels of meaningful information are to be noted.

The first is in the form of political mandate. If political authorities state that the number of rural health posts must be doubled within five years or that a cardiac care unit is needed in the capital city, planners, cannot afford to ignore this information.

The second level of information is expert judgment. While its objectivity may be a suspect, we must recognize the fact that the experience of experts generally includes important qualitative aspects of a situation that cannot be captured in quantitative data.

The third level of information is existing records and reports. In principle these should be readily available at little cost and should reflect important trends and emerging problems.

The fourth level of information is data collected specifically as a part of the planning process, usually through special surveys, properly designed surveys can produce relevant and accurate information, but they require skilled professionals and they can be costly and time-consuming.

Thus, each level of information has its values and limitations. In considering the limitations, it is well to recognize that precise data are not as important in planning as in implementation and evaluation.

Although the practical importance of qualitative considerations must not be underestimated, sound planning is ultimately dependent upon a solid base of factual data.

Population Censuses

Most countries periodically publish census information which is an invaluable source of data on population size, distribution, and characteristics. The frequency, and therefore, accuracy of censuses varies, however, along with the degree of detail provided. In particular, needed information about population characteristics may be unavailable for small areas. Even under the most favorable circumstances, some under reporting is inevitable, and it is likely to be more severe among certain groups, such as nomads or certain racial minorities.

Vital Registration Systems

Provision for registration of vital events is generally made, but completeness of reporting varies by country and by region within a country. An important consideration is the convenience and motivation for reporting births and deaths in a particular setting. If the health care system has responsibility for vital registration, motivation for reporting is likely to be low, and convenience likely to be variable. Thus, reporting tends to be more complete in urban areas, where a relatively large proportion of births occur in health facilities and deaths are more likely to occur in association with physician care. A common problem is the failure to report either the birth or death of a child who fails to survive the first week or two of life. This leads to an underestimation of the birth rate and the neonatal mortality rate, both of which are important for planning purposes.

Government Reports

Ministries of health and other public agencies invariably produce voluminous statistical reports. However, quality control over data is generally poor or nonexistent, and the data assembled are often of limited value for planning. Moreover, delays in collecting and processing the data frequently jeopardize the timeliness of the information assembled.

Professional Associations

Medical, nursing, hospital, and other professional associations are a rich source of data with decided limitations. Labour force registration statistics can be useful, but they may not indicate the number of personnel currently active or their location and type of employment. Hospital statistics on numbers of facilities and beds generally do not indicate their quality or service capabilities.

National Surveys

The Health Interview Survey (HIS) conducted continuously by the National Center for Health Statistics in the United States produces a wealth of information on health problems and patterns of health services utilization. The national sample is generally inadequate. However, to provide definitive data for state and regional planning, such surveys, in other countries are even more limited in size or nonexistent. In any event of household surveys such as these are based upon population perceptions of illness rather than medical diagnoses.

FURTHER READING

1. Djuikanovic V, EP Mach: Alternative Approaches to Meeting Basic Health Needs in Developing Countries. Geneva. and World Health organization 1975.
2. Hochbaum GM: "Consumer Participation in Health Planning: Toward conceptual Clarification," *American Journal of Public Health*, **59**: 1698-1705, 1969.
3. Blendon RJ, CR Gaus: "Problems in Developing Health Services in Poverty Areas: The Johns Hopkins Experience," *Journal of Medical Education*, **46**: 477-84, 1971.
4. National Health Planning in Developing Countries: WHO Technical Report Series No. 350, Geneva: World Health Organization, 1967.
5. Arnold MF: "Basic Concepts and Crucial Issues in Health Planning," *American Journal for Public Health*, **59**: 1686-97, 1969.
6. Kissick. WL(Ed.): "Dimensions and Determinants of Health Policy," Milbank Memorial Fund Quarterly, 46, No.1, part 2, January 1968.
7. Kleczkowski BM: "Matching Goals and Health Care Systems: "An International Perspective," *Social Science and Medicine*, **14A**: 391-95, 1980.
8. Michael JM, Spatafore G, Williams ER: "An Approach to Health Planning," *Public Health Reports*, **82**: 1063-70, 1967.

11 Towards Total Health Care

With spectacular advances in computers and telecommunications, it is easy to overlook the remarkable triumph of medicine and their contribution to our quality of life. The benefits are easy to measure. We are living longer and few die in their early years. But this very success is putting health care systems under pressure. The rapidly rising numbers of the elderly, together with new, expensive treatments have caused the cost of care to spiral. Information technology is, however, coming to the rescue by helping hospitals make better use of their resources and those unfortunate enough to need a stay in one can look forward to continually improving comfort and care.

It is, of course, a political matter how much society wishes to spend on health care, but it has become increasingly apparent during the past decade that providing more does not really ease the growing pressure on resources. Whatever, the governments provide is all too easily spent. A line must be drawn somewhere. So the actual level of services, hospitals and doctors can provide ulti mately depends on how wisely and efficiently they use their finite resources.

Efficiency is important for other reason too. In a hospital, where time is often precious, having the right people in the right place with the right information even faster than today would mean less suffering and a greater chance of successful treatment.

Patients in many countries are being given more choice about where they go. Hotel aspects are gaining greater significance as hospitals realise that the number and quality of additional services they provide can make the difference between whether a potential patient chooses them or goes elsewhere. Patients can expect greater comfort and relief from the tedium that a long stay in bed involves.

Integrated Care

The hospital's desire for improved efficiency and facilities is not so different from that of many other enterprises which are finding the answer in integrated computer systems and networks. And this is the route that hospitals have begun to follow. Indeed, they are becoming pioneers in adopting information technology and are reaping major benefits from the rapid exchange of and access to information.

Hospitals already have a variety of computer and communication systems. Apart from internal and external telephones, they have intercoms, paging systems for summoning doctors and nurses and fire alarm, heating, lighting, security and TV systems as well as diagnostic equipment and computers for analysis and administration.

Hosptials bringing together many of these systems into one powerful integrated network running throughout their buildings will not only bring immediate benefits by giving doctors and nurses more rapid access to the information then need; it will also help with monitoring and controlling costs and enhancing the efficiency of the whole organization.

Controlling Costs

Hospitals require an enormous amount of organisation, so it is hardly surprising that administration is a major cost. Yet administration does not directly benefit patients, so the more costs can be kept down, the more money is ultimately available for treatment. At the same time, it is vital to know what is being spent on what to provide the good housekeeping necessary to ensure that money is well spent.

Manufacturers are helping tackle both of these issues by supplying sophisticated computer systems in countries such as Austria, Spain, Switzerland, Italy and the Netherlands.

On arrival, patients are entered onto the system which then logs the medicine, treatment and other services they receive. When the patients' stay is over, the system produces invoices for sending either to the individual or the appropriate insurance company.

Medicines in the hospitals' pharmacy have a limited life, so effective stock control is vital to ensure that wastage is kept to a minimum, yet stocks are always immediately available on the shelves. The computer system also helps handle this, along with a staff salaries, room reservations and many other general administration tasks. Apart from greatly improving general efficiency such systems give detailed statistical information on precisely how much money goes where, enabling costs to be closely monitored and controlled.

In Switzerland's exclusive private clinics, a wide range of hotel-like services are provided. Guests can order newspapers, meals and other comforts. The computer system keeps track of exactly what each has received, ready to provide itemised bills when the patients leave.

Instant Access

But computer technology is making another major contribution to better health care by speeding the flow of information around the hospital. With major advances in medical equipment over recent years, doctors now have many more tools to help them make the right decisions on treatment as soon as possible. But information such as X-ray pictures is both difficult to get to the doctors and to store so it can be retired quickly. Much better if diagnostic information can be sent over a network so the doctors have instant access to whatever they need directly on their desks, or wherever else they may be.

Sophisticated high speed fibre-optic networks and storage systems are proving a boon to moving such vital information around the hospital, and giving patients more rapid and effective treatment. Apart from such diagnostic data, the hospital must also hold a variety of general information on patients such as age, address and next of kin, while they are in hospital and file this away when they leave. A hospital information system will help handle all this and archive it. The data will be made available on the same network as the diagnostic information so anyone who needs to, can access it.

This will mean the efficient and speedy handling of all the administrative details which patients are seldom in the mood for and also keeping, the worried relatives as uptodate as possible on all developments. There are also a number of other computer systems appearing in hospitals. Diagnostic equipment is increasingly being linked to computers to provide further analysis. Laboratories now also have their own special computers, and expert systems are starting to be used. All these can also be connected to the fibreoptic network.

Digital Switch

The new digital private automatic branch exchanges (PABXs) that emerged during the past decade are also of great benefit to hospitals. When installing a new phone system, hospitals almost invariably now opt for an integrated services digital network (ISDN) switch. Hospitals can make full use of the modern digital switch's ability to handle text and data as well as voice. It cannot cope with the large amounts of data from images such as X-ray picture, but certainly PC networking, small file transfers and electronic mail, for example.

Yet another wiring system allows patients to summon nurses. By pressing a button from their bed they can alert the nurse who will then, through an intercom system, ask the matter. If it is serious, the hospital's paging system will call for assistance. So far, this type of system has remained largely tailor-made for each ward with cables to every bed. But a far more flexible system is being developed which dispenses with the wires and provides a more direct link to the hospital's paging system.

Hospitality

Information technology entering hospitals will help doctors and nurses provide better clinical care. But for patients, the most obvious effects of this revolution will be very different, as the hospital resembles a high-class hotel more and more

As part of their drive to improve services, hospitals will provide more bedside TVs. To give every patient a choice even when they are not alone in the ward, they will have their own TVs with headsets. Cable and satellite TV programmes will give a wide-viewing choice, augmented by a hospital channel with programmes made from a small TV studio within the building. Videotext will provide day-to-day information such as visiting times and what is on the menu for lunch.

As in a hotel, each bed will have an intelligent telephone—a terminal to give patients access to a wide variety of services without leaving their beds. They will, for example, be able to order meals and newspapers, select movies on the television, even connect themselves to a computer at home.

The building itself will also incorporate many systems. The lighting, for example, will be controlled by computer. Using infrared signalling will remove the need for wiring light switches, again increasing flexibility. The very frail will benefit the most from even more tightly for personnel and accounts. The result will be the unprecedented integration of virtually all the information and control systems within the hospital.

Health Care Outside

Links to the outside are in some ways just as important for hospitals as communications within its walls. General practioners will have easy access through their own personal computer to data within the hospital, to receive the results of a blood test for example. Through the hospital's digital PABX, computer can be linked directly to computer, reducing the agonising wait for test results that patients can face.

Another advanced development will link clinics and hospitals by broadband cables, allowing doctors in different parts of the country to access data. Colleagues with common interests in a patient will be able to call up the same X-ray picture on their computer screens and discuss the case over the phone.

Specialists are in short supply and very busy people. It makes little sense for them to spend long hours travelling between hospitals for meetings. Video conferencing can ease the burden of travel, allowing them to use more of their time helping patients.

Understandably, the elderly wish to stay at their own homes as long as possible, but if something happens, they need to raise the alarm. Special alarm systems for this purpose are already available. The elderly need only push a button on their wrist or around their neck to summon help the system automatically calls the local doctor or hospital.

Total Responsibility

Advances in information and communications along with medical technology will further improve health care by allowing hospitals to have an intelligent telephone at every bed and allow the staff access to the databases of clinical and patient information from every work station. Electronic mail, voice mail, fax, telex, teletext, mobile telephones, paging, and more, will be incorporated within the hospital's system. Of course, it will take time to adopt the technology now available. Hospitals already have a variety of working systems that it would be difficult to justify replacing so quickly. But, as new hospitals are built, it will be possible to build-in virtually all the latest technology from the start.

HOSPITAL OF THE FUTURE

Medicine has benefitted greatly from recent advances in diagnostic equipment. X-ray, machines have been joined by CT (computer tomography-a sophisticated form of advanced X-ray analysis), digital vascular imaging (DVI) equipment and magnetic resonance (MR) systems. Most of these stand alone and produce images in the form a of photographic film. But such pictures are not easy to store or get to the specialists who need to see them.

A single X-ray photography contains the equivalent of several million bits of data, so a high speed network is needed along with a high capacity electronic filing system able to retrieve any one of thousands of images virtually instantly. The answers to both these stringent demands come from optics. Fibre optic cables can carry the data and an advanced optical filing system store the digitised images.

The latest diagnostic systems already generate digital outputs to allow further analysis, but film from older machines must first be scanned and converted to digital form. This image data is then passed to a system known as picture and data communication system (PACS). This handles the storage and retrieval of the images and makes them available on the backbone fibre optic network which runs throughout the hospital. Diagnostic information can then be viewed at any terminal connected to this network.

In fact, the fibre optic cable can carry much more than this. It consists of several strands, each of which can transport a large amount of data. One can carry PACS data, another general patient information, another data files and so on. The twisted-wirecabling used in the PABX system will run alongside the fibre optic cable in the backbone network. Patch panels can connect the terminals to a PABX line or to the fibre optic net work. If a nurse using a PC connected to the PABX requires infor mation on a patient, they can make a connection to the patient information network through the PABX. If the terminal is regular ly used for this purpose, it can easily (in less than a minute) be connected through the patch panel direct to the appropriate network. This approach gives much needed flexibility and leads to an extremely powerful series of interlinked networks which run throughout the hospital.

Resources must be Patien-focused

Our human resources, which represent over a half of operating expenses, spend more time coordinating care activities, waiting to deliver care, and writing about care than they do actually providing patient care. And not by a small percentage but by a factor of three or four.

In fact, staff under-utilisation is the single greatest consumer of resources. The majority of our health care expenses have nothing to do with patient care.

Clearly, our resources are not as patient-focussed and utilized as we would like them to be.

The Patient-Focused Hospital programme is changing all of this by increasing the effectiveness of our resources through breaking down the traditional walls separating departments from each other and from the patients they serve, staff are cross-trained across functions, thereby reducing hand-offs and overall cost.

In essence, Patient-Focussed Hospital programme structures the operations around the needs of the patients rather than the needs of departments. These care givers have more than doubled the amount of time they spend providing direct care to their patients' operations must be responsive to patient and physician needs. In addition to increasing costs, compartmentalisation also constrains our ability to provide good service to our patients and physicians.

The Patient-Focussed Hospital programme is putting patient-related information in the clinical decision-makers' hands in a fraction of today's time. It is accomplished by redeploying services, such as X-ray, lab and pharmacy closer to the patients' bedsides. This boils down the delivery process to its clinical essence-eliminating or shortening process steps, such as scheduling and transportation. Thus, turnaound times are measured in minutes rather than hours.

Individuals at all levels must be accountable and satisfied. It is easy to see how, within todays compartmentalized operating structure, no one is or can be truely accountable for the entire patient care process.

Traditionally, the doctor has looked to the nurse as the individual accountable for his patient's care. However, the nurse actually controls only a limited position of the care of her patients. She has to rely on others (such as therapists, technicians, and even other nurses on her) to provide the rest. In fact, much of her day is spent coordinating and following up on their activities.

Today's operating structure fails to match control with responsibility.

The Patient-Focussed Hospital progamme is empowering staff with far greater control over the entire patient care process. Cross-trained care givers are far more autonomous in their ownership of their patients "care. Unit managers oversee the great majority of services their patient consume and can therefore make explicit trade-offs across functions which are in the overall best interests of the patient the matching of control with responsibility strengthens accountability which enhances satisfaction. Patients must readily perceive value in their care.

12 The Patient–Centred Approach

Health care cannot be separated from the buildings in which it is delivered. The quality of space in such buildings affects the outcome of patient care, and architectural design is thus an important part of the healing process.

Hospital design has begun to focus on patients and their families—the consumers of hospital service. This redirected focus has resulted from the increasing competitiveness of the healthcare marketplace and the realisation that pleasant, user-friendly facilites can help attract patients.

Many of the qualities of space that are pleasing in hospitals are fundamental to good design in all types of buildings. A well-designed health facility reflects the art and skill of architects in the practice of their craft. The emergence of these qualities in new hospitals thus represents a maturing of hospital design from its focus on functional efficiency to a balance between function and aesthetics.

Undertaking the spatial qualities that make a successful hospital, is important to healthcare providers for two reasons. First, providers should be aware of the effects of spatial considerations on healing in order to manage patient care better. Second, informed providers can be advocates for good design in the planning and construction of health facilities, the qualities of space that characterise good architecture include: orientation, connection, scale, and symbolic meaning.

Orientation is the property of space that communicates to the user its physical relations to other spaces. It includes access, the ability to find and gain entrance to a building, and internal orientation, the ability to locate a destination within a building

Successful orientation begins with a clearly identifiable, legible entrance. The ability of patients and visitors to see where they are heading increases the sense of orientation. Proper signs are of course important, but direct visual cues transmit information better than signs. Another important device in orientation is the use of landmarks-easily identified and remembered objects that can be used as points of reference along patties. Sculptures, fountains, and gazebos often serve this purpose.

Connection describes the quality of the interaction between people and their environment. Connection with people is a continuum from community to privacy; good design allows a gradual transition between these extremes. This transition begins in the lobby. A successful lobby is an open, welcoming area, quieter and less busy than the street outside. From lobbies, more private hallways lead to patient areas. Within hallways, alcoves can provide private space for confidential discussions.

Connection with the nature is highly valued. Views of nature are associated with reduced stress and cause health-related complaints among employees obtaining views of nature requires both the appropriate placement of windows and the availability of nature requires both the appropriate placement of windows and the avail ability of natural views. The windowsills should be lower in patient rooms so that the landscape outside can be seen by patient lying in bed. The introduction of natural light into the center of the hospital contributes to the popularity of atrium hospitals. Windows admit natural light, which is more changeable, interesting, and informative than artificial illumination.

Architectural scale refers to the relation of sizes to one another, and particularly to the relation between the size of architectural forms and spaces and that of the human figure. Hospital's character must have a subtle balance of human scale and community scale the quality of the surrounding of the sick person may be as important in the cure as the specific therapeutic measures themselves. A hospital of about 180 beds permits the integration of the hospital function without sacrificing human scale. Large hospitals have difficulty in preserving a balance between human scale and community scale. Scale within a hospital should be modulated to provide variety, to accentuate change in function and ambience, and to help define the progression from public to private space.

Buildings also convey symbolic meaning by visual reference to cultural icons. Since patients and their families need to concentrate their energies on healing, architects often design the hospitals to provide an atmosphere of security, cleanliness, and physical comfort. In this way patients are encouraged not to worry about safety, sanitation, or physical discomfort. Making the hospital more home-like and less impersonal, is an important way to indicate that the focus in the hospital is on the individual patient. Familiar surrounding is an important adjunct to the healing process. Hospital patients should never be imbued with the idea that they are sick-health.

Hospitals are space for healing. Good architecture can be created in expansion or renovation projects, as well as in new facilities.

FURTHER READING

1. Corpman JR, Grant MA: *Design that Cares: Planning Health Facilities for Patients and Visitors*. 2nd ed. Chicago. American Hospital Publishing, 1993.
2. Horsburgh CR Jr.: Healing By Design. *N. Eng J Med* **11**: 735-40, 1996.

13 Patient-Focussed Hospital

All around the world, the cost of hospital care is rising to such an extent that government and the public are demanding the cost-effectiveness of hospital care.

Patient-Focused Hospital is an approach that involves a new way of structuring the current structural arrangements of the conventional hospital in the areas of staffing, management and hospital design in order to provide cost-effective service and better patient care.

The fundamental obstacle in the current structure is the compartmentalisation of each service. For example, if you examined the current structure of a 500 bed acute General Hospital in the USA or Europe, you would find that there are 16 to 20 separate departments and 18 to 20 nursing units. (Fig. 13.1) Each department and some nursing units would need to be specially designed, staffed and managed to suit individual functions: the result being that it takes approximately 35,000 to 40,000 sq. metres floor areas, 1500 to 2,000 staff and 350 different job classifications and constant movement of patients, staff and supplies. Furthermore, that over-specialization compartmentalizes jobs to such an extent that it can turn a simple task into a costly nightmare. For example, a routine in-patient X-ray can involve 15 to 20 employees and 30 to 40 different tasks. Only a small percentage of the total effort is related directly to the clinical aspect of Radiology.

Due to compartmentalisation and job classification, 50 to 55 percent of staff time is devoted to activities such as documentation, scheduling, co-ordination, transportation and management 15 to 20 per cent is used up as "idle time", and only 25 to 30 percent of staff time is spent on medical and clinical activities.

In fact, only a small portion of staff structure is directly related to actual delivery of medical or clinical care. Scheduling and documentation have become the primary operation functions of today's hospital. There is no wonder that it is proving extremely difficult to provide cost effective patient care let alone better patient care.

With this in mind, the aims of the Patient-Focused Hospital are:

- To provide better patient care;
- To increase the staff time spent directly on patient care;
- To simplify jobs classification and management structure;
- To simplify planning and designing;
- To reduce capital and running cost of the hospital.

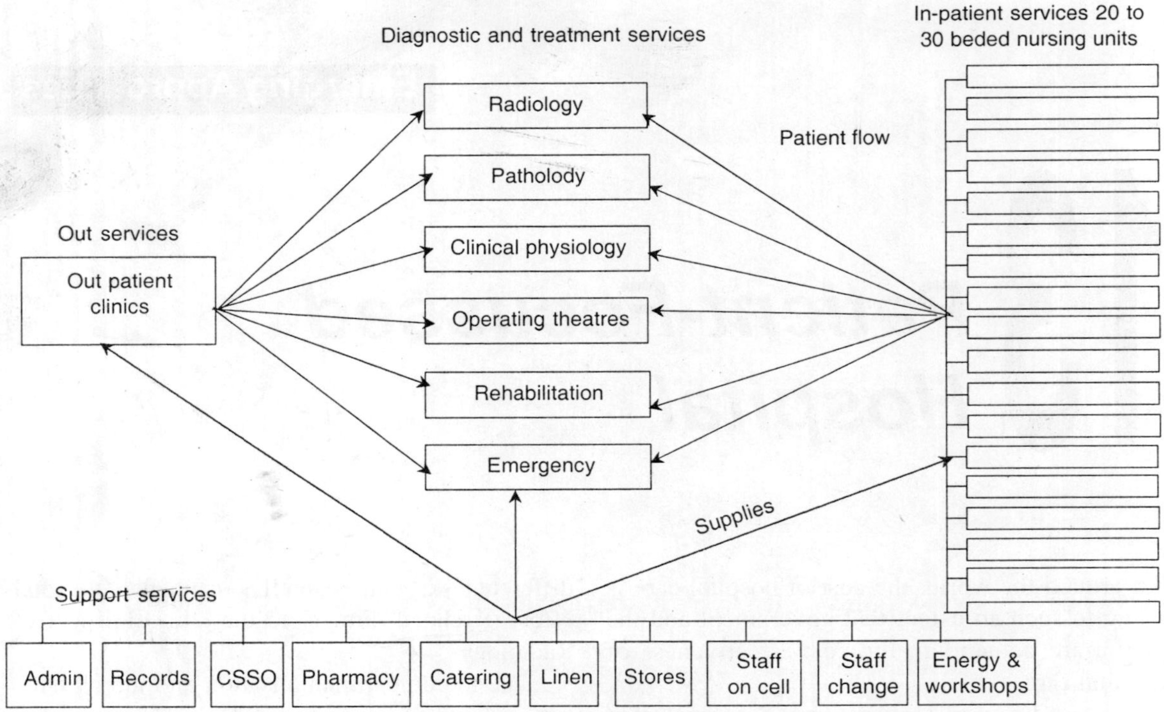

Fig. 13.1: Each department and some nursing units would need to be specially designed, staffed and suite individual functions

The major characteristics of the Patient-Focused Hospital are:

- Patients are grouped according to care requirements rather than clinical specialities;
- Decentralized and decompartmentalized diagnostics, treatment and support services;
- Operational units of 120 to 130 beds each with its own diagnostics treatment and support facilities in place of conventional 30 bed nursing units;
- Small care teams responsible for total patient care;
- Multi-skilled staff in place of many specialist practitioners;
- A flat management organisation;
- Tilization of available medical and information technology.

Figure 13.2 illustrates the basic operating structure of a 500 bed patient-focused hospital. This consists of three distinct centres, i.e. Day care and diagnostic centre, acute care centre and support centre. Key physical differences are in the Acute care centre when compared to conventional hospitals: here there will be four 120 to 130 bed operating units in place of 18 to 20 wards. Each operating unit will incorporate expanded functions: each will house its own operating theatres, intensive care, radiology, ultrasound, laboratory, pharmacy, administration and support facilities. Jobs in the units will be structured to directly involve care givers in all aspects of patient care (Fig. 13.3). Staff will be cross-trained to achieve a high level of multi-skills in order to improve continuity of care, increase autonomy of the unit and ensure maximum utlisation of resources.

While the aim of the Patient-Focused Hospital is to decentralize as much as possible, some functions such as those that exhibit demonstrable

Suplemenatry of radiology schedule and worksteps

Process tasks

	Cleark	Technition	Supervisor	Nurses	Physician	Total
Move	5	3				8
Support Activity		1				1
Data entry/Clerical	8	1	1		1	11
Communicate	8	2	1			11
Technical		2	1			3
Clinical patient care				2	2	4
Total	21	9	3	2	3	38

20 of 20 process tasks are to move things, records information or coordinate the activity

Process minutes

	Cleark	Technition	Supervisor	Nurses	Physician	Total
Move	35	7				42
Support Activity		4				4
Date entry/Clerical	25	2	1		2	28
Communicate	18	5	2			25
Technical		5	3			8
Clinical patient care				5	8	13
Total	78	23	6	5	10	120

These tasks represent 70% of total effort required to perform an X-ray

Fig. 13.2: This compartmentalized approach turns even the most routine tasks into operational nightmares-in which medical technical and clinical activities account for only a small portion of the overall effort

LPMC value-added (% Minimums)

Activity	....	....	Support	Administration	Total ($)	Total (%)
Medical and Clinical	$ 4.8	$ 2.7	$ 0.1	$ 0.5	8.1	10
Hotal and Patient services	0.4	0.3	3.3	0.2	4.2	8
Documentation						
Medical	6.2	2.9		0.7	9.3	19
Miscellaneous	1.0	1.4	0.8	2.4	5.7	11
Scheduling and co-ordination	3.2	2.1	1.2	0.9	7.4	14
Transpotation						
Patient	0.2	1.2	0.2	0.1	1.7	3
Staff	—	0.5	1.0	—	1.5	3
Management and Supervision	0.4	0.7	0.6	1.3	3.5	7
Ready for action	5.8	2.8	1.2	0.5	9.9	19
Total	$21.3	$ 14.4	$ 8.4	$ 7.2	31.3	100

Only a small portion of a hospital's value-added structure is directly related to the actual delivery of medical or clinical care. Scheduling and documentation are the primary operation functions of today's hospital

- Operating structure and approach, not the demand for or performance of clinical services, establish the cost and service effectiveness of most large, acute care hospitals today
- Structural idle time is the largest consumer of hospital resources. "Ready-for care" seems to be confused with "quailty of care"

Fig. 13.3: Hospital-wide aggregation of these findings revealed some startling conclusion about the drivers of personnel-related expenses and service performance in the healthcare industry

scale and those requiring very expensive equipment will be centralized or have a centralized component. The space required for the centralized functions is much reduced in the Patient-Focused Hospital, occupying approximately two-thirds of the space provided in a conventional hospital. The result of this decentralized approach is the radical reduction in scheduling, documentation and coordination and a reduction in the movement of staff and supplies. The Patient-Focused Hospital will entail.

Less Floor Area

Here the savings are of the order of 15 to 18 percent less floor space than the conventional hospital (Fig. 13.4). This is because:

a. With the decompartmentalisation of services such as nursing units operating theatre, radiology, labs and support departments, etc., there is less multiplication of support spaces such as clean utilities, dirty utilities, supplies, room equipment rooms, pantries, staff rooms and admininstration offices.
b. A reduction in communication space because fewer people and goods will need to be moved around.

Less Capital Costs

Saving in capital costs are of the order of 10 to 11 percent. Although the capital equipment cost increases by almost 40 percent because of decentralisation, still the total capital cost to 10 to 11 percent less than conventional hospital. (Fig. 13.5) This is due to 5 to 8% reduction in floor area.

Birth of an Idea

Almost every large hospital complex is in a permanent state of development and redevelopment. A hospital has to respond to so many constantly changing factors that a tour of the site and buildings provides an education in medical, social and

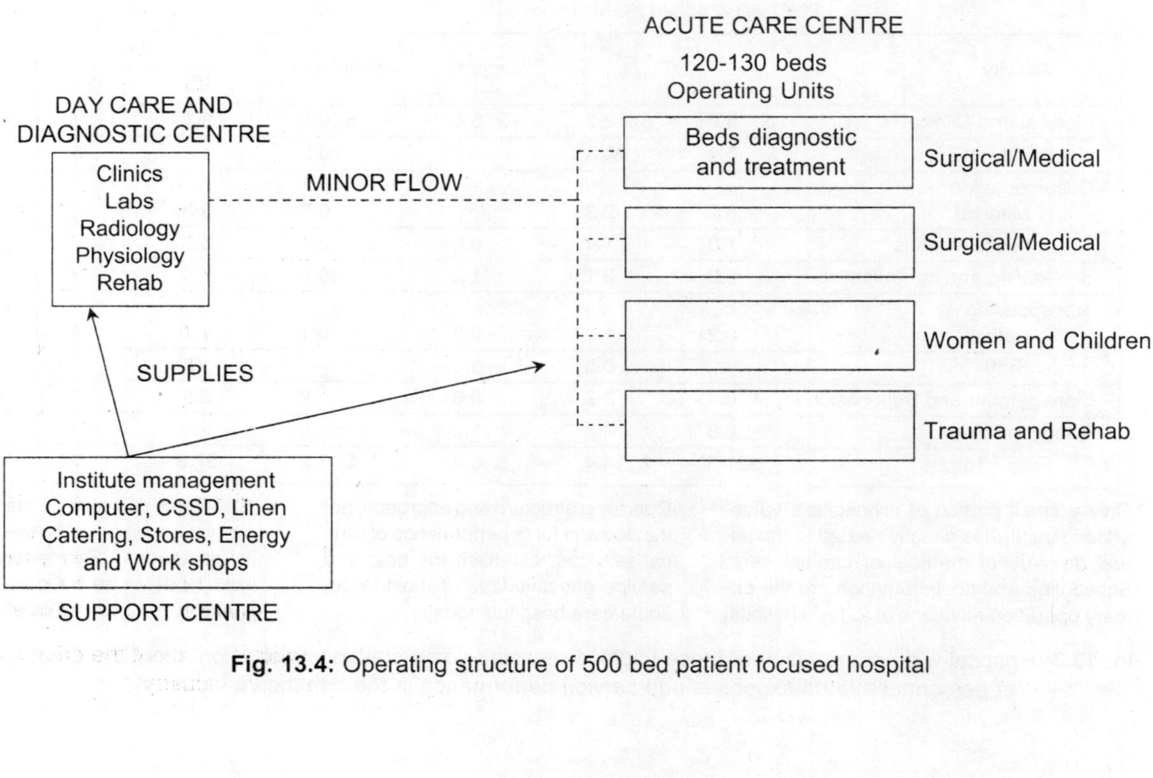

Fig. 13.4: Operating structure of 500 bed patient focused hospital

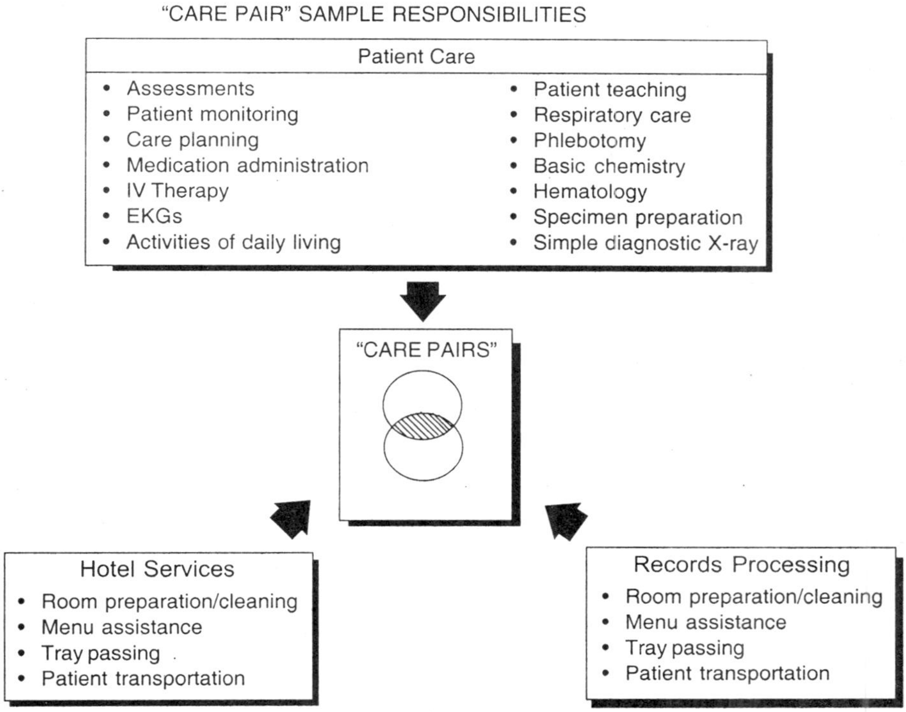

Fig. 13.5: Jobs on the units will be structured to directly involve care givers in all facets of patient care

architectural history from the date of its foundation. Kingston Hospital (England) is a typical example and its most recent building is a two-storey rectangular block measuring 67 meters by 47 metres. It fills a space on the entrance side of the site facing Galsworthy Road and it has other hospital buildings of several ages and styles close to its other three sides.

Limited Envelope

Apart from a small lightwell for the upper floor this building comprises a solid block of rooms and only those on the perimeter can have windows to outside. All others including circulation corridors are entirely internal and it does look as though no other arrangement of these two units was practical within the area available at this site. The departmental accommodation has had to be planned within the limits of this envelope. The plans appear to be technically satisfactory and there is certainly adequate space for the wrok. With very few exceptions, the rooms and circulation areas seem comfortably sized.

Adequate space, however, does not compensate for the dull, unvaried experiences obtained in all those internal rooms and corridors. Without windows, and with very little in the design quality of the environment to stimulate or distract users, these interiors could be anywhere.

The rooms on the perimeter are a most important exception to this. The curved feature at the entrance corner has a two-storey glazed facade to very pleasant offices on the ground floor and to mothers' and staffrooms above. Returns on each side of the curve accommodate separate canopied entrances for the two departments. The symmetrical entrances

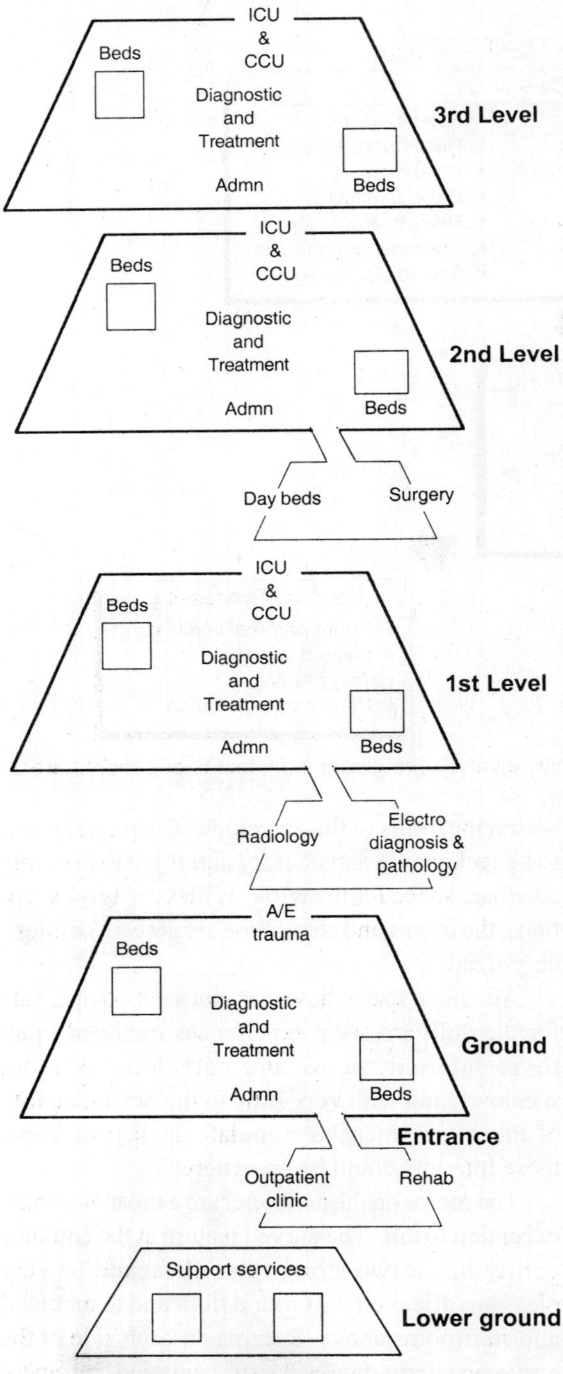

Fig. 13.6: Illustration of physical interpretation of patient-focused hospital

serve roughly symmetrical arrangements for reception and waiting on each side of a diagonally placed divide. Waiting areas for day surgery and for antenatal clinics are situated in the middle of the block underneath a first floor lightwell and they have perimeter roof glazing.

Surgical Day Unit

Staff take the patients for day surgery from the waiting area to changing rooms off a dayroom in which they remain prior to the procedure. A wood-frame translucent glass screen between the day-room and the waiting area has been provided to steal a little day light for this buried facility and this is most effective when direct sunshine occurs.

A double-width exit door leads to the theatre corridor and after their surgery patients go to one of three recovery areas. One is immediately outside the two main theatres where general anaesthetics may be used; the very large main recovery area has curtained bays for 23 trollies, and at one end, two cubicles; a smaller open area with four trolley bays and a cubicle has been designated for children.

The main recovery area, which is 25 meters long, is placed on the perimeter of the building enabling a continuous high-level window to admit some daylight. Some art work is being obtained for the waiting area but the environment of this day surgery unit lacks the positive qualities that design can bring.

Maternity Unit-LDRP Rooms

On entry to the maternity unit, the lifts and stair are to the right and ahead is the antenatal reception and the attractive toplit waiting area with the consulting/examination suites off it. Beyond the clinic, on the perimeter of the plan, are the unit's offices. Arriving upstairs, one enters a spacious reception area. There is an open reception desk, pictures on the walls and plenty of daylight from the glazed external walling.

Conventional hospital		Patient focused hospital	
	Gross m²		*Gross m²*
Inpatient nursing care	12,820	Operating units	13,900
Outpatient, day patient	4,960	Outpatient, day patient	3,660
Diagnostic and treatment	5,760	Diagnostic and treatment	3,110
Support services	4,230	Support services	2,930
Total functional space	27,770	**Total functional space**	23,600
Communication space (12%)	3,330	Communication space	2,830
Energy plant, air handling (6%)	1,860	Energy plant, air handling	1,590
Total	32,960	**Total**	28,020

Fig. 13.7: Spatial requirements for conventional and patient-focused hospital

	Conventional hospital	*Patient-focused hospital*	*Variance*		*Annual depreciation (1)*	
			£MM	*%*	*CH*	*PFH*
Construction	54.4	45.3	(9.1)	(17)	0.91	0.76
Equipment	7.1	9.7	2.6	37	1.01	1.39
	61.5	55.1	(6.5)	11	1.92	2.15

Notes: (1) Useful life—construction-60 years; equipment-7 years

Fig. 13.8: Summary of estimated capital costs: 1991 (£ Sterling, Million)

Expense category	*Variance*			
	CH	*PFH*	*£mill*	*%*
Staff	£ 19.3	£ 17.2	(2.1)	(11)
Non staff	6.4	6.4	—	—
Capital costs				
• depreciation	1.9	2.1	0.2	11
• capital charge	3.7	3.3	(0.4)	(11)
Total	£ 31.3	£ 29.0	(2.3)	(7)

Fig. 13.9: Summary of estimated annual expenses (£mill sterling)

The accommodation has been designed to suit an innovative approach to childbirth (for the NHS) in hospital. On admission for the birth, the mother-to-be is placed in a single bedroom where she remains for labour, delivery, recovery and post-partum care (hence 'LDRP' rooms) until she returns home with her new baby. This is a far cry from the old 'flow-system' from first-stage labour room, delivery room, to recovery bay, to lying-in ward with separate nursery for the babies. It is as near as a hospital can get to what happens in a home birth.

The unit has the usual provisions for abnormal birhts and cesarean sections—six single bedrooms for pre- and post-operative patients and a self-

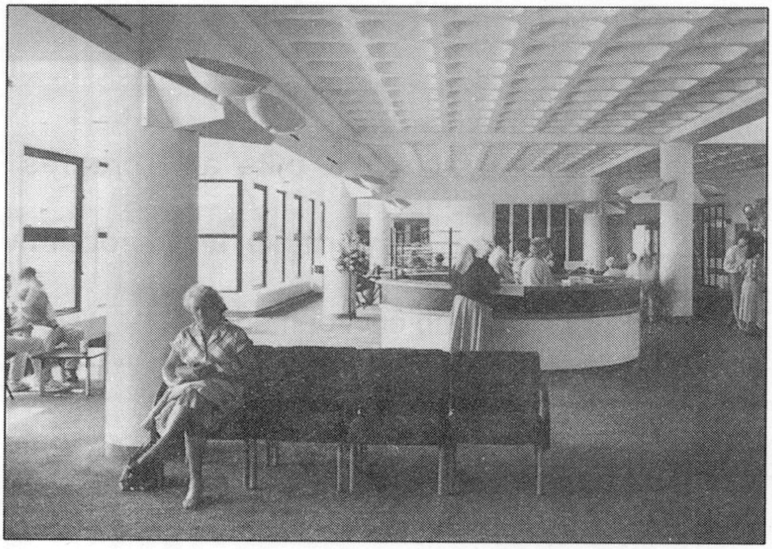

Fig. 13.10: An interior to 'lift the spirits' at the conquest hospital, Hastings

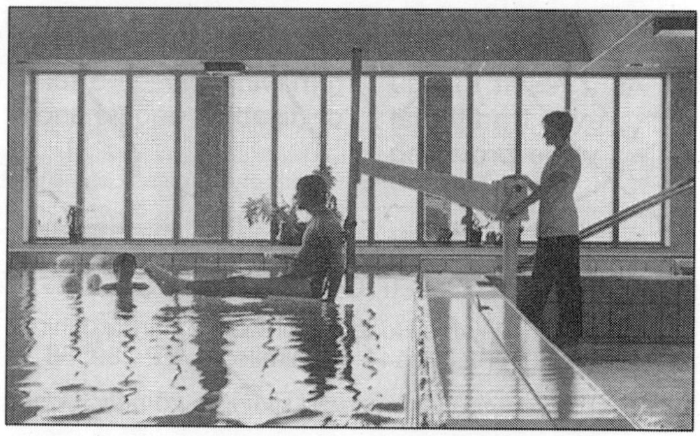

Fig. 13.11: Interior of 'echelon' ward at Chirk Community Hospital

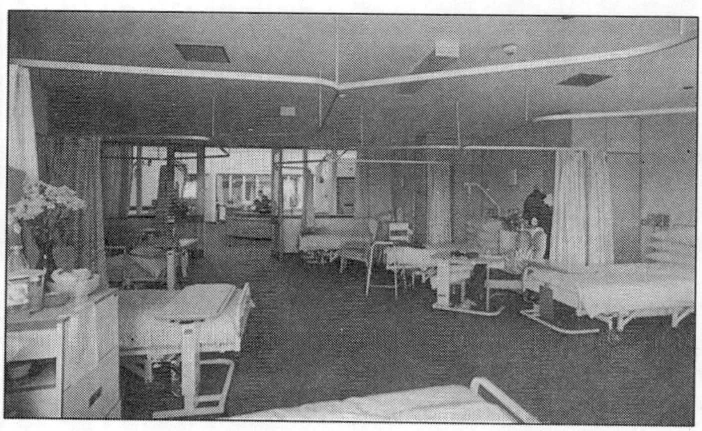

Fig. 13.12: The architecture of healing and caring for patients with spinal injury

First floor

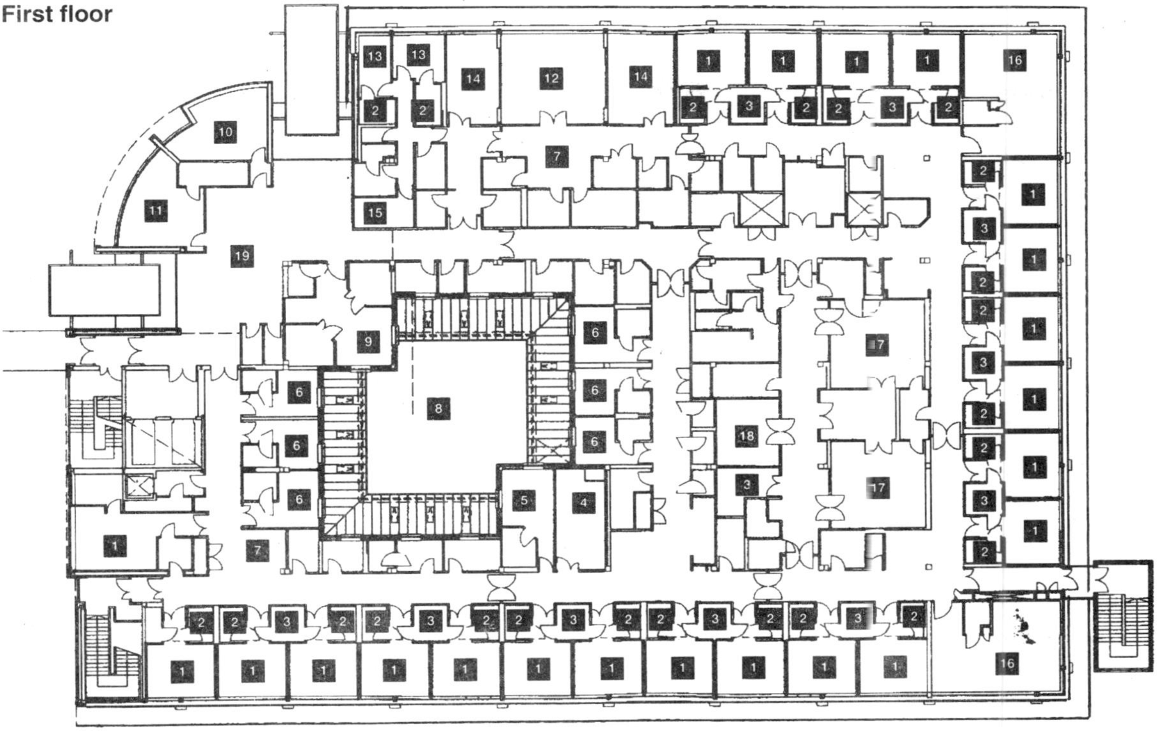

1. LDRP (labour, delivery, recovery, post-partum) room
2. Bathroom
3. Equipment room
4. Birthingroom
5. Day room
6. Single bed bay
7. Work-station
8. Flat-roof to waiting areas below
9. Day assessment
10. Patients dayroom
11. Staff restroom
12. ITU cots
13. Parent room
14. Cots
15. Quiet room
16. Five-bed bay
17. Theatre
18. Recovery
19. Reception

Fig. 13.13a

contained twin operating theatre suite. There are also two five-bed bays for 'long-stay' antenatal patients and women who would prefer not to be in a single room.

These five-bed bays are the only rooms in the building that are patently undersized. To design a single room that satisfies both the 'clinical' preferences of obstetricians and pathologists at delivery, and the 'domestic' preferences of mothers (and their partners) in all the stages of childbirth (labour, recovery, infant care and entertaining visitior) is no easy task. The innovation originated in US hospitals where some extraordinary transformations have been engineered at 'birthing centres'. Rooms that could be featured in 'Homes and Gardens' become high-tech delivery theatres by manipulating concealed retractable medical gear, lighting and very fancy beds-cum-operating tables.

Only a mother can say whether witnessing this mechanised scene-shifting as the labour sets in is preferable to being wheeled from one room to another. At Kingston, however, architects Llewelyn-Davies have balanced the conflicting requirements rather well. The design is entirely satisfactory for normal delivery, having the requisite space, services, cleanable surfaces and privacy. For

Ground floor

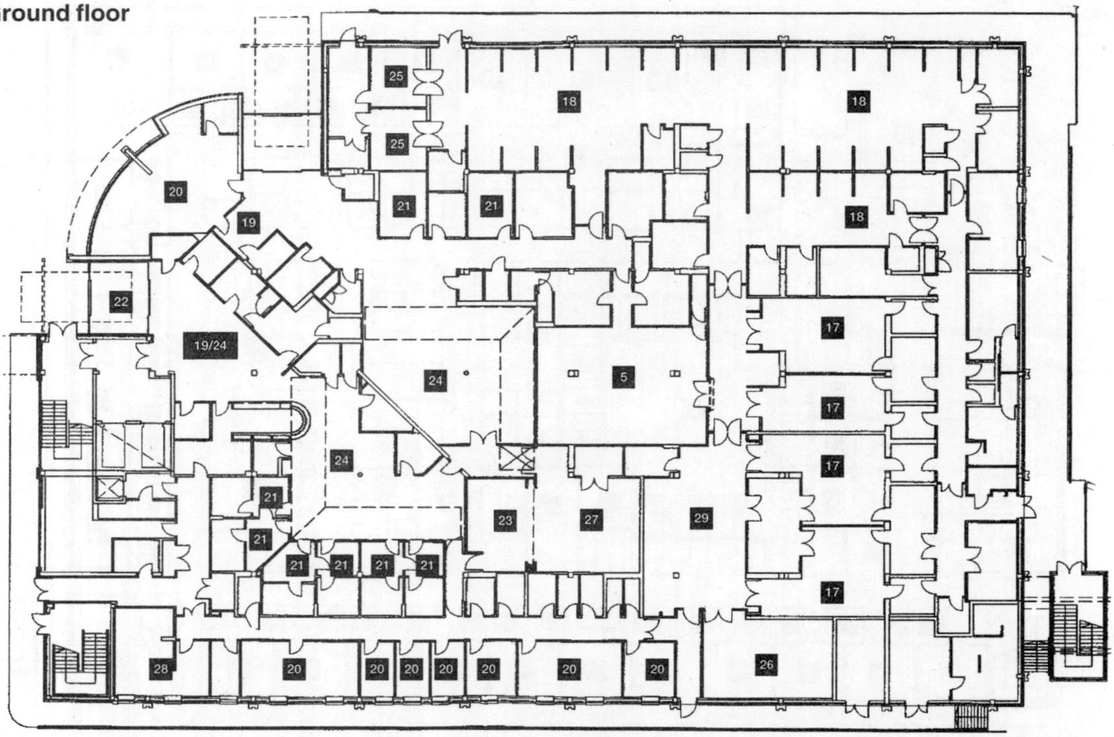

Key (Continued):	21.Consultant examination	23. Seminar	25. Endoscopy	27. Seminar	29. Staff base
20. Office	22. Entrance	24. Waiting	26. Store	28. Community midwives	

Fig. 13.13b

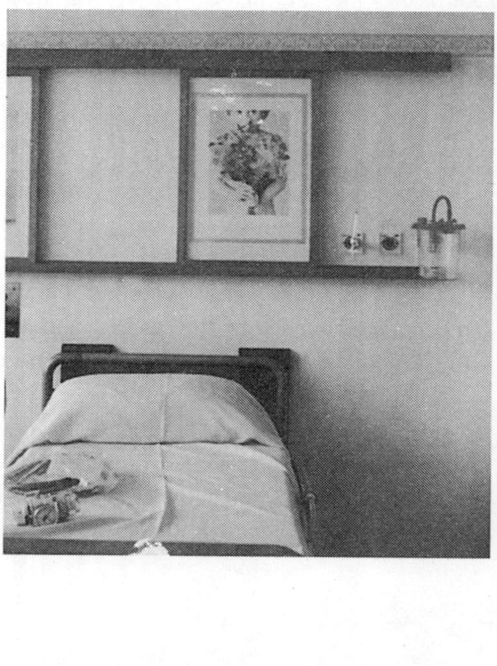

Fig. 13.14: LDRP room showing artwork covering medical gas outlets

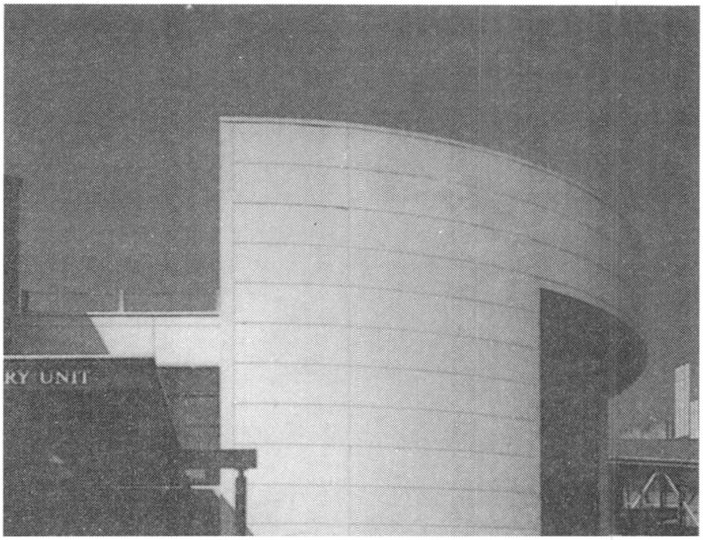

Fig. 13.15: Side view of day surgery entrance

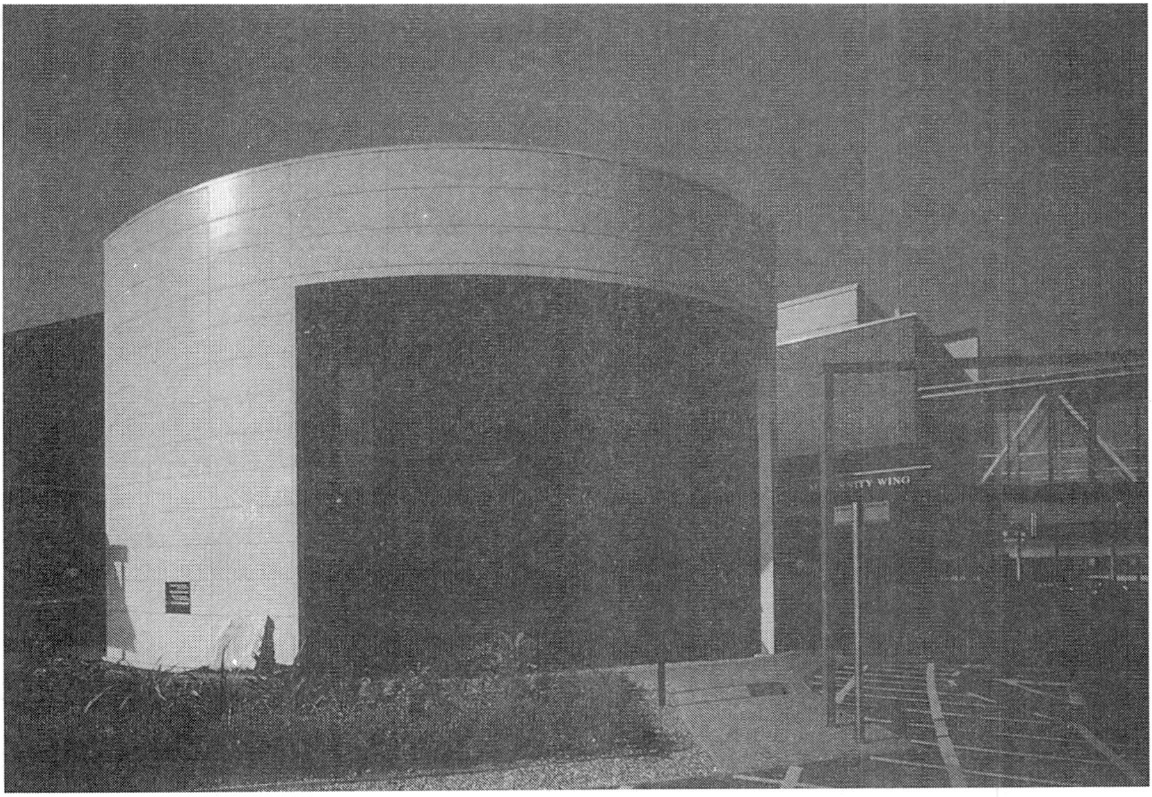

Fig. 13.16: Kingston Hospital's maternity unit, one of the first UK healthcare schemes to pilot the 'patient-focused' credo

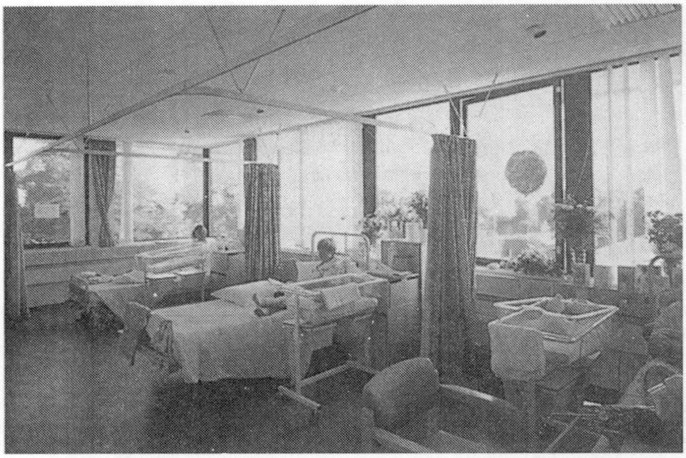

Fig. 13.17: Five-bed ward in maternity unit

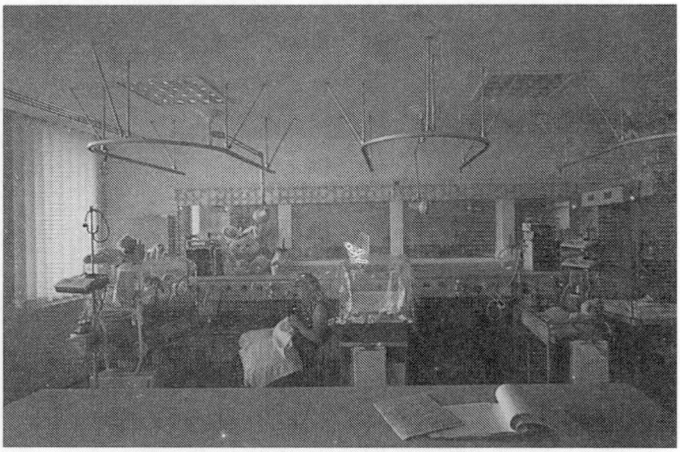

Fig. 13.18: Special baby unit

mother, baby, partner and visitors each room is very pleasant and agreeable while making no pretence at being a 'domestic' or 'non-hospital' interior with fatuous design gestures.

Each LDRP room has a private toilet, bidet and shower and each pair of rooms share a small equipment room. For this upper floor there is a continuous perimeter band of windows providing excellent daylight and views to the outside world. These can be enjoyed by all the LDRP rooms and the neonatal unit's nurseries.

Vertical louvre blinds control daylight and privacy and decorative curtains can be drawn across the windows at night. There is space in the LDRP room for a partner to stay with the mother throughout labour and birth. Above the bedhead, there is a polished timber frame in which two mounted prints are positioned to slide horizontally. They can thus conceal the medical gas outlets which are available if needed during delivery.

The latter seems an extravagant device to cover the outlets, which are relatively unobtrusive in comparison with the unusually large, prominent, and unconcealed aluminium plate of the bedhead unit. It also seems thoughtless to deny the mother in bed the pleasure of seeing the pictures which are

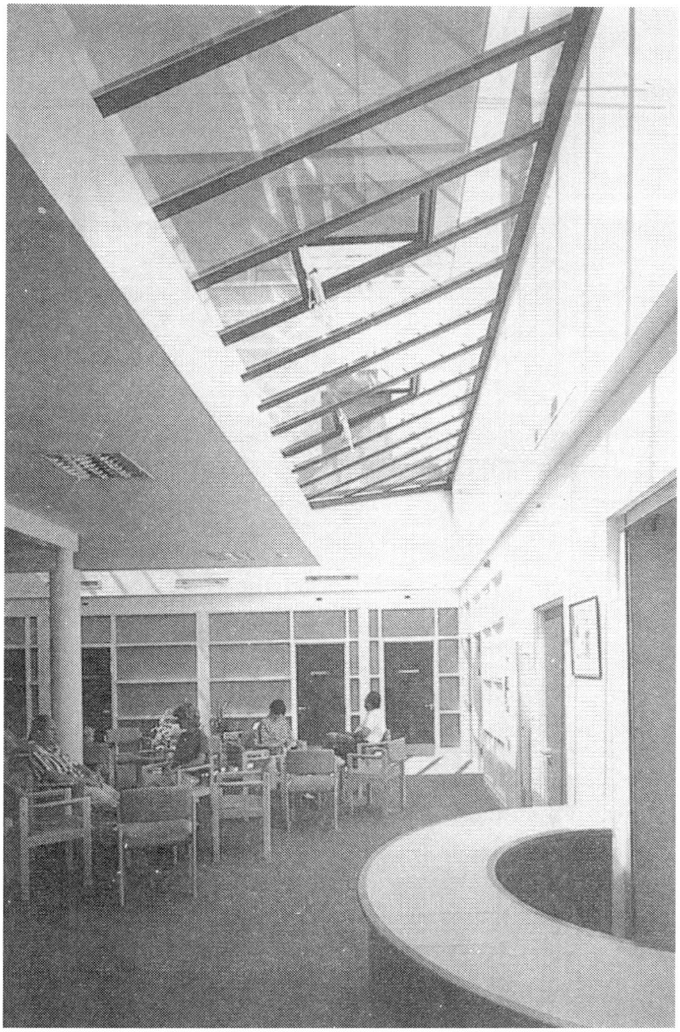

Fig. 13.19: Maternity unit reception

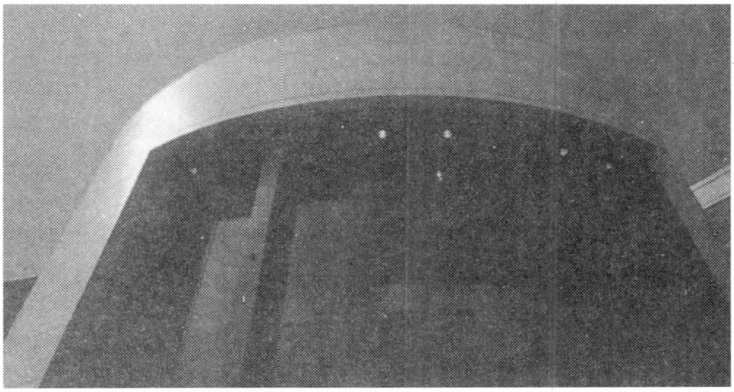

Fig. 13.20: Main entrance-close up

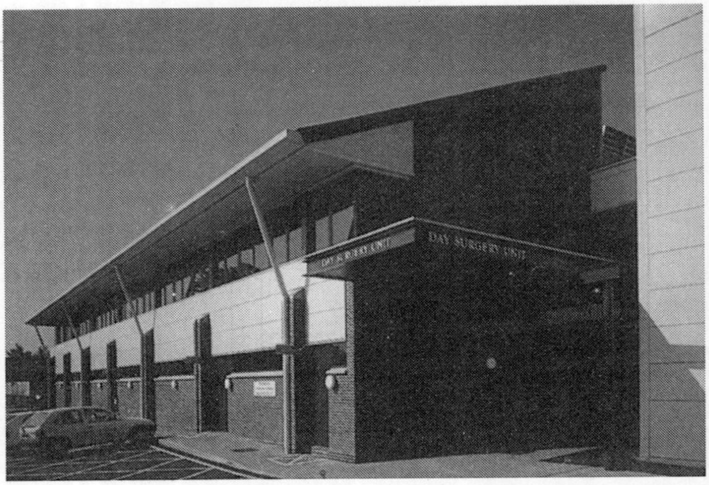

Fig. 13.21: Entrance to the day surgery

behind her while she is faced with the blank wall at the other end of the room. However, the fitting for interchangeable pictures is an excellent idea and a positive benefit for all users of these rooms.

Social Environment

Having LDRP rooms created a markedly different social environment from the typical NHS maternity ward, most mothers are in the unit for the very minimum stay and spend very little time without the company of partners or visitors. With individual ensuite facilities and trayed meals a mother need hardly leave her own room at all. Consequently, they have little need to socialise with other mothers or opportunities to discuss their mutual experiences and see each others' new babies.

There are two dayrooms, one off the recepiton area on the curved facade and the other looking into the lightwell via sealed windows. The latter is quite small and has a tiny beverage pantry but it is not comfortable and appears rarely used. Circumstances and tastes change and one need not doubt that Kingston's new maternity unit and the way it operates is very much liked. It is fascinating to compare it with the new Liverpool Women's Hospital where the delivery unit and lying-in ward are separated conventionally. There, too, the users are said to be delighted with the hospital.

Exterior

The other elements of the plan are readily grasped and fit neatly into the rectangular outline. External treatment is organised rationally and with few complications. Plain brickwork is used to clad the ground floor up to the narrow strip windows; above this the continuous horizontal spandrel is white coated-aluminium panels surrounded by the unbroken band of first floor windows. This treatment, which is completed with a large monopitch roof and wide eaves, wraps round three sides of the block. Brick-clad projecting piers pierce the spandrel and anchor back the angled downpipes from the eaves. The curved corner feature and the fourth evaluation where the main stairs are placed has more exotic composition.

As a whole, the building design is unremarkable in a setting at present almost devoid of trees, plants or attractive outdoor spaces. No room in the building has direct access to any outdoor space. It appears to be the outcome of happenstance—the content, the site, the imposition of stringent fire-code measures (an extra stair was added, windows had to be sealed), the need for a link corridor and the availability of development funding. The latter was given to Kingston by the Department of Health for piloting one of seven 'patient-focused care' sites (in this case for the maternity unit). Undoubtedly, the design of the LDRP rooms is the outcome of focusing on the needs of mothers and must certainly be the main reason for the maternity unit's popularity with its users.

14 Emerging Approaches in Hospital Design

Everybody is aware that there is a great need for change in the world of hospitals. We have reached the point where it is clear that the hospital system has changed and that it and its interdependencies have been thrown out of balance.

Financial limitations compel us to set priorities. For example, between ambulatory and in-house treatment, the trend is toward more ambulatory care. Technical, and scientifically-oriented medicine raises major ethical questions.

No healthcare system in the world is stable and are likely to undergo considerable change in the next 10 years. The drivers of change in deeloped economies are reaching the limits of the welfare state, exhausting traditional methods and tools for containing cost, and experiencing increasing consumer sophistication and demands. Change in the developing world is being driven by the growth of the middle class, greater demands, and the globalisation of economies. Some aproaches in the field of hospital design that could bring maximum of innovation include.

Network Management

A short analysis of a relatively simple network leads to the following reflections.

Owner/community relationship: because of the financial limitations of the public sector we know that there are more private investments. This has the great advantage that bureaucratic structures can be boycotted and that investment and exploitation are brought closer.

Even for health facilities, an investment is meant of producing results at the lowest possible cost. Private investors have to avoid risks, because they have to pay back their debts—a simple fact which might not always apply to the public sector. Such conflict can have the effect that good risks are covered by the private sector and bad risks remain on the government side or are even not covered at all.

One of the major achievements of the European health system is that anybody has access to it if they really need it. Thus, government should frame the conditions, but also should refrain from doing everything alone. It should engage persons with entrepreneurial skills.

It would be wise to set the frame from top to bottom but delegate responsibilities and authority for specific solutions to the lowest possible levels.

Relationship between hospital facilities and medical needs: Let us briefly analyse changes in hospital life during the past 50 years. For a given number of beds, the number of patients has at least doubled, the number of diagnostic tests has multiplied by 20, the average stay of patients dropped by half or more, the number of staff tripled and the standard of personal comfort increased substantially, All this, together with the technical equipment evolution, has led to more square meters per bed.

Our buildings should be designed in order to undergo changes.

In the world of hospital construction, everybody has to cope with a flood of new and sophisticated prescriptions. Normally, they also involve higher cost. Would it not be a good idea, therefore, before implementing new regulations, to examine the existing one and to cancel an old one for each new regulation? Government prescriptions should protect the public

Hospitals and hospital facilities are a part of a complex network. They can only play their role efficiently if the are aware of the ever-changing main relationships. These relationships are sometimes so strong however, that it is unwise to oppose them.

Problem-solving Process

Problem solving is a process which has to be done in different cycles. The cause not only influences the effect, the effect also influences the cause. It is a matter for all the people involved and ideally the task will be done within a team.

Problem solving has to be structured into phases, for example master-planning phase, design phase and execution phase. In every phase, we have to deal with all parameters, especially quality, cost and time. The results of a finished and accepted phase from the parameters of the next one.

It needs project management skills and an experienced and highly qualified specialist to handle a problem-solving process in consideration of all parts of a complex network.

Decisions to be taken at the begining of the project are usually more important than decisions to be taken in the course of execution. Unfortunately, our knowledge is less at the beginning, Feedback methods and experience can minimize such gaps.

Questions need to be addressed as to whether or not the architects as main players in a team are aware of their role, and if the standard curriculum at our universities takes such facts into account.

Emerging Hospital Design of Tomorrow

There is a considerable need to change our attitude to hospital design. A new approach can be summarized in 10 points:

1. Hospitals should not harm the patients.
2. Hospital facilities should be designed in such a way that they can be changed later.
3. When designing hospital facilities, the whole life cycle of the different systems involved should be taken into account.
4. Take into account the recycling process of building materials.
5. Take into account as a main design criterion-energy consumption: design intelligent buildings.
6. Changing, re-modeling and re-use of existing facilities become more important than dealing with totally new constructions.
7. Keep it simple. Specialization is the basis of modern life, but let us try to find simple solutions to avoid complicated technical means.
8. Architects' means are form, space, material and colours, but the architects are also responsible for function, time and cost.
9. Our facilities should be integrated into an existing net work. Location, surroundings and acceptance are also design criteria.
10. Support team work and innovation. Hospital buildings are complicated systems serving various purposes, which have to be integrated in an optimised facility. This will have to be integrated in an optimised facility. This can

only be done by team work between architect and engineer, architect and owner and architect and user.

In recent years, hospital architecture has not produced very many buildings of high architectural design quality compared with that in other fields of architecture. Some of the reasons require further study and elaboration.

Towards the middle of the nineteenth century, the monumental centre of Helsinki was erected. This took place at a time when Finland was an autonomous part of the Russian Empire. The archi tects were French and German, as well as finishing, and several enormous buildings were completed, including the university library, government palace and Russian military hospital, which today is an essential part of the university clinics in Helsinki. The hospital building represents the same level of architecture as the other public buildings of the same period.

The hospitals built between 1890-1910 are good example of the architecture of this time. They are pavilion hospitals with several building parts connected to each other with light corridors. These hospitals were typical solutions for the needs of that time, both architecturally and functionally.

Around 1930, Finnish hospital architecture was very creative and represented functionalism at its best, The buildings of this period, like the pavimion Sanatory and Kiljava Sanatory are top examples of global architecture and on par with other achieve ments of that era.

When hospital design from the 1940s and 1950s is studied, the buildings no longer represent the top architectural level of the time. It is possible that the functional demands become too difficult and in this situation architectural values were put aside or, after fulfilling the hospital's functional demands, nothing was left for architecture. The results of hospital design were poor and their scale was inhuman. The building structure was very simple and it led in the 1950s and 1960s to big impersonal hospital complexes with no relation to global architecture.

The planning of a hospital is lengthy and complex task, which demands a thorough knowledge of building technology, A multidisciplinary approach is required. Balanced attention must be allocated to various areas of specialized knowledge, such as economical building design, functionality for both patients and employees, architectural aims and so on. The field is broad and demands great effort, especially at the initial stage.

Today's Hospital Design

The preliminary planning where the volume, time schedule and initial cost forecasts are determined, is done by the client, and draws from information provided by individual hospital personnel.

The planning group is employed after this preliminary work to complete the project and to create the building, but the planning group often lacks the knowledge of functional requirements. The illusion still exists that hospital personnel have all the expertise, although in fact a building and planning project is usually a unique experience for them. This situation results in the fact that most of the responsibility for a balanced hospital solution lies with the architect.

Building Techniques

Architects and engineers involved in hospital design have several years of experience in planning projects of different volume. The technical possibilities have become familiar and additional feasibility studies are no longer carried out.

The functional demands of health care and hospital buildings have, during years of planning, become familiar to architects and the requirement for functional planning is usually fulfilled. The changes concerning the development of diagnostic and treatment departments have been adopted too. Hospital design groups have concentrated on realising functional demands, whereas the creation of pleasant working environment has been neglected.

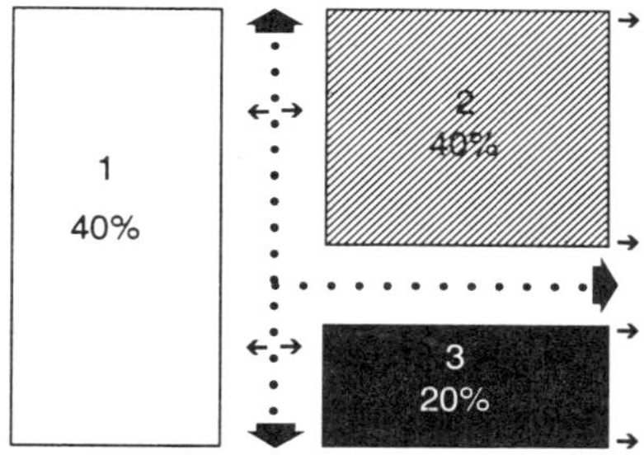

Fig. 14.1: Diagram showing the relationships between the three zones and indicating approximate proportions of space allocations in a typical modern general hospital

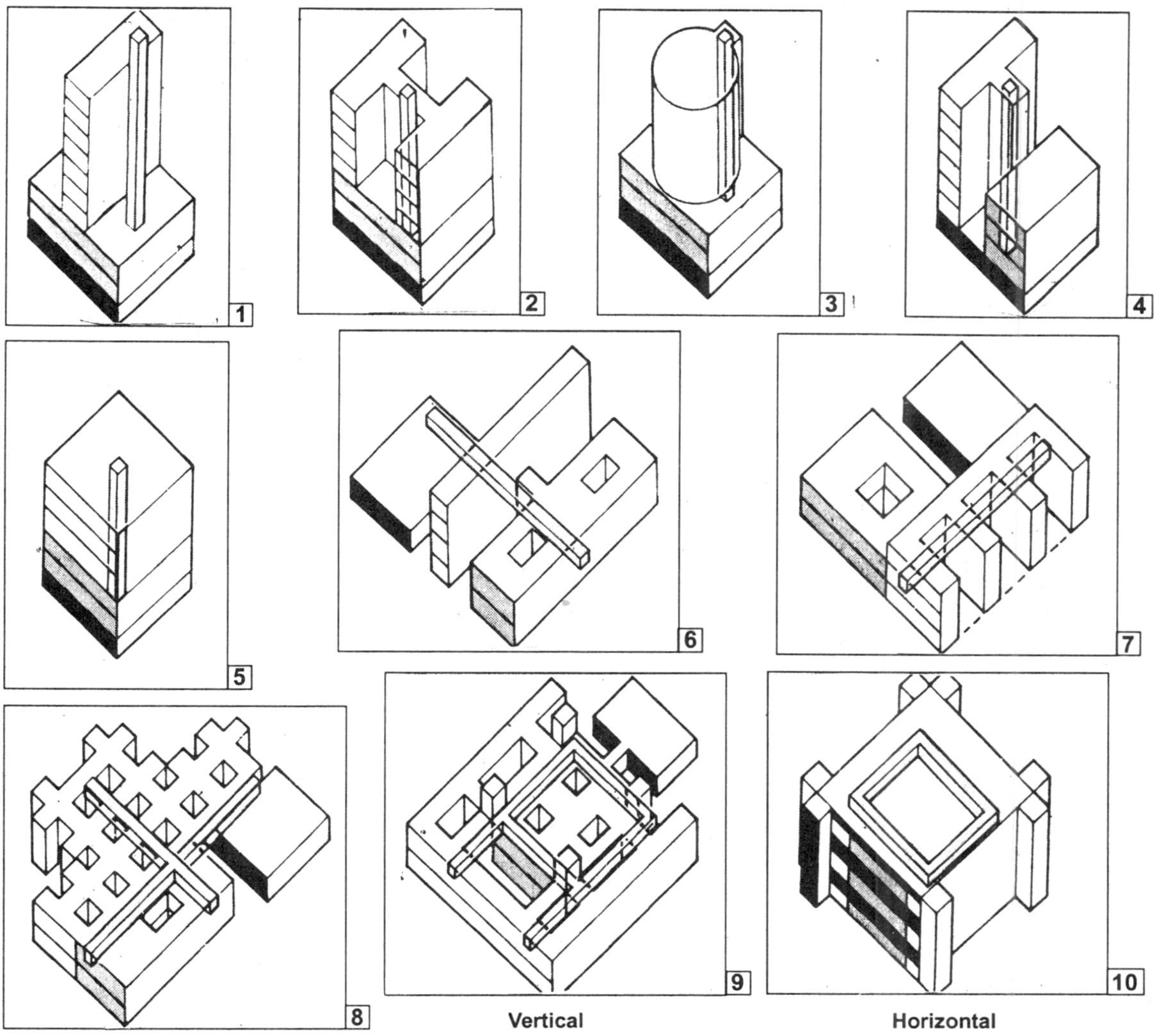

Fig. 14.2: Most of planning strategies can be classified into two main groups—vertical strategies (1-5) and horizontal strategies (6-10)

Vertical

1. Simple tower-on-podium
2. Complex tower-on-podium
3. Radial tower-on-podium
4. Articulated slabs-on-podium
5. Vertical monolith

Horizontal

6. Independent linked slabs
7. Spine and pavilion
8. Extended courtyard
9. Compact courtyard
10. Horizontal monolith

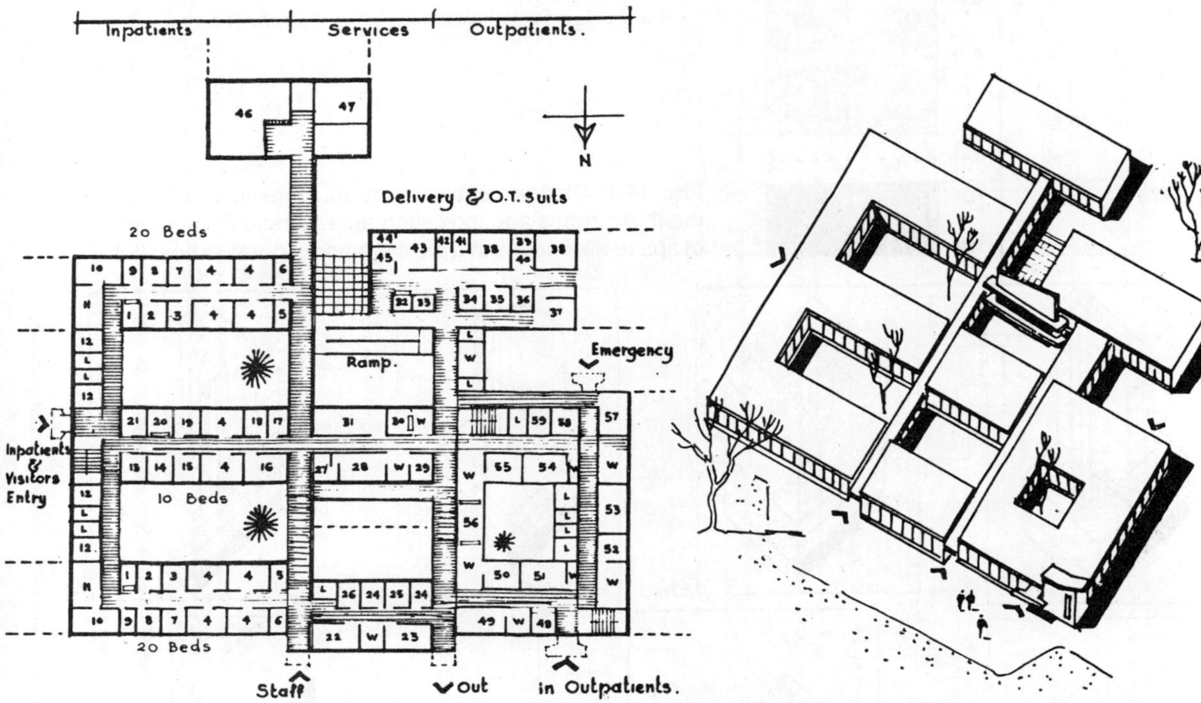

Inpatients

1. Duty
2. Serious patient
3. 2-beds
4. 4-beds
5. Store
6. Linen
7. 2-beds
8. Treatment
9. Pantry
10. Lav & stuice
11. Day space
12. Special bed
13. Admission
14. Treatment
15. 2-beds
16. Lav & stuice
17. Store
18. Linen
19. Serious patient
20. Duty
21. Sister

Services

22. Medical supdt.
23. Office & records
24. Store
25. Store keeper
26. Matron
27. Developing
28. X-ray
29. Radiologist
30. Specimen. rec.
31. Laboratory

Delivery and OTs

32. Duty
33. Linen & st.
34. Preporation
35. Changing
36. Sister
37. Recovery
38. OT
39. Sub-ster
40. Scrub
41. Linen
42. Stores
43. Delivery
44. Wash
45. Prep.
46. Kitchen
47. Store

OPD & Emergency

48. Registration
49. Med. clinic
50. Injection
51. Lady doctor
52. Health visitor
53. Eye-ENT
54. Surg. clinic
55. Dressing
56. Disp/pharmacy
57. Emergency. adm.
58. Minor OT
59. Obs. beds

L Lays
W Waiting
--- Future
— — — Expansion

Fig. 14.3: Basic layout for an intermediate hospital of 50-100 beds

The most important phase in hospital planning is to determine the basic solution, which means the organisation of external traffic and internal connections between the departments. As a result of the preliminary planning there will be several alternative solutions for the whole project. The planning group including the client medical expertise, should analyze these alternative and study the strong and weak points of each. A basic model for the next working period has to be drawn up by combining the solutions. Assuming that future hospital projects will involve more and more extensions and rebuilding, it is essential to concentrate on the so-called building grouping very seriously.

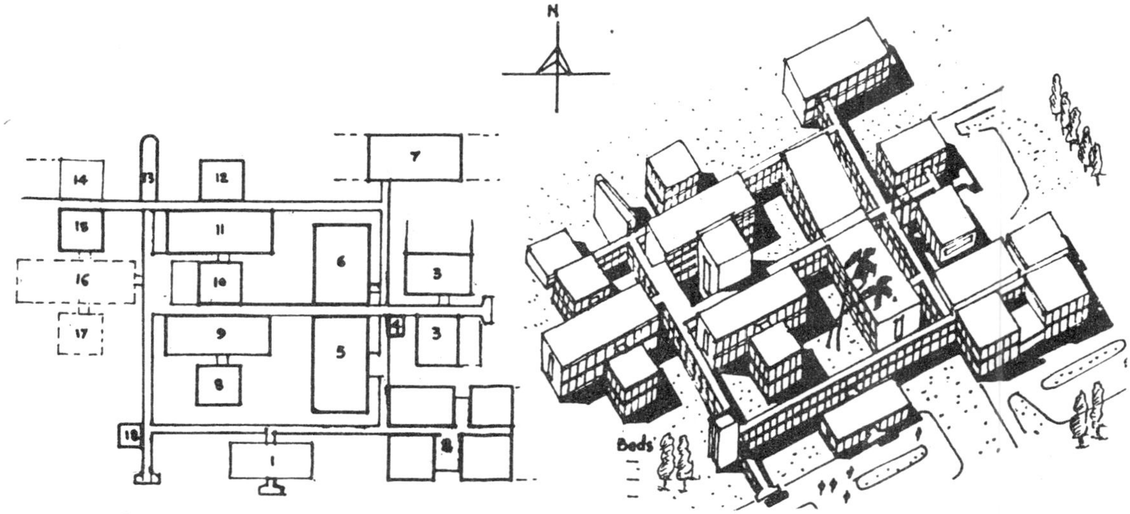

	Ground floor		First floor		Second floor	
	Facilities	*Beds*	*Facilities*	*Beds*	*Facilities*	*Beds*
1.	Administration	—	Future expansion	—	—	—
2.	OPD & Rehabilitation	—	OPD	—	—	—
3.	Emergency	—	Post operative & Int. care	20	—	—
4.	**Vertical Circulation**					
5.	X-ray & Therapy	—	Operation theatres	—	Future expansion	—
6.	Laboratory & Blood bank	—	Delivery suite	—	Future expansion	—
7.	Paying beds	5	Paying beds	5		
8.	Ward	14a	Ward	14a	Ward	14c
9.	Ward	26a	Ward	26a	Ward	26c
10.	**Vertical Circulation**					
11.	Medical stores	—	Ward	26a	Ward	26c
12.	Central sterilising	—	Ward	26a	Ward	26c
13.	**Ramp**					
14.	Kitchen		Ward	14b	Ward	14b
15.	Bulk store	—	Ward	26b	Ward	26b
16.	Ward	26a	Ward	14b	Ward	14b
17.	Ward	14b				
18.	**Visitors Vertical Circulation**					
Total beds/floor		80		146		146

Possible phases of construction	a	b	c	Total
	80/132	40/94	32/146	372

Fig. 14.4: Basic layout for a referral hospital of 100-350 beds

In modern designs there are indications that a lot of attention will be paid to interior design, with pleasant atmosphere and social implications according to different health care and hospital building requirements.

Health care facilities have several tasks. It is obvious that the treatment environment must relate to the functional aims. Facilities with long-stay terminal wards must differ from general hospital regarding their interior character, Hospitals or

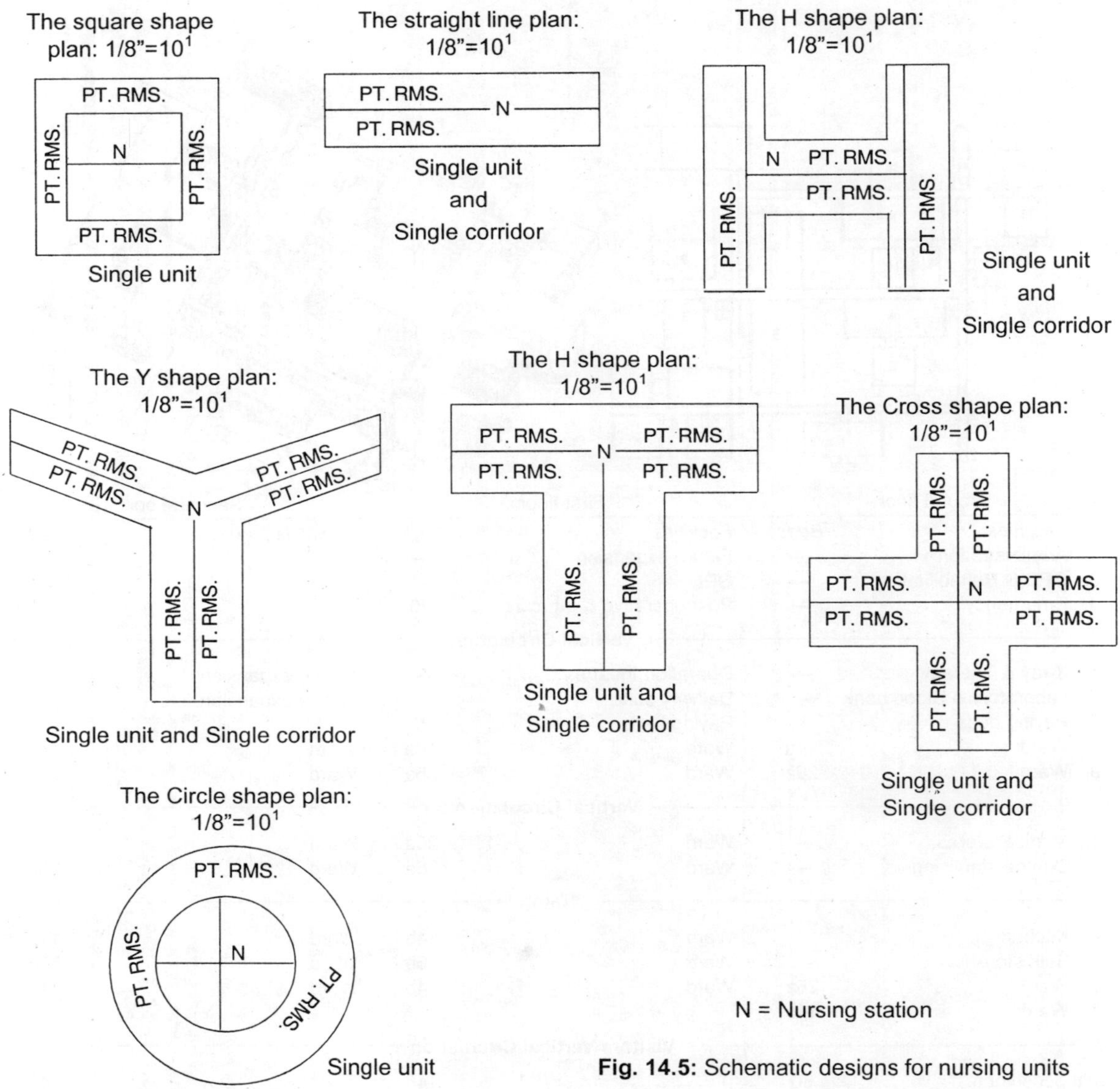

Fig. 14.5: Schematic designs for nursing units

therapeutic institutions for mental care undoubtedly have their own special demands. The theory is that the treatment environment relates strongly to the results achieved.

The latest trends in some European hospital designs show that great effort has been put into designing certain defined areas in a hospital such as entrance halls, waiting halls, offices and so on, to make them different from the normal hospital atmosphere. Only the diagnostic and treatment departments have the traditional technical standards and materials. The result of this planning principle leads to a pleasant atmosphere in the hospital building and perhaps provides guidelines for future planning.

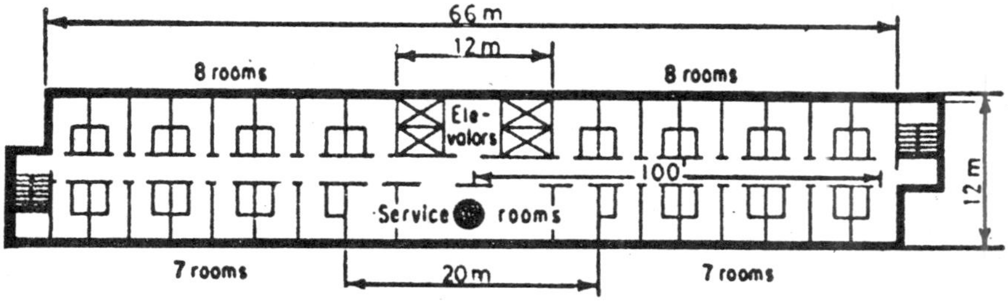

(A) All single bed rooms

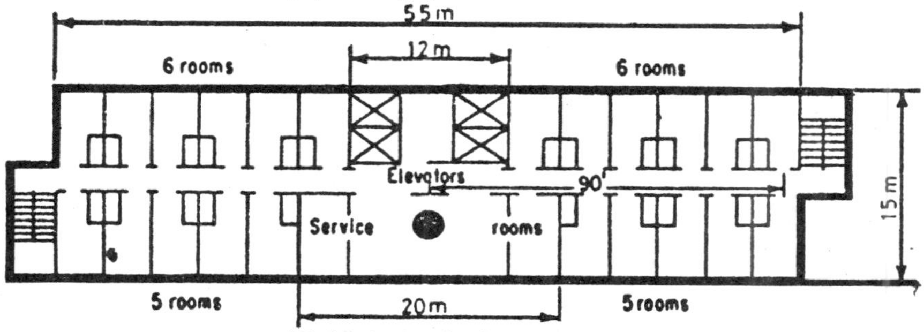

(B) All double bed rooms

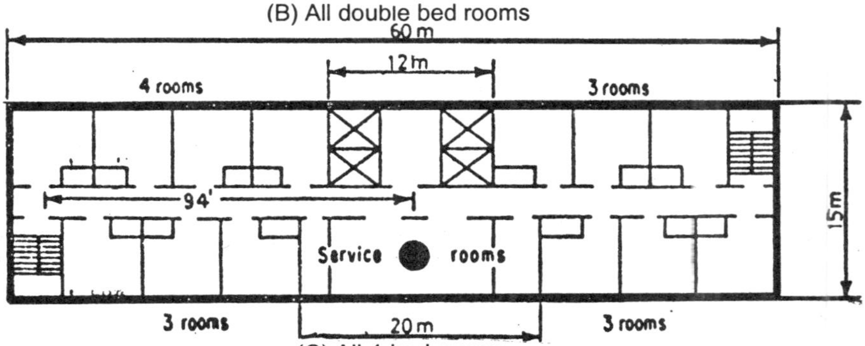

(C) All 4-bed rooms

Comparison

Itme	A	B	C
a. Total beds	30	44	52
b. Total rooms	30	22	13
c. Net area/bed	11.25	9.5	8
d. Tot gross area	870	930	915
e. Gross area/bed	29	21	17.5
f. Max nursing run	30	27.5	27.5

Fig. 14.6: For simplicity of comparison, three plans are illustrated, each an extreme of its kind. All plans are single corridor plans with a maximum run of 30m (100ft). Each room has access to a toilet and same central services are provided in each

Looking Ahead

The future aims of health care facility design will broaden as the demands of the community increase. The age structure of the population is changing, Attitudes concerning illness are developing and there are new expectations of interior and architectural design.

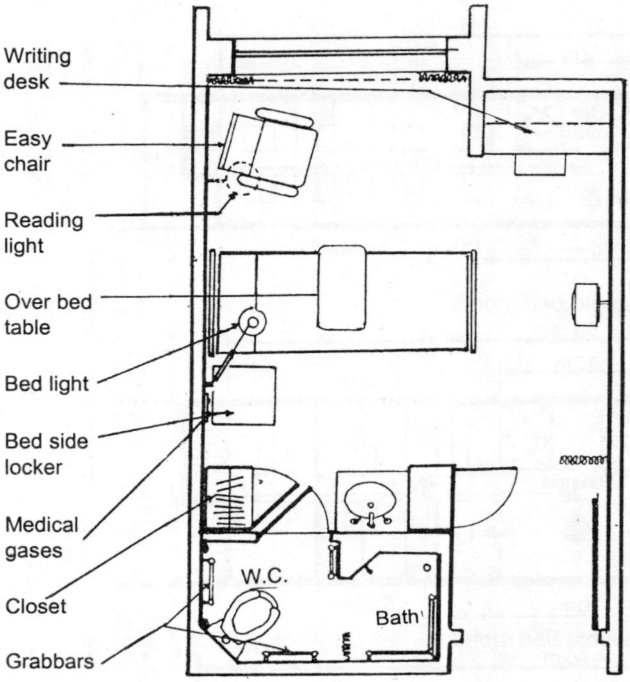

Fig. 14.7: Room layout

There will be more functional planning directed to certain hospital departments, the technical standard decreased and areas requiring high standard building technology limited, especially where ventilation and electrical services are concerned.

The human atmosphere and human scale of interiors will be the aim for future designers. The size of a hospital building will be smaller. Instead of one enormous complex it may be sensible to appreciate the human scale and build several smaller units. The human demands will have priority and the equipment,as well as the technology, will take second place.

Structural Planning

The diagram is showing the relationships between the three zones and indicating approximate proportions of space allocations in a typical modern general hospital

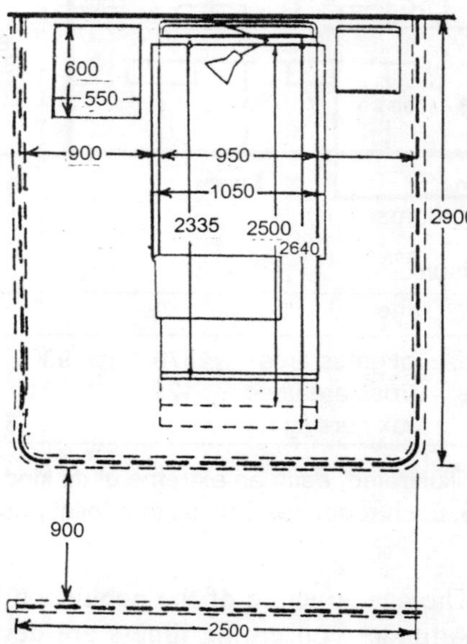

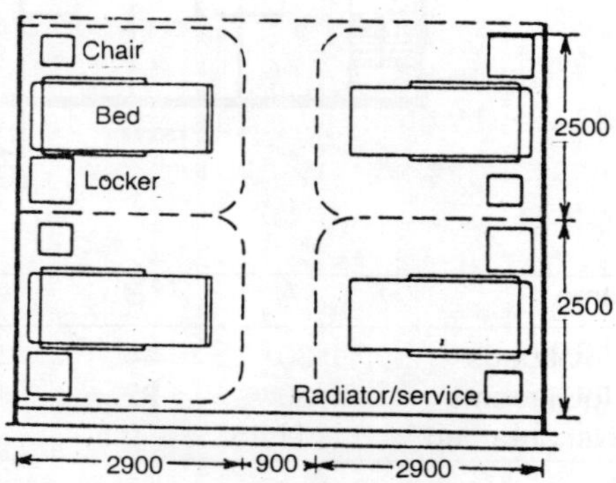

Although the bare minimum spacing between the beds can be 1.6 m c/c, it is hardly used (except in extreme shortage of space) for the reasons of cross infection. A more generous spacing of 2.5 m allows room for a locker, a chair and premits the use of cubicle curtains

Fig. 14.8: Space requirements of bed

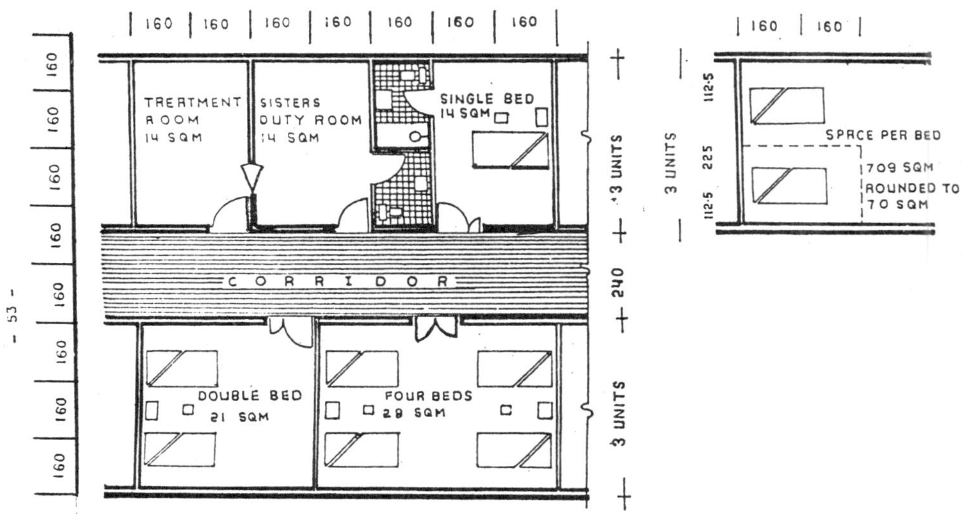

Fig. 14.9: Rationalization of floor spaces

(Fig. 14.1). Hospital planning is primarily concerned with putting together the 30 or more separate departments to form a functional and viable whole. Functional zoning can facilitate this process. It will permit the tailoring of plan shape, volume, structure and environmental services to suit the needs of groups of departments with similar characteristics. The clinical zone requires deep-planned, high volume, uncluttered and hygienically finished spaces suitable for sophisticated equipment and support systems. The nursing zone needs an appropriate environment for fostering sick people duirng their brief stay in hospital. Storage and processing areas can be housed in separate structures with industrial standard finishes, to form the support zone. Fire safety may require the separation of such high life-risk areas as the nursing zone from other high fire-risk areas such as the support zone. Each zone should be free to grow and change without affecting the integrity of the other zones.

Since the beginning of twentieth century various planning stategies have been devised to meet the requirements of differing health needs, cultures, climates, sites and budgets. Most of these can be classified into two main groups: vertical and horizontal (Fig. 14.2).

In vertical strategies (1-5 inclusive) the zones are arranged one above the other so that the movement pattern is mainly vertical.

In horizontal strategies (6-10 inclusive) the zones are linked together laterally, so that movement is mainly horizontal.

FURTHER READING

1. Kekalainen R: Hospital Architecture of the Future. Hospital Management International, London 1992.

Emerging Approaches

15 Nucleus Concept

INTRODUCTION

Developed by the Department of Health and Social Security in the UK from the Best Buy and Harness Programmes, the Nucleus Hospital has been around for three decades. The success and limitation of the design system is often argued and debated, but the fact remains that numerous nucleus schemes of one shape or another are now in existence up and down the country, offering healthcare facilities which arguably, without the system, could not have been provided within the same time scale and economy. More recently, extensive application of the planning system is also starting in other parts of the world.

During the period of development and application of the nucleus system, health care facilities in Hong Kong have been expanded with an incomparable ambition and scale in an effort to match the equally incomparable population explosion. (For the period between 1958 and the late 1980s, the population in Hong Kong increased from 3 million to over 6 million, while the number of hospital beds provided increased from 7500 to over 30,000, inclusive of nursing home and convalescent beds).

To maintain such a programme, Hong Kong has depended heavily on planning expertise from overseas, and up to now at least, from the UK in particular. In this context, one cannot help noticing that while various UK standards have been adopted and adapted to meet local hospital planning requirements, the Nucleus system has been singularly bypassed. Logically, a system which offers standardized briefing and design must be highly applicable and relevant to a rapidly expanding health care building programme.

The Nucleus departments are designed in two basic building forms: first, a clinical template containing whole departments or clusters of smaller departments; and second, service/ industrial areas in low-cost building envelopes.

The design system covers philosophy of service; phasing and expansion; design solutions; staffing; list of activity spaces; functional units; and optional assemblies and relationships.

Briefing

The Nucleus data pack offers ready-made design data, formulated through years of experience and research. It represents nationally-agreed policies and designs which can be relied upon by project teams.

The actual data contained the Nucleus system are obviously tailor-made for the UK, with due reference to staffing levels, health care standards, working procedures, economy, and so on. Needless to say, the system needs to be adapted before the data can be made applicable to other countries.

This would cut down on the often time consuming meetings and debates during the briefing process, as well as ensuring that necessary requirements are met by the project and design teams.

When the health authority which sets out to regularise the various categories of hospitals is fully established in Hong Kong, much can be gained by examining the relevance of the Nucleus data packs.

Design

Nucleus offers a series of templates linked to form a main street, capable of horizontal expansion resulting from phasing requirements of general expansion of workload. It is the outcome of considerable research into standardisation and departmental relationship. An attractive feature of the nucleus templates is the embracing of courtyard views. This permits more external elevation for natural light and ventilation, as well as landscaping potentials, However, the same idea also restricts the building height to preferably no more than three or four storeys.

Another feature is the linear style of development of cluster units and consideration of horizontal future expansion, offering a human scale and low-rise criteria which is ideal for a green field situation.

Both the above features assume that ample land is available for the hospital site. The system is therefore more suited to rural areas, rather than urban/inner city use. This may explain why although all new UK hospital schemes must seek to utilise the principle of Nucleus, few if any new city hospitals have so far introduced the system due to the uneconomic land use.

The same features become even more limiting in a place like Hong Kong, where lack of space and high land cost all add up to a need to assume high-rise/high-density design solutions. The often inclined topography of Hong Kong also negates the adaptation of the horizontal design concept.

Economy

One of the chief objectives of any form of standarisation is to achieve cost saving. In this respect, used in the right place and circumstance, Nucleus hospitals have proved to accomplish economy in capital and running costs without sacrificing acceptable clinical and service standards.

By providing readily available data, nucleus also offers the best opportunity to cut down on the planning and design time. This leads to a reduction in the fees paid to consultants, and a reduction in the involvement of expensive project team personnel who otherwise will have to be engaged in repetitive and time-consuming meetings during the briefing stage.

Adaptability

The functional content, services planning strategy and hospital policies upon which the nucleus design is based have all been researched in depth and developed through experience. So have the suitability of the template shapes for standardisation, and the departmental layout relationships. In application in the UK, the end products have, to a large degree, allayed fear of stifled inventiveness through standardisation, as designers and consultants often manage to adapt the system to respond not only to various siting, but to their own esthetic inclination in the creation of a sensitive environment. Indeed, it has been argued that having the mundane aspect of the design process taken care of, both the designers and the project team can concentrate on other issues of importance.

That the system adapts well in the UK is not surprising since it has been tailored to meet the country's health care policy and requirements. Its universal acceptance, however, will depend on its adaptability to suit the indigenous requirements of the particular region.

Development of the Brief

An architect-led multi-disciplinary team in the Department of Health (UK) to set work to produce a more detailed brief for agreement by ministers. The brief that emerged was in the form of eight aims and objectives. These were:

- To produce designs for a first phase nucleus hospital of about 300 beds, with capability for growth and change upto 900 beds
- To provide sufficient, limited, choice of content so that first phase could be tailored to different service planning priorities.
- To seek the utmost economic capital and running costs, consistent with acceptable clinical and service standards
- To keep the works cost of the nucleus hospital low
- To limit the provision in the first phase to what is needed to sustain the service provided in that phase
- To achieve maximum use of space by good functional relationships and clustering of departments, avoiding fixed specific equipment wherever possible; avoiding provision for exceptional demand, occurrences or procedures
- To cater for a reasonable range of sites, including sloping sites, to plan for two storeys preferably, but with a maximum of three; to make maximum use of natural light and ventilation; to meet fire and escape requirements, and
- To make the fullest use of experience, material and techniques already available from earlier development work, particularly 'Best Buy' and 'Harness'.

Development of Design

Quite quickly three important decisions were taken and these have shaped the design process from the beginning; Nucleus would be a briefing and design system and not a constructional system. The structure and fabric design would be left to design teams.

The concept of universal space would be followed, so that all hospital departments would conform to a common geometry, and all design work would be carried out within a fixed set of whole hospital policies.

It was realised that if simple standard shape could be found which would accommodate all hospital, then a hospital of any size analysis and content could readily be designed simply by plugging the standard shapes into a hospital street. It had, after all, worked for Florence Nightingale, so why not for us?

Many configurations were tested out against the requirements of certain key hospital departments, and what emerged from these studies was the now familiar cruciform template of about 1000 m^2. It was found that this size and shape most closely matched the patients' requirements of either single departments, or clusters of small departments, with a natural locational affinity. The shape had a beneficial wall-to-floor ratio, which meant that it was energy efficient, and the travel distance from its farthest point complied with fire escape requirements.

Once the decision on template size and shape had been taken, work started on the preparation of departmental and whole hospital operation policies, and the architectural and engineering designs for a range of departments. Design data began to appear in 1978. All building and engineering data relating each cruciform template is contained in data packs, the architectural pack consists of planning principles and design descriptions, a key plan, activity data (A, B, C, D and G sheet), a 1:50 scale detailed plan of the department, and a fire plan.

The engineering pack consists of a design description, a schedule of connected loads; and 1:50 scale plans of engineering services and drainage within the template.

Thus for every hospital department, there exists a complete brief and a very detailed design solution. The hospital design team still has to put the whole hospital together, and it still has to determine the structure and appearance of the buildings, but it is relieved of the time-consuming chore of designing each department in detail. The saving in time is considerable.

Since the first project in 1980, there has been an extremely encouraging uptake of the system in the NHS in the UK. There are 130 projects completed. It is axiomatic that the larger the programme the more benefit is derived from standardisation. The UK programme of nucleus hospitals represents a capital investment of some £ 2 billion (US$ 3.4 billion), and as a result, very considerable saving have been made. But even more modest programmes can produce every worth while financial benefits. It has been calculated, given the lower capital cost, the considerable savings in professional fees, and then much lower cost of client input, that for every ten nucleus hospitals built the client gets one free.

Updating the System

Two factors have driven updating programme forward, the first is the evaluation programme of completed nucleus hospitals, and the second is need to accommodate the rapid change in medical technology, nursing techniques and demography. More design-in-use evaluations have been carried out on Nucleus hospitals than on any other hospital design system. Weaknesses that have been identified in the course of these evaluation have been corrected, and revised designs issued to NHS users.

During the1980s there has been a considerable change in requirements for district hospital caused by factors such as reduced length of stay, an increase in the average age of patients, new developments in non-invasive surgery, and general increase in the expectations of patients with regard to the standard of the facilities in which they are treated. For example, as nearly all patients in acute beds are now in the high dependency category,the size of the original nursing section of 28 beds has been reduced to the new standard of 24 beds.

FURTHER READING

1. Chan W: The Nucleus Hospital: Pros and Cons Hospital Management International.1992.
2. Ward PL: The Nucleus concept. Hospital management International London, 1992.

16 Modular Building Concept

When the health care facilities are looking to expand, the modular building concept offers many major benefits. These advantages are flexibility, speed and lower cost can often satisfy health care facilities' requirements perfectly.

Flexibility

When ongoing construction requires temporary space, modular buildings can easily shrink or expand later as space needs change, modules can be easily moved to another site even when assembled as a one or two storey bukling. As a permanent solution, modular buildings provide custom-made facilities to satisfy customers' unique specifications. Site limitations, special operational uses of specific requirement of any nature present no problems with the flexibility of modular buildings.

Speed

When a new building has to be operational quickly to avoid down time in providing patient care, teaching or conducting research, a modular building can be on site within 8-12 weeks of order. By fabricating modular units off site and within a controlled factory environment, delays often associated with conventional construction are circumvented. Modular suppliers adhere to a stringent three-step monitoring process of inspecting buildings during and after fabrication and at installation on the site. All buildings are constructed from the highest quality materials that are energy efficient and require little maintenance.

Modulars are designed and manufactured to meet all applicable building codes. Wiring and plumbing, installed at the factory, are easily hooked up at the final building site, stud framing, floor joints and roof rafters are supported on steel I-beam frames. The unit is then placed on its foundation. Nearly all system components are installed at the factory, including heating, cooling and ventilation equipment. In many cases, furnishings, fire sprinklers and security systems are also factory installed. Claddings, exterior and interior wall finishings, door and window types, floor finishes and envelope thermal insulation levels can be specified to order. Site grading, foundation work, connection of utilities and services, landscaping and interconnection of the modular unit are the only on-site activities required.

Cost

Modular buildings provide significant cost savings. The cost of modular construction is often one-third

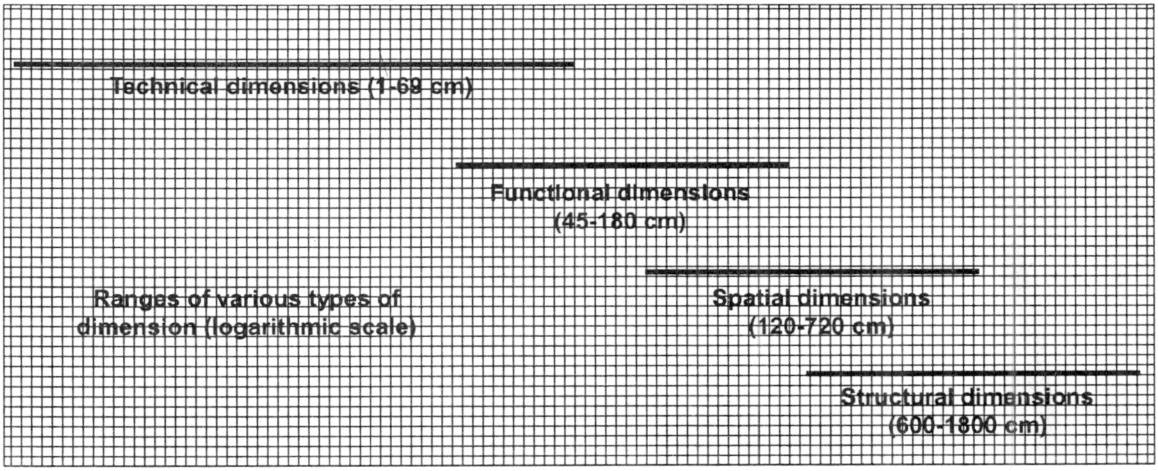

Fig. 16.1: To obtain full benefit from the modular discipline in medical-care building construction, the following comprehensive scheme is proposed. A modular discipline for the diverse building products (prefabricated elements) can be built up, starting from the characteristic dimensions of each product. In each architectural design these dimensions belong to one of the following types: (1) Technical dimensions result from technical consideration requirements. For instance the bearing capacity dictates column sections; sound insulation influences the wall thickness, etc. (2) Functional dimensions, such as door width, bench height, and length of working surfaces. These dimensions are the result of functional, anthropometric or ergonomic data, (3) Spatial dimensions: the dimensions of the various rooms, ceiling height, corridor width, etc., and (4) Structural dimensions, for spans, distances between beams and between columns, etc

less than conventional construction. In additional on-site labour requirements are minimal. Modular building suppliers can also act as financial analysis to help health-care facility planners choose the appropriate financing method to fit specific budgets and space requirements.

Applications

Modular hospital space can serve the needs of many areas, including space for research, teaching, surgery and clinical functions, registration/reception, laboratory frozen section rooms, examination rooms, phototherapy suites, nursing stations, physical/resident work and office areas, break rooms, cafeterias, equipment and record storage, rest rooms and child-care (day-care) facilities. In addition to functional requirements, modular buildings satisfy the special requirements of both patients and staff. Modular space is comfortable, quiet, climate controlled, private and secure

Interior and Exterior Considerations

Many exterior treatments are also available. Aluminum or wood siding or pleko, a stucco-like materiel, can easily be applied to match existing structures or can blend in with landscape environments. Tinted double-glazed windows can create privacy and add energy efficiency, as can optional rubber roof systems, which help to conserve energy inside the modular facilities.

Inside, a modular facility can feature 8 ft or higher dry wall ceilings that can be constructed to support specialised lighting fixtures needed for surgical suites. Customised air conditioning systems can be installed to continually pump in fresh air. For safety, Sprinkler and fire-alarm systems can be installed throughout the buildings.

17 Hospital Modernization

The procedures for planning new construction can all be applied equally well to planning for modernization and expansion, but in addition certain other methods must be used if there is to be achieved a balanced final plan. These include surveys of existing facilities, both as to their condition and their intensity of use; assembly of data on the known needs and desires for spacific improvements; analysis of existing floor areas by departments and comparison with known standards as a measure of space adequacy; and the projection of a functional program, including floor areas, through the stage immediately proposed and into succeeding future stages as far as may be desired. These methods do not replace other methods already discussed. But they offer additional guides to planning for modernization and expansion. It is assumed that the functional programme will have been derived from the long-range plan.

Existing Facilities

Fundamental to planning for expansion are the surveys of existing physical facilites. It may be found, for example, that limitations of the existing building site may be insurmountable, ruling out consideration of expansion at the existing location and forcing selection of a new site. But where existing site limitations are not the determining factor, it may still be necessary to relocate, considering existing land and the possibilities of acquiring additional land adjoining it. Steps in modernisation and expansion include:

A. Functional programme states needs. Schematic and site studies determine future location.
B. Gross floor area analysis reveals space deficiencies. Engineering studies and economic analysis determine future use of existing buildings.
C. From these studies the long-range plan for growth can be established three stages ten years each.
D. For state I, designs and drawings are made: schematic-detailed basics. Working drawings and specification. Bids, contracts and construction.
E. Phasing the work-operations-equipping activating.

The total space requirement will be a combination of these calculations and is certain to be more than what is needed simply to take care of the additional hospital beds. A table can best illustrate this.

Total gross area for stage I (200 beds)

Existing buildings	47,600 SFG
Deduct for buildings which are to be replaced	18,000
Net remaining area	29,600
Total floor area as programmed	129,900 SFG

Net building area required (use in budget) 100,300 SFG. This shows that a balanced hospital calls for much more new space than required for beds only, which might be 30,000 SFG.

Equipment and Utilities

Nowhere do the problems of expansion reveal more surpises than in equipment and utilities. A sterilizer which was quite adequate yesterday suddenly is revealed as unacceptable for use in the new buildings. Similarly piping, wiring, fixtures, fans, pumps, boilers, elevators, and even the whole heating system may undergo a sudden and painful downgrading when requiremtns of the future load are calculated. Such findings are normal and not serious if there has been proper physical maintenance and if they are discovered and included before the poject budget has been fixed, but too often they are overlooked or not fully explored until the scheme of expansion has been set and the budget established. Findings of inadequacy are then droped like a bomb on the planning team, and if the budget cannot be adjusted upward, some other needed and by then cherished improvements must be deferred.

One reason this happens with utilities is that it costs serious money to make an engineering survey of utilities and mechanical plant, and the architect is properly careful to have this work done only when needed; yet if it is not done well on advance of the final schematics, there can be painful results. Sometimes a preliminary engineering review will give sufficient guidance until the detailed survey is done.

With hospital equipment the psychology is little different, but the results are often the same. Equipment can be appraised more readilly than mechanical systems. But the planning team, always hopeful in the early stages, is prone to pass over the true condition of equipment on the assumption that what has been useful can continue in use. Often it is not until some equipment has actually been relocated that the folly of puttng old pieces into a new building becomes evident. Such a situation is not without its own advantages. Even through the discovery described is a painful one, in that it does seem easier to raise extra money for equipment when the building is well along than in the planning stages. Furthermore, the installation of an old piece does not necessarily preclude its later replacement.

Orderly planning and budgeting, however, call for a careful survey of both utilities and equipment and the inclusion of funds for modernization or replacement. The evaluation of movable equipment is the task of the hospital administrator and his staff or of the hospital consultant, but the architect should consult them so that utilities requirements for all equipment which are to be replaced can be calculated and included in the building modernization budget.

Utility Expansion

A related engineering problem is that utilities expansion may call for sizing certain main feeders to carry future loads as well as those presently planned. The engineer should be instructed to do this within reason; but care should be exercised that this not be overdone, particularly with standby elements. Cases have been known in which so much of the budget was required for replacement of utilities and mechanical systems on one hand and to carry future loads on the other that the remaining funds were inadequate for the prime functional needs. This is like building a complete boiler plant sized for the ultimate hosptial and having no funds left to build the patient beds.

Movable Partitions

The movable partition may be useable in the plan if you expect to move it three times:

1. There is little or no plumbing in it.
2. Electrical requirements are normal.
3. Only modest sound deadening is needed.

Advantages

- Dry construction—quick alterations—clean.
- Makes possible office rearrangements.

Disadvantages

- Costs more than most conventional partitions
- Does not lend itself well to special conditions
- Factory units may not fit existing spaces, even with and fillers
- Transmits some sound—often via the ceiling
- Encourages changes which may not be essential.

Mobility is not important along corridors, around stairs and elevators, in some bedrooms, in surgery, delivery, kitchen, laundry, central stores, central supply. Wherever movable partitions are considered for economy, they must be moved three times to show a saving two times to break even.

Phasing the Improvement

If site conditions permit, the new building should be completed and occupied before modernisation of existing buildings is undertaken.

In preparing the phasing schedules, there must be multiple studies of the various possible shifts. Taking into account both cost and time involved and making certain that hospital operations can be maintained at an acceptable level, the best solution is often that in which the bed units are the last to be fully occupied after the several steps have been completed for the essential supporting departments.

Any expansion and modernisation programme will require 2-4 years of actual construction time after work starts. Time for planning will be prior to this.

Some departments by their nature cannot easily be expanded in small increments. These are the kitchen, laundry, boiler plant, delivery suite, operating suite, and central sterile supply. In varying degrees they require large steps or none at all. Other departments are more easily expanded by adding whatever space is called for. The nursing services should generally be expanded by adding whole patient divisions rather than small groups of beds.

The problems of planning for future, expansion can be solved in various ways. For those departments which can easily be expanded or moved, the problem is only room for growth. For the nursing services there should be a long-range plan recording the various stages by which the ultimate number of beds is to be reached and maintaining at each stage workable sizes for all patient divisions. It usually better to plan for the addition of bed floors on top of existing floors. This is largely because of the relatively greater inconvience and somewhat greater cost is maintaining lower floors in use while construction is going on above, and because the extension of utilities and elevators upward poses many problems. Nevertheless, if site limitations compel and structure permits, it is not impossible to add floor on top of existing buildings.

Increments

It is the most difficult problem existing in those departments which cannot be expanded in small increments. Here the solution varies with the programmme conditions, and many variables will be encountered. If the existing hosptial is small say 40 beds, and the first stage is another 40 beds, and if the second stage of another 40 beds is anticipated fairly early, say in five years, then it is probably wise to plan kitchen, laundry, power plant, operating rooms, delivery rooms, and central supply to care for the second stage total of 120 beds instead of 80 beds. The total extra space in the departments thus planned would probably not exceed by more than 30 percent the area that would be planned for the 80 beds only. This is because the minimum size for these departments will support more than 80 beds and because unit sizes decrease slightly as the number of beds increases. But with a larger stage 2, this is not equally true.

An empirical rule is that a far future expansion of less than 30 percent may justify oversizing the supporting departments but that greater than 30 percent future expansion calls for the supporting departments to be sized for stage-1 loads only.

Why oversize? The argument is sometimes given that experience shows that it is gratifying to have oversized spaces into which the hosptial can grow. The only possible answer to this is that it may be done if the board can afford it, but how can they be assured that the right department will be chosen for oversizing? Is the whole hospital to be oversized for this reason? This line of argument discounts the conviction that careful programming and planning can produce an adequate but not oversized building, without which there is little point in making the calculations described.

Regardless of the approach, each expansion should be tested for each department by making actual plan layouts. In the case of an operating suite, such plans would show the possibility of adding the two operating rooms called for in the stage-2 expansion simply by extending the state-I surgical wing by another 30 feet. This would avoid oversizing surgery in stage I to provide for the stage 2 loads. But a similar expansion of the kitchen would probably be uneconomical, and the stage-1 kitchen should therefore be designed for the stage-2 load of 250 beds. The general rule is not to build excess size in any department if it can be avoided. This rule presumes adequate programming and preliminary planning in stage 1 and careful studies of the direction of expansion for stage 2.

The converse of this problem arises from the practice, too often followed, of adding hospital beds without increasing the supporting services. In this case the result is to overload the non-bed departments and create serious impediments to effective hospital operation. Only through a careful analysis of the size of existing departments and an equaily carefrul programming of those sizes for each stage of expansion can a suitable balance be maintained and the necessary oversizing be justified. Plans for present facilities should not be compromised for the sake of an uncertain future in which the requirments may be materially changed. Thus, the main problem is to estimate the likelihood of expansion being needed and make plans accordingly, if the future brings as many changes in pattern of hospital care as are predicted, even the most prescient plans will probably be absolete when the time comes for stage 2.

The point has been made that the tremendous investment in existing hospital facilities, plus continuing obsolescence, will assure the need for modernization in the future. In addition, population growth and the trend toward enlargment of existing hospitals and further concentration of education and research activities imply corresponding expansion.

Forces in the contrary direction are the growing dispersion of services into the field and to ambulant patients and the growth limitations imposed upon many hospitals by the size of site. The first of these would tend to lessen the requirements for floor space but would, if anything, greatly increase the need for alteration and modernization of exiting spaces to accommodate new functions. The second will be critical in many cases, but it seems probable that the one force most demanding of grounds area now, namely, automobile parking, will be removed in the future by exclusion or radical modification of private transport. If this happens, the chances are that many existing metropolitan sites will again be adquate even for the increased activity in future.

A second serious question about the future relates to the salvage of existing plant. If changes are as radical as predicted, there will be strong forces in motion to replace absolete buildings. For this, the architect can render great service by using his imagination to devise ways to continue old buildings in use at least for a portion of their remaining physical life. Failing this, there is bound to be extensive replacement of plant, as is seen currently in office buildings.

METHODOLOGY FOR HOSPITAL MODERNISATION

The methodology for, and attitudes towards, modernising and expanding a hospital include:

- *Step I:* make a thorough survey (drawings, prictures) of the full hospital premises and the relevant nearby surroundings.

  Draw an accurate site plan to scale with all main buildings, ancillary buildings, other facilities, circulation paths, special networks, access roads.
- *Step 2:* discover and understand the circulation pattern linking and crossing all the buildings.

  Pay special attention to: circulation outside (trucks, cars, people): horizontal circulation in all buildings: vertical circulation to buildings, separately by stairs and elevators; special main engineering networks covering the site (heating steam, power) and actual segregation of traffic (in-patients, out-patients, visitors, staff, goods, waste).
- *Step 3:* Improve and strengthen this pattern by opening up bottle-necks; adding staircases and /or elevators, and by-passes.
- *Step 4:* make a thorough survey of all existing buildings; structural survey; technical survey, and equipment survey.
- *Step 5:* develop a long-range masterplan beyond your immediate expansion needs. Even if there is no apparent need now, consider anyhow a growth in bed capacity and in size per bed standard. In case of a specialised hospital, investigate the expansion with other specialisations or even the transformation into a general hospital.

  Consider and evaluate alternative masterplans. In such evaluations, two major attitudes should prevail

  — *Attitude 1:* The next extension will be the last one. Any addition or growth has to fit into a scheme of long range open-ended planning, and

  — *Attitude 2:* When modernising, consider three aspects simultaneously: functional upgrading; safety improvements, and energy conservation.

  Compare upgrading with replacement or growth: in this latter case, consider three possible alternatives; growth and addition of new buildings; expansion by extension of existing buildings, and expansion by repetition of buildings.
- *Step 6:* Compare alternative circulation patterns too, even beyond measures proposed in step 3. Develop proposals for efficient segregation of traffic, the degree of segregation depending on the size and the nature of the hospital.

  Divide all valuable masterplans into feasible phase, paying attention to the functional continuity of the hospital as a whole and of critical departments separately.

  Consider eventually temporary measures for circulation (for example, 'dummy' corridors) during specific building phases.

  If needed give feed-back to step 5
- *Step 7:* Decide on your best masterplan, based on time, including phasing possibilities; costs, both building and running costs, and continuity of functions during building works in consecutive plans.
- *Step 8:* Decide on a phase-one project, checking in detail the functional continuity of the hospital during execution of that first phase.
- *Step 9:* and onwards; as for new construction, but with continuous feedback to step 5 phase after phase.

FURTHER READING

1. Delrue J: Hospital Modernisation and expansion. Hospital Management International. IHF. London 1992.
2. Wheeler TE Hospital Design and Function. McGraw Hill 1964.

18 Cutting Construction Costs

The cost of getting a new hospital designed and built, has as of now been soared. Driven by fluctuating economic conditions, technological advances, extensive legal requirements, and a level-developing awareness of the proper priority of health care, the design and construction of a modern hospital have become a more complex and difficult task. Because of this, it is time to re-examine the traditional approach to designing and building new healthcare facilities.

In the traditional approach, an owner retains design consultants to develop the design and then invites general contractors to submit competitive prices for the work. The design consultants evaluate these prices and make recommendations to the owner for selection. A prime contractor is chosen and given notice to proceed.

The decisions which have most effect on costs are made during design, and there has been no expert construction input during that phase. This approach also consumes valuable time and tends to develop an adverse relationship because the designer and contractor are dealing with what they view as separate and distinct pieces of the project and there is little incentive for co-operation.

After the contract award, there are often many claims for extras, and disputes from both parties. Schedule delays and cost overruns are a frequent consequence.

If an experienced contractor/construction manager is engaged at the same time as the design consultants are selected, several important cost and time-saving services become available to the owner. The key to the success of this approach is that a team is formed at the bagging of the project.

This team consists of the owner, the design consultants and a knowledgeable contractor/ construction manager. If the owner is not a health care professional involved in the operation of the hospital, representatives from the hospital administration and medical staff may be added to the team.

Estimates

The result is that the design and construction process is addressed in its entirety rather than in its separate parts. All aspects of the project are analysed during design development for potential effects on overall cost, schedule, and quality objectives.

Reliable preliminary cost estimates and planning are crucial in arranging project financing. An experienced contractor/construction manager is ideally suited to develop these preliminary data.

If engaged early enough, the contractor/construction manager will review the preliminary architectural documents and provide a realistic construction cost project based on both functional and parameter estimates. A functional area estimate provides a projection of cost-by-space allocation in various hospital departments. A parameter estimate defines, in cost per square meter, the actual building components.

To arrive at the parameter estimate, the project is divided into building elements: foundation, structural frame, plumbing, electrical, heating, air-conditioning, and so on. Thus, the hospital owner can get accurate projections of anticipated space use and cost per square meter. By analysing the design and construction sequence, the contractor/construction manager develops preliminary schedules and cash-flow requirements.

The early availability of this reliable preliminary information on cost, cash-fellow, and schedule, may help the owner finalise financial arrangements and overcome problems associated with cash-flow restrictions.

Value Engineering Principles

Once the preliminary information has been developed, the constructor/construction manager uses value engineering principles and works within the team to determine cost-effective solutions to the choice of equipment, system materials, and construction methods. Primarily, this is the valuation of life cycle costs—the costs of design, procurement, installation, operations, maintenance, and replacement over the entire projected use of the item.

For example, the relative prices of energy and labour, have a profound effect on operations and maintenance costs and can influence selection. Other questions to be asked include: Will the project benefit by modularization and pre-assembly to mini mize on-site skilled labour or special equipment requirements? Will alternate selections permit more participation by local firms?

The result of this process is that during the preliminary design stage, the team arrrives at the most effective solutions for the specific needs of the hospital. All the disciplines have co-operated in developing them, and the spirit of working together to achieve the owner's goals become the primary objective.

During this period the contractor/construction manager also uses his abilities and experience to help define the long-lead items, and ensures that they are given the appropriate priorities. These long-lead items such as elevators and special electrical equipment, require the longest times for design, procurement, and delivery to the site.

Identification of long-lead items is part of the continuing development of a comprehensive project schedule which includes the needs and activities to which the owner, the design professionals, suppliers congnizant authorities, and the construction constractors are (or will be) committed to achieve the owner's goals. This becomes a vital control document, expanding in detail as different aspects of the project are developed. Ideally, it will use the critical path-method which shows activity interrelationships so that potential problems can be more easily identified.

It is important to remember that pre-construction activity also needs to be monitored and controlled. For example, delays in approvals by congnisant authorities or in final design availability can produce overall project effects which can far outweigh their immediate impact. There are also continuing development and refinement of the cost and cash-flow estimates during this period.

A very important result of this team approach is that the contractor/construction manager can establish a guaranteed maximum price (GMP) before the final design is completed. Subject to the owner's agreement, site work can then commence. If it is decided to adopt the GMP approach and fast-tract the project (schedule design and construction so that site and structural work begin before the detail design and working drawings are complete), the planning, scheduling, field construction capability, and co-ordinating skill of an experienced contractor/construction manager is invaluable.

His first-hand knowledge in dividing the work, minimizing interferences, providing solutions to problems resulting from changing field conditions, and managing complex projects are essential to the success of this approach. The result is a completed revenue-earning facility several months earlier than would have been possible with the traditional approach.

Primary Responsibility

During the construction phase, the constractors/ construction manager assumes primary responsibility for completing the procurement and constructing the facility. He is also responsible for any costs which exceed the limit established by the guaranteed maximum price.

Because the total project is team effort, the many factors unique to constructing the specific hospital have been continually considered, and at this point, the most appropriate construction methods have been identified. The contractor/construction manager will generally invite the maximum participation of qualified local subcontractors and suppliers. This often helps the transfer of technology and encourages the development of local industry.

Selection of a contractor/construction anager should be done with the same care and judgment used in selecting design professionals. The criteria are similar, and include:

Experience on projects of a similar size and type:

- Identification of key individuals who will be responsible for overseeing the project,
- Favorable references from former and current health-care facility clients,
- Assurance of financial responsibility and stability,
- Successfully demonstrated a management systems,
- Experience working with an owner and professional design consultants during the early stages of design development,
- Knowledge of business conditions and economic indicators that can have adverse effects on the project,
- Knowledge of the construction market, including subcontractors and material suppliers,
- Knowledge of the building systems and experience in applying value engineering analysis.

The primary remaining factor in selecting the contractor/construction manager is the fee arrangement. Since he is being brought on board long before final plans are approved, it is not possible to set a fixed price. Therefore, the owner should negotiate a professional fee which is usually based on overlay project cost estimates. It can range from 2 to 4 percent on very large projects to 8 to 10 percent on small ones or those with special complications or extraordinary risks. Next, the contractor's general conditions or job management costs are established. The professional fee and general conditions costs combine with the construction cost estimates to establish the guaranteed maximum price for the project.

The team is the key. From the beginning, it helps the owner develop a working relationship in which all disciplines become involved and all parties benefit by co-operation and the free exchange of ideas, information, and prompt decision making. Establishing the team at the beginning of the health care facility project will be of great value in achieving cost savings and schedule improvements while maintaining quality objectives.

The objective of good hospital design is to produce buildings that respond to the operational policy objectives stated by the initial users, but which are capable of subsequent alteration and addition to meet the needs of an unknown future. The application of building guidance, the judicious use of standard designs and a continuing programme of evaluation, are excellent ways of achieving this aim.

FURTHER READING

1. Russel RM, Pasquale RW: Cutting construction costs. Hospital Management International IHF. London 1988.

19 Humanising Health Care Facilities

Architecture for humanising hospitals depends a lot on the nature of the building we are dealing with.

The historical hospital is in most cases in a building with architectural, cultural or historical value, and these factors have an impact on any necessary renovation, or architectural change intended for the updating of the building.

The emerging hospital is where medical treatment is performed in temporary structures, a cluster of dilapidated buildings adapted or improvised for hospitalization and medical services. In some cases a permanent building or a medical complex emerges in phases to replace the barracks.

The exploding hospital is an over-populated health care facility. To the chagrin of everybody, patient's beds spill from wards to corridors, and occupy crowded spaces everywhere.

The emergency hospital is used in cases of catastrophe and for war casualties. It includes stretcher wards, operating theatres and essential medical services. Operations in these facilities are carried out under severe tense conditions. This fact has its impact on the design of the emergency hospital.

Newly built hospital in most cases comprises only the nucleus of the future hospital. At this stage, it is very important to establish the master plan of the future medical complex.

The developing hospital is a functioning hospital or health care facility which is expanding and only ingenius architectural innovations can overcome construction disturbance in operating departments.

The consolidating medical complex in a health care facility in the state of transition between a newly built institute and a permanent running organisation. In this period, what was right and what was wrong in the original design becomes apparent.

The Need for Reassurance

Hospital architecture deals with the medical complex as a whole and with numerous details concerning humanising the building. Most important in this connection, is the avoidance of architectural barriers which upset human communication or movement:

- A patient talking to hospital personnel through a hatch or barred by a physical obstacle or clumsy furniture.
- A patient in a wheelchair or with walking difficulties trying to overcome stairs.
- A patient confined to his bed, unable to see what is going on outside because the windows were built to the wrong dimensions.

- Violation of privacy add to the patient suffering and occurs when he has the feeling of being exposed:
  — Personal details are disclosed to unauthorized people
  — Conversation with a physician is heard by others
  — Treatment is seen by others, not concerned.

Architects should use architectural means to minimize violation of privacy.

Patient care using sophisticated technology, should be delivered in a reassuring environment. Architectural innovations for humanising health care facilities must concern themselves with this need for reassurance.

FURTHER READING

1. Zarhy M: Humanizing health care facilities International Hospital Federation Year Book 99-100 1988.

20 Autonomous Health Care Facilities

Establishing autonomous healthcare facilities can help to improve the present health situation in underdeveloped areas, not only by providing health services and reducing costs, but also by demonstrating good examples for most basic functions of life, from which the local population may learn. Showing the people how to improve their living conditions, nutrition, hygiene and general life styles can in itself eliminate most of the causes of the disease, environmental pollution and poverty.

The buildings and their supporting facilities must be designed to suit the local medical requirements, guarantee maximum efficiency, create acceptable environments for patients and staff, correspond to traditional building constructions, and keep maintenance requirements to a minimum. Adequate facilities for accompanying relatives of the patients must not be forgotten, as their services form the backbone of the model.

Of all the building parts, the roof must be given maximum attention, and as far as possible, all major outdoor activities should take place under large roofs, in order to:

- Function at all times, irrespective of weather conditions.
- Achieve tolerable temperatures, despite the tropical climate.
- Collect as much rainwater as possible.

The energy supply could consist of the following:

- Solar systems for heating water, drying farm products and cooling, and if possible, for lighting operating theatres, refrigeration and autoclaving.
- Firewood from fast-growing plants for cooking on special energy-stoves.
- Windmills for pumping water, generating electricity, driving grinders and so forth.
- Biogas units for lighting rather than for cooking.
- Water power, if natural water courses are close by, for power generation, operation of grinders and so forth.
- Animal power for farming activities and transportation.
- Emergency power generators to run cooling systems, medical equipment and so forth.

The water supply should comprise of:

- Large reservoirs, above or below the ground, fed by rainwater.
- Pumping systems, wind, manual and other means.
- Water purification units for sedimentation, filtration and boiling.
- Tube wells and collection of surface water, from rivers or lakes for reserve supplies.

Waste and sewage disposal is most critical and could involve:

- Septic tanks combined with biogas units.
- Production of natural fertilizers by anaerobic or aerobic digestion of liquid waste, or by composting solid organic waste.
- Waste-water ponds, in which aquatic flora and fauna purify the water.
- Reuse of partially soiled water for flushing toilets.
- Incineration of dangerous wastes, utilizing the omitted heat to produce hot water.

Self-sufficiency in food supplies would mean:

- Extensive plantation of vegetables, fruits and grains, together with the necessary drying and cooling units, silos, stores and so forth.
- Livestock and poultry farming for production of milk, eggs and meat, not to speak of leather, wood, feathers and so on, needed for other purposes.
- Aquaculture in waste-water ponds, producing algae, fish and ducks for consumption.
- Production units for bread, cheese, juices, honey oils and other foodstuffs and local delicacies.

For building improvements, repairs or new construction a variety of materials should be produced on the site. For example.

- Building components and furniture from fast-growing timber and bamboo,
- Mats, baskets, sacking material from fibrous plants,
- Soil blocks and several other items made from materials found on the site.

FURTHER READING

1. Mukharji K: Healthcare Facilities for Developing Countries Hospital Management International Year Book, London 91-92, 1985.

21 Recent Trends in Hospital Architecture

A hospital is a human invention, and as such can be reinvented at any time. Patient care of high quality should be achieved by the hospital through provision of competent professional and technical staff and of the equipment of facilities necessary to support the hospital's patient care objective, and enforcement of standards and provision of programmes for patient care that are considered desirable by various health professionals.

A standard architectural plan should be achieved through determination of facility size appropriate to the projected service demands of the hospital service areas and of departmental areas large enough to provide the diagnostic and treatment services—an architectural design that will permit efficient use of hospital personnel, place departments with complementary activities conveniently together, anticipate future departmental expansion, provide privacy and flexibility, and adequate work space on patient units, adequate attention to infection control and emergency preparedness. The hospital as a key institution in the community health care systems, should recognise the public nature of its services and that its primary objectives should be to render an essential community services. Continuing advances in medicine and society impose great demands on the planning team. The planners must be aware of the ideology of the community. Attitudes and aspirations must be clearly understood. The role of the hospital architect and planner in an ever-more intricate interweaving of factors that form the framework of the society which has become very complicated.

The design can only be as good as the experience and research upon which it has been based. Planning involves and requires understanding and evaluation of the current cultural mainstreams, the economic and technological conditions, and the goals of the community.

There is need for innovations and creativity in the planning and design of healthcare facilities.

Construction Basics

A cost-benefit analysis should be undertaken as regards the polyvalence of the design and construction and the length of the building life. It would be a false economy to reduce construction costs, if it would result in increased operating costs. The hospital construction must be adjusted to the functional needs, be simple, rapidly executable and economical. These aims have to be controlled by the safety of the structure, the site conditions, and usual local requirements. The design of all technical components and installations must be balanced. Examples of over-design in hospitals include refrigration equipment covering twice the actual needs and lighting levels upto four times in excess of that necessary. The life length aspect of the hospital should be weighed in at the beginning of a planning process, when the economic life of the hospital and the implications of its change and growth are considered. The lifetime of a hospital building as a whole is frequently estimated to about 65 years. It may be convenient to assume that hospital buildings should be replaced after 60-90 years, but the chronological age cannot be used to determine the functional suitability of hospital building. Hospital should be used until their usefulness has been truly exhausted. There is no society which can afford to replace hospitals after every 50 or 60 years.

Generally, the supporting physical structure has a lifetime of more than 100 years, the basic installations such as wiring, and plumbing last 20-30 years. The elevators last 15-25 years: oxygen vacum and compressed air plants 20-30 years. The general domestic hospital equipment will last 5-20 years, the medicare technical equipment 7-12 years.

Energy Conservation

By adopting a range of technologies, the amount of energy used for environmental as well as functional services could be reduced.

The choice of level of technology depends on: low technology solutions are less financially demanding and easy to maintain.

High technology equipment ensures the precised control of environmental conditions necessary for some hospital procedures but demands a high level of maintenance and spare parts inventory.

The designer has the option of combining high and low level technology.

Some departments in hospital, such as laundry, kitchen and wards, need a constant supply of hot water. The hot water supply in a hospital not only requires the consumption of large amounts of conventional energy but also frequently fails, owing to lack of proper, timely maintenance and lack of availability of spare parts.

Use of simple, solar heating devices can avoid most such problems and ensure a reliable supply of hot water. It is aided by the orientation of the buildings. This almost maintenance-free system can provide hospitals with hot water at a very low cost. Solar energy can also be made use of for natural lighting windows to provide maximal lighting against the inner wall: the angle of incidence of light from the window to the inner working areas should be not less than 27°. Special inlets with translucent covers can be placed at various places in the roof to supply glare-free light during the day in various areas (corridors, waiting areas, etc.). Building design itself can reduce the capital and operating costs. Windows that open are the best means of ventilating most parts of the hospital. Air conditioning is necessary in operation theaters, intensive care units and imaging facilities, but not in routine nursing units (wards) or service departments. The use of high efficiency light sources, energy officient ventilation systems, the provision for local humidifiers for zones requiring this facility and higher levels of thermal insulation for heating and hot water distribution mains can be used as energy-conserving measures. The common practice of keeping steam mains alive even when the load is small are intermittent, has been found to be very wasteful in energy terms and the use of variable speed pumps has been found to be cost-effective.

Heat is available in the air extracted from a hospital and could be recovered either by run-around coils or by operating refrigeration plant in a heat pump made. The incinerator also can contribute a significant amount of energy greater than 0.5 million kWh annually in a 300-bedded hospital. The boiler plant is another area where recuperators can be used to recover some of the heat in the flue gases.

A carefully thought-out site energy strategy is an essential pre-requisite for a hospital. The significance of fuel types, the synchronisation of heat reclaim with demand, thermal storage and the relevance of combined heat and power cannot be overemphasized. The integration of these factors in determining an overall site strategy has to be considered in addition to exploring how thermal energy and power might be provided to the hospi tal other than by traditional means.

Other measures that can be adopted to conserve energy include micro-loss control gear and automatic switching for lighting circuits, motors for fancy pumps and fuel-less incinerators. By adopting different methods of cooking and by the use of more energy efficient appliances energy can be reduced.
Achieving Energy Efficiency:

1. By conservation methods
   - air-tightness thermal insulation
   - optimisation of glazing ratios
   - air-treatment systems
   - catering services
2. By heat reclaim from:
   - incinerator
   - boiler exhaust
   - exhaust air
   - refrigeration

A standardised system of hospital planning and design known as nucleus is considered to be efficient in energy terms. The estimated level of total energy consumption is 75 GJ/100 m^3 of building volume and compares favourably well with a figure of 90 GJ/100 m^3 for other present-day hospitals.

Economy in Construction

Use of value engineering The initial cost of construction of hospital with all supportive services-electric, mechnical, air-conditioning, water supply and sewerage is very high due to factors such as:

- Escalation in costs of labour and materials as a result of global inflation.

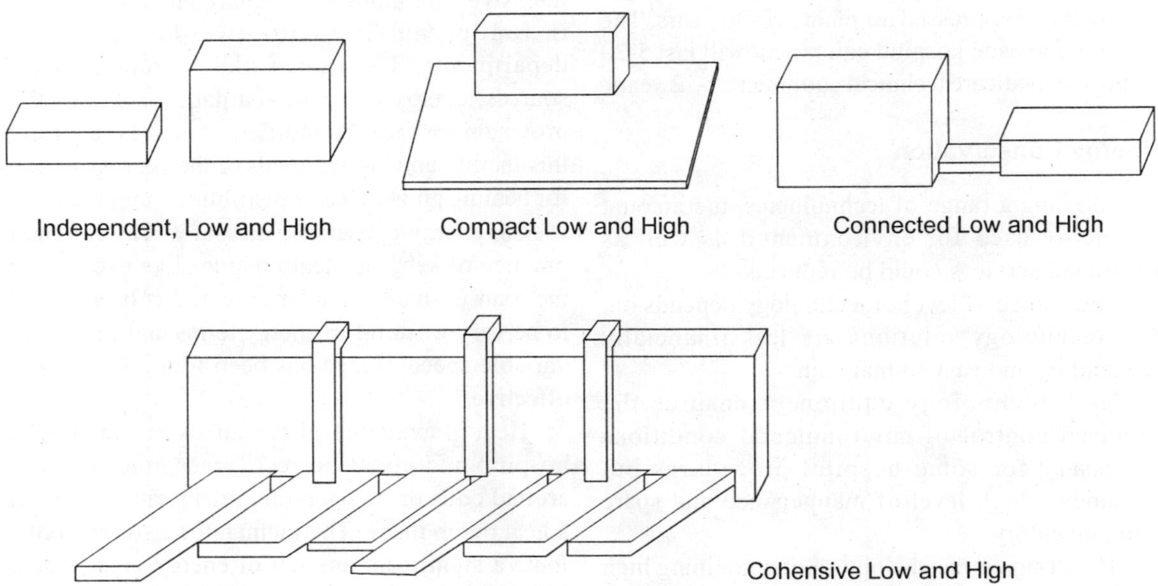

Fig. 21.1: Variations in existing hospital shapes are almost unlimited. Basically four groups could be identitied, most of them belonging to the artistic approaches. The cohesive group includes the hospitals based on biologic design

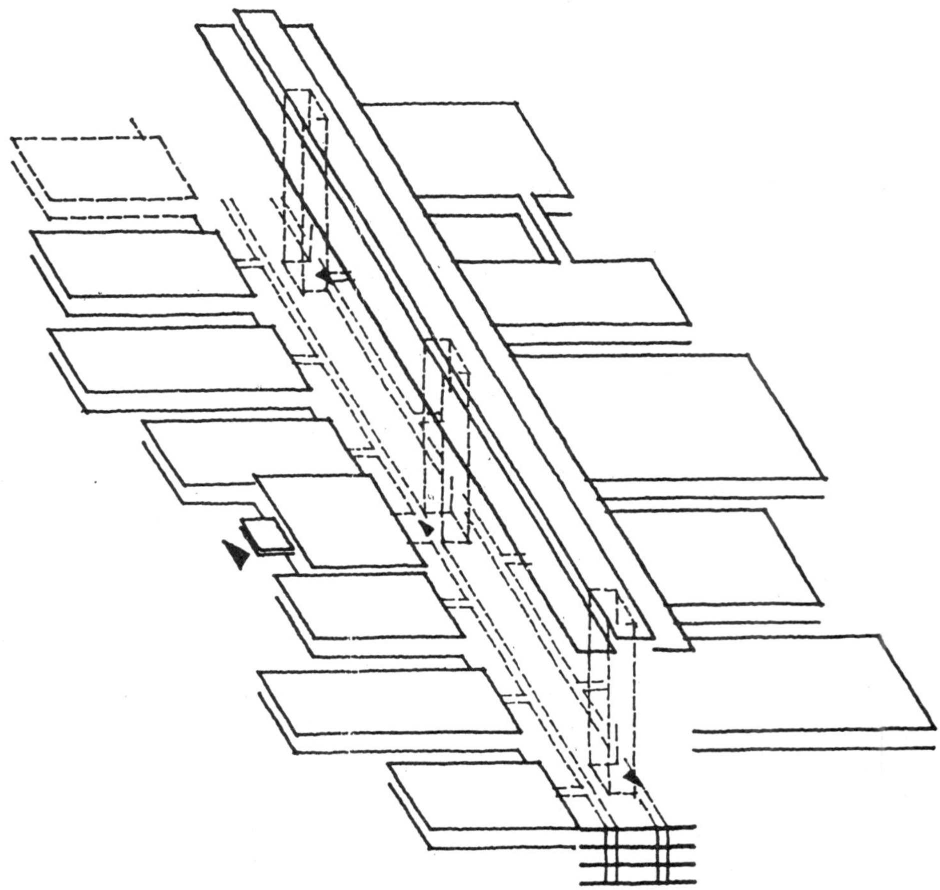

Fig. 21.2: Principle for a lienar 1000-bed hospital from 1968. On one side out-patient departments, on the other medical performance areas. Segregated elevator systems. Pütsep International

- Lesser of flattened productibility of labour
- Increased requirements for use of high technology equipment
- Greater preparation of total construction cost-electrical,
- .Air conditioning and ventilation systems.
- Non-availability of urban land necessiating high rise structures involving extra cost of foundations, lifts, fire fighting and fire alarm systems.
- Need for nursing home of private ward attached to the hospital.

There is scope for use of value-engineering techniques scientifically to reduce the costs without affecting the performance. The main advantages of value engineering are greater interaction between the user and the designer at the earliest stage, a better understanding of various aspects of the projects and the functional requirements, an open approach to meeting the requirements at minimum cost without sacrificing the function.

Value Engineering Principles

Once the preliminary information has been developed, the construction manager/contractor uses value engineering principles and works within the

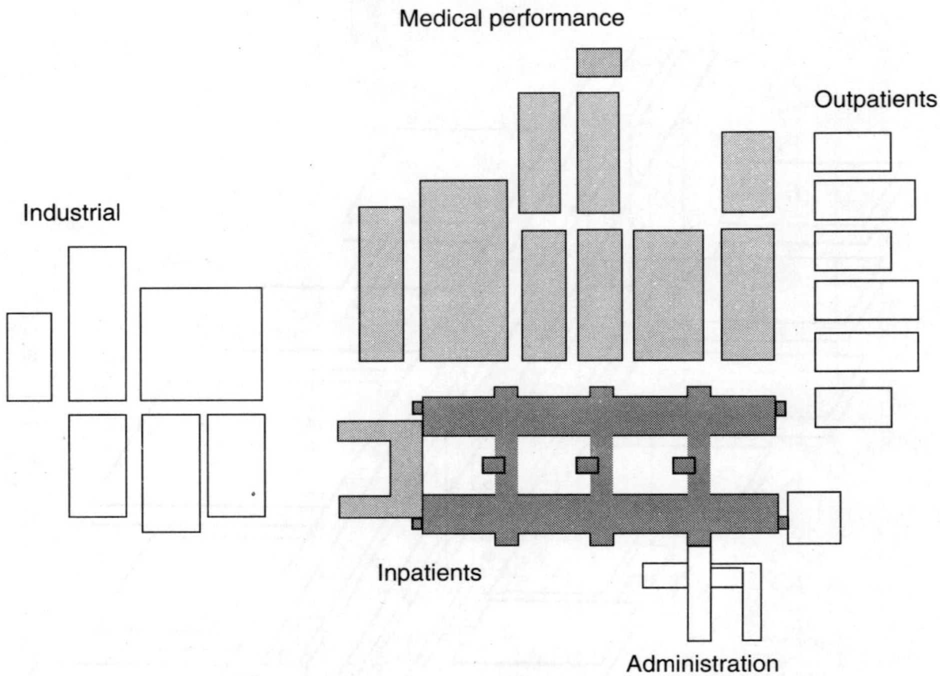

Fig. 21.3: Basic areas in a large hospital. Pütsep International

team to determine cost-effective solutions to the choice of equipment, systems, materials and construction methods. Primarily, this is the evaluation of life-cycle costs-the costs of design, precurement, installation, oerations, main tenance, and replacement over the entire projected use of the item.

The result of this process is that during the preliminary design stage, the team arrives at the most effective solutions for specific needs of the hospital. All the disciplines have cooperated in developing them, and the spirit of working together to achieve the owner's goals become the primary objective.

Identification of long lead items (elevators, special electric equipment) is part of the continuing development of a comprehensive project schedule which includes the events and activities to which the owner, the design professionals, suppliers, cognizant authorities, and the construction contractors are commited to achieve the owner's goals. This becomes a vital control document, expanding in detail as different aspects of the project are developed. Ideally, it will use the critical path method which can be more easily identified.

Preconstruction activity also needs to be monitoered and controlled.

Better value for money. The UK Best Buy hospitals cost two thirds the price of the average hositals being built at that time in Britain. The intention of the planners was not to aim at producing the best possible hospital, but while maintaining acceptable medical and nursing standars, to produce the best value for money: the bulk of the savings were made in medical planning. But important economies were made in every field. The reduction in on-coists (the percentage addition which has to be made to take account of pecularities of site, additional foundations, height allownace, air conditioning, etc.) at Best Buy hospitals was 50 percent.

Careful choice of site meant that the building could be contained in two storeys, courtyards

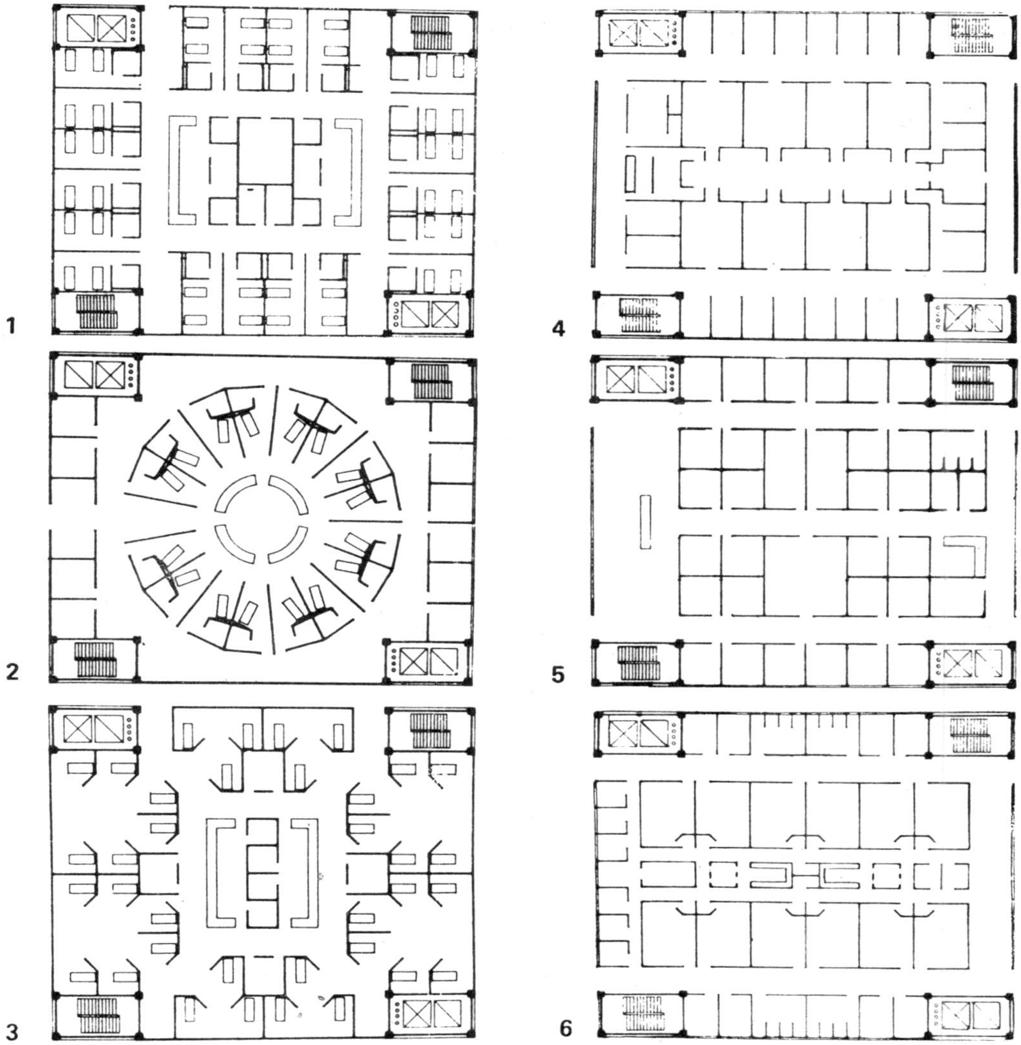

Fig. 21.4: CF Murphy Associates, Chicago, believe that a uniform module of 813 m^2 (30.5 by 26.6 m) satisfies the spatial needs of various nursing units (1-3) as well as the needs in therapy and diagnostics (4-6)

provide natural light and ventilation. Communications—the corridors and ducts linking the departments together are reduced. Instead of a conventional Boiler House with its factory chimney, distributing steam to all parts of the hospital, small interconnection roof-top boiler houses are located near the centers of demand. Artificial ventilations is restricted to the clincial zone at the core of the hospital.

Estimates

All aspects of the project are analysed during design development for potential effects on overall cost, schedule and quality objectives.

Reliable preliminary cost estimates and planning are crucial in arranging project financing. An experienced contractor/construction manager is ideally suited to develop these preliminary data.

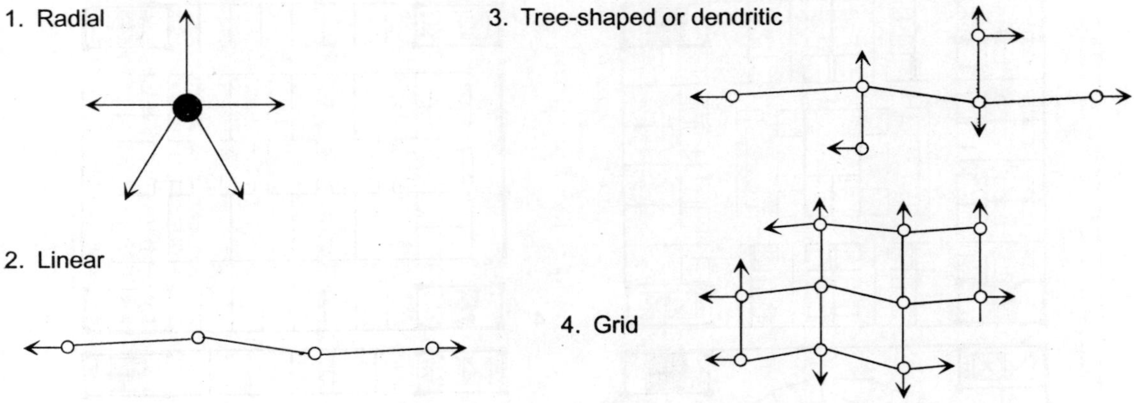

Fig. 21.5: Basic circulation patterns

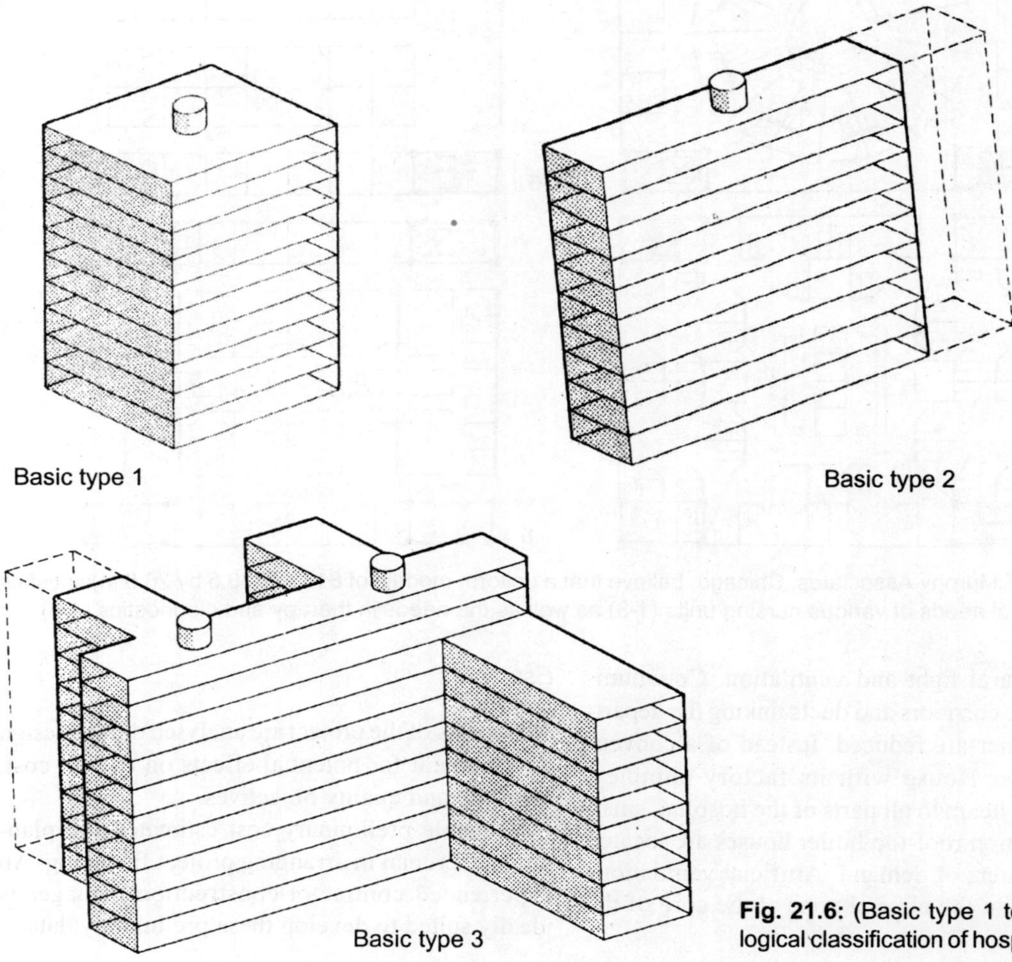

Fig. 21.6: (Basic type 1 to 3) Morphological classification of hospital buildings

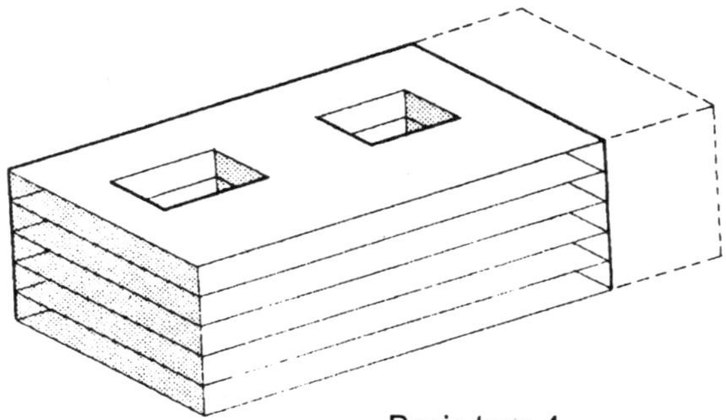

Basic type 4

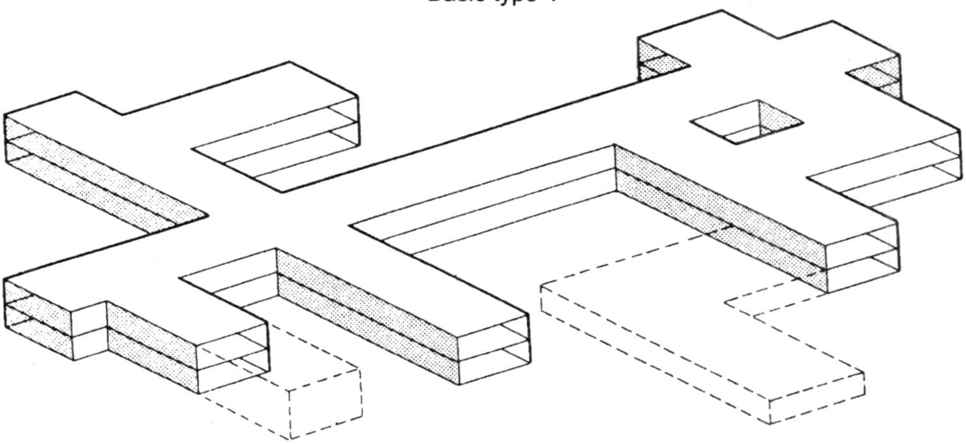

Basic type 5

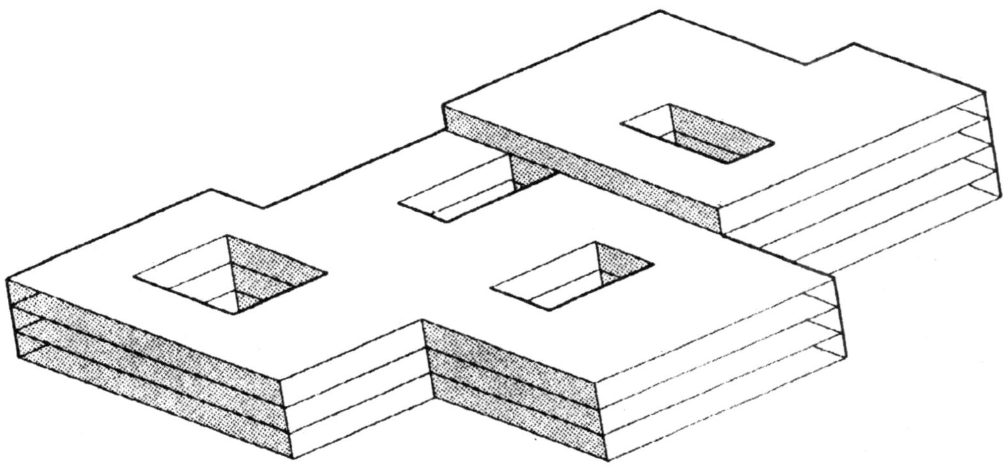

Basic type 6

Fig. 21.6: (Basic type 4 to 6) Morphological classification of hospital buildings

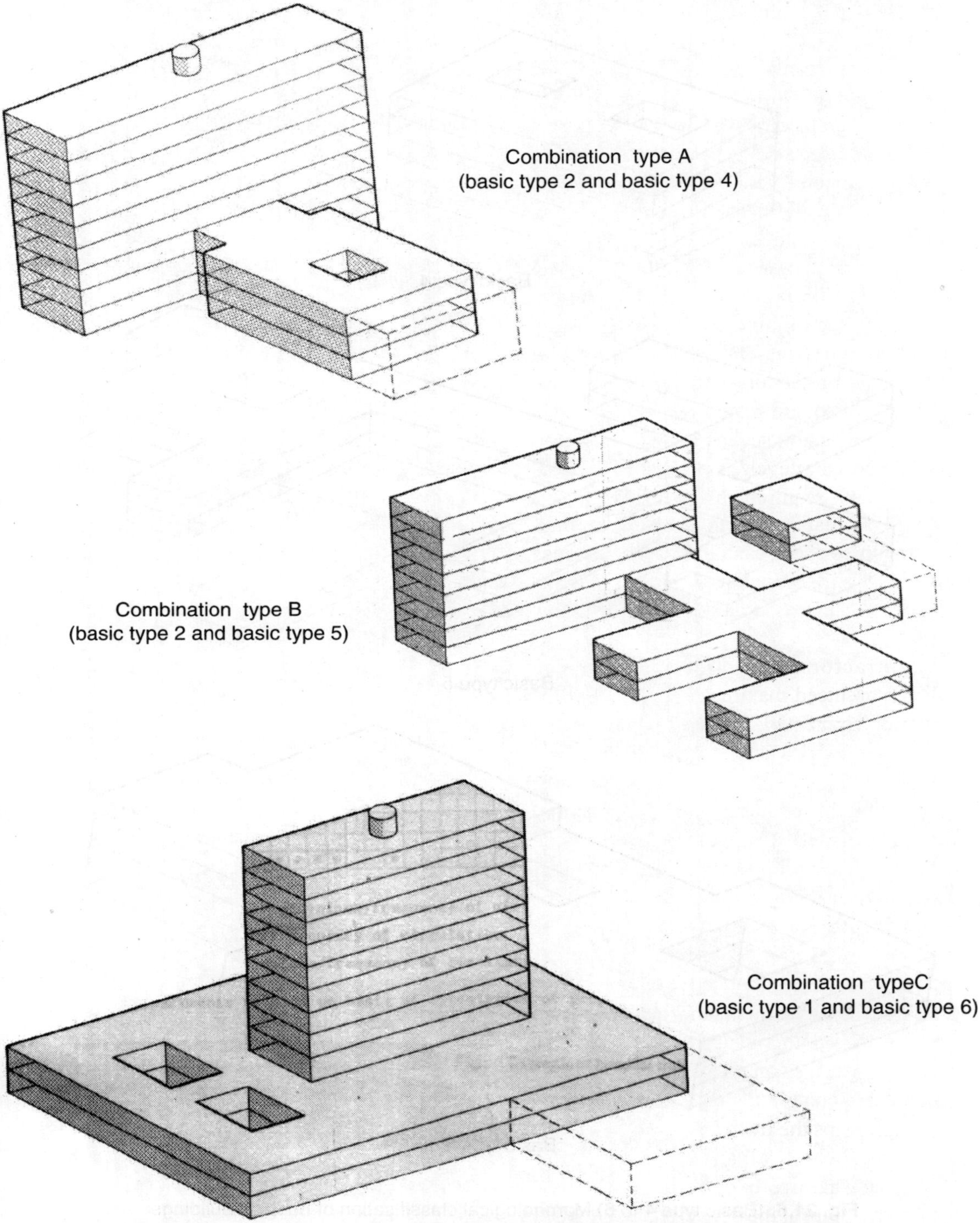

Fig. 21.6: (Combination type A to C) Morphological classification of hospital buildings

If engaged early enough, the contractor/construction manager will review the preliminary architectural documents and provide a realistic construction cost projection based on both functional and parameter estimates. A functional area estimate provides a projection of cost-by-space allocation in various hospital departments. A parameter estimate defines, in cost per square-meter, the actual building components.

To arrive at the parameter estimate, the project is divided into building elements; foundation, structural frame, plumbing, electrical, heating, airconditioning and so on. Thus, the hospital owner can get accurate projections of anticipated space use and cost per square meter. By analysing the design and construction sequence, the contractor/constuction manager develops preliminary schedules and cost-flow requirements.

The early availability of this reliable priliminary information on cost, cash flow, schedule, may help the owner finalise financial arrangements and overcome probblem associated with cash flow restrictions.

The contractor/costruction manager can establish a guarenteed maximum price before the final design is completed. Subject to the owner's agreement, site work can then commence. The planning, scheduling, field construction capability, and coordinating skill of an experienced contractor/construction manager is valnerable. His firsthand knowledge in dividing the work, minimising interference, providing solutions to problems resulting from changing field conditions, and managing complex projects are essential to the success of this approach. The result is completed revenue-earning facility several months earlier than would have been possible with the traditional approach. During the construction phase, the contractor assumes primary responsibility for completing the precurement and constructing it helps the owner develop a working relationship in whcih all disciplines become involved and all parties benefit by cooperation. Establishing the team at the begining of the facility project will be of great value in achieving cost savings and schedule improvements while maintaining quality objectives.

Approaches to Standardisation

The first approach is to produce standard plans (whole buildings). The second is to produce standard components (the bits and pieces). With a rapidly changing brief, uneven contours, irregular terrain and complex medical requirements, it is not difficult for a skilled designer to earn his fee producing a purpose-made hospital to solve a particular problem.

When standard designs are of evaluation and updating, the result is a highly efficient and statisfactory building.

The objective of good hospital design is to produce building that respond to the operational policy objectives stated by the initial users, but which are capable of subsequent modification to meet the needs of an unknown future. The application of building guidance, the judicious use of standard designs, and continuing programming of evaluation are excellent ways of achieving this aim.

Nucleus Hospital

One of the chief objectives of any form of standardisation is to achieve cost saving. In this respect, used in the right place and circumstances, Nucleus Hospital has provided to accomplish economy in capital and running costs without sacrificing acceptable clinical and service standards. By providing readily available data, nucleus also offers the best opportunity to cut down on the planning and design time. This leads to a reduction in the fees paid to consultants, and a reduction in the involvement of expensive project team personnel who otherwise will have to be engaged in repetitive and time-consuming meetings during the briefing stage. The advantages of nucleus are that more time and research have been put into the design of each department than would be possible with a one-off design. It does, however, require that the users' operational policy is fully thought-out, and tested for compatibility with both the whole hospital and departmental operational policies of nucleus. It is much easier to make an early assessment of site selection and development central plan options if the nucleus configuration is employed, as compared with the more time consuming early design studies on a non-standard basis.

Nucleus hospital is considered to be efficient in energy terms. In geometric assembly of cruciferm shaped templete and resulting courtryards maximises use of natural ventilation and daylight without compromising wall to floor ratio. The level of mechanical ventilation and air conditioning is kept to a minimum by judicious planning and by arranging for sanitary and storage accomdation transient areas and similar spaces to be deep planned however, possible.

Patient-focussed Hospital

Patient-focussed hospital is an approach that involves the new way of structuring the current structural arrangements of the conventional hospital in the areas of staffing, management and hospital design in order to provide cost-effective service, better patient care, to increase the staff time spent directly on patient care, to simplify job classification and management structure, to simplify planning and design and to reduce the capital and operating cost of the hospital. The major characteristics of patient-focussed hospital include:

- Patients are grouped according to care requirements (rather than clinical specialities).
- Decentralised and decompartmentalised diagnostic, treatment and support services.
- Operational units of 120 to 130 beds each with its own diagnostics, treatment and support facilities (in place of conventional 30 beds nursing units).
- Small care teams responsible for total patient care
- Multi-skilled staff in place of many specialist practitioners
- A flat management organisation
- Utlisation of available medical and information technology

The decentralised hospital is used on the new user-friendly technology which allows the training of multiskilled staff with a corresponding reduction in the number of specialist job titles. From the patient point of view the advantages are more personalised beside care and from staff point of view more effective control and responsiveness to patient care and consiquent heightened job satisfaction.

Adoptable Hospital Architecture

The needs for functional and/or technical changes in hospitals are not frequent. It is believed that within 10 years only 1 to 2 percent of the hospital areas require a technical re-equipping or shifting of functions.

A functional administrative grouping localities within a health care facility may remain wholly acceptable upto 20 years.

More or less sophisticated systems of movable partitions for room size and function flexibility and interstitial engineering floors for exchange and growth of engineering service.

The movable partitions in hospitals are regarded as essence of new architecture. There are movable furniture and wall partitions which are part of the system of modular seamless plastic containers, frames, carts, panels and rails. All space is considered capable of housing any activity until specialised equipment is moved to create a tailor-made environment. The use of movable panels and panel-hung work surfaces may enable to dispense with most fixed case work and achieve an anonymity in various rooms.

The interstitial spaces are for the mechanical discipline and can accomodate air handling equipment; transformer room; plumbing; fire stand pipe; domestic hot and cold water; acid waste piping; vacuum for cleaning, medical vacuum high and low pressure compressed air: oxygen, nitrous

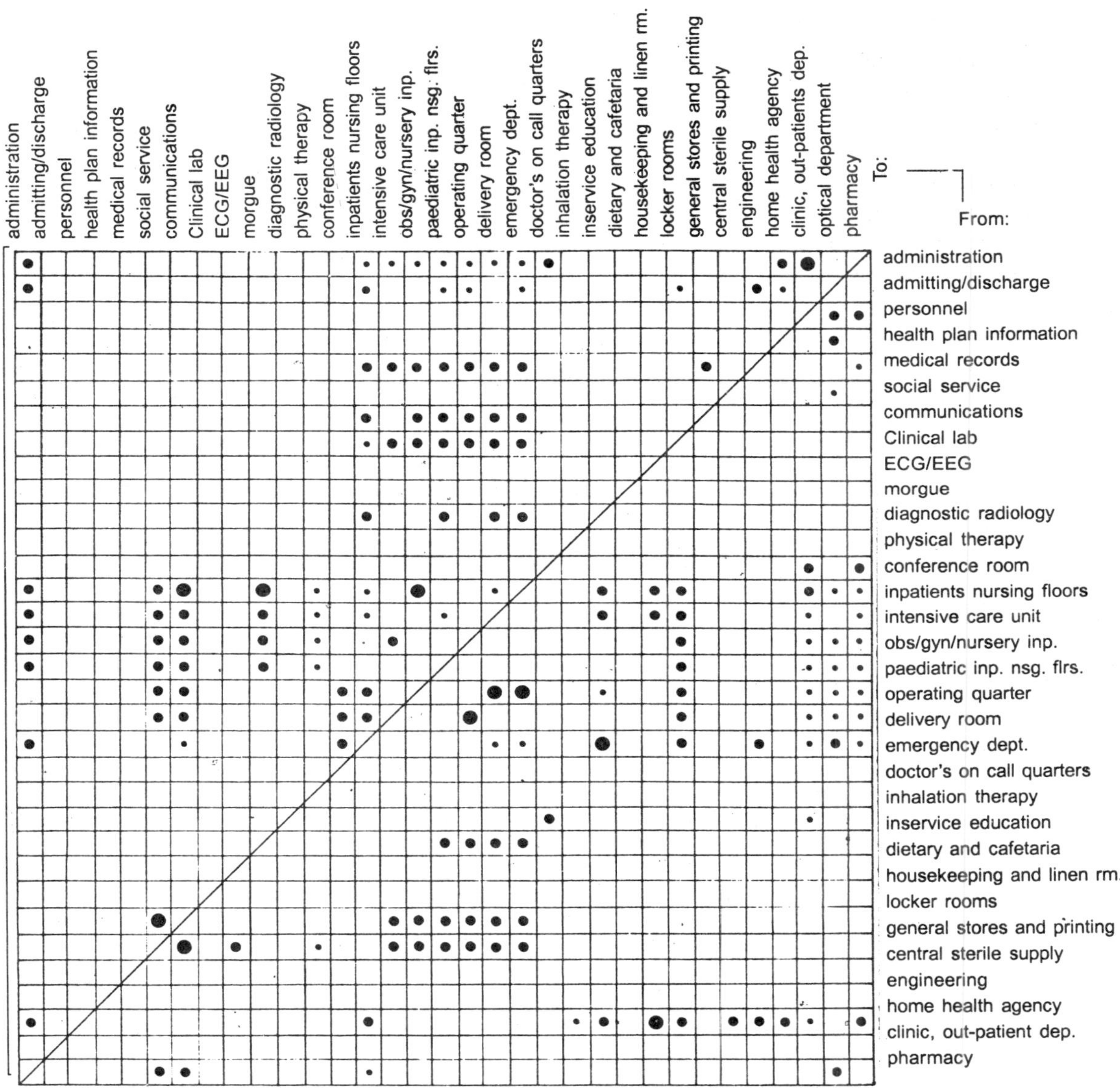

- Extremely high volume/frequency of circulation
- High volume/frequency of circulation
- Important volume/frequency of circulation

Departments related on basis of circulation of people, goods and/or information

Fig. 21.7: Example of hospital traffic matrix

oxide and natural gas pneumatic chutes for moving sealed bags of trash and soiled laundry to disposal areas: film and document conveyors, and other distribution systems. Upto 30 m long interstitial trusses to permit widespread columns have been used in connection with interstitial floors.

Other Techniques

Planners should be familiar with new techniques in hospital architecture such as:

- The computer design for similar health facilities,
- The "fast tract" system for initiating construction before design is complete (to prevent increased construction costs from inflation),
- The use of traffic models for hospital design, and
- The use of flexible designs with open options for expansion or change of facilities.

Planners must build for the future, not the past, anticipating worldwide trends, such as urbanisation, and plan for facilities to meet these major trends.

FURTHER READING

1. District Hospitals: Guideline for Development. WHO Regional Publications, Western Pacific Series No.4, 1992.
2. Ervin Putsep: Modern Hospital: International Planning Practices, Llyord-Luke Ltd., Londong, 1979.

22 Future Trends

INTRODUCTION

The role of the hospital has changed dramatically over the last two centuries. In the beginning the hospitals were mainly associated with death. The aim was to isolate the sick and to protect the healthy from infection. By the nineteenth century-with the development of anesthetic, and antiseptics—the idea that hospitals were about life, care and cure began to dawn.

The practice of medicine and surgery have manifestly made an impact on the layout and design of hospitals. However, the corollary is also true that hospital design affects the way medicine, surgery and nursing care is conducted. Buildings are occasionally modified to reflect a new device, technique or practice, but, once in a greatwhile, dramatic changes in health care delivery force major changes on the design of hospitals. We are currently on the threshold of such a change in the management of health care and this will render all hospitals of today, even those on the drawing board, obsolete.

Four major events have occurred to bring about this dramatic change in the delivery of health care:

- Economic and evolving payment mechanisms for health care.
- The explosive development in the knowledge base of the basic sciences upon which medicine rests
- Rapid advances in medical technology
- The increased sophistication, knowledge and behaviour of patients.

There are a number of change factors that will have a significant impact on the provision of health facilities in future such as: biotechnology; information technology; medical technology; consumer expectations; and new diseases. The likely impact of these change factors can be explored at the level of individual hospital departments, for example inpatient wards, hospital level or local district health authority level. The extent of change created by these factors, and the time scale over which changes will occur are uncertain. Nevertheless, it is possible to identify key issues at each of the three levels that should be considered now if health services are to develop in a way that will respond to future needs:

- Individual departments-inpatient wards
- Changing patterns of demand
- Changing patterns of care
- Reallocation of space to meet changing needs
- New objectives for ward design.

Whole Hospital

- Decentralisation of some services into the community
- Shift from inpatient to day-patient care
- Organisation of services around specialist equipment/expertise
- Shift to high-technology, short-stay, high-dependency inpatient care.
- Effect of information technology of hospital layout.

District Level

- Shift from acute hospital care to acute care in the community/primary care/self care.
- New models for acute care in the community.
- Enhanced role for general medical practitioners.

The change factors operating inpatient wards will change patterns of demand and care, and the pressure for re-allocation of space that these changes are likely to generate. As more procedures are undertaken on a day basis and as a result of developments in medical technology, inpatients in the future will be predominantly in the high-dependency category. This will create an increased need for continuous monitoring by a variety of monitors at the bedside and the staff base.

Bedside Tests

Developments in biotechnology and information technology will result in more tests being carried out and interpreted at the bedside. Test results and other monitoring information may be recorded at the bedside using hand-held terminals for later transfer of information into electronically-held patients' records.

These changing patterns of demand and health care will create a need for bed spaces larger than those currently provided but perhaps varying from patient to patient, depending on the equipment in use. Therefore, an arrangement, more like that of intensive therapy units at present, with movable screens rather than fixed curtains may be appropriate.

Larger bed spaces means fewer beds in a multi-bed bay and therefore a reduction in the overall size of a ward. This overall reduction in acute bed capacity might, to some extent, be offset by increased throughput arising from early discharge of patient's home or, more likely, into acute care beds in the community.

A variety of factors may create an increased future demand on wards for single rooms with integral bathroom facilities, including for example, care of patients with HIV infection and aids and increased consumer expectations. It may not always be easy to adapt existing wards to provide more single rooms without moving other functions into internal spaces without daylight.

Some modern hospitals in the UK currently provide centralized treatment facilities for use by inpatients as well as day and outpatients, instead of local treatment facilities on each ward. In future, with predominantly high-dependency patients on acute wards, centralized treatment provision will become less appropriate. Treatment space will, therefore, have to be provided on wards though not necessarily for all specialties.

Observation by Machine

If almost all patients in a ward are highly dependent the need for dayrooms for use by inpatients will be reduced. It may be more appropriate to provide sitting space within each multibed bay. At the same time, there may be an increased need for sitting and overnight stay facilities for relatives either in or close to a ward or group of wards. A ward containing all high-dependency patients may be more stressful environment for staff, creating a need for a restroom on the ward for staff to withdraw to, but in reach of the bed areas.

Modern ward designs are based on a series of planning principles. One principle that has had a significant effect on the overall shape and layout of modern wards is the need to provide good observation of patients, especially high-dependency patients, by nursing staff. This has led to ward designs that groups both single rooms and multibed bays around the nurse base for ease of observation. In future, increased need or preference for single rooms,more sophisticated monitoring equipment, continuing financial pressures, and so on, could lead to a more depersonalized style of inpatient care in which the emphasis shifts from direct nurse observation to monitoring and observation by machine. This pattern is already the norm in other cultures. Some existing ward designs may be easier to adapt than others. Future ward designs will need to be based on a different set of principles to reflect these changed requirements.

Decentralisation

At whole hospital level, a major focus will be the decentralisation of a variety of routine procedures and investigations and some acute inpatient care, to acute care facilities in the community. This emphasis on keeping out of an acute district general hospital whatever could be done effectiely and perhaps more safely elsewhere, will have a significant effect on services remaining in the district general hospital. Effects would include.

- A reduced outpatint department, specialised outpatient services including those for peopole with HIV infections would remain in the hospital
- A significant increase in the number of surigcal and endoscopic procedures that can be carried out on a day-basis will be created by developments in medical technology. Space no longer required for outpatients could, for example be used as an expanded day surgery, investigation and treatment suite. Treatment for inpatients would, in future, be carried out at ward level.
- Reduced casual patient workload in the accident and emergency department on the basis of drop-in casualty provision in the community.
- Reduced demand for routine X-ray, the spare capacity generated being absorbed by increase in interventional radiology for treatment purposes.
- Increased use of information technology meaning that some departments no longer need to be located adjacent to each other. For example, the medical records department could be relocated elsewhere in the hospital away from patient areas.
- Increased sophistication and use of diagnositic and monitoring kits, bringing about a reduction in routine labartory tests. Current pathology space provision may be overgenerous in relation to future needs. Future options for some pathology services include privatisation or provision on a regional basis.
- Any spare space created by the above changes could provide an opportunity to develop income-generating schemes, for example health screening, shopping facilities, health promotion activities and staff recreational activities.

Acute medical/surgical wards will be used intensively essentially for high-dependency patients with early discharge home or to acute care facilities in the community.

In parallel with increase in day surgery and in non-invasie procedures, there may also be an increase in major surgery procedures such as transplant/spare part surgery. This, in turn, could lead to an increased requireent for intensive care and to an expansion of the intensive therapy unit.

The implications of the changes for acute care that will need to be provided in the community are:

- Provision of more localised outpatient and casualty services.
- Decentralisation of routine tests, investigations and procedures.
- Provision of acute psychiatric services off the district general hospital site.

Focusing first on primary health care, it is clear that developments in both biotechnology and information technology will create the possibility of a considerably enhanced role for general medical practitioners (GPs), enabling them to diagnose, monitor and treat a wilder range of conditions than at present.

This, in turn, could result in a significant reduction in routine pathology workload, in fewer referrals to outpatient clinics and in fewer referrals for tests and investigations that have negative outcome. This enhanced role is dependent on the increased use of biosensors for testing purposes, the provision of computers for GPs, and the linking of these computers to hospital information systems, to expert systems and to outside databases.

Consumer Choice

These developments should also facilitate early discharge of patients from hospital, by providing GPs with immediate access to information on which to plan any necessary follow-up care and support.

These developments will require a long-term strategy for the future provision and improvement of primary care premises in a district. This may involve a combination of improving existing premises, relocating premises of provision of primary care facilities in conjunction with other community health facilities. Funding, incentives and training of GPs to carry out this enhanced role will also need to be addressed. It will also be necessary to co-ordinate more closely the planning of primary and secondary health care service and facilities.

From the consumers' viewpoint, there is likely to be an increasing emphasis on consumer choice and on the quality of services provided. This covers where services are provided (their location and accessibility), when services are provided (speed and timing) and the quality of the health care environment. The aim should be to keep people out of hospitals as far as possible and to provide more locally accessible services to cater to a wider range of acute health care needs than at present.

This examination of future changes in acute hospital care and primary care still leaves a gap that may require a new model of acute care in the community more appropriate for the health care needs of the twenty-first century. To fill this gap and to respond to the health care shifts outlined, the development of Community Health Units (CHU) has been suggested. It is envisaged that each CHU would serve geographical patch of 50-70,000 people. It would be a major focus for acute health care and health promotion in the area served, providing locally accessible services in a domestic environment and aiming to keep consumers out of more specialised district general hospital services as far as possible.

A CHU might provide the following range of services:

- Approximately 30-60 beds for medium/low dependency, convalescent, respite, terminal care
- Day hospital facilities
- Occupational therapy and physiotherapy
- Limited radiology service
- Outpatient and community health clinics
- Drop-in casualty service
- Minor operations and investigation service
- GP practice premises, and
- Base for neighbourhood nurses and community mental health professionals.

The range and mix of services offered by a particular CHU would reflect the particular needs of the geographical population served and would vary in detail from one to another. The CHU would be a new model of acute care in the community, providing a wide range of services to a wide range of consumers, It calls for innvoations in service organisation, in who is responsible for them and in how these services are integrated with each other, with other primary and community services and with secondary district general hospital services.

The choice of sites for CHUs should take into account not only their size, availability and cost of acquisition but also the accessibility of these sites to the population served. A facility close to where people shop, for example,may be as accessible as one close to where people live. Development of suitable site on a planning gain basis could also be considered.

The hospital of the future may not look very different from hospitals of today but what goes on inside it and where activities occur may be different.

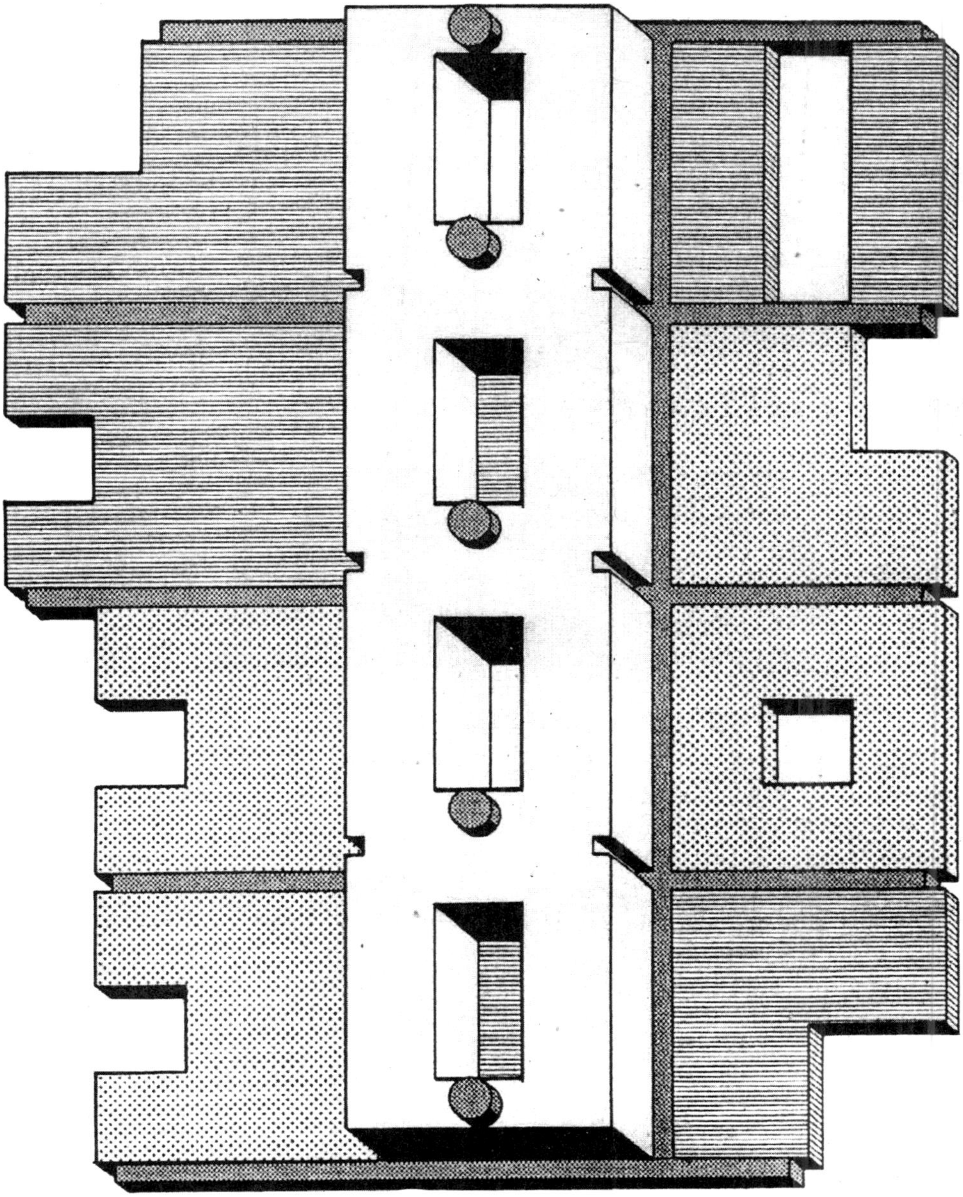

Fig. 22.1: Model hospital development plan (Generic model for a Low-rise 450 bed hospital)

To prepare for the future, it is necessary to consider the many different factors that will help to shape it and to plan facilities accordingly.

FURTHER READING

1. Rawlison C: A hospital for the future. Hospital Managment International IHF, London, 1989.

Recent Trends

23 The Hospital of Tomorrow

INTRODUCTION

Emerging trends in science and technology are likely to have a strong influence on the health care delivery system.

Breakthroughs in basic sciences including molecular biology, evidence based medicine, outcome of interventions, health services research, healthcare financing, demographic and epidemiological pressures, quality of care, consumerism information superhighway and value for money will transform the medical care in the future

Planning must become integrated in the health environment permitting coordination between hospital and non-hospital sectors, and between primary, secondary and tertiary health care. The different phases of planning are:

First Phase

Definition of needs and objectives. This phase comprises several stages of analysis.

Review of Current Strategy and of the Hospital's Image

In particular, this includes a review of goals and results, of sources projected and those actually used, and of the tasks assigned to the hospital.

Analysis of the Environment (Threats and Opportunities)

Some useful indicators are:

Current and foreseeable morbidity, incidence and prevalence rates, severity and type of emergency, methods of management of emergencies, etc.

Characteristics of the Beneficiaries

Demographic Age pyramid, extent of dependence of old people, of young people; birth rates, mortality rates (by age group, specific mortality by cause of disease, etc); natural growth rate, etc.

Socio-economic Mean income, poverty rate, unemployment rate, savings rate, patterns of consumption of house holds, literacy rate, educational levels, possible sources of information, etc.

Geographical Actual and optimum sitting of the health care system, present and future; catchment area of the hospital; specific location of various risk populations; means of access to the hospital; town planning constraints, etc.

Psychosocial Attitudes of the general public towards disease, death, welfare facilities for the handicapped, the dying (do people die in hospital or in the family setting), old people, etc.

Institutional factors

- Existence (or otherwise) of comparable care structures, location, size, share and type of specialist practice, competing sectors, forms of funding, etc.
- Existence of a health care service run by professionals or paraprofessionals, method of practice (alone or as a group, specialist or otherwise), form of remuneration.
- Health insurance scheme, rules governing professional practice (legislation regulations, customs), amounts and types of resources available, and local/regional economy.

Analysis of Organization (Strengths and Weaknesses)

In the analysis of organization, the following headings can be developed taking into account the strengths (centres of excellence, reputation of the hospital, promising sectors, etc) and weaknesses (sectors experiencing change of uncertain outcome, "pockets" of underproductivity, etc.).

Professionals and paraprofessionals: Age, Sex data of qualification or data of entry into the establishment, forms of continuous training, distribution by speciality, the various occupations, adaptability, geographical location of workplace, density by sector, etc.

Health care units: Number of beds, with breakdown by short-term, medium-term and long-term stays, by speciality and by disease; number of hospital bed days, bed occupancy rate, number or admissions (or discharges), re-admission (more or less long-term), mean length of stay, analysis of very long stays (over 30 days for example) or very short stays (less than 24 hours, except for day hospitals), turnover rate (mean period for which a bed remains unoccupied between a discharge and an admission), Patient renewal rate (number of new patients) by care sector, catchment areas of the different health care sectors, relationship between the potential for service delivery and the services actually delivered; number of outpatient clinics, with details of their staff and their resources; existence of non-traditional hospital sectors (day hospital, etc); dispensary activity, involvement in domiciliary care.

Technical Facilities

These are becoming increasingly important, Equipment present, quantity, age, working condition, utilization rate, intermediate supplies required for its operation, distribution by sector (imaging, biology); turnover rate of equipment, ratio between operating budget and capital investment budge, qualifications of staff using equipment, opportunities for training in new techniques, maintenance problems, amount of supplementary tests performed outside the facility, and types of such tests, means of communication with the patient-care units, etc.

Service Facilities

Logistic and general services: quality of accommodation, number and quality of meals, hygienes circuits (separate circuits for wastes, treatment of contaminated wastes, etc.), use of linen, disposable items, stock levels and stock management (food miscellaneous items, drugs), delivery periods for orders, location of the various stores, distribution of the various stores, procedures for communication with users, for distribution of drugs, existence of a central store; need for heating, lighting, to run operating theatres, types of energy used and feasible, etc.

Which of these activities need to be developed, concentrated, decentralized, contracted out?

Possible integration with the training, research and health education sectors; existence of a school of nursing, school for health workers, continuous postgraduate training, etc.

Evaluation of Challenges and Definition of Objectives

The preceding analyses can be used to identify and evaluate the major challenges for the period covered by the plan and to define objectives adapted to those challenges in the light of the cultural environment, the image and major areas of activity of the hospital concerned.

Second Phase

Formulation of the master plan Following the definition of the objectives, the resources, their location in time and space, starting from what already exists and knowing what is wanted, we arrive at what is possible, defined in terms of capital investment and operation. In the awareness that for every dollar spent on capital investment another dollar will need to be spent on operation every two or three years. This phase follows several stages: formulation of options and choices, which are looked at in the light of the expectations of those taking action and in terms of responsibilities towards society, and arriving finally at the refinement of strategic choices, on the basis of the dialogue between the various partners, by identifying a certain number of consensus objectives.

Third Phase

Defining the pathway This phase is concerned with defining the pathway from what already exists to what is desirable and possible, which means specifically:

- Defining the priorities for the plan and selecting the genuine emergencies that need to be dealt with rapidly, establishing an order of precedence for the various operations (e.g. there is no point in repairing an out-dated department that needs to be rebuilt); and
- Incorporating the constraints of feasibility (in the context of renovation it must be borne in mind that the hospital can be "moved" but must not close) and the financial constraints.

COMPONENTS OF A HOSPITAL STRATEGY

The various ideas on the future of the hospital and its components include:

- Hospital users
- Demographic Factors
- The drop in the birth rate

This concerns all countries to a varying extent. In Eastern and Western Europe and in North America, it takes the form (with a few exceptions) of a population decrease (total fertility rates below 2). The number of births will remain almost identical or will decrease. The marked decline in infant mortality is largely over, and each pregnancy is now a "wanted" pregnancy with a heavy demand for medical care and safety.

In most other parts of the world, especially in Africa and the Middle East, birth rates are falling because of wider spacing of births, but are still high (total fertility rates higher than 4). Because of the structure of the age pyramid, the number of births will continue to show a sharp increase.

Infant mortality rates are tending to fall and simple preventive measures (tetanus prevention, nutrition education, etc) can still be highly effective.

Ageing of the Population

While it is proportionally higher and of longer duration in Europe, the USA or Japan, it also affects most of the developing countries which will see increase (in absolute numbers) in age groups that are now often almost non-existent: the over 60s and the over-75s. This irregular increase between countries and between regions needs to be assessed in the light of the demographic indicators.

The relative importance of the very old (the over-80) also depends on sociocultural factors, but it must be noted that the greater the increase in the number of very old people, the more these people tend to be poor and isolated.

Internal Migrations

Such migrations within a country follow two patterns:

- Continued urbanization through drift from the land
- Trend towards special zoing of towns, breaking with the traditional mix of activities and populations whereby poor or very poor housing areas, either in the city centre (North American model, Cf. Chicago) or at the fringe (slumns or shanty towns as in Latin America, Africa, Asia), are separated from rich residential areas in the city centre (Cf. Paris) or in

certain neighbourhoods (cf. Lima). Moreover, the area of large cities is tending to increase sharply everywhere.

External Migration

Migration to another country has little influence on the demography of the country of origin. On the other hand, whatever the policies applied to curb the flow of migration by the receiving countries, immigration continues to take place, bringing with it the specific problems of migrants.

Morbidity

Certain overall changes are taking place:

Reduction of accidents Accident rates of all kinds (road, occupational, domestic), at any rate in most of the industrialized countries.

Reduction in cardiovascular diseases While these remain the leading cause of death in the industrialised countries, there is a downward trend on account of changes in lifestyle (diet, etc) and prevention. In these countries, there is a possibility of over-capacity for heart transplants and coronary surgery, but undercapacity for the fitting of pacemakers. The developing countries, have the double burden alongside the "traditional" types of diseases (infectious, parasitic, etc) the so-called disease of affluence (cardiovascular, tobacco-induced, etc.) are on the increase.

Later onset of disease of old age Although the symptoms of old age will appear later, very old age will become an increasingly heavy burden because the number of people reaching it will be larger. The average age of dependent persons will therefore increase. Even so, life expectancy will hardly rise at all (78 years for women, 70 years for men) and the age at death will probably not increase.

The hospitals can therefore expect a substantial growth of every day care for 60 to 80 year-olds (care that will increasingly resemble care for the working population) and of specific care for the very old (senile dementia).

The workload that old people will represent for the hospitals will depend upon the following:

- To some extent on their number which will certainly be high;
- To a great extent on society's attitude towards them, on the resources for accommodation or home help, and on the efforts made to develop their independence and to shorten the present waiting lists.

The diseases whose treatment requires the most resources Everything will depend on progress in medicine with the decrease in other causes of death, more and more cancers will appear and their detection will progressively improve until the day when they can be prevented.

The infectious diseases are likely to increase, together with their short-term and long-term consequences. We must expect the appearance of new, hitherto unknown viruses, as occurred with AIDS. The rate of increase of the disease will slow down for three reasons!

The AIDS/HIV infection will spread more slowly among heterosexuals. Uptil now, it has mainly affected homosexuals, hemophiliacs and drug addicts. The conditions for spread among these groups (number of partners, injections) were particularly favourable.

The increase in cases will follow a logistic curve, not an exponential curve. These forecasts show that the hospitals will need to have enough flexibility to be able to adapt to severe epidemics, the consequences of which will be felt in the fairly short term (5-10 years).

Although these diseases are very expensive, their individual weight is limited, No disease accounts for more than 2 percent of total expenditure cancers as a whole represent 13 percent. In the long term, the structure of hospital morbidity changes will vary slowly and its influence on expenditure is moderate (except in the current case of AIDS).

The changes in morbidity will principally affect the way care is organized.

The Selective Clientele

In developed countries, income has little influence on the consumption of medical care. Educational level, on the other hand, divides patients into two groups. The better educated select their system of care. They give precedence to prevention, make more call on specialists than on general practitioners, and keep hospitalization for acute and serious diseases. The less educated consult general practitioners and call very readily upon the hospital. There is therefore a selective clientele and there are passive users. The difference between the expectations and demands of these two groups of patients will increase.

New Expectations of the Selective Clientele

These are the clients with a high level of education who have developed new forms of behaviour. The middle class is diversifying; it is becoming structured in networks, where everyone is looking for personal growth. Individuals will need opportunities for personal expression, warm and trusting relationships, and will need to find their way within an increasingly complex system of relationships. "Health" shares priority among their concerns with education and the family but the needs will change. It will no longer just be matter of "repairing" observed damage. This clientele will demand.

Everything that will permit a "normal" family, occupational and cultural life, areas where advance in genetics, biology and minimization of equipment will bring supply closer to demand. The later onset of senility will increase the number of repairable disabilities; cataracts, hearing defects, hip fractures rehumatism, etc. There will be an increase in the number of prostheses and in surgery to "keep the body in working order".

Rapid and effective care. Society as a whole is becoming more professional. Advance in medical technology and information provided by the media will increase the demands. In particular, people will want to evaluate the results. Well-informed patients will want to choose their surgeon and their hospital on the basis of past performance. They will want to be treated quickly and well, to keep their stay in hospital as short as possible and not waste their time there.

Only specialist departments, which confer a high status on the patient, can hope to meet these expectations. Hospital departments also need to improve their relations with patients who are still denied information about their condition and their treatment.

A wide gap could form between these new expectations and the patient's actual experience in many cases. The public hospital is in great danger of losing some of these patients, who are becoming clients of other health facilities, and its respective share could fall as a result.

The needs of "captive" users These are the casualty patients, the badly informed, the drug addicts, and many old people of slender means. Those who fall ill will not make the same demands for speed and professionalism. The professionals and para-professionals of non-hospital medicine.

Physicians and other health workers outside the hospital often make use of the hospital for diagnosis and more specialized therapy and for part of their continuous training. In the future their relationship with the hospital will be decisive factor.

If it is good, hospital and non-hospital doctors will complement each other, leading to rapid diagnosis, short hospital stays, and the spread of better care techniques.

If it is bad, the hospital and the non-hospital practitioners will be in competition with each other, depriving patients of the benefits of the quickest, simplest and most effective care.

Information technology will transform exchange of information and the methods of communication between general practitioners or specialists in private practice and the hospital departments. Patients referred to a more specialized level will no longer take a letter with them. The patient's file will be transferred from one microcomputer to another and feedback will follow the same route.

HOSPITAL STAFF

Recognition of the usefulness and efficacy of non-medical staff is essential. Here the management of human resources plays a central role.

Good relationships between nursing staff and medical staff, on professional matters but also in terms of communication and support, are needed in order to achieve care of satisfactory quality.

In all countries, patients treated in hospital are increasingly demanding more than goodquality medical and nursing care. They want to be treated as users and their satisfaction also depends on the quality of the accommodation, the catering, and the human relations between staff and patients and motivation of the staff. The hospital world is spilt into two.

Motivating organizational settings This is the world of specialist departments, intensive care, fighting for patient's lives, research, children, cancer patients, transplants, etc. The organization complies with a scientific logic. The staff can take action. There is a belief in the ability to care and to cure. The results can be measured and can be improved. The staff are motivated despite being under stress. Interest in the work is high. The authority of the head of department is backed up by his medical skills and is exercised in units of human size. This is also the world of clinical research.

Demotivating organizational settings This is often the world of general medicine departments, emergency, long-stay patients. The logic is more humanistic. The objectives are poorly defined, hence not measurable. The organizational structure, inherited from the days when the hospital was a place of shelter, is no longer in keeping with users' needs. The real problems are not faced up to; death, pain, distress. Whose task is it to disclose them? should the patient know? The staff are often demotivated and are given little responsibility in over large departments. The overall result depends on the moral presence and involvement of the head of department. There is an immense gap between the aspirations of the staff and their job satisfaction.

Strategic Options

Hospital staff distinguish three such options

- Improving collaboration with colleagues outside the hospital. These colleagues can no longer do without the hospital. It could well be easy to establish good relations with them; many of them were trained at the hospital, many of them work there part-time.

  Developing a personal and lasting relationship with them is one way of improving the quality of the care provided for the patient.
- Exercising control over the process of patient admission and discharge. Many patients receive no outpatient or community medical care. The hospital staff should help them to make the best possible use of very short hospital stays.
- Seeking ways to provide fresh motivation for non-specialist departments.

How can objectives and responsibilities be redefined, and how can performance indicators be created? What new units should be organized to meet the real needs of users? These non-specialist departments, in particular, need to be run on business lines. The evaluation of care should make a major contribution to motivating these services, for the quality of the care they provide is the "only" thing they have to offer, yet they are essential to the smooth running of the entire hospital.

Economic and Financial Environment

The factors of production are plentiful. The resources of high-quality trained manpower are constantly increasing in the industrialized countries and in the developing countries. The resources of energy and raw materials are plentiful (particularly on account of the growing importance of the tertiary sector of the economy, energy savings and the recycling of wastes).

A wave of technical progress is spreading (information technology, communications, biotechnologies, etc). and should become a vital factor via the industrial and geographical changes.

The Leisure Society

The job structure presents a major risk: society will split into two groups:

- An educated middle-class who use modern forms of communication (information technology, media, etc), have well-paid but often stressful jobs, and accept the economic logic of open frontiers.
- An excluded group who are left with insecure jobs, who are no longer protected against all risks by social security, and whose attitudes or living and housing conditions gradually alienate them.

These prospects concern all the industrialized countries and the developing countries. The United States of America and Sweden have made a start with job-sharing and income-sharing (drop in wages, part-time work).

Controlled privatization With economic activity having picked up in the early 1990s, the financial context becomes difficult but not enough to undermine the structure of social security. Because pensions, unemployment benefits and health expenditure are not regulated, they continue to increase faster than the revenues of the social insurance funds. The chronic dificit is made up from year to year by a creeping privatization that leads insidiously to "two level"security.

Creating a sense of responsibility No solution is found to the international financial crises. Growth has slowed right down, but society agrees to give upon adjustments and to reconstruct solidarity on a new basis:

- sharing of available jobs and corresponding income.
- productive use of spare time.
- definition of a "right to health "which is exercised through the free choice of a protection scheme. The poor are issued with a "health care voucher," people in employment pay part of the cost.

It cannot be predicted with any certainty what will happen in the next 20 years, but in practically all countries, whether developed or developing, the provision of totally free health care, entirely financed by the state or by community mechanisms, is being called into question, and ways of making individuals (partially) responsible and getting them to participate directly in financing their protection against disease are now being considered.

HEALTH EXPENDITURE

From 1960 to the late 1970s, hospitals in the industrialised countries were able to spend a great deal of money; they were expanded, modernized, equipped, humanised, made open to all. Three factors were conductive to this:

- They derived virtually all their resources from health insurance schemes (or other systems of collective funding);
- Economic growth was high (average of 5 percent up to 1974); and the income of health insurance and social security schemes was adjusted to expenditure each year.

These financing conditions were the factor that permitted the expansion of public hospitals. The volume of hospital expenditure increased each year by between 8 percent and more than 10 percent form 1960 to 1980.

This period now seems to be over. Hospitals, which account for 50-80 percent of health expenditure depending on the country, will see this share level off or decline.

Blind Rationing or a Budget Linked to Level of Medical Activity? Funding could be based on an identical annual rate of increase for all hospitals or on an indicator of medical activity. The latter system is applied in the United States of America, and various European countries are moving in the same direction (Portugal, United Kingdom). This system will make funding more flexible. Success will depend on the use made of the project for medical applications of informations systems and on the quality attained by the hospital information system, the key problem is the hospital management of tomorrow.

It is reasonable to suppose that the annual rates of increase will be in line with economic growth. The future will therefore be in striking contrast with the recent past.

Unregulated expenditure Fees are paid according to the procedure and reimbursed in the same way. International experience shows that none of the conventional regulating mechanisms have much effect on overall expenditure (proportion of cost paid by the insured, agreements fixing unit charges). The volume of consumption is continuing to increase everywhere, especially where the unit prices are controlled.

The health insurance systems Its expenditure, if left unchecked, increases faster than its income. What can it consider doing? There are four possible approaches:

- Restrict private hospitals to a total budget or a flat rate per patient depending on the diagnostic group to which the patient belongs. But the latter system does not solve the problems of appropriateness of medical treatment.
- Restrict the medical profession to a total budget for out-patient expenditure. This calls into question the fee for service and what we call liberal medicine.
- Negotiate with non-hospital practitioners a flat rate for expenditure per patient (as in the Republic of Germany).
- Allow the proportion paid by the patient to increase gradually and partly privatize non-hospital expenditure.

It takes about five years after the introduction of a new mechanism before the effect is felt.

Pressure of Medical Demography

In many countries the number of doctors will certainly increase. This raises two major questions:

Where will these new doctors set up their practices? Density varies widely from one region to another, so some areas are likely to reach a virtual saturation point.

Will density stimulate consumption? It will increase the proportion of specialists and practitioners of alternative medicine (acupuncturists, naturopathy, etc.) and the charging of fees in excess of the reimbursible limit, i.e. the privatized sector. But on the other hand, the more doctors there are, the less they will have to do. Consumption will not grow as fast as the number of doctors. However, a large body of private practitioners will be prepared to accept patients who used to be treated in hospital to the non-hospital sector seems to be already under way in countries (such as France) where a total budget has been set.

The New Needs

New needs will have to be satisfied: artifical procreation, organ transplants, compensation for the deficiencies of old age, etc,. These needs are shifting the borderline between medical demand and social demand and are liable to endanger the different types of collective funding of care: some categories of care would no longer be regarded as medical and would involve households in additional expenditure, if indeed they could afford such care at all.

Two quite different situations, are therefore, appearing:

- A dwindling market for the hospital, which virtually has to deal with only one buyer, the social security system. Free hospital care cannot be called into question if the hospital's mission does not change, because its clientele is not well off. Its resources will be rationed. Its only way out seems to be to exploit untapped resources of productivity.

- An increasing market for non-hospital medicine: increasing because it is expanding, diversifying and because patients expenditure will be covered by social security, by themselves or by their insurance,

These future prospects are throwing the organization of health care and the relationship between hospitals and non-hospital medicine into the melting pot. In an expanding market, it is the producer which offers the best quality/price ratio which should grow the fastest. This is true with or without the involvement of private insurance. Advances in productivity will play a central role. The public authorities might seek partners with whom they can renegotiate the outdate terms of financing (private hospitals, biomedical laboratories). This would mean the public hospitals losing some of their clientele.

The teaching hospitals might turn to the private sector to find more varied training grounds for students. This would mean the public hospitals losing resources associated with teaching.

Non-hospital practitioners might become associated with hospitals through interfaces that improve the arrangements for care (emergencies, local hospitals, networks of coordinated care). This would mean the hospitals losing a lot of bed days and perhaps admissions.

The contrast between a hospital sector whose traditional market is shrinking and a non-hospital medicine bursting free of the financial constraints of the post-crisis period could render obsolete the old contest between "public and private" and replace it with a new contest in which the best would win, regardless of its legal status. Here, the only way out for the public hospitals would be to become more professional and effective and to extend their services towards expanding "markets".

Productivity at the Hospital

Increasingly, productivity means improving the ratio between the quality produced and the factors of production used. In a hospital, this ratio is measured by:

- the improvement in the health status of patients; and
- the hospital resources used.

In the future, if financial resources increase by from 0 to 2.5% at constant Prices), increase in productivity will be the main means of engaging in new medical activities and keeping up with technical progress.

A clear and original view of the sources of producitivity is needed, perhaps based on the nature of hospital costs.

Variable Costs and Structural Costs

The variable costs are the tip of the iceberg: approximately 15 percent of the total, covering medical expenses, food, labour. They increase quickly (more than 5 percent per annum). These are the only costs that can be reduced in the short term. It would seem desirable to avoid certain types of wastage in medical examinations (duplication between hospital and non-hospital medicine) and to develop consensus on diagnostic and treatment strategies and on systems for assisting with medical decision-making.

The structural costs,which are fixed (85%), are mainly staff costs (70%). They comprise: general hospital departments, 27 percent of expenditure and 19 percent of staff, technical departments (where part of the variable costs arise: films, medical equipment, transfusions, etc) and medical departments for short-medium-term and long stays. The structural costs change more slowly, but it is here that progress in productivity lies in the long terms, through adaptation of the structure to needs.

In general hospital departments, analytical book keeping can be used to identify the cost prices, it is known that these cost prices (for meals, cubic metres heated, tonne of laundry washed) vary widely from one establishment to another and are often higher than those for comparable industrial or commercial establishments. The question then arises whether to transfer some functions not directly related to care to outside contractors.

In specialist medical departments the practitioners suggest the general application of less expensive formulas that cater for the needs more effectively. A day hospital costs only 40-50 percent as much for the same disease, while scheduled admissions always cost less than emergency admissions. The change has got off to a good start with domicilary care and above all with the day hospital, which between them account for one patient in nine (one admission in three).

Prevention and a sensible sharing of the market with non-hospital medicine would make it possible to reduce the number of patients and the severity of some cases.

Measures to reduce queuing times (for performing technical medical tests whose results are required for taking case management decisions) can reduce the period between admission and initiation of treatment.

The teaching of patients and their relatives has the same effect (such as " cooperative care" in the United States of America). Part of the responsibility for this is borne by the patients, associations, which at present are not sufficiently developed.

In order to exploit these untapped seams of productivity, there is a need for restructuring, for getting rid of some beds,for creating facilities for rapid diagnosis, for day care, for weekday care and for coordinating this action with non-hospital medicine.

In surgery, the approach is similar. It seems certain that competition with private hospitals will play a cardinal role and stimulate advances in productivity.

In internal medicine, some departments receive or keep between 20 and 40 percent of patients who do not belong there. Either they are awaiting admission to a specialist department or to a medium-stay or long-stay hospital, or they are admitted by the emergency department because there are no social structures to meet their needs. Advances in productivity will be achieved by converting a lot more "acute" or short-stay beds into medium-stay and above all long-stay beds and by reorganizing emergency departments.

Adjustment of work timetables Hospital tasks are now changing: they are more concentrated in the daytime, a trend that will become accentuated. Adjustments to timetables should make it possible to adapt staffing levels to the "peaks" and "lows" or day-time activity. Substantial increases in productivity will be possible. The development of part-time or "selected time" work is a step in this direction.

Advances in productivity can be expected in the short terms from the control of variable costs. However, most such advances will come in the long term from a restructuring of the pattern of care between hospital and non-hospital medicine, and within the hospitals themselves, whereby the means will be strictly adapted to the needs. Taking the available techniques into account, a substantial part of these advances will come from fresh thinking about the borderline between the hospital and non-hospital medicine and about transfers of responsibility from the hospital to ambulatory medicine of severely-ill patients.

FUTURE TRENDS

Hospital Activities

Hospital activities will become increasingly specialized and diversified. This is the historical trend. New specialities arise through the fragmentation of disciplines. For example, hematology has given rise to hematological oncology, immunohematology and the study of blood clotting disorders. The gynaecology/obstetrics of the post-war period that has been transformed in the last 15 years into gynaecological oncology, obstetrics fertility and assisted reproduction, and non-surgical gynaecology. Finally, pediatrics is splitting up into pediatric nephrology, pediatric oncology, pediatric dermatology and so on.

The specialists expect the traditional tasks of the hospitals principally curative, to be extended to certain aspects of prevention and information.

In the next 20 years, progress in molecular biology and genetic engineering will transform prevention, which will become based on the evaluation of risk factors and on a genuine predictive approach. Molecular genetics can already detect pseudohypertrophic muscular dystrophy, soon it will be able to detect cystic fibrosis of the pancrease, followed in the no-too-distant future by common polygenic diseases, "predisposing genes", the risk of cancers developing, etc. These discoveries will lead on to predictive medicine and to gene therapy. Here, highly specialized and expensive techniques are involved, which initially will not pay their way. Such techniques will be developed in research laboratories and-quite apart from the ethical problems. Before they can be made available to the population it will be necessary to integrate molecular biology with clinical hospital medicine, evaluate it, then provide training, and organize relations with industry, other disciplines and prevention agencies. The expansion of molecular biology and the attendant needs for training and evaluation could be very considerable indeed.

A passive hospital medicine is likely to devote all its resources to expensive equipment (surgery, transplants), whereas a simple effort to reduce the waiting periods for specialist departments would lighten its workload. An active hospital medicine could devote more resources to speeding up the transfer of laboratory technology to non-hospital medicine and to prevention, instead of the costly and complex present-day methods. This activity would be more effective and in the long term less expensive as well. Active hospital medicine ought to play a leading role in the two-way transfer of technologies, a role that could extend to providing information for the media and the general public. Failing that, every-day medical practice could fall a long way behind the optimum practice as defined by the rapid and widespread use of the best available technology. And this backwardness would be expensive. The hospital must continue to take part in developing therapeutic procedures.

The example of cancer is often mentioned, as an example of "terminal" care. It is known that some forms of care do not lengthen the survival period of patients. How should we confront this reality? Should we spend money on this kind of care? Is it up to doctors or society to take the decision?

Specialist Activities

Specialist activities will need to be rationalized. The rapid growth of genuine prevention, the increased efficacy of drugs and ways of distributing them, and the increase in less expensive facilities (day hospital) will to a very large extent, replace traditional hospitalization. A specialty is likely to be defined in future as a cohesive set of skills, human and technological resources, which if need be, can call upon accommodation and catering facilities, close-in terms of access and time-to technical facilities, and flexible enough to permit frequent regroupings. In this area, a large number of changes are foreseen.

Specialties could regroup or become increasingly interdependent for example, psychiatry, neurology, gerontology and internal medicine or again, pediatrics, obstetrics, neonatology and specialist surgery of the fetus. Less invasive cardiological and radiological procedures would increasingly replace the traditional heart surgery techniques.

A new kind of organization should make it possible to integrate the work of the horizontal disciplines; immunology, molecular biology, invasive radiology. The technical facilities will become more resources-intensive and specialized, and at the same time some miniaturized and less expensive equipment will make its appearance in the clinical departments. In automation will lead to a tremendous increase in biogenetics laboratories, which will be used to deal with polygenic diseases.

Rationalization should lead to the elimination of about two-thirds of specialist beds. The majority of beds in psychiatric hospitals will disappear in the next 20 years, to be replaced by a few psychiatric departments within polyvalent hospitals and by more open facilities such as day or night hospitals or half-way houses.

In pediatrics and common hematology, most of the present beds are expected to become unnecessary, In pneumology and cancerology, a large number of beds will also be eliminated.

Many common procedures in conventional radiology and functional explorations should be performed outside the hospital, at lower cost, more quickly, with no waiting. These changes should be accompanied by constant measurement and optimization of the quality of care.

New Tasks for the Hospital

The hospital ought to create friendly environments to cater for its clients who are not ill (those admitted for childbirth, preventive care, etc), improve its staff recruitment and update its image for chronic patients (psychiatry, long-stay) in order to motivate its staff. These "friendly environments" should halt the deterioration in relationships between the general public, the hospital staff and the hospital management. Some experts analyze them in terms of "image and product". They see them as a way to escape from the image of the hospital as a place of disease and death, a source of anxiety, and transform the hospital into creation, acute diseases in adulthood, aging and death. This approach already exists in the areas of pediatrics and maternity and ought to be applied more generally. The experts believe it is vital for the public hospital to change its image in this way.

The hospital may develop epidemiological statistics centres, which are a novelty and a necessity. The epidemiological approach will lead to a better understanding of the risk factors and subsequently to ad hoc preventive attitudes. It calls for rigorous method, trained staff, and data-processing facilities.

The hospital should have flexible outpatient departments. It might almost be said that these departments should no longer be used to fill hospital beds but to empty them. They should be highly specialized, organized on the principle of programmed examinations as in the day hospital, and should make specialist skills and technical facilities readily accessible. The running of outpatient departments will call for well-organized appointment systems.

The hospital could define diagnostic and therapeutic strategies. Evaluation of the efficacy and cost of new treatments will be essential. The spread of new strategies will be a necessity for hospitals. This will raise ethical problems, for in medicine it is difficult to reach a consensus on "a" strategy, which often remains valid only for a short time. Evaluation of protocols ought to make it possible to give preference to the strategies with the best cost-efficacy ration. Once defined, these strategies should be disseminated and their every-day application should be evaluated.

There is a need for flexibility—in human relations and information. Medical teaching and the assignment of practitioners to hospital duties should be organized in such a way as to be conducive to regroupings, multidisciplinary work and the spread of new ideas. Some aspects of medical studies ought very soon to be redesigned in this direction, which is essential for the future. Flexibility is needed in capital expenditure as well. Equipment also ought to be the source of flexible organization.

Maternity and Pediatrics

These two disciplines have undergone considerable modifications in recent years.

In the last 40 years, in most countries the maternity units of public hospitals have been modernized and have gained a reputation for quality. Far-reaching changes have been observed in pediatrics, involving a new kind of hospital organization that is better suited to the needs of paediatric patients'- consultation, functional exploration, daytime hospitalization substantial efforts have been made to make the children feel more at home—architectural adaptation, appropriate decoration, development of cultural and recreational activities. This should lead to better acceptance of the hospital by child and family. The future introduction of family accommodation in pediatric hospitals should still further strengthen the concept of "home at hospital"

Preventive approaches will become increasingly refined. With the general improvement in living standards, and with the availability of vaccinations and antibiotic therapy, activities to prevent infectious diseases will probably be carried out at an increasingly early stage. The prenatal diagnosis already performed in many situations will extend further as a result of technical progress, understanding of the mechanisms of genetic diseases, and the discovery of new early indicators of anomalies detectable in the gene or gene product. Prenatal diagnosis will be performed by non-invasive methods or methods that entail the least risk for the woman and the fetus. Detection of certain malformations by echography or by other imaging methods applied to study of the fetus will become widespread. Some forms of treatment *in utero* and some reparative surgical therapies (for congenital cardiopathies) and the application of complex techniques such as bone marrow transplants will be introduced. Molecular biology techniques applied to the diagnosis of genetic diseases, or even treatment of these diseases, by "gene transplants", will develop in the centres with the best design and technology. All these developments will call for multi-disciplinary approaches covering genetics, immunology, biology and modern imaging techniques. Some hospital maternity units and some pediatric departments will be designed, so that they can benefit from all these technologies that are a direct outcome of research.

Pediatric departments will devote the majority of their efforts to severe or complex diseases requiring increasingly precise care administered according to a strict protocol. These include cancers, infections with an immunological component, and genetic diseases not diagnosed during intra-uterine life or infancy. The therapies will generally be expensive, as in the case of marrow or organ transplants which will increase in number initially, then level off and diminish as prevention improves. New kinds of transplant can be expected in bone marrow transplants after manipulation of cells *in vitro* to permit the replacement of organs affected by malignant disease (leukemia and cancer), or genetic (stress diseases and hematological conditions) or acquired disorders (medullary aplasia). Uptil now, these organ transplants have rarely been performed on account of the difficulties in ensuring survival of the transplant.

This kind of highly specialized medicine will require a large number of doctors, multidiscplinary organization, and teamwork whereby general practitioners and specialists will work in harmony paying great attention to diagnostic and therapeutic requirements, to human relations with patients and their relatives, and to ethical issues.

Psychiatry and Gerontology

The psychiatric hospitals will complete the process of giving way to district pychiatric services, community-based services, etc.

In gerontology, the deterioration of physical and intellectual capacity is occurring later and later with each generation. Old people will become dependent at a greater age. The "risk population" will be the age group over 85 years, 20 percent of whom suffer from senile dementia. Fewer old people will be admitted to hospital, but those admitted will on average have more serious conditions. They will require specific case management, and will no longer be able to remain in departments for "acute" patients, as is still often the case. It will be necessary to train geriatricians, offer them career prospects and organize suitable structure in which facilities for diagnosis, intensive care, reduction, rehabilitation and long-term care are all present. In both these disciplines "friendly environments" of human dimension should avoid concentration, promote sociotherapy and the "real life" approach, initiate the return to independences, and encourage the use of the alternatives to the conventional hospital.

Pneumology

This is a fast-developing discipline. It is now much closer to cancerology, haematology, infectious diseases and clinical immunology.

Diseases on the Increase

Bronchial cancer is mainly associated with tobacco consumption. Its frequency doubles every twenty years. It will take forty years before the effects of any reduction in smoking are felt. Rationalized screening should make it possible to recognize cases earlier and increase the indications for surgery, which will long remain the most effective treatment. Chemotherapy will become more costly and resources-intensive. Active and/or selective immunotherapy could produce prolonged stabilisation of cases.

Severe pneumonopathies of immunodepressive origin (chemotherapy, AIDS) will increase dramatically.

Transplantations of both lungs and above all of one lung will increase substantially.

Conditions in Decline at the Hospital

Although asthma is on the increase among the population, patients will less often be admitted to hospital since their condition will be controlled outside by prophylactic drugs. Mortality could be greatly reduced through better education of doctors and patients and through more appropriate facilities for care.

With the reduction in smoking and in occupational exposure to pollutants, chronic bronchitis and emphysema should follow the same trend, with a re-education in the number of patients and less severe disease that can be attended to outside the hospital.

More effective screening for thromboembolic conditions, which are still a cause of death on account of late diagnosis, should reduce cases by half. The genetic defects that lead to them are beginning to become known. It can be expected that physicians will receive better training in diagnosis, in prevention, and in ten years time in the control of thrombolysis new structures

Pneumologists will work in three directions: cancerology and severe immunodepressive disorders; asthma and allergies; respiratory insufficiency and occupational diseases. Pneumology units should be linked with the units for neoplastic blood disorders, clinical immunology, infectious diseases and intensive care, one-third to one-half of conventional beds should disappear, as should pulmonary surgery as an independent and exclusive entity. Laboratories for exploratory function tests should largely be replaced, at lower cost, by automatic devices.

Neurology

Advances in neurosciences and molecular biology (particularly mapping of human genome is likely to transform the care and cure. Efforts are on to identify the genes and/or molecules responsible for many diseases. A preventive approach would then become possible.

Neurologists essentially treat five types of disease:

- Genetic diseases, which are rare. They will be detected *in utero* in near future and may be subsequently treated by genetic manipulation in this century. These possibilities will present serious ethical problems and treatment will be resource-intensive.

- Degenerative diseases—some will be given symptomatic treatment (Parkinson's disease), Others (Alzheimer's disease) will be improved within five to ten years. We may hope to know the causes by about the year 2010. The effect of any preventive techniques would not be felt for 30-40 years. Priority therefore needs to be given to developing symptomatic treatments.
- Inflammatory diseases of the nervous system (multiple sclerosis) could become preventable at the same time as the diseases just mentioned.
- Cerebrovascular accidents require resource-intensive emergency care followed by functional reduction. Hope lies in prevention and in the long-term treatment of atherosclerosis.
- Knowledge of cancer has been improved by widespread use of the scanner and of nuclear resonance imaging. But the therapeutic protocols are still resource-intensive and not very effective. Hope lies in selective chemotherapies. More specific treatments are expected within ten to twenty years.
- Hospital neurology will be resource-intensive, and confined to diagnosis or to treatment of short-lived acute phases. It offers possibilities for rationalization and for protocols well suited to the day or short-stay hospital. It will need to be practiced in continuity with care by the family or by the patient himself (associations, hotels). A heavy demand will develop for structured organization of post-hospital care (postgraduate teaching, secretarial services, communication with the hospital, etc). This demand could be met by external facilities or domiciliary care. Severely handicapped patients and their dependents require special skills (psychological attitude, availability, pressence). Hospital departments respond poorly to their needs.

To optimize the methods of care, it will be necessary to encourage close contact with geneticists, cardiologists and hematologists. Neurologists should be given the resources to practice rapid and resources-intensive medicine in areas where this has proved its efficacy. Finally, where medicine is powerless, places where the patient can live and be looked after until death should be created.

Specialist Surgery

The decision-making approach will in future lead to two types of protocol and should provide a better cost/efficacy ration

- Reparative surgery and symptomatic medicine for old people or those who cannot receive transplants; and
- Preparatory medicine followed by transplant for younger people.

In this scenario, a separation between medical and surgical departments would be regrettable. The trend should be towards a small number of departments dealing with one organ or several organs (kidney, liver, pancreas), which would include an internal medicine unit, a surgery unit and a bioimmunology unit.

Day-case surgery could develop substantially along the American lines (30 percent of operations). With this system the patient's family bears part of the cost of care. The prospects depend on the attitude of the medical professional and old people the public hospital receives, the less it will be able to develop this kind of surgery.

The future of organ transplants raises three questions:

- Little is known about the cost/efficacy ratio. It is easy to list the advantages of this technique (life expectancy, quality of life) and to measure its cost. This ratio ought to be a good indicator of future trends.
- The supply of organs is still inadequate in quantity (kidney) or in quality (lung) compared with demand. If xenografts should become possible (grafting of organs of animal origin), the prospects would be greatly improved.

- A risk of over-equipment in twenty years time, when progress in prevention may well lead to a decrease in the use of this resource-intensive technology.

Transplantaton could increase substantially over ten years, then undergo regression. in any case it will only be carried out in a small number of specialized centres in the rich countries.

Heart and Blood Vessels

During the last four decades cardiology has benefited greatly from advances in electronics and information technology, together with the development of invasive techniques and increasingly effective imaging techniques.

However, epidemiology is undergoing a transformation, and conditions requiring post-rheumatismal valvuloplasty are becoming less common, to be replaced in part by degenerative valvular conditions. Congenital cardiopathies will decrease as a result of advances in prenatal diagnosis. Myocardiopathies, primary muscle diseases, will undoubtedly become more common. Indeed, the cardiology of tomorrow will be dominated by coronary ischemia, i.e. atherosclerosis and thrombosis. Prevention may reduce the frequency, but there is no prospect of genuine regression without effecttive research on atheroma.

Surgery will continue to be a growth area, with new appliances and prostheses. But radiologically controlled cardiological techniques will become increasingly effective at correcting certain anomalies without recourse to surgery. For example, stenoses or coronary occlusions will commonly be treated by angioplasty or by laser, under direct visualization of the lesions by angioscopy.

What treatment will be given for the cardiac consequences of arterial diseases associasted with smoking, arterial hypertension, lipids and platelet deposits? Drugs that block interactions are making their appearance. Efforts are being made to identify the subjects at risk who are more likely to develop a hyperlipidemia.

In the near future, prevention through drugs is likely to bring about a sharp decrease in cardiology needs as one generation succeeds another.

Hematology

Non-cancerous conditions account for only a small part of this field. Malignant hematological diseases will continue to be diagnosed in private practice and treated in hospital. A few beds will still be needed for severe hematological conditions (acute leukemias, lymphomas, marrow transplants). The traditional beds will disappear. All the other patients can be treated in a day hospital or outpatient clinic. A very small number of highly specialized centres could become responsible for all hematology cases, taking over from the internal medicine departments.

Molecular Genetics

The methodology of genetic engineering first appeared in 1972 and its medical implications are immense:

— *In "predictive"medicine* Progress in the prenatal and postnatal diagnosis of hereditary diseases. A highly original aspect will be the development of presymptomatic diagnoses, with screening for predisposition, so that measures can be taken to prevent morbidity.

— *In cancerology* Spectacular improvement in the resources for detection and prognostic evaluation of neoplastic and pre-neoplastic cells. and discovery of treatments designed not only to destroy cancer cells but also to correct cellular maladjustment.

— In diseases associated with invasion by a viral, bacterial or parasitic microorganism: improvements in detection, eradication and protection through the tools of molecular biology, and particularly through the development of new vaccines in the therapy of genetic diseases

— In the therapy of genetic disease: substitutive gene therapy through reprogramming of somatic cells could be made available in certain special cases.

Internal Medicine and General Surgery

Internal medicine fulfills the function of a "general hospital" in the major hospital complex. A substantial proporation of its clientele could now be handled by non-hospital medicine, social services, long-stay establishments. Its activity and patients' length of stay will therefore depend in future on initiatives by private practitioners and on the facilities available for the old or needy. Medical technology does not seem to be involved very much.

The long-term clientele of internal medicine at present includes subjects who have:

- multiple disease involving several organs, often young or old people;
- fever, weight loss, pain syndromes, unexplained fatigue-peripheral vascular conditions;
- non-localized or generalized cancers-disabilities due to the use of drugs; or
- "difficult" diseaes that need to be explored and not at first sight fall under any speciality.

These patients will continue to require care and long-term observation. Their length of stay will be reduced somewhat further, but not much.

The clientele on the decrease include, in particular, patients with:

- diseases associated with psychiatric problems; Acute cerebrovascular accidents; or
- bacterial diseases.

The new clientele includes patients with:

- viral diseases, with their concurrent and later complications;
- complex diseases of affluence; or
- conditions associated with pollution and accidents.

Internal medicine would become the focal point for specialities. The breeding ground from which specialists would branch out and to which they would return. It would give up its social function and become integrated with vast groupings coordinated either by a specialist or by an internist. This development would enable the hospital to remain an initial recourse for patients and would assist it is classifying patients. It would probably add flexibility. It would enable specialists whose work is on the decrease to acquire new skills and would enable disciplines that wish to become individualized to do so.

In the United States of America, hospital departments are general purpose. Each practitioner belongs to a speciality. Beds are not assigned to any particular speciality. Doctors working partly in private practice and partly in the hospital attend to admissions, information and discharges. This kind of organization has proved conducive to a fairly-specialized form of medicine.

In the United Kingdom, all patients are seen by their General Practitioner before being admitted to hospital and return to him on discharge. At the hospital they see the internist before being referred to a specialist.

There is also the problem of patients in the terminal phase of care. A corollary to society's increasing use of medical care is that deaths more and more frequently take place in hospital, which is becoming the natural place for life to end, a function it is not always suited to fulfil. Death is thus being excluded from the day-to-day pattern of society, and this trend seems difficult to reverse in the medium term. Should units for palliative care be developed? And if so, within which departments?

General surgery in public hositals will be subjected to two influences for change:

- Medical technology: and
- Competition from private hospitals.

Technological progress (praticularly in anaesthesia) will make it possible to reduce the length of stay still further.

Some activities are on the decline and whole areas of current surgery could disappear:

- Heart surgery (coronary and valvular);

- Common visceral surgery (prevention of cancers of the colon by detection of polyps, gall-bladder surgery);
- Removal of severe tumors; and
- Removal of renal calculi,

New activities will include:

- Partial organ prostheses (major organs, pancrease, joints, intraocular implants);
- Transplants;
- Intensive care and specific surgery for old people (replacement surgery to improve the quality of life);
- Cosmetic and plastic surgery; and
- Invasive endoscopy, laser surgery (opthalmology, cancerology).

Departments will need very few beds, but there should be comfortable and friendly hotels nearby.

Surgeons, like specialists, wil need continuing education to keep up with technology and needs.

Internists and surgeons have identified some major options on which their work in the twenty-first century will depend:

A National Prevention Policy

A national prevention policy will profoundly modify the demand for hospital care, especially in the following cases:

- Senile dementia;
- Road accidents;
- Sexually transmitted disease;
- Alcoholism and smoking; and
- Cardiovascular diseases and cancer (through the development of knowledge about the HLA (human leukocyte antigen complex).

This comment raises the fundamental question: if there is no external initiative, should the hospital itself take the initiative, i.e.get involved in providing information, whether alone or in partnership with others.

General Practitioners

The introduction of communications systems could modify the pattern of work of internists and surgeons through:

- Data banks, expert systems;
- Aids to the monitoring of treatment, message services for the chronically ill;
- Aids to the monitoring of treatment, message services for the chronically ill;
- Training in decison-making, software for computer-assisted teaching of diagnostic, therapeutic and preventive strategies;
- Epidemiological studies; and
- Teleconferences with general practitioners, doctors in other countries, etc.

Flexibility in all things This will include premises, staffing, subspecialties, response to clientele, etc.

Increased Productivity

This seems potentially possible everywhere; for example:

- Definition of protocols for care, so as to reduce the cost of equipments, improve the organisation of work, training and speed of the staff, evaluation of their application;
- Improved coordination between specialities (biology, endoscopy, radiology, and surgery; psychiatry, social services and internal medicine, etc);
- Improvements of emergency services and the classification of emergency patients;
- Programming of admissions to reduce length of stay;
- Professional management of accommodation and catering services, personnel and reception;
- Use of business techniquesfor management of services (management secretariate, quality control, queue management, etc); and
- Attempts to find appropriate ways of catering for the needs of very old people, patients in the terminal phase, the very poor.

Imaging and Radiology

This is one of the areas where the spread of technologies is most rapid. any forecast is therefore hazardous. What is certain is that major advances, unimaginable today, will appear in the next 20 years and will spread rapidly.

The CT scanner and MRI will reach the phase of maturity. The very high-performance scanners will level off by 2000 to make way for small scanners. The unit cost of procedures will drop. Three-dimensional MRI will be very widespread.

Ultrasonography and micro-endoscopy: Processing of the image will improve, the appliances will be smaller and will become generally available.

Expert systems, automated interpretation of negatives from banks of reference images, will make it easier to learn and use the technologies.

Digitisation of images will lead to the disappearance of films as the resolution on screen and paper improves. It will permit networks for transmitting images within the hospital and between the hospital and external practitioners.

Invasive radiology, will continue to develop and is really taking off from 2000 onward—intraluminal dilatations, transcutaneous biopsies, chemonucleolysis, catheterisation and embolisation, drug delivery to specific sites, etc. Automation of surgery under radiological surveillance has prospects which are full of promise and difficult to imagine. Scintigraphy with specific radio-immunological markers could make it possible to detect and then treat metastases. The first successful treatments could quickly lead to a large number of diagnostic examinations and subsequent therapy.

Very costly and resource-intensive equipment (Scanner, MRI) has led to centralized and multipurpose structures. Like all disciplines, imaging will specialize. Two factors contribute to this:

- more appropriate and less expensive appliances will appear.
- examinations are becoming more and more specific to clinical problems. The experts consider two extreme hypotheses.
- specialisation by machine (MRI, ultrasound, scanner). This is the "imaging departments" option.
- specialisation by organ (neuroradiology, urinary radiology, etc.), which is easy to develop in organ establishments or clinical departments. Clinicians will increasingly gain control over imaging for their own specialty in order to perform percutaneous procedures (uurology, obstetrics). Alongside the heavily equipped centres, miniaturised and less expensive appliances will become widespread in the clinical departments themselves.

The first hypothesis seems conducive to extendig the possibilities of the equipment. It could prevail in an initial phase where research predominates. The second hypothesis would be more appropriate for recognition of and ready access to the technology by patients. It seems more conducive to the extensive spread of these new technologies.

Imaging at the Service of Outpatients Clinics

This would reduce length of stay in hospital if there is an improvement in waiting and transmission periods, and could eliminate the need for many hospital admissions.

Decision trees, strategies and protocols The necessary equipment will be expensive, even if its unit price comes down. Heath insurance funds, hospitals and patients will demand in return:

- Avoidance of pointless examinations;
- Reduction in hospital admissions; and
- Less aggressive and more effective treatments.

The imaging experts will need to develop decisions with the clinicians and get general practitioners to comply with them by means of access criteria or control over the quantity of examinations requested. In return, they will have to agree to ensure the optimum use of the appliances and to supply the requesting physicians with reports in statisfactory from and within a satisfactory period.

Agreements between public hospitals and the private sector These are sure to develop. High-performance and up-to-date equipment are scarce.

The supply of examinations will remain limited by comparison with a highly expandable demand on account of lack of funds, restrictive regulations and bottlenecks in the public sector (limited recruitment, staffing difficulties). Efforts will need to be made to optimize the use of expensive equipment;

- Groupings in order to reach a sufficiently large local clientele;
- Private capital to increase funding; and
- Joint management of equipment so that it is used to its maximum technical capacity (increase in the number of teams)

General or Logistic Services

Providing accommodation, heating, laundry services, catering are not the real functions of the hospital. Methods of production are changing very fast from cottage industry to a genuine professional business (accommodation, mass catering). People are becoming aware of the need to modernize and of the possibilities of obtaining better service at lower cost. The extent of the human problems of reconversion is realized. But people often only consider two oiptions—should the hospital do it or get someone else to do it? Whereas the solution for the future is more flexible and more diversified.

Catering

Current advances offer hope of substantial increase in productivity and of improved quality. The new technologies (free-dried or frozen foods ready to serve) can eliminate three functions in hospitals:

Shopping

Preparation (peeling and cleaning fruit and vegetables, preparing meat, pastry-making).

Cooking

They could reduce the number of time-consuming, unskilled jobs, and staff could be redeployed in the health sector. The service offered to patients could be improved by:

- Packaging and reheating; and
- Distribution.

The "clients" will become more demanding and the quality of the meals will be an improtant factor in their assessment of the hospital. If they are to be treated as clients, technology will have to privide them with:

- Variety and choice of meals; and
- Quality, pleasant service, hot disheds.

Central Kitchens and Ward Pantries

The future chain of operations will be much simpler:

- Assembly of dishes in a central kitchen from ready-to-serve products, and transfer to the wards for distribution; or
- Assembly in the pantries, whose function will be upgradation.

It would seem that the service techniques (washable or disposables plates, etc.) should determine how serving is organized. Should the packaged food be transported to the patient while hot or cold, and what will become of the central kitchens and ward pantries?

Should the hospital do its own catering or contract it out?

- The real question is how to obtain a high-quality service, varied according to the patients' needs at a competitive price:
- Some of the productions are already within the public sector: premises, knowledge of the patient; while
- Others lie more in the private sector: know-how, organizational ability, capital.
- The "all public" and "all private"formulas may well belong to the past. For each problem there can be a flexible and adapted formula:
- Mixed investment company, whereby the capital and managerial ability of the private sector are combined with the medical and dietetic skills of the public sector; and

- Technical assistance contracts giving responsibility for organization, supervision and staff training to outside professionals. This solution has been tried. It preserves the hospital's independence and is reversible.

Laundry

Disposable bed-linen is rapidly becoming common. Various studies have shown that for the incontinent and severely ill, it is less expensive. It reduces laundry work, sterilization and sorting. It makes it easier to keep clean and dirty linen apart. It will require increased incinerator capacity, from which energy recovery is possible.

Unwoven fabrics, highly specialized and adapted to needs, will replace cotton. They already account for 60 to 70 percent of fabrics used in operating theatres in the USA. They are 40 percent cheaper and provide much higher quality. They present problems of storage and specific distribution.

Information Technology and Communications

The new technologies can be subdivided into four groups:

- Home and office information systems—message services, teletext, automated office services, working at home via a terminal;
- Man—machine interfaces through use of keyboard, optical character reader or voice recognition, translation of technical texts;
- Smart cards, magnetic or laser—read, for storage and dissemination of information, which are becoming widely used in patient management; and
- Expert systems are now being tried out, and added value systems.

  Some technologies have now become routine in industry and the service sector.

  Office information systems already lead to improvements in everyday work-management of the department, access to data banks, epidemiological statistics, they will soon provide:

- "annotated prescription" explaining the method of use of the prescription, the precautions, but excluding the contra-indications and drug interactions;
- spreadsheets on which reports of tests and hospital treatment will be directly recorded:
- list of available beds, waiting periods and criteria for access to medical and technical procedures;
- interactive message services for appointments, reports on hospitalization, exchange of files, test results, etc and
- teleconference with hospital doctors in order to determine therapies or for continuous training.

The Expert Systems Comprise

- Operation of data banks, computer-assisted design, computer-assisted data processing, image processing, etc.;
- Consultation of encyclopaedia with memorization of findings, scanning of data banks;
- Computer-assisted instruction for initial learning of diagnoses, and especially of the new treatments that will result from molecular biology;
- Automatic interpretation of routine technical procedures such as electrocardiagrams;
- Aid to diagnosis;
- Mutual information networks for specialists of the same discipline (e.g. nephrologists), these networks developing around a hospital diagnostic centre; and
- International data banks.

As an aid to diagnosis, the computer should not alter the medical procedure. It will be an "intellectual adjunct". It will remind the doctor of known facts, suggest a list of questions for him to ask the patient, then suggest a list of diagnostic hypotheses and therapeutic proposals. It can improve patient-doctor dialogue but not transform it. For patients:

- A user information service;
- Guidance on outpatient clinics, waiting lists, records to be brought by the patient, etc.
- An appointments system; and
- In the wards, videotex terminals can be used for selection of meals and explanation of treatment.

In the internal organisation of the hospital many applications are already operationzal:

- Appointments management:
- Circulation of reports on technical examinations by telefax or an added value system that provides an interpretation;
- Queuing occurs at the start of the chain of operations (registration, admission formalities) and at the time of discharge (payment), and could be reduced by means of a card system-transaction cards could eliminate some of the tasks of billing;

The Strategic Choices

Networks could be formed for a particular neighbourhood, for a particular speciality, around private clinics or group practices. They would be organised around a central computer linked to the doctor's microcomputers. Each patient would receive an individual card, filled in by the practitioner.

The hospitals choose cards for internal use, of the credit card type, which cannot be used outside the hospital. Microprocessor cards (smart cards) can be read by a microcomputer or by a videotex terminal equipped with reader. The system can be used for storing and processing information. The cards must be protected. They may contain administrative information, information on social insurance status, and a brief report on hospitalization. These systems will be flexible and inexpensive. They will be very well suited to the chronically ill, old people and pregnant women, who are admitted to hospital several times or are transferred from one department to another.

The information should focus on the patient, so that insurance coverage can be verified, records updated, and prescriptions read, etc.

THE HOSPITAL FOR ACUTELY ILL PATIENTS

The hard core of the hospital in the beginning of 21st century will be a set of technical facilities including large departments for diagnostic and therapeutic imaging, equipped with large and very advanced machines, located close to the emergency unit and the operating theatre.

Around these technical facilities there will be large polyclinics with specialist outpatient departments, day beds, intensive care units and only a few conventional beds for certain chronic or disabling disease and for the dying (palliative care units).

The centralization of expensive and resource-intensive equipment, which is common nowdays, will change because the equipment currently described as expensive and resource-intensive will be transferred to the specialist departments, whereas new technologies will remain centralized in the technical facilities and will be used jointly by several public and private hospitals.

Architecture will have two characteristics; horizontality and flexibility.

- Horizontality will mean no more 1500 bed tower hospitals, instead, there will be more horizontal 300 to 400 bed hospitals, more accessible to the outside world, with various shops and video room and public transport stopping at the hospital entrance.
- Flexibility has become necessary because we do not yet know what the future technologies will be. Since hospitals are built of concrete, the whole of the inside will need to be made suitable for extensive modification, for example, by siting all the piping and cables along the outside walls or above false ceilings.

- One floor of the hospital, with virtually no beds or medical services, will be set aside for education in chronic disease for patients and their families and friends (cooperative care in the United States of America).
- A good-quality hotel will be attached to the hospital for patients who live far away or in isolated place, who need to visit the hospital several times in succession but do not require medical care at night.

THE LIMITS OF PLANNING

Planning for the hospital is limited in two ways:

There is uncertainty about the forecasts made and of the risks taken on the basis of guesses about the future. Forecasting is a difficult exercise, but not to forecast at all means certain deterioraton. So it is important to be able to revise in good times a decision that proves not to be the right one and to avoid all-or-nothing situations. It is most important to evaluate the results of planning at regular intervals and to compare the forecasts upon which the plans are based with the trends actually observed.

The hospital planner does not have control over all the constraints, for example:

- Medical constraints, especially changes in the role of the hospital, the speed of scientific progress and the ability of the medical staff to keep up with such progress;
- Psychosocial constraints, which raise the problem of decision-making at the hospital and the relationships between the various centres of power (staff, trade unions, doctors, management, governing board, political authorities, etc), together with society's perception of the hospital, disease and death;
- Constraints resulting from health policies;
- Constraints arising from town planning and local geography; and financial constraints.

The plan must be adapted to these limiting factors, which means planning without undue rigidity.

It is important to develop "sliding" plans that can be updated and revised annually, to preserve the utmost external flexibility (for example, a reserve of spare land to meet urgent and unforeseeable needs), and internal flexibility (for example, the ability to convert a medical department rapidly into a surgical department or a technical unit, by using systems of movable partitions around a central core).

THE PLACE OF THE FIRST REFERRAL HOSPITAL

More than half of the world's people live in villages, where the organization of health services may be hampered by remoteness, adverse climatic conditions, poor communications, and poverty, and perhaps by illiteracy and superstition. The first referral hospital may be very small, with a tiny staff that is limited in experience and expertise. The other half of the world's people live in cities, some of enormous size, where poverty is again a factor, and where overcrowding, pollution, and stress may be overwhelming. The problems that city hospitals must face are different from those of village hospitals, yet both types of hospital provide essential services and it is important to see how they can be incorporated into the district health system.

In the past century, medicine has grown increasingly scientific and hospitals have tended to become technological workshops for the diagnosis and treatment of disease. This trend will undoubtedly continue, but at the same time the functional integration of hospitals into district health services is of vital importance, if they are to provide efficient. effective, affordable, and equitable services to their communities. This is not to underrate good clinical care and diagnosis, which are still the bedrock of hospital practice at the first referral level, but rather to emphasize the importance of making such care available to those most in need of it.

Within a district health system, there has to be a place where patients with complex medical conditions can be referred for diagnosis, treatment, and care, and which can act as a resource centre for the health work of the district. This place is the first referral hospital.

A hospital at the first referral level has the following characteristics.

- It has a place in the national system of health services:
  - It is recognized by its national authority as a hospital providing 24-hour clinical care;
  - It has a capacity for diagnosis, treatment, institutional care, and rehabilitation that represents a higher level of competence that the source of the referral.
- It can relate effictively to the district health system:
  - It recognizes itself as an integral part of a district heatlh system, and of the larger health system beyond;
  - It shares in district-wide information gathering and in the planning, implementation, and evaluation of health service programmes (including budget reviews and the monitoring of programmes through management information systems and quality-assurance programmes);
  - It is concerned with the health and well-being of the entire population of the area it serves;
  - It is a resource centre that is open at all times to requests for help from the district health council and the staff of the district health system;
  - It seeks to understand the practice of traditional medicine in the district and its contribution to the health of the community.
- It supports primary health care:
  - It is capable of supporting the development of primary health care services (such as antenatal and maternity care, growth monitoring, and immunisations), and ensuring appropriate linkages, referrals, and continuity of care between the primary health care services and the hospital;
  - It is also capable of providing support to primary health care services, including assistance in general management, procurement. supply, storage, maintenance, and transport.
- It can be related effectively to communities:
  - It has the capacity to interact with community members and their organizations through the primary health care services, and with community representatives on matters of concern to the whole area that the hospital serves, and is committed to the enhancement of community self-reliance and independence.
  - It shares with community members and their re-organizations in the planning, implementation, and evaluation of hospital-and community-related programmes.
- It has referral functions:
  - It is capable of responding appropriately to the needs of all patients referred form health facilities at first contact level, or of referring them safely to more complex levels of care;
  - It has responsibility for referring patients back to the source of referral with appropirate information;
  - It offers a reliable channel for the referral of laboratory specimens from the district and the speedy transmission of the results of the relevant tests.
- It has a training function:
  - It develops training and continuing education programmes for all levels of its own staff;
  - With staff at all levels of the district health system, it shares an interest in developing training programmes both for these groups and for the community.;
- It is a problem-solving resource:
  - It has the opportunity and need, in common with the community and staff at all levels

of the district health system, to address problems that have a bearing on the health of the people and the effectiveness of the health services.

– The hospital should promote the primary health care strategy for the district by helping improve the skills of health workers at first contact level and by concentrating on tasks that cannot be performed adequately at first contact level.

The hospital should continuously monitor and evaluate its overall performance, admission, policies and criteria, and particularly its quality of care in terms of humanity, effectiveness, and efficiency, taking local resources and ethical traditions into account. The hospital should develop standard treatment protocols. It should be equipped for effective clinical management with appropriate diagnostic services.

Thus, the hospital at first referral level is much more than a curative facility functioning at a single level in a health system, it is in fact closely linked with every aspect of health development within its district. With the community, the primary health care services, and other sectors of development, it shares the opportunity and obligation to provide effective and affordable health services to the entire population and to involve the community in their planning, implementation, and evaluation.

Hospital will have a changing role in near future–from the center of excellence to community support.

FURTHER READING

1. The Hospital in Rural and Urban Districts. Report of a WHO study Group on the Functions of Hospitals at the First Referral Level. TRS No. 819. WHO, Geneva, 1992.
2. Paine LHW, Siem Tjam F: Hospitals and Health care Revolution. World Health Organisation, Geneva, 1988.
3. WHO Commission on Health and Environment. Our Planet, Our Health. WHO, Geneva 1992.

All knowledge, which you seek for working in the service of humanity and for the uplifting of the world, brings you a step forward.

The journey of a thousand miles begins with one step. It takes a great team to scale the heights of success.
What is 'Today' becomes 'Yesterday' and what is 'Tomorrow' becomes 'Today'.
Give your best today, be it in your tiniest of duty performances, in practicing values and ethics, in fulfilling all big or small commitments. The best will come to you tomorrow. Grow with best of the traditions.
The world steps aside for the man who never stops.
Leave an indelible mark in history.

Part Two

Hospital: Design and Development

✍ From "An" Idea to "The" Idea

✍ Design and Construction

24 Hospital: From The Center of Excellence to Community Support

Hospitals arouse strong emotions. Doctors, nurses, paramedics, remembering the excitement of their early training years, associate hospitals with youth, vigour and the possibilities presented by a new carrier. The heady mixture of large numbers of young men and women exploring new ideas together remains as an affectionate memory with most medical professionals for the next of their working lives.

For the general public, the perception is different. Most people fear the prospect of entering a hospital, even as a visitor. This is ultimately because numbers of people who enter hospitals die there. Hospitals have an alien feel for most members of the general public. Which is not understood by people who work in them.

FROM 'AN' IDEA TO 'THE' IDEA

Balancing needs, desires, costs and regulations in the construction of a new health care facility, an addition, or a major renovation of an existing facility requires knowledge of a host of the complicated and inter-related activities. These include, finance, economics, medical practices, enforcement requirements, public relations, etc.

A person's ability to work under the constraints imposed on health care facilities today is directly related to his ability to know how to make the necessary activities happen, and happen at the right time.

Defining the Project

In defining what is to be built one needs to consider and thoroughly analyze five questions, documenting answers for each.

WHY – is it necessary to build?
– What is the need?

WHAT – should be built
– type (the basic structure envisioned: a new hospital, a new nursing home).
– size (depend on the functions and their number being proposed function (activities that take place in the new structure surgery gynaecology, maternity, pediatrics, cardiology, etc.)
– style (of the new structure describes the facade of the structure; brick, block or wood, depends on the location in the country).

HOW – Operation (a new, separate structure, adding onto an existing structure)

– Finance (initial capital in order to build).
– Health care delivery is very competitive today.

WHERE – Determining the geographic location of the structure.

Factors Influencing the Location

External

a. Environmental considerations (hills, rocks, rivers, soil, substrate).
b. Traffic and access.
c. Location of the nearest fire departments.
d. Utility capabilities—electricity, water, gas, sewage.
e. Public transport.
f. Parking.

Internal

For existing facilities (the overall flow of the people and goods must be reviewed).

WHEN – to build?
– balancing how well an institution can complete what is needed against how soon the project is needed by the community.

Certificate of Need (CON)

From the Government agencies certificate of need approval is obtained.

Financing

Building a hospital is a costly endeavor. Money to finance a project can be obtained from several sources:
- Grants
- Fund raising /Donations
- Issuance of Stocks or Bonds
- Conventional Borrowing via a mortgage.

Estimating Costs

- Estimating the cost of building
  - rough estimates are possible and necessary.
  - receive assistance from professional cost estimators.

The Land

Information about the land must be known before the piece of land can be considered acceptable for a new structure. Factors that influence affect the selection of a particular parcel of land:
- environmental
- geological configuration and activities
- foundation pre-requisites societal influences.

Environmental

Nature has the first dibs on what can be built anywhere on this earth.
- The terrain of the land as level as possible for as much as possible is desirable.
- Water condition: what has the water table been like over the past 25 years? Has it remained relatively stable? Is it raising or it dropping?

Because natural weather conditions (rain, snow) cannot be changed, the environment cannot be ignored when building a facility.

Geological Configuration

- Subsoil data must be obtained from a professional involved in this field prior to any design work.
- Test borings or sonic soundings are necessary to learn what exists 10,50,100 feet below the surface.

Foundation Prerequisites

There are many types of foundation solutions:
- Piles
- Floating foundation
- Variations of common foundations.

The possible types of foundations can be studied and calculations made based on the geology and weight or loads of the proposed structure.

Environmental Data

- What conditions exist below the land
- What conditions prevail above the land.

Societal Influences

Human condition related to the land

i. Vehicular access and expandability
ii. Potential patients
   - catchment area
   - health care needs assessment
iii. Potential staff
   - Quantity and type of staff needed (are there good schools, colleges, universities in the area?)
iv. Competition (the delivery of medical service is a business).

Structural Considerations

The structure of a building is the basic skeleton upon which the entire facility is erected. A great deal of consideration must go into deciding which system is best for the particular project.

Factors affecting the type and extent of the structure that can be built indlude:

***A.* Common to any Structure**

1. Subsoil level
2. Foundation
3. Proneness to earthquakes
4. Fire-resistive classification
5. Occupancy classification
6. Fire proofing requirements
7. Structural loading requirements.

Subsoil level The status of the subsoil below the site of the proposed structure is most necessary, because it determines how heavy (large a structure) can be erected on the site.

Foundation The subsoil data must be obtained prior to any decision about the type of structure desired. Such items as rock, water, sand, swamp, gravel and artificial fill will determine what type of foundation is possible and appropriate. Foundations that can handle future floors, will be well worth the investment.

Fire rating Fire and building codes specify what fire-resistive rating each type of structure is required to meet this specification in terms of the fire-resistive rating for the structural frame, walls and floor and ceiling assemblies.

Structural loading requirements structural configuration will vary between an auditorium, library, a hydrotherapy room a cobalt treatment room and a row of patient rooms.

B. A New Structure

Local traditions or preference may also affect the type or style of structure that can be built in a particular area.

Types of Structure

1. Concrete (poured in place), most versatile material (gives good fire-proofing)
2. Steel (steel-skeleton) is the next best selection It can be erected relatively fast.
3. Concrete (precast)
   - Precast column and beams
   - Precast and prestressed floor and root slabs.
4. Wood
   - Very easy to build
   - Fire safety restrictions.
5. Masonary structure (concrete block or brick) for 1, 2, 3, storey buildings
6. Combinations
   - One or more of preceding types can be combined. A structural engineer must be consulted.

The Skeleton

- The structure - the framing.
- The right method of structure for a particular building is essential.
- Should be functional and esthetic as well.

Factors Affecting

- size of the building
- subground conditions
- use of the building
- availability and cost of material
- space available
- time requirement to build.

All of the preceding factors must be taken into consideration before a particular design is selected.

The Skin

The outer walls or skin, that envelopes the skeleton of the structure may vary with location, esthetic nature and desire of the owner and with the skill of the architect.

Selecting the Consultants

During the building of healthcare facility four major consultants are required:

- the healthcare facility consultant
- the financial consultant
- the architectural consultant
- the construction consultant (contractor).

Contracts, fees and details of a contract are generally negotiated in which the following are specified

- a description and extent of work to be performed when reports, if any, will be due
- when work is to be completed
- the amount of money that will be paid for work and when and how remuneration for such work will be paid order of selection of consultant

Traditional Bid Method

The financial consultant and architect should be selected at approximately the same time. The contractor is selected by the bid process.

Construction Manager Method

The manager (the builder) the Architect and the financial consultant should be selected at approximately the same time.

- The construction manager to advise and monitor the physical building costs.
- The architect and engineer to determine programme (physical and operational parameters).
- The financial consultant to determine overall financial constraints if the project is to go to bid, the contractor is selected at this time as well.

"Fast-Track" Method

The contractor, the financial consultant and architect are all hired at the same time.

The method allows the construction to proceed without a bid system. It also allows construction to start prior to completion of all architectural and engineering documents.

"Not to Exceed Price" Method"

The contractor, financial consultant and architect and engineer are all hired at the same time. However, the contractor will exert the most pressure because he, as the price setter, has to control the financial level of the project in greater detail.

Fees

There are several ways in which fees can be paid. A flat, agreed upon fee for all work to be performed. A second is a percentage free based on the cost of the project. A third method is an upset fee based on the cost of the project. Construction management fee will vary between 6-10 percent of the cost of the project.

The Design Stage

For evaluation of facilities and operations the combined expertise and views of following are necessary and should be solicited for projected healthcare facility evaluation:

- the owner
- the financial consultant
- the architect/engineer

It takes many persons doing different tasks, in addition to treating patients, directly to make any hospital facility operate efficiently and effectively.

These activities range from regulating building temperature and humidity, maintaining surgical supplies, and preventing infections through washing and cleaning of the facility to ensuring the functioning of the physiological monitors and sending out accurate statements of accounts.

When should the Evaluation be Done?

1. An informal evaluation period can be considered during the planning phase of a long range plan (5-10 years plan) of what should be built.

   Estimate what services and thus what facilities a community needs and approximately when the community needs them.
2. A formal indepth evaluation:
   What is currently taking place and what is possible to undertake will be conducted.

What Should be Evaluated?

- The adequacy of the site in terms of the needed size can be decided. The ease of access can be studied.
- The fire, safety, building and health codes, the newest structural technologies can be followed. A more accurate cost estimate is possible.

What is to be Built?

i. Whatever is needed most and is affordable.
ii. Community needs.
iii. What is affordable, both to build and to operate?
   - Financial capabilities to be matched against the costs of several options that are usually generated from the evaluation.
iv. Facility needs (structural and operational)

This is a matter of setting priorities, developing various options against those priorities, deciding which option can be implemented to meet the most needs.

ARCHITECTURE

Preliminary ideas can be put to paper very easily in the project, but serious designs should not be finalised until everyone has approved design.

General Considerations

Design can be divided into two major categories exterior and interior.

Possibilities and Constraints

- geography
- regulations
- existing facilities
- CON approval
- money
- needs
- priorities
- structural factors.

Factors Affecting the Design

- the number of elevators and stairways necessary
- energy conversion techniques/requirements
- owner's/administrator's preferences
- the amount and shape of land available
- zoning height regulations

- corridor width enabling patient beds to be turned around
- special air circulation requirements
- a defend-in-place concept (as opposed to immediate exiting in the emergency but also for continuing certain essential activities during emergency).

The Exterior

It is a functioning element of the building concerned with what takes place inside the building in addition to keeping out, or allowing in, the weather (e.g. fresh air, sunlight).

It is an envelope that everyone approaching the structure will see.

Planning the exterior of a new structure is thus an exercise in unlimited possibilities tempered by reality and economics.

The Interior

Interior design itself falls into two categories:

Function and esthetics.

- The traffic flow within the building is of prime importance. The public (i.e. visitors) must not interfere with inhouse functions. The public must have direct and quick access to the areas they seek—mainly inpatient bed areas, without crossing the other facility paths of travel. This can be accomplished by:
- dedicated corridors or elevators that provide a path to an area reducing the chance of getting lost.

A designer's ability to create a feeling of modern, clean, and trustworthy facility meets its first test in the public lobby. Colour, furniture, plantings, skylights, wall materials and lighting are equally important. This space should not be cramped to save few bucks.

Great thought should be given to often over looked "patient approach" spaces.

A clearly defined path of travel should be indicated so that the patient knows where to go upon entering. Outpatient and emergency should be adjunctive, as should associated radiology and lab services. These three areas are interconnected by function, since both patients and staff may flow from one to the other as a matter of daily use.

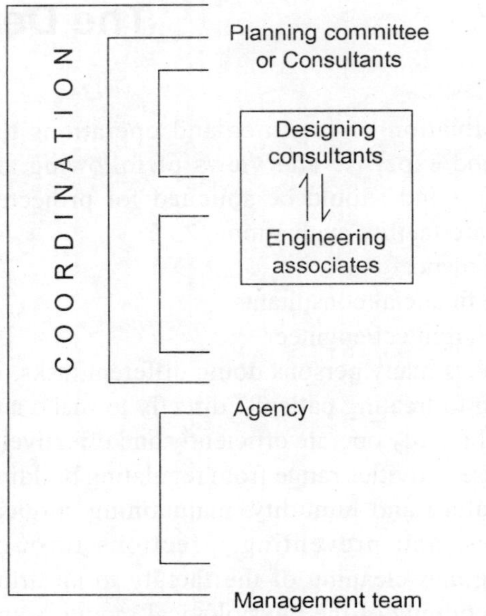

Fig. 24.1: Project development process

Simple, understandable signage, with print of readable size, should be incorporated in the decor.

The color and material of furniture and decoration, as well as the arrangements of lighting are important in creating a feeling of trust and claim in the patient. Corridors can be colour coded.

Good interior space planning is important to avoid cross traffic and long, roundabout corridors.

Internal Operational Requirements

What needs to the reviewed:

- Number of beds.
- Number of private rooms
- Number of treatment rooms
- Number of operating rooms and their type
- Number of consultant offices. Description of operational practices
- Description of services to be provided

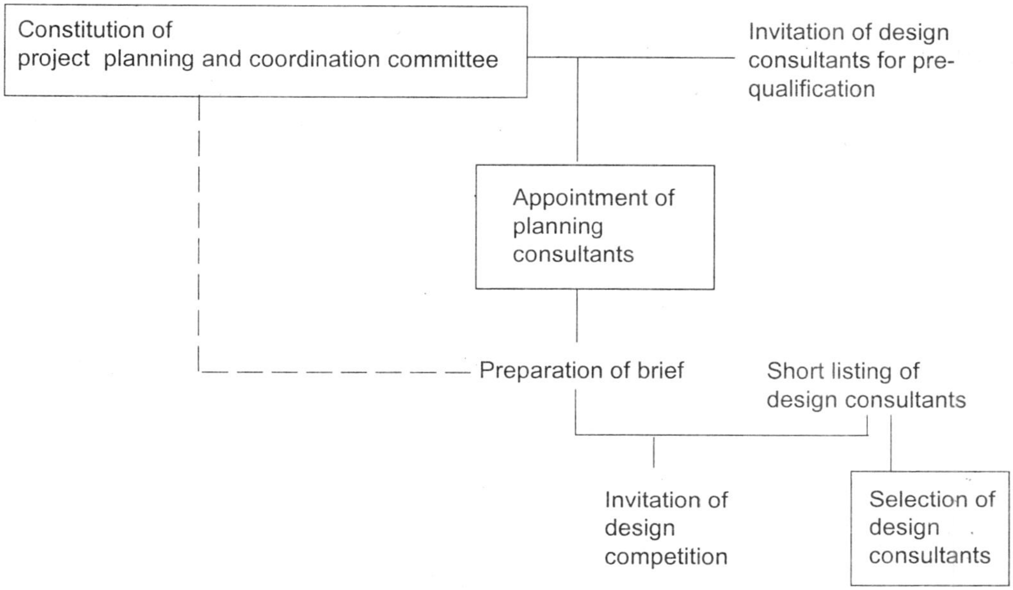

Fig. 24.2: Project management—selection process for design consultants

- Administrative functions to take place in that area
- The anticipated material and goods for the new area.

All these items have to be translated by the architect from items on a list to a drawing showing where items will be located, from individual drawings of areas to complete layouts of each floor to complete drawing of the entire building. All these internal operational factors become firm, a space verse function (programme) can be analyzed. Initially, this is done on a room by room basis but eventually this analysis has to consider entire floors and even the whole building.

All this effort is aimed at producing an internal design that maximises space and function in order to meet the prime purpose of a healthcare facility: medical service to patients.

Some Specifics: From the Outside to the Inside

A facility should have a well-defined entrance and exit roadways. There should be a separate service and delivery roadway and an easy turnaround for large trucks. There should be additional space for snow to be piled, if the facility is in the snow region.

Adequate parking is necessary to accomodate employees, visitors, patients, etc.

Inside a Facility:

- the main lobby should contain information and directional facilities, waiting space, gift and

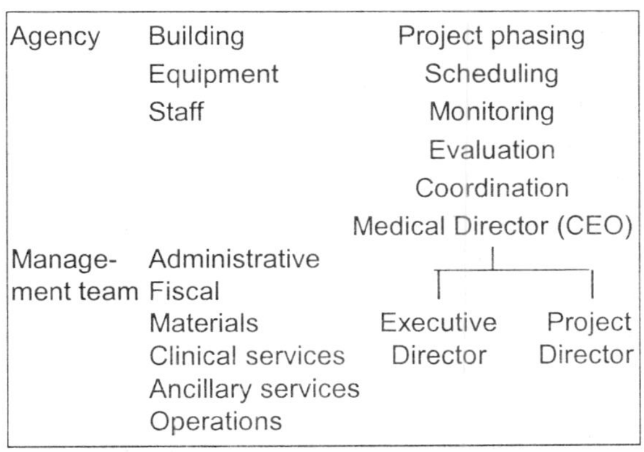

Fig. 24.3

Planning Committee or Consultants	*Developmental* *Functional* Physical Equipment Manpower Systems	Brief preparation Pre-qualification Competetion Selection of consultants for Design/Engineer
Designing consultants	*Master planning* Architectural Interior Landscape	Concept drawing Submission drawings Tender documents Assistance in selection of contractors Working drawings Supervision/coordination
Engineering associates	Structural Electrical Mechanical HVAC Public health Bio-medical	

Fig. 24.4

coffee shops, telephone spaces and public rest rooms.

- any emergency and outpatient lobby should have complete access (no barriers) for fast entrance.
- for emergency facilities, adequate ambulance spaces and technician areas must be provided.

The radiology and laboratory areas needed to service outpatient and emergency should be adjacent, with an easy path to each established and identified. Both outpatient and emergency areas should have a direct path to such place as admiting for surgery, coronary care, special care, etc. The delivery room access for emergency maternity patients should also be a direct path from the emergency area. In essence, patients must go by the shortest and most direct path without going through or into departments.

Delivery of portable equipment to inpatient bedroom floors must be considered.

Physical medicine and hydrotherapy, if used in conjunction with outpatient spaces, should also have direct access for the outpatient area to the department.

Elevators should be dedicated, to specific uses: public visitors, surgery patients, food and service. Sterile supplies must have a direct path to surgical areas, yet care must be taken that soiled material has no cross traffic with clean supplies, direct paths (without cross traffic) from the patient bed and return are absolute requirements.

Day Surgery

An evergrowing department in hospitals is day surgery, where patients are operated on and released in the same day. This area should be adjacent to outpatient area.

Food It must have good delivery access from the outside, combined with proper and adequate storage space.

Services

Ceiling height is an important consideration. Most will require a minimum of 10 feet, with storage provided on interior mezzanine levels. Environmental control spaces (e.g. boiler plants), electrical emergency spaces, electric power distribution panels and pumps may be isolated.

Disposal Incinerator spaces may be isolated spaces with proper access for disposal of ash or unburnable trash.

Patient Versus Nonpatient Areas

It is worth some thought to divide patient care and services into two non-crossing sections, so that all service spaces are on one side and patient-oriented spaces are on the other.

Requisite Items

In space planning, the one common oversight is forgetting in the initial programme, the requisite items which include:

- Janitor closets
- Duct Space allowance (vertical/horizontal)
- Plumbing run outs (require depths and add ceiling problems)

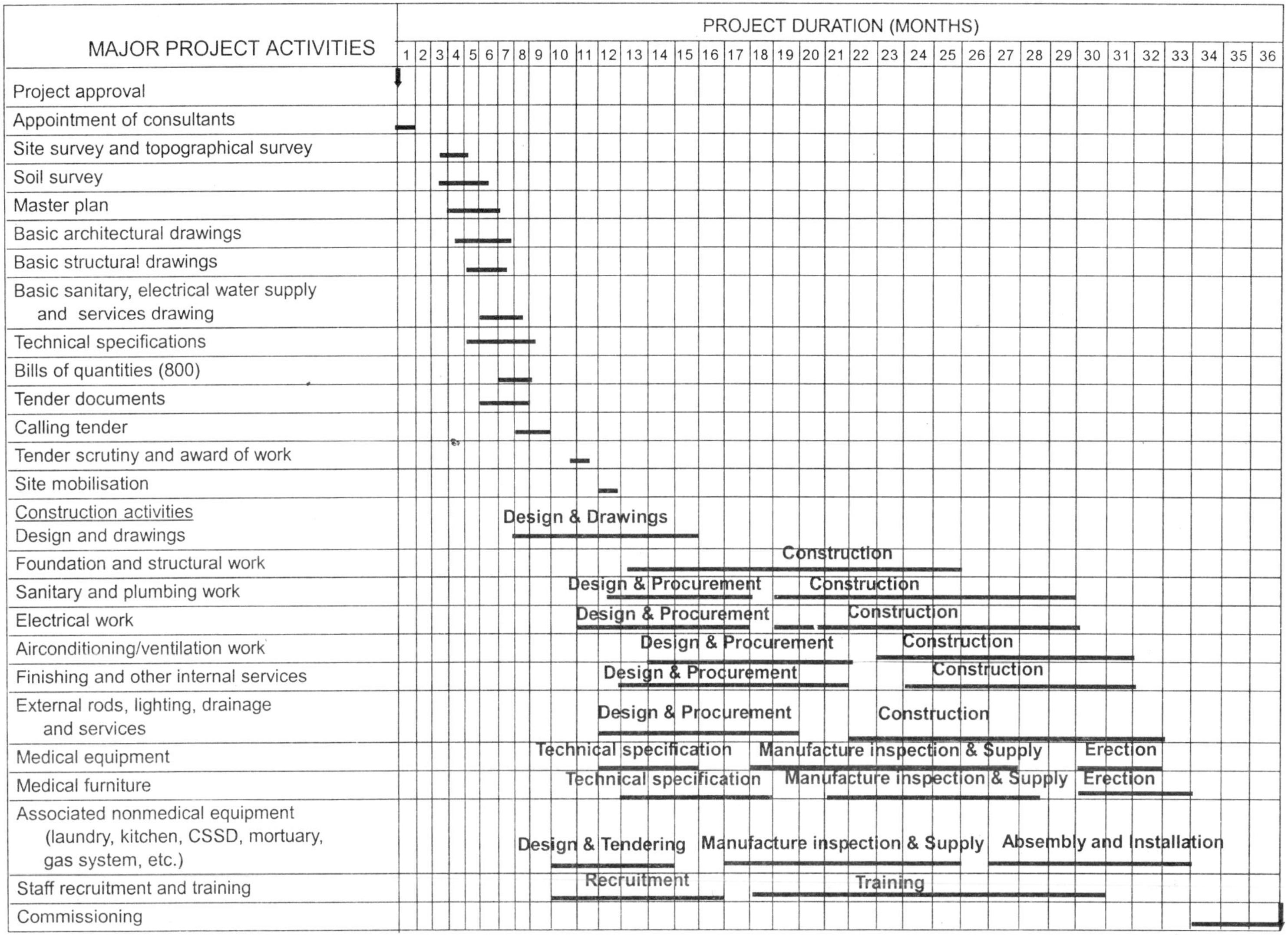

Fig. 24.5: Project implementation scheme for a typical district hospital

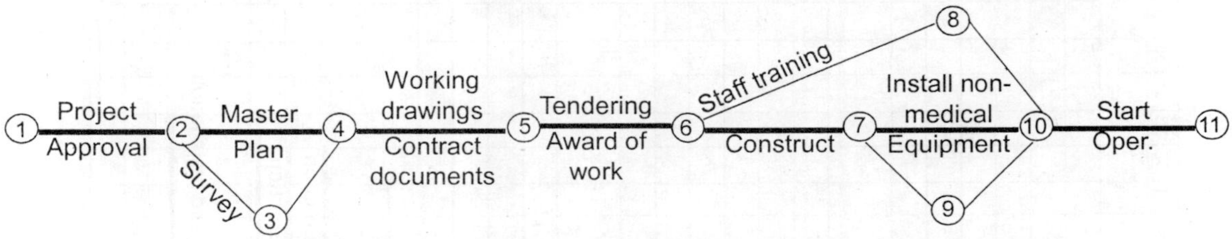

Fig. 24.6: Critical path analysis

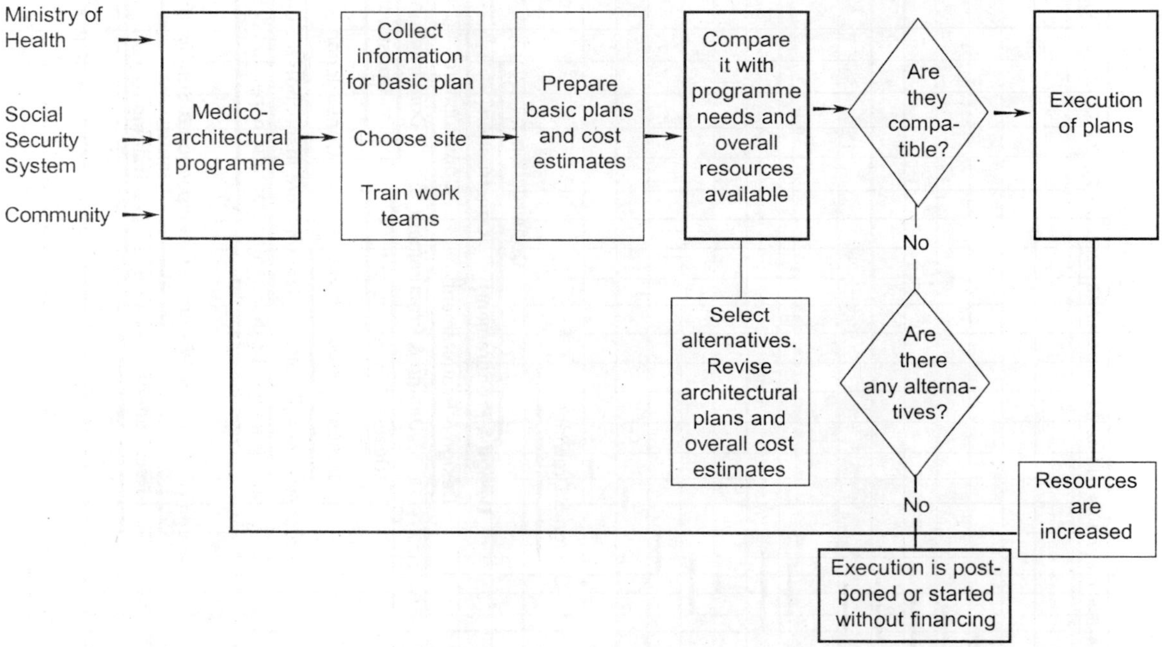

Fig. 24.7: System for evaluating preliminary stages of a project

- Stairway space
- Interconnection passage and corridors
- Storage space
- Employee lockers, rest rooms, toilets
- Door swing interference
- Electric closets
- Telephone equipment rooms
- Data processing rooms
- Drinking fountains
- Special equipment storage for intensive care and cardiac care units.
- Wheelchair space
- Handicapped toilets
- Main room.

Public Relations Office

- Patient record room
- Engineer's office.

A room-by-room or space-by-space interview with all pertinent and affected personnel in the facility must be conducted.

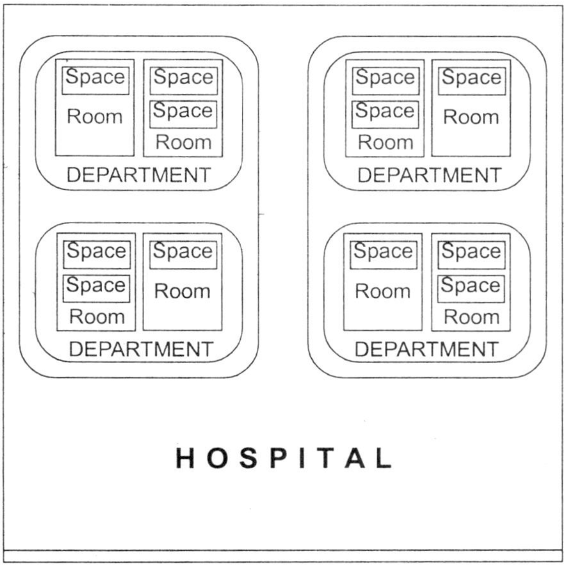

Fig. 24.8: Organization of zones and spaces

MEETING THE CODES

Codes are a set of parameters, such as specifications, performance criteria, or installation requirements, that have been developed and judged as acceptable boundaries and minimum levels for safety and/or efficacy. Codes reflect what society's attitudes, economies, and values evolve.

The knowledge and use of codes are important factors in producing a structure that will protect the lives of the people within and around it. The codes can be divided into two major groups: Those strictly related to the structure (facility codes) and those related to activities once the structure is built (operational codes).

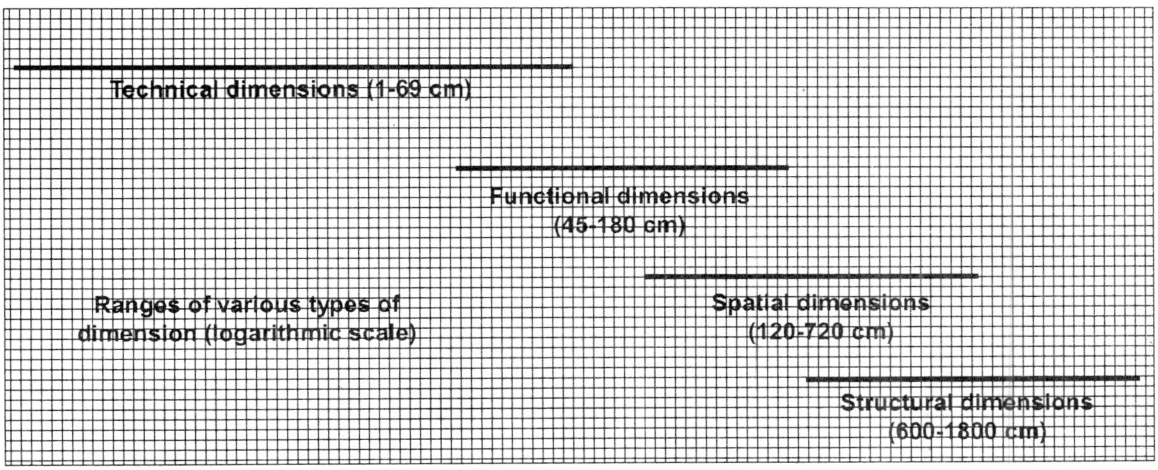

Fig. 24.9: Ranges of various types of dimensions—to obtain full benefit from the modular discipline in medical-care building construction, the following comprehensive scheme is proposed. A modular discipline for the diverse building products (prefabricated elements) can be built up, starting from the characteristic dimensions of each product. In each architectural lesign these dimensions belong to one of the following types:

1. Technical dimensions result from technical considerations requirements. For instance, the bearing capacity dictates column sections; sound insulation influence's the wall thickness, etc.
2. Functional dimensions, such as door width, bench height, and length of working surfaces. These dimensions are the result of functional, anthropometric or ergonomic data,
3. Spatial dimensions: the dimensions of the various rooms, ceiling height, corridor width etc., and
4. Structural dimensions, for spans, distances between beams and between columns, etc.

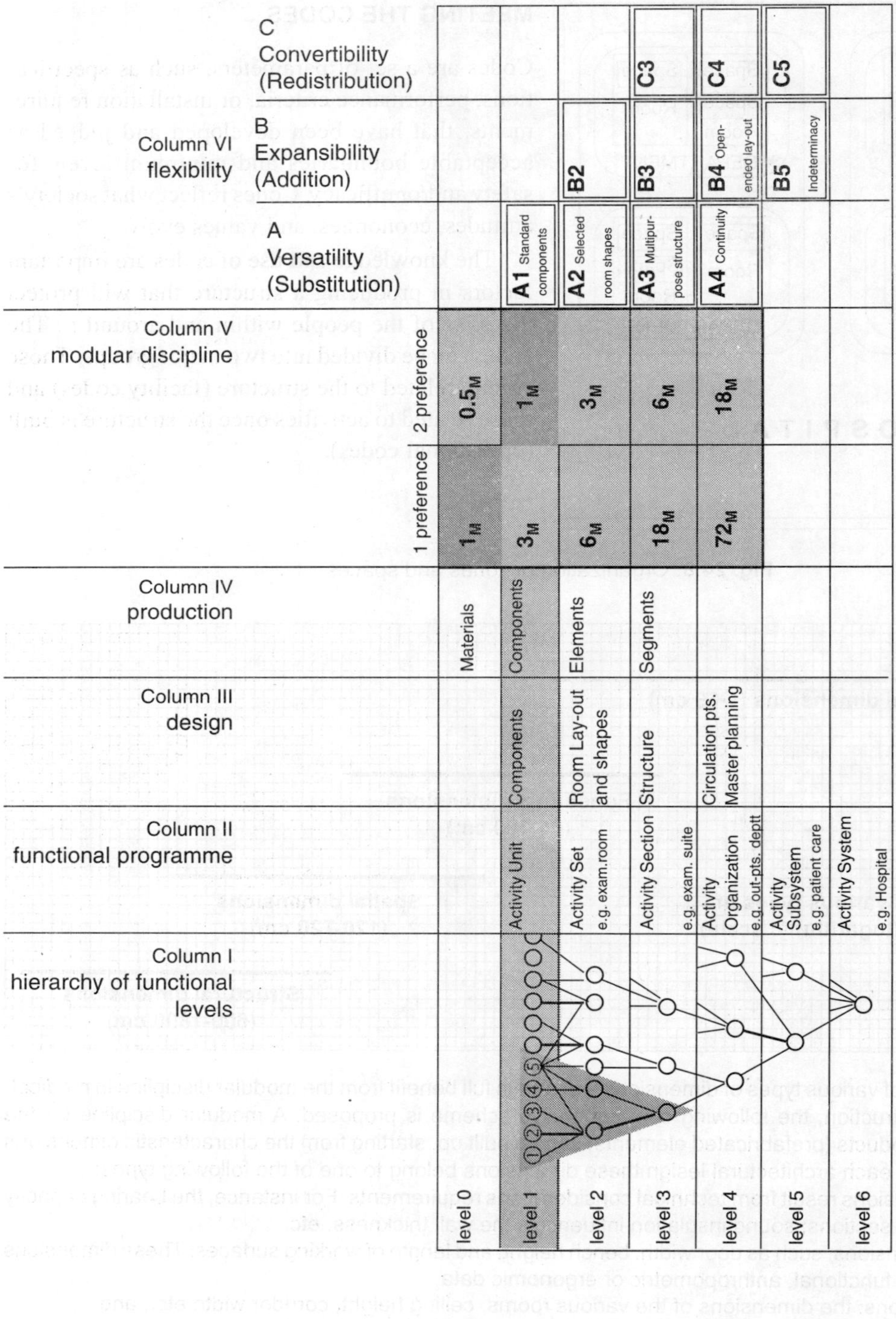

Fig. 24.10: Synoptic table

SPECIMEN	DATA BANK ACTIVITY UNIT DATA SHEET	Updated
ACTIVITY UNIT	Bedside activity in high nursing dependency	retrieval index AOI.A.

ACTIVITIES: To accomodate a patient who will need basic nursing care and supervision.
Nursing procedures will be performed by 2 staff from the side of the bed.
No special equipment is provided for.
The patient may leave the bed to sit in an easy chair.

Minimum space for this activity: 240 × 300 cm.

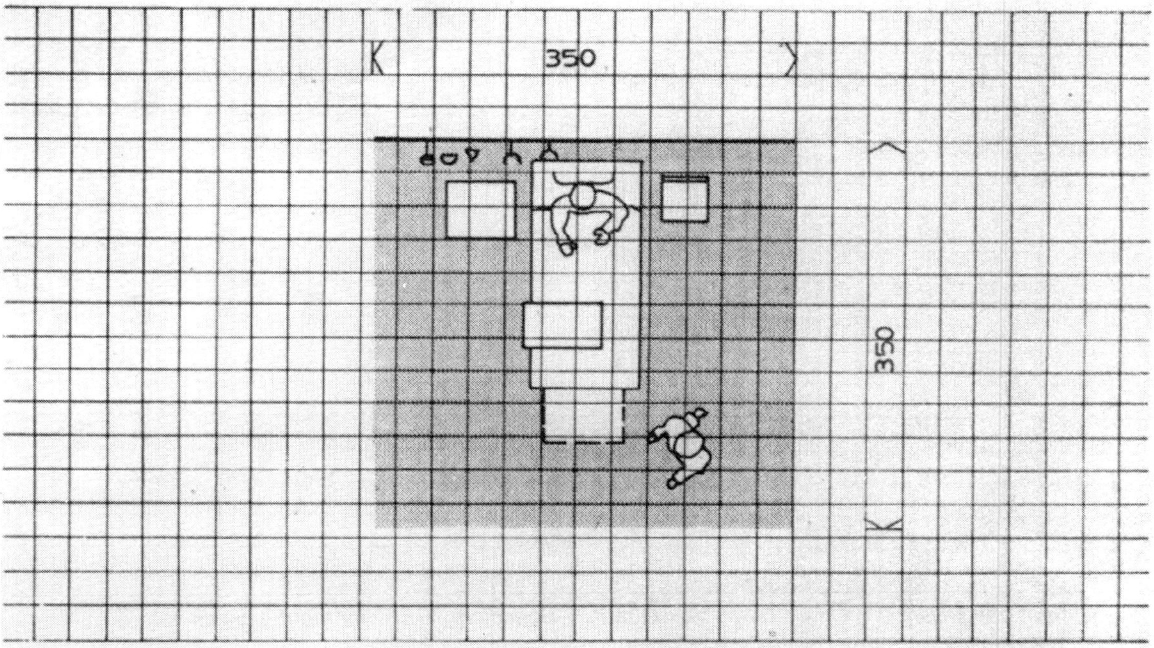

Hook; coat	1		Temperature	: natural.
Light; bedhead, wall mounted	1		Summer/Dry season	:
Patient handset; with nurse call button	1		Winter/Wet season	:
Socket outlet; 8 amp.	1			
			Air changes:	
Bed; hospital	1		– Natural	: 3/h
Chair; upright, stacking	1		– Mechanical	: no
Locker, bedside, wardrobe	1			
Holder; clinical thermometer, wall mounted	1		Lighting level:	
Mattress; bed, hospital	1		– General	: 50 lux
			– Local	: no
			– Night	: no

Fig. 24.11: Activity unit: bedside activity in high nursing dependency intermediate care

SPECIMEN	DATA BANK ACTIVITY UNIT DATA SHEET	Updated
ACTIVITY UNIT	Bedside activity in high nursing dependency	retrieval index AOI.A.

ACTIVITIES: To accomodate a patient who will need continuous basic and technical nursing care and observation and requires the use of oxygen, suction and associated equipment.

Medical and nursing procedures will be performed by up to 4 staff from the side or behind the bed using mobile equipment brought into the area. The patient will occasionally sit out in a easy chair brought into the bed area
Minimum space for this Activity Unit: 350 × 350 cm.

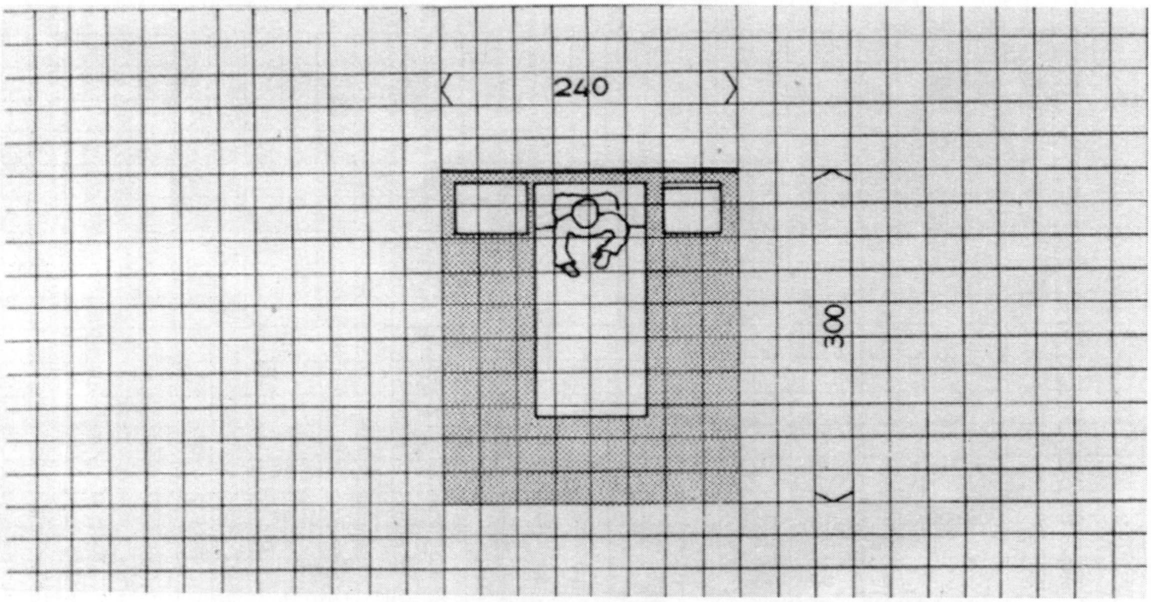

Equipment check-list	Quant.	Specific.	Environmental check-list
Hook; coat	1		Temperature:
Light; bedhead, wall mounted	1		– Dry season
Oxygen outlet; wall mounted	1		– Wet season
Suction outlet	1		
Bed head unit	1		Air changes:
Patient handset; with nurse call button	1		– Natural : 3/h
Socket outlet; 13 amp, switched double	1		– Mechanical : no
Bracket; suction bottle	1		
Holder; clinical thermometer, wall mounted	1		Lighting level:
Bed; hospital	1		– General : 32 lux
Chair; upright, stacking	1		– Local : 150 lux
Locker, bedside, wardrobe	1		– Night : 0, 1 lux
Mattress; bed, hospital	1		
Table; over bed	1		

Fig. 24.12: Activity unit: bedside activity in low dependency care

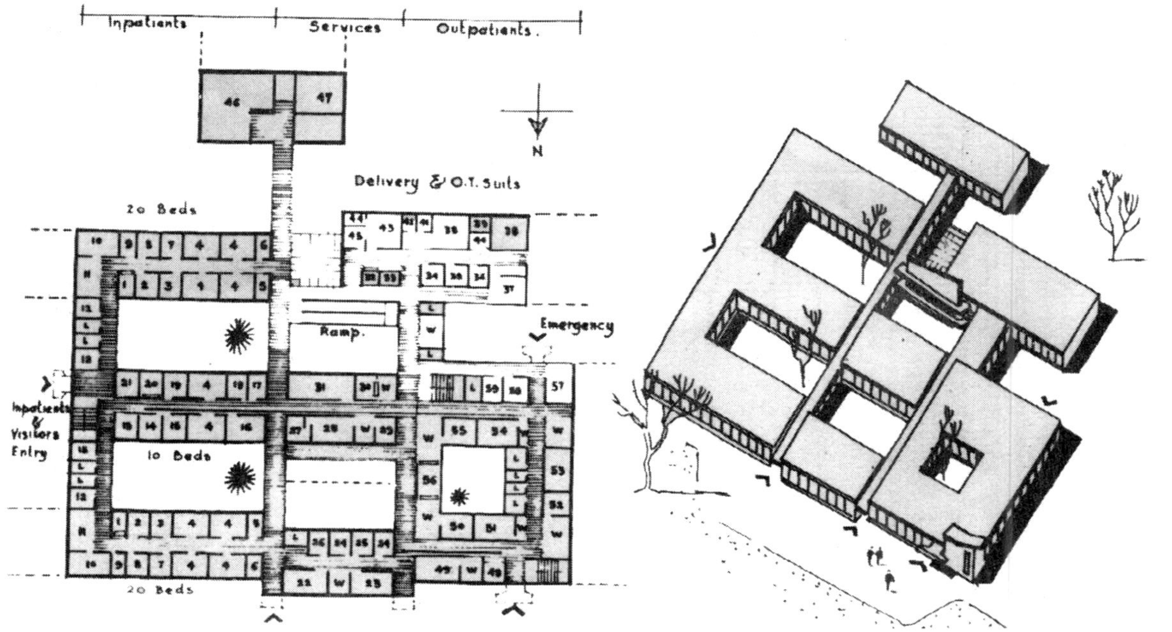

Inpatients

1. Duty
2. Serious patient
3. 2-beds
4. 4-beds
5. Store
6. Linen
7. 2-beds
8. Treatment
9. Pantry
10. Lav & sluice
11. Day space
12. Special bed
13. Admission
14. Treatment
15. 2-beds
16. Lav & sluice
17. Store
18. Linen
19. Serious patient
20. Duty
21. Sister

Services

22. Medical supdt.
23. Office & records
24. Store
25. Store keeper
26. Matron
27. Developing
28. X-ray
29. Radiologist
30. Specimen. rec.
31. Laboratory

Delivery and OTs

32. Duty
33. Linen & st.
34. Preporation
35. Changing
36. Sister
37. Recovery
38. OT
39. Sub-ster
40. Scrub
41. Linen
42. Stores
43. Delivery
44. Wash
45. Prep.
46. Kitchen
47. Store

OPD & Emergency

48. Registration
49. Med. clinic
50. Injection
51. Lady doctor
52. Health visitor
53. Eye-ENT
54. Surg. clinic
55. Dressing
56. Disp/pharmacy
57. Emergency. adm.
58. Minor OT
59. Obs. beds

L Lays
W Waiting
- - - Future
— — — Expansion

Fig. 24.13: Basic layout for an intermediate hospital of 50-100 beds

Facility codes

- Land codes
- Building codes
- Fire codes
- Mechanical codes (service within the building HVAC,. electricity, plumbing, elevators, fuel location, etc).

Building codes These are the generaic codes that cover general construction, and they include such items as structural integrity, material requirements, and HVAC. These codes are necessary for erecting a physically sound structure, model building codes include:

- basic building code

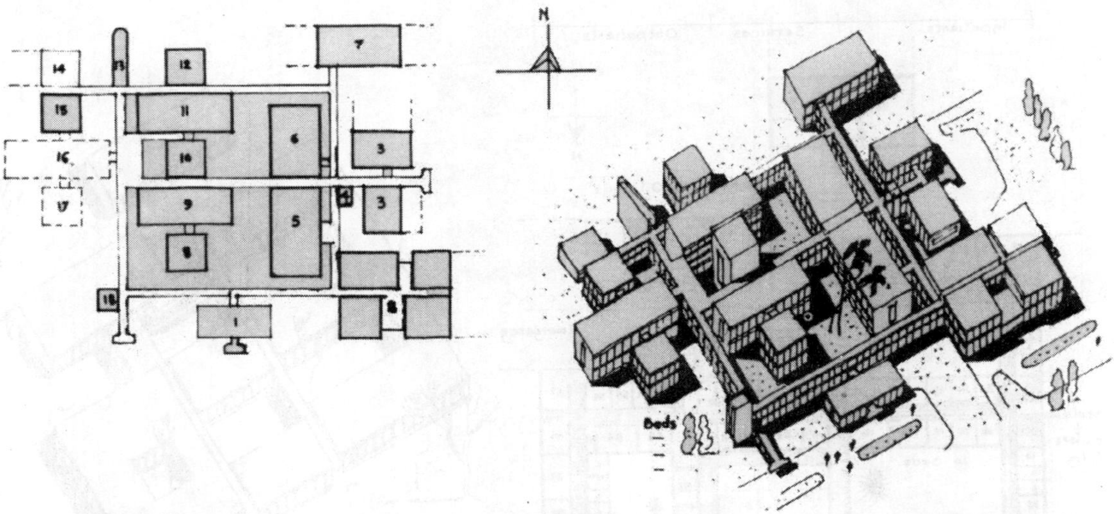

	Ground floor		First floor		Second floor	
	Facilities	*Beds*	*Facilities*	*Beds*	*Facilities*	*Beds*
1.	Administration	—	Future expansion	—		—
2.	OPD & Rehabilitation	—	OPD	—	—	—
3.	Emergency	—	Post operative & Int. care	20	—	—
4.	**Vertical Circulation**					
5.	X-ray & Therapy	—	Operation theatres	—	Future expansion	—
6.	Laboratory & Blood bank	—	Delivery suite	—	Future expansion	—
7.	Paying beds	5	Paying beds	5		
8.	Ward	14a	Ward	14a	Ward	14c
9.	Ward	26a	Ward	26a	Ward	26c
10.	**Vertical Circulation**					
11.	Medical stores	—	Ward	26a	Ward	26c
12.	Central sterilising	—	Ward	26a	Ward	26c
13.	**Ramp**					
14.	Kitchen		Ward	14b	Ward	14b
15.	Bulk store	—	Ward	26b	Ward	26b
16.	Ward	26a	Ward	14b	Ward	14b
17.	Ward	14b				
18.	**Visitors Vertical Circulation**					
Total beds/floor		80		146		146

Possible phases of construction	a	b	c	Total
	80/132	40/94	32/146	372

Fig. 24.14: Basic layout for a referral hospital of 100-350 beds

– standard building code.
– uniform building code.

Fire codes Fire codes set stamdards that attempt to prevent fires from occurring, suppress fires if they do start, or minimize the extent of damage until fire fighters arrive to extinguish the fire. Codes in these categories include the safety aspects of the followings:

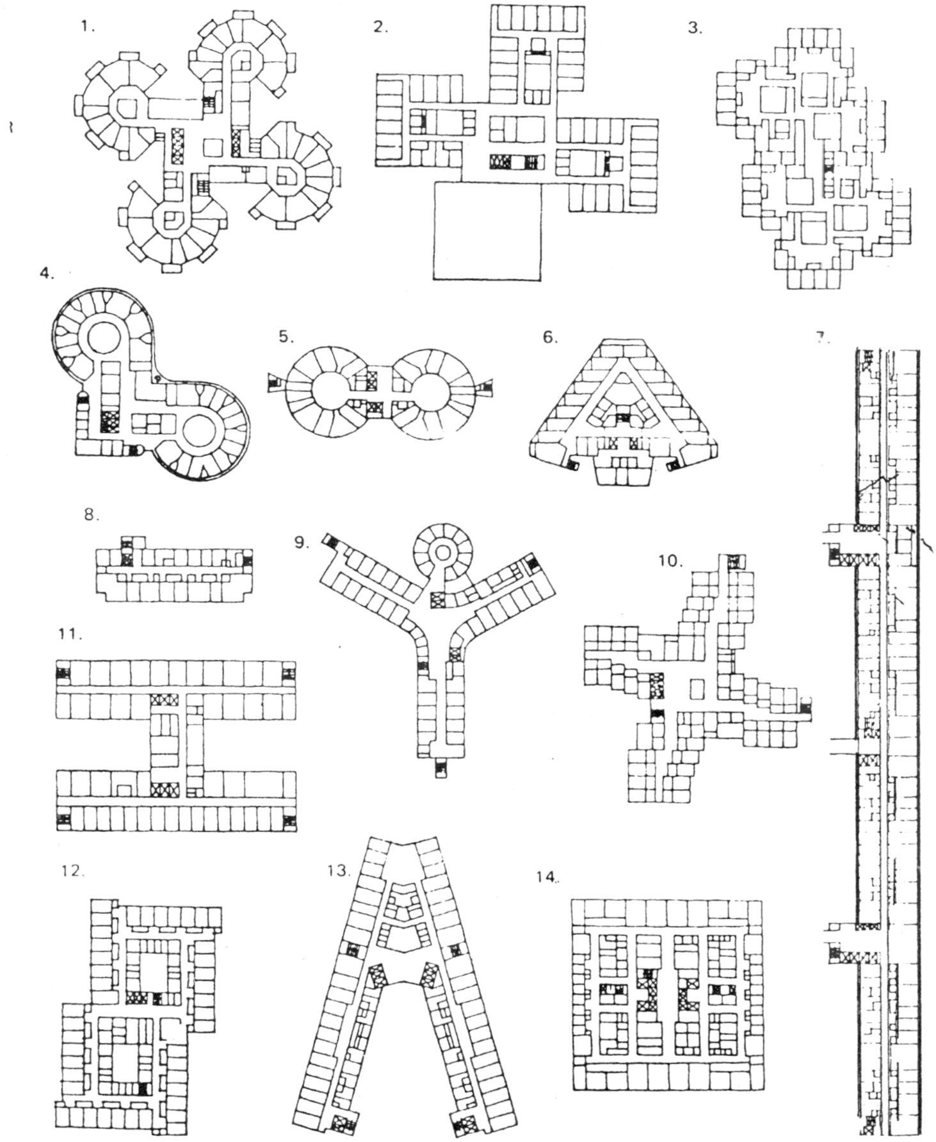

Fig. 24.15: The number of variations in ward unit design is almost limitless—(1) 80 bed unit-Göppingen, German Federal Republic (F Novotny, A Mähner), (2) 116 bed unit-Nuremberg, GFR (Walter Mayer), (3) 100 bed unit-Ravensburg, GFR (Hans Riempp), (4) 60 bed unit-Münster, GFR (Schachner, Weber, Brand), (5) 46 bed unit-Panorama City Calif. (CW Mayhew, LH Thiederman, SR Garfield), (6) 48 bed unit-Sulzam Neckar, GFR (Franz Brümmendorf), (7) 136 bed unit-Hannover, GFR (Gutschow, Nissen), (8) 30 Bed unit-Wolhusen (Brechbühl, Itten), (9) 44 bed unit-Louisiana US (Perry Segura), (10) 80 bed unit-Freudenstadt, GFR (Hans Egon Hahn, Werner K Hahn), (11)72 bed unit-Carmichael, Calif, (Rex Whitaker Allen), (12) 105 bed unit-Nagold, GFR (Hans Egon Hahn), (13) 100 bed unit-Berlin-Kreuzberg, GFR (Peter Poelzig), (14) 112 bed unit-London (Yorke, Rosenberg, Mardall).

- Location of the structure with respect to adjacent buildings
- Area around building
- Structural protection
- Life safety considerations (means existing compartmentalisation of building).
- Detection and extinguishment systems.
- Fixed building wide service systems (fuel and heating systems: electrical service: chutes for waste: elevators: piped gas, etc.).
- Fixed localized system (storage areas; kitchen cooking equipment).

Operational Codes

They are generally intended to be utilized by health care staff as they go about business of caring for patient, as well as the architects/engineers as they design a building:

- The size of the emergency generator depends on what is to be connected to the generator in the emergency.
- Areas that will be used as disaster control need the capability for rapid expansion.
- If electronic equipment to be maintained in-home, a space must be provided.
- Isolation policy.
- Radioactive materials to be used.
- Disposal of hazardous waste.
- Flamable and combustible liquids and gases on site.

If codes pertinent to the project are used from the beginning, a functionally esthetic building is quite possible and will still be within the bounds of the codes.

CONSTRUCTION AND BEYOND

Drawings

Drawings indicate specifically what is to be built and where. It is also through the development of drawing that firm and reasonably accurate cost estimates can be established since the drawings data for actual construction.

Drawing start with sketches formulated in the minds of the owners, can be developed long before any formal plans for building are raised. This will be followed by architect's home work phase when he or she will be starting the process of translating desires and dreams into real designs. Programmes and studies will now be reviewed in great depth for space and functioning aspects reduced to lines on paper. A composite of the results can be generated in the form of scale drawings. This will determine the medical, supportive, and administrative activities able to take place in the new building, as well as the space necessary for mechanical systems (boilers, air-conditioning) storage areas, stains, vents, and structural members.

Basic Scale Stage

- Design development drawings are generated.
- Involves appropriate plans of building, elevations and site work.
- Engineering assistance is necessary to advise enspace requirements of heating, ventillation, and air conditioning and utility restrictions and availability. The persons who do this type of work are called structural, HVAC, plumbing, and electrical engineers.
- A specification work is started at this time which describes the parts of the project in a detailed technical way.

For more accurate costing, more detailed drawings must be developed. A review with owners should be conducted at least several times.

- Drawings are made by various people.
- Architect does the concept drawings. Most drawings are done by skilled drafters. Techniques (computers now available allow them to produce multicolour, shaded and superimposed drawings).
- The final set of drawings for a project are made on fine-grade drafting paper, mylar plastic or cloth with ink or pencil.
- Drawings are printed by a process that results in blue-line or black-line prints on a white background. Computers are being used to generate

drawings as the technology becomes more sophisticated and enables them storage and access of larger quantities of data.

- New form of drawing:

  With the Mylar overlay system prints are placed on top of each other, the system will appear as if only one drawing were made of all the systems.

Workings Drawing Stage

These drawings represent what is actually to be built. When complete they are considered ready for:

- Final approval by owner
- Final approval by enforcement agencies (CON, Fire department, health department, etc.)
- Submission for bid in order to obtain a price to carry out the project construction
- Final cost estimate.

Types of working drawings The various types of drawings and their components are:

1. Title sheet.
2. Abbreviations.
3. Site survey.
4. Subsoil data.
5. Site plan
   - It should indicate all details appropriate to the work: sections of grading, light pole details, patios, roads, curbs, curb cuts, ramps, steps, flag poles, walks, parking, layouts, drainage, hydrants and site utilities.
6. Planting plan indicates planting and landscape decoration.
7. Existing buildings (demolition plan).
8. Existing building (elevation).
9. Floor plans.
   - Room names, dimension, door swing, smoke partition and fire partitions. A floor plan of each floor must be drawn.
10. Elevations
    - Materials, dimensions, window locations, doors, canopies, and all features required to complete the desired architectural complex.
11. Wall sections and details
    - exterior walls, window and door details.
12. Interior details.
13. Reflected ceiling plans.
14. Casework (built-in cabinetary).
15. Room finish schedules and colour material layouts including furniture layouts.
16. Fire and safety plans.
17. HVAC site plan.
18. HVAC floor plan.
19. HVAC details.
20. HVAC riser diagrams.
21. Plumbing site work.
22. Plumbing floor plans.
23. Plumbing riser diagrams.
24. Pulumbing details.
25. Electrical site plan.
26. Electrical floor plan.
27. Electrical details.
28. Electrical riser diagram.
29. Special Drawings
    - Asbestos removal
    - Radiation protection
    - Radiofrequency interference.
30. Shop drawings (details).
31. Detailed drawings.

The change-order drawings

- The change, the drawing reflecting the changes, and the sign-off must be accomplished before any work associated with the change is started.
- It should usually be avoided, as it is the least desired by all parties and involve cost and time, both of which must be justified.

GROUND BREAKING

A ground-breaking ceremony requires planning. This planning can start as early as when it is certain that construction will take place.

One person should be designated as the coordinator of the event. The media coverage is necessary. The administrator should state the purpose of the process (project).

The Construction Process

The many facets of construction process from obtaining permits to having inspection done need consideration.

The contractor is required to obtain various permits needed to build (necessary to erect a building).

Types of permits

- General building permit
- Foundation permit
- Crane operation permit
- Elevator permit
- Gas installation permit
- Oil tank installation permit
- Electric wiring installation permit
- Plumbing installation permit
- Oil or gas heating permit
- HVAC permit.

Construction methods

1. Straight-bid construction.
2. Cost-plus method is used when the contractor is selected without going through the bid process but does agree to submit all costs involved as work progresses. A base figure of 10 percent is added to the base cost as the contractor's profit.
3. *Fast-Track method* It is used by construction management groups to start construction before drawings and specification have been completed.
4. *Construction management method* This method brings construction firm on board early in the process. Its purpose is the use of consultant who has actual cost experience in the field, in order to avoid overrun and underruns in construction cost. A fee is charged for this service.
5. *Turnkey (Design/Build)* This method is used to design and build a project as a package. One company will design and then build new structure.
6. Owner-Build method. This method best suit very small in-house projects.

Mid-course corrections The subject of changes after a contract has been signed is the least desired problem of a project. Minor changes are almost always expected/anticipated. Major changes is expensive. Careful planning will reduce the impact.

Inspections along the way

- As work on a project takes place, various inspections for different purposes will also take place. Are the specifications, being followed? Are the various items being installed in the correct sequence. Are all the various items being installed in the correct sequence. Are all the materials being stored correctly? Another is a check on the quality of workmanship for safety purposes. What is the integrity of welds and flooring? Has the heating system been checked for clean ducts, leaks, and proper air supply and exhaust?
- Check whether items, equipment and systems have been installed correctly and are operating, as intended.
- Check the quality of the workmanship for appearance (finishing work quality).

Maintain safety during construction is contractor's responsibility. The safety of persons in and around the job site needs inspection.

Final approval and start-up Construction is now complete. All inspections and reviews have been completed. There are two government agencies whose approval must be obtained in order to occupy and operate a new hospital. One is the licensure agency which issues a license, stating what type of health activity is permitted in the structure. The other agency is the local building department, which issues an occupancy permit.

Documentation It provides a record of exactly what was built and how it was accomplished.

Documentation can consist of the following:

- construction photographs
- copies of studies or planning conducted in connection with the project.
- copy of any feasibility studies.

CON

- set of all contracts
- full set of updated as—built drawings reflecting actual construction
- copy of the daily log kept by clerk of the works
- record of external costs
- records of all payments
- set of approvals from all agencies
- set of all warranty agreements
- set of instructions for all equipment
- file of all correspondence, meetings, etc.
- addresses of all agencies involved

A well-organised file and filing system will save time and money in later years when trying to locate information for internal needs as well for external audits.

FURTHER READING

1. Klein, Burton R, Albert J Platt: Health care Facility planning and construction. Van Nostrand Reinhold, New York, 1989.

25 Fundamentals of Design

For hospital design biologic and artistic approaches are used.

The biologic approach bases the design on the functional needs and on the balance of the hospital organization with its environment. In this philosophy, the lower boundaries of functions are represented by certified facts, the upper by pure, rationally manipulative concepts.

The hospital development model incorporates the elements of growth, aggregation, formation, differentiation, regrouping, and separation. The increasingly distinct functions, capabilities, and organizational clusters grow until a further differentiation into specialities and sub-specialities occurs which requires new units or departments. Aggregation of specialities produces cross-professional teams with their own requirements on hospital space and the consequent need of regrouping.

A hospital, which imposes a rigid pattern of work on its users, no matter how excellent that pattern might have been theoretically at the time of its conception, is in the long run far less appreciated than the one which may be used in a couple of ways and is extendible. A design anticipating change means design for stability.

The general requirements of the anticipatory planning, which could also be called the open-end planning are:

- Each functional unit of the organization should be expandable at different rates, or replaceable
- The circulation and transport patterns should enable extension without disturbing the basic connections
- The structural systems should be coordinated.

A distinct plan must be provided. Every possible parameter and continuum has to be rigorously planned and systematized, so that a total system and order can be maintained. Somehow the greatness of a plan seems to be poised between absolute determinism and absolute freedom.

Linearity suggests itself immediately as an anticipatory form, which exhibits a high degree of stability with reasonable adaptability.

In the linear spine system, additive departments are entered from a central spine, which may have several levels. It steers the circulation and may house the mechanical service mains. The circulation and energy routes run past the departments and units they serve. There are no thoroughfare departments. This system takes the hospital growth easily, as the departments linked to the linear spine cannot strangle themselves. Labyrinthine paths are avoided. The linear spine system is a straight line arrangement, but it could be bent through 90° or in other geometrical configurations generated by the peculiarities of a site. All deviations from the straight line cause restrictions in the freedom of planning. The linear circulation core in a large hospital has similarities with the main street of a small town. In this area the medical and paramedical activities meet other activities of the society. It is also the meeting area for the outer and inner hospital communities. Diversity without diffusion can be assured by giving different segments of the main corridor some specific character. The higher density of visual elements along the spinal circulation system heightens its image quality and increases its memorability, which is intensified by the awareness of time and weather, if natural light and outside views are available. In the preconception of linear spines, the final configuration of the hospital is not the dominant criterion for design. The functional departmental volumes attached to the linear core are independent, non-permanent, expandable or interchangeable components. A basically linear communication system also simplifies the development of the site in stages.

The image of large hospitals designed linearly will be low, irregular and not monumental. Purposefully-designed spaces and gardens around the hospital would contribute to the well-being of the people in the hospital. Variations in existing hospital shapes are almost unlimited.

The artistic design approach The creative impulse in the artistic approach is based primarily on forms, patterns, and predetermined spaces in the creation of a hospital building. Even in cases, when it is emphasized that structural and mechanical modules have been developed to accommodate a variety of functions and to ease building rehabilitation, the buildings are meant to keep their shape, their original artistic totality and wholeness.

These overtly monumental and systematic hospital buildings are generally much more admirable as pieces of large-scale sculpture than the common, older hospitals.

Most of the artistic forms exhibit poor focus expansion values. No matter how efficiently they may expand their perimeters, their forms will build up internal stress, which results in either a reactionary self-limiting situation, or a high cost and functional disturbances when the central focus is to be renewed. The principle of the qualified, functionally developed shape instead of the a prior determination of shape, the search for the essence of an architectural assignment have to loosen up the one-sided, overhasty, formal dogmatism that has formed like a rigid crust over architectural thinking. To make independent growth of the various units and departments possible, the medical performance areas have to be at the ground level. The anticipatory approach requires generous sites.

Site limitations have been a frequent restraint. When a limited site is the inevitable choice for a new hospital, also the hospital size has to be limited. Large hospitals containing all specialities should give way to some kind of programme-orientated clinics such as human growth and development clinic including pediatrics, obstetrics and gynecology, and musculosketal clinic including rheumatology and orthopedics. Separate specialized clinics need to be less anticipatory than large complex hospitals.

Architectural Qualities

Architecture as the art and science of building the entire man-made environment, in terms of the way it works as much as the way it looks, is like everything else always in the state of metamorphosis. Also a hospital expresses the period-bound requirements of a health cure and care organization, its management system, and the creative architectural ambitions of the same era.

A building, being an embodiment of life, should be conceived as a living entity where form follows function. The function is the sum of all material and spiritual, intellectual and emotional activities within the building. It could be added that a building without comfort, safety, and inviting quality, peace silence, beauty and proper atmosphere have no significance as architecture.

The essence of architectural design include: respect for function, structural integrity, awareness of time, integration with environment, expression of meaning, and unity of design. In outstanding health care facility solutions global experience has to be merged with the local wisdom.

The art and sciences of medicine, concerned with man-as-man, require an environment that is pleasant and peaceful, an environment that will help to restore, as far as environment can keep up the dignity of a man who has lost his own on the bedpan or in the operation room

Bricks and mortar alone do not make an outstanding hospital. High creative work probably needs both time and waste. Good science emerges from dull science, and good literature from a mass of valueless staff. Hospital development is no exception.

The hospital architecture's strength must come out of the intense regard for the needs of patients, staff and visitors. Solutions derived by minds which are both trained and experiences in the specific discipline of hospital design could be expected to be logical and effective. Sensitive architects produce balanced, unconcerned architects dehumanizing buildings. Therefore, the choice of the designer is of a great importance.

Much of hospital architecture affects people from beyond the focus of awareness. They are not sure what it is about a building or room that affects them. This may explain the use of the hospital. Architectural layout is one factor among many that affects communication and morale. A building can make a good situation better or a bad situation worse. Thus, a good hospital not only permits, but actually stimulates good hospital care. An inadequate care creates direct and almost unsurmountable limitations on its personnel. It should always be insisted on quality of the built environment. No opportunity to develop a design should be missed, nothing should be left to chance. Design quality cannot be added to a hospital, which is finished.

Material difficulties must not be allowed to impoverish the human spirit.

People with Disabilities, Personal Privacy

All the known functional needs of the hospital must be satisfied. This is achieved by creating proper spaces in an adequate technological framework. Both recongnized and emerging trends in environmental requirements and needs must be observed. After the general design characteristics have been determined the nature of functions to transpire in each individual space must be determined. Minute attention has to be directed to the fixed and major movable equipment, wall finishing, ceiling finishes, floor coverings, the placement and seeing direction of doors, and the size and position of windows.

The order in which different requirements and components of the hospital are considered, determineds very greatly the physical character of the finished facility.

Most buildings, facilities, and equipment are traditionally designed for the average adult of average weight, height, stamina, agility, reaction time, eyesight, and hearing. The problems of wide variations in agility, stamina, and reaction time are not often seen and understood by the able-bodied population and even by the planners and designers. Consequently the requirements of these people-they may have locomotor, manipulatory or sensory disabilities, or a combination of these are rarely considered during the design process. Lack of these considerations in the health care facility planning process is highly regrettable.

In itself, the current concepts of personal privacy are a relatively recent development, which explains the sometimes-surprising lack of respect for basic sanitation. Degrees of privacy, either desired or possible, are also a function of family values and of socio-economic or other status. In societies with resources on the increase, the respect for the patients' private life and the shift to more private and personal facilities is inevitable as well as the adoption of individualized care.

In groups, where crowded living conditions force a lack of privacy or where privacy has never been experienced, privacy norms are much less severe than they are in situations where they are realistic societal requirements. High densities associated with choice present no problems, but crowding people against their will gives rise to endless difficulties. Possession of territory helps the patient meet a need for security and identity, loss of it can upset psychological homeostasis. Use of space, could be regarded as a non-verbal communication. Where people sit and stand in relation to each other reflects how they feel about one another. The predisposition towards personal territory determines how much intrusion by other a patient could accept. Personal space is an invisible boundary around the body. It is said that it is the area immediately surrounding the individual in which the majority of his interactions takes places. It has no fixed or geographic reference points, moves about with the individual, and expands and contracts under varying situation. It does not extend uniformly in all directions.

The human being is surrounded by four distances zones which differ in sensory input. Intimate distance—0 to 45 cm—allows for the adults the most bodily contact for perception of breath and odour. Visual distortions are present. Personal distance—45 to 120 cm—means that the self of the person is extended and surrounded by a small protective sphere. Voice is kept moderate, body odour is not apparent, and visual distortion is gone. Social distance—120 to 360 cm—is for impersonal transactions. Perceptual information is not complete, as many details are lost public distance—more than 360 cms—means that individuals are not personally involved, only subtle facial expressions are lost. Voices must be projected. It is common under certain conditions for one person to react to another as an object or part of the background. The interpretation and the use of space are derived from past experiences and are influenced by both cultural and social expectations. People from different cultures not only inhabit different sensory worlds and structure space differently, they also experience it differently.

Basic Hospital Areas

In general hospital, there are five rather characteristic and homogenous areas, which have to be arranged so that the interdepartmental circulation flow is kept reasonable. *The in-patient area houses the* residential patients and here their medicoclinical routines are followed. *The clinical service areas* contains the surgical department, including the maternity section, diagnostic and therapeutical X-ray units, pathological laboratories, and the physiotherapy unit, used both by residential and non-residential patients. In *the out-patient area,* which includes the independent emergency department, non-residential patients are admitted for consultation, examination, diagnosis, and treatment.

These three areas are subdivided, articulated and organized to respond to the various requirements, patterns and aspects of the medical work. *The industrial or non-clinical service area* includes catering, house-keeping, maintenance, and central supply services, and the laundry. *Administration,* public and staff facilities form another group. In large hospitals, facilities for research, and in teaching hospitals units for teaching are added.

The main hospital component areas have different development and change rates.

The basic in-patient area—the nursing units—still dominate the hospital set-up. For some time transition from in-patient treatment to out-patient-treatment with the intention to relieve the pressure on the in-patient beds has been observed. Certain economies of cost and energy conservation can be attained by separating hospitals into component buildings that have systems and construction suited to their use.

To zone, the component areas may ease some of the technical problems. There are sub-areas with windows for long-lasting activities and low dependency on service ducts; sub-areas with windows for long-lasting activities and high dependency on service ducts; sub-areas without windows and high dependency on service ducts; circulation areas; and service ducts.

A tight fit between the abstract space demands set out in a brief and the reality of the actual provision might mean an initially more economic building. This would be at the expense of some buffer space to hedge against changes

For hospitals a small range of room sizes appears to accommodate the great majority of activities; the majority of these rooms—70 per cent—are between 5 and 25 m^2, not more than 15 percent are larger than 20 m^2. It is still quite reasonable to suppose that rooms of 15m^2 will serve a very large proportion of hospital needs and would guarantee, if technically properly equipped and prepared, a good degree of interchangeability in use.

CONSTRUCTION BASICS

The hospital construction must be adjusted to the functional needs, be simple, rapidly executable and economical. It should agree with the particular materials it is made of. The limits of these aims have to be controlled by the safety of the structure, the site conditions, and unusual local requirements. The transport requirements play a considerable part in the hospital generation process.

The hospital transport system must be so simple to operate that it can be used by all groups. It must manage all loading conditions. There must be no disturbing noise. The system should not contribute towards spreading nosocomial infections. Passenger transport accounts for 90 percent of hospital transports. The remaining 10 percent account for goods and food transport. Goods transport can be carried out during periods of minimal loading of the hospital's general lift-based transport system, even at night.

The life-length aspect of the hospital should be weighed in at the beginning of a planning process, when the economic life of the hospital and the implications of its change and growth are considered. Various design concepts are being suggested to offset the energy crisis. They include using solar energy systems, using windmills, tapping underground geothermal and acquifer steams, recycling heat generated by incineration of waste, and returning to use of natural resources such as wood and coal. Through careful design, considerable savings can be achieved. The life time of a hospital building as a whole is frequently estimated to about 65 years. It may be convenient to assume that hospital buildings should be replaced after 60 to 90 years, but the chronological age cannot be used to determine the functional suitability of hospital building. Hospital should be used until their usefulness has been truly exhausted. There is no society, which can afford to replace hospitals every 50 to 60 years. Usually, when the supporting physical structure is replaced massive investment is involved. Therefore, supporting physical structure should not be integrated with other building elements. Service systems should be easily replaceable, and accessible for new tappings throughout their whole length. It should be easy to accommodate installations and add new lines.

Generally the supporting physical structure of a building has a life-time of more than 100 years, the basic installations, such as wiring and plumbing, last 20 to 30 years. The elevators last 15 to 25 years, oxygen, vaccum and compressed air plants 20 to 30 years. Mechanical equipment becomes obsolete within 10 years.

Macroelements, Universal Envelopes

Functional and esthetic design considerations have to respect well-motivated requirements of production. However, long-term determination of the shape of a hospital building by the short-term technical and economic conditions imposed by the construction process without understanding the basic needs of the hospital would amount to manufacturing cars without wheels. Construction should be the consequence and not the cause of planning. Huge cube-shaped containers believed to be less expensive to design and build than buildings with identations still catch considerable attention in hospital production as they are believed to solve the problems of perpetual contemporaneity's three variables: time, content and place.

In the Germany, a macroelement of $1200m^2$—5 by 7.2 m in one direction and 5 by 6 m in the other—has been made the basis of a whole hospital set-up. This area's size was greatly determined by the that time fire regulations. The chosen macro-element was expected to house 54 to 60 regular beds or 16 to 22 intensive care beds or 36 to 38 obstetric beds or 60 pediatric beds or 40 beds for infectious patients or a maternity with 18 prepartum beds, 4 labour rooms and 7 delivery rooms or an operation unit of 4 operation rooms and 6 recovery beds or a six room X-ray diagnostic unit including an angiography unit or an out-patient unit for 9 to 12 physicians or a unit for physiotheraphy or a pathological laboratory or an emergency unit or a catering unit for 1500 people. In the US, a uniform module planning unit of $812m^2$ (30.5 by 26.6) has been proposed.

The transport requirements play a considerable part in the hospital generation process.

As a complement to the hospital lift systems, automatic internal distribution systems in all sizes have been introduced. Their merits must be evaluated at an early stage, as their installation is not always justified.

The smallest scale systems relate to materials which would otherwise be transported by the human hand. The largest demand usually a mechanical lift to transport vertically or a cart or a wagon and sometimes special corridors. There are automatic cart inject-eject lifts, which have been in use for some time in spite of the fact that time is wasted waiting and nursing the cart on and off the lift. Electrically-guided vehicles for food trays or supplies, rely on wire-guided paths in the floor and can travel up a 6 percent grade. They can follow paths which are generated in minutes by spraying on the carpet. These tracks remain invisible to the naked eye. Large-scale pneumatic tubes are used to transport bags of soiled linen and trash.

The design of all technical components and installations must be balanced. Examples of over-design in hospitals include refrigeration equipment covering twice the actual needs and lighting levels upto four times in excess of that necessary.

In the Germany Federal Republic, a basic unit of about $1,000m^2$ was made a basic of various nursing units and even for a whole hospital.

In Switzerland a 22-floor hospital tower is based on an almost square shape containing $560m^2$ functional area, when elevators, stairs and waiting areas have been excluded. The floors house a pharmacy, an institution for clinical chemistry and hematology, ward units with 18 respective 28 beds an ENT clinic on three floors and an eye-clinic on three floors.

All universal envelope hospitals conceal enormous stresses as departments attempt to find their size without bursting the envelope. Also high-rise buildings limit the scope of adaptability to functional changes and have a higher percentage of non-usable areas. In Netherlands, about 8.5 percent of the areas in low-rise constructions, but 12 percent in the high-rise constructions are needed for walls, columns and mains shafts. An air-handling system in a high-rise building is less flexible in coping with change, the horizontal building requires less duct shaft area-3 percent versus 8 percent for the high rise—that the horizontal building requires less equipment room space 2.6 percent versus 9 percent and that energy costs be lower in the low-rise building, However, a low rise building requires more ceiling space and their duct work distribution costs and maintenance costs are higher.

Unlimited Adaptability

There are movable furniture and wall partitions which are part of a system of modular seamless plastic containers, frames, carts, panels and rails. All space is considered capable of housing any activity until specialized equipment is moved in to create a tailor-made environment.

The use of movable panels and panel-hug work surfaces may enable to dispense with most fixed casework and achieve an anonymity the various rooms. Rails can be placed at various heights on walls and working surface modules hung from them to set up "action office stations". Movable walls and partitions by themselves are no guarantee for making variability in functions easy. These and similar provisions for change to the inside of build ings are expensive. The kinds of change that most often happen are additions and minor modifications in existing area. These occur in a random way that make demountable partitions almost useless and not cost-effective.

An Interstitial Space

Interstitial space is defined as a space above the ceiling and below the floor of two adjacent stories measuring not less than 1.5 m in height and of not less than one-hour fire-resistive noncombustible construction. Its free height varies between 2.2 and 2.8 m.

. The interstitial spaces are for the mechanical discipline and can accommodate air handling equipment; transformer rooms; plumbing; fire stand pipe; domestic hot and cold water; acid waste piping, vacuum for cleaning; medical vacuum, high and low pressure compressed air oxygen, nitrogen, nitrous oxide and natural gas; pneumatic chutes for moving sealed bags of trash and soiled laundry to disposal areas; film and document conveyers, and other distribution systems.

In the US, the building standards require in interstitial space exhaust ventilation at the rate of not less than two air changes hourly. The fire alarm system, including wiring, has to be insulated against fire. The real needs for interstitial accommodations are very limited. The part of a hospital mechanical system which requires maintenance on a continuing basis tends to be the fans, which are most easily dealt with if they are located in an easily accessible fan room, which can be located on the roof or on the same floor level as everything else. The true potentials of the interstitial floor system in all hospital areas, have not yet been thoroughly exploited. This concept would be best used when all parts of the facility have equal perennial requirements of considerable changes. The interstitial spaces are initially very expensive and not particularly amenable to growth. The interstitial space with long-span construction increases initial construction costs.

DESIGN CONSIDERATIONS

Single Storey vs Multistorey

Hospitals have been and continue to be planned in a variety of forms. The form varies from-open, low density plan to the monolithic, air-conditioned tower-giving high-density site coverage.

Low density developments are more easily ventilated naturally, need no lifts, are more easily extended and can be evacuated easily in case of fire. It is also easier to build both in terms of money and energy.

The ward buildings must be at least 9 m apart to prevent conversation in one building being overheard in the other. Higher buildings should have adequate spacing in between (at least equal to its hight).

In hot dry climate, building with small windows insulated walls, deep shady internal courts may be used to keep the building cool.

Fire Safety

Fire safety is very important while planning a building. Means of escape must be provided at the ends and the center. There should be fire-resisting doors, which may be used to divide the floor into fire-resistant compartments.

Orientation

View is the most important criteria for deciding the orientation of ward buildings. Since the patient is confined to his bed for nearly 24 hours a day during his stay, the view he gets is his only link with the outside. The wards should be so planned as to have maximum number of patients getting a good view.

Acoustics

Though certain sounds can be comforting, excessive noise causes irritation, distraction and fatigue. The ways in which noise can be controlled or reduced are:

- controlling noise at its source, by using silent machines,
- maintaining the equipment, closing doors softly, etc.
- site planning—buildings should be away from noisy streets.
- architectural design—building elements should be divided into quite and noisy groups, both horizontally and vertically to prevent transmission of sound noise and vibrations producing equipment should be placed in the basement or isolated from the rest of the building.
- sound can be absorbed by using acoustical material on the walls and ceilings and inside the walls surrounding the source.

Climate Control

The comfort criteria is not limited to temperature alone but must also include control of humidity in order to avoid respiratory illness, dehydration, and static electricity as well as good quality air sanitation to prevent the spread of odors, air pollutants and bacteria. The comfort range lies between 22°C to 26°C with the relative humidity varying between 30-60 percent. The system should be selected so as to minimize noise.

Since air-borne infection is a major problem in hospitals, ventilation system should be designed to control this problem by the clean areas like the clean utility, operation rooms, ICUs, etc. should be maintained at a higher pressure than the adjoining areas so that the infected or dirty air cannot leak into them through the openings. Filters should be provided at the diffusers in clean areas and also at the inlet of fresh air.

Ward Access

The following points are important about the entrance to the wards:

No ward should form a passage-way into the other.

- Where more than one entrance is provided the main entrance should be clearly identifiable.
- For security reasons the entrance should be visible from the nurses' station.

Plumbing

The plumbing should be capable of providing the water at the required temperature at various points i.e. 110°F or 43°C for washing and 180°F or 83°C for sterilizing. The system should be capable of delivering 300 lit/bed/day. Fixtures include:

- Lavatories: Goose-neck facets for all hand washing lavatories. The valves should be controlled by foot, knee or wrist to prevent contamination.
- Toilet fixtures: Bedpan washer and a WC.
- Bathing facilities: Elevated bath tub or shower fitted with spray head.
- Clinical service sink: Similar to a WC, used for emptying liquid waste from a bedpan.

Auxiliary Electrical Systems

Several auxiliary systems must be incorporated in order to provide safety and security:

1. Fire alarm system capable of:
   - detecting smoke, fire.
   - locating its origin and automatically inform the fire station.
   - activate prevention systems like the sprinkler system.
2. Nurse call system: This allows for a relatively small number of staff to be on call to a large number of patients, it should have the following features:

It should be capable of two-way communication.
   - The call button should be located in the toilet and bath also.
   - The pannel at the nurse's station should indicate the origin of the call.
3. TV antenna system: if televisions are provided for the patients, a central television antenna will be required. An empty conduit system should be provided in the building with outlets in room, launges, day rooms, etc.
4. Telephone network capable of handling:
   - internal communication within the building and
   - external to and from calls should be provided. The dusting should be provided for the same.

Doors

Clear openings required in a doorway is for:
- Stretcher 110 cm
- Wheelchairs 86cms
- General purposes-80cms

Door hardware should be designed with a single lever action. A device which holds the door open must be provided.

Doors subject to heavy traffic must be protected upto a height of 125cm with rubber, PVC or stainless steel, kick-plates should be sound absorbent.

Windows

The ability to look out is extremely important. A good view consists of a portion of both ground and the sky. The view should change with a change in the viewer's position. Window size is a compromise between a satisfying view and the need to conserve energy used in air conditioning, if provided. Otherwise windows are a means of providing natural ventilation in buildings. Near views require about 3.1 sq. mts opening and distant views require about 2.4 sq. mts. Generally, window area is about 20-30 percent of the floor area.

Metal casement windows often made from standard steel sections provide a long-lasting window. These windows are quite effective ventilators since they can scoop air into the building if they are opened in the right direction. However, there is no vertical control of the air movement and often large panes reduce the effective open area.

Insect-proofing can be achieved by using a mesh of appropriate size.

The use of adjustable louvers has the following advantages:
- It is cheaper than wood or metal
- Allows for variable ventilation upto nearly 100 percent of the opening.
- Can control the vertical movement of the breeze.
- It can be adapted to any width of the opening simply by cutting the glass lower blades to the required length.
- They can be easily burglar proofed by fixing horizontal bars between them.

Finishes

Carefully-chosen colour schemes not only contributes to the beauty of the patient care facility, but will also create a beneficial psychological effect on the patient. There is evidence of increased activity and alertness in the presence of warm and luminous colour, thus creating an environment conducive to muscular effort, action and cheerful well-being. Colour treatment should be based on the use of the room. The size of the surface area to be coloured should also be considered. Large surfaces should be in pastel and soft shades, while small surfaces areas could be strong bright colour.

Interior Surfaces

Interior surfaces are an important aspect of the environment in stimulating vision and the sense of touch. The materials should be selected after considering their hygienic qualities, colour, reflect, acoustical qualities, insulation, texture and durability.

The usage of the walls should be kept in mind while deciding its surface materials. Walls and doors should be easily maintainable. Glossy surfaces should not be used in order to avoid glare. Vinyl wall covering is excellent in areas, which need frequent cleaning, The material chosen for floors should have smoothness , warmth, resilience, ease of maintenance.

Other factors like wheelchair or stretcher maneuverability should also be considered.

Ceilings can be more textured than the walls or floors since they don't come in physical contact. They are maintained for thermal insulation and sound distribution and absorption. Other surfaces like the built in equipment, furniture, etc, should have flats, non-glossy finish with low reflectance.

Resident furnishings must be of sufficient variety to appeal to different tastes and must always be residential looking. The beds may be adjustable in height through a certain range. The height adjustments may be manually or electrically operated. Beds should also be provided with other accessories like side rails, TV stands, and frames for suspension of arms and legs in cast. The head panel should be collapsible in order to give aid to the patient from the side near his head in case of emergencies. Recent scientific developments have made it possible to use a special material in the manufacture of beds which is radiolucent to X-rays. The chair should have a high back, be water-proof, and easily cleanable. Reclining chairs with footrest adds to the comfort of the patient's visitor who may stay for long periods. Sleeper chairs can be used by patients visitors intending to stay overnight. A bedside cabinet is necessary for the storage of patient's belongings. The cabinet should have lockable drawers and an acid resistant top for keeping drinking water and medicine. An overbed table should be provided for the purpose of reading, writing or feeding. The top can be modified to have a built in vanity storage with a mirror for the grooming of the patient.

Signposting

Signposting, identification sings and graphics is a must for proper orientation of an individual. Signage must be clear and consistant. It is generally recommended to have the characters in white set against a dark background. Signage is of two types:

Interior signs—needed to identify the building, entrance, parking and exits include:

Directory or layout plan is the first reference point showing various departments in the building.

- "Road sign" is used for directing people to proper areas.
- Room identification are signs placed outside the door to be identified.
- Emergency exit direction should be prominently displayed showing the nearest emergency exit.

Well designed lighting is essential to create a positive and esthetically pleasing environment for the patients, staff and visitors. Both natural and artificial lighting should be designed against the same criteria. General room lighting should come from several sources as it is fatiguing to have to work between areas of greatly varying intensity. Direct lighting is important for special tasks like-examination, writing, reading, etc. It can be improved by the use of polarising panel or with high angle cut off diffusers. Abrupt changes in lighting levels or types must be avoided. The source should provide high, glare free, lighting level which is necessary for the safety of the people in the building and also keep the operating costs minimum.

The levels of lighting must be sufficient for instrument reading, charting and patient examination. Illumination must not distort colour and complexion. Attention must be given to the reflectance value of walls, ceilings and floors. Reflectance value depends upon colour and texture. Recommended reflectance values are:

Ceilings	80-95 percent
Upper walls	40-60 percent
Floors and lower walls	15-25 percent
Furniture	25-40 percent

General illumination level of 300 lux has been recommended. Night light should be variable and controlled by a dimmer. Lighting in intensive care and cornary care unit must not produce any electrical noise in monitoring equipment.

Lighting arrangements in wards must not disturb the patient continuously.

In corridors, continuous lighting e.g. continuously mounted flourescent tubes in or on the ceiling adjacent to one of the walls are used. The reasonable levels of illumination are about 300 lux at daytime 200 lux in evening 20-40 lux at night.

There should be minimal glare from the fluorescent tubes when viewed by patients on bed or trollies.

General room lighting should come from several sources. Light quantities should be about 750 lux with dimmer. Task lighting of 2,000 to 10,000 lux is required.

Uniform indirect lighting with the level of 400 lux is recommended, in emergency department supported by special examination lamps.

Lighting in corridors should be continuous and along the walls.

26 Functional Design

Architecture uses space and materials to create a permanent structure as a framework for action, so fitness for purpose is of primary importance. Architectural forms are according to the building purposes. Typically, architacture serves different forms of action and takes their specific needs into account. Foreseeable changes should also be given consideration.

Architectural technology has many parts contributing more or less equaly to the final result. They include construction techniques, harmonious arrangement of building massas and spaces, typical of architacture is the cooperation with other planning groups concerned with building elements. thermal, water, ventilation and electrical services, aconstics, and indoor decoration—all integral parts of a project. The most important and earliest phase of cooperation is with the future users of the building, to achieve a detailed analysis of its final use.

Research is Vital

All research in these fields must be considered basic architectural research. The purpose of all such research and practical study is to encourage constantly progressive techniques that will contribute to improved architactural art.

Functional research is indispensable to any architect if his building is to fulfil the practical demands of its users. Functional and architectural harmony must exist together. Once functional demands have been clarified, the architect, should be able to show how modifications will influence a total design. Research in architectural technology should be thorough since building techniques and materials, as well as basic functions, are constantly changing. The individual planner should be able to take advantage of modern architectural technology by having available a source of up-to-date information resulting from basic research.

This is particularly nacessary for hospital building something that many architects have not found particularly interesting, in spite of the opportunities a big general hospital offers. The size of the project, its high standard, and the variety of available building elements and materials all offer scope for creativity. Generally, in hospital, architecture, big entries are concieved and handled vary freely as far as block and space arrangements are concerned. On the other hand, very specific functional demands in certain parts of the building bring discipline to the planning work.

Hospital building can claim many projects of high architectural merit, which incorporate interesting details and a feeling for atmosphere despite the large size of the building. Good hospital planning must be scaled to human needs.

Planning a hospital building is a vast multi-dimensional task which demands an all-round knowladge of building technology and a multi-disciplinary approach. It is necessary to have adequate understanding of basic medical aspects, such as examination, treatment and a major consideration underlying all architectural design is the fulfilment of human needs, but hospital buildings must cater for a changing population of patients, who all need secure and encouraging conditions in which to improve their health. There is also a permanent population of staff who require the basic possible environment in which one finds it difficult to perform and do arduous duties efficiently and happily. Hospital buildings often risk being intimidating in scale and institutional in character, and architectural delight often becomes overclaimed by technical planning issues in the design stage.

Maximum Flexibility

Datailed user studies of function often prove to be misleading, inadequate and of no help to the designer when functional requirements change rapidly.

The user studies of function are not in themselves a sound basis for hospital design. Functions change so rapidly that designers should no longar aim for an optimum fit between building and function, the real requirement is to design a building, which will inhibit change of function least and not one that will fit a specific function best. One means of accommodating changes in function and technology has been to design a high quality, fully-serviced building shell that offers the maximum amount of flexibility in the three main operating zones: nursing, clinical and support. The nursing zone deals primarily with patient care, and should have as much natural light and ventilation as far as possible. The clinical zone consisting of diagnostic and treatment facilities, is largely associated with technical equipment and is often artifically ventilated. Finally the support zone comprises kitchens, stores, laundry, building services and all the other facilities required to run the hospital. On the basis of this interpretation, successful hospital planning relies on the manipulation of the three zones and the relationship created between them.

In order to provide a caring environment on a human scale, there has been a move away from very large centralized hospitals. This has many advant–ages to staff as well as patients and has dictated a closer network of community health care. health care planners are now avoiding specialized treat–ment centres where patients are treated in unfmiliar surroundings away from their community and providing an affective system of primary medical care. This filters patients to the appropriate local treatment centre from general practitioner and community health center upto district general hospitals and the large city teaching hospitals.

Hospital designers have also responded to a problem of built-in obsolescence that finds any large hospital buildings out of date by the time their complex planning and building programme attempt to contain the cost and scale of acute care hospitals it provides for an initial phase or nucleus of a general hospital, which can subsequently be extended if required. The first phase is limited to about 300 beds and is fully operational in its own right, it is a highly versatile and economical answer to the problem of growth and change. In design terms, the nucleus hospital has best been conceived as a modular development of linked, low rise buildings which relate to the local community and allow maximum flexibility of function. This care of buildings may be expanded over a pariod of time as the requirement limited capital investment, responds quickly to new medical needs and forms a strong base to the national healthcare service. The clinical designs of a cancer centre must address the needs of the patients and their families and encourage joint efforts with the professional staff to form a common therapeutic and supportive bone. The design focus must concentrate on crucial human values, such as control of disease, pain and disability. Life must include psychological, as well as physical health. Today's cancer centre must be designed for such fulfilments, not efficiency in patient care alone. The management of cancer has changed dramatically during the past three decades and is becoming increasingly individualized and complex both in diagnostic procedures and in treatment and costs. Advances in treatment have produced a steady increase in the number of cancer patients cured or living with stabilized disease. These patients require physical and psychological rehabilitation and support. The advances in treatment, the increased surival rate, along with skyrocketing health care costs, mandate, change in the design of buildings that provide care to the cancer patient. In the past two decades more hospitals have developed outpatient services, to compete with inpatient services.

The shift from inpatient to outpatient care has resulted from a number of factors: rising health care costs, patient satisfaction, demands for cancer care that is convenient and accessible, family involvement, and evolving and everimproving technology, including interlocking pharmacy and drug delivery systems.

Plot Ratios

Examples of plot ratios and subsequent possible schemes for distributing the required areas in the hospital are as follows (Figs 26.1a to d).

In the suburbs, where population densities are low and land can be obtained easily, a plot ratio of not more than 0.5 should be sought. In the center of a town, no more than 2 should be provided.

Orientation

The orientation with regard to the sun and prevailing winds must be checked (Fig. 26.2). It has been found that orientating buildings along an east-west axis, giving the longer sides of the building northen and southern exposures, is the most desirable. In areas where the major climatic problem is humidity rather than heat, buildings should be sited at a slight angle, either towards the east or the west, depending on the direction of the prevailing wind.

In order to overcome severe aspects of the climate at the building site, a favorable microclimate

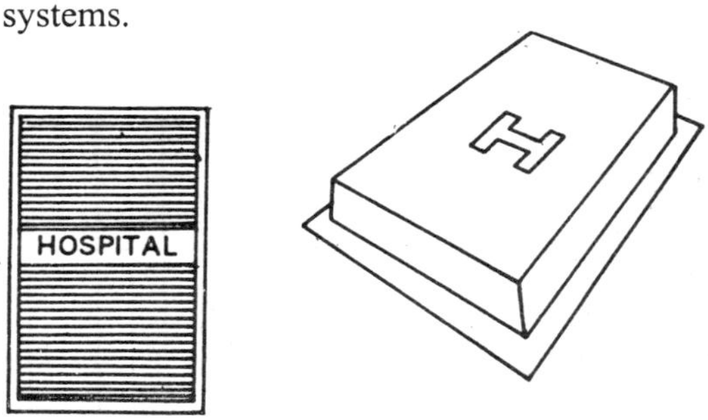

Fig. 26.1a: A plot ratio of 1 means that one-storey building will cover the entire area of the site

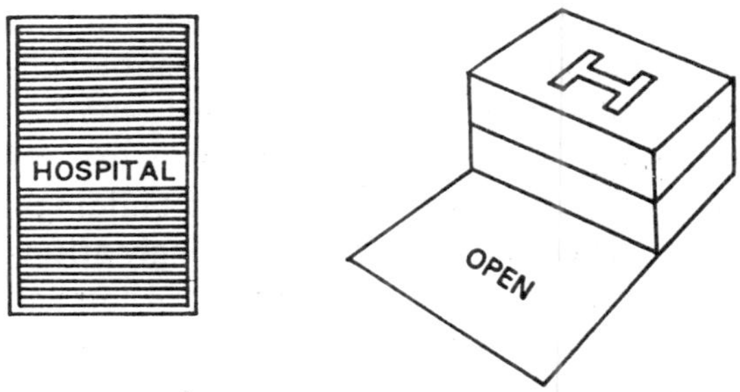

Fig. 26.1b: Since it is recommended that 50% of a site area be left open for roads, other circulation routes, parking and landscaping, a plot ratio of 1 would require a solution in which the area requirements are distributed in a two-storey building

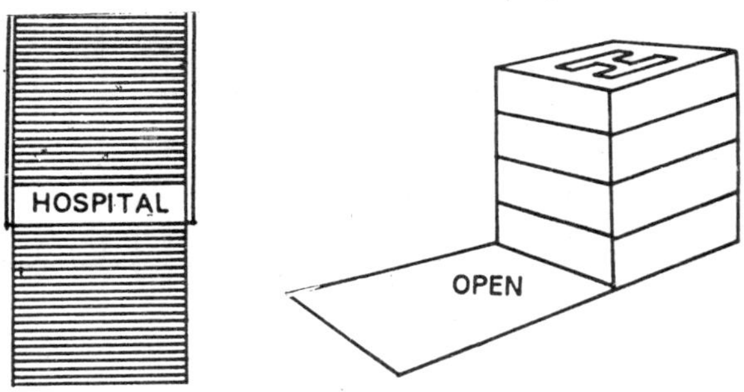

Fig. 26.1c: Similarly, a plot ratio of 2 would lead to a four storey solution

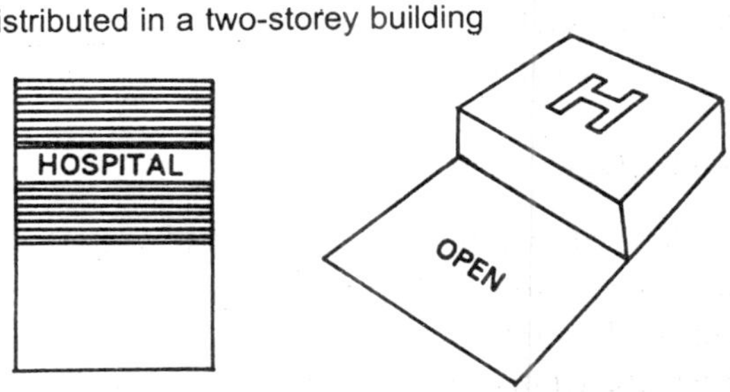

Fig. 26.1d: A plot ratio of 0.5 would lead to a one-storey

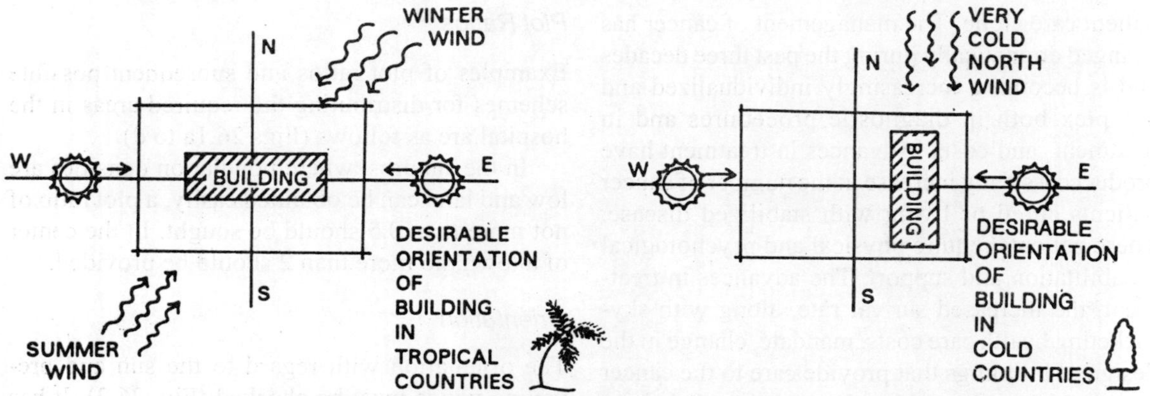

Fig. 26.2: Orientation of sun and wind (conditions in northern hemisphere)

should be provided through landscaping, lawns, paving and planting trees and shrubs as well as constructing ornamental bodies of water and creating sunny and shady areas.

Illumination and ventilation are major problems in hospitals, and these are further aggravated by modern trends to construct 'deep' buildings using steel and reinforced concrete. Good ventilation in tropical climates ideally requires long, narrow buildings; but this is not always feasible, and a compromise must be found by separating activities and orientating builodings or wings of buildings. Incorrect orientation of buildings strongly affects the consumption of energy in the finished hospital.

In areas where there are heavy rains accompanied by wind, all openings should be protected against wind-driven rain. In hot, humid areas, the external surface should reflect as much solar radiation as possible, and the walls and roof should, as far as possible, be made of lightweight material with low thermal capacity.

Slope Study

On sites with steep slopes, the best areas for building must be found. As a rule, slopes of 0-10 percent are desirable and easy to build on (Fig. 26.3); slopes greater than these require either massive cuts or massive fill or a combination of the two.

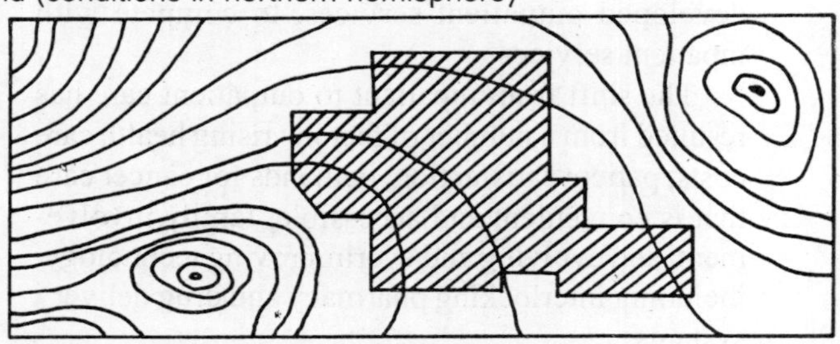

Fig. 26.3: Slope map

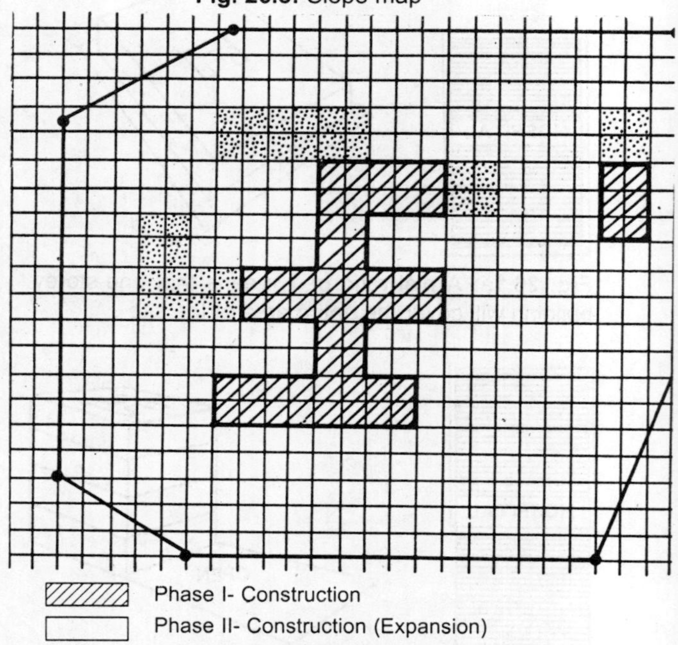

Fig. 26.4: Independent expansion of separate components

Upwards (Vertical) Growth

This direction of growth is the option for block forms on very limited sites (Fig. 26.5). It disrupts operations, particularly on the top floor of the hospital; construction materials are difficult to transport, requiring an elaborate system of scaffoldings and hoists. Excess material, although initially expensive, must be installed ahead of time, in:

- foundations that will accommodate the future load of additional floors;
- sanitary, electrical and mechanical systems that will accommodate future requirements;
- a strong roof slab on the top floor that can be converted to a future floor slab that will support the projected load of patients and equipment; and
- special and sometimes costly provisions to ensure that the building remains waterproof throughout the period of extension.

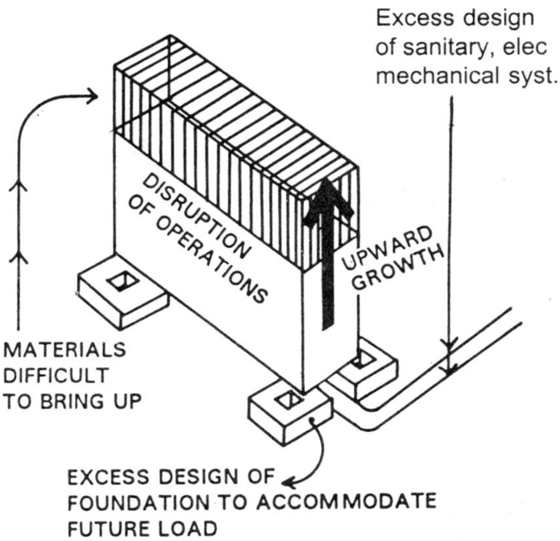

Fig. 26.5: Upward growth

Master Plan

The master plan of a hospital is the basis for present and future decisions on the layout of buildings and services, changes in needs and phasing.

The master plan consists of two elements: determination of circulation routes and corridor system, and location of elements on the site in relation to one another.

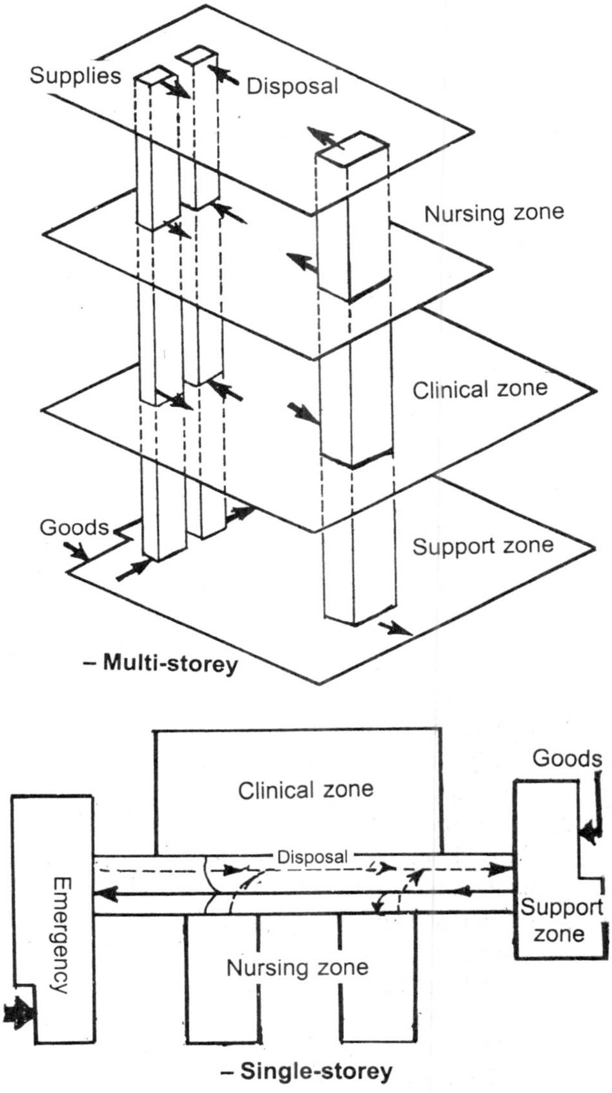

Fig. 26.6: Circulation in Multi- and Single-storey

The placing of elements and departments on a site should result in an optimal interrelationship among departments and provide room for expansion (Fig. 26.7). Some principles and guidlines for the disposition of the units of a hospital are as follows:

1. Departments that are most closely linked to the community should be closest to the main

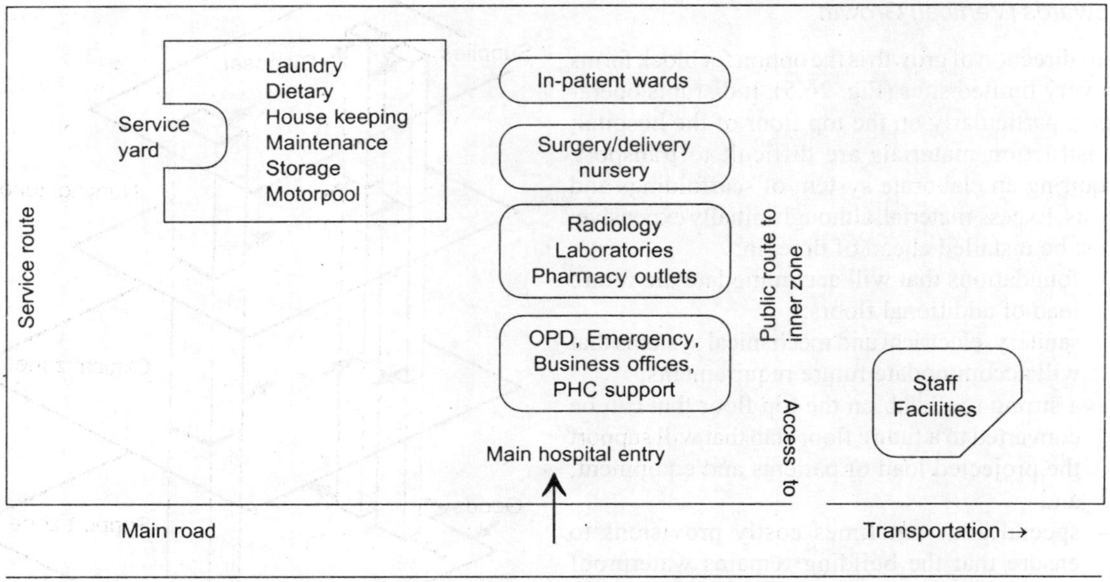

Fig. 26.7: Zoning of elements on a site

entrance: out-patient department, emergency, administration (especially business sections), family planning clinic and other primary health care support.

2. Departments that receive their workload from those described above should be next closest to the entrance: X-ray, laboratories, dispensary.
3. In-patient departments should be in the interior zones, or wards.
4. Operating theatres, the delivery department and the nursery should have (1) and (2) on one side and (3) on the other, e.g., to provide easy access from the emergency and accident.

The modular *village form* (Fig. 26.8) is similar to the village concept except that the departments must fil into a predetermined form. This form is useful when repeated modules are used. It results, however, in forced planning of departments to fit within the same shape: some will fit just right, others will be 'bursting at the seams' and others will have wasted space.

The *finger* plan consists of a central corridor and side corridors, which link various departments branching out in 'finger'. It is a development of the train corridor form (Fig. 26.9), in which one must pass through one compartment to reach the next. Since the corridors in the finger plan have single function, this form lends itself to the provision of abundant natural ventilation and lighting.

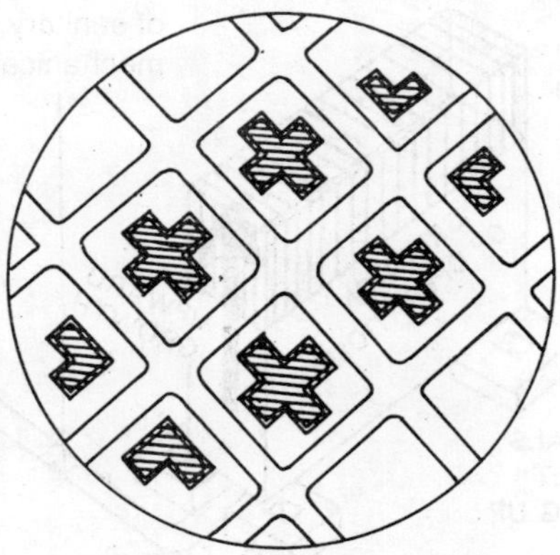

Fig. 26.8: Modular village form

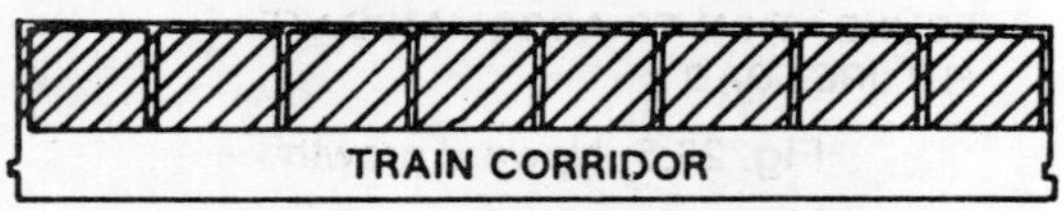

Fig. 26.9: Train corridor plan

An *open-ended finger* development plan (Fig. 26.10) can allow for the expansion of individual

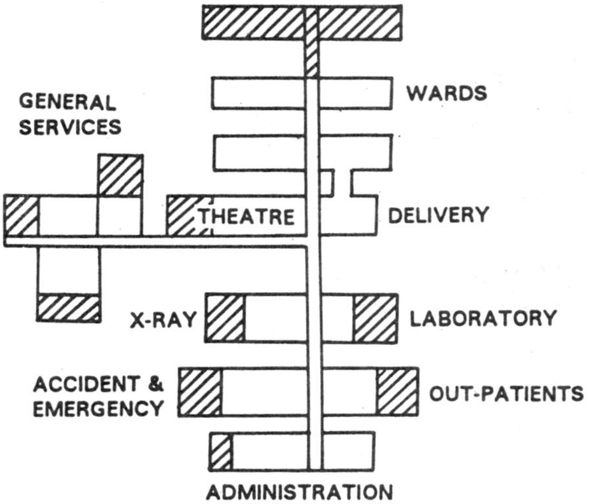

development, by progressive extension of the main corridor as further components are required.

The *block* (Fig. 26.11) is a form for sites where the ground area is limited. As the hospital is developed vertically, optimal relationships between departments may be difficult to achieve and one department may be disposed on two levels. It is also a form that is difficult to expand later. It is appropriate for designing wards, since wards have generally similar floor plans; however, structural costs are likely to be higher than those for a similar number of wards in a single-storey construction.

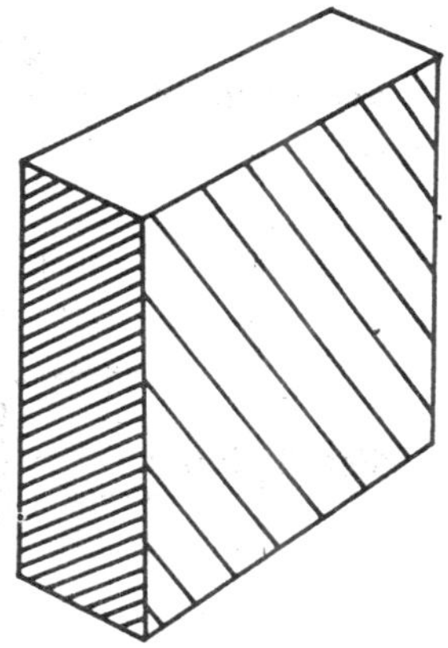

Fig. 26.11: Block form

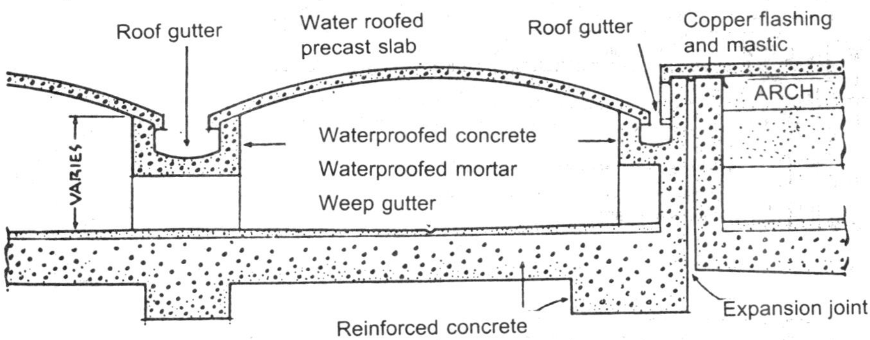

Fig. 26.12: Detail of double concrete roof construction

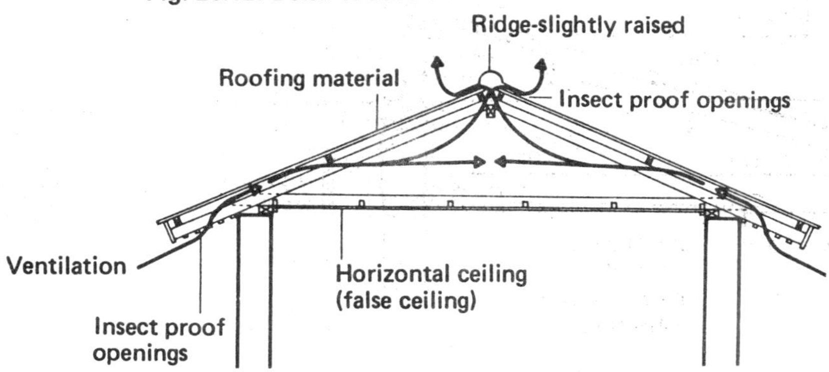

Fig. 26.13: Ventilation of roof space in a building provided with a false ceiling

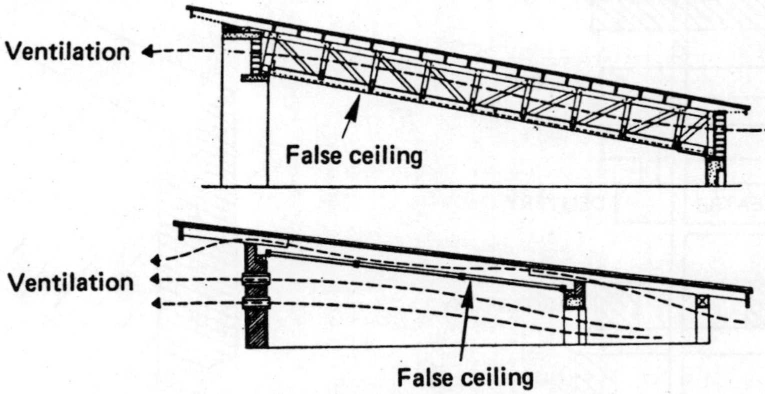

Fig. 26.14: Ventilation of roof space in buildings with a sloping roof and false ceiling

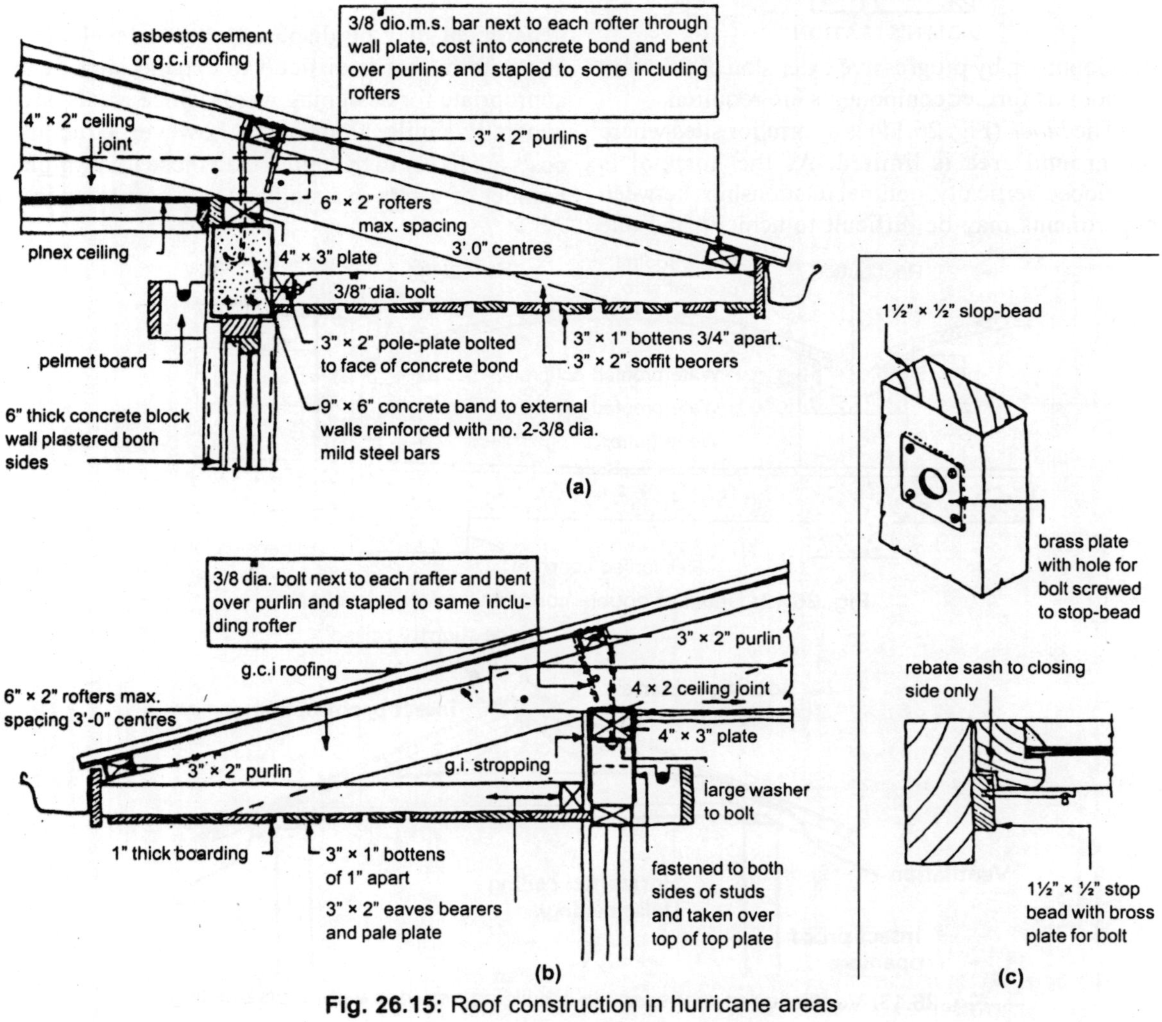

Fig. 26.15: Roof construction in hurricane areas

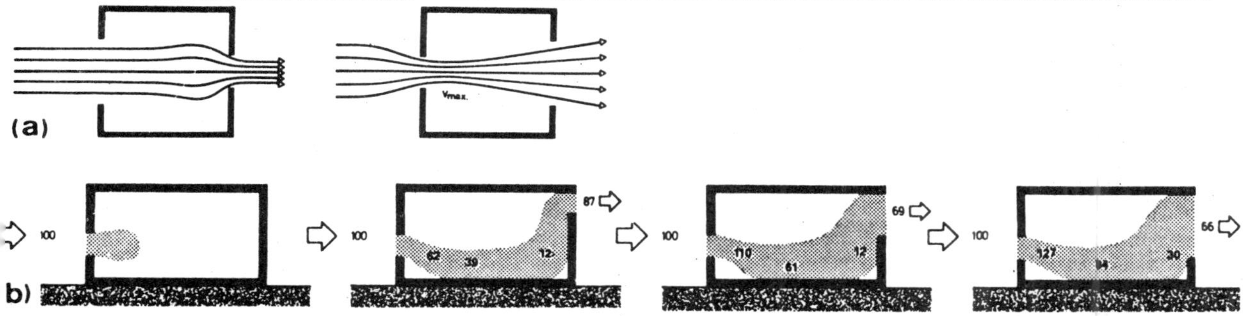

Fig. 26.16: Air flow patterns for various sizes and patterns of openings and partitions (a) the velocity of air flow is increased if the inlet is made smaller than the outlet, and (b) the size of the outlet compared with that of the inlet is critical; if the initial air velocity outside the building is taken as 100 (left), the other figures represent percentages of the initial velocity

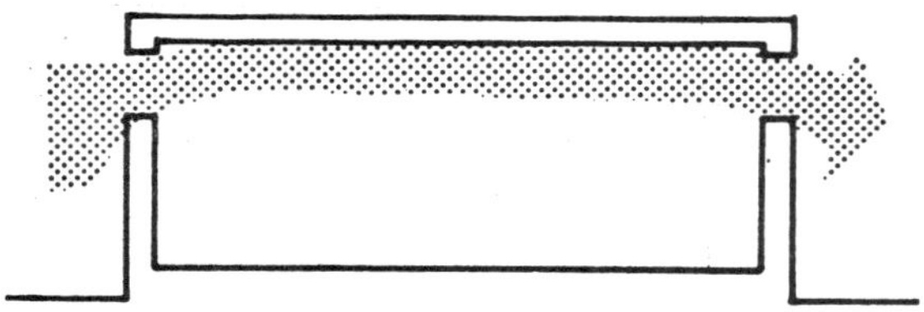

A. High inlet and outlet do not produce good air movement at body level

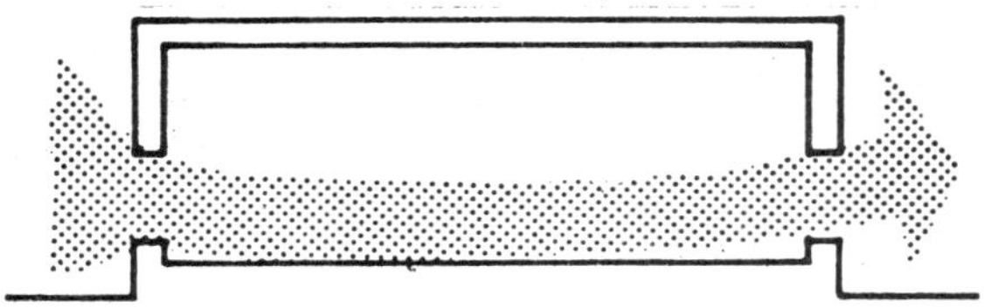

B. Low inlet and outlet produce a beneficial low-level wind pattern

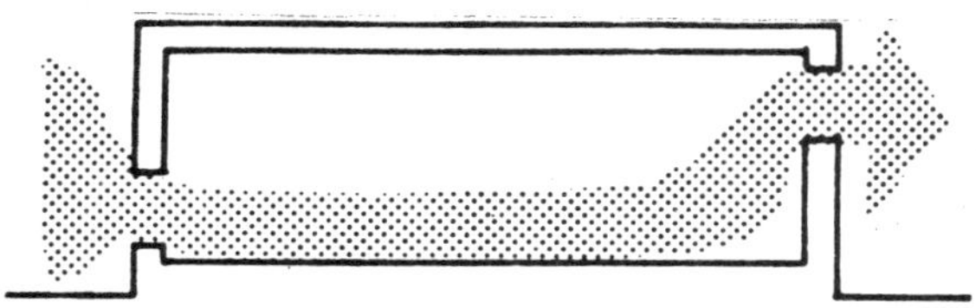

C. Low inlet and high outlet produce a good pattern of air movement

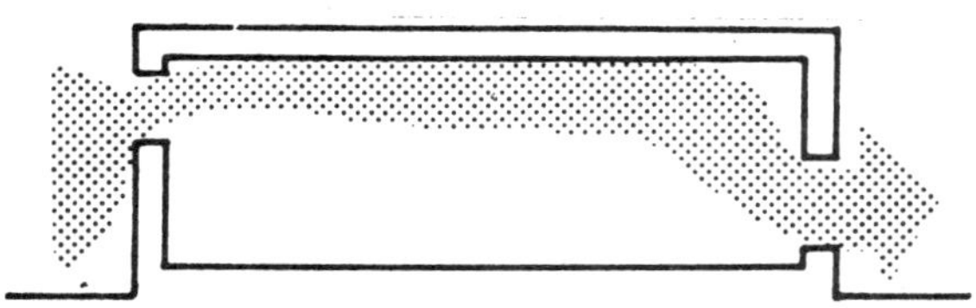

D. The bad pattern caused by a high inlet is not corrected by a low outlet

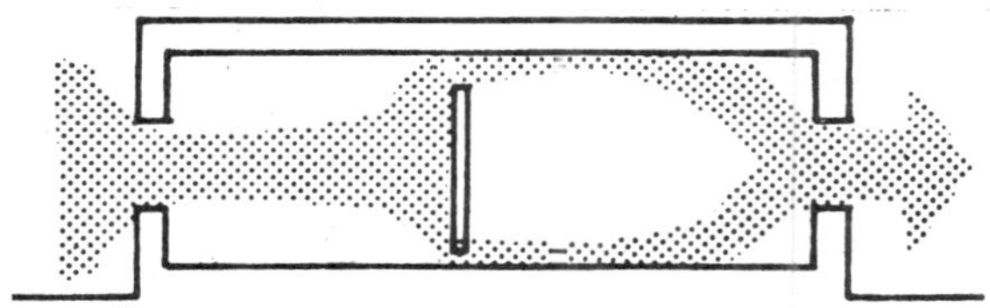

E. Internal walls obstruct wind

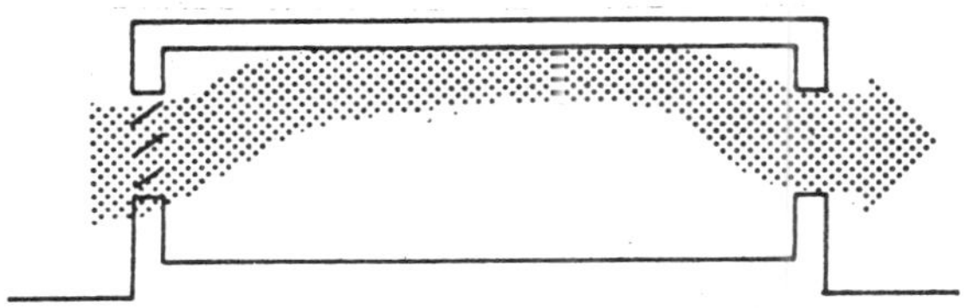

F. Louvers can deflect the air stream up to the ceiling....

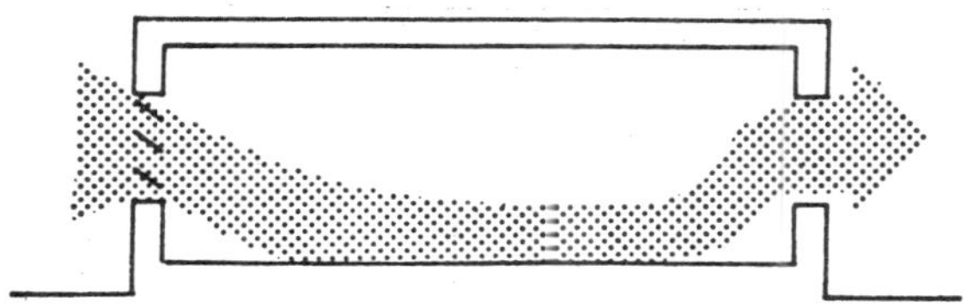

G. ...or down to the floor

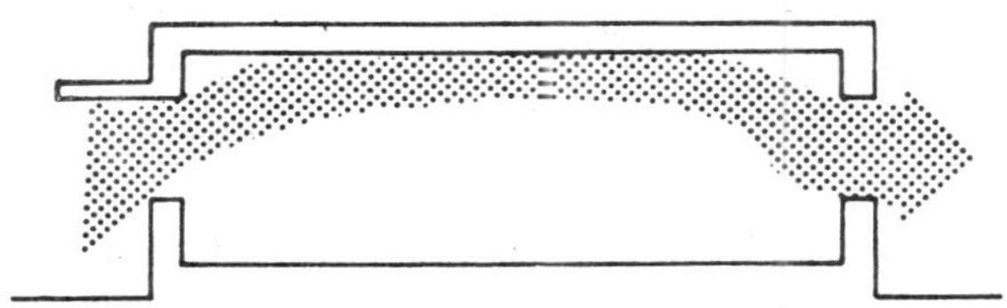

H. Projecting sunshades produce a bad upward air flow...

Fig. 26.17

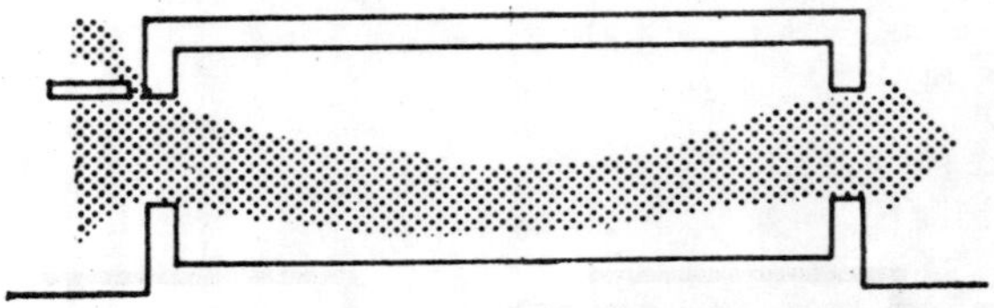

I. ... this can be corrected by slots in the projection

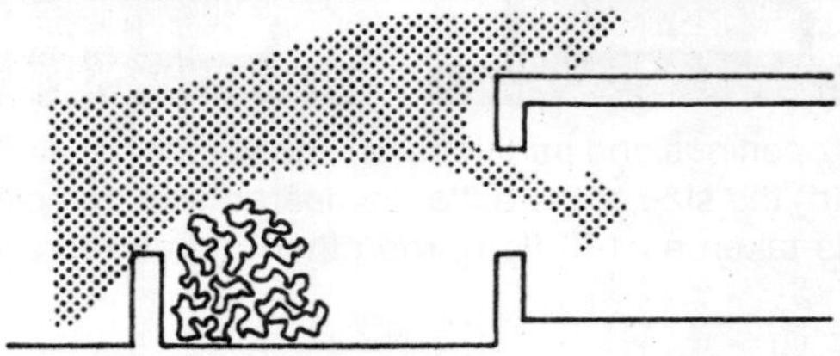

J. Bushes and other external obstructions can reduce the air flow

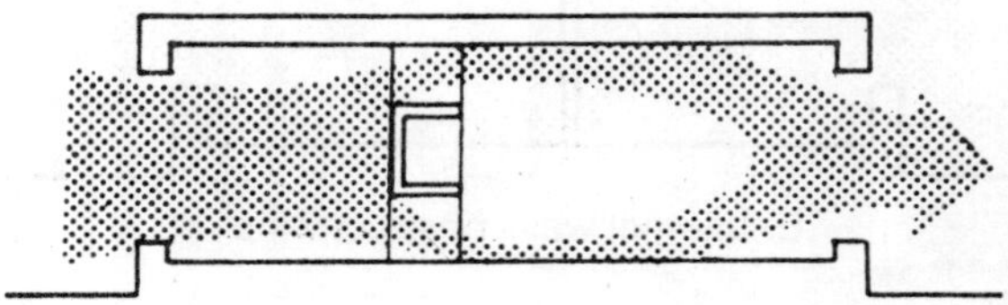

K. Internal partitions and room dividers can create large still areas

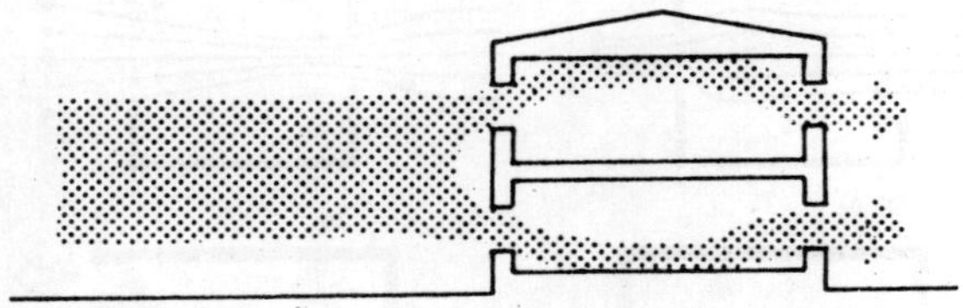

L. Air flows differ on different levels

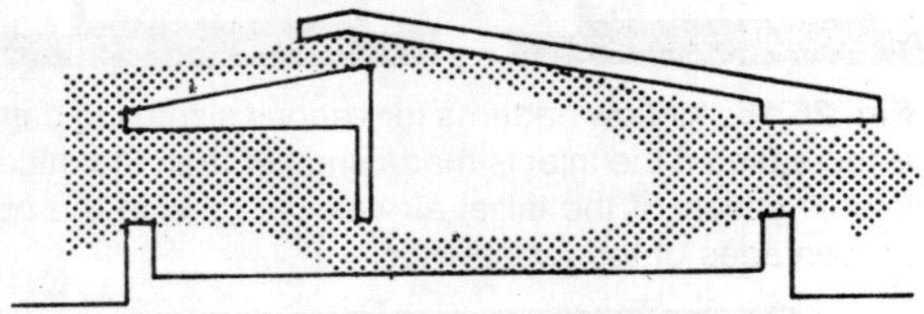

M. Clear-storey ventilation will not improve air movement of low level

A to E—Sections showing cross-ventilation patterns

F to I—Sections showing the effect of louveres and sunbreakers on air movement

J to M—Sections showing the effect of obstructions on air movement

Fig. 26.17: (A to M) Effects of size of air inlets and outlets on wind speed inside a building

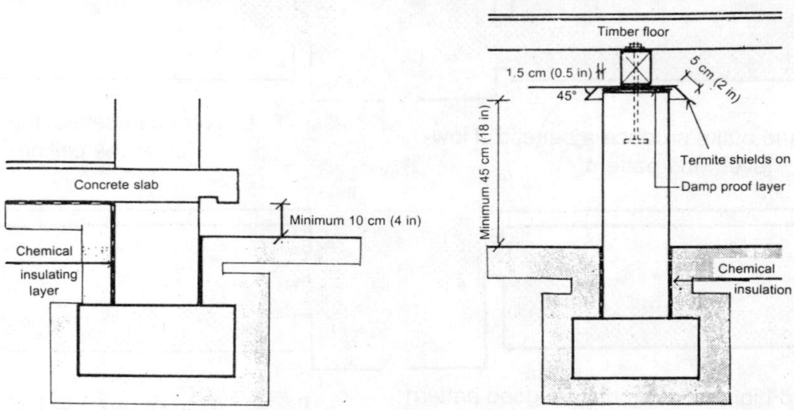

Fig. 26.18: Measures for protecting buildings against termite attack

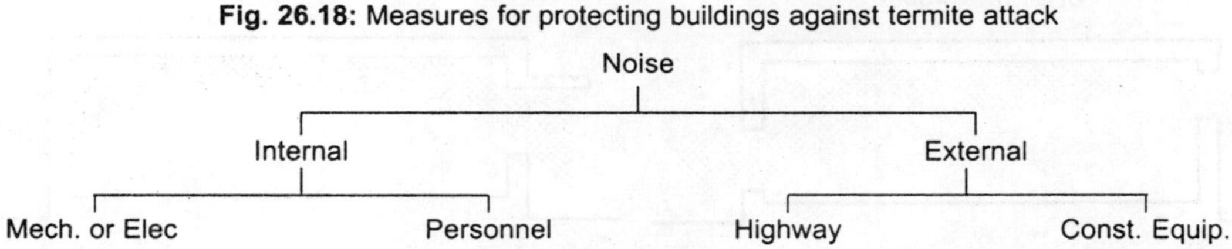

Fig. 26.19 contd...

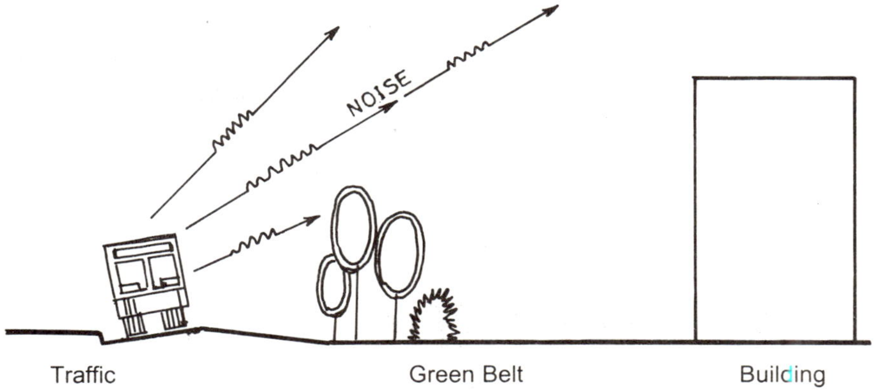

Fig. 26.19: Noise control

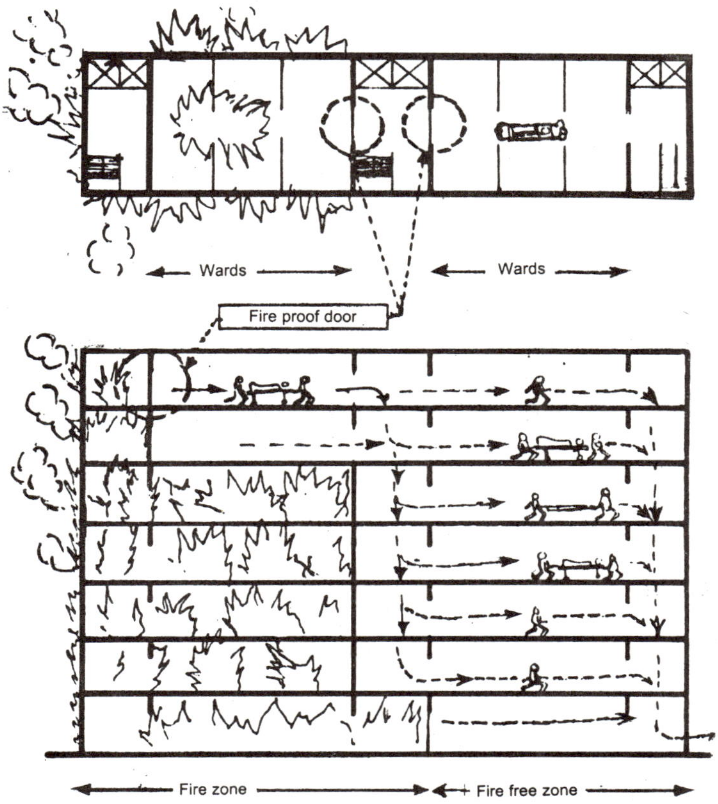

Fig. 26.20: Fire safety

FURTHER READING

1. Kakalainan R: Functional Hospital Design. International Hospital Federation year book, London, 1988.
2. Wood Read T: Trands in Hospital Design. Hospital Management International, London, 1988.

27 Profile of the Hospital Environment

The hospital is a complex organization utilizing combinations of intricate, specialized scientific equipment, and functioning through a corps of trained people educated to the problems of modern medical science. These are all welded together in the common purpose of restoration and maintenance of good health.

The hospital, as an organization, provides special facilities and trained personnel to facilitate the work of the physician in his primary position involving care of the patient who is the focal point about which all activities of the hospital revolve. In the delivery of medical services to patients, therefore, the medical and associated technical staff of nurses, dieticians, etc. become a most important factor. The character and extent of hospital services are adjusted to continuously to keep abreast of changes and advances in medical science.

Although primary emphasis is placed on the care of bed patients, the frontier of the hospital in recent years has been extended from the sick person in the hospital bed, to the potentially-sick person in his normal living situation. Hospitals have been assuming more and more responsibility for programmes of preventive medicine. They serve as the medium in many communities through which the professional staffs and official health agencies pool their efforts for improvement of the public health.

The Old Paradigm of Medicine vs the New Paradigm of Health

Old paradigm of Medicine	*New paradigm of Health*
• Treatment of symptoms • Specialization by disease • Emphasis on efficiency • Intervention with all drugs and therapies available until death • Body as a machine in good or energy, bad repair • Goal to eliminate disease • Patient as dependent, professional as the authority	• Search for patterns and causes integrated, concerned with the whole patient; emphasis on customer satisfaction • Intervention with the minimum appropriate therapies • Body as process, field or context, dynamic system • Goal to promote maximum health and well-being

Old paradigm of Medicine	*New paradigm of Health*
• Body and mind separate; psychosomatic illness mental, treated separetely • Primary reliance on quantitative data; defensive medicine, batteries of tests • Centralized regional health facilities and services providers • Isolation of the patient from home and family in a hospital for treatment • Physician's total control over patient's care	• Patient independent; professional as a therapeutic partner • Body and mind connection recognized and utilized in therapeutic approach • Major reliance on subjective data from patient and professional intuition to comprehend test data • Widely decentralized service with many types of care • Treatment of the patient in the context of home and family • Patient's assumption of the responsibility for their own health

Table 27.1: Tensions and Trends in the Changing Health Care System

Tension shaping the system		*Resulting organizational trends*
• Specialized care	Primary care	Health services gatekeepers restructuring, re-engieering
• Technologically driven	Humanely balanced	Patient-focused care client satisfaction
• Cost unaware	Cost accountable	Economic alignment
• Institution focused	Ambulatory/community focused	Integrated delivery systems, decentralized
• Service professionally	Managerially governed	Benchmarking, performance
• Acute care	Chronic care	Cost containment
• Individual patient	Population perspective	Clinical outcome assessment, patient-care plans
• Curative care	Preventive orientation	• wellness and total care
• Content master	Process mastery	• systems thinking, learning organizations
• Individual provider	Team provider	• self-directed team
• Competition	Cooperation	• consolidations, mergers, partnerships, acquitance
• Current regulation	Re-regulation	Multiskilled providers

Dominance of Medicine

Health services provide the service itself (e.g., consultations, operations), employ staff, have an effect on the country (e.g. fitter people) and have an effect on patients (they live longer and feel better).

The demands on health services are always greater than the supply. An efficient hospital requires a well-balanced organisation for compassionate care within an adequate technical and environmental framework.

The activity of assessing the operating environment which is increasingly complex is a fundamental step in the strategic management process.

The Assement Process

The key to any successful planning process (Fig. 27.1) and to the survival and success of the organization is the timely identification of both trends in the environment which are likely to impinge on current organizational operations and opportunities for change in the organization's direction positioning the organization strategically relies on accurate information about the organization's market and competitors and sound judgements on future external conditions which will affect it.

The environmental assessment process, at the organizational level can be defined as a continuing

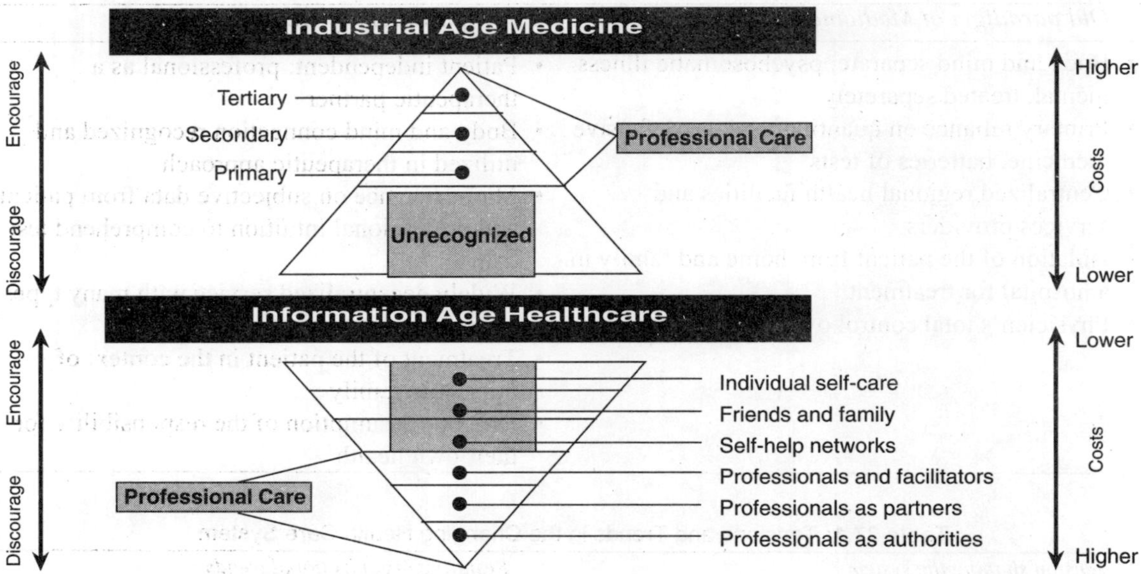

Fig. 27.1: Transformation of patients into consumers

process providing management with a timely analysis of events and trends in the external environment in which the organization exists with associated potential implications for operating units.

The environmental process, or environment scanning is the cornerstone of the generic strategic planning process, however, complex that process may be. The timing of the activity in terms of the planning process is at the initiation point of the strategic planning cycle: although fundamental to successful environmental scanning is that the activity continues throughout that year, or cycle.

The logical activities following the assessment of the external environment are the competitor assessment and the internal assessment within the organization followed by the the generally accepted sequence of events in the planning process.

If the purpose of strategic planning and indeed strategic management is to provide a framework within which decisions throughout an organization can be made, then the environmental assessment must provide a framework of trend-analysis and forces for the future, rather than a straight line extrapolation of single trends and how these trends and forces may change over time.

It is this framework and the way in which it is structured which is so important to the success of the strategic process.

The components that make up the environment assessment process as it is applied at the operating level are as follows:

- Analysis of the broad trends identified on a national or regional level.
- Identification of those trends that have particular application at the local level.
- Market analysis of the market in which the local hospital or health care organization operates.
- Analysis of the competition organizations operating in the local hospital market.
- Analysis of the broad trends identified on a national or regional level. The first step in any environmental assessment process at the local operating unit level is to acquire or produce a high quality environmental assessment of the trends and forces affecting the health care environment at a national and regional level.

This analysis should include: key trends affecting the hospital industry and identification of key issues such as:

- The national or regional economy

- Demographics of the population
- Medical technology
- Human resources
- Private and public finance and payment
- Government regulation and other policies
- Implications of these trends and issues for the hospital field
- Strategies that might be employed by the local operating units.

This national or regional environmental assessment should then be used by the local hospital and its management staff to study thoroughly and understand the trends and forces that are likely to affect all hospitals throughout the next planning cycle. These trends, forces and their implications should be presented and discussed in a planning session solely devoted to their understanding and consideration. This will allow the participants to focus their attention solely on these broad trends rather than skipping over them quickly to get to those issues which will affect them on a local level. All too often this component of the environmental assessment process is not done thoroughly or well by the local hospital.

The next step is to identify those trends that will have particular application and impact at the local hospital level. The primary source for identifying these trends should be the national and regional assessment which was used in the first step of the process. In addition, a hospital management should be developing its own local assessment with particular attention to the following local trends:

- Changes in the demographics of the population of the local service area.
- Trends in the economy of the local area.
- Specific changes in the application of medical technology by competitor organizations.
- Availability of human resources and the cost of those resources to the local organization.
- Trends in the private and public finance and payment through such organizations as HMOs. PPOs, state and local government.
- New or different government regulation or other policies that will affect directly the local organization.

Again, a separate planning session devoted to the local area trends and their impact on the local hospital should be established by senior management of the organization. This session should be expanded to include key medical staff leaders, department managers of the organization, and the senior administrative management of the hospital. Market analysis of the local market in which the hospital operates expands upon trend identification described in the earlier component. The components of this particular segment of the planning process include the following:

Market Definition or Segmentation

In this section of the market analysis, management should attempt to define clearly their market or service area. It must not be assumed that this market definition is static and once established never changes. It does change with the addition of the new providers: the introduction of new technology; changes in the population: changes in government regulation: and all of the other trends identified in the local trend analysis.

It is important that the local hospital management, medical staff and governing board agree on the definition of their market and the various segments which make up that market. The market definition might be broadly defined as the geographic area in which the hospital operates. However, it is far more important to describe the various segments of the market such as its demographic make up and how each of the services of the hospital has a different component of this defined market.

- *Evolutionary changes in the market* Hospital management should attempt to describe how the current market definition has changed over the past five or six years and how the trends identified both nationally, regionally and locally are likely to change the hospital's market definition on the future.

  Attempting to demonstrate how the hospitals market will be defined five years in the future, will begin to lay the base for the organizations understanding of how it must change to adapt to that market or how it must put in place strategies to expand its market or change its focus.

- *Size and growth of market segments* Hospital management must segment the hospital's market and attempt to define the size of each segment along with its growth or decline during the next planning cycle.

  This description of the size and growth of the market segments will be particularly important to various parts of the hospital's medical staff, to different departments in the hospital, and will be viewed as particularly important by many departmental mangers, since it will affect them differently from the broad market analysis

- *Health care needs of each market segment* In this componant, the planning staff should have prepared an analysis of each market segment and what they anticipate will be the needs of each segment over the next planning cycle. These needs can be defined differently for each market segment, but generally could include the volume of services, the ability to pay for those services, and how the local hospital has previously related to each of these segments.

- *How each of the market segments is changing* It is important for the planning staff to project how the needs of each of those market segments identification of those needs and how they are changing that will greatly influence how the hospital should go about attempting to meet those needs.

- *Identification of which market segments are unreserved now and likely to be in the future.* A particular analysis of the changing needs, as identified above, will be a specific identification of those market segments which are undeserved at the present time or are projected to be undeserved in the future. These represent the opportunity segments of the market that the hospital might wish to address more aggressively.

The market analysis discussion can and should be conducted in the same session in which the local market trends have been identified. This will allow the audience to tie together in their minds the trends at the local level and how those trends will influence the particular market segment in which they are most interested.

The competitor analysis segment of the assessment process includes the following components:

- Who are the existing competitors?
- What are their past objectives, key resources, strengths and weakness?
- What are their likely future objectives and strategies?

Gathering the information on competitors is one of the most difficult components of applying the environmental assessment. In many cases, the information is not readily available or the information is not felt to be reliable. The competitors' analysis must be completed as critical part of the environmental assessment. The definition of who are the existing competitors should be done by market segment rather than only by the broad total organization. It is possible, therefore, that the organization will identify widely differing competitors for each market segment. It will be most important to conclude at the end of the total analysis, who are the prime competitors. The prime competitor's past objective should be agreed upon, as much as possible by senior management of the hospital. The competitor's key resources, strengths and weakness should be identified and should be particularly compared to your own hospital's resources, strengths and weakness. Areas of deficiency, as compared with the competitors should be clearly identified and set aside for particular attention by the hospital staff. The last component of the compatitor analysis is estimation of the competitor's likely future objectives and strategies. Of course, this is not likely to be based on accurate internal information from the competitor organisation but rather medical staff who may be practicing also at that competitor hospital: on information gathered from the hospital, departmental plans: and from general data publications of the competing organisation. A profile should result from completing this competitor analysis which should then be compared with the profile of your own organisation. This profile comparison should attempt to identify areas of strength and weakness that can be a part of the planning process for the organisation.

The key to the results of strategic management and to the effective control of resources is in the initial and continuing determination of the way in which the changing environment is and will effect the organisation. The environmental assessment should strike a balance between an asoteric future analysis and pragmatic short-term operational projections. It provides an essential strategic management tool enabling the organisation to be proactive rather than reactive to forces in the environment.

The process and result of going through the market testing of a service can result in a wide range of benefits. Conducted well it can be useful refocusing exercise resulting in qualitative and financial benefits.

28 Environment

Environment has a tremendous influence on planning and design of a health facility. Development of reliable bio-climatic indices is a basic necessity for effective climate control. Without such indices far more effort/energy and equipment than necessary is put into climate control engineering.

The adult human body hemostatic theramoregulatory mechanism—maintains temperatures within the limits of 36.0°C to 37.5°C. Its entire resources may be throum into an effort to restore the disturbed thermal equilibrium. Within limits, the healthy human body can adjust its heat production to thermal conditions. Females and males respond differently to dynamic changes in the thermal conditions. Males in general tend to feel hotter and react more rapidly. The indoor comfort levels of the humans vary considerably. There has been a trend towards higher temperatures in the industrially developed countries. A generally preferred indoor temperature for healthy adults seems to be in the region of 22 to 23°C. When the mean night temperature rises above 24°C, the percentage of those whose sleep is disturbed, increases.

The influence of temperature on the viability of microorganisms is small as compared to the effects of relative humidity.

Temperature and infants Maintenance of an optimal thermal condition is one of the most important aspects of effective neonatal care.

Environmental temperature of 30°C, which might be considered excessively hot to adults, may be too cold for a naked infant. This is due to a small amount of subcutaneous tissue and a large surface in relation to body mass in the newborn infant. Naked babies in incubator are exposed to serious and unnecessary risks of cooling when the temperature is less than 27 to 30°C. For older infants temperatures of 26.5 to 28°C have been required. On the other hand, temperatures hotter than the baby are dangerous. A temperature between 32°C and 34°C has been suggested as a proper range of air temperature for the newborn infant, as then his oxygen consumption is minimal. For pre-term infants 35 to 36°C has been suggested as a range of thermal neutrality in the environmental temperature within which the boys' normal body temperature is kept without extra heat production. Bathing during the first hour after birth appears to decrease body temperature significantly despite previous stabilization of temperature. Defying the bath would minimize instability of temperature.

Temperature in Operation-Room

The character of the thermal environment of the operation-room and the anesthetic room is determined by the need to protect the patient's physical resources—more aberrations of body temperature are seen in the surgical practice than in any other branch of medicine—and to ensure good working conditions for the operating staff.

The thermal environment has some effect on the efficiency and accuracy of surgical procedures. However, the extent of this effect is still to be determined. Whatever the season or the weather, adequate comfort conditions, for the surgical team and patient are to be maintained. The temperature at which unclothed man at rest achieves thermal neutrality with his surroundings is in the *British Isles* between 24 and 27°C at the relative humidity of 50 percent. When conditions change beyond these limits then the body's own temperature control mechanisms are called into play. Heat loss during anesthesia occurs not only because of low environmental temperatures and humidity but also because of the infusion of cold fluidis, ventilation with cold gases, the exposure of body cavities, the absence of muscle movement and subcutaneous vasodilation.

Already a 0.5°C fall in body temperature can result in a doubling of the rate of the patient's energy expenditure. This constitutes an enormous stress on a sick elderly patient undergoing a major operation. From the age of 70 years onward the body's ability to adjust to changes in thermal conditions decreases progressively. There are indications that in operation rooms cooler than 21°C all patients will become hypothermia unless the procedure is very short. In operation rooms with the temperature between 21°C and 24°C about a third of patients will become hypothermia when operations last more than an hour.

In operations lasting a couple of hours, the greatest patient temperature drop usually occurs in the first 30 minutes. This is because of the effect of anesthesia induction, exposure to cold ambient temperature, and preparation of the operative site. Patients undergoing intra-abdominal or intra-thoracic operations loss more heat than others because of more exposed surface. Irrigation of these surfaces with cold fluids adds to the heat loss. Patients kept at 24°C or warmer will retain their normal body temperature. There is a large decrease in skin temperature during transfer to the recovery room, despite the beginning of patient's activity and maintenance of the environmental temperature. Hypothermia has been found in 11 percent of surgical patients—especially in young children and the aged, admitted to the recovery room. This can only be accounted for by the removal of the drapes from the patient. This decrease is larger than the hourly loss during anesthesia and, in view of the detrimental effects of hypothermia, should be prevented by suitable covering.

In burned patients, hypothermia is often initiated by the administration of an anesthetic and perpetuated by exposed wounds and donor sites. The application of dressings lessens the loss of heat by convection and evaporation. However, hypo-dressings lessens the loss of heat by convection and evaporation. Hypothermia in itself is not an indication to dress the patients wounds or donor sites. It is preferred to warm the patient by a source of radiant heat, such as heat lamp.

Temperature Control in Pediatric Surgery

Temperature control of the infant is an essential component of pediatric surgery. The responses of infants under general anesthesia are poikilothermic in character, because shivering is abolished—it appears between the third and sixth month of life-and there is peripheral vasodilation. The effect is greater than in the adult because of the infant's larger body surface in comparison to its total bulk. Also radiation loss from limbs, head and face is relatively greater.

Low temperature, particularly for patients less than one year old, as well as high temperature, may be gravely injurious. The hypothermia produced in the air-conditioned operation room in the absence of any heat source has been associated with increased risk of cardiac arrest, morbidity and mortality for the babies. Low weight newborns have great tendency to hypothermy although there are wide variations in cold resistance among neonates. The greatest drop in baby temperatures occurs when the baby is removed naked from an incubator, placed on an operation table and left during induction of anesthesia exposed to a cold environment.

The newborn undergoing operation should be kept warm and the patient placed on some warming device, e.g. the water blanket, thermostatically controlled to 37°C. Operation room tables with a source of radiant heat are in use to provide a temperature of 27 to newborns and infants and to burn patients. This radiant heat and high temperature may be uncomfortable to the surgical team. However, since most heat loss from a child occurs early during anaesthesia induction and preparation for surgery, the room temperature could be lowered and radiant heat turned off later if the child temperature is stable.

If the control mechanisms are not in good order, refrigeration and air-conditioning increase considerably the risk of overcooling the patient. When air-conditioning and refrigeration are not available, there is a risk of overheating the patient if the weather suddenly turns hot and reasonable precautions are not taken. Excessive external heat tends to produce undesirable vasodilation with a further decrease of the circulating blood volume. As the patient is usually unconscious, this is potentially more hazardous than any situation encountered in hot industries.

Thermal Comfort Requirements for Surgical Teams

During operations, heat is released according to the activity of the human body. The heat gain from senior members of the operating team owing to the nervous energy released is as follows

Surgeon, Assistant, Operation-Room Sister	640 kJ/h at 21°C
Anesthesiologist	420 kJ/h at 21°C
Other team members	320 kJ/h at 21°C

The total heat production per hour caused by the staff, OP-lighting and equipment may be about 2 kW or 1750 kcal/h.

Thermal comfort requirements for the surgical team vary in different parts of the world. Requirement changes may be caused also by the seasons. Views and opinions on what constitutes a comfortable working temperature for the staff in an operation room have changed considerably during the last decades. There has been a reduction of temperature from the general standard of 28 to 30°C and 19 to 24°C. However, temperatures of 25 to 37°C within the operation area are still being measured.

Thermal conditions which satisfy the surgeon may lead to the anesthesiologist complaining of cold. The highest number of so-called scrubbed staff have been comfortable at temperature between 21°C and 23°C, and so-called unscrubbed staff between 22°C and 25°C, the average for the former being 22.4°C and for the latter 23.3°C.

It is difficult to produce a working environment that is comfortable for all parties involved in an operation without changes in operation room clothing or developing selective air-conditioned zones in the room.

Acrylic Cements in Operation-Room

The use of acrylic cements is well established in orthopedic surgery, but few data appear to have been published on the acceleration of the setting-time as a function of increasing the operation room ambient temperature. The time to set varies with temperature of polymerization: 15°C-21.6 min, 20°C-4.9 min, 30°C-3.3 min. Thus, between 20° and 25°C there is a reduction in setting-time of about 34 percent. This may be vital during the manipulation and insertion of the cement into the prepared bone cavity. In order to achieve a desirable extension of setting-time, the unmixed components of the cement should not be stored in the operation room, but be refrigerated to approximately 0°C for period of 10 minutes before mixing.

Temperature in Delivery-Room

The most important aspect of newborn care is the maintenance of normal body temperature. The environmental temperature in an airconditioned delivery room is frequently maintained around 23°C, midway in the thermal, comfort zone for lightly-dressed adults, but more than 10°C below the critical environmental temperature for the newborn.

Although full-term as well as pre-term newborn infants have, already at birth, developed mechanisms to maintain normal deep body temperature, in the wet newborn infant exposed at birth to the room temperature the deep body temperature can fall 2 to 3°C unless special precautions are taken. The heat loss that occurs during the first few minutes of life when the infant is exposed to the delivery room environment is significant. Even one minute of delay may cost the infant considerable loss of heat by condition, convection, radiation, and, most significantly, by evaporation of moisture from its skin. Action taken or not taken during the first five minutes of life can greatly influence the baby's entire future.

All infants in the delivery room should be provided with a micro-environment which eliminates or reduces body heat loss and minimizes associated metabolic acidosis. Radiant heating devices are sufficient to reduce the baby's body heat loss during the initial examination, cleaning, suction, and performance of other routine procedures. The facilities for supplying adequate warmth to perinatally asphyxiated and other newborns in need to resuscitation measures are sometimes not satisfactory. Several cases of injuries due to excessive heat have been reported. An extended stay in the delivery room means that for the infant temperature control and monitoring should be provided. Final value judgements concerning the optimal thermal environment for the newborn infant must await further investigation not only of acute physiologic responses to thermal stimuli but also of their effect on growth and development of the newborn.

Temperature in Intensive Care Units

Uncomplicated recovery from anesthesia and a surgical operation requires control of heat loss. Close control of air temperatures and environmental conditions in general is important in intensive care and resuscitation units.

A temperature of 22 to 23°C and humidity at 50 to 60 percent have been found appropriate in the intensive care and treatment units as well as in isolation rooms.

Temperature in Radiodiagnostic Department

Some heating design temperatures for the radiodiagnostic department:

- Waiting area 19°C
- Patients changing room 22°C
- Lavage room 21°C
- Recovery bay 19°C
- Diagnostic X-ray room 22°C
- Thermography room 21°C
- Processing area 19°C
- Viewing area 19°C
- Demonstration room 19°C
- Records 19°C
- Office 19°C
- Chemical and film stores 16°C
- Staff cloak room 17°C
- Disposal room 17°C

Temperature in Laboratories

For laboratories an average temperature of 20°C has been recommended. The importance of air humidity for a comfortable indoor climate has long been the subject of divergent opinions. In the zone of thermal comfort, the effect of humidity seems to be negligible for grown-ups. The acceptable limits for relative humidity as regards static electricity are 45 to 60 percent. For newborns and premature infants, a 55 to 65 percent relative humidity has been considered to be desirable. One of the aspects of humidity is bacteriological. Microorganisms ride on dust particles whose attractability to one another is favoured by low relative humidity resulting in increased static electricity. Low relative humidity has been reported to be an optimal condition for *Klebsiella pneumoniae* type A. A threefold decrease in the biological decay of a hospital strain of *Staphylococcus* at 75 percent relative humidity as compared to 39 percent relative humidity has been reported. High humidity in the hospital enhances the danger of growth of *Pseudomonas*. Humidity in the operation room is believed to cotribute to the prevention of dehydration of exposed tissue.

To minimize the explosion risk it has been suggested that a standard of relative humidity be fixed for the anesthetic locations. Recommendations have varied between 40 and 65 percent. For the prevention of electrostatic changing the relative humidity should be maintained at 70 percent. However, when the temperature is allowed to rise above the normal, this degree of humidity is hardly bearable for the patient and the staff. An authorized standard of relative humidity might give a false sense of security concerning the explosion risks. No device can substitute for the constant alertness of the anesthesiologist and his awareness of the hazards associated with explosive agents.

When the flammable anesthetics are not used, it is not necessary to maintain a 50 percent or greater relative humidity in the whole surgical department. A reduction of humidity in general conditions to more acceptable 40 percent would be possible. Only when very young children are involved the humidity should be increased.

Temperature-Humidity

The majority of the investigations in hospitals has tried to find the values, which offer the patients and the staff most comfortable conditions. In the British Isles the preference in the ward areas is for an air temperature of between 21.5°C and 22°C and a relative humidity of between 30 percent and 70 percent, with the air velocity less than 0.1 m/s and the mean radiant temperature close to air temperature. In Western Europe 21 to 24°C and 50 to 60 percent relative humidity has been recommended. Thirty-five percent humidity and 22 to 24°C and 50 to 60 percent relative humidity have been recommended. In the Baltic area, the liked winter room temperature is 18 to 20°C and in summer 20°C with a relative humidity of 55 percent. In the US an individual room temperature control range of 21 to 26.5°C and the relative humidity of 30 to 60 percent has been recommended. In Mexico, the favored temperature range is 22 to 24°C and the relative humidity 50 to 60 percent. In South Africa, a temperature of 18 to 23°C and relative humidity of 50 to 60 percent have been found well tolerable.

There is a range of air temperature within which any individual doing light work or similar conditions will be reasonably comfortable. The permissible tolerance in relative humidity is even wider.

In the UK operation rooms the temperatures 20 to 22°C and 50 to 60 percent relative humidity and in other sections of the operation department 18 to 24°C and 45 to 60 percent relative humidity have been favored. In the United States the air temperature of 21 to 24.5°C with 50 to 60 percent relative humidity in the operation room has provided a compromise between the supposed requirements of the patient and those of the surgeon. A following recommendation for operation rooms of highest quality in Scandinavia and areas with similar climate could be made: A fully air-conditioning equipment with control mechanisms for variations in temperatures from 19 to 26°C and in relative humidity between 40 and 55 percent.

- In laboratories, a fairly stable temperature between 21°C and 22°C and in relative humidity between 40 and 55 percent.
- In laboratories, a fairly stable temperature between 21° and 22°C and a relative humidity between 40 and 60 percent should be maintained.

Color

Color is a sensation, which creates an instant impact. A humanity does not respond equally to all colours. The response is more to green, yellow, and orange than to red or blue. The individual variations are considerable. One and the same color evokes innumerable readings. Communication of colour is seriously inhibited by the inability of man to describe in sufficient detail the visual attribute which precisely characterize the object. Colour can delight and soothe, provoke and disturb. A very personal sensitivity to color is active from the moment of birth. Likes and dislikes regarding colors are strong.

The positive visual appearance of an environment where much time is spent may reduce absenteeism, rejection rates and increase productivity by 15 percent.

Unpleasant colours can be a psychic burden to those who are particularly sensitive.

Bright reds, oranges and yellow are believed to be attention—getting white, light green, light blue would create spaciousness and red-organs, red, orange stimulation and excitement. Distraction prevention is achieved by soft, gray colors, eye and bodily fatigue reduction by use of colour contrasts. Green, blue and violet are for tranquilization; blues and greens for coolness, and red-orange, red, orange, yellow for warmth. Violet is the color of highest tension. Many of the orange, yellow, and light green colors attract the attention of people with limited visual abilities. The reds and violets are, for them, difficult to distinguish.

Infants can see, process, remember and act on chromatic information in their environment. Much of the young infant's behavior parallels mature behavior and conforms with expectancies of a trichromatic model of color vision. The young child is early adapted to process and use the chromatic information in his environment in reasonably sophisticated ways. His first knowledge of the world grows out of the distribution of his visual attention, and the child differentiates and responds to different features in his world according to their color, organizes his world by color, just as he may remember different aspects of it on the basis of their color.

Just as infants appear to follow patterns rather than color, the design of the wall-paper or curtains appears to be of significance to the aged or senile. The choice of color should make it easier for the cleaners to discover dirt and substances capable of transmitting infections.

Frequently, white is used in a hospital widely as this colour carries the message of cleanliness. However, ophthalmologists have warned about interiors with large areas of bright white, which may cause an effect similar to snow blindness.

In floor colors brown tending towards red and other brown tinges may give a feeling of safety and peacefulness. A dark green tinge may lead to the association of moss or a soft lawn. Light and vague colours should not be used. They may be associated with slipping and falling and produce of feeling of insecurity.

Color in Surgical Department

The color of the drapes should be somewhere between that of the skin and the incision or wound so that the retina need for extra adjustments when the eye moves between the drape and the wound, reduces. Also the strict application of Schonfelder's law to the problem of choice of the color of surgical drapes and sponges leads to the choice of color of raw beefsteak. The medical staff has also to observe the color of the patient's skins, as any change from the normal could indicate impending surgical shock, respiratory obstruction, of sudden hemorrhage.

The tones of operation room wall and ceiling colours have to be determined in relation to operation room lighting intensities. With high levels of illumination and luminous and warm colours such as yellow, orange, and pink, the body tends to increase its activation in general. With soften surroundings, lower brightness and cooler hues such as grey, blue, green and turquoise there is less distraction, and good inward orientation is furthered. Instead of the surgeons green on the operation room walls beige, coral, taupe peach, part gray, terra cotta, avocado, aqua rose, sapphire blue, or pale gold would be suitable. In the UK, generally pale blue, grey and green have been found to be the most suitable. Avoid blues and yellows. A light grey color for the operation room floor has been recommended. The use of patterns on the walls may provide visual response for the strenuous visual task. In the color scheme of the scrub-up room there have been some trends towards the use of yellowish or red shades. The color of the anesthetic rooms ought to be chosen so that the reflections on the patients face would not obstruct the anesthesiologist's judgment of the patient's condition. The color scheme in the anesthetic room may be the same as that for the operation room, possible softer and warmer.

The observation of the patient's color is frequently of importance also in the post-anesthetic recovery unit and in the newborn suite. Patient care areas of these units must have white or slightly off-white walls and ceilings. Use of any other colur will distort true skin tones though reflection of light possible, will delay early detection of some of the irregularities.

Color in Other Hospital Areas

For intensive treatment area cool pure gray, and warm grayed terra-cotta walls have been used. Blues and greens should be avoided in the intensive care rooms 28. As about 50 percent of the light reflects from the walls the green and blue colors may make the patients to appear cyanotic blue or blue-green shades should be used in waiting and holding areas where they are calming. When choosing the colors in the laboratories, there are in principle no restrictions.

Signposting, Identification Signs

Signposting is a systematic arrangement of visual to help the individual to reach a particular destination. The size of the letters, words, and lines have to be chosen for optimal readability. Choice of a typestyle should take into account legibility and compatibility with the pictographs and the environment. The signposting contents must be clear and consistent. Consistency means that the text and the pictograph must be identical from the starting point to destination to make it easier for some deaf people who have difficulties taking and being understood. General signs lettered in blue and underlined with a brown stripe have helped persons with vision problems to read each line. Some investigators recommend that the characters should be hide set against a dark background. One of the most important aspects of good signing is siting. The closer to one's natural line of vision, the better. Exceeding a 10° angle from this line should be avoided. Uniform terminology for signposting ought to be established at least by nations. Also colors of signs and other makings ought to be determinate by national standards associations.

As the ability to remember picture images usually surpasses the ability to retain word messages, pictographs can transcend the language and education barriers. It is important that the picture image always be dark on a light symbol field.

When planning a signposting system, the character of the exterior and interior of the particular health care facility should be considered. To ensure integration of the graphic elements with other architectural features, lighting and color schemes, the signposting system ought to be developed already at the preliminary design stage.

Although visual acuity diminishes with age, the sight elderly people retain is almost always adequate for the more limited range of activities that characterizes their time of life. However, about 30 percent of the elderly sustain a gradual loss of central vision while retaining periphera vision. They will continue to see well enough to move around and to take care of themselves, but their ability to read, to write, to enjoy art and to watch television or a movie may be severely impaired. Diagrams and maps put up to help people find their way around often fail to help because of too small lettering or surface glare. When patients with limited or blurred vision are involved, intense colors, which can be perceived easily, should be used to indicate doors to stairways, public facilities, elevators, and emergency exits. The doors should be labelled in large typography for easier identification.

In some US institutions all identification signs have recessed white letters on a black background with Braille beneath. For the 85 percent of the blind who do not read Braille and for the partially sighted, standards in the US require that identification signs for the general public have letter and numbers of contrasting colours that are raised or recessed. The American Foundation for the Blind recommended that letter and numbers be 15 cm high and 9 cm wide. For identification of hospital rooms, offices, and so on identification plaques with raised or recessed letters or numerals should be used. They should be mounted about 1.5 m on the handle side of the door opening. Coloured lines on the floor to direct the people to a hospital destination are not very effective in a crowded corridor.

Sings for Accident Prevention, Safety Color Codes

Red danger signs with white and black lettering may be used only where immediate hazard exists. Caution signs are required as warning of potential danger. They are yellow with black letters.

Radiation warning signs are yellow with magenta lettering and standard symbols. Safety signs must be safe—i.e. not stick out or cause an obstruction. Safety color codes are used for marking caution and physical hazards: red identifies fire protection equipment, danger and stop, green safety and first aid equipment, purple caution of radiation, yellow caution for physical hazards, orange, dangerous parts of machinery, blue caution limited to starting and using equipment, such as lifts under repair.

Art in Hospital

Architecture is an event itself. It can exist quite independently, and it may have no need either of sculpture or of painting.

The societies are for the most part visually illiterate. It has been stressed that the visual memory is very poor in comparison with the auditory memory. The hospital could provide an environment for people to come to some terms with art at a time when many of their connections with the outside world have been severed. This task should, as in museums, not be regarded as a primarily educational function, but as a possibility of providing visual delight. However, the education of the spectator's eye must be taken into consideration. A lot of art in hospital is for seeing while moving. Visual pollution of any kind must be avoided in hospitals as well as the cosmetic approach. Usually, the decorated hospital areas have been in and outside of the main entrance, regular nursing units and cultural and worship areas. To these children wards, pediatric out patient areas, nursing units for infectious diseases and some circulation areas have been added. The hospital areas demanding least attention from the art point of view, are technical areas, industrial areas, administration and out-patient areas.

Art in hospitals is part of a non-regular milieu. The conditions for it are not yet firmly established. A fact which eases amateurish ideas—they may even be official or semi-official—to gain superiority in determining the character of art for hospitals.

An imaginative application of art can contribute greatly to the attractiveness of the hospitals, but it should not turn hospitals to some kind of prestige loaded mini museums.

To create an artistic hospital milieu is to have a clear aim for interior quality during the whole planning and construction procedure and to secure the solidarity of all involved towards that aim.

In their attempt to be sure that what they are doing is satisfactory, architects make models, perspectives and drawings, of parts of the buildings, interiors and details. In order to gain something from these drawings they must be in a total involvement. The artists would agree that mostly they would prefer the space to be there, built, before they started work. The artist has to know for whom, what and for which spaces he has to create. Art placed in the hospital milieu, particularly in its focal points, should have the same qualities as art placed in civic site. It must be decorative, commanding, easy to take in at a glance, but difficult, stimulating, various enough in receiving light change to provoke continued pleasure, engagement and surprise. One of the most profound qualities of sculpture is scale. It can only be perceived intuitively because it is entirely a quality of thought and vision. To become some kind of landmark rather than an indistinguishable of the hospital college, scultipute must retain its autonomy, involve it environment enough to augment but not be absorbed by it.

INTERNAL TRANSPORT SYSTEM

AUTOMATED TRANSPORT SYSTEM

The hospital environment is characterised by a tremendous range of items, which must be transported throughout a facility. Among many examples, medical supplies move between various units, food is transported form central preparation areas to individual patient rooms and clean linens must be delivered. Traditionally, each functional area of the hospital has addressed its transportation needs through manual labor and performed its respective functions independently of each other. However, such traditional approaches are expensive and labor intensive. Concerned with steaming operations to maintain profitability, many hospital administrators are looking for better ways to control the transpiration of all goods and supplies internally.

When setting out to design and construct a new government army hospital facility, officials at Madigan Army Medical Center in Fort Lewis, Washington, USA, sought to increase cost efficiently through centralized control of transpotation of supplies. A comprehensive automated transpiration system (ATS) was proposed to be integrated into the hospital layout and poor plan. The ATS would use automated guided vehicles (AGVs) for transportation of materials to fulfill a variety of operational and support functions in all areas of the new medical centre.

The ATS system provides transportation of closed stainless steel logistic carts containing medical/surgical supplies, contaminated reprocessibles, trash and sterile material. The entire system includes 23 AGVs which transport these items among several functional units, including centralized processing, distribution points and user units. Three buildings, seven elevators, nine patient floors and a controlled, dedicated crawl space are serviced by the system.

Turnkey System

A complete, turnkey ATS system was provided, including ATS, AGs, guidepath, carts, elevator interface, facility co-ordination and interfacing, twenty-three AGVs transport goods throughout the system. The AGVs are fully automatic, computer-controlled vehicles, featuring bi-directional, driver-less capability. The AGVs can also be bi-directional, driven manually. All AGs in the system are electronically guided and battery powered. System maintenance features are provided for the AGV fleet, including battery chargers and a test loop. The system features include warming signs and alarms, automatic doors, and a five-minute uninterruptible power supply. Each AGV also has important user safety features for the operators. Other system-wide user safety devices include an AGV master console, cart arrival indicators and remote cart present indicators.

The entire ATS system is controlled by a Microvax configuration. This incorporates two Microvax computers with an automatic fail-over capability.

Microcomputer aboard each of the AGs work in tandem with the systems central host computer and input/output devices through a continuous communications linkage. Low-power radio signals are transmitted to and from the vehicles through the system guidepath.

The AGVs travel along horizontal guidepaths, which are defined through the use of conductive wires embedded in the building's floors. In addition to determining the AGV's travel path, the guidepath supports the communication's link between the AGVs and the host computer, providing continuous traffic monitoring and control vertical movement of the vehicles is accomplished by seven dedicated, single cab, single and double-entry elevators and one surgical cart lift. Both the horizontal and vertical systems share the same computer to control and co-ordinate the linkage between the AGVs and the elevators. A graphics package is also supplied with the system, which is composed of a computer with a 19-inch high resolution color monitor. The primary display consists of two windows, one for the system and one for the guidepath. The status window contains a system wide alarm indicator, power source indicators and the computer connection. A pull-down menu creates a window that permits the user to monitor and control the system. Functions included in the operator interface are executable from the graphic's monitor work station, allowing immediate access to information needed for problem resolution. The guidepath window displays, to scale, the system layout by individual floor or elevator, enabling the user to see the exact position and status of the AGVs and associated system equipment. A command menu is provided, which allows the user to zoom for an enlarged view of a portion of the guidepath. Successive zoom commands are permitted on already enlarged displays.

The ATS system serves functions hospital-wide which are grouped under three operational components: user units, distribution centres and processing points.

Hospital-wide Services

User units are individual activity centres which use medical supplies, linens, or sterile materials, or generate trash, or both. Examples of supported functions include the blood banks, chemical laboratories, emergency, intensive care units, labour/delivery, medical records, nuclear medicine, nursing units, outpatient clinics, outpatient pharmacy, pathology, patient administration, rehabilitation, physical rehabilitation, radiology, radiation therapy and surgery.

Distribution centres are locations where medical/surgical supplies, case or clean carts are stocked or restocked and prepared for transport to a user unit. Examples include clean stores/distribution, sterile stores and clean linen/distribution.

Processing points represent areas where carts containing soiled linens, trash or reprocessibles are emptied and sanitized.

Carts move from one location to another according to the facility requirements. They are initially placed manually at a pick-up station. The operator enters the carts distention into the host computer through wall-mounted data terminal. Through the systems linkage with the host computer, an AGV is selected to move the cart's by using the fastest available guidepath route within the facility. The selected AG then moves to the carts location and picks up the cart. The cart is transported by the AGV to the selected destination and switches on the appropriate arrival indicators. A technician manually removes the cart from the drop-off point, completing the cycle, which automatically turns off the appropriate arrival indicator.

The entire system permits an AGV to be queued anywhere along the guidepath and used as required.

Applications

Immediately prior to a "send cycle", the CPD technicians review an ATS computer-generated manifest to identify the carts to be sent during the cycle, and the sequence in which they are to be sent. Technicians move the loaded carts from the holding area and place them in four detents located at pick-up points. The carts designated for first pick-up sequence are placed on the pick-up points and then the remaining carts are placed on the pick-up points as required in the manifest.

The technician then uses the areas wall-mounted data terminal to enter the cart's destination. The terminal will display a message such as "Pick-up Station" which is triggered by the cart being set upon the detent. This message remains active until a valid destination is entered. Active messages may be scrolled so that a technician may enter cart destinations in any sequence. The technician enters a numeric destination code and presses the enter key. If the code is an invalid destination, the data terminal displays "invalid destination" another destination code may be entered. If the code destination is valid, the message will express the correct destination, which is verified when the technician presses the enter key. The host computer immediately updates it active order list. During the send cycle, the computer locates the available AGV from the area nearest to the pick-up point, determines the fastest route to that location and instructs the AGV to proceed to the cart pick-up point. The AGV moves to the cart, rolls under it, stops, raises its deck and picks up the cart. The host computer determines the fastest route and instructs the AGV to proceed to the drop-off point. The AGV uses the system guidepaths to sense low frequency, local range radio signals being broadcast from the embedded wires in the floor and uses the signals to guide it along the route.

The built-in safety horn sounds as the AGV begins to move. While the cart is being transported, the host computer linkage assures that there is a smooth traffic flow. Warnings are provided at pedestrian crossings that an AGV is approaching. In case the AGV is moved off the guidepath, it stops and the computer will automatically signal the master console. The AGV can also signal an automatic door to open as it approaches, if an open door cannot be confirmed the AGV stops and waits until the condition changes, or reports the conditions for operator action.

At an elevator tower, the host computer will call the next available elevator, based on system functional criteria. The AGV will approach the elevator and position itself for entry. At the same time, the host computer provides an interface command to the elevator for its destination. The elevator travels to the destination floor and an "automatic transporter approach" light illuminates, warning pedestrians that an AGV is approaching. At the door open command, the AGV will leave the elevator, follow the guidepath and centre itself over an available drop-off point, lower its deck and position the cart on the clean receiving detents. Once the deck is lowered, the AGV will back out from under the cart and proceed on the guidepath. The AGV communicates with the host computer to receive the next assignment. The AGV's arrival is signalled by a "cart arrival"indicator immediately adjacent to the corridor entrance door to the arrival station and activates the remote "cart present" indicator at the cart's destination. The technician comes to the drop-off point and manually moves the cart to its point of use.

Carts also may fit the unscheduled category, if necessary, when there is an unexpected increase in the workload. The CPD technician prepares the unscheduled cart and places the cart on the pick-up station. The technician then uses the data terminal and enters the destination into the host computer. The host computer acknowledges the entry by showing the destination on the display. The rest of the procedure is the same as for scheduled carts.

PNEUMATIC TUBE TRANSPORT SYSTEM

Pneunaatic tube system connects separate buildings as well as departments and offices located at different ends of on different floors of a large building.

In spite of modern communication system such as telephones, fax machines, electronic mail and so on, a personal porter system is still necessary. In hospitals the movement of medical reports, X-rays, documents, drugs, laboratory samples and blood bags normally requires personal delivery by hospital staff. This leads to interruptions in individuals on duties, unanswered telephones calls, overuse of lifts and general time wastage. Hospital management is now striving to use personnel in the most efficient way possible to achieve cost-effeciency. One means of achieving this is through the installation of a pneumatic tube system.

Hospitals which already have a pneumatic tube system use them to transport:

- Medical reports, test result and computer print-outs

- laboratory samples, such as blood, tissue and urine sample plasma
- Prescriptions and drugs
- X-ray plant's
- Menus
- Patient's mail and newspapers, and
- Generally anything that fits into a carrier.

There are many different sorts of pneumatic tube systems. It may be large, covering virtually the whole of the hospital, or just a small point-to point system, consisting of only two stations connecting, for example, the main reception to the administration office, or a special system connecting the central laboratories to various sample reception areas.

The size of a pneumatic tube system, that is, the diameter of the tube and the departments, connected to it, is determined by the load also determines the size of the carrier, as this restricts the type and size of the sample or item transported. There are standard carriers for sending reports and documents and special carriers for various other tasks. For example, long carriers for the transport of X-ray, carriers with a special protective insert for the transport of laboratory samples or extra large carriers for the transport of blood bags.

The tubes are normally made from U-PVC, aluminium or steel, for economic reasons most customers decide to use U-PVC tubes, which have been designed specifically for use in pneumatic tube systems. The popular tube sizes are either 90, 110 or 160 m diameter, but other sizes are available, For example, a 250 m diameter system has been installed in a UK hospital to transport complete medical records, including X-ray reports. It is possible nowadays to link buildings with underground tubes. These have a protective outerskin, which protects the inner tube from natural distortion or from damage caused by heavy vehicles crossing the ground above. It also acts as a perfect weather seal. An important factor in the installation of a pneumatic tube system is the radius of the bends. Formerly the bend radius had to be between 1.5 and 3. In modern system, the bend radius has been reduced to 0.65 to 0.80 for the same tube and carrier size. The data cable is part of the tube installation. It is attached to the tube using cable ties.

When a tube passes through a firebreak wall, special sleeves are fitted. The fire sleeve is made up of intumescent material, which expands when heated, thereby crushing the tube and maintaining the integrity of the fire compartment. The material is, naturally, fire resistant. At the heart of every system is the main controller. Point-to-point systems are controlled by a simple relay. For larger systems however, the main controller contains a microprocessor, where all the data of the system is received, analyzed and processed. A built-in record printer offers the facility of logging all or selected data and operating conditions with a real-tie clock. It is also possible to print out programmes and data on this printer. A pneumatic tube system can be compared with a train set. There is only one train travelling on each line, passing over points before finally reaching its destination. There are central stations where trains can switch lines or where they can wait until oncoming traffic has passed.

In pneumatic tube system the points are called diverters and come in 2-, 3- or 4- way versions. Diverters can be arranged so that upto eight separate circuits can be linked together and carriers can wait in a siding before passing through the diverters into another circuit. These separate circuits are called zones.

A pneumatic tube station consists of an entry tube, either top or bottom loading, a dispatch tube and a swivel tube, which maintains the integrity of the station. The swivel tube rotates to accept a carrier into the system or to eject a carrier out of the system.

The destination address is entered in the programme at the sending station. The address consists of upto four figures, and can be identical to the internal telephone numbers of departments. The stations themselves are easy to use. After entering the address on a keypad, the carrier is put into the dispatch tube. Delivery is then carried out automatically by the system.

Each station can be programmed with a priority which will queue-barge lesser priority stations. This can be determined by the users. A damping arrangement is attached to every station, which slows the carrier down on arrival to ensure a smooth landing. The carrier is then ejected out of the station into a basket, ready for collection. Audible or visible remote indicators can be used, if several departments or wards share a tube station. The indicators would be activated through the address entered by the sender and would tell the addresses to go to the station and pick up the carrier.

A pneumatic tube system is powered by one, or several side channel blowers. The carrier is either sucked or blown, depending on the direction of travel. The carrier is transported on an airflow, which means there is no real pressure or vacuum. A large blower would only have the capability of 300 m bar pressure maximum, with 3-4 m^3 of air per minute. The installation of pneumatic tube system during the construction of a new hospital, or conversion or modernization of an existing hospital causes no particular difficulty.

Things are slightly different if a system is to be installed when a hospital is running normally and no other building work is being undertaken. There are, however, fewer problems than one might expect. Wherever possible, the tubes are installed in service ducts and risers, or hidden by suspended ceilings. Therefore, only limited drilling is necessary in patient or administrative areas and disturbance, dust and dirt can be kept to a minimum planning. Modern pneumatic tube systems operate quietly, even though the carriers travel at a speed of 6-8 m/sec. The reason lies in the special felt rings around the carriers, and the air cushion they are transported on. The air is not expelled from the system with the carrier, so no hygiene problems are caused. In operating theatres, where hygiene is critical, the pneumatic tube system can be operated by suction alone. This way, the system can become an ideal "porter" for supplies of plasma and other item.

For the optimum transport of laboratory samples, systems have been developed that can send carriers at various speeds. Robust loads and empty carriers usually travel at 6-8m/sec, whereas more sensitive loads, such as blood samples, can be sent at 3m/sec. Research has shown that samples transported by pneumatic tube systems suffer no greater damage than samples carried by porters.

The servicing requirements of a pneuatic tube system depend largely on its size and usage, In normal circumstance, 2-3 preventative service visits, per year are recommended. Minor faults that occur within the system can frequently be corrected by the main controller through special programmes in its microprocessor. The problem can also be traced by an engineer from the information displayed on the main controller. As in other fields microcomputers have led to a vast improvement in the technology of pneumatic tube systems.

The cost of a system varies enormously, and depends on the number of stations, the distances involved and the type of system chosen. But a 1100"-bed hospital took the following into account before purchasing a system with 70 stations divided into four zones with a total tube length of more than 3000 m.

Average time needed for transportation by hand = 10 mins.

Therefore:

$$1350 \times 10 = 13500/60$$

$$225 \text{ hrs} \times 365 = 82125 \text{ hrs pa}$$

This means that staff spent 82125 hours a year hand-delivering items that could have been sent in a pneumatic tube system. Staff costs for 82125 hours will vary from country to country, but one thing that is true for all is that this tie could be used more efficiently—especially if this tie is made up not only of porters' but also nurse's; doctors' and office staff's time, too. In the example above, the cost of installing the system was lower than the staffing costs for the 82125 hours. The system was therefore, amortized within one year. A pneumatic tube system may not sound like an exciting piece of equipment. Apart from the cost saving shown above, however, for the everyday user in the hospital it soon becomes a vital piece of equipment.

The speed with which samples and results can be sent to and received from laboratories by, for example, accident and emergency units or operating threatres can make the difference between success and failure.

THE HOSPITAL TROLLEYS

Trolleys perform a vast number of tasks within the hospital-transporting supplies around the building; delivering food to patients; moving patients themselves; providing speciality functions within departments; safe storage and distribution of drugs to patients; and the provision of mobile emergency 'equipment 'packages' for situations where seconds count if a patient is to be saved.

Transport of supplies and equipment by the modern hospital trolley has greatly enhanced patient care. One area of improvement is drug and medication distribution. An entirely new approach to what was once thought of as a very simple function has become an integral part of patient care. The complexity of medications available for prescription by doctors to patients, the potency of these drugs, and their costs have increased dramatically in the past three decades. The result is that four important factors have become highlighted in the drug's path from pharmacy to patient:

- *Security* Many drugs are of significant interest to people other than the patient for whom they were prescribed; a system must be devised to prevent pilfering between the security-conscious pharmacy department and the patient's stomach.
- *Waste* In a state health system or in private practice, accountability of drugs has become vital, as astronomical sums are spent each year on medications.
- *Reduction in dispensing errors* This means ensuring that the patient receives the correct drug, in the appropriate dosage, at the prescribed time.
- *Enhanced quality of patient care* Nursing staff can give more time to patients.

The Purpose Built Trolley

These problems can be solved by using the purpose-built ward medicine trolley. This trolley, also known as a medication cart, should include features to cope with:

- A means of rapidly and effectively securing the contents of the trolley. This means a central lock should be applied when the trolley is not in use or has to be left unsupervised for a short time. A simple means of locking the trolley itself to a specified location is also a desirable feature. If you cannot steal from locked drawer, why not take the trolley?
- With the advent of individual patient medication and unit dose systems in hospitals, the modern trolley will need provisions for individual storage of patients medicines. These must be easy to get at when needed but well secured when not in use. A method for safe transportation of the patient bin between ward and pharmacy is also desirable. A cassette, removable from the trolley but easily secured in it, is one answer, and a number of medicine trolleys now include this feature.
- The trolley must, of course be easy to move, easy to clean (particularly the top work surface), and have provisions for accessories such as waste disposal bins, flashlight, and drinking-cup holders. The trolley must be flexible enough in design to be easily adapted to different drug administration systems and to varying ward or hospital requirements. For example, it must be suitable for use in the large 40-bed ward or the single-patient room.
- Another important use for a trolley is in emergencies. There are different names—emergency trolley, resuscitation trolley, crash cart and so on, but the equipment's function is generally the same. This is to get immediate help to a patient-or, indeed, staff or visitors in a movement of special crisis anywhere inside the hospital or in its immediate vicinity, including the carpark. This trolley must carry all the vital immediate

life-support systems. These could include a heart monitor and defibrillator; breathing equipment; an oxygen supply; drugs and accessories; intubation equipment; instrument; swabs and bandages.

- In the past (and unfortunately in the present too) this equipment was stored on the conventional trolley, or trolleys, usually consisting of open shelving on four wheels. Too often in an emergency, an item was found to be missing-usually because it had been borrowed and not returned. These trolleys often lacked inventory control measures and compactness. Sometimes more than one mobile device was needed to transport all support equipment.

Special Requirements

The modern hospital emergency trolley is purposely built to cope with the special requirements. It has a large, easily cleaned work surface, quickly expandable by means of a fold-down shelf. It has drawers with compartments for storage of all the needed supplies, drugs, and dressings; a large compartment for bulky items, including suction pumps; and most important, the means of ensuring that these material cannot be removed without its being obvious that the trolley has been tampered with. There is storage for a oxygen cylinder, a retractable IV pole, and a bank of electrical sockets with a cable and plug so that individual electricity powered items can be kept plugged in at all times.

A new generation of emergency trolleys have been designed to afford all code members constant, simultaneous full-view access to every compartment in and on the trolley. This advanced concept offers everything a code team needs for an efficient and immediate response.

Doors swing open instantly and lock in place. Trays lift out without tools. All critical supplies can be placed at bedside where they are needed the most. Since all trays are interchangeable, restocking and exchanges are more efficient. The trolley can be ready for another code in minutes. All this adds up to time saved, not for one or two procedures, but every procedure. We all know that one of the most critical factors in saving a life is time. An advanced-design emergency trolley can become an important member of a hospital's code team.

Other features found in today's new breed of emergency trolleys include removable ABS tops, reinforced side rails, easy-access cardiac boards, oxygen tank holders, slide out work surfaces, retractable IV poles, full-swivel dual locking casters for easy manoeuvrability, plus a variety of options for tailoring the trolley to individual hospital needs.

Treatment, Procedure and Infection Control

Rounding out a hospitals choice in purpose-designed trolleys are those for treatment and procedure, and infection control. Treatment and procedure trolleys are highly versatile units providing organization and bulk storage for a variety of procedures. These include arthroscopy, laparoscopy, broinchoscopy, and endoscopy, Treatment trolleys also make ideal cast trolleys, as well as dressing and bandage trolleys. You will find them at home in cardiac catheter laboratories. They are also used extensively as open heart trolleys.

Infection control trolleys are distinguished by their bright yellow warning color. IFC trolleys address a hospitals concern in containing the spread of infectious disease within the healthcare environment. Three large bulk-storage drawers are designed to store caps, gowns, goggles, and disinfectant supplies for the containment of infectious disease. Collection trolleys help promote hospital asepsis by effectively preventing microbial dissemination. A well-designed collection trolley includes a cover that automatically closes under the weight of materials placed in the trolley. Red collection bags identify contents. The color red also indicates that caution should be practised in handling the bag and it contents.

Other Uses

Other uses for purpose-designed trolleys include anesthetics; instrument storage, particularly expensive optical instruments; storage of sterile packs in isolation wards; and they can be used as treatment trolleys in consulting rooms, out-patient departments, or wards. The humble trolley has now grown into a vital piece of equipment in its own right.

FURTHER READING

1. Bartlett D: The Hospital Trolley and Patient care. Hospital Management International. London **58**: 1989.
2. Dancer GE: Automated Transport system, Hospital Management Internationa , London, 264-65, 1997.
3. Ewertowski J, Basten J Beska J: Pneumatic tube transport system Hospital Management International London, 171-72, 1997.

29 Influence of Climate on Buildings

The main climatic elements that determine the climatic characteristics of an area include:

1. Solar radiation and temperature;
2. Humidity;
3. Prevailing winds;
4. Clouds, rain, and snow.

Solar Radiation and Temperature

Solar radiation and temperature are interrelated. The intensity and amount of radiation depends on the movement of the sun, its varying horizontal direction and vertical height. In the northern hemisphere the apparent movement of the sun is from north-east to north-west in summer and from south-east to south-west in winter. In summer the sun attains its maximum elevation, but in winter it remains at a comparatively low elevation. This explains why, again in the northern hemisphere, there is more direct sunshine on the east and west sides of a building in summer but more on the south side in winter.

The roof of a building receives a much greater amount of solar radiation than any of the vertical walls and there is comparatively little variation during the day. Where day temperatures are high, therefore, the construction of the roof should receive special attention.

Temperatures are directly related to solar radiation. However, temperatures are always higher in the afternoon when the sun is in the west because as the temperature rises in the morning, heat accumulates and is not dissipated into space as long as there is continuing solar and radiation input of heat. Temperatures are lowest in the second half of the night and early morning. They gradually increase at sunrise, reach their peak in the afternoon, and start to fall after sunset.

Clouds limit the amount of solar radiation reaching the earth's surface and therefore the temperature. Objects, natural or man-made, that provide shade also affect temperature and produce cooler conditions. Trees provide natural shade but when used to protect buildings, their shape and volume should be taken into account. Trees that shade walls in summer may act as barriers to sunshine in winter. However, deciduous trees that lose their leaves in winter and have abundant foliage in summer would be suitble for both seasons.

Temperatures can be roughly classified into ranges to decide whether, for comfort, sunlight should be admitted to buildings or excluded. These ranges, in round figures, are given below.

Cold — below 10°C (below 50°F)
Cool — 10°-15°C (50°-60°F)

Temperate	15°-27°C (60°-80°F)
Hot	27°-38°C (80°-100°F)
Very hot	above 38°C (above 100°F)

The body mechanism functions normally in the temperate range of temperatures but would be under stress in both cool and cold conditions as well as in the hot and very hot ranges. In the cold and cool ranges it is advantageous to allow sunlight into the building while in the hot and very hot ranges it should be kept out. The questions of light intensity and glare are dealt with later.

Humidity

Humidity refers to the amount of water vapour suspended in the air. The ratio between the amount of water vapour actually present in the air and the maximum amount the air can carry at the prevailing temperature and pressure is called "relative humidity". The temperature-regulating mechanism of the body operates through the release of moisture from the skin (sweating) and evaportive coating. If there is already a considerble amount of moisture in the atmosphere (high relative humidity) evaporation from the body is feeble and the person experiences a feeling of discomfort. It is therefore vital to study the relative humidity inside a building.

Data for relative humidity generally relate to two periods of the day: morning (08 hoo) and evening (17 hoo). The two sets of data indicate fluctuations during night and day and help to decide the critical periods for comfort.

Relative humidity can also be classified into ranges for study in relation to temperature:

Very dry	0-25%
Dry	25-50%
Humid	50-75%
Very humid	75-100%

The "comfort range" lies mainly between 22.5° and 29.5°C (72.5°-85°F) at a relative humidity of 20-25%, i.e., in the "dry temperate" type of climate.

In climates of the "hot, dry" and "hot, very dry" types it is possible to take advantge of evaporative cooling when water is in sufficient supply. In "hot, humid" or "hot, very humid" conditions air movement is very important in relation to comfort. During warm weather man experiences no discomfort as long as there is evaporation of perspiration into the atmosphere. When there is no air movement the air around the body becomes saturated with mositure, producing a sensation of discomfort. Movements of air during periods of high relative humidity remove saturated air from the vicinity of the body, bringing fresh air into contact with the body and providing relief although there may not be any change in the room temperature. For this reason movements of air inside buildings are essential and as much use as possible should be made of prevailing winds as a means of achieving these movements.

Discomfort due to high relative humidity can be overcome to a large extent also through use of electric fans or mechanical ventilation. It is therefore necessary to know which aspect of climate, solar heating or high relative humidity, is most troublesome in a building. If it is the former, the building should be protected primarily against solar radiation and electrical or mechanical means should be used to provide relief against humidity. When the diurnal variation of temperature is small and the heat problem less buildings may be oriented to obtain maximum benefit from the prevailing winds. In rural areas where electric power is not available, decisions regarding the construction and orientation of buildings have to be based on natural factors alone.

For comfort it is essential to provide partial or through ventilation by taking advantage of the prevailing winds. When there is extreme heat in summer and it is necessary to avoid heat and glare close to opernings in buildings it would be avangtageous to orient buildings to face the winds of the humid months instead of the average prevailing wind, which may be from another direction. It is not, howoever, necessary to place the building at right angles to the direction of the prevailing wind because wind velocity is not greatly reduced up to an angle of 60° from the perpendicular.

Precipitation

Rainfall influences both temperature and humidity and also poses problems of protecting buildings and disposing of drainage water. The shape of the roof and the materials of which it is constructed are important in relation to protection and drainage. Information on the duration of the rains and the amount of precipitation is available for various regions in the meteorological data.

Snowfall will generally be limited to hilly areas. When there is snow the shape of the roof and the construction materials are again important. The problem of glare is accentuated by snow.

Meterological data provide a generalized picture of the climate of a region or a fairly large area. This is a macroclimate. In designing building, however, microclimates should be taken into account. Microclimate refers to the climatic conditions in and around the health facility.

- Ventilation pattern in absence of trees and hedges;
- increased ventilation through proper positioning of hedges;
- incorrect positioning of tree and hedge in relation to a low buiding
- correct positioning of tree and hedge to provide good ventilation in a low building.

Tall buildings or a cluster of buildings affect the temperature either by casting shade or by radiating and reflecting heat. In large urban areas temperature differences of 3°C (5°F) have been observed between the congested central area and the open outskirts.

On a large campus differences in ground level, the character of the surface, whether covered with vegetation or bare and rocky, and presence of lakes or rivers or other bodies of water, make for considerable temperature variations. A low-lying area is likely to contain a pool of cooler air, as cool, heavier air tends to settle or gravitate at night, like water, in the lower areas.

The conditions that produce microclimates outside buildings can also be used to create microclimates in and around buildings. In hot climates, courtyards protected from direct sunlight, shaded during day, and planted with flowers and greenery offer a pleasing outlook during the day and a cool sitting-out area in the evening. Alternatively, in winter, courts receiving direct sunlight during day would store heat and radiate it into the surrounding rooms.

Landscaping and surface treatment of the land surrounding buildings can help to create, to some extent, a suitble microclimate.

Most of the developing countries lie within the tropics and subtropics. In these areas four main climatic types can be distinguished for our purposes, each of which poses specific problems in relation to building design and the provision of comfortable conditions. The four types are as follows:

- cool
- hot, dry
- hot, humid
- warm, humid

Cool Climates

Cool areas in the tropics are found in hilly regions. The main problem in these areas is to capture the maximum amount of heat during day and to conserve it for the night. Heat from solar radiation is most readily absorbed by buildings oriented along an east-west axis. Walls and roofs should be heavy enough to absorb and store a large amount of heat, while air movements and ventilation should be restricted to the minimum.

A compact building with few openings is most suitable for cold areas. Protection from rain and snow and drainage for rain water and melted snow should also reeive attention.

Hot, Dry Climates

The temperature range in this type of climate is from about 27° to 38°C (80°-100°F) or even higher.

Maximum temperatures are experienced for three to four months of the year. The relative humidity is generally below 50%.

The main problem in these climates is to exclude daytime heat and solar radiation. The most efective method is correct orientation of the building in relation to the sun. The location of a building with the long side facing south and with minimum exposure to the west would be most appropriate.

Thus in the northern hemisphere, if a building is oriented east-west, its south side remains comfortable during both summer and winter.

In hot and dry climates the question of walls and, especially, roofs is of particular importance since these are heated by the sun's radiation. They have to act as heat barriers. Since they cannot reflect all the heat received they must also function as heat reservoirs, the main requirement being that they should accumulate heat without allowing it to reach the interior of the building, as long as there is sunshine outside, i.e., the build-up of heat continues. This will depend on outside and inside temperatures and on the nature and thickness of the materials used for construction.

The walls and roofs of buildings are exposed to solar radiation during the day; some of this radiation is absorbed and some is reflected, the proportions being determined by the construction materials and the surface finish and colour.

Through judicious choice of materials or combinations of materials and wall thickness the internal temperature of a building can be controlled to a considerble extent.

Insulation is very helpful in cold climates where buildings are mechanically heated and it is necessary to restrict the escape of internal heat, but in hot, dry climates insultation acts at night as a trap, retaining the accumulated daytime heat inside the building. Insulation is useful only for parts of a building that are air-conditioned. It remains useful if there is a substantial temperature difference between the outside and inside of the building but insulation only retards conduction, and if there is no temperature, difference between inner and outer wall surfaces there is no conduction.

There are two methods of reducing heat intake by walls and roofs. The outer surfaces may be given a white or near-white finish, and they may be shaded as far as possible. Overhangs are generally provided for window openings only, leaving other parts of the walls exposed. In fact, all sunlit surfaces should be shaded. For this purpose trees are very suitble.

Hot, Humid Climates

The temperature range in this type of climate is about 27°-38°C (80°-100°F). High temperatures persist during the greater part of the year. Afternoon temperatures are higher throughout most of the year except for two or three winter months (December to February in the northern hemisphere, June to September in the southern hemisphere). Day and night temperatures in the summer months are high with very little fluctuation.

Relative humidity is generally higher than 50%, especially during the rainy season. The main problem of this type of climate is to provide the maximum possible natural ventilation in order to counteract discomfort due to high humidity.

Maximum use should be made of prevailing winds for this purpose. Glare is generally a problem. Vertical fins and perforated screens or walls shield off light from a bright sky but allow breezes to pass through.

In hot, humid climates an effort should be made to maintain indoor temperatures as near as posible to outside shade temperatures. The walls and roofs should, if possible, be of light-weight construction with low thermal capacity. The external surface should reflect as much solar radiation as possible.

Heavy rains accompanied by wind generally persist for three to four months. Rain should be excluded from the building and all openings should be protected against wind-driven rain. Winds required for counteracting humidity often coincide with the direction of the rain. The answer is then to provide adequate adjustable covers or temporary awnings to protect openings.

A rectangular building with courtyards and openings on the windward side is suitable for these climates.

Warm, Humid Climates

This type of climate is often found near a river or the sea. River and sea breezes are useful for overcoming high humidity. Unless river banks and coastal areas are properly planned and their development regulated there is danger of tall buildings blocking the view and blanketing air currents from the buildings behind them.

Generally, open and low-rise structures are most suited to this type of climate.

BUILDINGS

A building is composed of elements which together give it a form, shape, and appearance. These elements are the floors, walls with openings for doors and windows, and roof. Each element is protective: the floor protects the building from influences underneath while the walls enclose the building laterally and the roof provides protection from above.

The climatic conditions determine the general form of the building but its overall volume and shape depend to a great extent on the kinds and volume of activity it houses.

Floors

In humid areas the problem arises of moisture from the ground entering the building. Damp-proof courses are introduced below floors, and special care is needed if the water level of the soil is very near the surface.

Floors should be stable, hard-faced, and washable. Paved floors are recommended for naturally ventilated buildings exposed to external climatic conditions, pests and considerable dirt. The requirements for easy care and simple cleaning are best met by smooth artificial stone (terrazzo). For strict, hygienic requirements, such as in hospitals or laboratories, it can be laid almost without joints and taken up as skirting.

For reasons of economy, poured cement floors or pressed cement tiles are mostly used, but the quality and color of the cement affect the appearance of the floor. Locally manufactured cement varies in color, not only as between brands but also within different batches of the same brand. Color matching is therefore difficult and special care is necessary.

Linoleum and plastic floors are common in developed countries but they are suitable only for air-conditioned buildings. In tropical climate they warp and become uneven in a short time, and maintenance costs are very high.

Walls

Walls are of three types: solid, light, and cavity. Solid walls store heat during the day in hot climates. Light walls, particularly in humid areas, dissipate heat as soon as outside temperatures fall, but during the day they should be adequately shaded to avoid high inside temperatures. Cavity walls are useful only if the air in the cavities is free to escape, thereby helping to keep the inner wall comparatively cool. Sealed-in air, even in hollow building blocks, does not help in cooling a building; on the contrary, it may retard reverse flow, as explained previously.

Brick is used almost universally for constructing walls. Where cement and sand are easily obtained, hollow concrete blocks can be used. However, brick retains its predominance on account of the simplicity of production, the wide availability of clay, and, in developing countries, the existence of cheap labor.

In cold climates, as well as in hot, dry areas, walls are generally made thick for the dual purpose of retaining heat inside the building in cold weather and keeping interiors cool in summer. In cold areas the finish and color treatment of walls can be designed to absorb heat, but in hot zones the sunlit faces of walls should have reflective surfaces. Roofs and walls with non-reflective surfaces may attain a temperature as high as 70°C (160°F), or even higher, and they should therefore have adequate thermal capacity and time lag to provide comfortable indoor living during the daytime.

In humid areas also wall surfaces should be reflective. Where there is not much difference between day and night temperatures a long time lag is not necessary. Walls need not be thick; thin and light walls would be adequate. However, dampness may be a problem when walls are thin. Waterproof plaster finish and other forms of external protection may be necessary.

Roofs

Roofs are subject to greater climatic stress than any other building element. However, the same basic ideas apply to both the roof and the walls. The traditional shapes of roofs or coverings for shelters clearly indicate how the problem of protection against the natural elements has been overcome in different areas.

Flat roofs are now very widely used, irrespective of climate, because construction methods employing reinforced concrete are simple and versatile and because of improved methods for disposing of rainwater and snow have been developed. However, the value of this trend is questionable. Many of the roof shapes have also been involved in the light of advanced structural design knowledge, but specialist builders are needed here and such construction may not be feasible in some places, at least, for smaller hospital schemes. In national and large-scale projects, when expertise is available, these advanced designs could be adopted.

In cold climates a thick roof stores heat during the day and helps to maintain the internal temperature at night when outside temperatures may be very low. In very cold areas roofs of adequate thickness may be a handicap because of their weight; to reduce the load some type of insultation would be necessary. In areas where there is snow the additional weight load on the roof and the disposal of snow and water are important considerations.

In hot areas also roofs should be solid and have a high heat capacity but should be as reflective as possible. The cheapest and simplest way of making a roof surface highly reflective is to paint it white. A white-painted roof would be around 15°C (25°F) cooler than a roof with the usual dark, dull finish. A roof in the tropics can be heat insulated, but with questionable success, since the insulating material prevents heat that has already penetrated, from escaping.

Where the air is not almost saturated with moisture, particularly in the hot, dry regions, the roof can be covered with water and benefit can be obtained from the cooling efffect of evaporation. Two methods are available. The first method is to create a pond of water on the roof terrace; the other method is to arrange for water to be sprayed on to the roof automatically when the roof surface temperature reaches a critical limit. Yet another method adopted for cooling the roof is to fill the terrace with earth and grow grass and flowers. It should be noted that both water and earth on the roof would increase design loads.

A further method of keeping the roof cool is to use a double-layered construction.

"Double roofs" are made of both light and heavy materials; a combination of the two is also feasible. The main principle is to provide shade over the inner skin and minimize heat gain and storage in it. Provision of additional or "false" ceilings below the main roof and ventilation of the gap between the two also helps to reduce inside temperatrures.

In humid areas roofs should be thin, light, and have a reflective surface. In rural areas, especially, pitched or sloping roofs covered with corrugated iron, aluminium, or asbestos-cement sheets are not only logical and convenient but also resistant to prolonged rain.

A sloping roof is amenable to simplification; for smaller span, which are quite adequate for rural health buildings, "ridges", "valley", and "hip" construction can easily be avoided by sloping roofs in one direction only. This not only helps to dispose of rainwater on one side but also facilitates the escape of heated air from the higher end of the roof.

The materials used for covering flat roofs in the tropics are also important. They provide protection against the weather and have to remain impermeable, not only when there is high humidity and heavy rainfall but also when surface temperatures are high and there is less humidity, as in hot, arid climates where sudden drenching storms may occur. Roofing materials such as tiles, asbestos, cement, metal, etc., are suitable for tropics. Misgivings must, nonetheless, be expressed at the excessive spread of corrugated metal roofing which is often insufficiently galvanised and inadequately maintained, especially in coastal regions and so they rust quickly.

Bituminous roofing felt, guaranteed suitable for tropical use and plastic foil are used for flat roofs, as in the temperate zones. Excessive heating of the material can be prevented simply by whitewashing. A layer of gravel pressed into the material is even better because the durability of the roofing is improved and it is protected from mechanical damage. A particularly good material for hot arid regions near the coast is crushed shells, because its sterility in sunshine prevents all plant growth on the roof, it stores heat and insulates against it, while reflecting solar radiation well, due to its whiteness.

The roof is frequently used as a terrace in hot regions, especially the arid zones. The surface is best finished accordingly, with a screed or paving laid on sand to prevent damage to the roofing.

Openings: Windows and Doors

Openings in buildings exist primarily to provide daylight and ventilation. Some aspects of natural lighting must be considered along with the design of openings.

Daylight is received from two sources of illumination: direct and reflected (specular, spread, semi-diffuse, diffuse). The sun is the direct source; this is called the "sky component". The diffuse source (or "reflected component") is the light reflected from objects outside and inside the building. Scientific methods have been evolved for calculating windows size, but a rough and ready rule is to make the window area equivalent to a certain proportion of the floor area of the room or space to be illuminated, having regard to the type of activity carried out in the room. This proportion will vary from 15 to 25%. In both, cold and hot, arid area's proportion of window area to floor area will be smaller than in humid areas, where more ventilation is desirable.

Glare This is a troublesome aspect of natural lighting. The sky is the main source of glare but other buildings and surrounding areas are secondary sources. Excessive contrast and abrupt and large changes in brightness produce the effect of glare. When glare is present the eficiency of vision is reduced and small details or suitable changes in tone cannot be perceived.

Ventilation openings in buildings are the usual means of ventilation.

Interior air movements are encouraged by providing larger outlets for air than inlet openings, and the movements of air can be guided by the correct positioning of air inlets and outlets. Effective ventilation needs openings on opposite sides of a room, preferably a low-level air inlet and a high-level outlet.

Cooling by ventilation is only possible when the air temperature is below that of human skin (95°-97°F or 35°-36°C). Though ventilation does facilitate evaporation if the air temperature is higher, the resultant cooling does not balance the higher heat intake. This explains why the interior climate can be modified by ventilation only in the humid tropics; since the air temperature is never as high as that of skin.

Ventilation has a special significance in hospital buildings. The spread of infections is a very great hazard in hospitals but this can be combated successfully by providing proper and adequate cross-ventilation.

Windows and doors Wooden window and door frames have long been common in the developing countries. In urban areas, however, steel and aluminium are replacing wood. Lack of seasoned timber and its high cost are largely responsible for the change. Doors are, to a large extent, made of wood with facings of artificial wood or plywood. Veneered block board is also used, but is unfit for external use as the thin veneer cannot withstand wet conditions or wide variations of temperature. The application of good quality paints to those doors would be helpful but it is preferable to avoid the use of such material for doors in exposed places.

Use of reinforce concrete for building construction has encouraged the construction of large door openings and these need more shading as protection from the sun. When the doors are glazed, which is usual, they are sources of glare and allow incerased heat intake.

Insects

Tropical climates and associated environmental factors encourge the presence of termites, flies, and mosquitos. Buildings have to be safequarded against such pests.

Against termites, chemical treatment of the soil and certain structural measures such as metal shields are in use.

Openings are provided with wire gauze screens as a protection against flies, mosquitos, and other insects. Unfortunately, fly-wire gauze restricts the amount of light considerbly and, moreover, it collects a lot of dust. Fly barriers should therefore be used intelligently so that crucial entry sources are protected, and where posible a certain amount of fixed glazing should be employed to reduce the area of gauze screening required. Anti-mosquito screening restricts light even more than fly-wire gauze.

That the most effective way of reducing fly hazard is to maintain a high standard of hygiene. Areas surrounding buildings and also interiors should be kept as clean as possible, and the usual prophylactic precautions should be taken.

Comfort in Buildings

It has long been thought that high ceilings in buildings are desirable for comfort in tropical climates. Temperature in an enclosed space is influenced more by ventilation and air changes in that space than by the volume of the space and that there is no physical principle which would lead us directly to think that the temperature of an object should depend on any of its dimentions whether it be brick, or a stone, or a hollow structure.

The Environmental Settings

Orienting buildings along an east-west long axis, giving northern and southern exposures for the longer sides of the building, is most valuable except in cold and hilly ares, where more exposure to the sun or eastern and western aspects might be desirble.

In areas where the major climatic problem is humidity rather than heat, locating the buildings at a slight angle, either towards the east or the west, depending on the direction of the useful wind, would be beneficial.

The most severe aspects of the climate and the handicaps specific to the building site should then be observed in order to provide, as far as possible, a favorble microclimate through landscaping, grassing, paving, planting of trees and shrubs, constructing ornamental bodies of water, and creating sunny or shady areas.

The plan adopted for the building, whether a large, single block, a building with many wings, or a cluster of small blocks, should be considered with the environmental setting and achieve the best possible microclimate. For smaller schemes it might not be economical to divide buildings into smaller units. In such cases the plan most suitable for the particular climate should be chosen: square and compact for hot and arid areas, rectangular with wings and courtyards open to the wind for hot, humid areas, etc. As far as the actual construction is concerned, thick walls and roofs, small openings, and minimum exposure to the west are appropriate for hot, arid areas. Light, thin walls and a similar kind of roof are better for humid areas. However, a composite solution will be necesary in most situations because a uniform climate throughout the year is rare.

Hospitals, which provide many different services need to be planned within a compact area but should also have scope for expansion. Risks of cross-infection are minimized when activities are kept separate. In terms of building, this suggests the distribution of medical and other activities in different wings of a building or in a cluster of small blocks, both arrangements being suitable for providing a favoralbe microclimate.

Separation of beds or ward units (nursing units) has further advantages. Climatically, both day and night conditions can be easily taken into account to give maximum comfort to the sick in contrast to accepting unsatisfactory compromies when various activities are mixed in a composite building. Incidentally, this arrangement assures more privacy and greater accessibility of nursing units, and independent access to wards may also be feasible.

Similar climatic considerations can be applied to other hospital activities. X-ray units and operating theatres do not need natural illumination and laboratories can forego natural ventilation.

Illumination and ventilation are major problems in hospitals and these are aggravated by the trend towards deep buildings, which has followed the constructional use of reinforced concrete and steel. There is no problem if deep buildings are air-conditioned or mechanically ventilated, but this will not be possible in most developing countries for a long time. Therefore, double internal corridor buildings are not suitble for developing countries unless they are strictly limited in length. Even in plans utilizing single corridor with rooms on both sides, the length of the building should be limited to ensure illumination and ventilation from the two ends. Open-ended corridors or cross corridors are essential.

To accomodate beds placed 2 or 3 deep, ward units should be, respectively, about 4.25 m and 6.10 m (14 feet and 20 feet) wide. Such units situated on either side of a corridor are best treated as general wards with columns and very low partitions. A sense of privacy can be created with partitions. Patients lying in bed would not see other patients in adjacent beds if partitions are about 1.05 m (3.5 feet) high. Such partitions can be built between beds and along the sides of corridors. This arrangement not only helps ventilation and illumination but also facilitates observtion and supervision of patients by nurses.

FURTHER READING

1. J. Shastri: Influence of climate on buildings. Approaches to Planning and Design of Health Care Facilities in Developing Areas. Kleczkowski, Pibouleau (Eds): World Health Organisation, Geneva, 1976.

30 Space Programming and Functional Systems

INTRODUCTION

The hospital building should be attractive, dignified, of good quality without appearing extravagant, human in scale and appeal, and efficient, for the building speaks to the public as often as does the staff, though in a different language.

There have been tremendous and revolutionary advances in the field of medicine, and hospital, as it represents the nucleus of medical care, has been effected by each of these changes. Each advancement in medical field has constantly forced the planners and designers to evolve continuously. The hospital structure and its design, its basic concepts and configuration's structure and its design, its basic concepts and configurations have been following a dynamic course. The architects have to continuously work with the thought of absolecence lurking in their minds. On an average, it should take three to five years for planning, building and commissioning a reasonably large, say 750-bedded or more, hospital. And when it throws its gates open to the patients, one finds to his dismay that part of its structure, design and space programming is already outdated. This is where planning and building a hospital distinguishes itself from constructing skyscrapers, bridges or the highways. Hospital architecture has been continuously evolving itself due to the dynamic and ever-changing requirements of the hospital.

Another factor in hospital building is that it does not lend itself for modification or expansion as easily as other buildings Vertical expansion of a hospital building is a nightmare for patients as well as the staff and the administrators. It can completely cripple the functioning of floors below and can throw the whole block out of gear, functionally. The dust, the noise, the seepage are dreadful to the patients and doctors alike. Removal of overhead water tanks for construction purpose can in itself be something unacceptable.

Open-ended construction is too simplistic a concept. The land in most countries is at a premium and a untilised space is a burden on the financial commitments of that hospital.

Keeping in view the shortcomings of vertical expansion and open-ended construction of a hospital, scientific planning and space programming are important, which should be based on:

- Perception of need for building programme
- Need survey and feasibility evaluation
- Determining the planning design and construction approach
- Scheduling, planning, design and construction
- Opening the completed project

Space Programming

One of the vital steps in hospital planning is space programming. It includes room programme, which consists of listing of every room or area in a proposed construction to which an operational function is assigned. It is a direct derivative of the master programme wherein each room named is discussed with regard to function, functional relationships, and certain environmental characteristics.

Net Space Programme

A net space programme is a room programme, together with an assignment of square feet of space for each room or other functional area.

Gross Space Programme

A gross space programme is a conversion of net space to gross space, most commonly accomplished by applying empirical conversion factors to net space by department and/or functional entity.

Assignment of Net Spaces

While assigning spaces for various areas of the hospital, the criteria for space assignment, should be mentioned in reasonable details. This is where the team effort of architect, clinician and hospital administrator becomes vital. For example, if one has to plan a family waiting room of a surgical suit, the criteria could be laid down as:

- Assume (i) Average of 1½ family members awaiting surgery and recovery, (ii) peaks of four patients awaiting surgery, six weekly, (iii) provide for 80 percent of peak. Thus

Total number of patients	26
Family number	26 × 1½
80 percent of this	26 × 1½ × 80% = 32

- Allow 15 sq. ft per person waiting, thus the space requirement would be 15 × 32 = 480 sq. ft.

Similar technique should be applied for all the areas where space assignment is to be done.

For practical reasons, the net space is converted to gross space. The net to gross ratio should normally be around 66 percent as more than 40 percent gross space would be taken up by corridors, verandahs, wall thickness, etc.

For assessment of plinth area, a conversion factor of 120 percent is to be added to total floor area requirement. This is to cater for circulation area including stairs, lifts, ramps and wall thickness.

Steps in the Planning and Building Process

The actual construction of a new hospital or an addition can be achieved only through a well-developed pattern of organization. All administrative and medical elements of the hospital structure—the board of trustees, the executive committee, the administrator, the medical staff, and many key employees—are involved in this kind of programme. Their beliefs, suggestions, and criticisms must be made known to the professionals who are working on the building project, primarily the hospital architect and the hospital consultant. At a later date, the contractor would also be involved as one of the professionals. The assumption is made that certain prior steps will have been taken by the hospital, as follows:

- A community survey has been made to determine the need for the new facility
- The specific hospital has determined and accepted the role it will play in serving total community needs
- A decision has been made by regarding the scope of service, this particular hospital will carry out in-patient care, and research.
- A site has been selected for the new hospital, if it is a new facility, or in the case of an addition, the general site location has been chosen.
- A tentative budget (in gross figures) for construction has been established and this budget is within the foreseeable funds that may be available.

The building committee is the direct representative of the board of trustees in this building programme and it is the committee's job to work closely with the consultant, the architect, and the administrator and to give necessary approval, within the limits established by the board of trustees, for each step in the construction process.

It is expected that the administrator will reflect the point of view of the respective departments within the hospital, that he will seek counsel with department heads on programme and plans.

Preparation of Working Drawings

Before the architect can proceed with schematic approaches to the solution of the problem or the preparation of preliminary drawings, it is necessary that a functional or architectural programme be developed. This *functional programme* would list the facilities to be constructed or remodelled and determine the space required for each one of these facilities. This determination will indicate in net square feet the requirements for each department and for each room within the department. It should also indicate the relationship between the various hospital departments and, within the department, between the various segments or the various rooms of the department. For example, whether the emergency room should be located near the surgical suite, near the diagnostic radiology suite, or near the clinical laboratory should be decided. Within the surgical suite, the relationship of the doctors, and nurses, lounges to the control areas, to the operating rooms themselves, to the patient transfer rooms, and to the recovery room should be established as a matter of record.

The special features to be embodied in the hospital, such as air conditioning, lighting, patient-nurse communication, physician communication, finishes, monitoring devices, and mechanical services should also be indicated. From the point of view of economy of operation, it is most important that the relationship of departments be fully delineated for the architect and that the size of nursing units (the number of beds per unit) be established. This latter factor may require considerable research and analysis by the department of nursing and by the medical staff. The transportation to be utilized in the hospital is of paramount importance, as it has an effect on economy of capital construction and also on economy of operating cost.

The *functional or architectural programme* is a formal document prepared by the consultant with the assistance of the hospital administrator, the medical staff, and the building committee. It is possible, after preparation of the functional programme, to prepare a very rough preliminary cost estimate for construction and fixed equipment, and for the movable equipment and supplies that will be required in the construction programme. This cost estimate is prepared by the consultant in collaboration with the architect, if one has been appointed, and with the advice of the administrator on movable equipment and supply items.

After this functional programme has been approved by the building committee, *Schematic plans* can be started. If the cost of the programme deviates markedly from the orginal proposals approved by the board, it should go to the board of trustees for their concurrance. The programme is then referred to the architects, so that they may start on their work. The architects are expected to produce some preliminary schematics indicating how the problem can be solved from an architectural point of view.

Most architects will prepare a number of different approaches. These will indicate in general design, location, and shape the approach to solving the problem. There will be block space assignment for each department. The shape by floors, including the shape of the various nursing units, will be clearly delineated. It will be possible to review and appraise.

The different designs from the point of view of economy of construction cost, economy of operations, separation of service from visitor travel, privacy and quietness, balance, and esthetic qualities. Usually these schematics will indicate the number of floors, the degree of air conditioning, the relationship with other buildings on the site and the relationship with future buildings not to be a part of the immediate construction programme. A general impression of the exterior design will be included with this proposal.

After the review and analysis of the various schematic plans, the decision is made to pursue one specific plan. Upon approval of the plan by the building committee, the architects and the consultants are empowered to proceed with preliminary plans. The preliminary plans are a further extension of one of the orginal schematics, and single-line drawings will be drawn to scale at either one-sixteenth or one-eighth of an inch. These plans will indicate the departmental layouts within the blocks previously assigned to the departments. It will be possible to define and review the relationship between the individual rooms and subsections of each department. As a part of this step, a set of outline specifications will be furnished. It is most important for the building committee to know at this stage exactly what the architect has in mind of the construction. Therefore, the specifications will include the following:

1. Number of stories.
2. How future expansion is to be provided.
3. Whether the foundations and footings will be able to carry additional stories and, if so, how many.
4. Materials to be used in foundations, structure, walls, partitions, roofs, etc.
5. Materials to be used for floor coverings.
6. Materials to be used for ceilings.
7. Kinds of windows to be used.
8. Kinds of doors to be used.
9. Stairs.
10. Incinerator.
11. Chutes.
12. Site work to be included.
13. General statement on the quality and materials to be used for built-in equipment such as cabinets, laboratory cabinets, kitchen equipment, laundry equipment, power plant equipment, etc.
14. Transportation system, elevators, dumbwaiters, escelators, pneumatic tubes, and conveyors.
15. Electrical work.
16. Plumbing work, including vacuum, gas compressed air, oxygen, nitrous oxide, etc.
17. Heating.
18. Ventilation
19. Air conditioning. The degrees and the kind of air conditioning are most important. The inclusion of separate systems for air conditioning surgical operating suites and obstetric delivery suites should be noted.
20. Power plant requirements, including the emergency power requirement.

The preliminary plans will show the locations of all fixed equipment in each room. Some plans will show outlet locations for telephone, power, oxygen, etc. and in addition will indicate elevations in some of the essential rooms the elevation of the head wall in patient bedrooms, for example. The consultant will be working very closely with the architect during this stage. His knowledge will supplement the knowledge of the architect and the hospital personnel in matters of technical operation. It will also be possible for the architect, at this stage of development, to prepare more refined cost estimates for the building committee. Such cost estimates should include the cost of land, the cost of construction and built-in equipment, the cost of movable equipment, the fees for the consultant, architect, and engineers, the site development cost, the cost of any extra utility work, the cost for surveys, the cost factor to be used for contingencies, the cost of the clerk-of-the works, and the cost of insurance (builders, risk, fire insurance, liability insurance), in addition, it is expected that the administrator and the consultant will be able to furnish the cost of interest on loans or mortgages during the construction period, the cost of moving into the new facility, and any operating deficit that might accure during the first year of operation.

The next step is the preparation of final *Working drawings* and specifications by the architects. This step projects the preliminary architectural drawings and adds all the required dimensions for the finished set of "double-line" architectural drawings. Concurrent with this, the architect will translate this information to the mechanical and structural drawings. The work involves the presentation of the detailed room and department drawings. Elevation of the building, and elevations and sections of many rooms and many items of equipment. It involves detailed finish and floor schedules and detailed specifications for all fixed equipemnt and materials to be utilized. During this process, it is the hospital's responsibility to furnish the architect with information on all movable equipment for each room, including the name, use the catelogue number of the equipment and the electrical, plumbing, and any other utility requirments. It is important to know at this stage whether all movable equipment can be fitted into the allocated rooms.

The consultant, the administrator and, at times, the building committee will review all detailed schedules and room layouts. The adminsitrator will have his department heads, review all drawings as they relate to each department. The hospital engineer must be brought into this planning review; his knowledge of operation, equipment, and systems will be of great benefit to the entire process.

It is also important that the final drawings be reviewed for the locations and the operation of the following systems:

1. Piped oxygen
2. Suction
3. Nitrous oxide
4. Compressed air
5. Gas
6. Pneumatic tube
7. Nurse call
8. Doctor paging
9. Emergency call system in operating suites, delivery suites emergency rooms
10. Fire alram system
11. Intercom system for administration, X-ray, laboratory, physical medicine, dietary, etc.
12. Telephone system
13. Music, radio, TV system
14. Remote control TV of ambulance or emergency entrance, or of specific patient rooms or diagnostic or therapeutic areas such as cobalt therapy and deep X-ray
15. Clock system
16. Fire detection systems
17. Watchman system.

Decisions to be made by the building committee during this period include the approval of the brick (sample) to be used for the exterior, the use of any special consultants (such as kitchen, elevator, or interior decorating), any alternates to be taken as part of the bid, and the method of setting up bids. The methods could be as follows:

- Separate bids on all major phases of the construction, such as general, electrical, mechanical, plumbing, air conditioning, heating, ventilation, etc.
- All-inclusive bid from the general contractor, to include all phases of construction.
- Separate bids on major phases and then a price from the general contractor for assuming responsibility for the other contractor for assuming, responsibility for the other contractors.
- Cost-plus contract with selected contractor.
- Negotiated contract with established ceiling.

A decision must be made as to whether surgical lights, sterilizers, kitchen equipment, and laundry equipment will be part of the contract and included in the bids of the various contractors, or whether these fixtures and equipment will be purchased by the hospital and then installed by the contractors as part of their contract. Discussions should be held with the architect on the phasing of the project and the proper sequence of the phases should be determined, so that the construction may proceed with optimum efficiency and the least amount of interference with hospital operation.

The list of prospective bidders should be approved by the building committee, after recommendations of the architect. Hopefully, once a list is established, it will not be changed during the bidding process. In all instances the architect determines, by his specifications, the quality of manufactured goods that will be accepted. He may specify only one manufacturer and obtain the competition required under a government contract by having a number of general contractors or special contractors bid on the total job, using the manufacturers previously specified. The architect may establish three or more manufacturers, many of whose products will be acceptable, thereby obtaining the necessary competition.

One of the largest problems in hospital construction is the pressure brought on board of trustees by local manufacturers who indicate that they will make some kind of donation to the hospital if their product is utilized. The best practice is to have the ultimate decision on the quality of products to be used, remain exclusively with the hospital architect.

The project is advertised for bid, and the contract documents are distributed to the various contractors who desire to bid on the project. These contract documents are very specific in the sense that they include all the general conditions for construction, the bid proposals, the alternates, and any ajenda, which have been sent out during the bidding period. The required guarantees on the part of contractors and manufacturers for equipment to be furnished are also listed. The working drawings and specifications are integral part of the contract documents.

Functional System

Hospital

- Segregate paying and non-paying patients
- Segregate male and female patients
- Segragate male and female staff changing and rest facilities
- Use higher proportion of staff doctors.

General Wards

- Do not dadicate wards to spacific single speciality care i.e. each ward will be managed in a way that permits two surgical specialities to be nursed.
- Designate wards for specific specialities.
- Apply progressive patient care concept i.e. designate high dependancy nursing unit within each ward.
- Functional nursing i.e. each nurse has responsibility for the full range of care, within the scope of his/her qualifications and competence level activities related to a specified number of patients.

Pediatric Wards

- Separate pediatric patients from adults.
- Separate surgical and medical pediatric nursing units. Provide sanitary where installation for dedicated pediatric use.
- Encourage maximum parental participation in the care regime.

Obstetrics and Gynecology Ward

Separate obstetrics and gynecology from other patients.

i. Accommodate obstetrics and gynecology patients in general wards. Saperate obstetric in patients from gynecology in patients.
ii. Obstetric patients have their baby (a) rooming in with them, (b) accommadated in a nursary.
iii. A flexible combination of (i) and (ii) to optimise mother baby contact but provide period or rest for the mother.
iv. Assessment and admission to be undertaken in the ward.
v. Assessment and admission to be undertaken in four separate obstetrics admission suites.

Intensive Therapy Unit (ITU)

- Utilize the intensive therapy unit (ITU) for adult patients requiring life support from surgical and medical specialities.
- Saparate ITU care for medical and surgical adult patients requiring life support.
- Accommodate 25 percent of patients in single rooms and the 75% in multi-bedded area.
- Patient allocation.
- Separate staff location system.
- Central monitoring of vital signs.

Neonatal intensive therapy unit:

i. Care for all critically ill neonates within the centre.
ii. Provide emergency, stabilizing care for critically ill neonates and transport to another institution for intensive care.
iii. Provide full range of neonatal care including intensive care, intermediate care, and isolation for immunocompromised.
iv. Provide spacial care for babies born outside the centre.
v. Separate special care from well baby care facilities.
vi. Provide all care (including transfusions) at the cot site.
vii. Develop breast milk bank supplemented by pre-prepared infant formulae.
viii. Encourage mothers to spend time with their babies including overnight stay.
ix. Teach parents baby care procedures.
x. Provide bedside and central monitoring system of cardiac function and vital signs.

Convalescent Unit/Paying Patients Ward

Manage a convalescent unit as a minimal care facility that supports the acute care activities.

Isolation Unit

- Patients who are infectious or immunocompromised.
- Traffic to the unit and within the unit to be strictly controlled. Parsonnel and visitors should gown upon entring the unit.
- Food to be prepared in the central kitchen. Use disposable or autoclavable cookery and cutlery.
- Traffic routes for clean and infected items to be seperate.

Acute Mental Health Unit

To be separately and securely managed. No intensive care rooms. Patient to be individually accommodated. Adopt a therapeutic community operational and care approach.

Emergency

i. Provide emergency care to all patients regardless of their ability to pay.
ii. Provide major trauma facilities for multiple injury and patients suffering from burns.
iii. Provide stabilizing emergency care and minor trauma care for patients to be transferred to a major trauma centre.
iv. Provide emergency ambulance care.
v. Provide 24-hours-trauma service.
vi. Provide setallite minor trauma care to surrounding rural areas.
vii. Provide day surgery for elective minor surgical procedures.
viii. Pool emergency and day surgery staff.
ix. Treat all minor elective surgery as an inpatient episode.
x. Planned programmed diagnostic investigation.

Outpatient

Physically separate consulting rooms from examining and appointment system is desirable.

- Pay individual payment for consultation, lab tests, X-rays, treatments, etc.
- Cumulative billing system i.e. provide services and bill subsequently.
- Provide diagnostic services on an out-patient basis e.g. ECG, EEG, X-ray, laboratory, etc.
- Staff doctors for outpatients i.e. directly employed by the hospital.
- Rent out consultation suites to independent physicians.
- Separate paying from non-paying patients.
- Provide antenatal care and family planning on a scheduled basis.
- Provide dental treatment.

Operating Theater Suite

i. Anesthetize patients in the operating suite.
ii. Anesthetize patients in a separate anesthetic-room adjacent to each OR.
iii. Recover post operative patients in a recovery area and not on the table.

iv. Recover postoparative patients in a recovery ward.
v. Prepare instrument sets for all theatres centrally
vi. Provide all sterile instruments in pre-prepared sets in a theatre sterile supply unit (separate from the CSSD).

Patient Transport

a. From ward to theatre suite (red line) by patient transport trolley, transfer to "clean theatre transport trolley" to *OR* (operationroom).
b. Postoperatively from *OR* to recovery on patient transport trolley.
c. From *OR* to recovery on transport trolley, transfer to recovery bed and then return to ward.
d. Recovery until vital signs are stablised but not fully conscious.
e. Dedicate operating rooms to specialities.
f. Seperate clean traffic routes from dirty..
g. Sex segregation of staff regardless of status for changing and rest facilities.
h. Undertake cesarean section in operating theatre suits.

Delivery Suite

- Provide cesarean section surgery as an integral part of the delivery suite.
- Seperate labor care from delivery.
- Combine first stage and delivery care in one space.
- Provide first stage care for each patient.
- Provide multi-patient rooms for first stage care of some mothers.
- Separate eclamptia patients
- Rasuscitate newborn babies in the SCBU.
- Scrub separately from normal delivery rooms and abnormal delivery.
- Obstetrician should be available in delivery suite round the clock.
- Fatal monitoring of 100 percent of deliveries.
- Natural child-birth procedures.
- Assess on admission in delivery suite.
- Seperate delivery suite staffing from other specialities.
- Telemetric monitoring to central nurse station.
- Tubal ligations and other clean gynecology procedures to be carried out in delivery rooms.

Radiology and Imaging

i. 24-emergency on call service.
ii. Special procedures by appointments.
iii. Collective sorting, viewing, reading and reporting procedures.
iv. Central radiology service for inpatients, outpatients and emergency room.
v. Store films for minimum of 6 years hospital ownership of exposed films.
vi. Frequency of obstetric ultrasound scanning.
vii. Automatic day light film processing.

Electro-medical Diagnosis

- Provide diagnostic facilities centrally for outpatient, inpatients, including executive screening.
- Provide cardiology, cardiac surgery, neurology, and neurosurgery facilities.
- Appointment system for paying patients.

Physiotherapy

- Provide hydrotherapy.
- Provide active gymnasia therapy.
- Manage a health club and executive screening follow-up as an integrated service.
- Brace and prosthetics making and filling facilities.
- Provide ultravoilet treatment for dermatological disorders.

Nuclear Medicine

i. International safety standards to be applied.
ii. Storage and disposal of isotopes.

iii. Commercial contract for maintenance.
iv. In vitro procedures.
v. In vivo procedures.

Central Sterile Supplies

- Centralized preparation of all sterile instruments, dressings and linen for the whole hospital.
- Centralized preparation of sterile sets, dressing and linen for wards, with separate preparation for theater suite.
- Centralize ethylene oxide sterilizing, formaldahyde disinfection or glutaraldehyde soaking.
- Working week of 7 days.
- Contract out sterilizing service to other hospital.
- Mechanized washing and manual washing of instruments.
- Central storage of material used by CSSD.
- Use commerically available disposables.
- Central storage of patient-related equipment e.g. suction machine, pumps, humidifiers.
- Use automatic programmable steam autoclaves.

Hospital Pharmacy

i. Unit dose system to be adopted.
ii. No pharmaceutical manufacturing to be undertaken.
iii. Pharmacy to dispense to both paying and non-paying in- and out-patients.
iv. Pharmacy supplies to be from on site pharmaceutical commerical company.
v. 24-hour on-call staff availability.
vi. Pharmacy to maintain and advise on ward stock drugs.
vii. Distribution of pharmaceutical products to wards to be on a central trolley system or exchange cart system (for unit dose distribution)
viii. Qualified chief pharmacist or a biomedical technologist to manage separate central medical gases store and inflammable goods store.
ix. Centralized water distillation unit to be controlled by the pharmacist.
x. Drug information service to be provided by the pharmacist.

Medical Records

- One patient should have one case sheet.
- Computarize patient master index.
- Diagnostic index to be recorded and computarized.
- Case note to be kept for a minimum of 6 years before miniaturizing or microfilming.
- Physician's secretaries to work on a pool basis.
- Outpatient to be administrated on a planned appointment system.
- Records for free patients to be the same as for paying patients.
- Centralize registration of patient for out- and in-patients.
- Centralise doctor dictating and transcribing system (medical transcription).
- Systematized patient record/chart filling for easy retrieval of each admission or out-patient visit.

Research Offices

1. Research staff to have access to computerized diagnostic index.
2. Research activities to be primarily administrative.

Laundry

- Topping up system of linen distribution to wards with lockable linen stores.
- Incinerate infected linen.
- Manufacture rapair and washing staff uniforms to be undertaken by the laundry.
- Mechanized washing, pressing and folding machinary.
- Contract out laundering services: sell spare capacity to other institutions.
- One week supply of unused linen to be held in store. Purchase ready-made staff uniforms.
- Daily exchange cort system of linen control and distribution.

- Patient purchases own pillow and takes home disposable pillow or washable pillow and blankets.

Kitchen

i. Plate meal distribution system
ii. Provide menu choice to patients, range of cultural diets
iii. Commercial restaurant facilities independent of hospital
iv. Centralisa washing up
v. Separate changing and rest facilities
vi. Traditional cooking methods
vii. Individually designed and prepared therapeutic diet regimns for patient's. Nutritional counselling and advice to patients
  - Use disposables only for isolation patients
  - Catering staff serve patient meals at ward level
  - 24 hour food service for staff

Maintenance and Biomedical Engineering

- Manufacturing of some spare parts
- Planned preventive maintenance programme.
- Minor construction works to be contracted out.
- Vehicle maintenance to be contracted out.
- Storage of spare to be controlled by the maintanance mangaer.
- High technology equipment maintanence to be contracted out.

Staff Dining

- Free meals to staff on duty, no collection of cash
- No segregation of staff by status
- Contract staff dinning to on-site restaurant
- Centralise washing up in main kitchen
- Limited menu choice and diet range
- Separate coffee area from main dining area
- Meals available for all shifts.

Administration

i. Autonomous management of site.
ii. Computerised billing system.
iii. Cashier for all paying.

Main Entrance and Communications

– Access to be available for the disabled.
– Centralised staff location control, telephone switchbord, alarms.
– Automatic PABX system for telephones.
– Automatic patient telephone billing system.

Conference and Seminar

i. Conference facilities to be commercially available
ii. Catering to be provided by main kitchen
iii. Regular medical staff saminers to be held
iv. Modern medical library to be available for physicians, nurses and other health care professionals
v. Nurses and other professional training facilities to be administered by the hospital
vi. Audio visual aids to be used for teaching
vii. Provide oriantation training for all new employees
viii. High provision of inservice and continuing education programmes for physicians, nurses and other professionals
ix. Entry level training to be provided for certain categories of ancillary and support staff.

Stores

- Economic inventory level to be held
- Secure receiving and storage arrangements
- Computerised stock control system
- Trolley distribution system of supplies to Wards
- Routinise requisitioning system
- Mechanised handling within stores
- Flexible segregation of stores by functional group.

Functional Programme

There is no formula which sets the proper size of division in every case, but if specific programme factors are analyzed, the range of choice can be set with assurance. The usual solution is a mixture of singles, doubles, and four-bedded cubicles within the following ranges, all according to local judgement.

Single : 15 to 30 percent of the beds in each unit
Double : 40 to 70 percent of the beds in each unit
Fours : 0 to 85 percent of the beds in each unit (Five and six bed rooms, favored by some, might vary also 0 to 85 percent). With such wide ranges it is apparent that no fixed patterns exist and each plan must be tailor-made to specific needs.

An example of a functional programme will illustrate many of the points mentioned.

Functional Programme of Beds for a 500-Bed Hospital

Total number of beds (excluding bassinets, recovery and emergency)	500	(16)
Medicine (often medical and surgical are listed together)	100	(3)
Surgery	115	(3)
Maternity	70	(2)
Pediatrics	70	(2)
Psychiatry	20	(1)
Intermediate care	60	(2)
Intensive care	25	(2)
(Figures in parenthesis show the desired number of patient care divisions).		
Convalescent and long term care	40	(1)

Programmes for the operating and delivery suites will list additional postoperative or post-partum recovery beds if desired. Such beds and those in emergency, PMR, EKG, injections, or other special services such as bassinets in pediatrics are included in the total but not those in obstetrics.

Desired Subdivision by Size of Rooms

The more highly specialized subdivision adds two nurisng stations, those reducing the average size of division from 39 to 36 beds and further lowering the potential efficiency by introducing speciality groups in place of general medical/surgical divisions. This is an unavoidable result of specia-lization.

Special requirements for teaching:

1. Adequate charting space for interns, residents and student nurses at the nursing station.
2. Separate routine lab at the station.
3. Conference room on each floor.
4. Treatment or examining room for each patient division.
5. An office for the floor supersvisor.
6. Offices for residants or paramedical instructors are desirable.

Facilities Desired in Patient Rooms

- Lavatory with wrist operated faucets in each room.
- Access to a private toilet for each room (with shower if budget permits).
- Shower baths in several delux rooms in medical units.
- Air conditioning of all patient rooms.
- A cheerful residential chartacter of interior design.
- An intercom system (nurse to patient).
- Provision for radio and TV reception.

From this functional programme, the architect can prepare the architectural programme listing each space in the division.

The functional programme for the surgical divisions will be similar, with necessary modi-fications for the number and distribution of beds as given in the programme.

In the maternity division there can be a much lower percentage of single rooms, as already indi-cated, but other elements will be similar.

Architectural Programme for Medical Patient Care Division

- Four divisions of 38 beds each (152 beds) ten single rooms with lavatory and private toilet.
- Two deluxe single rooms with lavatory, toilet, and shower.
- Two, four-bedded rooms with lavatory and toilet.
- Nursing station with charting and work space.
- Medication alcove and sink adjoining nurses station.
- Small office for supervisor.
- Separate charting space for house staff.
- Staff toilets one patient toilet.
- Two bath tubs and two sitz baths for patients.
- Utility room storage cabinets (clean and soiled).
- Treatment (examining) room.
- Solarium (may serve two divisions).
- Linen cart alcove (may be in utility room).
- Small lab.
- Elevator lobby (public phone), waiting.
- Storage alcove for stretchers.
- Serving pantry or kitchen.
- Storage closet.
- Conference or classroom.

Floor area The gross floor area requirements of the patient care divisions represent 40 to 50 percent of the total hospital area; yet it may vary considerably for a given number of hospoital beds, depending upon such factors as the number of single-bed rooms and the number of beds per division, the inclusion of private toilets, the extent of teaching space on the bed floors, the limitation of funds, and the methods used in nursing care.

The procedures for planning new construction can all be applied equally well to planning for modernization and expansion, but in addition certain other methods must be used if there is to be achieved a balanced final plan. These include surveys of existing facilities, both as to their condition and their intensity of use: assembly of data on the known needs and desires for specific improvements; analysis of existing floor areas by departments and comparison with known standards as a measure of space adequacy; and the projection of a functional programme, including floor areas, through the stage immediately proposed and into succeeding future stages as far as may be desired. These methods do not replace other methods already discussed, but they offer aditional guides to planning for modernization and expansion. It is assumed that the functional programme will have been derived from the long-range plan.

Existing Facilities

Fundamental to planning for expansion are the surveys of existing physical facilities. It may be found, for example, that limitations of the existing building site may be insurmountable, ruling out

Service	*Total number*		*In singles*		*In doubles*		*In fours*		*In multiples*	
			No.	*%*	*No.*	*%*	*No.*	*%*	*No.*	*%*
Medicine, acute	100	(3)	40	25	36	36	24	24		
Surgery, acute	115	(3)	47	41	44	38	24	21		
Maternity	70	(2)	6	9	40	57	24	34		
Pediatrics	70	(2)	6	9	12	17	40	57	12	17
Psychiatry	40	(1)	32	75	8	25				
Intensive care	25	(3)	3	12	—	—	—	—	(2 × 11 = 12)	80
Reduced care	40	(1)	28	70	—	—	12	30		
Convalescent	40	(1)	28	70	—	—	12	30		
Totals	500	(16)	190	38	140	28	136	27	34	7

Suggested subdivision of beds

consideration of expansion at the existing location and forcing selection of a new site. But where existing site limitations are not the determining factor, it may still be necessary to relocate, considering existing land and the possibilities of acquiring additional land adjoining it.

Steps in Modernization and Expansion Include

- Functional programme states needs
- Schematic and site studies determine future location
- Gross floor area analysis reveals space deficiencies
- Engineering studies and economic analysis determine future use of eaxisting buildings
- From these studies the long-range plan for growth can be established
- For stage 1, designs and drawings are made: Schematics-detailed basics
- Working drawings and specifications. Bids—Contracts—construction
- Phasing the work-operations-equipping-activating.

The total space requirement will be a combination of these calculations and is certain cases to be more than what is needed simply to take care of the additional hospital beds. A table can best illustrate this.

Table showing architectural programme (distribution of beds by services and size)

Service	*100*	*3*	*200*	*6*	*300*	*9*	*400*	*11*	*500*	*14*
Medical-surgical	80	2	150	4	165	4	209	5	215	6
In singles	32		64		65		89		87	
In doubles	32		54		68		80		80	
In fours	16		32		32		40		48	
Obstetrics	20	1	30	1	40	1	60	2	70	2
In singles	4		4		6		6		6	
In doubles	8		18		18		30		40	
In fours	8		8		16		24		24	
Bassinets	(25)		(36)		(47)		(67)		(78)	
Pediatrics	—	—	20	1	30	1	35	1	70	2
In singles	—	—	4	—	4		5		6	
In doubles	—	—	8	—	10		10		12	
In fours	—	—	8	—	16		20		52	
Psychiatry	—	—	—	—	30	1	35		40	1
Open	—	—	—	—	16		21		26	
In singles	—	—	—	—	12		15		18	
In doubles	—	—	—	—	4		6		8	
Quiet-singles	—	—	—	—	8		8		8	
Disturbed-singles	—	—	—	—	6		6		6	
Intensive care	—	—	—	—	15	1	21	1	25	1
In singles	—	—	—	—	3		3		3	
In doubles	—	—	—	—	—	—	—	—	—	—
In multiple	—	—	—	—	12		18		22	
Long-term	—	—	—	—	20	1	40	1	80	2
In singles	—	—	—	—	12	1	26		56	
In doubles	—	—	—	—	8		14		24	
In fours	—	—	—	—	—	—	—	—	—	—
Postanesthesia recovery	(6-10)		(14-20)		(18-30)		(24-40)		(26-42)	
Emergency observation	(4)		(6)		(8)		(10)		(12)	

(Beds shown in parenthesis are not in total bed count)

Departments	100 beds		200 beds		300 beds		400 beds		500 beds	
	Low	*High*	*Low*	*High*	*Low*	*High*	*Low*	*High*	*Low*	*High*
Total hospital	528	745	506	720	494	701	486	698	470	678
A. Nursing services	295	432	287	423	284	418	290	434	286	427
1. Patient care divisions	240	350	240	350	240	350	250	370	250	370
a. Medical and surgical	250	320								
b. Obstetrics, including nurseries	330	380								
c. Pediatrics	220	300								
d. Psychiatry	300	330								
e. Others	270	300								
2. Operating suite, recovery	35	50	30	45	28	42	25	40	22	35
3. Delivery suite including labor rooms	10	16	9	14	9	14	8	12	8	12
4. Emergency	10	16	8	14	7	12	7	12	6	10
B. Adjunct facilities	58	77	54	73	56	79	53	75	50	73
1. Laboratories	20	26	19	25	18	24	17	23	16	22
2. Radiology	24	30	23	29	22	28	21	27	20	26
a. Diagnosis	(24)	(30)	(22)	(27)	(21)	(26)	(20)	(24)	(19)	(23)
b. Therapy	0	0	(1)	(2)	(1)	(2)	(1)	(3)	(1)	(3)
3. Physical medicine	8	12	7	11	8	13	8	12	7	12
a. Physical medicine	(8)	(12)	(7)	(11)	(6)	(9)	(6)	(8)	(5)	(8)
b. Occupational therapy	0	0	0	0	(2)	(4)	(2)	(4)	(2)	(4)
4. Pharmacy	6	9	5	8	5	8	4	7	4	7
5. Medical social service	0	0	0	0	1	2	1	2	1	2
6. Medical illustration	0	0	0	0	2	4	2	4	2	4
C. Service departments	125	166	117	159	108	144	99	133	92	126
1. Dietary	35	45	33	43	30	38	26	33	24	30
2. Housekeeping	5	7	4	6	3	4	2	3	2	3
3. Laundry	12	15	10	14	9	13	9	13	8	12
4. Central sterile supply	9	12	8	11	8	11	7	10	7	10
5. Central general stores	25	35	25	35	24	32	23	30	22	30
6. Employee facilities	9	12	9	12	8	10	8	10	7	9
7. Building maintenance and operation	30	40	28	38	26	36	24	34	22	32
D. Administration	50	70	48	65	46	60	44	56	42	52
1. Offices	31	43	31	40	31	37	31	35	30	32
2. Medical records	8	10	7	9	7	9	6	8	6	8
3. Public space	6	10	6	10	5	9	5	9	4	8
4. Auxiliary	5	7	4	6	3	5	2	4	2	4
E. Ambulant patient facilities (not in hospital totals)	0	(40)	0	(40)	0	(35)	0	(50)	0	(60)

(Extra-educational facilities)

These units vary with the service— little with the size of hospital

Suggested ranges of gross floor area (SFG) per bed by departements

Total Gross Floor Area for Stage 1 (200 beds)		Net remaining area	29,600
Existing buildings	47,600 SFG	Total floor area as programmed	129,900 SFG
Deduct for buildings, which are to be replaced	18,000	Net building area required (use in budget)	100,300

A balanced hospital calls for much more new space than that required for beds only, which might be 30,000 SFG.

Equipment and Utilities

Nowhere do the problems of expansion reveal more surprises than in equipment and utilities. A sterilizer which was quite adequate yesterday suddenly is revealed as unacceptable for use in the new building; similarly piping, wiring, fixtures, fans, pumps, boilers, elevators, and even the whole heating system may undergo a sudden and painful downgrading when requirements of the future load are calculated. Such findings are normal and not serious if there has been proper physical maintenance and if they are discovered and included before the project budget has been fixed, but too often they are overlooked or not fully explored until the scheme of expansion has been set and the budget established. Findings of inadequacy then drop like a bomb on the planning team, and if the budget cannot be adjusted upward, some other needed and by then cherished improvements must be deferred.

One reason this happens with utilities is that it costs serious money to make an engineering survey of utilities and mechanical plant, and the architect is properly careful to have this work done only when needed; yet if it is not done well in advance of the final schematics, there can be painful results. Sometimes a preliminary engineering review will give sufficient guidance until the detailed survey is made.

With hospital equipment the psychology is a little different, but the results are often the same. Equipment can be appraised more readily than mechanical systems, but the planning team, always hopeful in the early stages, is prone to pass over the true condition of equipment on the assumption that what has been useful can continue in use. Often it is not until some equipment has actually been relocated that the folly of putting old pieces into a new building becomes evident. Such a situation is not without its own advantages, even though the discovery described is a painful one, in that it does seem easier to raise extra money for equipment when the building is well along than in the planning stages. Furthermore, the installation of an old piece does not necessarily preclude its later replacement.

Orderly planning and budgeting, however, call for a creful survey of both utilities and equipment and the inclusion of funds for modernization or replacement. The evaluation of movable equipment is the task of the hospital administrator and his staff or of the hospital consultant but the architect should consult with them so that utilities requirements for all equipment which is to be replaced can be calculated and included in the buiding modernization budget.

Utility Expansion

A related engineering problem is that utilities expansion may call for sizing certain main feeders to carry future loads as well as those presently planned. The engineer should be instructed to do this within reason, but care should be exercised that this is not overdone, particularly with standby elements. Cases have been known in which so much of the budget was required for replacement of utilities and mechanical systems on the one hand and to carry future loads on the other that the remaining funds were inadequate for the prime functional needs. This is like building a complete boiler plant sized for the ultimate hospital and having no funds left to build the patient beds.

Movable partitions The movable partition may be usable in the plan:

- You accept to move it three times
- There is little or no plumbing in it
- Electrical requirements are normal
- Only modest sound deadening is needed.
- *Advantages*
  - Dry construction-quick alterations-clean
  - Makes possible office rearrangements.
- *Disadvantages*
  - Costs more than most conventional partitions
  - Does not lend itself well to special conditions

- Factory units may not fit existing spaces, even with end fillers.
- Where plumbing is needed the mobility is greatly reduced.
- Transmits some sound—often via the ceiling.
- Encourages changes which may not be essential.
- Mobility is not important along corridors, around stairs and elevators, in some bedrooms, in surgery, delivery, kitchen, laundry, central stores, central supply.

Departments	*Existing 100 beds*		*Desirable 100 beds*		*Stage 1 200 beds*		*Stage 2 250 beds*		*Stage 3 400 beds*	
	Gross	*per bed*	*Gross*	*per bed*	*Gross*	*per bed*	*Gross*	*per bed*	*Gross*	*per bed*
A. Nursing services	29,600	296	35,400	354	69,800	349	83,800	339	134,800	337
1. Patient care divisions	24,000	240	29,000	290	58,000	290	72,000	290	116,000	290
2. Surgery	3,600	36	3,600	36	7,500	37	7,500	32	12,000	30
3. Delivery	1,800	18	1,800	18	2,500	13	2,500	10	4,000	10
4. Emergency	200	2	1,000	10	1,800	9	1,800	7	2,800	7
B. Adjuncts	4,900	49	7,100	71	15,400	77	16,500	66	24,800	62
1. Laboratory	1,600	16	2,600	26	5,700	28	5,700	23	8,800	22
2. X-ray	2,000	20	2,800	28	6,300	31	6,300	25	9,200	23
3. Physical therapy	600	6	1,000	10	1,800	9	2,300	9	3,200	8
4. Pharmacy	700	7	700	7	1,200	7	1,800	7	2,400	6
5. Social service	—	—	—	—	400	2	400	2	400	1
6. Medical illustration	—	—	—	—	—	—	—	—	800	2
C. Service departments	8,700	87	13,800	138	27,700	138	29,700	118	42,200	105
1. Dietary	2,800	28	3,500	35	7,500	37	7,500	30	11,000	27
2. Housekeeping	600	6	600	6	600	3	800	3	800	2
3. Laundry	—	—	1,200	12	2,800	14	2,800	11	4,000	10
4. CSS	600	6	1,000	10	2,300	11	2,300	9	3,200	8
5. CGS	2,000	20	3,000	30	5,400	28	6,700	27	10,000	25
6. Employees	600	6	1,000	10	1,800	9	2,300	9	3,200	8
7. Maintenance and equipment	2,100	21	3,500	35	7,300	36	7,300	29	10,000	25
D. Administration	4,400	44	5,300	53	10,000	50	12,100	48	18,000	45
1. Offices	2,600	26	3,100	31	6,000	30	7,500	30	12,000	30
2. Medical records	1,000	10	1,000	10	2,000	10	2,000	8	2,800	7
3. Public space	800	8	800	8	1,400	7	1,800	7	2,400	6
4. Auxillary	—	—	400	4	600	3	800	33	800	2
Subtotal hospital	47,600	476	61,600	616	122,900	613	142,200	57	219,800	549
E. Ambulant patient department	—	—	—	—	2,000	10	2,500	10	1,000	10
F. Housing	—	—	—	—	—	—	—	—	—	—
G. Education	—	—	—	—	3,000	15	3,000	23	5,000	12
H. Research	—	—	—	—	2,000	10	3,000	12	4,000	10
Total project	47,600	476	61,600	616	129,900	648	150,700	605	232,800	581

Certain departments are shown with stage I figures sized for stage 2 loads. These are : surgery, delivery, emergency, laboratory, X-ray, social service, dietary, laundry, CSS, maintenance and equipment, research and education. This results in a high unit for stage 1 but savings at the time stage 2 beds are added. This relatively large number reflects the fact that the increment from stage 1 to stage 2 is only 50 beds.

Certain departements are deficient in existing space. These are : the patient divisions, emergency, laboratory, X-ray, physical medicine, dietary, CSS, CGS, employees, maintenance and equipment and offices. To these must be added space for new and for deficiencies. Laundry, social service, medical illustration, and auxillary departments were added. Other departments are sized in stage 2 for stage 3 load (for example : social service, housekeeping, and auxillary).

Area analysis, existing and expanded, square feet gross floor area (SFG)

Wherever movable partitions are considered for economy, they must be moved three times to show a saving, two times to break even.

Phasing the Improvement

If site conditions permit, the new building should be completed and occupied before modernization of existing buildings is undertaken.

In preparing the phasing schedules, there must be multiple studies of the various possible shifts, taking into account both cost and time involved and making certain that hospital operations can be maintained at an acceptable level. The best solution is often that in which the bed units are the last to be fully occupied after the several steps have been completed for the essential suporting departments.

Any expansion and modernization programme will require 2-4 years of actual construction time after work starts. Time planning will be prior to this.

Providing for Future Expansion

Some departments by their nature cannot easily be expanded in small increments. These are the kitchen, laundry, boiler plant, delivery suite, operating suite, and central sterile supply. In varying degrees, they require large steps or none at all. Other departments are more easily expanded by adding whatever space is called for. The nursing services should generally be expanded by adding whole patient divisions rather than small groups of beds.

The problems of planning for future expansion can be solved in various ways. For those departments which can easily be expanded or moved, the problem is only room for growth. For the nursing services there should be a long-range plan recording the various stages by which the ultimate number of beds is to be reached and maintaining at each stage workable sizes for all patient divisions. It is usually better to plan for the addition of a separate wing with beds on several floors than to plan for the addition of bed floors on top of existing floors. This is largely because of the relatively greater inconvenience and somewhat greater cost in maintaining lower floors in use while construction is going on above, and because the extension of utilities and elevators upward poses many problems. Nevertheless, if site limitations compel and if structure permits, it is not impossible to add floors on top for existing buildings.

Increments

The most difficult problem exists in those departments which cannot be expanded in small increments. Here the solution varies with the programme conditions, and many variables will be encountered. If the existing hospital is small, say 40 beds, and the first stage is another 40 beds, and if the second stage of another 40 beds is anticipated fairly early, say in five years, then it is probably wise to plan kitchen, laundry, power plant, operating rooms, delivery rooms, and central supply to care for the second stage total of 120 beds instead of 80 beds. The total extra space in the departments, thus planned would probably not exceed by more than 30 per cent the area that would be planned for the 80 beds only. This is because the minimum size for these departments will support more than 80 beds and because unit sizes decrease slightly as the number of beds increases. But with a larger stage 2 this is not equally true. An empirical rule is that a far future expansion of less than 30 per cent may justify oversizing the supporting departments but that greater than 30 per cent future expansion calls for the supporting departments to be sized for stage 1 loads only.

Why Oversize ? This line of argument discounts the conviction that careful programming and planning can produce an adequate, but bot oversized, building, without which there is little point in making the calculations described.

Regardless of the approach, each espansion should be tested for each department by making actual plan layouts. In the case of an operating suite, such plans would show the possibility of adding

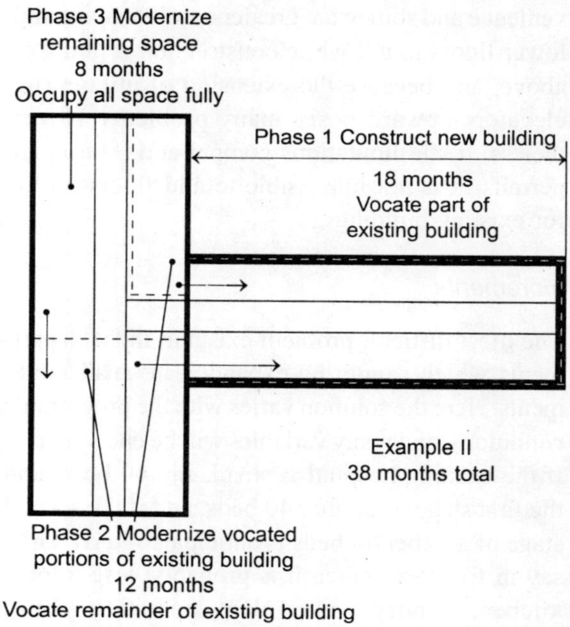

Phasing construction for expansion and modernization

the two operating rooms called for in the stage 2 expansion simply by extending the stage 1 surgical wing by antoher 30 ft. This would avoid oversizing surgery in stage 1 to provide for the stage 2 loads. But a similar expansion of the kitchen would probably be uneconomical, and the stage 1 kitchen should therefore be designed for the stage 2 load of 250 beds. The general rule is not to build excess size in any department if it can be avoided. This rule presumes adequate programming and preliminary planning in stage 1 and careful studies of the direction of expansion for stage 2.

The converse of this problem arises from the practice, too often followed, of adding hospital beds without increasing the supporting services. In this case the result is to overload the nonbed departments and create serious impediments to effective hospital operation. Only through a careful analysis of the size of existing departments and an equally careful programming of those sizes for each stage

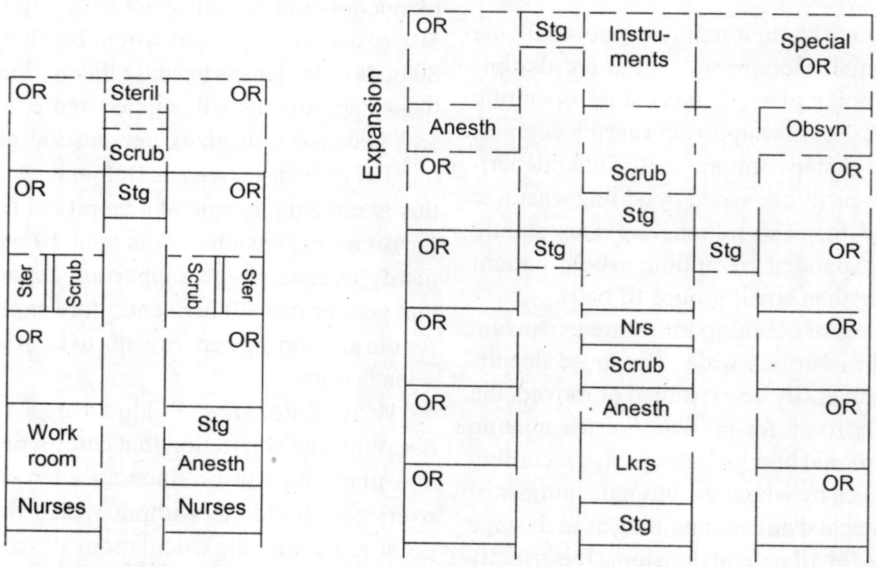

Expansion of operating suite. These schemes provide expansion up to 50 per cent

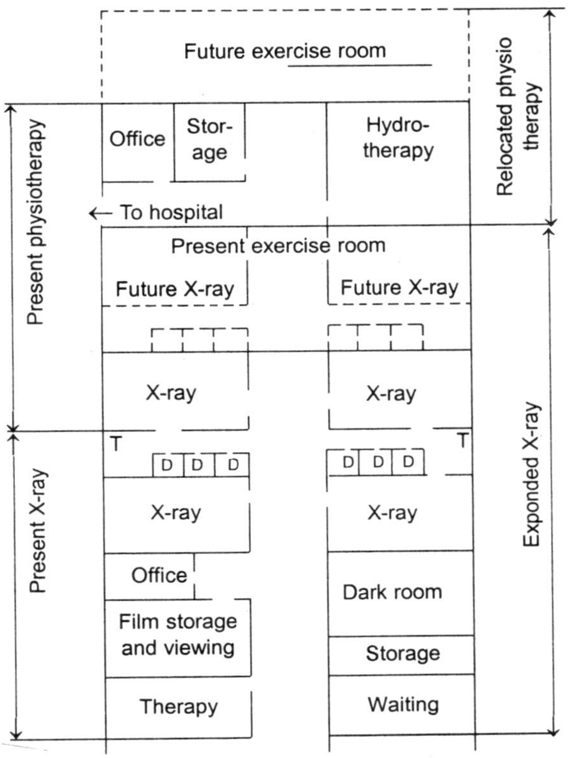

Expansion of X-ray and physical therapy

of expansion can be a suitable balance be maintained and the necessary oversizing be justified.

Plans for present facilities should not be compromised for the sake of an uncertain future in which the requirements may be materially changed. Thus, the main poroblem is to estimate the likelihood of expansion being needed and make plans accordingly. If the future brings as many changes in patterns of hospital care as are predicted, even the most prescient plans will probably be obsolete when the time comes for stage 2.

The Future

The point has been made that the tremendous investment in existing hospital facilities, plus continuing obsolescence, will assure the need for modernization in the future. In addition, population growth and the trend toward enlargement of existing hospitals and further concentration of educational and research activities imply corresponding expansion.

Forces in the contrary direction are the growing dispersion of services into the field and to ambulant patients and the growth limitations imposed upon many hospitals by the size of site. The first of these would tend to lessen the requirements for floor space but would, if anything, greatly increase the need for alteration and modernization of existing spaces to accommodate new functions. The second will be critical in many cases, but it seems probable that the one force most demanding of grounds area now, namely, automobile parking will be removed in the future by exclusion or radical modification of private transport. If this happens, the chances are that many existing metropolitan sites will again be adequate even for the future increased activity.

31 Hospital Patient

Hospital is for the patient where all activities are patient-focused and consumer-oriented. The patient is a member of the society under influence and care of a health organization. The word patient is derived from the Latin *patior*—to suffer. In many cases the character of the patient's demand for hospital care is both medical and socio-psychological.

The concept of the sick person is in the state of continuing evolution.

One of the most obvious facts about patients is their individuality. Each human is unique. The combination of circumstances that gives rise to her or him can never again be duplicated.

Also the ever-present difficulties in communication between planners and architects and representatives of other human sciences converge on the same central situation: the diversity of man. The scientists exploring the human being tend to build up unitary models of man from an all too narrow factual base, which is the limited segment under their particular attention.

All these and other models reflect a circumscribed professional experience of a specialist group. They do not give material for good overall planning purposes.

The authorities have to provide and maintain all the measures as may be necessary to obtain and support the patient's state of complete physical, mental, and social as well-being.

Respect of dignity is one of the most basic rights and needs of the patient. In spite of that most hospitals provide less than a minimum of normal privacy for the patient.

Entry into the hospital environment means entry into a system which the patient generally has less control of daily events than in the home environment. It is assumed that already this experience produces stress which requires a coping or adaptation procedure on the part of patients.

In fact, the patient enters frequently the hospital in a vulnerable state, being to some degree, incapacitated by disease and apprehensive about outcome. The hospital adds to this vulnerability by enforcing additional dependencies, intensifying the helplessness of patients and making them passive participants in drama in which they have little to say about events that are for them more than usually consequential.

The psychosocial stresses The stresses experienced by hospital patients are mainly stresses brought about mere fact of hospitalization, regardless of the nature of the illness or reason of hospitalization.

Growing evidence suggests that these stresses are measurable and associated with observable physiologic changes.

Many suffer in the hospital under unpleasatness caused by three forms of contemporary social behavior: togetherness, conformity and herd-mindedness. Each of these forms of behavior operates in direct opposition to the autonomy that almost all psychologists feel is a precondition of self-actualization.

Much unhappiness results from promulgating the concept that all people are equal, and that in instance where they are unequal they can be equalized.

In a diversified society everybody is right in his own way. This means that in any general hospital solution it will be at best a compromise–satisfactory to some, inconvenient to others.

Even the requirements of disabled people differ. What may help one person may sometimes hinder another. No arrangement will be perfect for people of every size and with every kind of disability.

Although one of the objects of hospital care is to decease stress and anxiety, many hospitals inadvertently decrease the patient's psychic strength by depersonalizing him. *TS Eliot* provided a deeply felt description of this aspect in act one of his play **The Cocktail Party**

You're suddenly reduced to the status of an object–
A living object, but no longer a person.
It's always happening, because one is an object
As well as a person. But we forget about it
As quickly as we can.

The main hospital stress factors are unfamiliarity of surroundings, loss of independence, separation from spouse, financial problems, isolation from other people, lack of information, threat of severe illness, separation from family, and problems with medications.

The effects of hospital stress on patients are not well understood, but they are thought to be both psychological and physical effects.

Higher stress scores for surgical patients compared with medical patients have been indicated.

Hospital personnel continue in their scientifically unsupported manner of perceiving patients behaving in an infantile way. It should be mentioned that not all patients feel this infantilization as disturbing or offending.

There still are remnants from the one-time philanthropic attitude of the medical body who received from the indigent nothing. In an extensive study of patient adjustment to hospitalization, *Hans Mauksch* observed that in addition to getting well, most patients must also strive for psychological survival in a power system where the rules for behavior are often ambiguous.

Patients, whom nurses dislike, are also discriminated by them. Most patients realize the power of the nurse and fear to anger her as they quickly learn that patients out of favor are ignored and hospital rules strictly enforced. They feel the need to show cooperation, trust and confidence, and not to be too demanding.

Patients with physical defects like deafness, obesity, or disfigurement, those of foreign nationality, and those whose hospitalization was longer than three months are significantly more unpopular among nurses.

Unpopular are also those that grumble, complain, and demand attention, and those the nurses think should not be in the hospital at all. A certain way to become an avoided patient was to have a terminal disease.

Age, sex, or illness—except for psychiatric and terminal illness appear not to be important in influencing the nurses' attitudes. Some patients are neither popular nor unpopular. They have virtually no verbal communication with nurses: routine tasks are carried out without exchange of a word. Although patients may prefer not to talk, it is more likely they are afraid to take the initiative.

Patient's nurses like best are those who know their nurse; are able to communicate readily with nurses; can joke and laugh with nurses, and co-operate in being helped to get well and express determination to do so.

Patients come to a hospital to be treated and not to be administered. Therefore, the regularity with which hospital routine takes precedence over the rest requirements of the patient is amazing.

The process that reduces a person to a patient, is only partly understood. This includes also the losing of confidence in the knowledge, which the patient was so sure about before entering the hospital.

One of the factors may be the objectivist type of medicine now being widely practiced, in which the disease and the patient is the object of care. The other may be the paradoxical situation that the patient who outside the hospital had been overflooded with general health information, suddenly is deprived of all information concerning his own health.

Anxiety and fear are the inevitable consequences of poor communication between doctors and patients. Frequently patients who complain about their doctors want two things: someone to give them a scientific explanation hedged with doubts and someone to do the magic and deal with the uncertainty.

The importance of the information factor should not be overestimated, as the average patient is generally ignorant in most of the health matters: anxiety, physiology, causes and symptoms of illness.

The medical staff should not regard the patient as a passive object who would be given all possible information. Delivering and receiving medical information is a delicate procedure.

Hospitalization may represent a crisis for both the patient and his family.

Hospitalization is a period of strain for patients, whose emotional needs probably vary as much as their physical emotions. Hospitalization for them is an uncommon, often unpleasant experience. The physical discomfort, environmental estrangement and forced isolation, together with the fears and anxieties associated with sickness, tend to threaten or weaken the patient's existing adaptive mechanisms and defenses.

Some patients can be alert, but as in the case of endotracheal respiration utterly frustrated for being unable to communicate. Apprehensions arise both from the patient's natural preoccupation with his own physical condition, and from his necessary dependence on the abilities of others to effect the treatment. In order to deal effectively with physical condition, the emotional factors involved must be recognized.

The patient may be affected by his pathophysiological status with its accompanying discomforts, mechanical apparatus, constant observation periods and therapies, lack of privacy, time disorientation, sensory monotony, sleep deprivation, as well as by his personal reactions to illness, life and family problems.

Vulnerable patients include those with high levels of anxiety and depression proneness, females under 40 years of age, those who have not been in hospital before, those admitted for a series of tests, and those with infective or undiagnosed illness.

Sleep is more than rest, it is a state of unresponsiveness brought about by active nervous mechanisms, a form of rest that ensures that the whole body, including the nervous system, can recuperate.

A study of hospital sleep patterns shows that the deficit is principally due to early awakening.

Sleep deprivation may actually improve some depressed and schizophrenic patients, at least briefly. This observation highlights general ignorance about the functions of sleep and the effects of sleep deprivation.

Patients in Wheel Chair

Wheelchair users have capabilities as varied as those of the ambulant population. Accidents, illness-related disability, and congenital defects affect all parts of the body leaving limbs in various stages of weakness, paralysis, of absence. The healing process is much longer in disabled than in able-bodied people.

The most common wheelchairs have a width of about 0.60 to 0.62 m, the seat being approximately 0.48 m above floor. A turn of 180 degrees should be possible in a 1.80 to 1.85 m diameter. A corridor width of 1.05 m is required to make also a turn into a 0.8 m clear door opening possible. Corridors with a width of 1.8 m allow wheelchairs to pass.

Reaching from a seated position is limited and depends on access to the location of the item being reached. If side approach to telephone or vending machine is possible then the highest operable part of the equipment can be located 1.35 m above the floor. If approach from the front is only means of access, then the highest operable part should not be higher than 1.2 m from the floor. In toilet rooms towel or tissue dispensers and other equipment must be located not higher than 1 m from the floor.

Intensive Care Unit Patients

The most common patient problem in a burn unit is the pain; in the surgical intensive-care unit, the delirium; in the respiratory intensive-care unit, the chronic depression; and in the cardiac-care unit, the anxiety.

Particularly the psychological problems in intensive care and treatment units represent a complex issue.

Death is a constant presence and threat. Patients are bound to be aware of it, often despite the efforts of the staff to screen them from it. Death figures in the fantasies of the patients despite denial either of its presence or of the intensity of its emotional impact.

Numerous cases have been reported of acute emotional distress in intensive care and treatment of patients, whose life is threatened.

There have been many demonstrations of the relationship between psychological states and physiological changes which could have an adverse effect on the coronary intensive care patient.

Most of the patients will have delusional states in varying degrees while on the unit. There might be psychological implications in a patient who is continuously reminded of being so seriously ill as having to be nursed in the strange environment of the ICTU. The importance of recognizing psychiatric disorders in severely ill patients has been stressed. The main psychosomatic aspects revolve around reactive psychic disorders and the states of delirium, clouding of consciousness, and confusion. Serious psychological breakdowns are rare–less than 0.5 per cent–of all patients admitted to the ICTU.

Of course, even within the same country the various types of ICTU cannot be easily compared. Numerous factors—psychological climate, design, discharge procedures, nature of the organic conditions involved, personnel—determine the specific character of a unit and in this way exert a particular influence on the patient. If only for this reason it is difficult to give a general description of the psychiatric or psychological problems, which can arise in various ICTUs. Moreover, interpretation of the various results is subject to limitations. One of these limitations lies in the fact that the behavior sciences deal with less factual, less sharply defined and more controversial events and acts that their practitioners would wish.

The intensive therapy patient is mostly conscious, and is disturbed by the activities, light and particularly by noise in an ICTU.

Homologous stimulation, solitude, confinement, isolation and invariant input predispose to illusions and hallucinations.

There is deterioration in intellectual performance with an increased susceptibility to influence and stimulus seeking behavior.

Patient stress is described in an account of the experience of Mr *Lawrie*, an analytical chemist, who was ventilated for nine days. He experienced discomfort related to lying in one position for any length of time and found himself looking forward to positional changes. He hallucinated when effects of his drugs subsided. He suffered from double vision and large objects seemed to be nearer than actually where the ceiling appeared to be only about 0.5 m above him. Therefore, he preferred not to be left on his back. His hearing was very acute: sounds were magnified and he heard most conversations in his vicinity, but his worst memories were when he could hear nothing.

Elderly Patients

The results of interdisciplinary research in gerontology in recent years–whether in the field of psychology or in medicine, psychiatry, sociology, or ecology–give added weight to the demand for a differential gerontology. It must be questioned whether psychological and physical aging processes conform to any universal laws.

In the aging process there are not only inter-individual differences–i.e. persons born in the same year may show marked differences in their 'biological', 'functions', 'social', and 'psychological' ages–but that there are also differences with regard to the intraindividual agingprocess, that there are patterns of intraindividual development which vary interindividually.

Psychological research in gerontology during past 20 years has been able to show that the 'deficit' model of aging, which is still widely entertained, is in need of revision or modification. There need not be an age–induced deterioration in the mental sphere. There is neither a general (i.e. affecting all fields) nor a universal (i.e. affecting all persons) aging deficit.

Elderly patients vary greatly in emotional stability and in mental acuity. The results of the research point to the primary significance of a personality structure characterized by a generally higher level of activity, which usually goes with a more elevated mood and more marked ability to adapt to, or to cope with, any given life situation.

Over 65 years old patients are considered to have the highest degree of individuality, in spite of the fact that measurable mental deterioration occurs in as many as 25 per cent of them. Many elderly patients easily lose contact with reality when placed in new surroundings. Disorientation and hallucinations may occur due to darkness, or after a minimal dose of drugs.

The sensory perceptions of aged people suffer under sensory understimulation and disengagement. Because of sensory impairment and the loss of vital, tactile, aural levels of perception, the environment will be for the aged increasingly confusing and frustrating.

The visual acuity of the eye influences perceiving objects at a distance. The capacity of the lens determines the way light is transmitted and affects perception of colors and textures. Elderly see colors almost 20 per cent less keenly than those with normal vision, particularly in the cold end of the spectrum. Colors too often blend, and closely related textures cannot be differentiated.

Glare is a major visual difficulty with elderly. Direct and indirect glare caused by shiny walls and floors, make it difficult to distinguish between rooms and cupboard doors. Shiny floor areas can be mistaken for openings in the floor. The perception of subtly shaded mural paintings and signs on doors is rendered impossible. Glare should not be confused with light level. The light level must be increased for the elderly.

The aural aspect should be mentioned. The elderly have trouble distinguishing meaningful sounds. The background hum of heating, ventilating and air conditioning systems, easy for younger people to adapt along with television notes, etc. need to be modified for the elderly.

Pediatric Patients

Children should be admitted to the hospital only if it is absolutely inevitable.

The infants must be treated as persons in their own right.

Children of all social groups suffer emotional stress when admitted to hospital. Many children do not master it without symptom formation.

Emergency hospitalization constitutes an even stress than elective admission for both children, parents and staff.

The most common cause of psychological disturbance in children in hospital is a sense of lost affection. Separation from the mother is felt most severely in the first three years of life, particularly between the sixteenth and fifteenth month. Only a day's separation from the mother would mean practically nothing to the child.

It has been found that children under three years may stop in their mental development when hospitalized and their games and play may be carried out on a lower intellectual level than before hospitalization.

Children under five years of age not only suffer from the separation from their parents and accustomed surroundings, but it is also difficult to explain to them the reasons for undergoing such unpleasant experiences as injections, intravenous therapy, gastric suctions and operations. Before the age of the five, the concerns commonly held by children are abandonment, pain and mutilation, invasion of body orifices, and loss of control over their usual routines.

Eleven to sixteen–year–olds usually dread leaving the hospital in a dependent position, and worry about their occupation choice.

The majority of children who undergo surgical procedures are able to differentiate and integrate their fairs and painful experiences, and psychopathology does not become a part of their clinical history. In 20 per cent of the cases, children's fears of operation have resulted in severe postoperative reactions. The extent of the surgery is not so important as the fact of interference with the child's body.

Children in hospitals appear to be less afraid than grown–ups, perhaps they are more trusting or naïve. However, the children are frequently more afraid of injections.

All periods of illness, whatever their length, seem painfully long to children because they differ from adults in their concepts of time and turn all periods of time into waiting times.

Time passes more slowly for the child than for the adult. Time for a middle–aged of 50 years flows about ten times as fast as it does for a child of five years, and for a young man of 20 four times as fast as 5-year old. This intellectual aspect of the child must be considered as a factor not least in planning units when pediatric patients are waiting to be operated or in an other way medically treated.

The child is more interested in activity involving people than in a distant view. Children in bed require something to hold their interest and compensate for their immobility. The ward should be so planned that the sick child always see an adult.

The children are sensitive to space and their response to it is strongly emotional, but any toys or other security objects seem to give the child more comfort than environment.

Playrooms and outdoor play areas for children must be provided. The child in hospital has a need to play out the anxieties and problems of being in a strange and frightening environment, and the hostile feelings he may harbour towards parents who seem to have abandoned him and staff who cause pain.

Play is essential for the children who have not the capacity to understand the procedures or the verbal language to express their feelings about the procedures. Play gives a child the assurance that he can still use his body and limbs normally. By occupying himself in creative activities he is, in a sense, repairing those parts of himself which he feels has been broken or damaged. Play is also a means of socializing the children with each other.

A full-time child-life worker should be responsible for the playroom programme. The playrooms should be in the sunny area accommodating about 25 children. It should be furnished with low stationary table and child-sized chairs.

One corner could be reserved for painting, another for child-sized playhouse furniture and the third for large construction trucks. Equipment which increases the mobility of already active children is disruptive and unsafe.

Puzzles of all types, tea sets, dolls, dishes, small blocks, and games all can be used in a supervised playroom. Hobby horses with springs and all forms of battery toys are impractical.

Neonates

From the moment of birth, the newborn is acutely aware of his surroundings. Newborn infants, with their relatively sophisticated sensory systems, response preferentially to the stimuli that occur in human social interaction. The infant's contribution has been woefully underestimated until recently.

At birth the neonate can see, focus, follow, and exhibit visual preferences. Further more, recent evidence suggests that newborn infants are especially interested in face-like configurations. Within minutes after birth, babies visually follows a face-like pattern more than others of similar brightness, complexity, and symmetry. Neonate can also interact with adults by imitating visually-presented behaviors.

Newborn infants do respond more to the female than to the male voice and will rapidly develop a preference for the mothers voice through her caregiving and interaction.

Auditory noise without signal value to the infant appears consistently hamper development. Repeated encounters with meaningless sound serve to habituate the attention and arousal of the orienting response to such sounds.

Perinatal medical care was introduced with the purpose of further decreasing mortality and morbidity by preventing infection and managing physical problems. However, maternity unit routines were established before research in pediatrics, anthropology, development psychology, ethology, and physiology created a new appreciation of the remarkable capacities of the neonate for social interaction and of the importance of the newborn period for a mutual parent–infant involvement.

In industrialized societies the previous pattern of frequent nursing and abundant physical interaction has been replaced by one of intermittent artificial feeding and minimal contact. Perinatal medical management has additionally imposed a pattern of early separation on mother and neonate.

Neonates may be upset by unusual maternal appearance or behavior. When bottle fed by their mothers wearing a mask, one-week-old infants become distressed, avoid their mothers physically and visually, feed poorly, and have disruptions in their sleep cycle. The social responses of healthy mothers and infants are also altered by hospital routines, which involve separation.

The infant more readily organizes his cycles of sleeping, waking, and crying if exposed to a single caregiver in the first ten days of life. Newborn infants who room in cry distinctly less and a establish a day-night rhythm more quickly than infants in a traditional nursery with multiple caregivers and four-hour feeding schedules.

It is inhuman to force on infant's artificial schedules based on the convenience of hospital's shifts. In particular, sleep cycles can be disrupted or months after the baby has spent a longer time in a brightly lit nursery. Equally cruel is the *neonatal exile*, the interrupted mother-child contact, caused by the assumption that the mothers are infection-risks.

Current programmes encourage the presence of both parents, their participation in feeding where this is practical, and an openness to inform them fully concerning their infant's condition. This interaction between the infant and his family is believed to safeguard the child's emotional, social and physical development. However, there is still need for some clear guidelines by which to determine the optimal amount of tactile, visual, auditory, and other forms of stimulation necessary for the early development of newborn, especially the immature infant.

There is no medical reason why healthy mothers and babies should not be together from the time of birth to the time of discharge from the hospital.

Situating the Department

It is advantageous to have the department easily accessible to other departments:

- Emergency department
- Outpatient clinics
- Surgery and cystoscopy

Economical considerations usually dictate that the department be located on the ground floor. Radiographic equipment, radiation protection and film storage increase floor loading substantially. This increase may require special construction if the department is on an upper floor. The department will eventually need expansion. The department should therefore be situated in a section of the building–proper where expansion is possible.

Room Dimensions

Some generally-accepted standards for various room sizes, dressing booths and control booths given below should only be used as guide:

Radiographic room	:	15' × 18'
Radiographic and fluoroscopic room	:	16' × 18' to 16' × 20'
Remote fluoroscopic room plus control space	:	16' × 20'
Special procedure room	:	20' × 25' to 20' × 28'
Automated chest room	:	11' × 15'
Head room	:	12' × 14'
Head and chest room	:	14' × 18'
Cytology room	:	12' × 16'
Cobalt room plus maze and wall thickness	:	16' × 17'
Simulator room plus control area	:	18' × 18'
Ultrasound rooms	:	12' × 14'
Mammography room	:	10' × 15'
Control booth for R and F	:	5' × 6' to 5' × 8'
Dressing Booths	:	3' × 3' to 6' × 6'

Construction Recommendation

Ceiling mounted equipment requires properly designed rigid support structures located above the finished ceiling. The bottom of the structure should be flush with the finished ceiling. Through–button or welding of these structures is recommended.

A light–out type ceiling is recommended in most radiological departments for ease of service, installation and remodeling. This may be a 60 × 60 cm or 60 × 120 cm grid system.

Room lighting requirements vary with the examination and equipment involved. Both general ceiling and cove lighting are recommended. Dimmer controls on lights are required in some rooms, particularly special procedure rooms and fluoroscopic rooms.

Trough or trench ducts with removable covers are recommended to facilitate the installation of the required cable connections between the various equipment components.

Trough or trench ducts simplify the equipment installation and permit plugged interconnecting cable type installation. This type of design dramatically reduces installation time and also allows future changes.

The ampacity (for the X–ray diagnostic rooms) of supply branch conductors and overcurrent protective devices shall not be less than 50 percent of the momentary rating or 100 percent of the long–time rating, whichever is the greater.

The rated ampacity of conductors and over-current devices of a feeder for a two or more branch supplying circuits supplying X–ray units shall not be less than 100 percent of the momentary demand rating of the momentary ratings of the X–ray apparatus.

Provisions should be made for emergency electrical power in the event of a power failure.

Specifications should be made 480V, 240V, and 208V three–phase 60Hz power supply. Delta and Wye type systems for single–phase equipment. A 480V system is recommended.

Voltage regulation must not exceed full momentary load of a specific KVA at a certain power factor percentage. The phase-to-phase utilization voltage has limited tolerance and daily voltage variation, due to causes other than X–ray equipment, and must not exceed a ± percentage factor (± 5 percent).

The relative humidity in all the examination rooms be maintained at between 35 to 60 percent. Air–charge rate should be received.

Rooms and corridors should be bright, cheerful, and habitable for staff and patients.

Diagnostic Radiology

Diagnostic X–ray rooms are grouped according to their specialty with the radiograph rooms located nearest the patient waiting areas. The rooms are also situated around the darkrooms in an effort to keep film cassettes carrying to a minimum.

Toilets serving the fluoroscopic rooms are designed so that the patient can enter the toilet directly from the diagnostic rooms and exit from the toilet without re-entering the X–ray room.

Adequate dressing booths must be provided. X–ray control booths should be designed to provide adequate radiation protection for the operator.

FURTHER READING

1. Putsep E: Modern Hospital International Planning Practices. Lloyd-Luke Ltd. London, 1979.

32 Floors, Walls and Installations

Flooring

Floors are one of the most important components of a hospital. Dominating hospital floor coverings are vinyl, resiliant shet vinyl, asbestos tiles, terazzo, terazzo tile, and carpeting.

The function of the floor should be the determining factor when choosing floor covering. The blind use sound reflected up from walking surfaces to orient themselves.

The vinyl asbestos tiles are cheapest. Demanding a quality carpet designed for health care-not to be used in potential high-spillage areas-will result in a higher initial cost than for vinyl, but the long-term maintenance costs are considerable lower.

Wheeled equipment, and carts will require third-generation nylon of low, thick pile, glued directly to the floor.

Considerations, such as acoustical quality, safety, comfort, and appearance could make *wall-to wall carpeting* an appropriate and perferred selection in carefully considered areas, not at least in the patient day areas and in the administrative section. Carpet tiles come in various styles and constructions, including velvets, tweeds, and prints.

Carpets in hospitals must be of low static resistance to avoid electric sparks. Caution in the use of carpeting and under carpet padding should be exercised both as to fire resistance and potential production of toxic fumes in case of fire.

Smells caused by bacteriological decomposition of spills on carpeted floors are a major drawback to the widespread use of carpets in patient-care areas of hospitals. Liquid spills on carpets are difficult to remove completely, because the liquid is absorbed by the fibres and soaks through the backing to the subfloor. The use of non-absorbent pile fibres and an impervious backing can prevent in this but necessitate the use of synthetic fibres. It is feasible to produce conventional, woven wool carpets, with a liquid-impervious back, but making wool non-absorbent for water and oil based liquids is almost certainly not an economical proposition.

It is inadvisable to instal carpets in critical care rooms and in spaces where stains from blood, vomitus, food, beverage, and clay can be produced. Moreover, the use of such carpeting is not recommended on floors which are subject to considerable wear, or where carpeting itself is a source of wear, for example, on children's clothing.

Resilant and accoustical foam-backed sheet vinyl would be a good substitute for carpeting.

To improve the floor cleanliness standards, colors and patterns that disguise uncleanliness and dirt should be avoided in hospitals.

For the flooring material in the operation rooms as well as in anesthetic and equivalent rooms, high demands are made.

The floors should be nonslippery, when wet withstand intensive application of water and disinfectants not absorb phyhsically, foreign molecules have a high resistnce to breakdown be elastic and recover after the removal of heavy objects be fire resistant, be color fast, not require treatment with wax or other preservatives.

Coved skirting with a minimum radius of 3 cm and a minimum height of 10 cm should be used for all floors, thereby eliminating junction between skirting and flooring.

PVC flooring is the floor finishing probably to satisfy the majority of the requirements of operation room flooring. If a minimum of seams is desirable, PVC should be heat-sealed.

Terazzo is completely satisfactory because of its hardness, noiseness and tendency to craze, and the time taken to repair it. Terazzo can be destroyed by wrong cleaning materials.

Precaution against explosions must be maintained in the operation room and where flammable anesthetics are stored. Also in teaching hospital areas when taught on flammable anesthetic agents, the flooring should be conductive. The operation rooms should be uniformly protected to avoid restrictions in their use.

The conductive floor finishes have to conform with the standards and requirements of national agencies.

During the lifetime of an antistatic floor, its resistance may change. The resistance of terazzo floors usually increase, whilst that of PVC floors decreases with time. Antistatic rubber has a somewhat limited life and is less convenient in other ways.

For *laboratories* special building adaptions, such as deep inserts in the floor, must be taken in planning considerations at an early stage. When heavy equipment might be used, attention has to be paid to floor loading.

All materials to be used for laboratory floors should be tested with strong acids, alkalis, water, solvents, and histological stains. The floors should be of non-slip quality, also when wet, easy to clean, hard wearing, and fire resistant.

Linoleum and tiles are widely used in laboratories. Linoleum floors are slippery, when wax-treated. In spite of that they have to be kept well polished in areas where decontamination occurs.

Asbestos vinyl tiles are hard wearing and not so slippery when wet. They are, however, attacked by some alkalis and acids. Flexible vinyl is preferred for laboratory floor covering because it is more impervious and therefore a little more resistant to chemical attack. Flexible vinyl is resistant to acids, but not to all solvents. Vinyl sheets should not be laid where it would be subjected to abrasive materials or to heavy point loads.

Floors which have to be hosed down should be laid with falls and the channels should discharge into sealed top back inlet gullies outside the building: if open floor channels cannot be avoided, they should have rust-proof, easily cleaned metal grids.

To reduce the noise level in the laboratory corridors to a minimum resilient and accoustical vinyl floor covering should come to use. More recently it has been recommended to use in laboratories caperting in as many areas as possible.

Conductive floors in rooms where electronic equipment is used on patients are needed. No appreciable charge should be allowed build up on the floor, which should have a resistance to limit the current from any defective equipment and simultaneously dissipate the energy through its conductivity.

Ramps, Steps, Stairs

If ramps are to be used by the ambulant disabled as the main means of entry, a minimum gradient of slope is best.

Pedestrian circulation on the site and in the building be no steeper than a 5 per cent gradation. Any length of circulation steeper than five per cent is considered a pedestrian ramp, the gradation of which may not be greater than 8.3 per cent (1:12). Pedestrian ramps must have handrails.

As minimum width of the slanting level 1.6 m could be accepted, all slanting levels should be slip-free and fitted with hand rails, one at the height of about 0.9 m and the other at the height of 0.5 m for the ease of visitors in wheel-chairs.

Many of the ambulant disabled find stairs easier to negotiate than ramps,which are necessary for the chairbound.

Staircases in health care facilities should have 0.15 m risers and 0.32 m treads.

Handrails should be positioned on both sides of stamps and stairs and should extend beyond the first and last steps on at least one side and preferably on both to allow people with long leg braces to pull themselves beyond these points.

Steps, stairs, and handrails should not be made of slippery material. Hard, level, non-skid surfaces are essential.

Walls, Ceilings

Wall materials in the high hygienic standard areas like the operation rooms should be hard, robust, impervious, jointless, non-absorbent, easily cleaned and decontaminated. Likewise, it has been recommended that the wall finishes should be unaffected by color change, staining and mildew.

These requirements in perfection are held too high as the hygienic hazards of the walls are extremely small.

Ceramic tile has been criticized because the rough surface of grouting may entrap bacteria. New, smooth grouting materials, suitable for operation room use are available. Other suitable surface materials include laminated polyesters with an epoxy finish and hard vinyl coverings which can be heat-sealed.

Good quality coating may be a less costly solution which can be accepted. The glossier the surface, the easier it is to keep clean. High-gloss speciality coating finishes are relatively impervious to stain penetration.

The corners in the operation room should be rounded and viewing cabinets, switches, plugs, cupboards and door frames in flush with the wall surfaces to make cleaning routines easier.

Factory-made wall units with equipment mounted on them so that they can be maintained from outside the operation room may simplify both maintenance and alteration works. The walls should not cause the build-up of a static electrical charge.

Primary protective barriers, rather than secondary, should be provided for all wall and floor areas likely to be exposed to the beam currently or in the future.

In all hospital areas where equipment is moved, protective guards against wall damage should be made of a very heavy material.

Partitions may be used to divide corridors from use areas. From the view-point of fire safety the normal requirement is continuous, slab-to-slab wall with at least-one hour resistance.

The choice of *ceiling* construction in the medical performance area, particularly in operation rooms and X-ray rooms depends on lighting, heating, and ventilating arrangements. Diversified demands for ceiling-mounted equipment require a careful programming.

Basically, the requirements for operation room ceiling surfaces from the view point of cleaning and decontamination are the same as for the walls.

As requirements concerning noise control in operation rooms have increased, the wall surface should be relatively non-reflecting.

Electronic measurement of a patient's heart, brain, and other potentials generated by the body involves extremely weak electrical signals. As the recordings on the instruments are obtained by a high degree of amplification of these signals, the physiological recording may be seriously distorted or degraded by interference in the surrounding area.

Electromagnetic interference should be eliminated from rooms in which electroencephalograph (EEG), electromyograph (EMG), or other equally sensitive equipment, but not electrocardiograph (ECG), is used or where the output of this kind of equipment is fed into a computer for comparison or analysis.

Among such rooms the following can be mentioned: intensive care and monitoring rooms operation rooms for catheterization rooms for angiographic techniques all rooms for measurements of bioelectric potentials.

The electrical installation on inside or both sides of walls, floor and ceiling of the room should be screened by means of ferrous metal shielding of cables resp metal conduits for cables and wiring. This shielding should be connected only at one point to the protective earth.

Shielding systems vary from copper-clad plywood and modular panels of galvanized steel with a plywood core to transparent vinyl sandwich constructions encasing sheets of bronze screen. The latter permit a visual check for breakages in the metal screen and simplify the location of holes to be cut in the panels to accommodate pipes, ducts, conduits, and equipment.

To ensure radio-frequency interference-proof environment when galvanized steel panels are used, seams and corners have to be tightly sealed with galvanized steel strips. As duct openings are a potential source of radio-frequency intrusion, supply air must enter the space through baffled wave-guide vents.

Any wire-power, telephone, and intercom penetrating the shield may act as an antenna to conduct radio frequency into the space. Every electrical wire must therefore enter through a radio-frequency electrical filter.

Because fluorescent lighting introduces its own electro-magnetic contamination into the shielded environment, lighting must be supplied by either incandescent or interference-free cold cathode fluorescent lamps.

The shielding of a radiation room shall protect occupationally exposed persons as well as non-radiation workers. It must not be impaired by joints, openings for pipes ducts, etc. passing through the barriers, or by conduits, service boxes, etc. embedded in the barriers.

Permanent wall radiation screening in X-ray department rooms, where the working capacity does not extend 150 kV and radiation is undirected, should comprise of a 2 mm thick sheet of lead or equivalent material. In the X-ray department shielded floors will be necessary if there are rooms below the X-ray rooms, particularly if tube, ceiling shielding will be necessary for rooms above. Concrete is likely to be the most effective shielding material.

Doors and other means of access to the room and observation windows also require special consideration to ensure adequate protection without sacrificing operational efficiency. The lead lining must also be sandwiched into the doors leading to the room.

For viewing openings between the operator and patient, at least 10 mm thickness shielding glass containing barium or lead should be used.

Similar requirements have been adapted on computer-assistant tomography units.

In operation rooms where X-ray equipment may have the same capacity as that in the X-ray department itself, it is essential to apply the X-ray department standards.

The radiation protection relates also to the walls of the rooms in the emergency and in the intesive care unit where X-ray equipment is used frequently.

In *nuclear medicine laboratories* safety precautions are much more important in in vivo than in in vitro studies. Shielding is required not only of the nuclides themselves, but of the surrounding room, so that the floors, walls, and ceilings adequately reduce radiation exposure.

OPENINGS

Doors must not constrict the space required in different rooms.

Doorways should have 86 cm clear opening width to allow easy passage also for a wheelchair. A level space of at least 152 cm wide should extend about 45 cm on either side of the doorway for opening and closing the door by a wheelchair patient.

Door hardware should be designed with single-lever action and should require no more than 4 kg of pressure to open the door.

In the operation department, staff dressed in sterilized garments need a minimum door opening width of 90 cm.

A clearance of about 10 cm on either side of the bed including special equipment is required to move it through an opening. A width of 150 cm for (two leaf) door openings can be recommended. If self-closing operation room doors are used they should preferably be surface sliding, power operated, and controlled by photoelectric cells.

Doors subject to heavy traffic should be protected at least up to a height of 125 cm with rubber, PVC or stainless steel. The sound insulation properties of the doors should be good.

Operation rooms and anesthetic rooms should be provided with safety glazed openings with blinds to save unnecessary opening.

Doors to fluoroscopic examination rooms should have no lightleaks into the examination room.

In the postoperative recovery area the doorways should pass beds easily. A door width of about 145 cm is recommended.

In the ICTUs handles can be omitted from doors, which can be pushed open. Also here the door width should be about 145 cm. In neonatal intensive care units the door width of 90 cm have been accepted.

X-ray doors can generally be shielded by sheet lead, possibly in the form of a wood-lead-wood sandwich. Shielded doors may need an automatic closure to ensure that they are normally shut.

In laboratories 120 cm is considered to be the minimum acceptable door width. For easy exit, doors should swing out from the laboratory. Secondary escape exists should be provided. There should be no windows in the doors to exit corridors.

Emergency exits must be clearly labelled. Exit signs may be designed to flash when the emergency alarm is on.

Farthest point from a room to the nearest exit should be less than 60 m, from a pateint-room less than 45 m in the US, in Sweden this distance in the nursing units is reduced to 30 m.

Windows

Attention to the outer world is essential to relieve the sense of enclosure and to provide muscular relief to the eye by allowing it to focus at a distance. A view may be judged to be 'good' if at least a small portion of each 'layer' ground, landscape, sky is visible and it changes as much as possible with each change of the viewing position of the subject.

Window size is a compromise between the need to afford a satisfying view and the need to conserve energy and afford privacy. When window size is reduced, the shape and position of windows ought to be adjusted to the view. Near objects seem to required wider windows 3.1 m and distant objects narrower by 2.4 m^3. Satisfaction is generally achieved when window area occupies 20 to 30 per cent of the window wall.

Windows in the medical performance area must be easily accessible for cleaning. If used for ventilation, they must be equipped with filter screens and looks requiring special keys as precaution against unintentional disturbance to the interior climate.

Special care is necessary in the placing of windows in the X-ray rooms. They may not look out onto areas outside the control of the X-ray department or onto public access areas outside the control of the hospital. Windows in the path of direct X-ray beam for lateral X-ray exposures are hazardous. Window glass is ineffective for X-ray absorption. Even lead glass would be unsatisfactory.

Blinds should be provided for shade and privacy in X-ray rooms which have windows.

Water Supply

The general estimate of water supply needs is about 400 to 650 litres per day and bed.

Basically, hospitals require a two-temperature range for hot water. Low temperature about 43.5°C is required for patient washrooms. For showers 38 to 40°C is appropriate. Higher temperature systems between 71 to 90°C account for the majority of a hospital's hot water requirements including physiotherapy, kitchen, and cafeteria requirements.

The temperature of hot water supplied to the surgical and similar departments should be regulated between 40°C and 44°C.

Drinking fountains should project out from the wall rather than be fully recessed. It is useful to have both hand and foot-operated controls.

There should be an arrangement for emergency cold water supply, which, on the failure of normal supply can be turned on.

Steam Supply

Steam should be piped only to departments where nonelectric sterilizers are used.

Sanitary Equipment

The nature of work in the hospital generally, and in the surgical and similar departments particularly, demands a very high standard of hand cleanliness, and easily accessible washbasins.

Washing should always be done in running water.

Warm water approximately 32 to 39°C is more comfortable than either hot or cold. In public facilities the provision of only fixed-temperature water at approximately 43°C could be considered.

The comfortable working height, when standing, can be set up at about 96 cm, with the water source at about 10 cm higher and the height of the washbasin rim at 91.5 to 96.5 cm. If the washbasin is used by both standing and sitting persons, the basin height has to be lowered to 80 to 85 cm. The minimum dimension of the washbasin from front to back would be 38 cm.

Most of the hospital washbasin water controls should either be self-activating or require minimal contact by the user and should automatically shut off after a predetermined interval of approximately 45 to 60 seconds. This might be accomplished by photoelectric cells, proximity sensors and electronic or pressure-operated timing valves.

Wall mounted *sinks* with double drainers, will be required also in the operation room disposal room, pantry, sterile service and endoscopy (cystoscopy) rooms.

In the patient areas now there is a general tendency to move in the direction of providing greater privacy for all personal hygiene functions.

Water closets should be wall-mounted and not foot-operated. Containers for paper seat protectors as well as soap and paper towel dispensers should be provided. There should be no water closet without a *washbasin*.

The minimum area for a wheelchair toilet is 2.9 m. If the wheelchair patient needs to be helped in the toilet, the toilet area has to be increased to 4.85 m. Circulation area outside the wheelchair toilet must be provided. In wheelchair-toilets grab-bars are a necessity. The space between the wall and the grab-bar is critical. About 3.5 to 4 cm must be adhered to it.

All toilets should have esthetic appeal and quality products to withstand normal hard use. Additional convenience are mirrors, shelves, coat and handbag hooks, and disposal containers. Proper height for toilet mirrors for wheelchair patients is 0.9 m above the floor. Toilet doors should be hung so that they open outwards.

Urinals in hospital setting are not recommended.

The basic *shower* container or enclosure should have the dimensions of 106.5 by 91.5 cm. The water source, which should be adjustable both to angle and coarseness of spray, should be set that at a height of 152.5 to 167.5 cm the centre of the stream would be 30.5 to 38 cm from the wall. The bottom of the shower head itself should be no less than 198 cm from the floor.

A 38 cm full bench should be added across the dry end of the enclosure. A positive non-slip surface should be provided. The minimum opening to the shower should be about 61 cm wide, the still height of not more than 10 cm.

Electrical Installations

Mains wiring should be arranged so that interference with patient monitoring and data transfer is minimal.

No patient should be permitted to come into direct contact with a potential electrical source. This requires non-electric controls for the nurse call, television, reading light, etc. All electrical power should be connected to an isolation transformer.

To meet future developments, space should be left in building ducts for additional services.

X-ray equipment may require an independent feeder not used for other branch circuits. In radiology departments the position of the switchboards should be chosen to facilitate the access of cables and to shorten the length of cabling to the radiodiagnostic units thus reducing voltage drop.

In several hospital areas a special or general emergency power supply has to be added to the ordinary main supply.

In operation rooms about 20 outlets are needed for avanced operations. Electrical outlets in the vicinity of the operation table could be combined in a control panel comprising switches, fuses, signal controls, and plug outlets for main voltage and low voltage for electronic appliances. It is prefered to have the control panel hanging from the ceiling.

In the *anesthetic room* provision should be made for at least six electrical outlets.

The anesthetic store light fittings must not produce sparks. The spine of the light fittings, and the transparent part in particular, must be of a material which will not spread flames. The light fittings should be protected from mechanical pressure.

In general *post-anesthetic units,* upto eight electrical points are necessary for each bed. In post anesthetic units for cardio-thoracic and similar surgery the number is up to ten. The outlets must be sparkproof and failsafe. Daily work is facilitated if fuses are placed over each bed.

In *intensive care* and treatment units 10 electrical points per bed are required.

In *neonatal intensive care* units 10 to 12 electrical outlets per infant are required.

In the *resuscitation-room* of the emergency department, there should be four equipment two twin sockets with indicating lights and switches, one general purpose socket outlet, one twin socket outlet for X-ray viewing and a provision for fixed electrical apparatus.

In *corridors* electrical outlets with protective ground should be spaced at 10 to 12.

Any building containing medically-used rooms shall have separated neutral and protective earth conductors throughout the building.

The protective earth conductors shall be marked green-yellow. At least inside medically-used rooms they shall be insulated.

Operation room doors and other doors in the surgical unit could be operated by compressed air devices controlled by photoelectric cells.

Ideally, all water controls of washbasins should be automatically controlled either by proximity sensors or photoelectric cells, or by electronic or pressure-operated timing valves.

Patient Calling and Paging

Patient calling systems include simple loudspeaker communicating directly by the doctor and the waiting patient, loudspeaker used by the receptionists after a request by the doctor, loudspeakers with simultaneously illuminated light above the door to consulting suite in question nameboard with a light opposite each doctor's name, illuminated and accompanied by a buzz signal when calling the patient, also color coded to match the color of the waiting room chairs and consulting room nameboards. Illuminated call board above the door to each consulting suite, and accompanying buzz.

Patient-nurse call systems in nursing units seem to give the patient a sense of security, which is for them more important than convenience. During the day, the staff initiates more calls than the pateints.

To meet the pateints' needs for security and control, a hard control made up of modules has been recommended. These modules, which include a nurse call, an emergency call, entertainment, window shade and temperature control, could be removed or added to, according to the patients' competencies.

Acoustic Staff Paging and Calling

In hospitals it is essential to be able to contact key personnel immediately and individually without disturbing others.

This can be achieved by installing a radio-paging system, which basically consists of a control-encoder, a transmiter with an antenna and a number of pocket receivers with different code numbers. The paged receiver emits an acoustic signal. All the other receivers remain silent because of the selectivity in the system. The system can function also as a group alarm facility,which makes it possible to alert groups of people, *e.g.* special emergency teams within seconds.

Normally the paging is handled by a central switch board telephonist. One way or two way speech system provides for the controller, the facility to speak directly to the paged individual.

Regular acoustic paging, which must be balanced is most needed in offices, lounges, changing rooms, etc. It should be avoided in operation rooms and anesthetic rooms.

Each bed in intensive care and therapy unit must be supplied with a call-system which patients or attendants can use to call the staff. A two-way nurse-to-nurse speech facility may sometimes be required.

A loud-speaking intercommunication system has been considered to have advantages in a radio-diagnostic department for location of staff, general enquiries and rapid reporting on results of films.

Sometimes visual display of information is given preference over audible systems.

Visual Staff Paging and Calling

The simplest form of visual paging is represented by annunciator lights which indicate that some specific action should be taken. More elaborate visual paging includes a message or instruction on a video display screen, where messages are entered by means of a keyboard. The message remains on the screen until the paged responds or the information remains valid.

Flashing or audible signals attract attention to the screen.

Centralized Supervisory System

In large hospitals a centralized control and supervisory system of the functioning of technical equipment for lighting, ventilation, heating-cooling, etc. can reduce the number of maintenance staff.

The various equipment for ventilation, lighting, heating, cooling, etc. are first connected to sub-panels, which in their turn are connected via coaxial or multiwire cables to a central panel.

From the central panel the equipment can be started and stopped automatically or manually. Temperature, pressure, humidity, etc. can be checked and set points adjusted.

Main alarm points are monitored. A printer will print out the time of the arriving alarm and the identification number of the locality. The maintenance staff is alerted simultaneously via the paging system and/or acoustic signals.

Telephones

Telephone facilities for internal and external calls are required in consulting rooms, nurses' room, appointments and reception rooms, and for ambulance drivers. Connections to the hospital telephone exchange are also needed for duty rooms, changing rooms, and staff lounges of the units belonging to the medical performance area.

Telephones should be of desk pattern. For nurses they should be fitted in parallel with an indicating light which is easily visible.

Public call boxes or booths should be sited adjacent to the waiting spaces and in the entrance lobby. The needs of wheel-chaired patients must be observed.

Bed and Service Elevators

Lifts are needed for moving beds, stretcher beds, and other wheeled carriers. *Bed and service lifts* should have the dimensions 3.3 by 2.7 m, the height of 2.3 m and the capacity of about 1800 kg. They should be equipped with normal controls and no landing call accumulation devices.

No single lifts should be provided, they should be arranged in groups of two or three.

The control system for a group of *staff and visitors' lifts* should be based on normal controls with call-accumulating devices to shorten waiting times. Car-start time should be less than one second.

Lifts must be accessible to handicapped persons on the same level on which they enter the building.

The minimum door opening should be 0.85 m and the minimum inside measurements 1.5 m. The control panel, including emergency buttons should not be higher than 1.1 m above floor.

Medical Gases, Piped Air, Vacuum

Oxygen is the best known of all medical gases, used primarily for inhalation therapy and for anesthesia. Constant supply and immediate availability throughout the hospital are esential. The non-interruption of oxygen supply is said to be more vital than any other service in the hospital.

Nitrous oxide has been described as the safest anesthetic known, provided it is administered with an adequate supply of oxygen. Together with oxygen it acts as the vehicle for stronger anesthetic vapours.

To maintain homeostasis the inspired gases should be warm and humidified. There are heated humidifiers which supply gases at 35°C and at 100 per cent relative humidity. The temperature of gases should be monitored to prevent tracheobronchial burn.

Piped breathing air may be needed in some hospital areas. The primary use of this air is for inhalation therapy, and in operation rooms and intensive care units for both adults and infants. Air must be both oil-free and dry.

Modern ventilators have built in mixers for oxygen and air whereby the final oxygen concentration can be varied according to the needs of the patient.

Air is also used in laboratories for a variety of purposes. Air is normally supplied from a cylinder manifold or from compressors.

Supply pipes from the gas centre should terminate with self-locking stop valves. Gas outlets points shall be at least 20 cm from electrical components which, correctly used or in case of a fault, could generate sparks.

Gas should be released only when an apparatus for its administration is connected to the valve. Plug-in for similar rapid-connection plugs must be used. Gas connections must be non-interchangeable.

Gas pipes must be identified by colours according to national or international standards. Anaesthetic gas termination points should be clearly marked.

In the preoperative waiting areas only outlets for oxygen are needed.

In all anesthetic rooms, operation rooms, plaster rooms, and recovery rooms outlets for oxygen, nitrous oxide, and compressed air are needed. In a preferable arrangement of operation room gas outlets, compressed air, and up to four suction pipes are laid in telescopic tubes which extend downward to about 2 m above the floor. The installation should allow variations in the placing of the operation table.

In the post-anesthetic area two outlets for oxygen, two suction points, and one outlet for compressed air are needed per bed.

In the intensive care and therapy units two outlets for oxygen, one for nitrous oxide, one outlet for compressed air and three suction points per bed are required.

Vacuum is used throughout hospitals in patient treatment areas and in laboratories. In the surgical, recovery and intensive care areas it serves to remove fluids from incisions and body cavities and is used in postoperative drainage. In the laboratory it is used for filtering, cleaning delicate apparatus, and transferring fluids from one container to another.

At least three vacuum points in an operation room should be provided for surgical equipment, pneumatic motors, suction pumps.

Surgical suction devices comprise injector pumps,water-jet pumps, and mobile electric suction pumps. Pneumatic injector suction pumps, which have a sealed extrctor is isolate contaminated air,are considerably most suitable.

Compressed air tubes or the installation of central compressors is required. Compressed air must be filtered and dry. Condensation moisture must be drawn off from the pipes.

Three outlets for compressed air are needed in the anesthetic room and in the operation room

To obtain a reserve of air and a drying effect simultaneously, an air-tank could be used. This reserve may provide safety margin during power failures.

The compressed air installation must not be placed in a room together with oxygen and nitrous oxide containers.

FURTHER READING

1. Ervin Putsep: The Modern Hospital: International Planning Practices. Lloyd Luke, London, 1979.

33 The Nursing Zone

THE NURSING UNIT

A nursing unit consists of three elements:
- Patient space
- Nursing space
- Corridors

Types of Nursing Units

- General wards
- Private/Isolation wards
- Recovery wards/rooms
- Intensive care/Emergency/Critical care
- Pediatric wards
- Maternity wards
- Psychiatric wards/De-addiction ward
- Geriatric wards
- Cardiology ward/ICCU
- Orthopedic ward
- Skin ward/Burn unit
- Neurology ward

The patient care unit provides accommodation for patients whose prescribed and routine care is the responsibility of one nurse. The number of patients whose care she can direct and the number of personnel she can supervise efficiently will depend upon:
- Her own characteristic (education, experience, temperament)
- Number, training and experience of the personnel working under her supervision.
- Efficiency of the patient care unit plan and hospital services.
- Degree to which nurses are freed from duties, which can be otherwise handled by ward clerks and other departments.
- Type of patients, rate of turnover and variety of patient health problems.
- Number of doctors and their standard of practice.
- Teaching and research programmes of the hospital

Information on all these questions is seldom available when a patient care unit is being planned. However, they should be borne in mind. In the absence of conclusive data and in the presence of strong convictions among nurses at all levels, nursing staff and administrators, about 30-35 appears to be the maximum number of patients whose care can be safely directed by one nurse even on the most efficiently designed unit.

After the total number of hospital beds is known, numerous other details relating to the patient care divisions must be determined. First is the number of beds to be nursed from each station. Factors affecting this include:
- The size of the hospital

- The types of services given
- The average length of patient stay
- The demands of the community
- The need for seregation by sex, medical service or otherwise
- The number of single rooms
- The type of floor plan

It is helpful to make a long range plan for growth.

The existing facilities are studied for their adequacy both physical and functional

The improvements needed to be known are determined, future growth is projected on the basis of community survey and a specific plan is prepared to guide such a growth.

An important finding taken from the long range plan is the number of hospital beds to be provided in each stage. The total number of beds for the first stage should be subdivided according to the type of care i.e. medicine, surgery, obstetrics,pediatrics and psychiatry; and also by the size of patient care divisions.

Unavoidably the size of the hospital and of each nursing unit affect this subdivision. In large hospitals it is common to separate medical and surgical patients for the ease of nursing care.

For a hospital of 100 beds or less the number of maternity beds is established usually from 15 to 20 percent of the total hospital beds, depending upon the local demands.

The remaining beds are designated as medical and surgical. Pediatric patients are cared for in a medical nursing unit and if necessary a separate nursing station is established for them.

This would give 20 maternity beds and 80 medical and surgical (and pediatric) which can be subdivided into two 40 bed patient divisions or three 27 bed divisions).

The choice depends upon the local preference of upon the number of single rooms needed or method of future expansion.

There is a movement towards larger patient care divisions for the sake of operating economy but that too depends in part upon the percentage of single bed rooms and the shape of the plan. These factors establish the maximum distance from the nursing station to the door of the patients room which should be no more than 100 ft. (30m).

In a 200-bedded hospital 20% of 200 is 40, which gives one division of 40 maternity beds.

The remaining 160 beds subdivided into four 40-bed medical and surgical divisions or five 32 bed division. A second division of 25-30 pediatric beds may be there. That would leave four medical surgical divisions of 37-38 beds each.

The objective is always to have as few patient care divisions as possible without losing flexibility or getting them oversized.

Provision of Intensive Care Beds

Intensive care patients, both medical and surgical are best accommodated in large well staffed hospitals, in special units of at least 6-8 beds with permanent allocation of skilled staff and with concentration of equipment and service. Where such accommodation is impossible, intensive medical care patients are better housed in a part of a general ward unit, as their complete separation is potentially dangerous.

Flexibility

Flexibility of nursing care may be achieved through management, by allocating beds to ensure the best use of all beds and also through planning. As far as possible, wards should not be specialized except where psychological or medical needs demand such segregation e.g. the maternity, psychiatry or isolation wards.

The Shape of the Nursing Floor

The use of the nursing space can be classified under 3 main headings:

- The bed area (including open wards for two or more beds, and single rooms)
- Ancillary rooms (including clean and dirty utility rooms, the ward kitchen, the treatment room, the day spaces, nurses station and patients WCs and bathrooms).
- Corridor space/circulation space.

The shape of the floor plan greatly affects the size of the patient care division and also the area per bed.

Here a prime consideration is the distance from the nursing station to the door of the remotest patient room which should not exceed 100 ft. (30 m). It is easy to visualize that in a single corridor plan within patient rooms on both sides of the corridor, this limitation of maximum travel distance would produce a smaller number of beds in each nursing unit than with a double corridor plan with central nursing stations.

An even greater difference will exist if the single -corridor plan has bed rooms on one side only or if the nursing station is at one end of division.

Thus, the shape of the patient floor plan and the number of divisions per floor have become critical planning elements.

A decision has to be taken whether to use a T Plan, H plan, Y plan, Cross plan, double T, double Cross or any other variation of these plans which are shown in the illustrations. With such wide variations, comparisons become questionable, and the shape of the plan is seen to be only one factor in evaluating its worth. The size and the working relationships of the departments and the amount of space devoted to stairs, corridors, and elevators in relation to the net assignable space becomes more important than the shape.

If the non-assignable space is more than one-third of the gross floor area, the efficiency of the plan should be questioned. Having two or more patient divisions per floor helps to keep this ratio low. Such factors, in addition to the shape, help establish the efficiency of the floor plan.

These shapes are modified and used to achieve the various layouts of wards. There are a number of different type of plans (derived from the previously mentioned forms) in which the 3 elements of the nursing unit can be layed out.

Starting from the simple open Nightingale form, changes have been incorporated in the pursuit of:

- More privacy (corridor or continental)
- Greater amenities for patients and staff (Duplex or Nuffield)
- Compactness (Racetrack or double corridor)
- Economy (Courtyard—a naturally ventilated version of the above)
- Better observation of all patients (cruciform or cluster)
- Shorter distance between patient and nurse (Radial)
- Duplex or Nuffield

The Nuffield studies published in 1955 questioned the economy of attendance principles (30 beds to one nurse). It proposed a new concept of team nursing, which would enable more patients to be nursed in one unit. This gave rise to duplex layout which splits the ward into two sections of upto 20 beds each with its own nurse's base. Nursing ancillary space is shared between the two sections.

Corridor or Continental

Beds were moved from the external walls and arranged in bays, usually of upto 4 beds, separated by cross walls or screens, a corridor is needed to gain access to the bays. Wards are fully compartmented, with beds arranged in rooms each with its own toilet facility and day space. Each suit has nursing ancillaries placed on both sides of its spine.

Race Track or Double Corridor

In the mid-twentieth century, modern frame structures, air conditioning and mechanical conveyer systems contributed to the development of the race-track or double corridor ward layouts. The plan is based completely on a grid which helps to solve the structural problems.

It provides for 50-60 beds in single and two bed rooms, each with attached toilets. Vertical conveyers deliver supplies direct from central storage and processing departments into the central staff core on each floor.

Courtyard

The development of a courtyard type of ward plan was brought about by a need for a change and also for the reasons of economy. The planners were reluctant to accept a totally artificial working environment for the staff. So courtyards of varying sizes were inserted into the core areas to provide natural light and ventilation. The natural light and ventilation also brought economy to the functioning of the unit.

Cruciform or Cluster

Although modern corridor ward plans did provide the patient with greater privacy and amenities, it took away the Nightingale goal of ease of supervision and access to the patients. The nurses not only had to travel more distances to reach the patients but also had more barriers, doors, walls, partitions, toilets between them and the patients. This problem was solved by manipulating the shape of the plan in order to group as many patients as possible around the nurses' base.

Radial

Though radial form circles, squares, polygons had been used in ward plans for many years, earlier examples were open layouts. However, in recent years these forms have been adopted for the modern corridor layouts.

The illustration shows a typical 28-bed ward unit. Observation of 24 beds is unobstructed by partitions, doors, etc.

Staff-Patient Contact

In ward design, an acceptable compromise between providing privacy and a high level of amenity with the ease of supervision, is required. Another important factor is the staff-patient contact which can be crudely measured by the distance between the bed and the nurses' base.

Economy

Every square meter of space should be efficiently used. A corridor is of course necessary, but is used intermittently. If the doors are kept closed, a nurse in a corridor is out of sight and out of touch. The number of beds per 3 meter run of the corridor is, therefore, a useful indicator. The higher the number, the more compact the plan.

Patient Space

The amount of space in a nursing unit which is allocated to accommodate the patients is influenced by:

- Open or corridor layouts
- Bed spacing
- Number of beds in a room
- Ratio of toilet accommodation
- Provision of day, space, etc.

Illustration

For simplicity of comparison, three plans are illustrated, each an extreme of its kind. All plans are single corridor plans with a maximum run of 30 m (100 ft.). Each room has access to a toilet and same central services are provided in each.

Comparison

Item	*A*	*B*	*C*
Total beds	30	44	52
Total rooms	30	22	13
Net area a bed	11.25	9.5	8
Total gross area	870	930	915
Gross are/bed	29	21	17.5
Max.nursing run	30	27.5	27.5

(all areas in sq. mtrs).

Patient Space Includes

- Multibed bays
- Patient rooms

Multibed Bays In multibed bays, the bed spacing is governed by nursing procedures requiring the circulation of treatment trollies, drip stands, wheel chairs,etc.

According to the room data sheets prepared by the World Health Organisation, area required for nursing procedures is:

a. High-dependecy Unit—3.5 m × 3.5 m This space allows for working of 4-staff members with all technical services like ECG, respiratory machines, etc.
b. Low-dependency Unit—2.4 m × 3.0 m This space allows for working of 2-staff members with normal nursing equipment like nursing trolley, IV stand, etc.

Although the bare minimum spacing between the beds can be 1.6 m. It is hardly used (except in extreme shortage of space) for the reasons of cross infection. A more generous spacing of 2.5 m allows room for a locker, a chair and permits the use of cubicle curtains.

Patient rooms The desirable number of beds in a room and the proportion of different size rooms in the unit will vary.

A unit made up of one-bed rooms offers maximum privacy. However, such a unit is more expensive to construct and also the greater distances between patients may result in a reduction of the time spent in bedside care.

A unit made up of multibed rooms has less flexibility and provides less privacy for the patient and the physician, but is less expensive to construct, provides more opportunity for observation of patients and saves nursing time because the distance between the patients is less.

Day Space

- Allows patients a change of environment.
- Encourages early ambulation.
- Provides for reading, writing, talking, listening to radio or watching TV.
- Provides for exercise under supervision.

It can be located so as to:

- Serve the ward nearest to ambulant patients.
- Be shared by two wards.
- Be near the elevator lobby so that the ambulant patients can meet their relatives without the latter having to unnecessarily cross the entire length of the ward.
- Be shared by a floor of upto 120 beds This will make it possible to be used as a dining area.

Patient's Relatives Room

This accommodation is used for relatives, allowing them to relax in comfort and sleep overnight. It need not be near the ward. All such rooms can be sited together so that they can be managed easily. In India usually a Sarai provides the accommodation to the patients, relatives which is generally located away from the hospital building. The accommodation varies from dormitories to two-room suites.

Visitors Waiting Area

Patients relatives and friends awaiting access to the patient wait here.

Location

Sited to serve one or more wards depending on proximity of ward entrances. It should be comfortable and reassuring.

Corridor Space

The amount of space required for corridors will depend upon the shape of the ward, the system of arrangement of rooms. The average width of the corridor should be such that two trolleys can pass simultaneously. It generally varies between 2.1-2.6 m, however the length depends on the room arrangement and nurse's travel distance.

Service Area

Size and location of a service depend upon the number and types of beds served. Each service area may be arranged and located to serve more than one nursing unit. The service area includes:
- Nurse's station.
- Administrator's office
- Treatment/Examination room
- Clean utility
- Dirty utility
- Storage
- Pantry
- Multipurpose room for conferences
- Janitor's closet
- Storage for stretchers, wheelchairs.

Nurses Station

Two systems of nursing are:
- Centralized system
- Decentralized system

The functions of nursing station include:
- Nursing, administrative and clerical control point for the ward.
- Storage of patient records
- Issuing and receiving point for all information
- May include a medicine storage and a beverage point.
- It is in use 24 hours a day.

It should be sited to give maximum visual control of the main patient activity zones, specially the ones with critically ill patients. A view of the ward entrance is important. Patient bedrooms should preferably not be sited behind the base to avoid disturbance to the patients.

Nurses Rest Room

It is generally shared between 2-3 wards.

Sister incharge office.

Functions
- Carrying out administrative duties. Interviewing relatives.
- Other functions which require talking, reading and telephoning.

Can be located in any one location:
- Near the ward entrance
- Near the nurses station
- Adjacent to a seminar room.

Clean Utility

Functions
- Reception and storage of sterile packs, syringes and needles, clean items such as bandages, external lotions and disinfectants.
- Preparing all clean and sterile materials used in treatment of patients.
- Heating of lotions, etc
- Washing hands.
- Reception, storage and preparation of drugs.
- The area required is about 12-15 sq.mtr.
- It should be directly associated with the staff base.
- Preferably adjoining the treatment room.

Treatment Room

Functions include:
- It provides for treatments and examinations to be carried out with greater safety and privacy, without disturbing the other patients.
- It helps to prevent the spread of infections.
- The area required for a treatment room is about 14-16 sq. mtr.

The provision for a treatment room depends upon the type of treatment and hospital policy. Therefore, the treatment room should be arranged in such a way so that it can be converted to another function if no longer required. It should be located preferably near the nurse's base and connected by means of a hatch to clean utility and disposal areas.

Dirty Utility/Sluice

Functions include
- Collection of dirty, foul and infected linen and holding mobile stands.

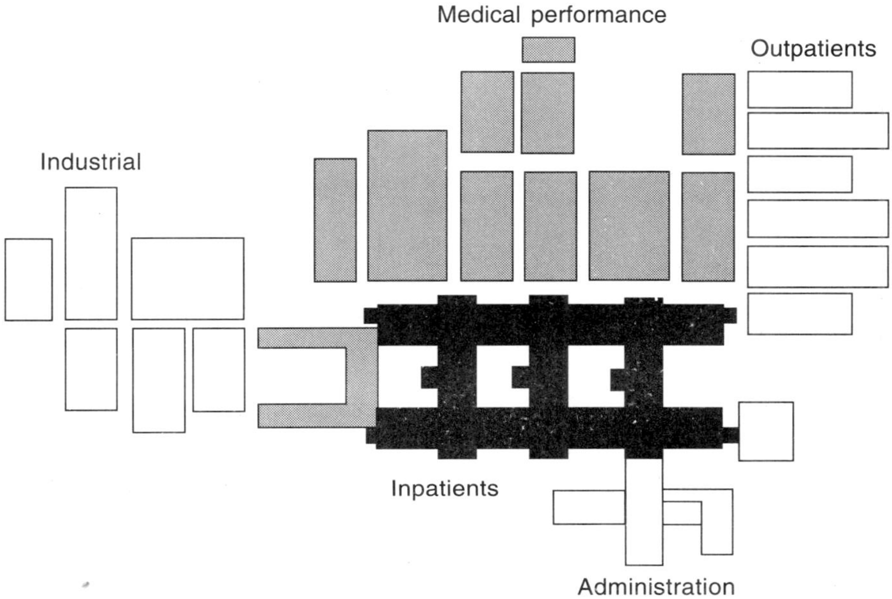

Fig. 33.1: Basic hospital areas, zoning of components, room sizes

- Clearing trays or trolleys used in treatments. Holding sacks containing dirty dressing and general waste.
- Holding return containers for central sterile supply department.
- Disposing of liquids.
- Washing and storage of bedpans.
- Holding and testing urine samples.
- Washing hands.
- The area required is about 10-12 sq mtr.

Should be located nearest to critically ill patients and adjacent to the treatment room if possible.

Storage

Functions and activities

- Storage of clean linen brought in from the laundry.
- Storage of other clean equipment which is used occasionally.
- The area required is about 15 sq.mts. The storage may be a part of the clean room or a separate space. This must be out of the path of normal traffic and under the superivison of the nurse on duty.

Pantry

Functions

- Provide a base for the service of meals to the patients, and
- Also used for storing ingredients and making snacks and beverages.
- Washing and storing crockery, cutlery and service equipment.
- Area required for pantry is about 2-4 sq.mts.
- A refrigerator and provision for heating food should be provided.

It should be located near the service corridor to facilitate supply and removal of food trays and trolleys.

Multipurpose Room

Functions

- Formal and informal teaching sessions by medical and nursing staff.
- Clinical demonstration involving a patient in bed or wheelchair.

It should be sited conveniently to serve adjacent nursing units also.

Janitor's Closet

One should be provided on each floor for storage of cleaning equipment.

Stretcher and Wheelchair Storage Facilities

These should be stored in the alcove of the corridor

Facilities for AIDS Patients

AIDS and HIV-infected patients may need hospitalization under the following 3 conditions:

1. Proper diagnosis of a clinical condition—any clinical situation where hospitalization is necessary for reaching a diagnosis.
2. Therapeutic hospitalization—patients require hospitalization at least on their first admission for treatment of opportunistic infection.
3. Acute emergencies—HIV infection can often lead to acute emergencies i.e. acute haemorrhage, respiratory distress, acute neuropsychiatric disorders, etc.

Physical set-up of an AIDS unit

The AIDS unit must consist of an

- Inpatient ward
- Out-patient clinic cum day care center.

AIDs Inpatient Ward

At some places AIDS patient is treated anywhere in a general medical ward. Whereas in other, a separate area identified an AIDS ward is in practice. Both the arrangements have some advantages and some disadvantages. However, the latter is being preferred due to the following reasons:

- It has the advantage of a willing, motivated, trained staff-team for managing an HIV infected patient, reducing the risk of accidental exposure.
- A trained team can provide better patient care and follow-up.
- Counselling and psycho-social aspects are also looked after in a much more effective way.

Initially six beds and one isolation room may be earmarked for AIDS and HIV infected patients within a general medicine/infectious disease/clinical immunology ward.

Physically it could be at one end of the ward. Four of these beds could be routine HIV beds and two beds could be converted into intensive care beds.

- *Routine beds* The four routine beds can be placed in one cubicle of a general ward. But, curtains, or preferably room dividers, would be essential for privacy of these patients.
- In each cubicle, a small wall-fixture to hold boxes of unsterile, disposable gloves is required.
- A waste disposal bucket or basket lined with plastic bag would be necessary. Each cubicle must have a puncture proof container specially designed for the safe disposal of any sharp items. Each bed should be provided with central oxygen and suction points. Adjustable beds are preferred over the ordinary beds. Each bed should have a cardiac table. Beds should have mattress covered with a mackintosh or heavy plastic and pillows should have polythene covers for frequent changing.

In addition to these specific requirements, the beds would have all the usual facilities of a general ward bed i.e. head light, bedside locker, chair or stool, IV stand, power points, etc.

Intensive Care Beds

The intensive care bed can be placed in one cubicle (which generally houses 4 beds). The cubicle may be separated for the rest of the ward by a room divider having swinging door large enough for getting through the portable X-ray machine. The following gadgets form a part of the special requirements:

- 2 monitoring units
- 1 resuscitation equipment complete with incubation equipment
- 2 respirators
- Adequate number of power points and extension boards.

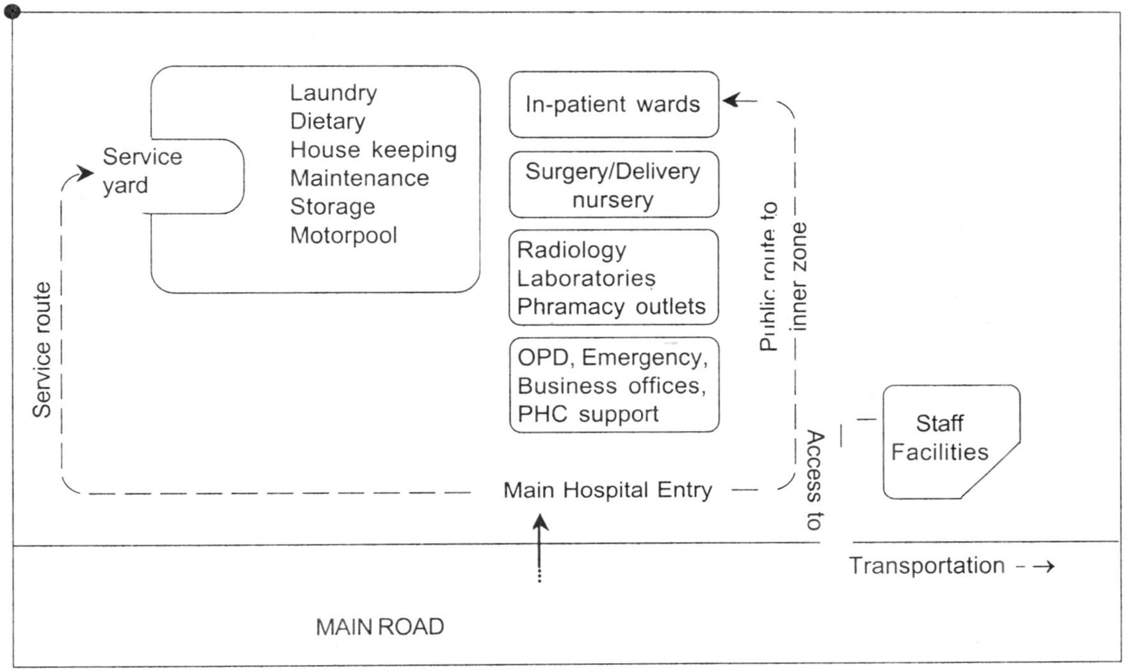

Fig. 33.2: Zoning of elements on a site

- Isolation rooms (with attached lavatory and bath rooms). The isolation room is used only for dying patients or those who would benefit from a quiet environment. The facilities are the same as for the routine HIV beds.

General Facilities for AIDS Ward

The area of six beds would require at least 2 lavatories and 1 bathroom separate from the general ward lavatories and bathrooms. It is essential because frequent loose motions is a major problem in AIDS.

- Two wash basins between 4 routine beds and one in the intensive care area.
- One waste disposal plastic lined bucket or basket next to each wash basin.
- One wall bracket for holding packets of disposable unsterile gloves and wall fixtures for liquid soap for each wash basin.

Procedure Room

The ward must have one procedure room where endoscopy, bronchoscopy, biopsies, aspiration, etc. can be carried out. This room would also require suction points, oxygen supply, pressurized air, special wall fixtures, power points, wash basin, shelves, and cupboards. Expert advice of specialist is required at the time of designing this room.

This whole inpatient area should be in an air conditioned part of the hospital. The windows should be adequately secured to reduce the possibility of patients jumping out in suicidal attempts. All the other services of these patients could be in common with the rest of the general wards. This includes a common utility room, store room and sluice room. It should be noted that sluice disposal of HIV infected and AIDS patient can be carried out exactly as for any other ordinary patient. If possible, a small autoclave should be provided in the sluice room itself so that after soap and water washing, bedpans, urine bottles, mugs, etc. can be auto-claved in the ward itself.

Out-patient Clinic and Day Care Center

Unlike the patients with other illnesses, it is advisable to keep the HIV patients at home rather than in the hospital as long and as often as possible. Psychologically, it is better for them to be at their home in an illness for which there is no cure.

The AIDS clinic or day care center would be exactly similar to any other clinic or day care center. There would be cubicles, examination couches, doctors desk, chairs, etc. There should be provision for keeping eye shields, goggles, plastic gown and puncture proof disposable containers.

For a day care center, 2-4 beds on the pattern of AIDS routine beds is required. The area should have an easy access to toilet facilities.

Major equipment required for AIDS unit.

- Respirators 2
- Monitoring units 2
- Ultrasonic nebulisers 1
- Complete set of endoscopes with light source
- Bronchoscope with light source
- Small autoclave for sluice room.

INPATIENT SERVICES

The inpatient service area forms approximately 1/3rd of whole hospital complex. The functions of inpatient services are:

- To render nursing care to all patients
- To provide necessary equipment, essential drugs and all other stores required for patient care in an organized manner in the ward.
- It serves as a temporary home for the patient and hence it is designed to accomodate all the needs of a patient.
- It provides opportunity for training medical, nursing and paramedical staff, besides conducting research work.

  The inpatient area can be:
  - *General ward*—where patients are admitted without any specific requirement.
  - *Specific ward*—where patients are admitted with the specific objective either by nature of disease or social reasons e.g. ICU, ICCU, Pediatric ward, maternity ward, isolation ward, etc.

Planning and Design

The planning and design of an inpatient unit is a very vital step in hospital planning. The hospoital policy based on community need and resource availability will effect directly the type of inpatient care units. However, following factors should be considered broadly, when planning is being done:

a. Policy
   - General or specific hospital
   - Bed strength of hospital

b. Physical facilities
   - Area
   - Location
   - Size
   - Shape
   - Ancillary accommodation
   - Water and electricity supplies
   - Communication
   - Air-conditioning
   - Auxiliary accommodation

c. Staffing
   - Medical
   - Nursing
   - Supportive.

Policy of Hospital

The policy of hospital is very important for designing inpatient care area. It should be considered whether the hospital will be a general with the facilities grouped into or it be a super-speciality or specific hospital, e.g. neurosciences, centre, maternity and child centre, cardiothoracic center, psychiatric hospital, etc. Bed strength of hospital influences on planning and designing of hospital structure. A hospital with less than 200 beds are generally planned as horizontal where it saves lot of time in internal movement than in vertical (multistorey complex) horizontal planning is usually considered upto 300-bedded hospital. However, hospitals of 300 and more beds require the inpatient care area planning on vertical expansion which is cost-effective and convenient for patient movement.

Physical Facilities

Inpatient care area covers approximately one-third of total hospital area. However, it can be increased to one half in specialized hospital where residential accomodation is limited. Approximately 70 to 90 sq. ft. (about 7 sq. m) area is required per bed.

The inpatient area should be located away from main roads and from out-patients department area to avoid disturbance, noise infection. However, the inpatient area should be approachable from supportive services (imaging, laboratory, blood bank, CSSD, etc.) and a good intramural transportation should be planned for effective and efficient movement of patient and staff within the hospital.

The limiting factor in the size of the ward unit is the capacity of the head nurse to supervise and know intimately the nursing care of each patient. Flornce Nightingale recommended a 30 beds ward and unitil now the same limit is more or less being followed. The capacity of the head nurse depends upon her personal ability and the type of patients under her care. The modern trend is to have bigger ward units of 40-50 beds. Two or three of such units are located on one floor with certain common essential service areas in the middle.

The rectangular pavilion type of ward was first constructed in 770 AD by a Frenchmen. About 80 years later Florence Nightingale adopted this design and it is still known after her name. This ward consisted of patients beds in two rows at right angles to the longitudinal walls with bathrooms and WC facilities at the other end. It was usual to house 30-35 patients in such wards of ward continued till 925 AD. Subsequently, the nurse had to walk long distance to attend to the patients. The bathrooms and WC facilities were also shifted in the centre in the form of a annexe. After some time this nurse's table was replaced by a proper nursing station consisting a few cubicles to house the various service facilities. A treatment room and an isolation room were also added. In tropical countries wide verandahs are placed on either side of the ward to protect it from direct sun light. This modified design had the advantages that it provided plenty of fresh air, cross ventilation, natural light and the nurses had direct observation of all the patients. But it had certain shortcomings which were:

- No privacy for patients
- No freedom from noise
- Danger of cross-infection
- Constant glare to the patients.

In order to overcome these shortcomings the ward unit has been divided into small compartments or cubicles for 1,2,3,4 or 6 beds each. This arrangement is called Riggs pattern and the beds are arranged parallel to the longitudinal walls. In Western countries, increasing number of ward units are being planned on one or two-bedded compartments. The Rigg's pattern has its own problems:

- Communication between nurses and the patient becomes more difficult
- The patients are deprived of direct observation by the nurse
- Wards become longer, consequently the nurse has to walk more
- More nurses are required
- Costly to build and maintain.

These shortcomings were overcome by artificial device like call bells, signal lights, two-way speakers and closed circuit television. These wards are designed in different shapes as T or Y-shaped semi-circular, and single or double corridor type.

The modern trend is to build the wards and the hospital in the form of multi-storeyed structure rather than the sprawling single storey construction which creates problems of communications and control. Verandahs are no longer in vogue as they are very costly.

Ancillary Accommodation

Nursing station is the nerve centre of the ward and should be so located that the nurses can keep watch over as many patients as possible and the distance to the farthest patient should not be too much. In the Riggs pattern the acute patients are housed on either side of the nursing station with provision of large glass windows for direct observation. The nursing station should be 20' × 20' and have the following essential components:

- Nurses room with attached bath and WC. This room should have a cupboard for medicines
- A counter in the open space outside the nurses room carry out work
- A built-in drug cupboard for daily use medicines. House physicians room: A suitable size room with examination couch and wash-hand basin is provided for the doctor on duty.

Clean Utility Room (100-200 sq ft)

It is used for clean storage, e.g. intravenous sets and solutions, CSSD articles, dressing, drugs and clean work like setting up a trolley or a treatment tray for a minor procedure and so on. This is sometimes combined with treatment room.

Treatment room including special examinations, minor dressings, lumber puncture, intravenous injections and so on are carried out in this room. This reduces the risk of cross infection, the patient and the doctor receive better facilities and privacy and other patients are not disturbed.

Ward Kitchen/Pantry

The major function of the ward kitchen is temporary storage and distribution of meals and the preparation of beverages. The kitchen should be equipped with facilities for hot water, refrigerator, hot case and facilities for storage of crockery and cutlery. This room should have a large sink for washing various articles.

Day Room

A place congenial for sitting and relaxing is provided in the ward unit with comfortable chairs and reading material. This place can also be used as dining place and for meeting visitors. A common day room can be provided for two adjacent wards.

Stores

A small store room for keeping linen and bulk supply of cleaning material is also provided. Attached to the stores, a space may be provided for patient's lockers where they can keep their personal articles.

Dirty utility or sluice room is provided in each ward for cleaning bed pans, urinals, sputum mugs and for storage of stool and urine specimens. It should be fitted with bedpans sink/washer.

Bath and WC

Bath rooms and WC are to be provided in adequate proportion:

- Urinal — One for 12 beds
- WC — One for 8 beds
- Bath — One for 12 beds
- Wash hand basin — One for 10 beds

The above scales are exclusive of WC, bath and wash hand basins provided for single and double-bedded rooms and staff toilets provided on floor basis.

Janitor's Room

A Janitor's room is provided in each ward for keeping cups, cleaning material and buckets. It should have a large sink for cleaning buckets and other equipment and adequate supply of hot and cold water.

Water and Electricity Supplies

Adequate round-the-clock water supply should be available for ward areas, approximately 300 liter of water is required per bed per day.

Light points for ward and ancillary accommodation should be carefully designed. There should not be any glare from the lights. Alternative source of sunlight should be planned. There should be one industry switch for portable X-ray and one each of 15 ampere and 5 ampere in each cubicle (1,2,4,6) for any contingency.

Communication

Effective two-way communication should be planned and provided. If hospital is 500 bedded with teaching and research activities, an alternative communication system of paging could also be planned for effective and prompt patient care.

Airconditioning

A centralized positive pressure air-conditioning of hospital inpatient area helps in patient comfort and reducing hospital infection rate.

Auxiliary Accommodation

This accommodation includes ward laboratory, seminar room, Nurse's rest room, Visitor's room, etc. This accommodation is usually, common between 2 and 3 wards or for each floor.

Staffing

An appropriate planning of hospital inpatient care area should be done well in time, so that user staff is recruited and trained before the ward unit is completed. The general staffing norms for ward are suggested (Tables 33.1 to 33.3).

Table 33.1: Norms for nursing staff

Nursing personnel	*Staffing norms*
Nursing superintendent	1 per hospital
Dy Nurisng Superindent	1 upto 400 beds 1 more for every 200 additional beds
Asstt Nursing Superindent	1 for 25-30 beds or one per ward
Teaching hospital	1 nurse for every 3 beds*
Non-teaching hospital	1 nurse for every 3 beds
For ICU/ICCU	1 nurse for every 1 bed*

* (+ 30 percent leave reserver)

- Extra nursing staff to be provided for departments and research functions
- It is suggested that for each 250 beds there should be one infection control nurse.

Space Requirement

Nursing services take place around the patient's bed and patient beds are the key to the entire hospital plan-(Hospital planning considering the size of hospital bed as 2 m × 1 m and allowing a minimum distance between the center of two beds as 2.25 meters, space at the foot-end 0.90 meters space at the head end 0.25 meters the space needed would be 3.15 × 2.25 = 7.09 sq mt or 75 sq ft. Half of this area i.e. 3.50 sq mt or 37.5 sq ft may be considered adequate for a toilet comprising two or three sanitary fittings, i.e. WC, Wash-hand basin and a shower.

Correlation of Bed Space with Hospital Engineering Grid

Half of space required for bed has been considered as hospital space module i.e. 3.5 sq m or 37.5 sq ft and this can be correlated with hospital Engineering Grid. Keeping in view the technological feasibility of construction. A planning grid of 1.6 meters is chosen out of many possible ones. One grid would give an area of 1.6 × 1.6 = 2.56 sq mt and 3 such grids would add upto 7.68 sq mt say 7 sq mt (ignoring 0.68 sq mt for wall thickness, etc.).

This correlates with hospital space module of 3.5 × 2 = 7 sq mt. The same grid can then be conveniently utilised to delineate width of doors, verandahs and corridors, etc.

Table 33.2: Nursing hours required

Category nature of illness patients	*Direct nursing hours per patient per day (24 hrs)*	*Nurse patient ratio*
A. Critically ill patient	8-10 hours	1 : 1 (Needing intensive care)
B. Moderately ill patient needing intermediate care	3-5 hours	1 : 3 (Teaching hospital) 1 : 5 (Non-teaching hospital)
C. Middly ill patients needing self care (Ambulatory)	1-2 hours	1 : 6 (Teaching hospital) 1 : 10 (Non-teaching hospital)
D. Chronically ill patient requiring skilled prolonged medical and nursing care	30 min to 1 hour	1 : 12 (Teaching hospital) 1 : 18 (Non-teaching hospital)

Table 33.3: Norms for nursing Aides/Assistants

Number of beds in the hospital	*Number of class D employees suggested*	*Suggested norms*
30-50	15-25	1 employee/2 beds
100	50	— Do —
200	100	— Do —
300	150	— Do —
500 and above	250	— Do —

Door = 1.2 m (3/4 grid)
Verandah = (1½ grid)
Windows = 1.2 to 1.6 m (3/4 to 1 grid)
Corridors = 2.4 m (½ grid)

Following space requirements are recommended:

- Distance between bed centers : 7 ft
  (in teaching hospital wards) : 8 ft
- Clearance between head end and wall : 1 ft

Clearance between wall and side of bed in respect of bed

- Closer to wall : 2 ft
- Isle between two rows of beds : 5 ft

Area per bed within the ward therefore need not be more than 70 sq ft.

Basic Types of Wards

Nightingale pattern—where the beds are arranged, head end towards the windows along both the walls. This is also called pavilion type. Rigg's pattern—is a modification in which beds are placed perallel with the windows (First followed at the Rigg's Hospital in Copenhagen, hence the name). In this pattern bays are often enclosed, so that they become rooms. There are many versions of the basic pattern and combine 4,5 and 6 beds rooms with single bed-rooms in varying proportion. In America, the supposed demand for privacy has led, in some cases, to the provision of all beds in single rooms. These are very costly and demand more staff and/or communication system. It is doubtful whether all patients desire and enjoy such total privacy. Space requirement bed is more in Rigg's pattern. It gives less busy appearance and more serious patients can be grouped near Nurse's Station.

The Nightingale ward is cheapest to construct and easy to supervise. But is has high noise level, more glare, and is not flexible. It provides better supervision and observation of patients by the staff but allows less privacy.

Single Occupancy Rooms

An increasing trend towards privacy in every aspect of life accounts in part, an emphasis on single occupancy room in hospitals. However, people who were alone in their lives, resent being left alone in a hospital. These are obviously costly to build and maintain. Nursing staff seems to like it for better personal rapport with patients. Less medication errors occur.

The patient's bed should be so placed that there is enough circulation space for doctor and nurse to be on either side of bed. The length of bed should not be close along any of the walls.

Attached WC, bath, washing facilities are essential in such rooms. A wardrobe and locker, a small table and one or two chairs are essential.

A minimum area of at least 125-150 sq ft with a minimum width of 12 ft has been suggested for a single occupancy room.

Double bed rooms have been recommended to have an area of 226 sq ft. Single occupancy room should be so designed that another bed can be accommodated in emergency. Hence, there should be two cup boards and two bed-side lockers in each room.

Multi-patient Room

Sharing a room in hospital is a source of some positive and some negative experiences. It is good to have a room-mate to talk to and room mates try to help each other but a very ill-room mate, or a very young or very old one or the one who has unending visitors may be difficult to put up with. Room-mates who would not snore, smell, smoke and have attractive quite visitors would be preferred by most.

Single and Multibed Accommodation Mix Wards

Another variety of wards is the mix of earlier two.

The proportion of single beds to multibed rooms would depend on preference of clinicians, number of sub-specialities and social and economical factors and 40 percent of ward unit beds should be provided as the single beds.

The combinations and their designs could be endless each having its own comparative advantages and drawbacks.

Besides these many other types of wards have been described, e.g. Linear ward, deep ward or race track ward and courtyard plan, etc. Each carries its own advantages and disadvantages.

While thinking and planning ward nursing unit, following factors may be kept in mind:

Walking Distance

It should be kept as short as possible for nurses and ambulent patients. Maximum distance from bed to WC should be 40 ft and from nurse room to farthest bed 60-65 ft.

Observation

A good design should allow 50 percent of beds to be observed directly from nurse's station.

Noise upto 40 DB during the day and less than 30 DB by night. Single bed units should have even less.

Daylight and glare Direct sun light and excessive glare should be avoided.

Ventilation Mechanical ventilation (ceiling, exhaust fans and air circulator, etc.) are noisy and air conditioning is very costly. If the hospital is located away from dusty and noisy surrounding, natural ventilation is most desirable.

Nurse call system: Close Circuit TV (CCTV) Ordinary call bell is most practical and reliable. Sophisticated devices are all liable of being misused and failure. In any case a seriously sick person cannot operate them and can be looked after mainly by observation.

Ancilliary Areas

1. *Nurse's room* The location should be such that maximum number of patients remain under direct observation of the nurse. The room would normally contain a cupboard, a drug cupboard, sink, chair table, telephone, call system signs and records. An area of 100-120 sq ft for this facility is required with additional 60 sq ft for toilet.

   Some have suggested an area of 110 to 170 sq ft depending on design.
2. *Clean utility room* used for sterilising instruments, packing of surgical drum, etc. An area of 100-120 sq ft is required.
3. *Dirty utility room (sluice room)* is used for emptying and cleaning bedpans, urine bottles sputum-mugs, storing stool and urine samples etc. space required 150-170 sq ft big.
4. *Treatment room* is used for carrying out minor procedures, dressings and administering injections, etc., space required is 120-150 sq ft.
5. *Ward kitchen/pantry* food is collected and distributed from here and beverages are also

prepared here. The room has refrigeator, hot case, water boiler and facilities for storing cutleries. An area of 100-120 sq ft is recommended.

6. *Stores* Linen and other requirements are drawn from main stores and kept here. An area of 80-130 sq ft is recommended.

7. *Bath and WC* Following scales are recommended:

Water closets	1 for every 8 beds
Ablution taps	1 for each w/c. +1 tap with draining arrangments near WC
Urinals	1 for every 12 beds
Wash basin	1 for every 12 beds
Bath	1 bath with shower for every 12 beds

Others recommend:

Urinals	1 for every 16 beds
WC	1 for every 8 beds
Bath	1 for every 8-16 beds
Wash basin	1 for per 10 beds excluding wash basin attached to single bed rooms.

The WCs are also exclusive of the ones attached to single bed rooms.

Other facilities required include:

Assisted bath room	110-130 sq ft
Bathroom	75 sq ft (for ambulant patients)
Washing and shower compartment	
WC with hand rinse basin	25-30 sq ft

8. *Janitors closet* an area of 40-60 sq ft

9. *Day-room or day-space* As early ambulation is the modern concept. Patients are encouraged to move about early but at the same time, it is not safe for them to move out of the ward. They have to be provided a place congenial for sitting and relaxing. An area of 15 percent of the area capacity or 180 sq ft per ward, is recommended.

10. *Circulation* The corridor should not be more than 8 ft wide. The circulation area should be optimum and not on higher side. Twenty percent of total floor area of ward as circulation area is recommended.

Ward Unit for Particular Specialities

These ward units have certain requirements additional to general wards, described above. These include:

Postoperatived Wards

It should be located close to operation theatre. The bed space required is more as the wheel chairs have to be manovoured and treatment appratus have to be accomodated. Space per bed 95 sq ft is required.

Pediatric Ward

Twenty five percent of patients in this ward have been recommended to be provided isolated cubicles, in single or two-bedded rooms.; Cubicles should be separated by glazed partition to allow observation. Each pair of cubicle may be provided with a common toilet of 56 sq ft having WC bath and wash basin.

Further 25 percent of beds should be in the form of cubicles of 4-6 beds to provide extra space for mother's bed along with sick pediatric cot. Floor-space per bed therefore works out to be about 112 sq ft. Auxillary facilities like, mother's halting and change room, mother's bath and WC, mother's dining, lecture room for health education, doctor's room are optional.

Some of urinals, basin, etc. are to be fitted at lower height and special care taken while fixing electric sockets, etc. to keep them out of reach of children.

Psychiatry Ward

All windows and verandahs opening should be protected with steel grill. The ward should be located preferably on ground floor or lower floors. All electrical fittings and fixtures shall also be suitably protected.

Dermatology

Twenty-five percent of beds in this ward have been recommended to be in the form of 2 and 4 bedded rooms for segregation.

Toilet for single-bedded rooms of dermatology ward is to have long bath arrangement in which case its floor space is to be 56 sq ft. One bath room in the laboratory block of dermatology ward is to have long bath arrangement.

Infectious Disease Ward

It may be located away from main ward blocks but connected with a covered passage. It may be put in the main block but separated by an air-gap of 4-6 ft.

It requires an additional sink room of about 115 sq ft two staff changing rooms of 115 sq ft each and a discharge room of same size.

Obstetrics and Gynaecology Ward

Maternity services includes antenatal care, delivery and post-natal care. Before and after child birth, the patient should be attended to in the out-patient department and during labour the patient is confined to bed in nursing unit. The lab investigations may preferably be done on out-patient basis. This area may be on the same floor and in close proximity with its out-patient component.

The in-patient unit should have following areas:

a. *Delivery suite unit* Following facilities are recommanded:

Ward unit of 750-bedded hospital	*Sq ft ward unit 24-30 beds*
• Reception and admission with waiting	450
• Examination and preparation room with toilet	230
• Nurse's change room	115
• Doctor's change room	115
• Staff change room	115
• Technician's change room	115
• Sterile storage	3000
• Instrument and linen store	5
• Trolley bay	115
• Switch room	115
• Recovery room	912
• Pack preoperation room	190
• Anesthesia room	230
• Labour room (divided into 7 cubicles)	800
• Delivery room	230
• Operating delivery room	380
• Instrument sterilizing	380
• Scrub up	115
• Children bath	115
• Eclampsia room	230
• Dirty utility	190
• Janitor's closet	75

Antenatal ward The pregnant women should be kept separate from the ones, who have delivered. It requires same facilities and areas as a general ward except that is should have its own well-equipped laboratory and a larger treatment room.

Enclampsia ward Number of beds one for every 20 postnatal beds. Single or two-bedded rooms with attached toilet.

Postnatal ward Women who have delivered healthy babies are kept here. Babies are in a cardle.

Formula room It is meant for preparing feeds for babies should be located loose to nurseries and larger room would be required if bottles are washed and sterilized here.

Postoperative ward It should be large enough to accomodate two beds per delivery room. Per-bed area requirement is 95 sq ft.

Neonatal Unit

This unit is for premature, high-risk babies and sick newborn. It should be established as independent unit under the care of pediatrician.

Area Requirement

a. Nursery
   - Premature 230 sq ft
   - Septic 150 sq ft
   - Normal 150 sq ft

b. Nurse's station with toilet 190 sq ft

c. Doctor's duty room 190 sq ft

d. Formula/breastfeeding room 115 sq ft

e. Store 115 sq ft

f. Phototherapy room 115 sq ft
   (Room with one transparent side wall for observation of babies in natural light)

g. Sluice room 115 sq ft

Gynecologiy Unit

The proporation of gynaecological beds should be 40 percent of maternity beds. Space requirement for various facilities remain the same as for a general ward described earlier.

Intensive Care Unit

This unit accomodates seriously ill patients requiring intensive life support measures and highly-skilled and specialized medical and nursing care. It should be ultimate quality care that a hospital can provide.

The number of patients requiring intensive care may be about 2-5 percent of total medical and surgical patients in a hospital. The unit should not have less than 4 beds and the number should not exceed 12 beds in an ICU. It should be close to X-ray, pathology and emergency and should have the best of engineering services that the hospital has to offer. All beds are to be enclosed in glazed cubicle with centrally-located nursing station. The per bed area should be 115 sq ft.

Following floor area is required.

- Patient relative waiting room 190 sq ft

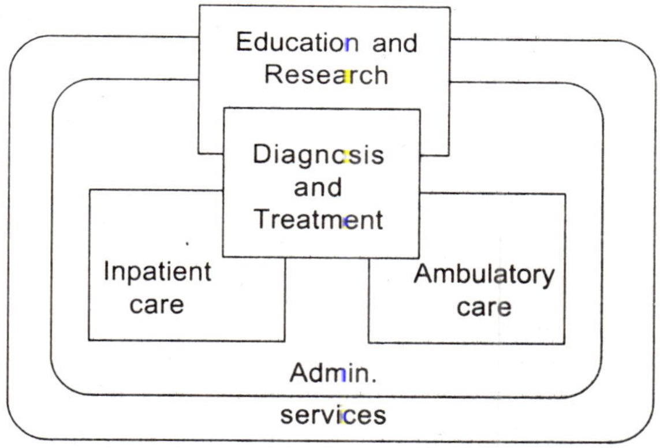

Fig. 33.3: Hospital sector (siagram of relationship)

- Nurse's station with toilet 190 sq ft
- Doctor's duty room 190 sq ft
- Intensive care laboratory 150 sq ft
- Equipment room 150 sq ft
- Stores rooms each 150 sq ft
- Pantry 115 sq ft
- Switch room 115 sq ft
- Trolley bay 115 sq ft
- Sluice room 115 sq ft
- Janitor's closet 37 sq ft

Coronary Intensive Care Unit (Cardiac Care Unit)

This unit should not be a part of general ICU. In this unit, there should be an intensive care zone or section (IC) and an intermediate care section (IMC) as significant risk continues beyond 12 days of hospitalisation of cardiac patient. Patient may saty 1-3 days in IC and thereafter 8-30 days in IMC.

Size 6-10 beds. Area required is 140 sq ft per patient room. In Sweden the recommended area is 190-240 sq ft and one of the rooms should be 300 sq ft as in case of cardiac arrest a physician and nurse may have to stand behind the head and of patient's bed, hence more clearance required between head-end of the bed and wall.

Besides, there should be a pulmonary intensive care unit, neurovascular unit, a burn unit, an obstetric intensive care unit, and neonatal intensive care unit.

WARD PLANNING

Wards form about 50 percent of a hospital so their importance is not in question. However, as spaces that provide accomodation for inpatients who are being assessed, treated and nursed, the reasons for the intensity of the debate are not immediately obvious. Many of the nursing and patient care functions have not changed much over the years and many wards in use today are well over 50 years old.

Functional and Managerial Units

Beds for inpatients can be grouped in wards in a number of different ways for various reasons. They may be grouped into wards to form functional units such as acute, long-stay psychiatric, maternity, medical or surgical. They may be grouped into management units responsible for the inpatient administration and the use of the hospital support services, such as supplies, linen, catering, building maintenance, or into units that relate to the organisation of the nursing staff and nursing duties. Alternatively, they may be grouped according to the characteristics of the patients—generally age and sex or by the way in which it is proposed that the patients will be treated. The allocation of beds to specialities or to particular types of patients may coincide with any of the above groupings, and may be a component of one ward or cover several. The beds may be in spaces that range from single bedrooms, to rooms containing more than 50 beds depending on which part of the world it is.

In the UK, for example, a 28-bed ward may have beds distributed into four single bedrooms, three-four bed rooms and two-six bed rooms. This is likely to be managed as one nursing unit but the nurses may work as two teams, each team responsible for half of the beds. In the ward, beds may be allocated between several different specialities or may be one of several 20-bed wards allocated for, say, acute surgical beds. Clearly, there are number of overlapping perspectives on such a ward: views on its location within the hospital, the number of beds, and its detailed planning will differ between a patient, a nurse managing the whole unit, a nurse working in a team within it, and a doctor to whose speciality some of the beds are allocated.

The number of inpatient bed places remain the fundamental means of defining the size of a hospital. It also determines a substantial part of the revenue expenditure of the facility in terms of staff, supplies and support facilities. A place on a ward is the necessary precondition for obtaining access to the assessment, nursing, medical and therapeutic facilities of the hospital. Beds are therefore the mechanism for controlling the access to the hospitals resources. inevitably much interest focuses on the number of beds in a hospital and in a ward, both in situations where the bed numbers cannot be exceeded and in those where it does and the resultant overcrowding means acceptable standards of good nursing practice cannot be achieved. One reason why large open wards were rejected in favour of compartmentalized ones was that it relieved nurses of the pressure to fit in additional beds.

The primary concern of patients is to obtain access to the medical and nursing care that they need. Within that context, patients have views about the particular bedroom and sanitary facilities that they are allocated but are not generally aware of any aspects of the ward outside their own immediate bedspace.

The planning and design of hospital wards over the years and in different countries have developed in relation to the role of the nurse and the pattern of nurses activities. The Nightingale open ward design provides the nurse with a central role; the

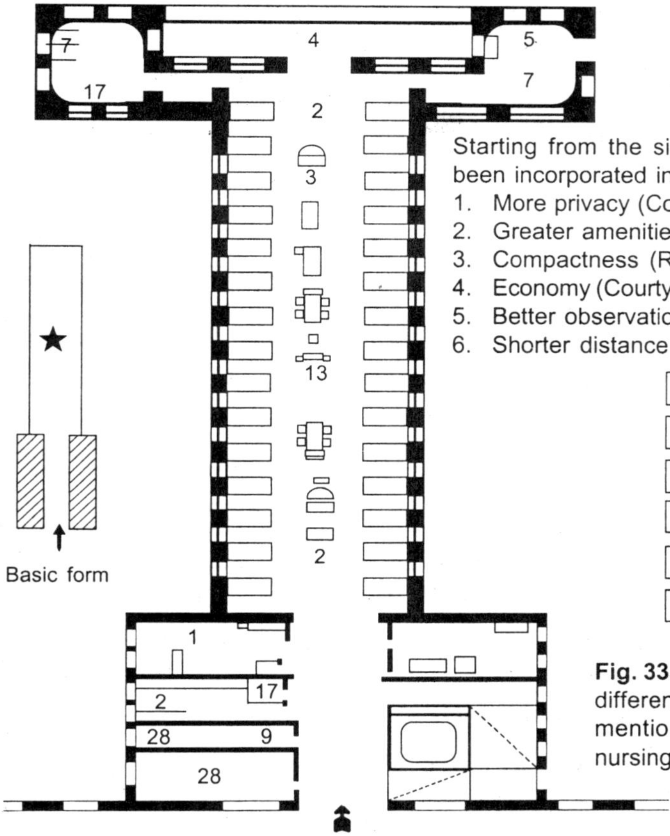

Starting from the simple open Nightingale form, changes have been incorporated in the pursuit of:

1. More privacy (Corridor or continental).
2. Greater amenities for patients and staff (Duplex or Nuffield).
3. Compactness (Recetrack or double corridor).
4. Economy (Courtyard-a naturally ventilated version of the above).
5. Better observation of all patients (Cruciform or cluster).
6. Shorter distance between patient and nurse (Radial).

3	Day space
5,6,7	Toilets
13	Nurses station
14	Treatment room
16	Clean utility
17	Dirty utility

Fig. 33.4 (Nightingale Ward): There are a number of different type of plans (derived from the previously mentioned forms) in which the 3 elements of the nursing unit can be layed out.

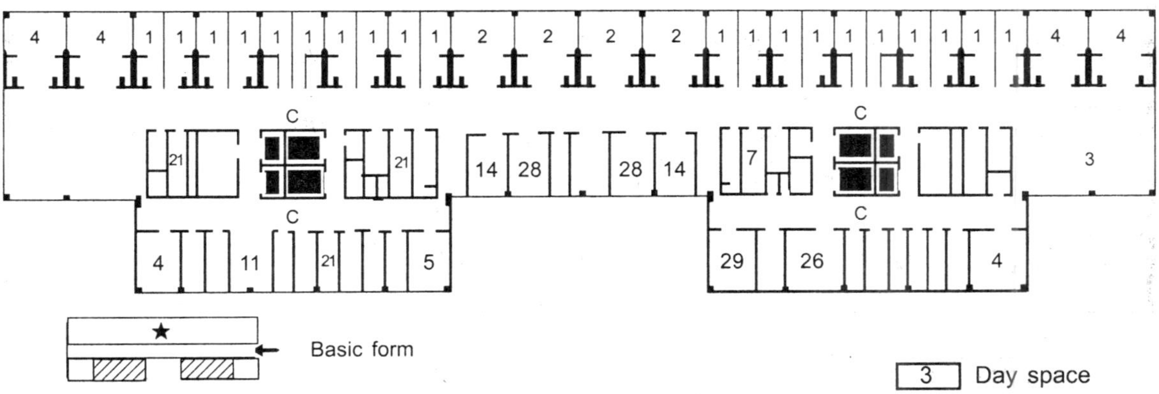

3	Day space
5,6,7	Toilets
13	Nurses station
14	Treatment room
16	Clean utility
17	Dirty utility

Fig. 33.5 Corridor: Corridor or continental–Beds were moved from the external walls and arranged in bays, usually of upto 4 beds, separated by crosswalls or screens. A corridor was needed to gain access to the bays.

Verburg Hospital—Sweden (1973) Wards are fully compartmentalized, with beds arranged in rooms each with its own toilet facility and day space. Each suit has nursing ancilliaries placed on both sides of its spine.

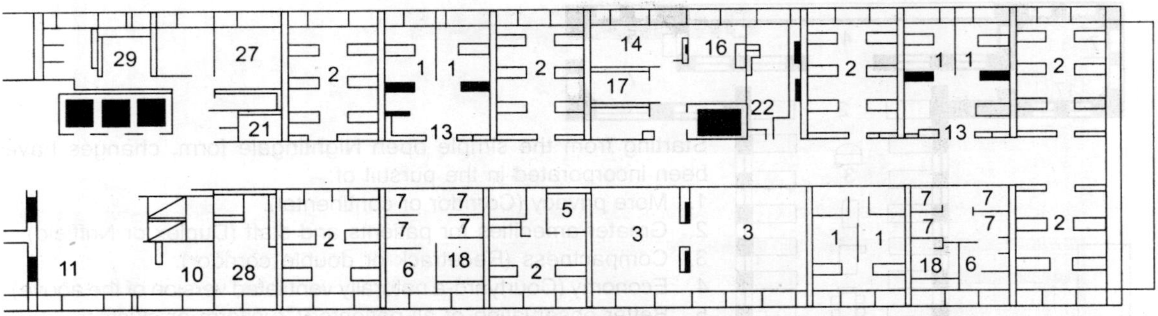

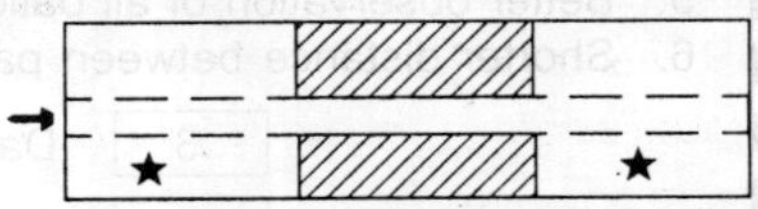

Basic form

Fig. 33.6 : Duplex or Nuffield—The Nuffield studied published in 1955 questioned the economy of attendance principles (30 beds to one sister). It proposed a new concept of team nursing which would enable more patients to be nursed in one unit. This gave rise to duplex layout which splits the ward into two sections of upto 20 beds each with its own nurses base. Nursing anciliary space is shared between the two sections.

Swindon Hospital: UK—shown below is a 40-bed unit using a mix of 6 bed bays on both sides to reduce the length of the coridor.

3	Day space
5,6,7	Toilets
13	Nurses' station
14	Treatment room
16	Clean utility
17	Dirty utility

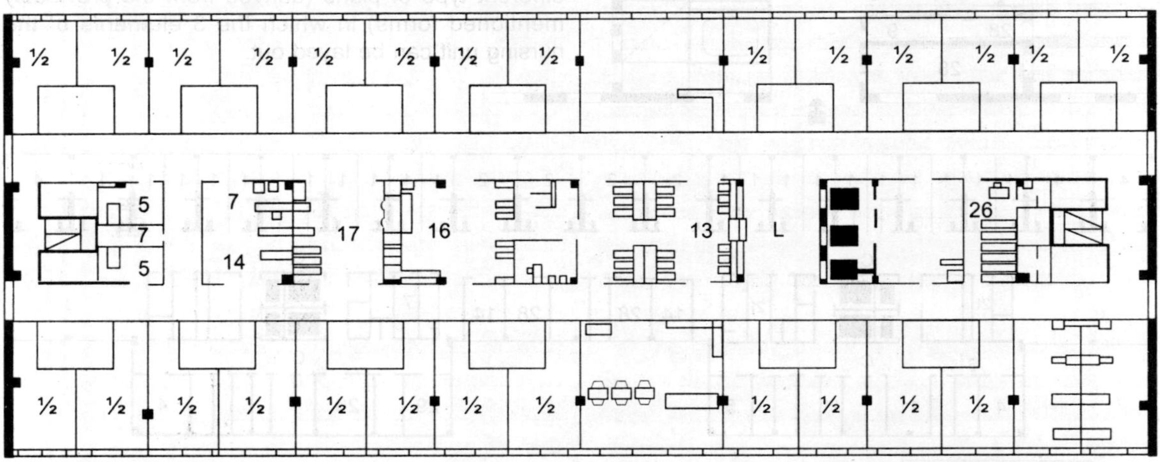

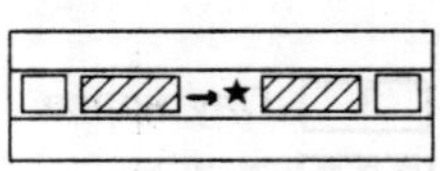

Basic form

3	Day space
5,6,7	Toilets
13	Nurses station
14	Treatment room
16	Clean utility
17	Dirty utility

Fig. 33.7: Race track or double corridor—In the mid-twentieth century, modern frame structures, air conditioning and mechanical conveyor systems contributed to the development of the racetrack or double corridor ward layouts. As event from the illustration below, the plan is based completely on a grid which helps to solve the structural problems.

Shown below is a typical racetrack plan developed by Gorden Friesen. It provides for 50-60 beds in single and two-bed rooms, each with attached toilets. Vertical conveyors deliver supplies direct from central storage and processing departments into the central staff core on each floor.

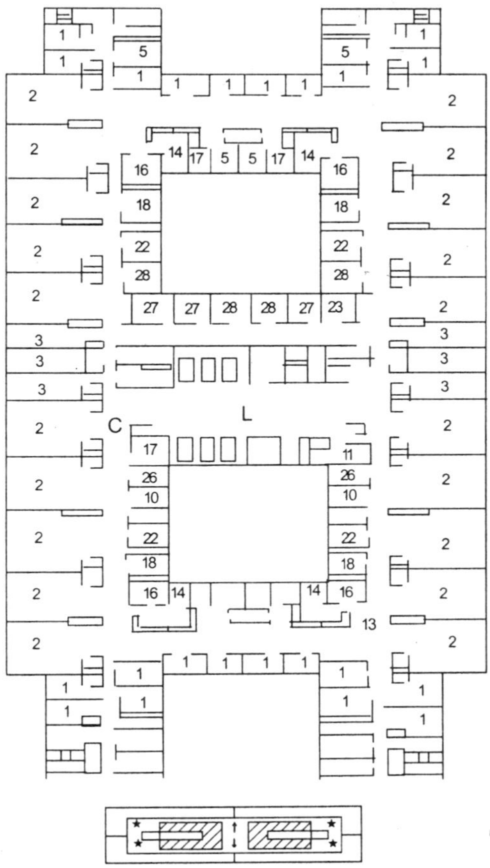

Basic form

Fig. 33.8: Courtyard:

3	Day space
5,6,7	Toilets
13	Nurses station
14	Treatment room
16	Clean utility
17	Dirty utility

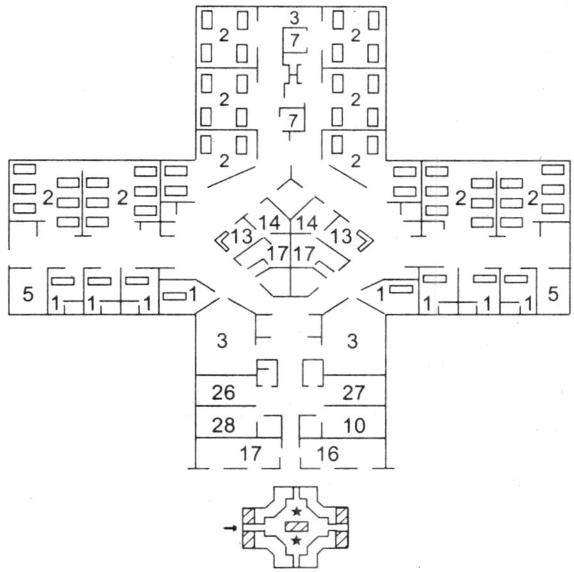

Basic form

Fig. 33.9: Cruciform:

3	Day space
5,6,7	Toilets
13	Nurses station
14	Treatment room
16	Clean utility
17	Dirty utility

nurse is visually and functionally at the centre of everything and the sister is in a position to control, monitor and direct all activities. Compartmentalized wards with separate bed areas, day areas, treatment areas, bases and utility rooms, reflect a move away from the centralized, generalized role of the nurse in accordance with the Nuffield studies, which divide the nurses work into separate, identificable tasks. Adoption of the progressive patient care approach of nursing, where nurses differentiate between highly dependent patients, is expressed in ward designs where some bed areas are close to the nurse base and others are not. In the USA, pattern of wards made up of single bedrooms, the nurse has a different role again, being besed in a separate office out of sight of the patients with the

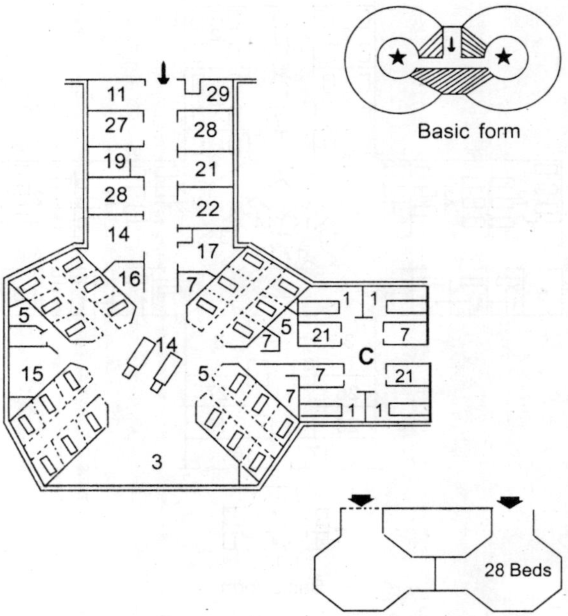

Fig. 33.10: Radial

3	Day space
5,6,7	Toilets
13	Nurses station
14	Treatment room
16	Clean utility
17	Dirty utility

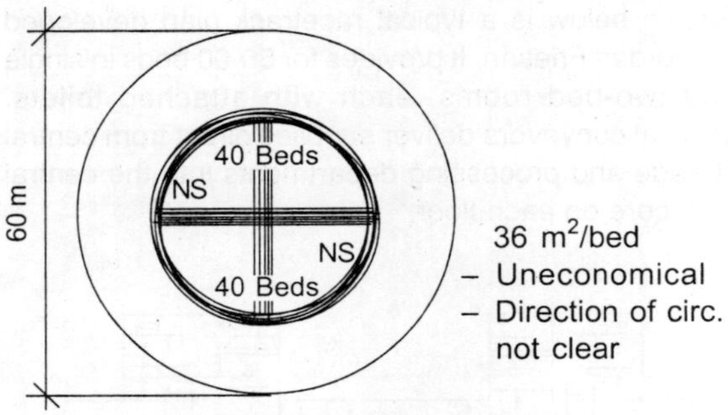

Fig. 33.11: Circular Plan

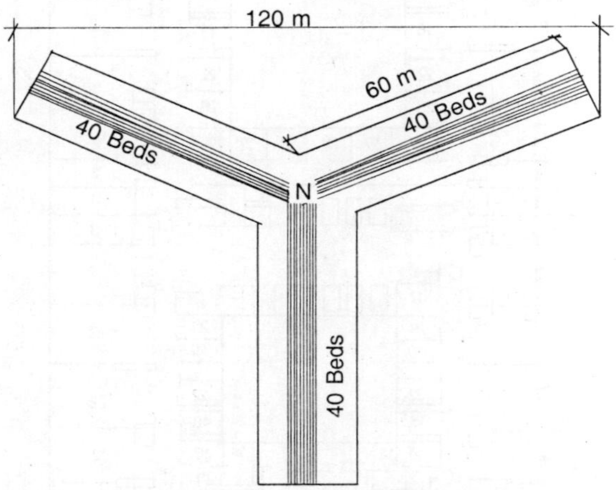

Fig. 33.12: Y plan

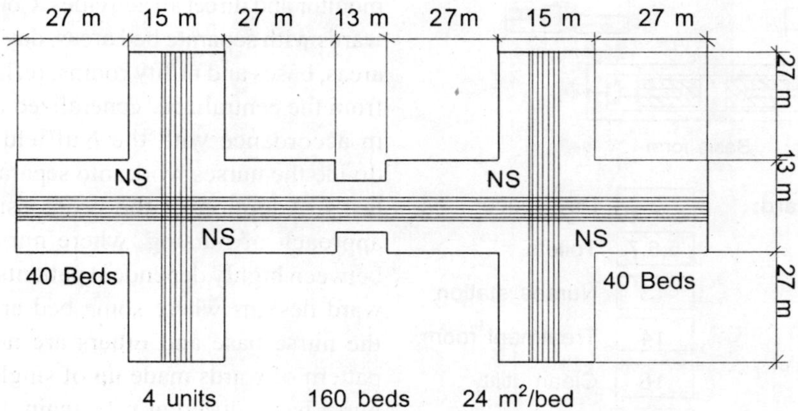

Fig. 33.13: Cross plan

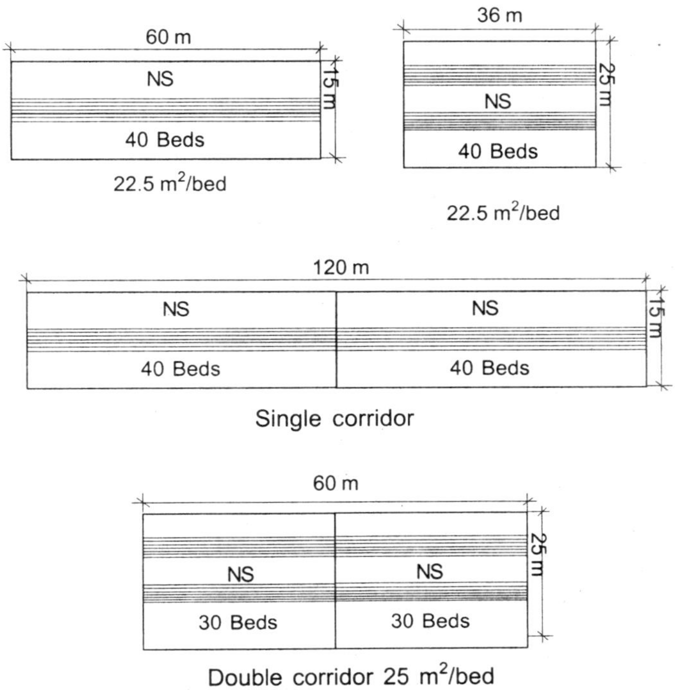

Fig. 33.14: Rectangular plan

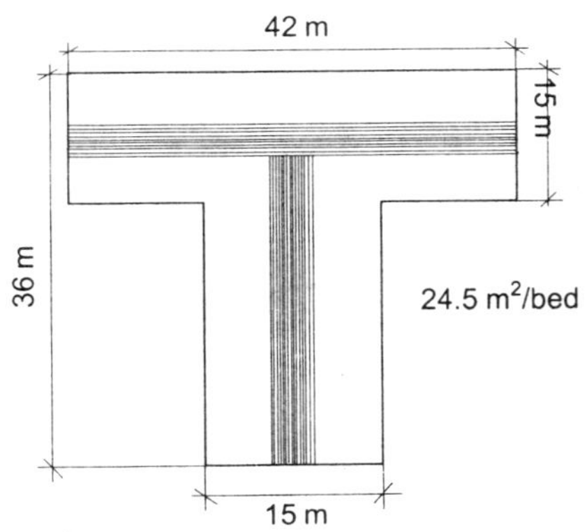

Fig. 33.15: `T' plan

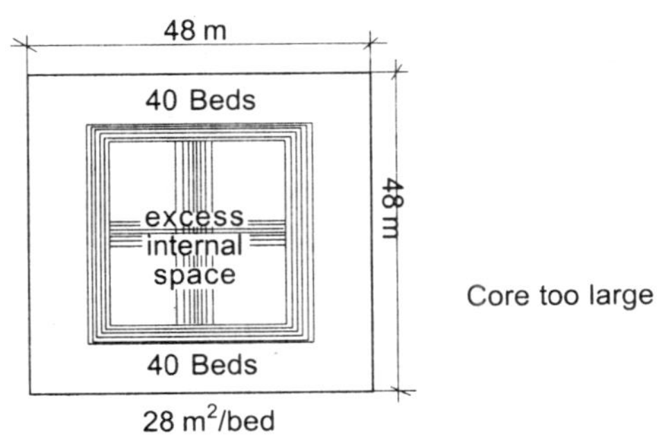

Fig. 33.16: Square plan

patients initiating most of the contact. Nurses in this situation have been compared to bell-hops by those who are used to a different role and to whom this one is unacceptable. There are countries with few nurses and others where the role is closer to that of a domestic help or an orderly. In these cases, the lack of a substantial nursing role is generally reflected in the complete lack of ward planning.

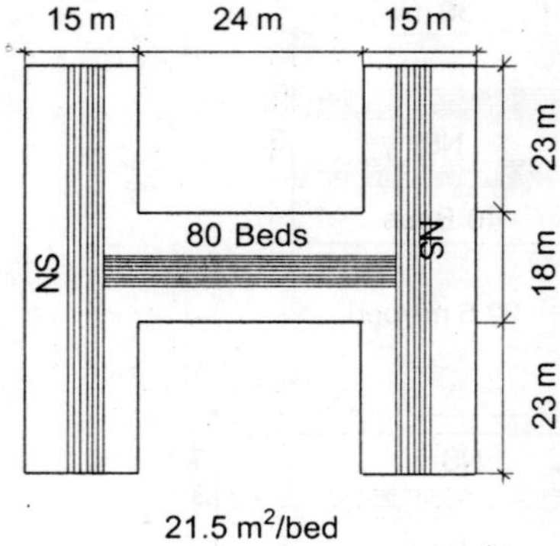

Fig. 33.17: H plan

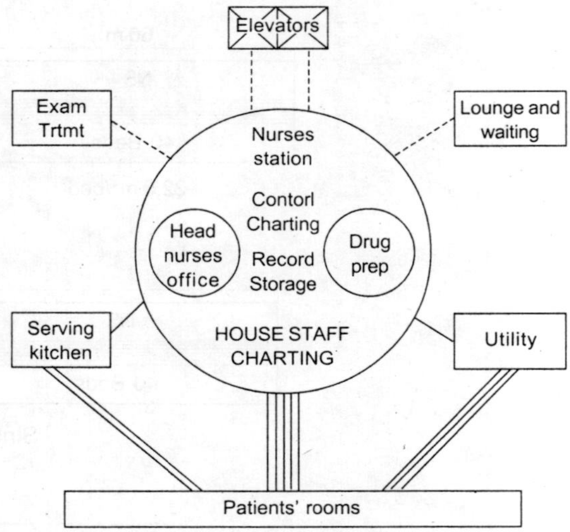

Fig. 33.19: Traffic to nurses' station

The two-ward planning issues that are most debated are the number of beds in a ward and the degree of openness or compartmentalisation of the design wards. Planners are trying to use staff and space as effectively as possible: at the same time they are trying to design that meet with their perception of good nursing practice and high standards of patient care. Integral to this perception are assumptions about the role of the sister and the role of the nurse on the ward. The strength of feeling about the role of the sister should not be underestimated. It is the basis on which the size (number of beds) of the ward is often decided. The amount of space required can be varied accoridng to the number of beds, the number of nurses allocated

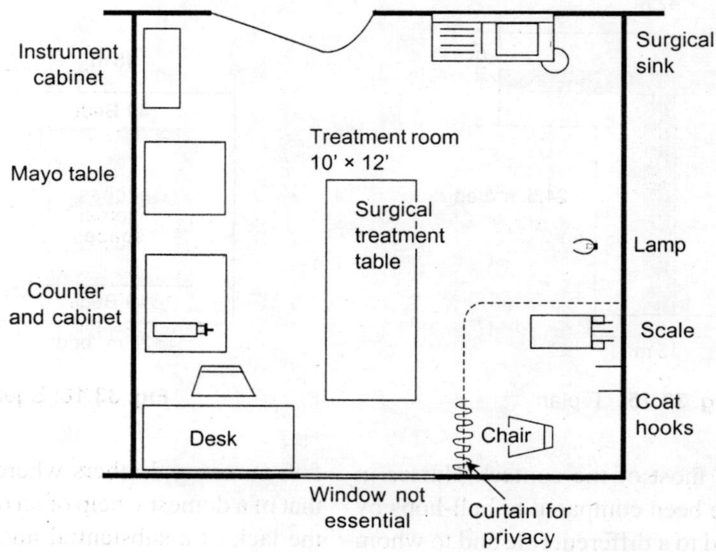

Fig. 33.18: The surgical treatment room

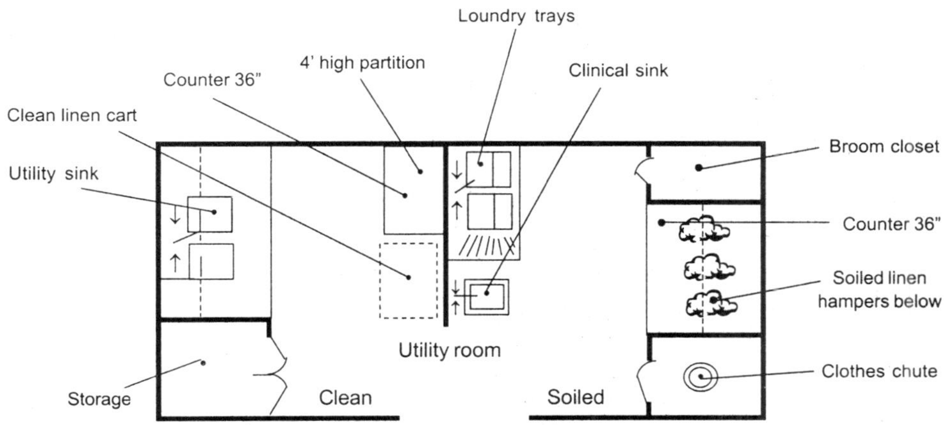

Fig. 33.20: The utility room

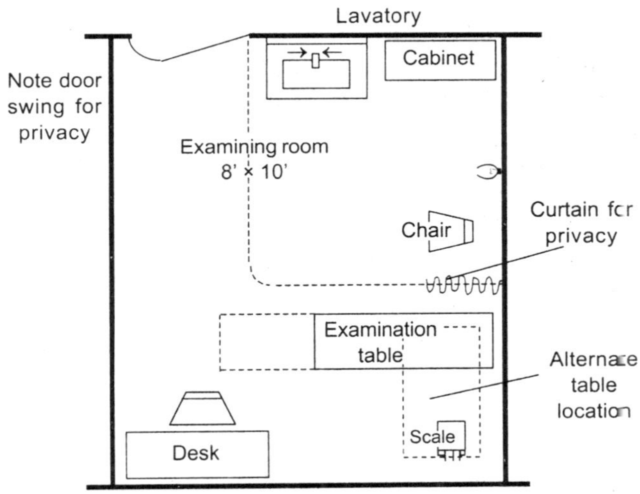

Fig. 33.21: The examining room

to a ward can be varied according to the work load associated with the number of beds but a sister's relationship with the patients and nurses on a ward is determined first by the number of beds, and second by the layout of the ward.

In such situations, where ward planning takes place within the context of proposed or anticipated levels of nurse staffing, emphasis is inevitably placed on their most efficient use.

Much of the debate that is apparently focused on the detailed design and planning of wards is really concerned with how to control access to hospital resources, fears about available staffing, anxieties about bed allocations, and strongly-held feelings about the sisters and nurses role.

It is important that they are not allowed to overwhelm consideration of other health buildings, good ward designs cannot ensure good practice

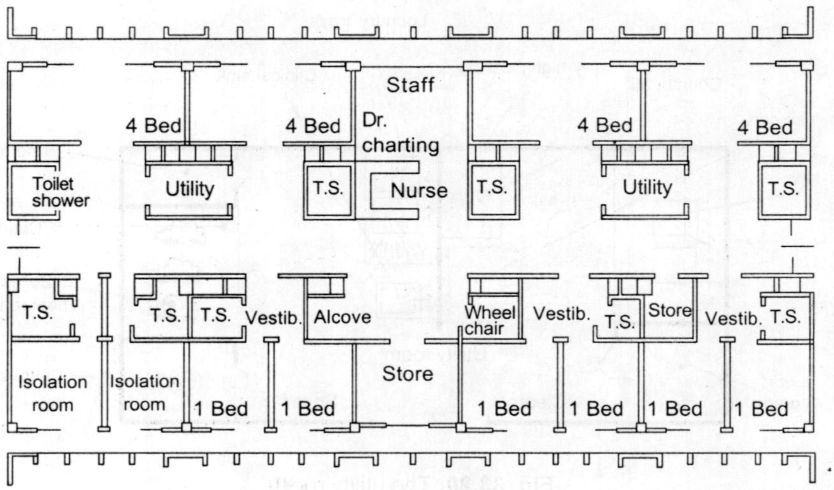

Fig. 33.22: A basic 24 bed ward unit with inner and peripheral corridors. Pütsep International

but can permit or encourage it and bad designs can prevent or discourage it. Much thought and skill is necessary to achieve ward designs that provide an appropriate therapeutic environemnt, that encourage and facilitate standards of good nursing practice and that offer physical, social and psychological comfort for both patients and staff.

FURTHER READING

1. Noble A: Ward planning. Hospital Management International. IHF London 250-53, 1989.
2. Porter DR: Hospital architecture: Guidelines for design and renovation. Health Administration Press, Ann Arbor, Richigan, 1982.
3. Putsep E: Modern Hospital: International planning Practices. Lyoyd-Luke Ltd. London 1979.

34 The Clinical Zone

PATIENT-FOCUSED EMERGENCY DEPARTMENT

The function of an emergency department is to evaluate and provide advice of initial treatment to anyone who comes there seeking medical assistance. In planning, a new or renovated emergency department for a hospital, it is necessary to realise that some well-defined trends are changing the character of emergency-care departments. The trends must be appreciated before specific programming for a given hospital is undertaken. It is necessary to have a clear idea of the kinds of services to be rendered, as well as projected patient loads, types of patient and son on. Analysis and development of planning factors will provide information on size, cost and functional characteristics of contemplated emergency department.

The concern of the hospital planning is the quality of medical care and the improvement of its standards. The planners must be aware of continuing advances in medicne, changes in society, ideology and attitudes of the community, and economic and technological conditions. An efficient hospital requires a well-balanced organization for compassionate care within an adequate technical and environmental framework. Emergency department is the shopwindow of a hospital. Adequate planning, design, management and maintenance of the facility and equipment of the Emergency Department is essential to ensure the high quality of services at a reasonable cost.

Planning Consideration

The concern of the hospital planning is the quality of medical care and the improvement of its standards. Continuing advances in medicine and society impose great demands on the planning and design of medical services. Community needs must form the basis for planning attitudes and aspirations must be clearly understood. Planning involves and requires understanding and evaluation of the current cultural mainstreams, the economic and technological conditions, and the goals of the community. Planning ought to be thinking in the probable terms of tomorrow. The long-term cost of operating a hospital can be greatly increased by the initial failure to plan proper systems and equipment. The objectives should be fully understood. The care needs of patients should directly dictate the character of every care function.

The hospital is for the patient. The patients and their needs must always be the point of focus when planning any facility. The constructed environment is to be designed with nursing and treatment in view.

There should be recognition of the fact that an active emergency service tends to embrace more than accident and true emergency functions and often assumes responsibility for admitting during the evening and night shifts.

Functions of Emergency Department

The function of emergency department is to evaluate and provide advice or initial treatment to any one who comes for medical assistance. The definition of an emergency has come to be determined by the needs and the perceptions of the general public. Owing to the increased specialization of medical services and the mobility of the population, the emergency department is increasingly being viewed as a place to get prompt medical attention for any condition. The emergency department must be designed and organized to handle this wide variety of expectations.

Every hospital must have a provision for receiving and dealing the "walking causalities" very simple fractures, cuts needing suturing, abscesses, and othe rminor conditons. Provision has to be made for dealing promptly and efficiently with medical and surgical emergencies, from whatever cause.

The future of the emergency may well lie in the field of automation. If automatic dispensing machines are to take the place of personal issue of supplies, and automatic analysers to take over the more painstaking diagnostic procedures, it is possible that the emergency department of the future will look a self contained, fully organised patient care service.

Facility Planning

Adequate Space

The department should be designed to allow ready expansion of space to accommodate future changes in the volumes of the patients. It should be large and constructed of materials that ware well. Twenty to twenty-five percent must be added to the present patient volume to approach the load at completion and another 25 percent should be added to avoid overcrowding in the first 4 or 5 years of operation.

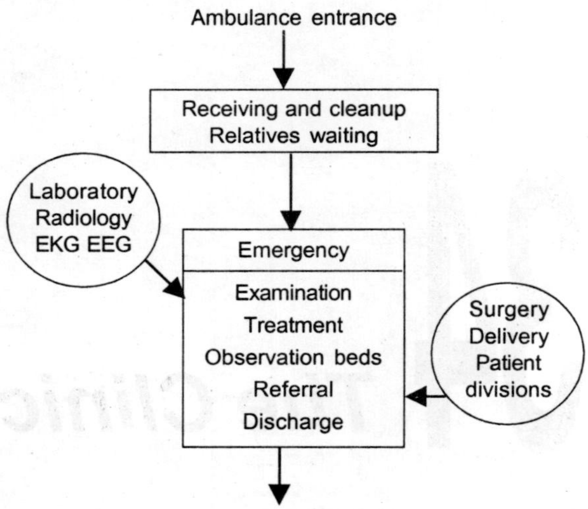

Fig. 34.1a: Functional relationships, emergency

Easy Access

The department should be located on the ground floor so that it is easily accessible to ambulances and ambulatory patients as well as to the rest of the hospital. There should be easy access to hospital and ambulance parking.

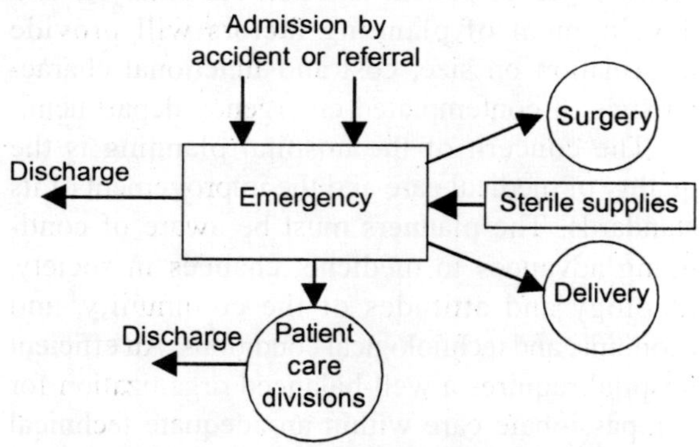

Fig. 34.1b: Functional relationships, emergency

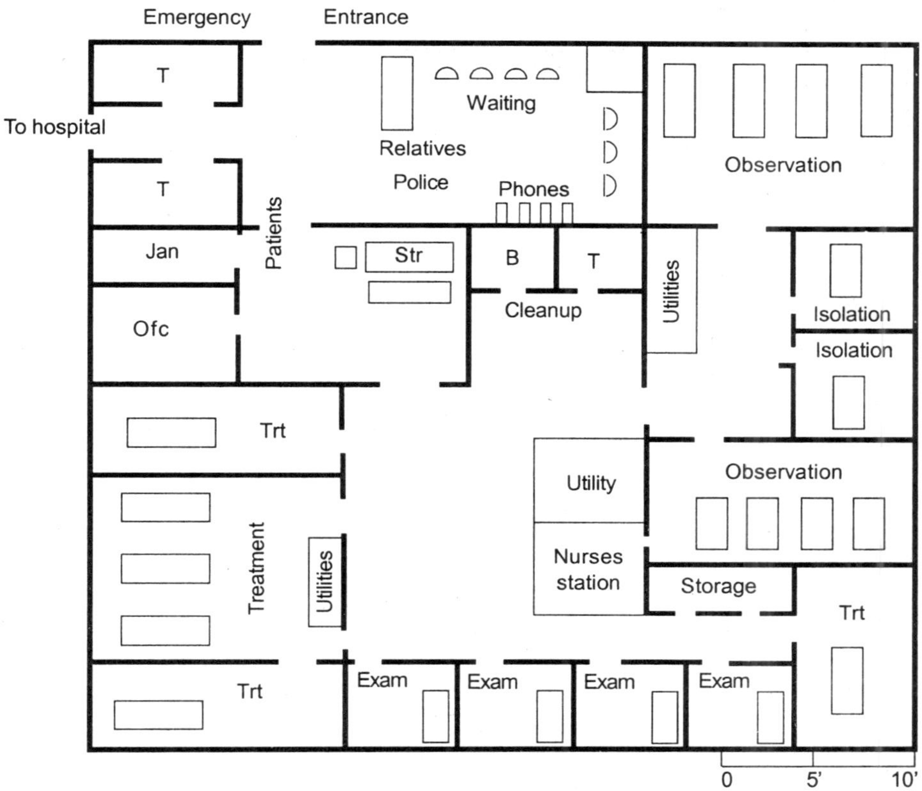

Fig. 34.2: Emergency patient's travel

Separate Entrances

Entrances to the department should be separate from those to the rest of the hospital so that they do not function as a corridor to the rest of the hospital. Directions to the Emergency should be well marked and clearly visible. The Ambulance Bay should be large enough to accommodate several ambulance simultaneously and should be covered and protected from inclement weather. An area just inside the entrance should be allocated for the storage of wheel chairs and stretchers. There should be separate entrance for ambulatory patients whenever possible.

Proximity to Other Hospital Services

The emergency department should have its own laboratory and Radio-diagnostic facilities, ECG room, drug counter and operation theater. Alternatively, the department should be located near the radiology services, laboratory, pharmacy and admitting office.

Adaptable Space

All area of the department should be equipped to handle seriously ill patients if the need arises. Rooms in the emergency department should be multipurpose so that depending on need, they can be converted from use by ambulatory patients to use by gurney patients and *vice versa*. An adequate number of oxygen, suction, and electric outlets must be available therefore.

Functional Rooms

Design of the department should make the most efficient use of staff and space while providing

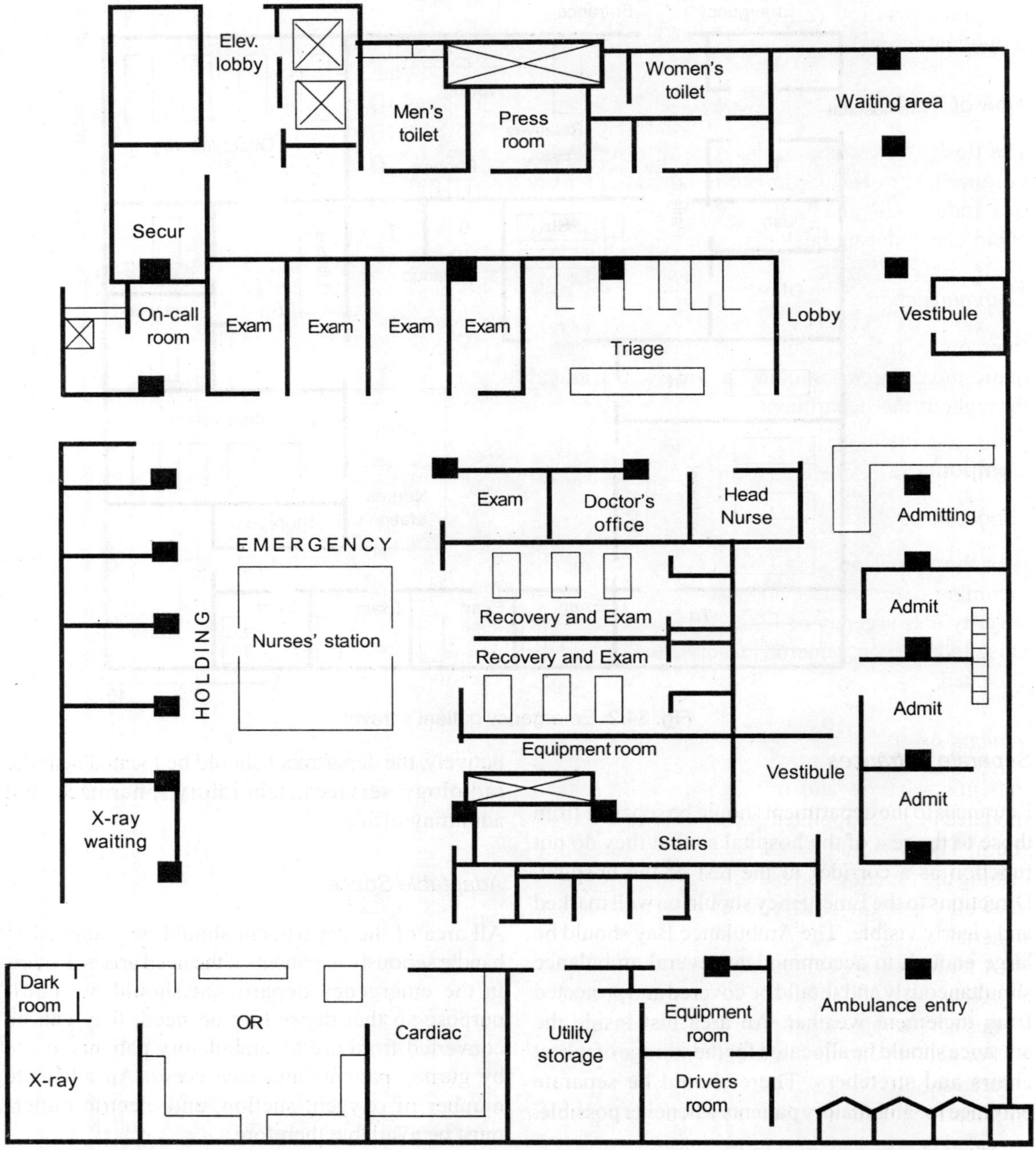

Fig. 34.3a: Emergency department layout for inner city hospital. Due to limited outside space, ambulance entry is within confines of the department area. Large triage area with holding cubicles adjacent to nurses desk is easily converted to mustering area in event of catastrophe

adequate privacy (curtained cubicles versus individual rooms).

Flow of Traffic

The floor plan must consider patient flow and the volume of traffic. Unidirectional patient flow (separate 'exit' and 'entrance') is preferable to avoid chaos during busy periods.

Communication

Intercoms, paging system, telephones, and pneumatic tube systems should be widely distributed throughout the department.

Components

Triage Area

It is the reception area (14 ft × 200 ft), where incoming patients are evaluated for the degree of severity and urgency of illness. It should be very close to entrance, generous floor space should be allocated.

Waiting Area

Patient's relatives and friends should be accommodated in well appointed and comfortable waiting room. There should be shelves for literature describing the function and the rules of the department as well as other well chosen current reading material.

- A television set may be an asset.
- Access to a tea or coffee bar or vending machines is valuable.
- For accompanying children, a separate waiting area should be provided.
- Clearly marked visitors' toilets should be provided near the main waiting space.

Admission Office

Admissions, discharges and record-keeping are carried out in a reception and registration room of about 15 m^2 size, located immediately adjacent to entrance. This office has to be manned on 24 hrs basis.

Care of Burns

A room of 20 m^2 size is needed for the immediate care of burn patients.

Staff Rooms

The nurses station should be adjoined by a work room for nursing personnel.

Miscellaneous Facilities

- Blood storage area
- Room for medico-social worker
- Drug dispensing facility
- Room for brought dead
- Room for Police personnel
- Room for class IV employees.

Operation Room

The emergency operation room should be self contained. It should be provided with conducting floors. Wall suction and oxygen are indispensable. Operation theater must be connected to emergency electric supply system.

Radio-diagnosis Room

There should be two or three diagnostic rooms, a dark room, a dry film room, a radiologist room, radiographer's room, a record office, store room and waiting area. A large X-ray room, may be divided by partition into two or three bays, each large enough to carry out X-ray examination of patient on a stretcher. The operator must be able to see into each bay from the contral cubicle.

Automatic film processing is of great advantage. In order to meet the increasing demand of trauma cases, a CT scan facility may be considered.

High resolution ultrasonography tests should be performed in the evaluation of acute surgical emergencies. Radiology section should be connected to emergency electric system.

Laboratory

It is preferable for the emergency department to have its own laboratory and technicians, so that the priority tests can be quickly communicated. Microscopes, centrifuges and a Bunsen burner are needed. Biochemistry autoanalyser, blood gas and electrolyte analysis facilities are desirable.

Observation Ward

This ward is used for patients who have been evaluated and need extended treatment, observation, re-evaluation, or other time-consuming procedures. The observation ward permits more efficient use of treatment rooms. It is desirable to establish and absolute time limit a patient may spend in this ward. Generally, 12-48 hours is reasonable depending on the size of the ward. The need of 1-2 observation bed per 100 in-patient beds in the catchment area has been indicated. The observation ward could be used as an acute treatment facility in times of mass casualties or when the patient load is exceptional.

Storage

Storage space must be provided for intravenous fluid drugs, clean linen and instruments. Plaster, larger mobile equipment (X-ray and ECG machines etc.), wheel chairs and stretchers. Life-saving equipment such as resuscitation sets, tracheotomy and other procedure sets should be made available.

Utility and Soiled Linen Room

Utility room for emptying, cleaning and storing of bedpans should be equipped with a bedpan washer, disinfector and cupboards. Soiled instruments and containers are rinsed and soiled linen stored in this room. Each room should have the size of about 7 m^2.

Staff-changing Room

Changing rooms for female staff should include lavatories, showers and lockers for personal possessions. There should be a retiring room. A lounge with pantry for the recreation of staff may be provided. Comfortable quarters for slack periods are required for doctors and nurses on duty. An on call room of 9 m^2 should be furnished.

Treatment Room/Examination Cubicles

- *For major emergency (20' × 20' or 6 m × 6 m)* The area should have ample floor space to accommodate several people and large pieces of equipment. Each room must be fully equipped to handle any major illness. There should be several wall-mounted suction units, electrical, oxygen and air outlets.
- *For intermediate emergency (12' × 14' or 12' × 16')* Rooms set aside for patients with illness or injury of moderate severity are used for stretcher patients (e.g., suture or fracture cases). Food lighting and wall-mounted suction and oxygen outlet facilities are required.
- *For minor problem (10' × 12')* Ambulatory patients with non-life threatening problems are treated in rooms set aside for this purpose. Curtained cubicle are both more efficient and safer than single rooms.

Special Treatment Rooms

- *ENT, eye and dental room* Equipment should include a dental chair, ENT chart, slit lamp, suction device and oxygen source.
- *Cast room* It should have a sink for mixing plaster, a cast saw, X-ray view boxes, ahnd storage for orthopaedic supplies.
- *Obstetric room* It should be equipped for pelvic examination, evaluation of patients in labour, and emergency delivery.
- *Psychiatric holding room*
- *Decontamination room* It should be tiled, with flexible-hose shower head for cleaning patients

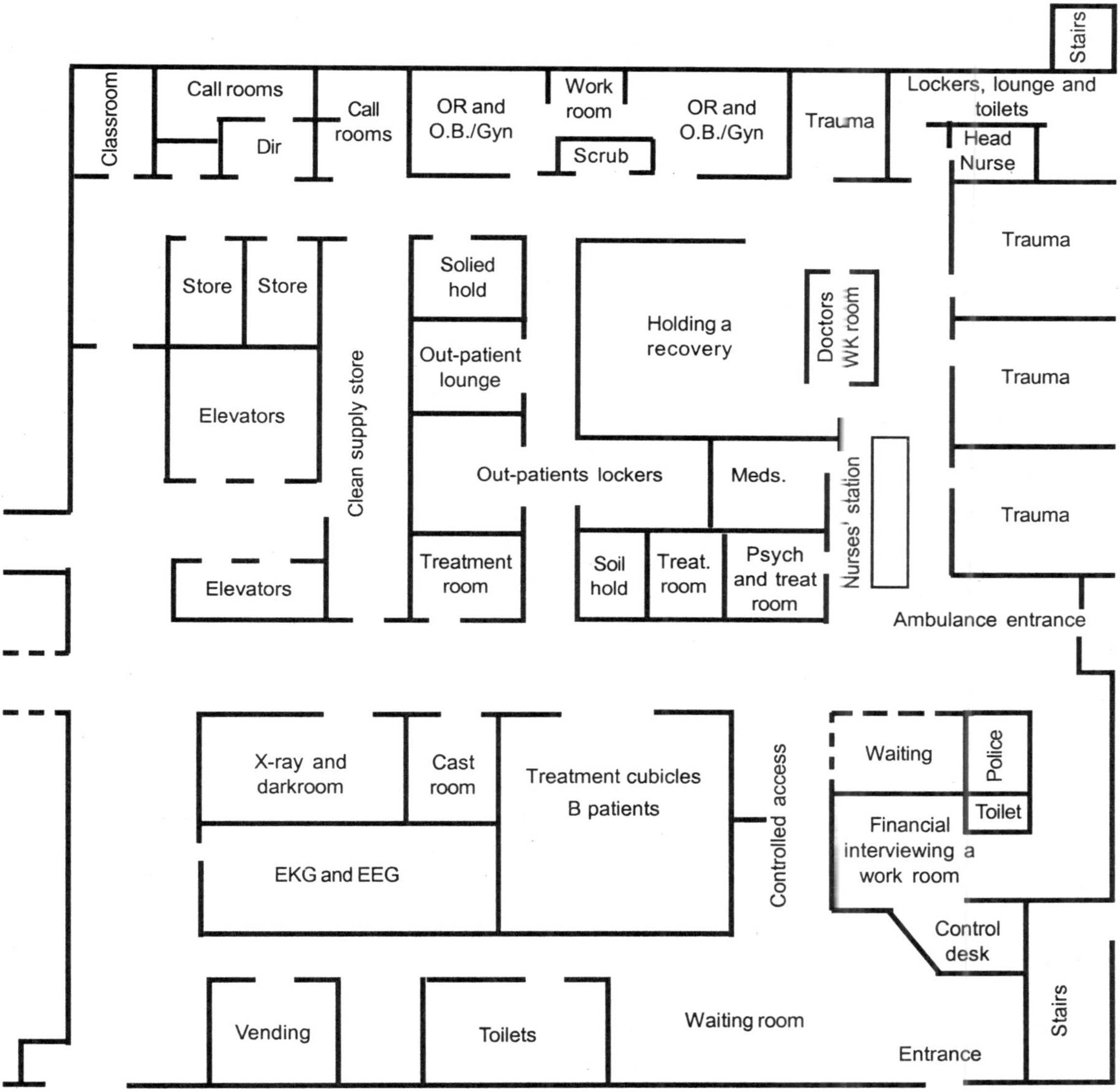

Fig. 34.3b: Example of emergency department layout of a suburban hospital showing efficient layout with such features as a room for police and press, trauma rooms immediately next to the ambulance entrance, separate obstertrical and gynecologic rooms, and a good-sized holding-recovery room area. Outside access is usually no problem in suburban areas where external space is usually plentiful

(radio-active decontamination, delousing) 13 m^2 size.

- *Suture room* It should be equipped for treatment of superficial wounds.
- *Resuscitation room* The patient is to be stabilized in this room. Immediate attention is given also to patients who need opening or cleaning of air passages and restoring the blood volume of the

body. All the equipment including ECG and medications for comprehensive cardiac area should be kept in this room so that the procedure could be immediately started. The equipment includes a treatment table or a patient's trolley, an oxygen outlet and a suction point, adjustable lamps (one of them for performing minor sugrical procedures), a lockup cupboard for respiratory equipment, an X-ray view box, a refrigerator for blood, a working top, shelves for balnkets, a wash basin and shelves for drugs and IV fluids. An area of 30 m^2 is required. This room must be connected to the emergency electric supply system.

- *Treatment room for burn patients* One air-conditioned dressing-room with a stainless steel bath and mechanical hoist should be provided. Plenum-Ventilation of dressing-room with an exhaust ventilated air lock has been shown to reduce infection in a burns unit. An operation room within the burn unit is frequently favored.

Other Facilities

If the departement is large there should be a centrally located nurses station with doctors' and nurses' charting area and dictating booths. An office for the emergency department supervisor is desirable. Public telephone booths within easy reach of waiting area should be provided.

General Consideration

The gross floor area to be assigned to the emergency department will vary from nothing to 15 sq ft per bed, according to programme requirements. The best test of size is to programme the department for local experience, determine the number of treatment rooms and supporting spaces and actually calculate the net and gross areas.

Functional Programme

For 500 bedded hospital, it will be as follows:

- Provide an emergency department for 24 hours operation.
- Include four surgical treatment-examination rooms.
- Include 4 additional examination rooms.
- Provide 12 observation beds and all necessary supporting spaces.
- The receiving and preparation room, 14 ft × 20 ft, shall adjoin a grade entrance with wide doors (leading immediately into the receiving corridor) and shall have facilities for taking care of at least 2 patients at a time. In a catastrophe, the adjoining space will have to be used as overflow receiving and first aid rooms.
- Public waiting (partially or wholly screened) with seats for 20 persons and access to toilets is to be provided.
- Provide 12 observation beds in four rooms with private toilet and shower adjoining each room, provide oxygen and suction and usual communications. Provide a nursing station for this unit.

Staffing

The staffing of emergency department will depend on its size, work-load, type of hospital, and the resources available. Depending upon the scope of the servies, the following personnel are essential to man the emergency services:

- General surgeon
- Orthopedic surgeon
- Medical specialist
- Anesthetist (on call)
- House surgeons/Junior residents
- General duty medical officers
- Obstetrician
- Nurisng staff
- Nursing orderlies
- Sanitation staff

The department needs to be staffed in its own right. From the consultant incharge downwards by personnel whose primary concern is to run it efficiently. It is no use leaving the department (that needs to be staffed throughout the 24 hours by specialists with a high degree of skills) in the hands

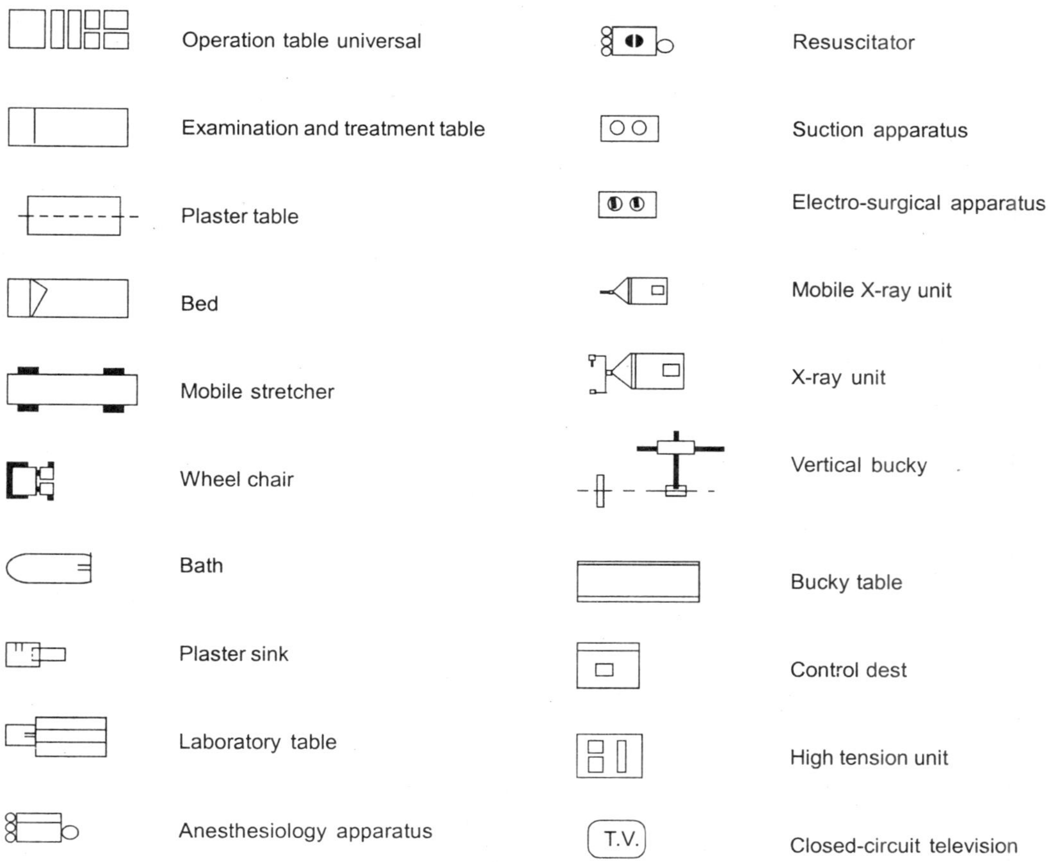

Fig. 34.4: Symbols of equipment for emergency department
(designed by Netherlands Hospital Planning Consultants)

of junior doctor, as is so often done, instructing him to call the specialist in case of difficulty.

The emergency department will function best if all personnel in the emergency area are directly responsible to its chief or officer in charge. The officer should be responsible to a policy committee consisting of the members of the medical staff and representative from hospital administration.

Emergency Preparedness

A mass casualty situation arises whenever a rapid influx of large number of critically injured people exceeds the capacity of the receiving facility to provide individualized medical care in the usual way. The objective in organising for mass casualities is to furnish care that benefits the greatest number of people.

Every year many places on our planet are struck by floods, earthquakes, landslides, house collapse, droughts, famines, vehicular accidents and other catastrophes.

Disasters

Any occurrence that causes damage, ecological disruption, loss of human life, deterioration of health and health services on a scale sufficient to warrant any extra-ordinary response from outside the affected community area are bound to be more frequent in the coming decades due to progressive deterioration of environment, deforestation, misuse of land, etc.

Though it is not possible to prevent most of the disasters, but still their worse effects can be alleviated or mitigated in magnitude by anticipated preparedness.

Disasters may be natural (earthquakes) or human (transportation accident, civil disturbance or terrorism) and the nature of injuries depends on the type of disaster.

Provisions must nonetheless be made to provide everyday emergency, medical surgical and obstetric services if no other medical facility is available. A plan for efficient management of mass casualities in times of disaster should ensure rapid organisation and expansion of community medical resources to maximum possible capacity (under emergency conditions). A plan for providing expanded medical and surgical services in disasters must be disseminated to all appropriate personnel. Emergency Medical Services is an essential element in the contribution of hsopital towards the total health care of the community. Providers of emergency services as well as the consumers should clearly define and understand the emergency medical care needs of their population and the facilities available in the hospital so that maximum benefit can be derived within limited resources available. Emergency department must be efficient at all the times and for all the purposes for which it is meant. It must be established on right cost benefit basis. Adequate physical facilities, equipment and stores should be available. An alert well-trained and sympathetic staff who can render prompt and correct medical care to the critically ill patients is desirable.

FURTHER READING

1. American college of surgeons. Committee on trauma: Advance trauma life support Course for physicians. Amercian College of Surgeons. 1996.
2. Tabish SA: Planning Tomorrow's Hospitals Today, *JAHA* **2**: 7-14, 1990.
3. Emergency medical system. In: Principles and practice of emergency medicine. Schwartz GR *et al* (Eds): Suanders 1371-1494, 1978.
4. Mills J *et al: Current Emergency Diagnosis and Treatment* (2nd edn.) USA, 1983.
5. Putsep E: Modern Hospital: International planning practice. Lloyed Luke Ltd. London 640-54, 1979.
6. Parker S: Emergency room utilitisations at Hermann Hospital. *Texas Medicine* **74**: **10**: 62-70, 1978.
7. Spencer JH: The hospital emergency department. Springfield, **III**: 38, 1972.

OUTPATIENT DEPARTMENT

The outpatient department is an ambulatory care centre (also called polyclinic) which provides to all members of a community the whole scope of services that are needed to keep them in good state of health, directly or by referral to more qualified institutions.

Patient care is the primary function of the outpatient department (OPD). It also functions as a centre for imparting education to professional staff as well as to patients and visitors. It provides medical students, house physicians, nurses and technicians with valuable and diversified clinical experience.

In light of changing role of hospitals following Alma Atta declaration (1978), primary health care being key to achieving health for all, outpatient department has a vital role to extend cost-effective services encompassing health promotion, preventive care, early diagnosis and treatment.

A health care–community centre (OPD) would be complete when it includes: medical and nursing care unit, dentistry service, social welfare office, work therapy and vocational therapy unit, pharmacy, optician service, chiropodist unit, health insurance office and health information office. An OPD should conduct ante-and post-natal as well as child welfare clinics. It is also the natural centre of probably active medicine for the community.

Planning Considerations

The out-patient services must enable the clinical and non-clinical staff to give their best service and the patients to receive the services without surrender of personal dignity.

The facilities have to be planned so that:

- Ease of access for patients is ensured
- The dignity and privacy of patients is respected
- A quite orderly pattern of work is achieved
- The requirements of handicapped are wholly satisfied.
- Some regrouping of functions within the centre is possible.
- En extension or expansion of the centre is possible without the need to rearrange its possible without the need rearrange its basic circulation system.

Designs characterized by simplicity can and ought to be produced.

Outpatient department has functional and administrative links with the hospital of which, it is a part. It may also be linked with health centers, satellite clinics and dispensaries dependent on it. Expected demand will have to be determined based on the hospital's catchment area and the population to be served. As a matter of policy, health promotion and preventive care should be provided with curative medical care.

Needs Assessment

An assessment of the expected demand for outpatient care must be made in the very beginning. Demand for care is computed as per capita per year basis.

According to an Estimate

- About 25 inpatients are given service per bed in a year
- With 6,19,433 beds in India, 1.54 crore inpatients are therefore served per year
- For each hospital bed, about 500 outpatients per year are given service
- More than 30 crore outpatients are treated in a year in the OPD.
- Cost to the patient—cost-effective

Other factors include:

- Distance
- Degree of urbanization
- Socio-economic status of community

- Level of facilities and staff, and
- Quality of care provided.

OPD is the patient's first point of contact with the hospital and entry point into the health care delivery system. It is a stepping stone for health promotion and disease prevention. It acts as a filter for inpatient admission. It contributes to the reduction in morbidity and mortality. It is the "shop window" of the hospital. On an average two to three outpatients per hospital bed attend to OPD per day. A 300-bedded hospital should expect to cater to 450 to 900 outpatients a day. As the strength of the hospital beds increases, the attendance in OPD tends to rise.

Design Considerations

After determining the expected need, following considerations should be taken into account:.

- Range of services to be provided
- Daily and hourly capacity required
- Number of staff required
- Possible service time per patient
- Flow diagram
- Holding capacity and lifting capacity
- Equipment and furniture required
- Layout of the department.

OPD is one of the rapidly growing services of the hospital. It must be planned for a substantial capacity for growth. Special. attention should be given to the following areas:

- Adequate parking facilities
- Storage area for wheelchairs and stretchers
- Lobby and lounge with seating accommodation
- Elevators easily accessible to lobby
- Minor operating room
- Waiting area and sub-waiting areas
- Consultation chamber.

Location

The outpatient department should be conveniently located adjacent or in close proximity to vital adjacent services such as registration and medical records, admitting, emergency, and social service. It should also be easily accessible and prompt services should be available from the laboratories, radiology, pharmacy, and physical medicine departments. Attention should be paid to circulation which should result in the smooth flow of the various traffic lines traversing the department.

Space Requirement

An average total area of 250 m^2 per doctor ought to be sufficient for rather complex outpatient care. In larger OPDs the accommodation for each separate and identifiable speciality or team should be closely associated with its own reception and waiting accommodations and visually recognisible. Easily understable signs should be used to identify destinations.

The grouping of OPD should preferably be at ground level to allow for future growth. The OPD should be on the ground floor in a multistoreyed building. The OPD should allow the majority of rooms the benefit of windows. Landscaped courtyards given frequently a pleasant touch to the building. Circulation routes along courtyards are attractive (Fig. 34.4).

Functional Zones

Generally, three functional zones in an OPD can be distinguished.

Public zone The entrance lobbies, waiting areas, public toilets, pram park.

Joint use zone The reception areas, individual clinical rooms, seminar rooms.

Staff zone The staff cloak rooms and toilets, work rooms, retirement rooms, communal rooms stores.

All separately operating functional entities should be approached by way of an administrative control centre.

The public entrance should be brought in near to the receptionist, so that he /she can handle enquiries she need no other services.

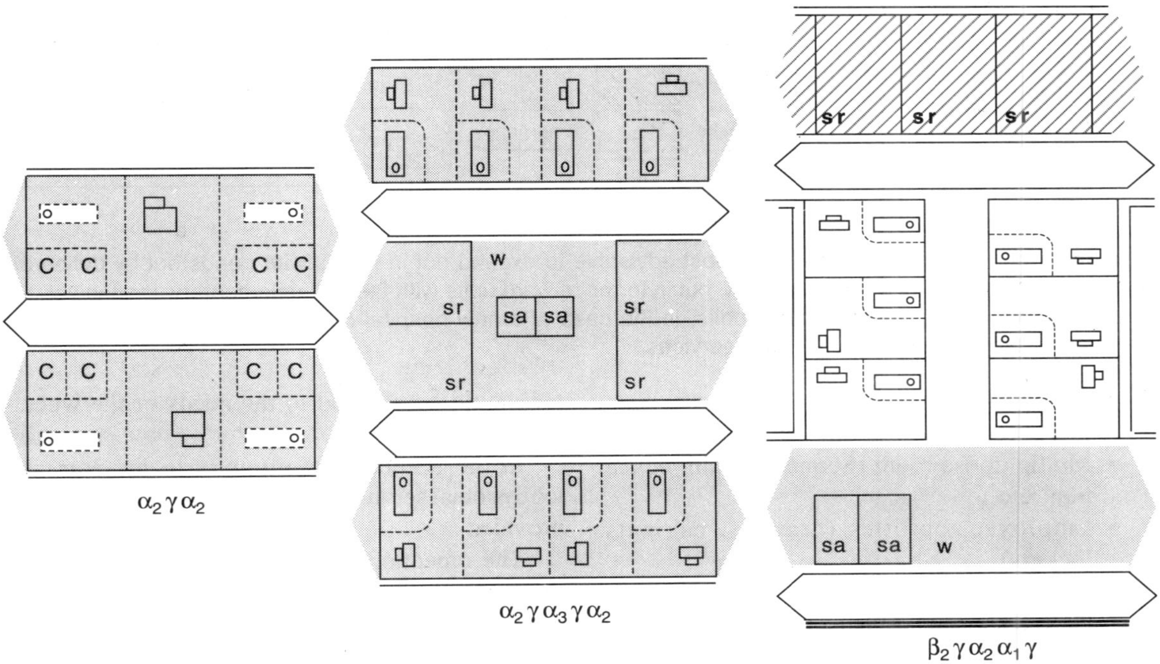

Fig. 34.5: Zonal combinations for outpatient departments; combined consulting/examination room system

The design of individual functional areas should not allow any extraneous traffic to penetrate any work area.

There may be separate entrances for staff and public, each giving access to the relevant zone.

Circulation routes must not pass through waiting areas, which should be screened both visually and acoustically.

Waiting areas must relate closely to their associated group of consultation chambers so that verbal systems of patient call remain possible and walking distance short.

Within the joint use zone standardized rooms should allow multifunctional usage and cater in detail for the needs of the patients, their comparisons and the staff.

Within the staff zone administrative patterns, role relationships and job description are frequently in a state of development and therefore room relationships must not impede development.

Entrance

An approach road from public transport with a wide footpath should lead to the entrance. The space around the entrance has to be slipfree and sized to allow the simultaneously setting down or picking up of infirm patients from two cars.

The ambulance entrance should be separate and covered. It should be possible to the vehicles of staff and patients near to OPD entrance.

Elements of Outpatient Facilities

The following facilities are required in the OPD (Fig. 34.5).

A. Public area and administration.
- Wheelchair and stretcher storage alcove
- Reception and information desk
- Registration counter and cubicles for staff to interview patients on one-to-one basis.
- Public toilet facilities.

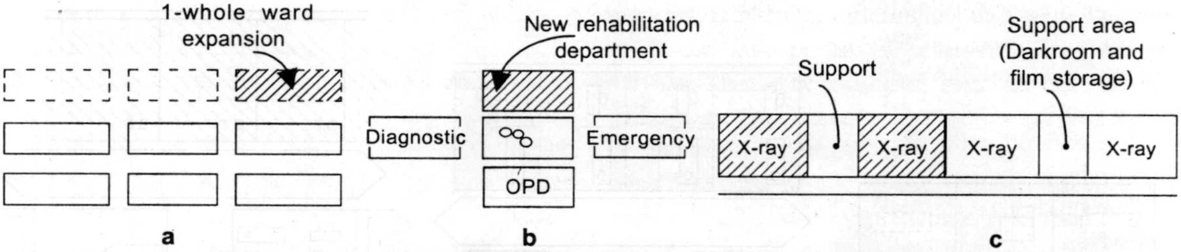

Fig. 34.6: Increments of growth—It is most advisable to expand not in spurts with needs but by deliberate increments, thus: (a) by number of beds, but in terms of ward units with their complementary manpower and supporting services (b) by functional units, in the case of a new hospital department, and (c) by specialist rooms and their supporting units and services

- Public telephones
- Water cooler or drinking fountains
- Multipurpose room (Seminar, health education, etc.)
- Employee facilities (drawers, cabinets, lockers)
- Stores for supplies and equipment
- Coffee shop/snack bar
- Gift shop
- Security post.

B. Clinical facilities
- Examination room
- Consultation chamber
- Treatment room
- Observation room
- Nurses' station
- Clean storage
- Dirty utility room
- Wheelchair storage space.

Enquiry and Reception

The workload at the enquiry desk includes.
- Receiving patients and directing them to reception stations
- Helping patients to complete forms
- Explaining the implications of advice just received by confused patients and providing instructions to them.
- Making appointments
- Supervising the entrance areas.

The needs of the privacy and dignity of the patient must be recognised. The height of the counter should be adapted to the needs of the wheelchair patients.

In the immediate contiguity to the entrance lobby social service and cashier facilities should be provided.

The receptionists have to be located close to the particular medical team's accommodation—each reception station should be distinct and separate. The main activities at reception station include:
- Receiving booked patients and directing them to subwaiting areas.
- Helping patients to fill forms
- Calling patients to consulting rooms
- Producing outpatient identity cards
- Supplying forms
- Making appointments

Each receptionist requires 1:2 m length of counter with drawers, and shelving space. An area of 6 m^2 is the minimum working space for each receptionist.

The reception area should have direct communication with an office and the medical record area.

Waiting

Appointment systems may reduce the lines of waiting patients and the waiting areas. If no appointment systems are used, the areas required for waiting is about twice as great than that required with an appointment system.

Frequently shared waiting areas have been advocated for several lines of persons ready for the various consulting suites in simultaneous use these lines may be differentiated by using color schemes or distinct labelling of the chairs. Up to six consulting suites running individual type sessions—roughly 30 waiting patients can share a single waiting area.

The patients calling system has to identify both the person and the room he is to go to.

The shared waiting area is determined by adding a basic size of about 7 m^2 for each participating doctor.

Waiting area should be screened, visually and acoustically, from areas used for any other activities.

The advantages of shared single area waiting have been assumed to include economy of space, ease of patient supervision, and maximum flexibility in use as peak loads of one consulting suite could spill over into the areas of a less hard-pressed suite.

Subwaiting (a waiting space near particular consultants room) is essential. A special waiting space for children is highly desirable.

An area of about 20 m^2 is required for a each pediatrician acting. A water closet and a washbasin are needed as a well room of about 4 m^2 for baby care.

Lavatories

The approximate provision is to allow a ratio of one water closet and lavatory basin for every 20 patients attending a session.

Toilets must be close to waiting areas and all examination rooms. Generally, the patient and staff toilets are separated. Toilet facilities, and the like must be designed with the comfort and convenience of the patient in mind.

Consultation Rooms, Examination Rooms

As consultation and examination suites must allow for multi-functionality of use, some standardization of consulting and examination rooms has to be adopted (Fig. 34.6).

Consultation room of about 12 m^2 is adequate for most activities performed within the room. Every consultation room should have a door to the corridor. A consultation room should be equipped with:

- A desk, 1.3 by 0.75 m, 0.8 high
- A swivel chair for consultant

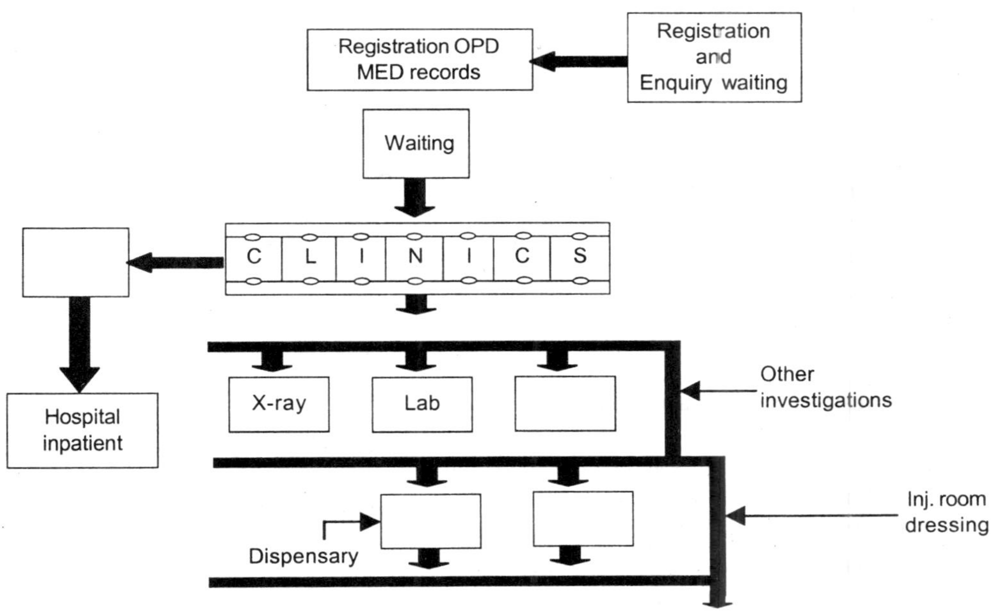

Fig. 34.7: Flowchart of outpatient department

- Two chairs for visitors
- About 4 m of bookshelves
- An X ray viewing screen
- A Dictaphone
- Desk telephone.

Each consultation-cum-examination room should have additionally an examination couch, a trolley for instruments, a washbasin, a soap dispenser, a paper towel dispenser, and a container for used towels.

For examination only a room of 8 m^2 is sufficient. All examination rooms require daylight with visual privacy. Acoustic control is important. The sound transmission rate should be no more than 55 decibels.

Local, control of heating and ventilation to meet intermit heavy demands is frequently essential.

When the diagnostic element has been chosen e.g. two examination rooms and one consulting room—the number of diagnostic elements need for each speciality — N — can be calculated.

$$N \frac{p}{D \times H \times V}$$

P = Number of patients visits per year,
D = The number of clinic days per year,
H = The number of clinic hours per day,
V = The number of visits per element per hour

Per 100 inhabitants there are about 35 estimated annual patient visits in the filled of internal medicine 30 in general surgery. and 15 in gynecology.

When the quality of medical services increases, the number of visits per element and per hour will be reduced.

Requirement of Examination Rooms

The number of patients that can be effectively handled by a clinician in the outpatient department time is difficult to establish. For a consultant it can be 6 active consultations per day. The number of visits per clement per hour is as follows:

- Internal medicine 3-4
- General surgery 7-8
- Gynecology 3-5
- Pediatrics 6-8
- Orthopedics 5-8
- Ophthalmology 4-6
- Otorhinolaryngeology 6-8
- Dermatology 6-8
- Psychiatry 2-4

The requirement of consultation cum examination room can be determined as follows.

Assumptions

Direct Population	200,000
Indirect Population	100,000
Consulting per person per year (direct population)	2
Consulting per person per year (indirect population)	0.5
Average first consultations	30 percent
Average subsequent consultations	70 percent
Time taken for first consultation/ exam time taken for subsequent consultation/exam	20 minutes
Time taken for subsequent consultation/Exam	10 minutes
Scheduled hours of OPD	6 hours

Procedure

Direct population × Consultation
200,000 × 2 = 400,000 Consultations

Indirect population × Consultations
100,000 × 5 = 500,000 Consultations

Total consultation/ examination per year = 450,000
450,000 ÷ 300 = 1500

$$\frac{\text{(Consultation per year)}}{\text{(Working days per year)}} \text{ Consultations/days}$$

First consultation/exam per day $\frac{1500 \times 30}{100} = 450$
(consultation per day × 30%)

Subsequent consultations/exam per day $\frac{1500 \times 70}{100} \times 1050$

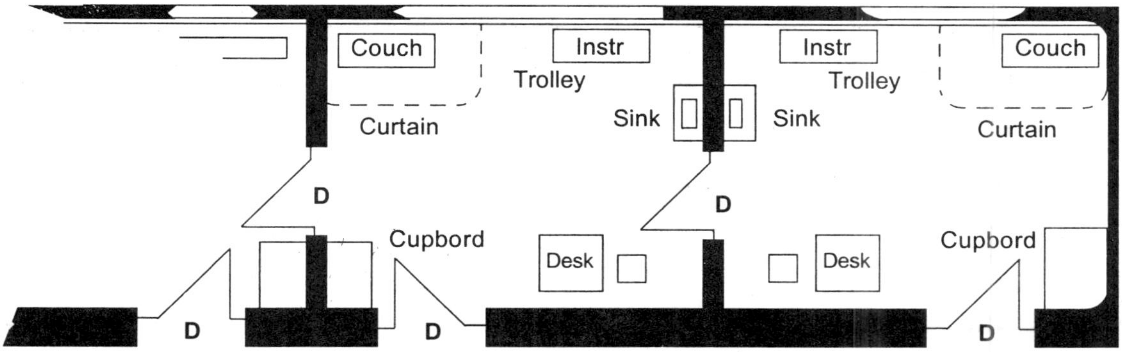

Fig. 34.8: Intercommucating consulting examination rooms

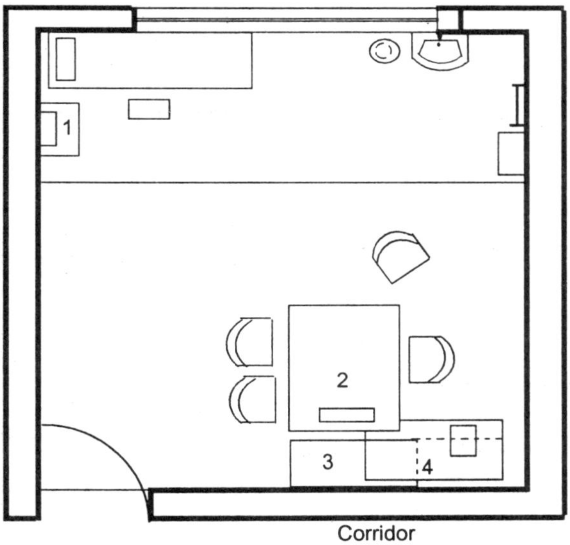

1. Work table
2. Physician's desk
3. Wall mounted cabinet
4. X-ray viewer

Fig. 34.9: A typical one-room outpatient consultation-cum-examination facility

(consultations per day 70%)

Time for first consultations exam 450 × 20 min = 9000 min

Time for subsequent consultations/exam 1050 × 10 min = 10500 min

Total time = 9750 mints

Consultation hours per day required

$$\frac{19500}{60} = 325 \text{ (hours)}$$

$$\frac{\text{(Total time minutes)}}{60}$$

Consulting rooms required

$$\frac{\text{(consulting room hrs per day}}{\text{(scheduled hours of OPD}} \quad \frac{325}{6} = 54 \text{ consulting rooms}$$

The average number of patient visits per doctor may be as follows:

General surgery	40
Orthopedics	30
ENT	30
Dermatology	30
Internal Medicine	15
Gynaecology	25
Pediatrics	15
Ophthalmology	20
Psychiatry	10

Treatment Room

A general purpose treatment room should be about 17m^2 in size with following equipment:

- An examination couch (1.9 by 0.6 m by 0.75 m high)
- Steps for examination couch
- An adjustable lamp over couch
- Oxygen and suction outlets (1 m above floor)
- A working top, length 1.2 m
- An upright chair

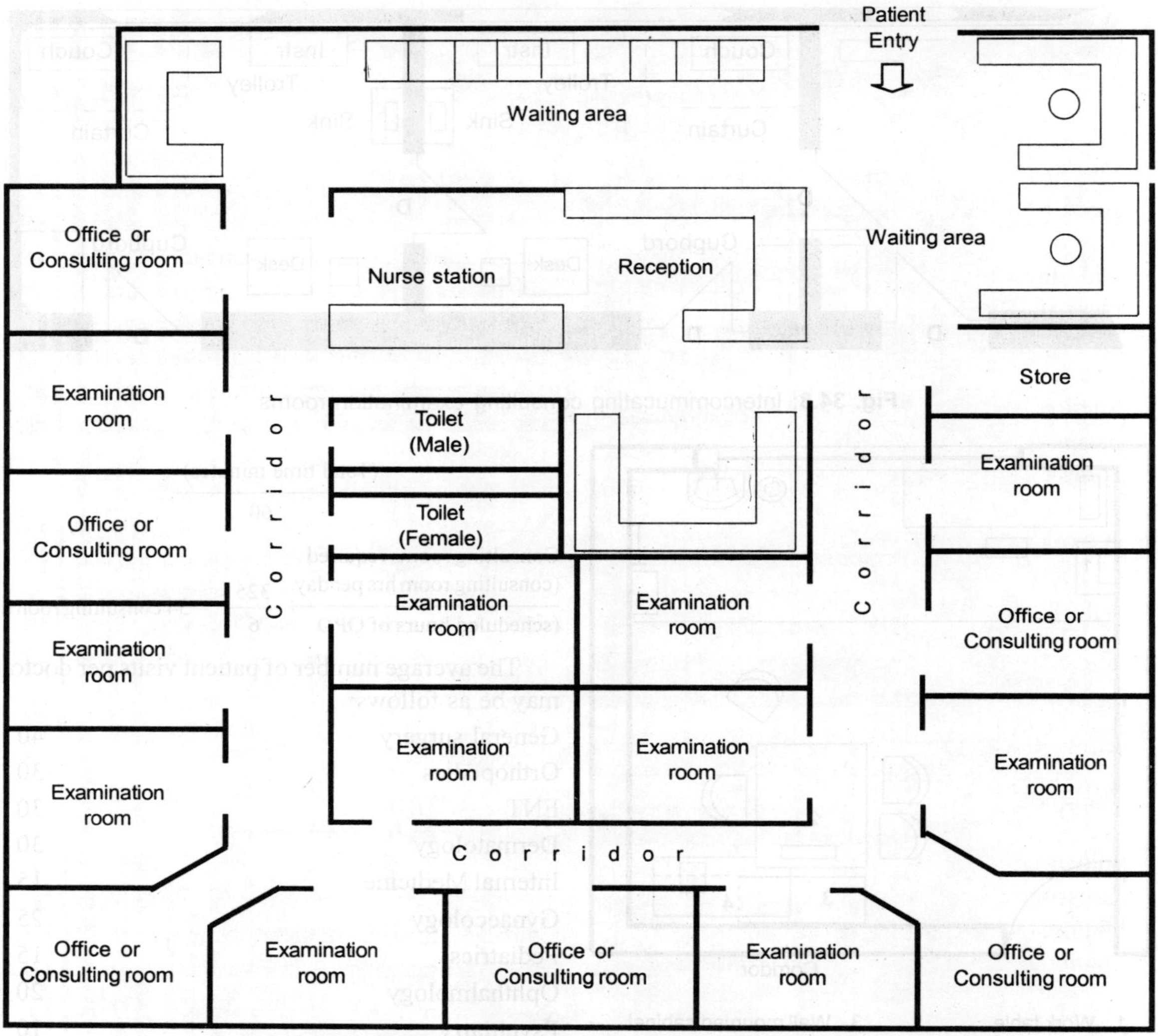

Fig. 34.10: Layout of a multi-pod outpatient clinic

- An instrument trolley
- Curtain
- A mirror
- A washbasin
- Containers

Limited surgical treatment under local anaesthesia is carried out here.

Special Facilities

- An ECG room of 20m^2 size
- In Opthalamic outpatient units

An additional examination room of 10m^2 size is needed for perimetry, slit lamp, etc. A room of 25 m^2 would adequately serve two refrectionists

- For an orthoptist a room of 12 m^2 equipped with desk, chairs, synotophose test types , and less screens
- In ENT, a sound insulated room of 6 m^2 for audiometer tests
- In Psychiatric outpatient units a room of 20m^2 for EEG machine

- A sample collection room or clinical chemistry room for blood and urine testing

Dental Clinic

- The first dental treatment room 18 m^2 waiting space is needed for each additional 6 m^2
- The operatory should not be less than 4.2 m wide and 3.6 m deep to accommodate the equipment and to leave space for movement of staff.
- 16 m^2 is recommended as a fully satisfactory size for the dental treatment room
- Suction, hot and cold water as well as sediment basins for plaster and wax
- A desk and a chair
- A recovery room of 7 m^2
- A work room mainly for adjusting and polishing of dentures should be equipped with a sink, work top with fitted cupboards, A room of 6 m^2 should be adequate for 2 operators.
- Separate bays or rooms should be provided for plaster work and polishing work.
- A room of 10 m^2 for Dental office

Ancillary Services

- Injection Room
- Dressing room
- Pharmacy (250 SFT)
- Radiodiagnosis unit
- Outpatient clerical work office, record stores (12 m^2)
- Staff changing rooms, cloak rooms and toilets
- Communal staff room (library, study)
- Catering facilities (10 m^2)

Supply room (Stock of linen, blankets and expendable items) each 10 examination and treatment rooms should be provided with a storage of 9 m^2 size.

Filter or Screening Clinics

All patients visiting OPD do not require care by specialists in the absence of screening, all patients tend to crowd the speciality clinics. Since many ailments can be tackled by House Officers, filter clinics manned by these doctors would be able to relieve congestion on speciality clinic

FURTHER READING

1. Kunders GD, Gopinath S, Katakam A: Hospital Planning, Design and Management Tata McGraw-Hill publishing Co. Ltd New Delhi 1998.
2. Putsep E: Modern Hospital: International Planning Practices Lloyd-Luke Ltd London 1979.
3. Rowland HS, Rowland BL: Hospital Management: A Guide to Departments. An Aspen Publication. Maryland, USA, 1984.
4. Sakharkar BM: Principles of Hospital Administration and Planning. Jaypee Brothers: Delhi 1998.

OPERATING DEPARTMENT

PLANNING PATIENT-FOCUSSED SURGICAL SUITE SYSTEM

Special care facilities in hospitals distinguish today's hospital from those of former decades. Many hospital care costs can be largely attributed to such facilities, generally the highest cost centers of any hospital. Technological advances, better understanding of physiological processes in the human body, and analysis of patient care requirements have resulted in quantum improvements in instrumentation and equipment which, in turn, necessiate special facilities.

With the advent of newer drugs, cardiac monitors, better anesthetic drugs and equipment, open heart surgery, neurological surgery, transplant surgery, joint replacement surgery, foetal surgery, cardiac pacemakers, laparascopes, etc., the percentage of surgical admission has substantially increased (from 30-40% in 1970s to more than 60% during the last decade of 20th century). Advances in technology have provided more precise monitoring of vital functions besides accurate and prompt diagnostic and therapeutic facilities.

These advances save lives and further broaden surgical horizons by helping poor-risk patients to withstand major definitive surgery through preoperative conditioning and postoperative therapeutic support. In light of many recent changes, programming and planning of special-care facilities must now be made on the basis of system analysis, and projections from a detailed programme that precisely defines the needs of a given hospital, the type of equipment and support services required, and the projected workload.

Proper application of programming methods to the design of a surgical suite requires a thorough understnading of the design criteria that are important to proper sizing and arrangement of the area.

The operating room system complex consists of four main systems:

- Surgical support system (the environment)
- Traffic and commerce (the activities)
- Communication and information (the record)
- Administration (the management).

By appropriate meshing and balance of these systems, the surgery is performed on the patients.

Basic Requirement for Design

- The design and performance criteria of the suite must be determined and defined for a given institution.
- The objectives of the surgical discipline of the institution must be kept in mind.
- A sensible traffic pattern should be provided.
- Specific requests of individual specialities should be given every consideration.
- Decisions must be made regarding location of the surgical suite in relation to other services (laboratories, surgical in patient areas, imaging department, etc).
- Caution should be exercised in design planning to accomodate fixed equipment. It is desirable

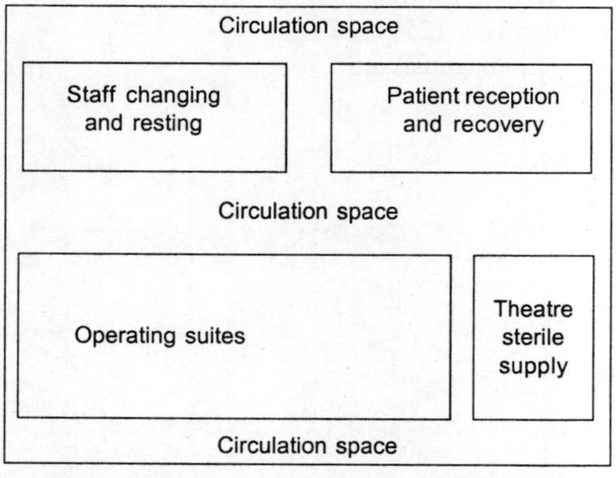

Fig. 34.11: Diagrammatic representation of an operating department showing optimum relationship between various functional zones

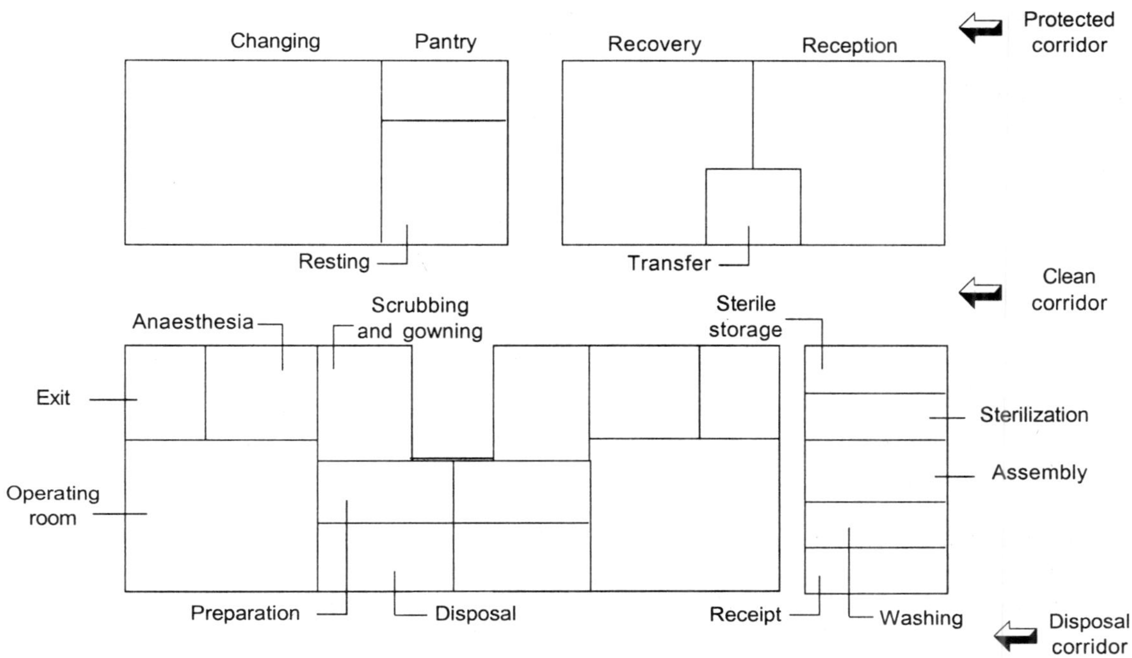

Fig. 34.12: Diagramatic representation of an ideal operating department showing breakup of each functional zone into facilities

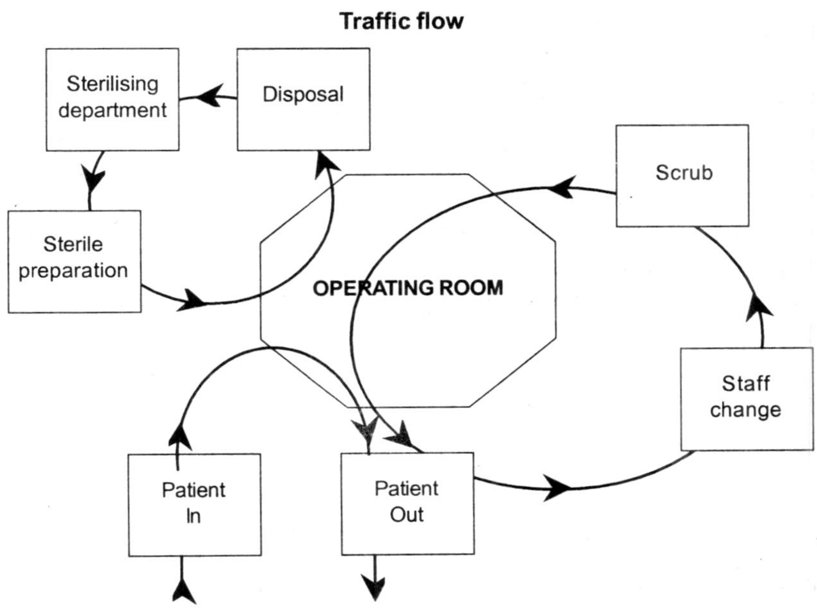

Fig. 34.13: Medic modular operating theatre showing traffic flows

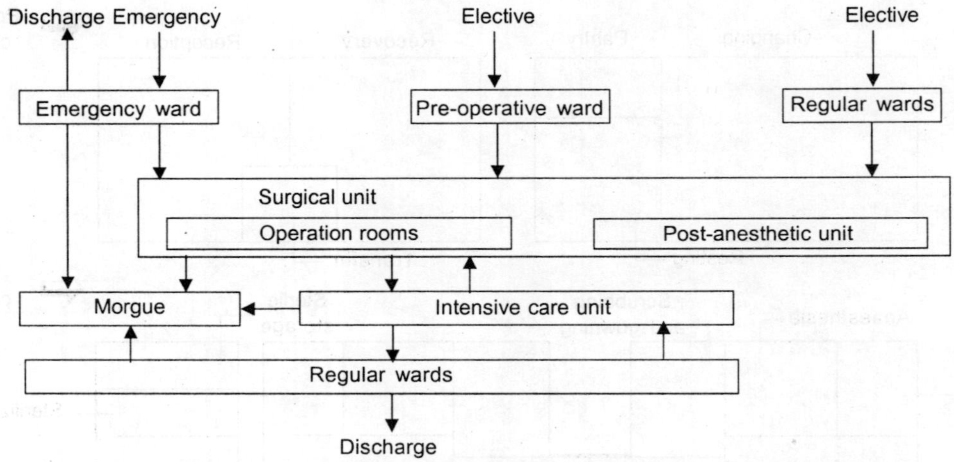

Fig. 34.14: Patient movements in the course of surgical operations

that the design provide for ease of installing and changing fixed equipment.

- Scope for further expansion and flexibility.

Utilization Analysis

The determination of the number of operating rooms, recovery beds, and all other support facilities is essential for the design of surgical suite. This involves a re view of surgical scheduling methods, instrument, sterilization techniques, storage space utilization, and equipment utilization. The planning factors that influence surgical suite size can be identified by hospital size, the proprtion of surgical beds in the hospital, and the types of patients seen in the hospital. Bed occupancy rate also affects size.

Planning Criteria

Functional Criteria

The design of the operating suites must follow the functional requirement of the operating department.

Ergonomic or Workflow Criteria

The flow of the patients, supplies and staff in an operating department is to be conceived and preplanned. This will ensure optimisation of relationship between various functional areas of the operating departments.

Environmental Criteria

The environmental aspects should also be considered for the safety and comfort of the patient and staff.

Planning Considerations

The essential planning considerations while designing an operating department are:

Zoning

It is universally agreed that surgery is to be performed under the most aseptic conditions. To ensure this aseptic condition, the operating department is divided into four distinct zones: protective zone, clean zone, sterile zone and disposal zone.

These zones are bacteriological zones of varying degrees of cleanliness. The bacteriological count diminishes from the outer to the inner zones. Hundred percent sterility must be ensured in the sterile zone. The zoning of the operating department has the following advantages:

- Minimises risk of hospital infection.
- Minimises unproductive movement of staff, supplies and patients.

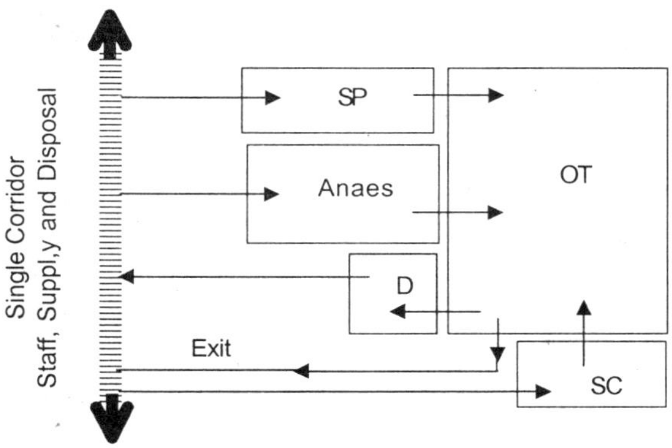

Fig. 34.15a: Suite with anesthetic room with or without shared facilities

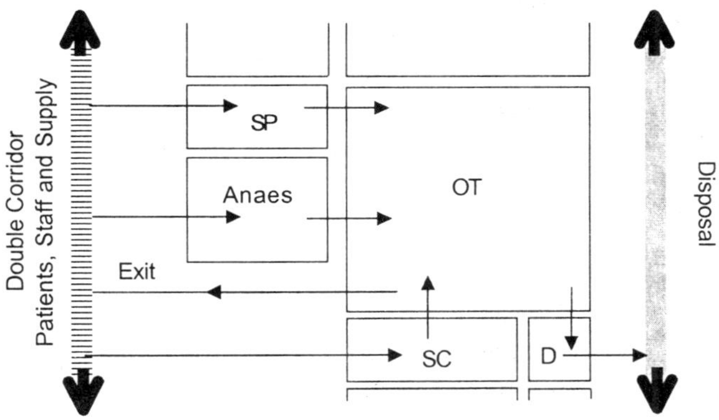

Fig. 34.15c: Suite with anesthetic room with or without shared facilities

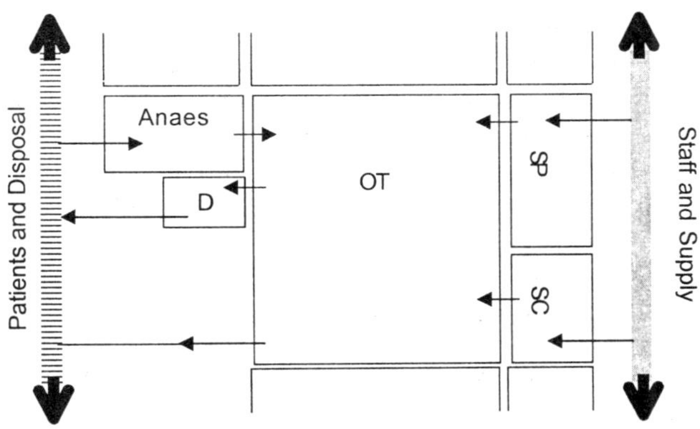

Fig. 34.15e: Suite with anesthetic room with or without shared facilities

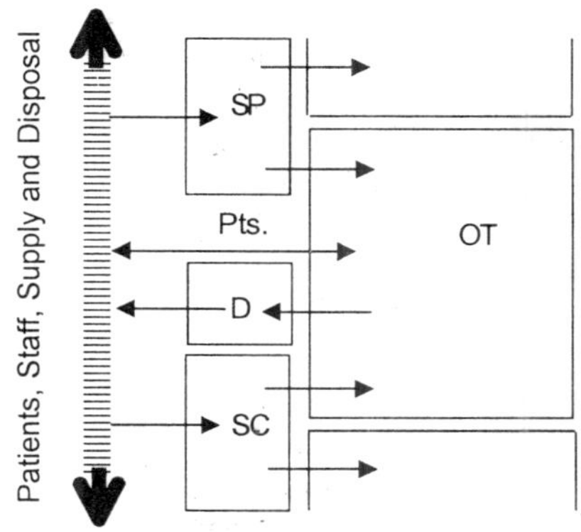

Fig. 34.15b: Suite without anesthetic room with shared facilities

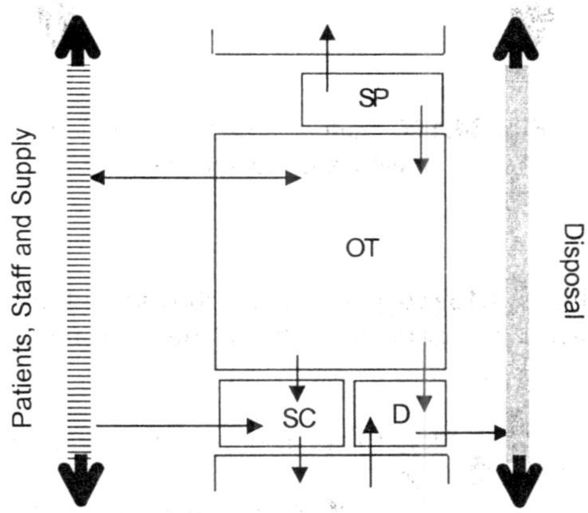

Fig. 34.15d: Suite without anesthetic room with shared facilities

- Increases efficiency of staff working in the operating suites.
- Ensures smooth workflow.
- Reduces hazards in the operating suites.
- Ensures proper positioning of the equipments.
- Ensures optimum utilization of the operating states.

Scales of Accommodations

1. *Protective zone* It usually provides facilities like (i) reception (ii) waiting room for patients relatives (iii) changing rooms (iv) autoclave (vii) trolley bay (viii) control area of electicity.

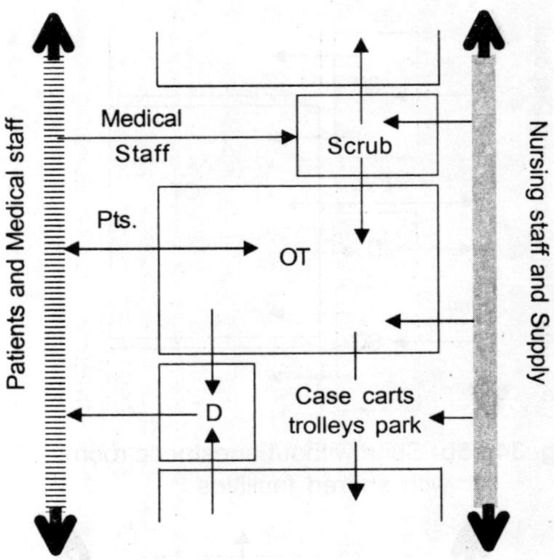

Fig. 34.15f: Suite without anesthetic room with shared facilities

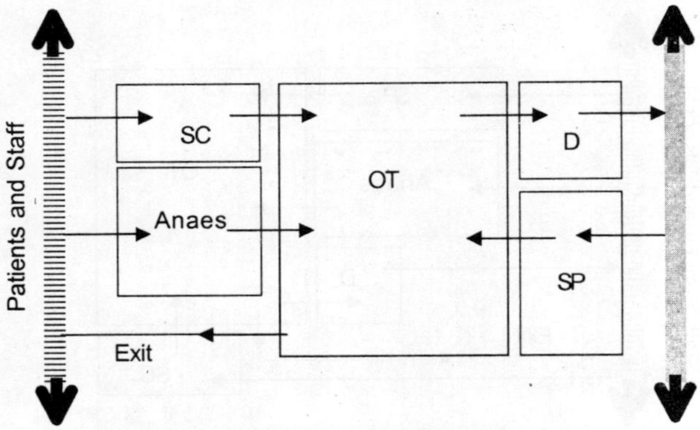

Fig. 34.15g: Suite with anesthetic room with or without shared facilities

Keys:

Pts.	Patients
OT	Operating Theatre
Anaes	Anesthetic Room
SP	Supply and Trolley Prep Room
SC	Scrub and Gowning
D	Disposal

Figs 34.15a to g: Illustration shows number of different ways of organising traffic in the main corridors

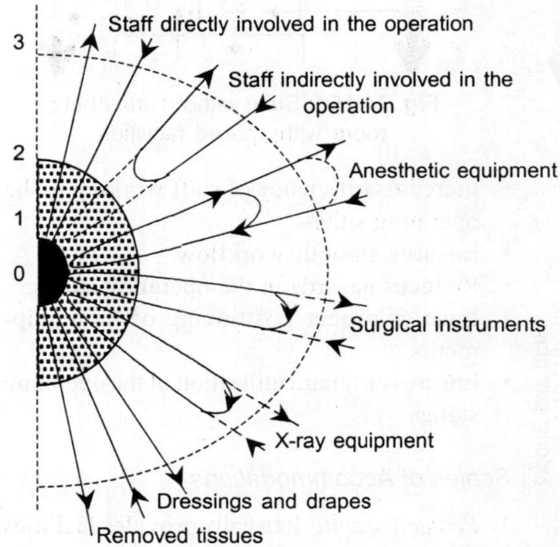

Fig. 34.16: Circulation in the cleanliness zones of an operation room. 0—aseptic zone; 1—ultra clean zone; 2—super clean zone; and 3—clean zone

2. *Clean zone* It provides facilities such as (i) pre-operating room (ii) recovery room (iii) theatre work room (iv) plaster room (v) blood storage and frozen section room (vi) plaster room (v) blood storage and frozen section room (vi) X-ray unit with dark room (vii) nurse's duty room (viii) doctor's work room (ix) anesthesia store.
3. *Sterile zone* This zone has facilities like (i) operating room (ii) scrub room (iii) anesthesia room (iv) instrument sterlization and trolly area.
4. *Disposal zone* This zone provides facilities like (i) dirty wash-up room (ii) disposal corridor (iii) Janiter's closet.

Number of Operating Suites

The number of operation theatres required for a particular hospital can be worked out by studying in great detaile the following factors which are more or less quantifiable.

Principle of air flow

↓

Lay up and operating theatre

↓

Scrub room anesthetic room, Clean movement, Clean rest area, sterile store

↓

Transfer, Changing rooms, Recovery plaster room

↓

Disposal and Dirty movement

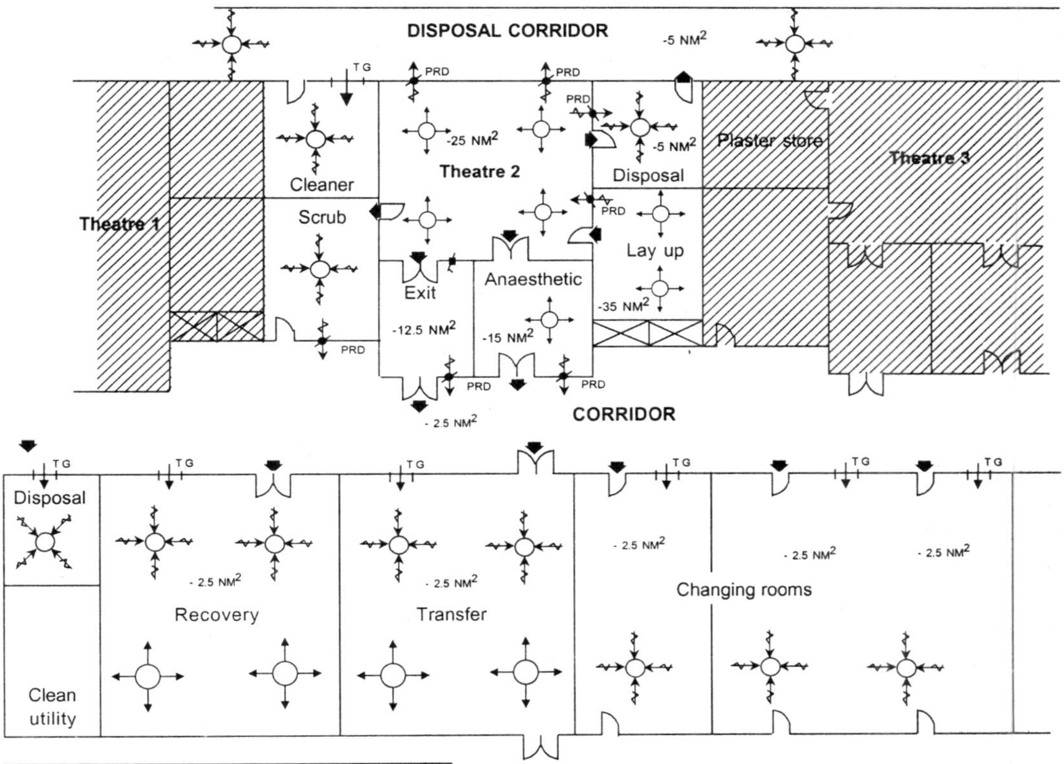

TG – Through grille

PDR – Pressure relief damper (Operates when doors are closed)

Supply diffuser

Extract diffuser

Direction of air flow

NM² Newton/Metre²

Typical airflow pattern for a theatre suite

Fig. 34.17: Standard theatre air flow

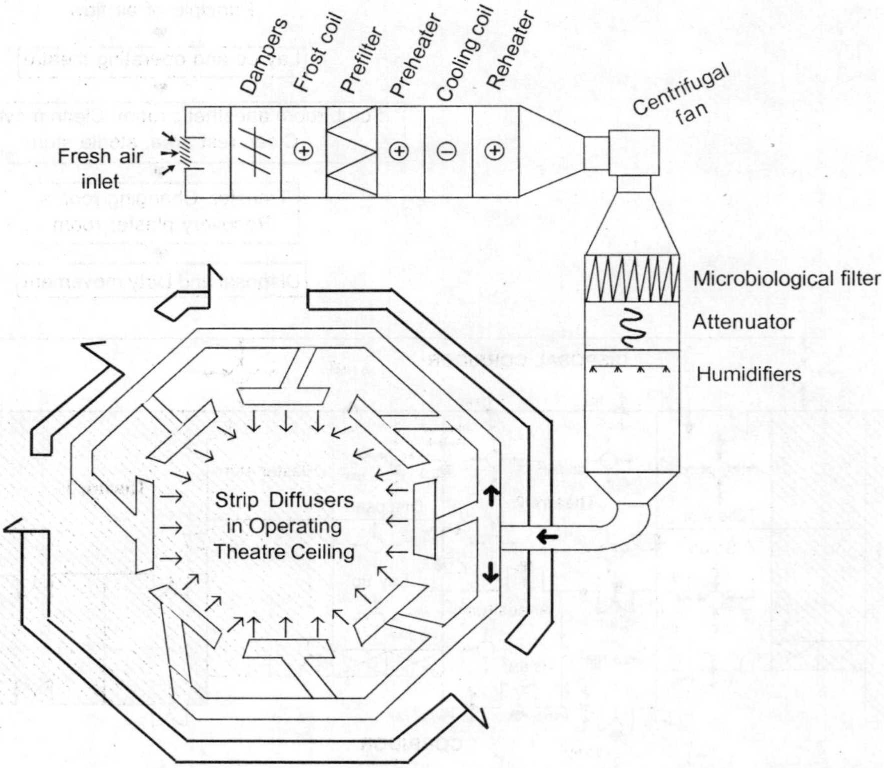

Fig. 34.18: Diagrammatic arrangement of filtered/treated air flow in medic modular operating theatre

- Number and type of surgeons
- Type of hospital
- Hospital policy and procedures
- Hospital bed complement
- Number and nature of elective and emergency surgery anticipated
- Number and type of surgical patients
- Number of operations per day
- Expected average length of stay of surgical patients
- Expected turn over interval in operation theatre
- Size of an average OT list
- Average time of operation
- Estimated time for cleaning between operations
- Time allowed for staff breaks
- Time allowed for maintenance of OT
- Amount of time operating suites can be equipped and staff available for use
- Amount of time reserved for emergency use
- Allowance for septic patients.

However, the number of operating suites can be conveniently worked out from the number of operations per day and number of hospital beds.

i. Number of operating suites and number of operations per day:

The number of operating suites can be found out from the predicted number of operations per day. The predicted number of operations can be calculated by dividing the number of surgical beds by the ALS (average length of stay) of surgical patients. Similarly, the number of operations per day.

$$\frac{\text{No. of surgical beds} \times \text{percent of BOR} \times 365}{\text{ALS} \times 100 \times \text{No. of working days in that hospital}}$$

The number of operations, which can be performed in each operating suite can be deter-

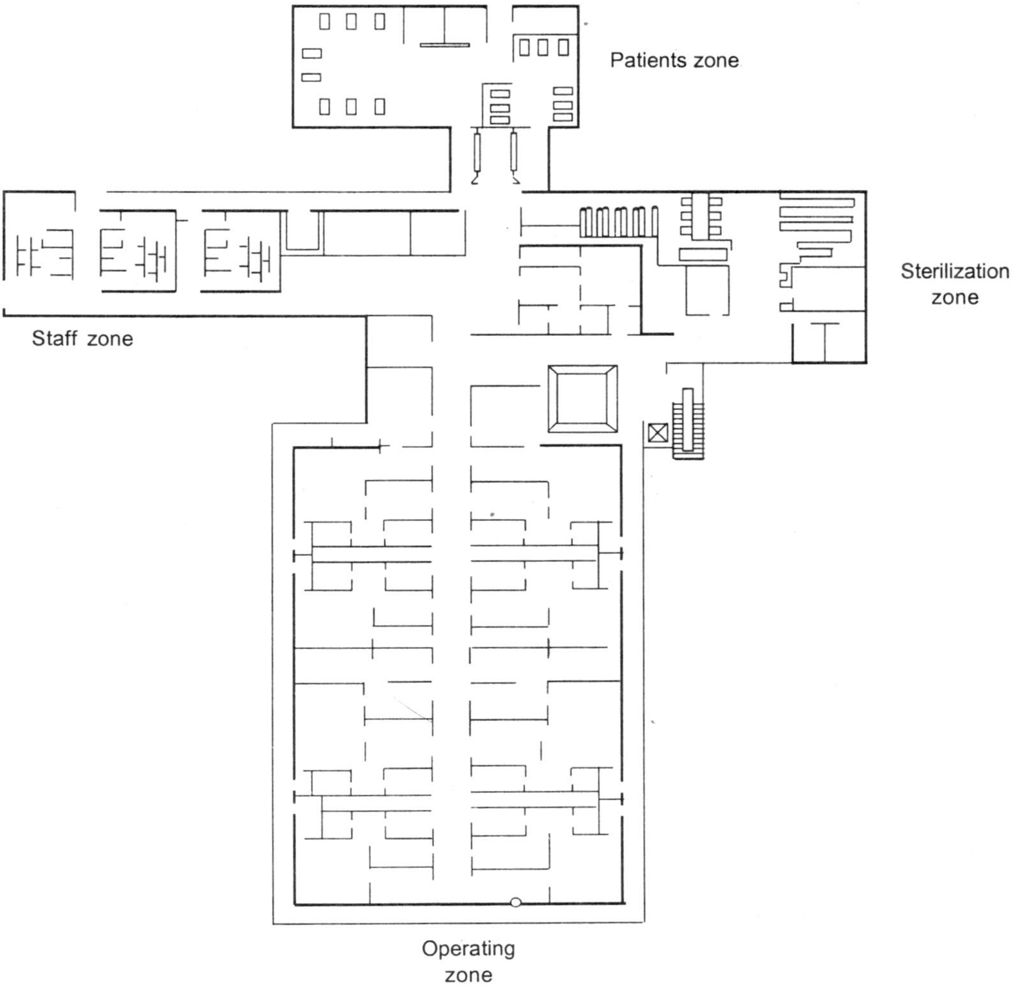

Fig. 34.19: Layout of operating department of a six hundred bed tertiary-care teaching hospital

mined by studying past trends and by conducting work studies or by making use of available standard norms. American authorities calculate one operating suite for two or three operations per day, while European authorities recommend that a minimum of six operations should be performed per day in one operating suite.

ii. Number of operating suites and hospital beds: According to American pattern, one operating suite is required for every 25 surgical beds while Europen authorities recommend one operating suite for every 50 surgical beds. Rao Committee (1968) recommended one operation theatre for every 50 surgical beds. However, the Committee On Planned Projects (COPP-1964) has given the following guidelines.

	Indoor	*Outdoor*	*Emergency*	
Number of Beds	*Minor*	*Major*	*Major*	*Minor*
300	2	3	—	1
500	2	5	1	1
750	2	8	1	1
1000	2	10	1	1

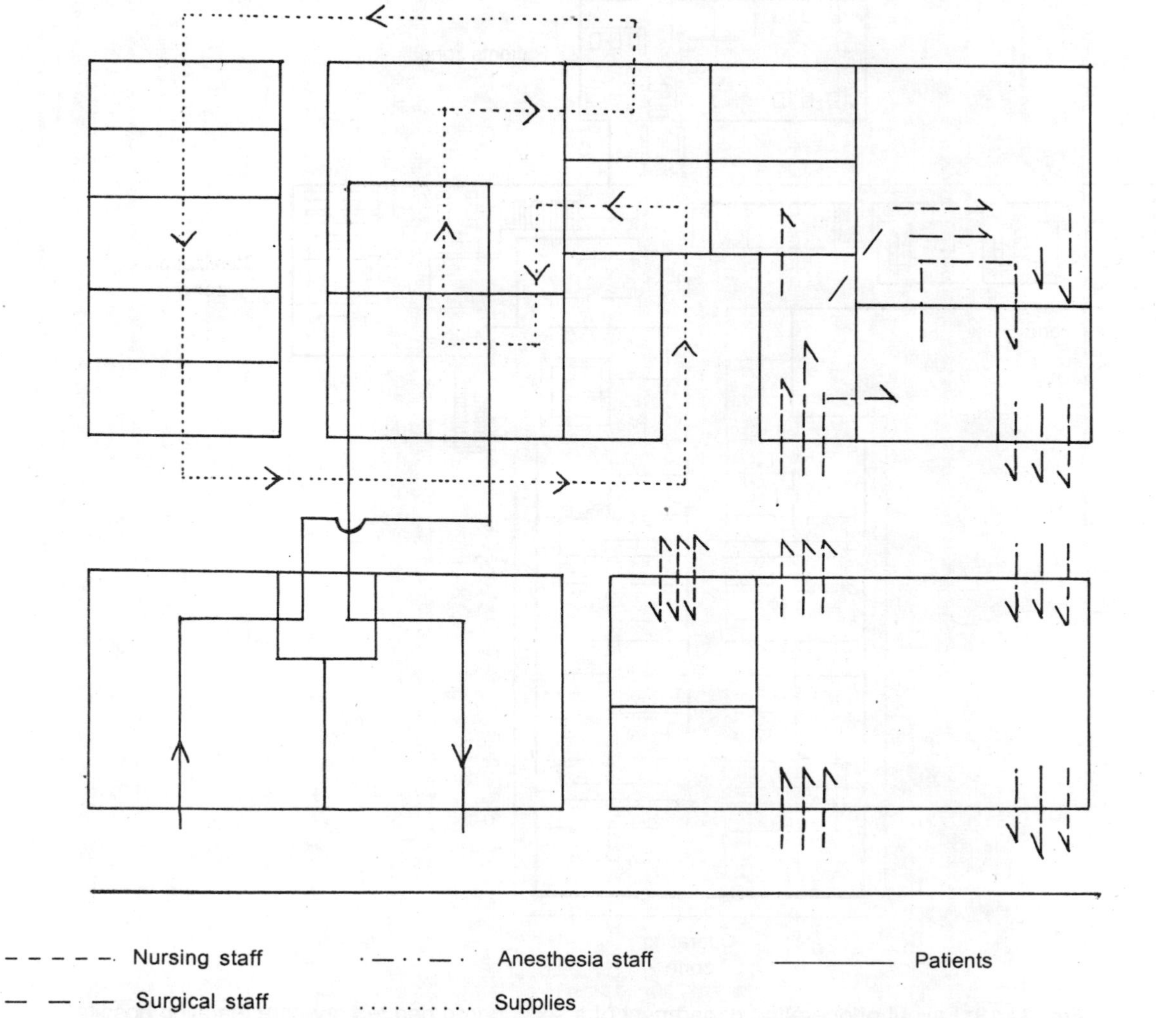

Fig. 34.20: Diagrammatic representation of flow of work through various functional zones of an operating department

Grouping of Operating Theatres

The centralization of major operating suites in one area to form a single surgical theatre complex has got definite advantage over individual operating theatre disturbuted close to the various surgical wards. These advantags are:

- Maximum flexibility in use
- Easy expansion at times of future demands
- Simplifies theatre staffing and better training centralization and standardization of procedures improving efficiency.
- Economic in common facilities such as men, material, machines and minutes.
- Flexibility in allocation of operating suites to various specialities
- Minimises infection and cross-infection
- Improves utilisation of operating suites

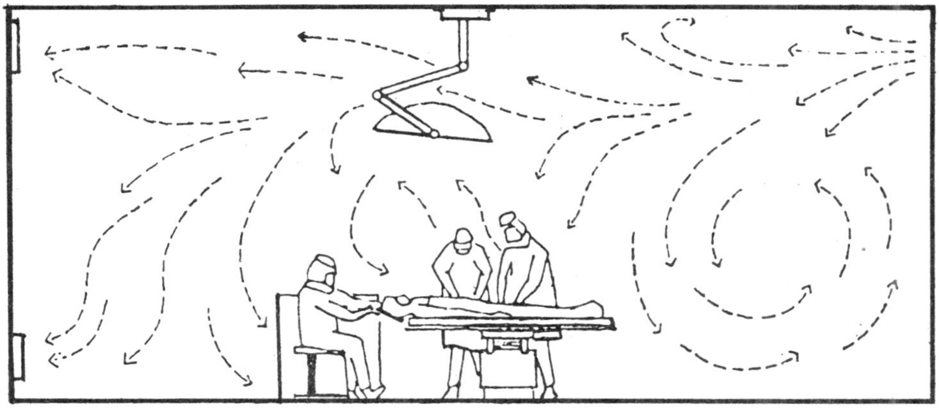

Fig. 34.21: Turbulent or mixing air distribution system

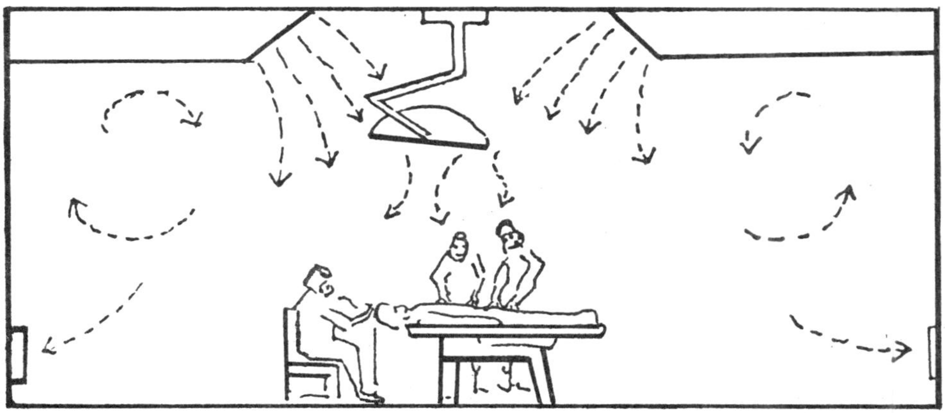

Fig. 34.22: Downward displacement piston air distribution system

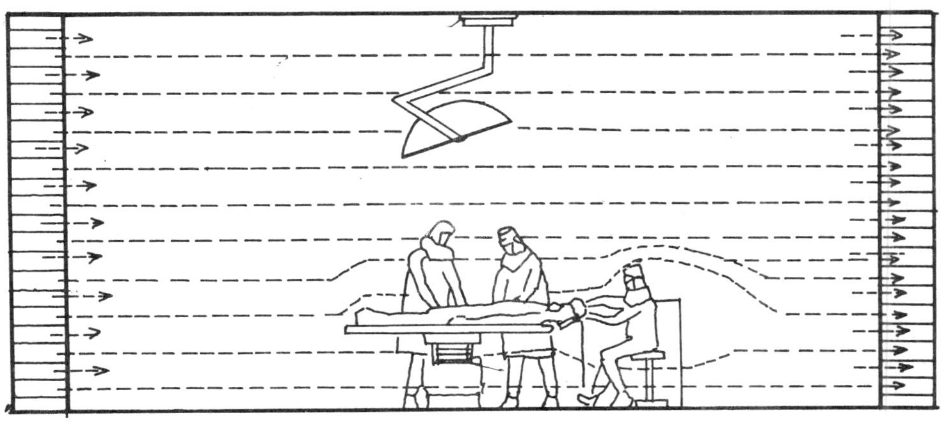

Fig. 34.23: Unidirectional horizontal air distribution system

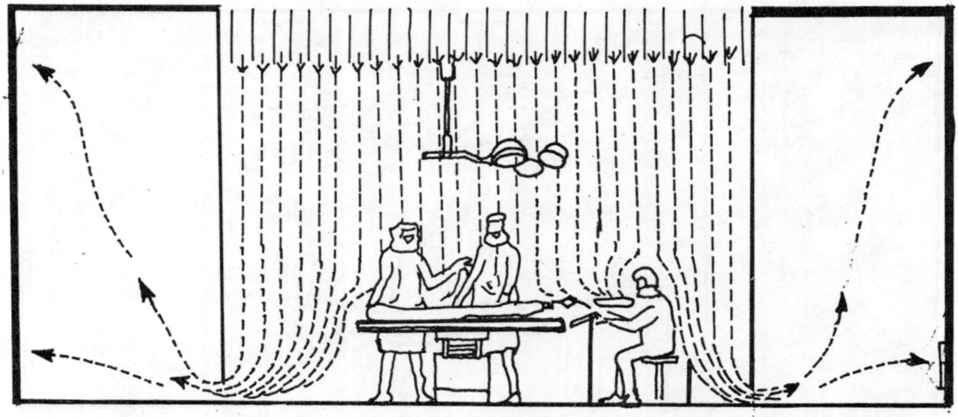

Fig. 34.24: Undirectional downflow air distribution system with partial wall enclosure

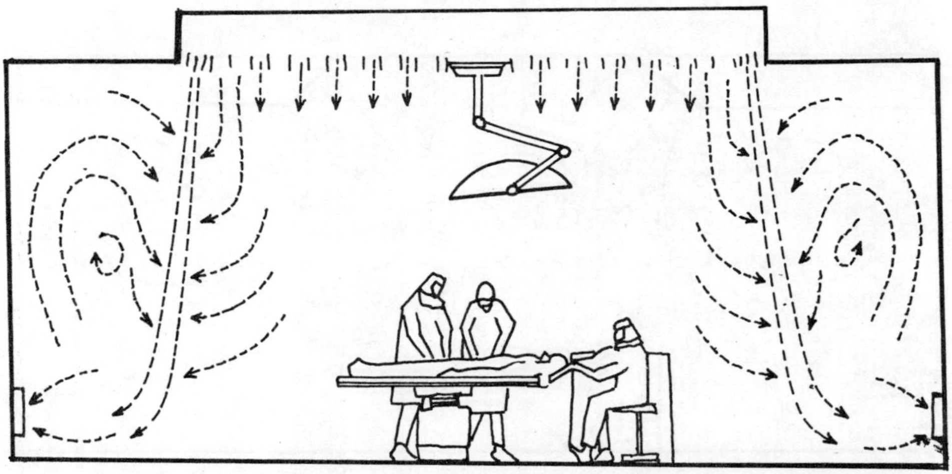

Fig. 34.25: Undirectional downflow air distribution system with air curtain

- Improves efficiency of staff
- Minimises cancellation of operating schedules.

Location

The location of operating suites is dictated by the number of suites to be provided. If the number of suites is more than six, it is better to distribute them into two locations. The operation theatre complex can be conveniently located in the ground floor. Sitting on other floors adds to design and communication problems. The operating department should be easily accessible to the Central Sterile Supply Department (CSSD)/Theatre Sterile Supply Unit (TSSU), emergency department and surgical wards. It should be independent of general traffic and should have maximum protection from sun, heat, noice, dust and wind. However, the most recent concept is that operating suites can be located anywhere as the atmosphere and environment of operating suites are under controlled conditions.

Size

The size of an operating suite should be restricted to what is functionally optimum. Large size

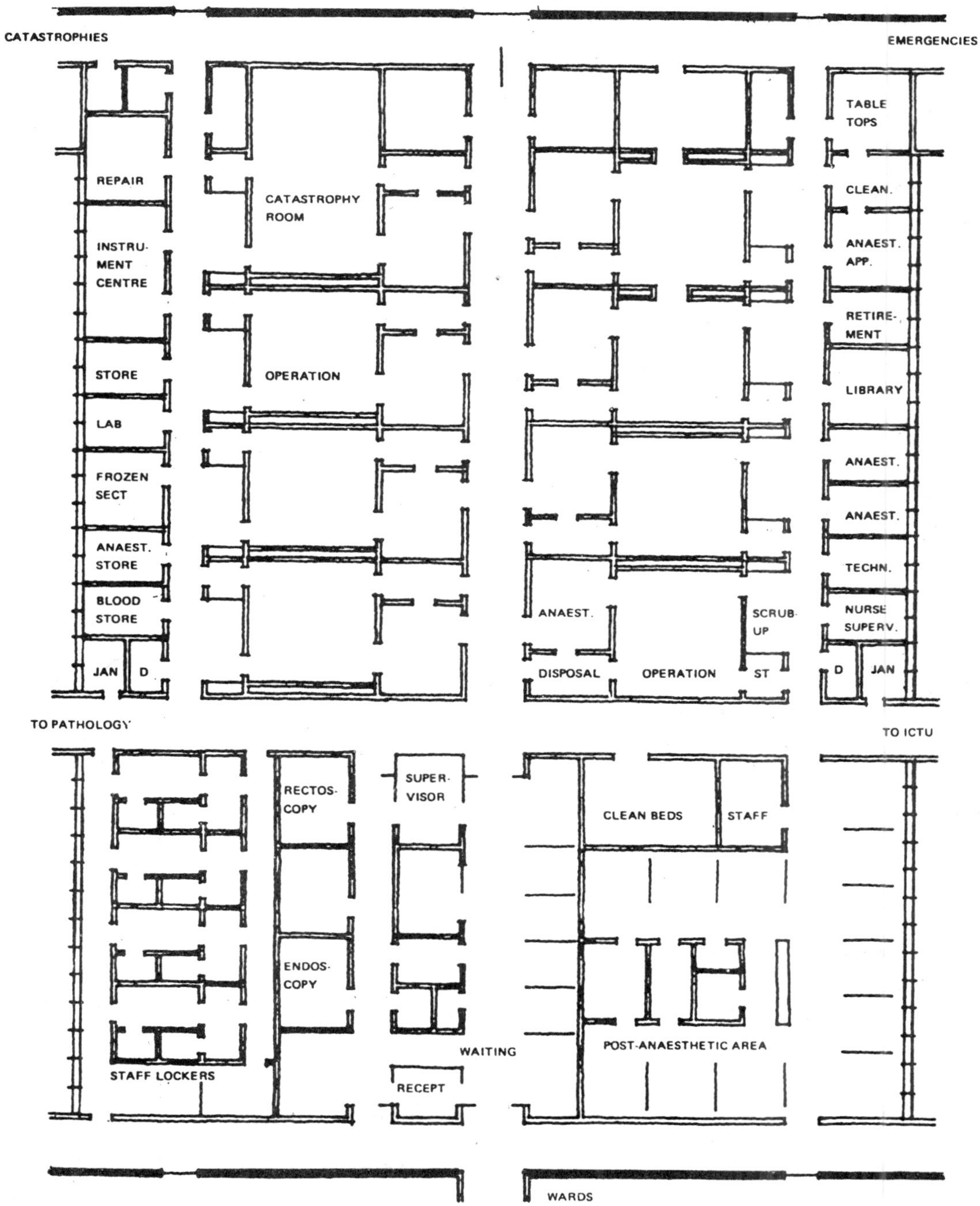

Fig. 34.26: Surgical department with 9 operation rooms, a section for endoscopies and a post-operative area for 12 patients. Pütsep International

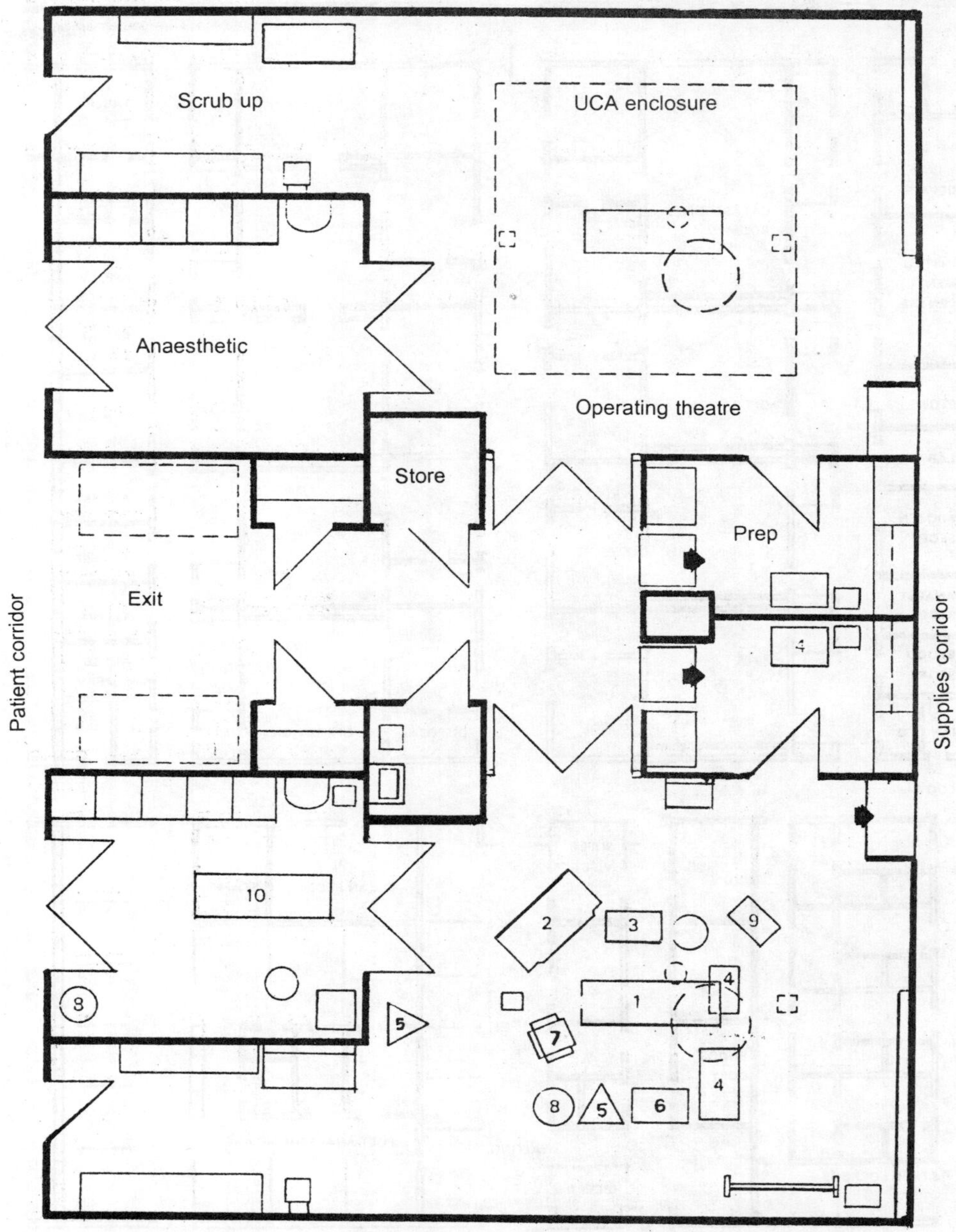

Fig. 34.27: Nucleus Hospital, UK: standard plan of typical twin operating suite showing layout of equipment. Each suite comprises four compartments: operating theatre, anesthetic room, scrub-up and preparation room. Most other countries in Western Europe follow this general arrangement. In recent years many theatres are being equipped with ultra clean air (UCA) enclosures. The use of UCA systems brings into question the need for multi-compartment layouts

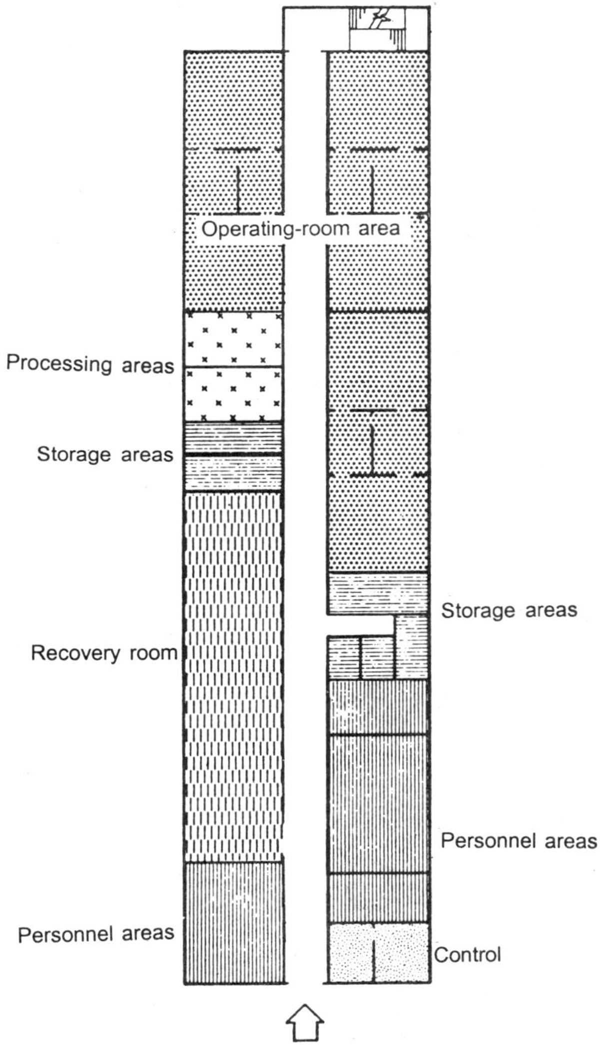

Fig. 34.28: A Single corridor layout extends the circulation distances. Control is more difficult, the corridor tends to be congested, and there is a greater danger of contamination. If the suite must cross the entrance or an elevator area, control of traffic and of contamination is still more difficult

operation suites give rise to problems in airconditioning, washing and cleaning. The size considered optimum is 18 × 18. In any case, it should not be more than 20 × 20. All operating suites should be of standard size and uniform design.The design should be flexible for use for general surgery. However, cardiothoracic and neurosurgery may require operating rooms of 500-600 square feet to accommodate large surgical team and special equipment.

Workflow

The assumption that "clean" and "dirty" streams of traffic should be segregated to control infections within the department is no longer justifiable. Recent research by the Department of Health and Social Security, UK, has proved that there is little difference in infection rates.

Whether one segregates "clean" and "dirty" traffic or not, there should be an efficient air handling system always. Staff discipline and traffic congestion normally determine single and double corridor systems.

Single Corridor System

Here all traffic: patients, staff, supply and disposal are circulated through a single corridor. This workflow requires a high degree of staff discipline. It is essential to have proper bagging of dirty instruments, dirty linen and disposable items and to clear away from the disposal room, out of the operating department, after each case.

Before the start of the operating session, a supply of sterilized instrument packs is delivered to each suite's supply room to cover the full session in order to minimise trolley traffic within the department.

The single corridor system is the most economical and efficient given good staff discipline standards, not only from the medical/nursing but also from ancillary staff. In the USA, the majority of hospitals are built this way; in UK recent hospitals, also, have adopted the single corridor system.

Double Corridor System

There are various schools of thought on which types of traffic should be segregated, depending

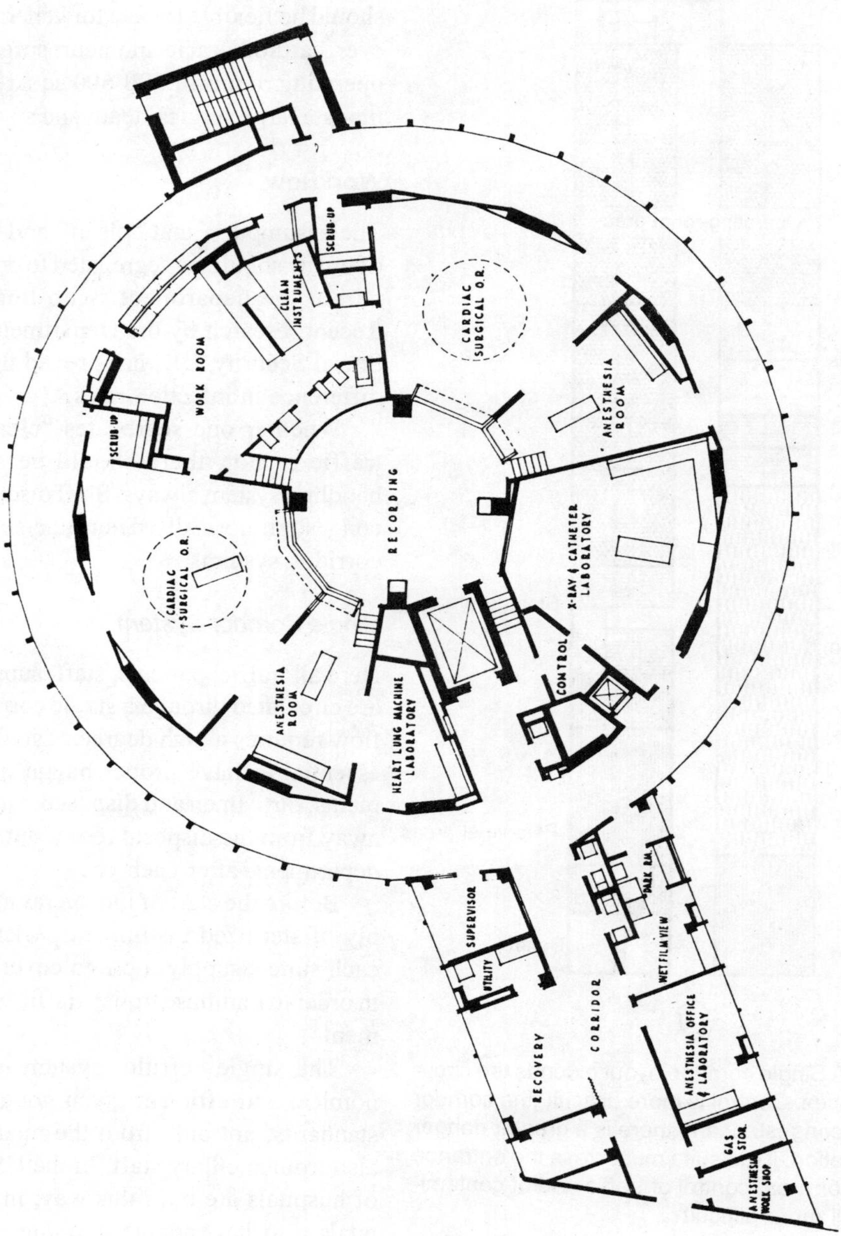

Fig. 34.29: Round plan is well adapted for small suite. (Cardiac Surgery Theaters at National Institutes of Health, Bethesda, Md.) This unit is for cardiac surgery with neurosurgery on another floor. Overhead observation behind glass and directly over the table is indicated by dotted lines

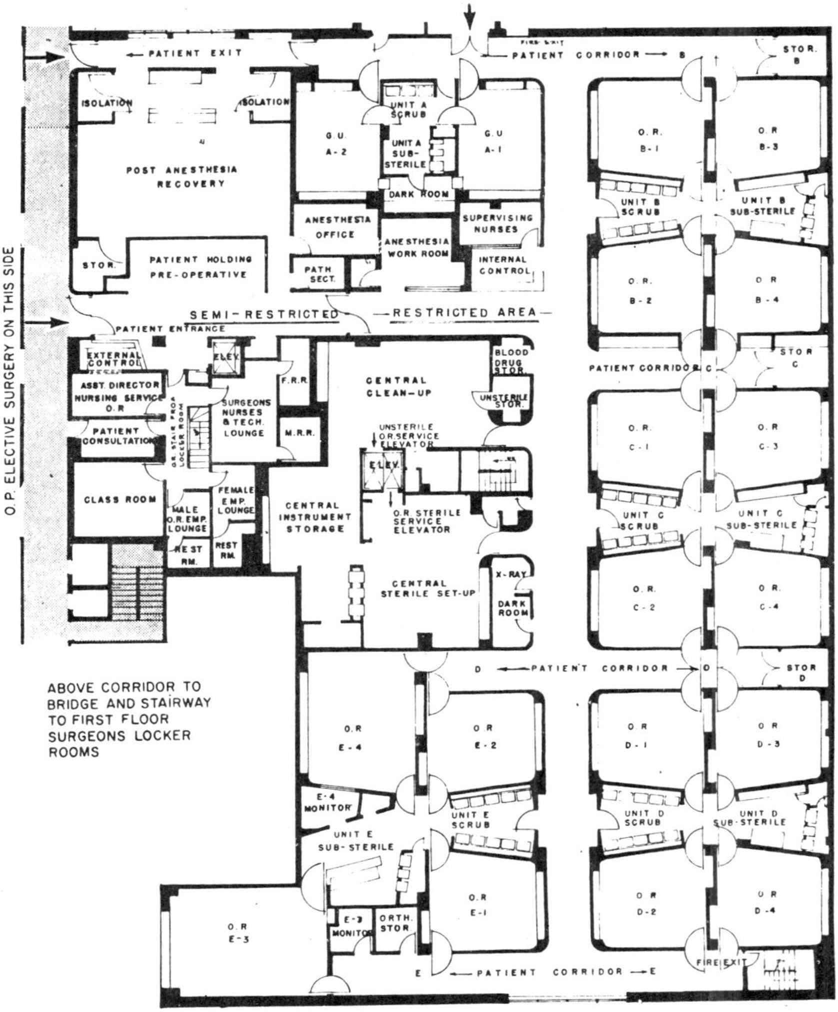

Fig. 34.30: At Michael Reese Hospital, Chicago, most of the eighteen new second-floor operating rooms are grouped in units of four, permitting surgeons to move readily from one room to another. Two rooms are 500 sq ft in size, with monitor satellite rooms. The nerve center is the central work area, with a central sterile setup, and sterile supply in the basement. Change areas for the surgeons and nurses, and the frozen section laboratory, are on the first floor. Note separate patient corridors. An outpatient surgical unit (on the left) is separate from the main suite. An intricate intercom system on the floor permits ready communication, replacing considerable movement of individuals with its associated contamination hazard

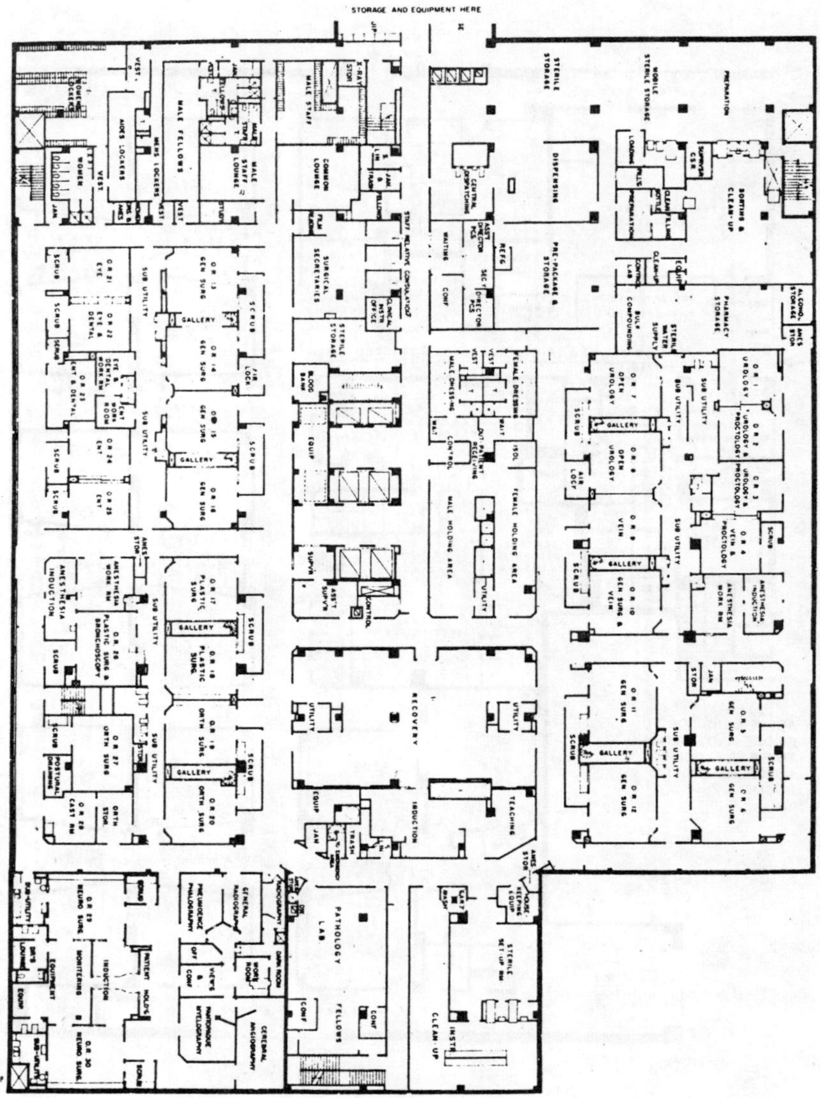

Fig. 34.31: At Rochester (Minn.) Methodist Hospital and fine suite of thirty operating rooms has a peripheral corridor for doctors and patients with a central corridor or subutility for the nursing staff. Several of the rooms are especially large. Male and female holding rooms are also large. Neurosurgery, cerebral angiography, and myelography have a separate suit (lower right). Elevator access is central and recovery is closeby

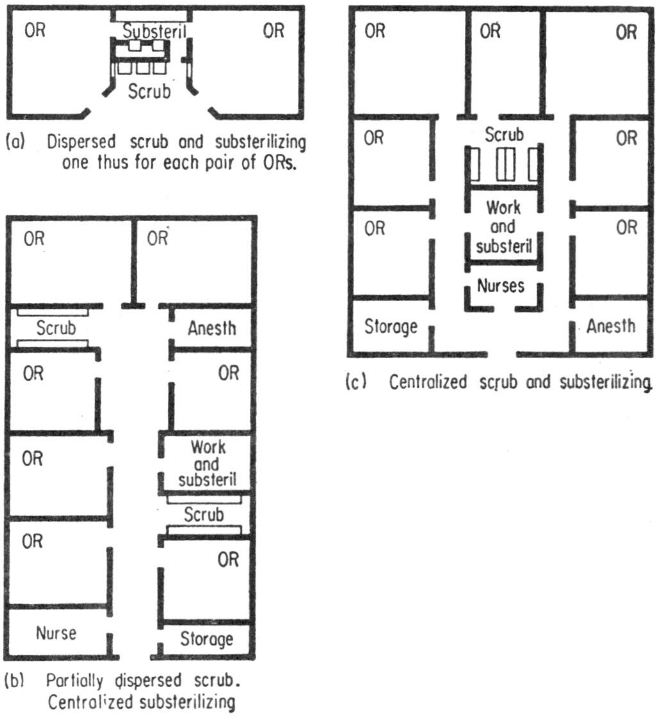

(a) Dispersed scrub and substerilizing one thus for each pair of ORs.

(b) Partially dispersed scrub. Centralized substerilizing

(c) Centralized scrub and substerilizing

Fig. 34.32: Scrub and substerilizing arrangements

upon the country and users' cultural behavior. The following types of traffic are most commonly in use:

Disposal traffic Here, patients, staff and supply traffic are segregated from disposal traffic. In the UK and most of the developing countries, the majority of hospitals built during the past 40 years have used this style.

It is still the most suitable system where it might be difficult to achieve a good standard of staff discipline especially from the ancillary staff here, by locating the disposal holdingroom in the outer zone of the department, the dirty items can be collected at regular intervals—or after each session—by ancillary staff of the CSSD or TSSU without entering the inner zone.

Patients and disposal traffic This system segregates patients and disposal from staff and supplies; it was developed by Mr E Pütsep of Sweden during the seventies and it is commonly used in Scandinavia and Germany. The discipline of clearing away used items from the disposal/exit bay after each surgical procedure is of the utmost importance.

Patients and staff traffic This plan segregates patients and staff from supplies and disposal traffic. The principle here is to separate trolley traffic from patients and staff areas to minimise traffic congestion. Some hospitals in the UK and the USA have been built following this system and they seem to work remarkably well.

Type of Suites

The first question to be considered here is: Is a separate anesthetic room necessary in a modern hospital? The UK and the USA have adopted different approaches to this question: in the USA separate anesthetic rooms were never considered

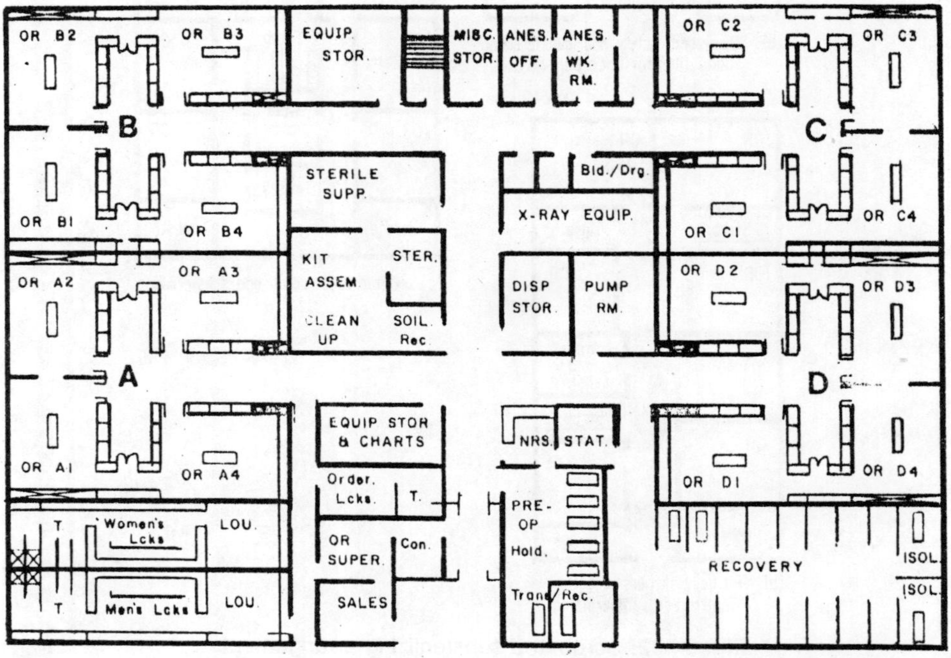

Fig. 34.33: Cluster plan variant for 16 operating rooms in a space allocation far below usual requirements (four clusters A-D). This surgical suite is working remarkably efficiently. Notice vestibular area inside entrance

necessary, while in the UK and Europe it becomes normal practice to provide them.

Separate anesthetic rooms were first introduced in the UK in the 1960s on the assumption that it was desirable, from patient's moral's point of view, to anesthetize him in a separate room rather than in the theatre; it also reduced the theatre's occupancy time. These are minor advantages however, when compared with the huge increase in capital as well as running costs incurred in providing an anesthetic room separate from the theatre. It can hardly be justified on the following grounds:

a. Additional anesthetists (highly trained and highly paid staff) would be required;
b. The area of an anesthetic room would be approximately half the size of the theatre's: this would constitute a considerable increase in the overall departmental area;
c. The additional equipment requirements of the anesthetic room: duplication of anesthetic apparatus, sanitary fittings, storage units, medical gas outlets, etc.
d. Low utilizing factor, as a patient could only be anesthetised a few minutes before surgery. In fact, while the patient is undergoing surgery, the room is not utilized for its proper function. Its major function has now become a patient-holding room while the operating theatre is occupied.

A second question in connection with the types of operating suites deals with the possibility of sharing scrub-areas, supplies and disposal facilities. Here also, different practices have emerged. In the

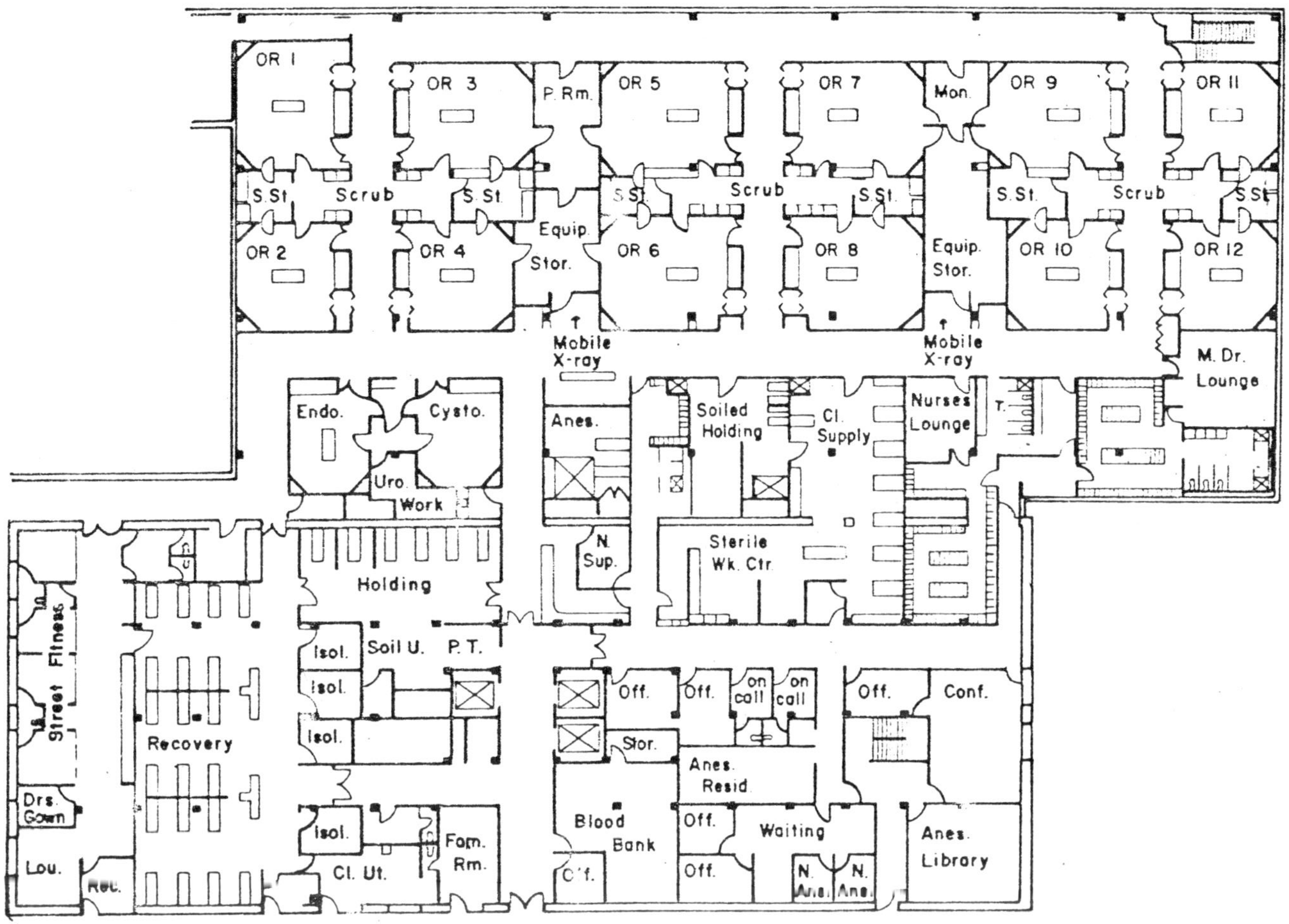

Fig. 34.34: Cluster plan variant for 12 operating rooms surgical suite plus two cystoscopy (or endoscopy) rooms showing wall assembly of door, pass-through cabinets, stretcher alcove, and cabinet for each room. Also shown are relationships between substerile areas and scrub stations within each cluster. Also note location of four isolation cubicles near the nurses' station and the 20 noncubicled beds in the recovery unit. Out-patients will use the street-fitness area after recovery when necessary

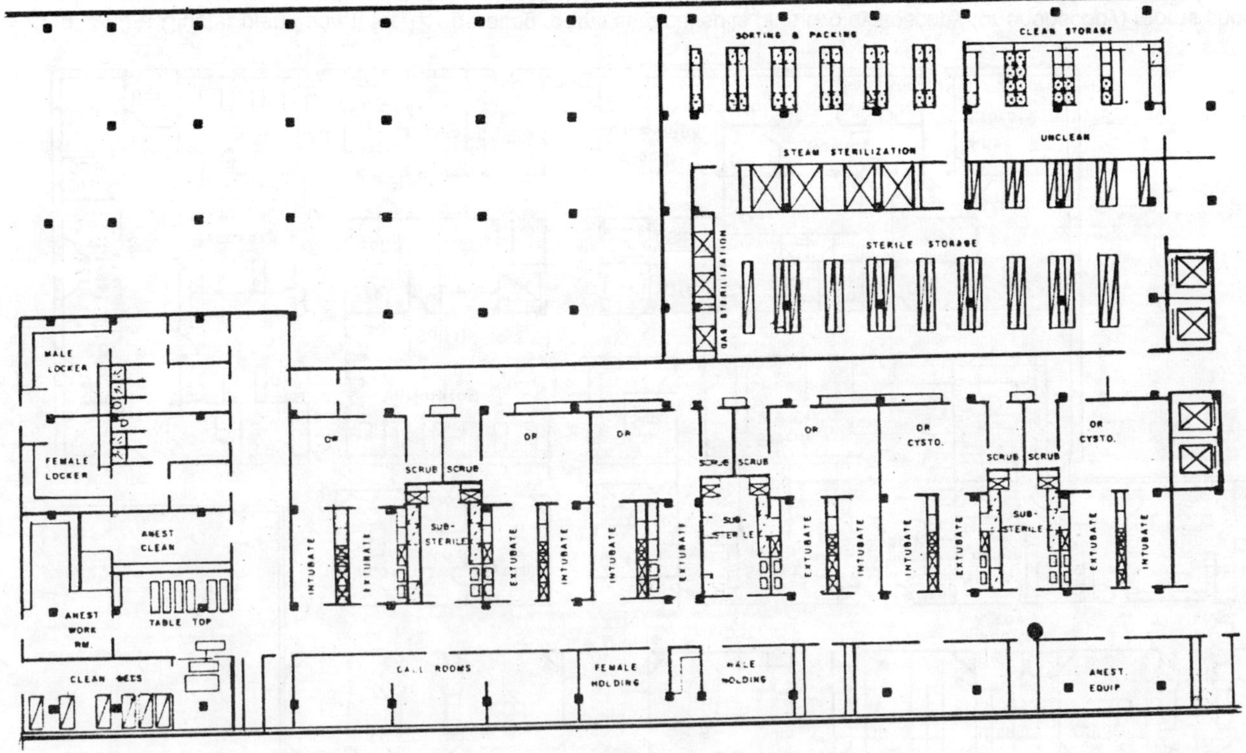

Fig. 34.35: Layout of a European surgical suite showing intubation (also known as preparation or induction rooms) and extubation rooms for every operating room. This double-corridor. Line or scheme occupies almost twice the square footage as it would if it were designed for an American hospital in which case the four operating rooms would be arranged in a cluster with only two induction rooms (if indeed, any) and no extubation rooms. The two cystoscopy rooms could be designed as a pair of rooms sharing a common X-ray control panel. The space allocated to instrument processing and sterile storage would be considered unnecessarily large for a suite of this size

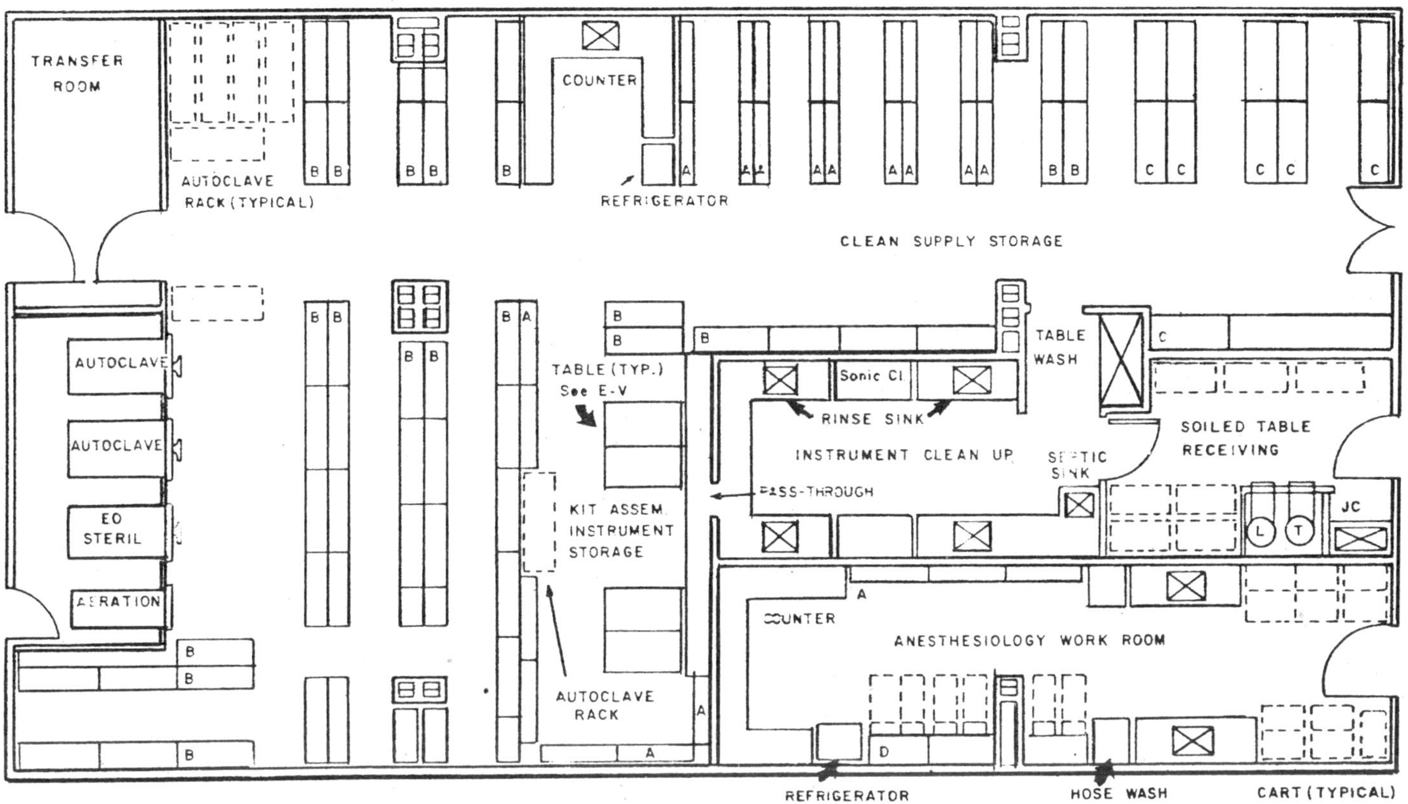

Fig. 34.36: Equipment layout for a typical instrument processing area of a surgical suite. The same type of flow should be maintained in the surgical instrument section of the CSS when the CSS, situated remote from the surgical suite, does all instrument processing for the surgical suite. The only difference is in the distance instruments and supplies must travel to and from the surgical suite. Disadvantages of a remote instrument processing operation are longer turn-around time between operations and the need to purchase many more instruments as compared to locating the surgical instrument processing operation in or near the surgical suite. According to all our studies, the capital expenditure of a sterilizer for the onsite processing area in the surgical suite in addition to the ones in CSS is more economical, by far, than the expenditures for a transport system additional personnel, and poor utilization of operating-room time when the entire instrument processing for the entire hospital is limited to the CSS

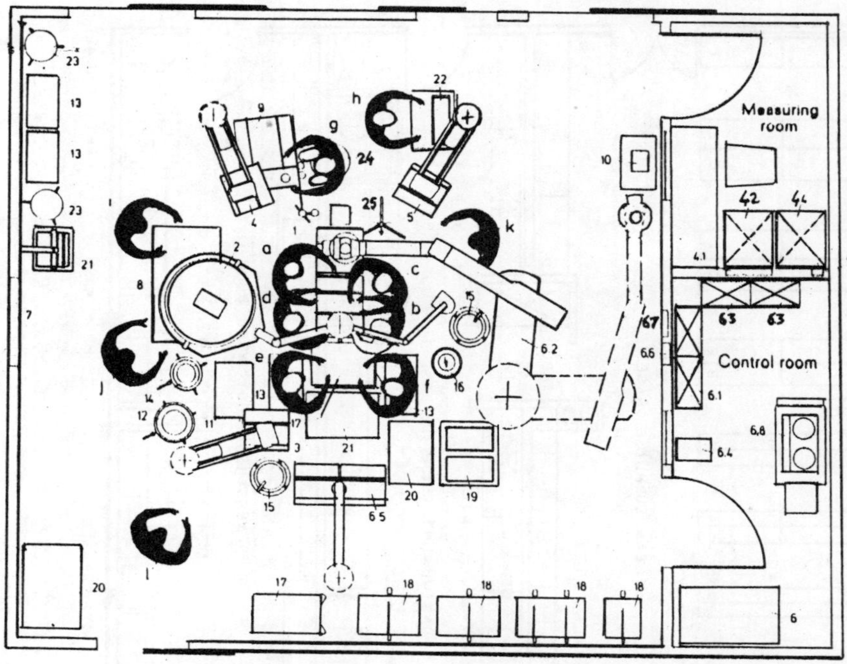

Fig. 34.37: Overhead view of cardiothoracic surgery operating room prepared as a service by equipment manufacturer, showing X-ray unit (6.2) in position of use over operating table. Large videomonitor (6.5) is mounted over foot of operating table. Also shown, electrosurgery unit with gases and power outlets (3), anesthesia monitoring unit with gases and power outlets (4), and cardiotherapy unit containing cardiac pacemaker and high-tension generator (5)

UK, each theatre has its own scrub-room, supply room and disposal room, whereas in the rest of Europe and the USA scrub facilities are provided in an open bay shared between two theatres, the supply room serving a number of theaters on the casecart system; disposal facilities are sometimes shared between two theatres or combined with the exit bay.

The most efficient type of operating suite in terms of maximum utilization of resources as well as the most cost-effective, will display the following characteristics:

a. It will be without a separate anesthetic room
b. It will have shared scrub facilities between theatres
c. It will have a disposal bay or room servicing two theatres
d. It will have a centrally located supply room servicing a number of theatres

- Special fixtures
  - Anesthesia cabinet
  - Instrument storage cabinet
  - Gowning cabinet
  - Scrub station
  - Macerator
  - X-ray viewing
  - Swab count rack
  - Writing board
  - Inter-communication
- Special furniture
  - Instrument trolley
  - Bowl stand
  - Infusion stand
  - Kick about

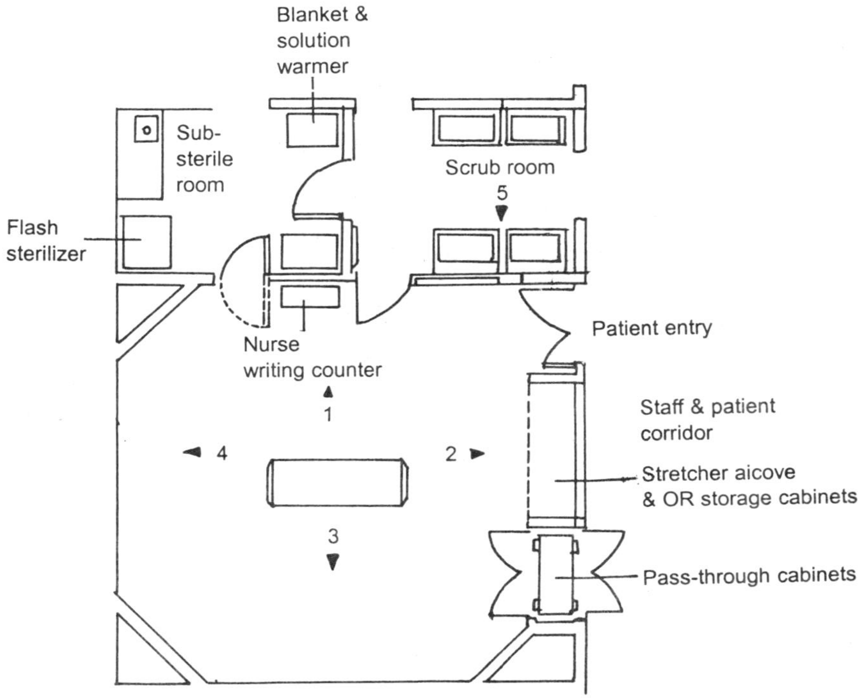

A

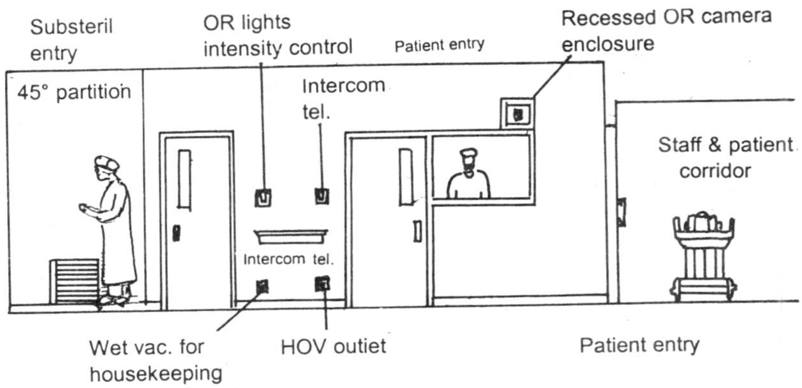

B

Contd...

  - Step stair
  - Disposal bag holder
  - Stool
- Surgical instruments and endoscopes
- CCTV system

ii. Sterilization zone

- Instrument washing/disinfection equipment
- Instrument inspection/repair equipment
- Assembly tables
- Multicycle sterilization equipment
- Sterile storage racks
- Furniture and fixtures

iii. Patient zone

- Patient monitoring and resuscitation equipment

ELEVATION 1

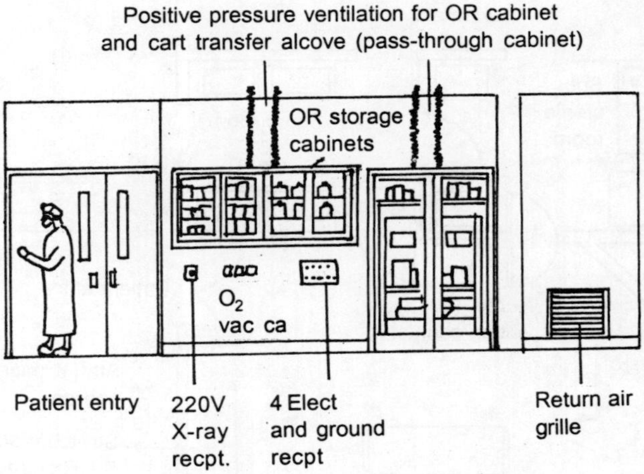

C

ELEVATION 2

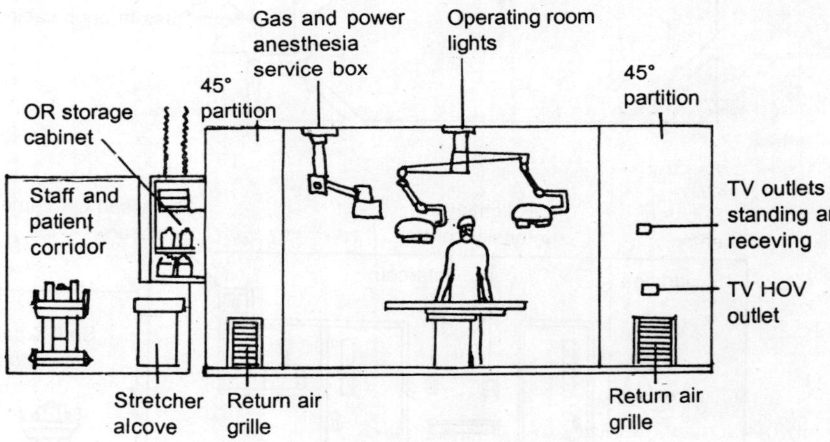

D

Fig. 34.38: (a) Layout of operating room showing wall assembly of door, pass-through cabinet, stretcher alcove, and operating room cabinet, as well as arrangement of scrub station and substerile area between operating rooms, (b) to (d) Elevations of walls of operating room and of scrub station

Fixed services
- Medical gases.

Equipment Planning

The equipment planning is determined, to a large extent, on the basis of the level of the hospital, the nature and eaxtent of surgical procedures are contemplated, and extent of and the constraints of financial, physical and human resources in their acquisition, installation and use.

While planning the equipment mix for an operating department therefore, it is necessary to match their characteristics and specification with the professional and technological requirments and other considerations of logistics and resources.

Following is the standard inventory of equipment required in a modern operating department:

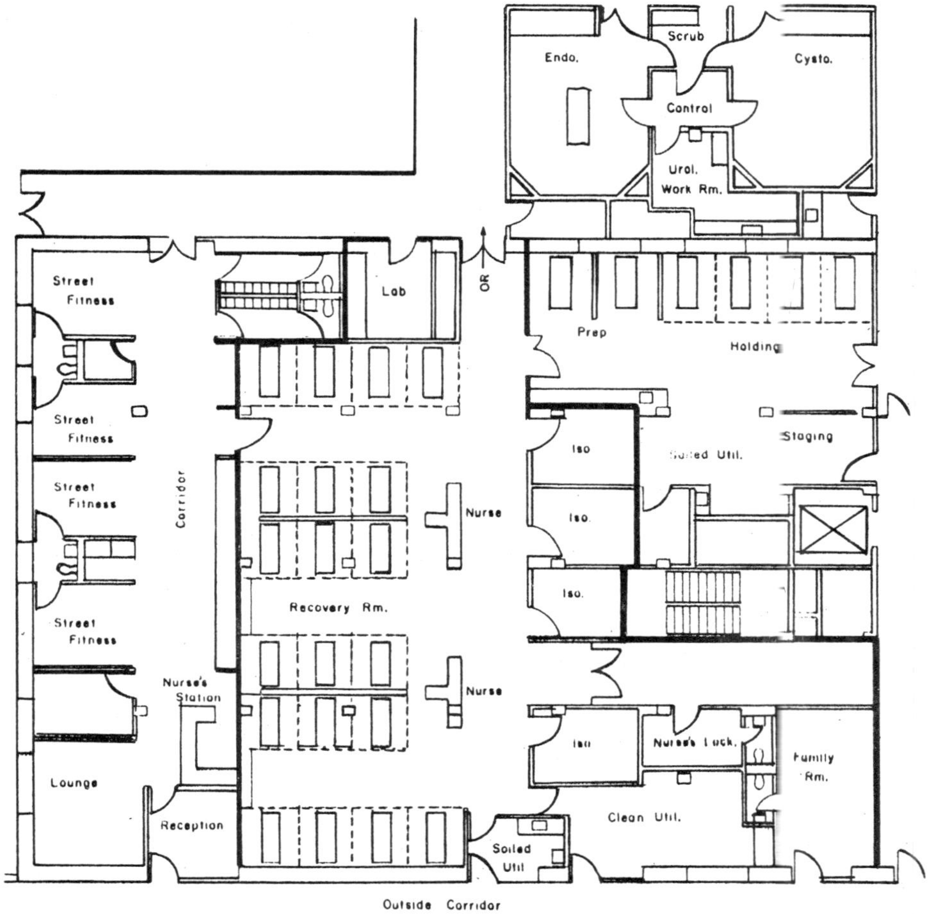

Fig. 34.39: Plan of recovery unit and holding area of a 14-room surgical suite including cystoscopy and cystoscopy-endoscopy rooms. The heavy line separates the recovery unit from the holding area on the right and an outpatient street fitness recovery area on the left. The operating rooms (not shown) are located above the sketched area. Note the four isolation cubicles in the recovery area, all located close to nurses desks. The total number of recovery beds is 24. The holding area has six-bed spots, two of which are isolated and can be used for prepping or isolation of preoperative patients

Operating Zone

- Operating table and transfer trolley system
- Operating light system
- Fixed services system
  - medical gases
  - vacuum
  - surgical diathermy
  - cold light
- Anesthesia equipment
- Patient monitoring and resuscitation equipment
- Operative radiography system
- Operating microscopy equipment
- Extra-corporial circulation equipment
- Patient heating and cooling equipment
- Laboratory support equipment
  - blood gases

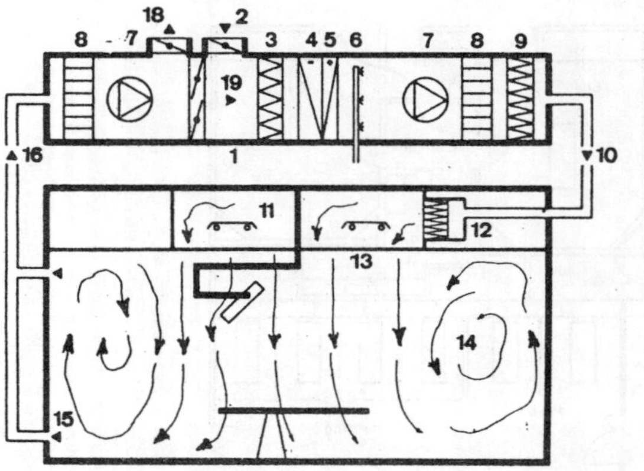

Fig. 34.40: Flow sheet of the airconditioning installation of an operating theatre using the spotprojection principle. (1) airhandling unit; (2) outside aire; (3) coarse filter; (4) air cooler; (5) air heater; (6) steam humidifier; (7) supply air fan; (8) sound attenuator; (9) fine filter; (10) supply air duct; (11) plenum box; (12) HEPA filter; (13) introduction of air via Luwa CG clean air distributor; (14) operating theatre; (15) extract air grille; (16) return air duct; (17) return air fan; (18) exhaust air; (19) recirculated air

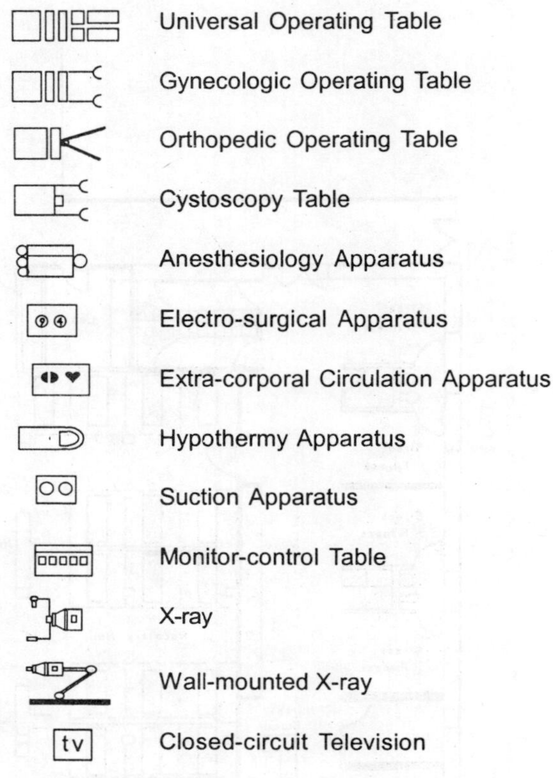

Fig. 34.41: Operation room equipment symbols

  - electrolytes
  - glucose
- Bedpan washer/disinfector
- Macerator
- Furniture and fixtures

Although adequate lighting, proper acoustics, safety against fire hazards, static charge and other risks in the use of electric equipment, etc, contribute towards the creation of an ideal operating room environment, stress must be laid on the following aspects of the physical environment:

i. Temperature
ii. Humidity
iii. Ventilation

A patient is generally compromised due to illness and is more vulnerable to thermal assault, more so during surgical intervention. The character of the thermal environment in an operating room, therefore, is determined by the need to protect physiological resources of the patient, while providing optimum working conditions to the operating staff.

An unclothed person at rest achieves thermal neutrality with one's surroundings at 24°-27°C at a relative humidity of 50°. When conditions vary the body's own temperature regulating mechanisms come into play.

During anesthesia patients lose body heat. This heat loss is due to the following factors, which are related to the surgical intervention as well as operating room environment:

- Low ambient temperature and high humidity
- Infusion with cold fluids
- Ventilation with cold anesthetics
- Exposure of body cavities
- Absence of muscular movement
- Subcutaneous vasodilatation

In an operating room environment, while high humidity enhances the growth and proliferation of pathogenic organisms such as *Pseudomonas aeruginosa,* there are obvious advnatages in preventing dehydration of exposed tissues and other hazards of static electric charge.

Under normal circumstances a relative humidity of 45 to 60° is recommended for operating rooms. When flamable anesthetic agents are not in use, a relative humidity of 40° is considered adequate. Further when young children and infants are involved, a higher range of 55° to 65° is recommended.

Documentation on temperature-humidity influence on postoperative recovery process is very limited and non-conclusive. The standards adopted for the operating room environment, therefore, vary between different countries. In the United Kindgom 20° to 22°C at 50 to 60 percent relative humidity is favored while in the United States 21° to 24.5°C at 50 to 60 percent relative humidity is recommended as a compromise between the optimum requirements of the patients and the surgical team staff. In Scandinavia, however, operating rooms are provided with air-conditioning control mechanisms to achieve variations in temperature from 19° to 26°C and in relative humidity from 40 to 55 percent at the operating staff.

A ventilation system essentially consists of two major components, namely, (i) an air moving device and (ii) a ducting system. Other components are added depending upon requirements such as heating, cooling, humidification, and air cleaning.

Air Changes

Ventilation at the rate of one change per hour will reduce the level of air contamination by 63 percent, two air changes per hour by 86 percent and ten air changes by about 99 percent. There are no clear indications of what an increase in air changes of 15 to 20 per hour or more would mean. In the US however, 25 air changes per hour are mandatory in newly-built facilities.

Air Distribution

Room air distribution systems used in operating room ventilation have many configurations and variations in air handling equipment and patterns of air flow. Some of the prevalent systems are as follows:

i. Turbulent or mixing air distribution system promotes uniform mixing of air including the airborne contraminants throughout the entire room.
ii. Downward displacement piston system, which takes air in the top of th operating room and exhausts at the lower levels, is highly effective and economical system and transports contaminants arising below the operating table out of the operating room environment.
iii. Unidirectional air flow system, sometimes popularly known as laminar flow ventilation system, is observed in literature with many modifications such as downflow, tunnel, horizontal, and crossflow patterns.

A horizontal airflow room offers 11 times efficiency in reducing airborn bacterial counts in the operating room environment when compared with conventional systems. Downflow (vertical) systems offer even a greater efficiency of 90 times.

Scavenging

Scavenging system essentially is a piped vacuum system which can be hooked onto the patient ventilators used in anesthesia practice so that the expired gases are sucked out of the operating room environment.

Although standards for scavenging system have not been formulated, the following guidelines have been offered.

i. The system must not require the attention of the anesthetists during the course of anesthesia;
ii. It must not interfere with the function of anesthetic apparatus and patient ventilator or influence patients respiration, and
iii. It must collect and transport all excessive gases expired by the patient quantitatively.

Many innovations have been reported in the literature for patient safety and low vacuum, high flow, low resistance systems with many protective devices have become available.

Cleanroom Technology

The principles of cleanroom technology, the task of which is to provide an environment with low concentrations of airborne particles and microorganisms, are gaining recognition in the surgical field. A number of different facts and trends influence the requirement profile to be met:

- The impressive advance of surgery: high-risk interventions of just a few years ago are now being performed routinely by hospitals all over the world.
- The increasing percentage of severe operations being performed on elderly patients with reduced infection resistance.
- The widespread use of immunosuppressive drugs, especially in transplantation surgery.
- The introduction of product liability legislation in many countries of the world according to which a person causing health damage or death to another person—whether through negligence or not—will be held liable for compensation of damages, and
- The continuing cost escalation of the public health system.

The challenge, therefore, is to offer a low–germ environment for surgical interventions for a minimum of expenditure, both regarding investment and operational cost.

Cleanliness Levels

Standards and guidelines published in Switzerland and Austria distinguish two quality classes of operating rooms: class I, with a miximum germ concentration of 10 colony-forming units (CFU) per m^3 of room air, and class II, with a maximum germ concentration of 200 CFU/m^3 of room air.

These concentration limits have to be observed during use of the room, that is during surgical interventions. The values refer to the room areas critical for the success of the operation: the compliance with an adequate level of discipline during the course of the operation is a complementary requirement to be met.

For class I operating rooms, both the Swiss and the Austrian rule require final filtration of the supply air with high-efficiency particulate air filters (HEPA filters) capable of eliminating microorganisms from the airstream with more than 99 percent separation efficiency, and supply air introduction into the room according to the principle of low-turbulence displacement airflow, with the air moving vertically downwards on parallel streamlines.

The Austrian standard recommends in addition that transplantations, heart surgery, arthroscopy and bone surgery be performed in a class I operating room. A similar recommendation can be found in the latest edition of the German hospital air conditioning standard which, however, gives no numerical limits as to the germ concentrations to be achieved in the so-called operating rooms for particularly high requirements concerning the absence of microorganisms.

The purchasing and operating costs of the air circulation systems for cleanrooms depend above all on the airflow rate in circulation. To minimise cost the aim must therefore be to minimize the area protected with low-turbulence displacement flow and to reduce, in paralled, the flow velocity to the lowest possible value compatible with the necessary stability of the airflow and with the air cleanliness level to be achieved.

The target, therefore, is the closest possible approximation to the airflow rates usual in conventional class II operating theaters with turbulent airflow. There, 1500 to 2000 m^3/h are typically required to fulfil the minimum air change rates given in the relevant standards and guideline, to compensate the heat load liberated in the room.

To be able to minimise the extension of the displacement flow areas, the spot protection principle must strictly be adhered to. Thus, protection must be limited to the true risk areas, that is the wound and, to a slightly lesser degree, the instrument table.

Comprehensive laboratory tests have shown that a supply air distribution area of 1.2 m × 2.4 m is normally sufficient to offer the necessary protection for both the operating zone and the instrument table. To complement this, it is possible to reduce the air velocity from 0.4 m/s, the value usually recommended in clean room technology, to a value of 0.25 to 0.3 m/s. These two measures together result in the air flow rate being reduced to less than 3000 m^3/h. This is a value which is only negligibly higher than that for a conventional operating theater with turbulent airflow.

Figure 34.19 shows schematically the complete air circuit for the air-conditioning system of an operating theater in accordance with the spot protection concept for the operating table and instrument table mentioned above. The air handling unit contains the necessary components for conveying the supply air and for controlling the temperature and relative humidity of the air.

Three-stage air filtration is provided. The principal task of the first filter stage is to prevent contamination of the air handling unit. The second filter stage, a fine dust filter positioned downstream of the last potential diffusion source for dust and microorganisms of the air handling system, ensures a good level of cleanliness for the supply air and prevents contamination of the ducts. The third filtration stage, the high-efficiency particulate air filter, or HEPA filer, removes any microorganisms which may still be present in the supply airstream, and is normally attached to the air distribution plenum box.

As a functional element for the establishment of the required vertical displacement airflow, a clean air distributor is fitted to the lower face of the plenum boz. It consists of two layers being positioned at a short distance from each other and fitted at high tension over a frame made of extruded aluminium section.

This device is capable of producing a practically turbulence-free displacement airflow of particularly high homogeneity and with very uniform air velocities. The low degree of turbulence efficiently supresses all transversal mixing tendencies, and also contributes to the hgih stability of the airflow. Due to the laminarity of the airflow through the fabric, the induction of impurities from the surrounding room areas into the clean zone is prevented with particular efficiency.

From the clean air distributor installed flush with the false ceiling of the operating room, the air moves vertically downwards as a true displacement airflow with parallel stremlines. Therefore, the wound area will continuously be flushed with clean, uncontaminated first air, practically devoid of microorganisms.

Upon meeting the flow obstacle presented by patient, operating table and instrument table, part of the airflow will be deflected into a horizontal direction. Thus, after flushing the wound, it is directed against the surgical team, so that it effectively sweeps sway all microbial contamination liberated by them into the background area of the operating room. There, of course, it can cause no danger, as re-entrainment of that contamination into the operating field is effectively prevented by the quasi-laminar displacement airflow effective there.

Turbulent airflow establishes itself in the peripheral areas of the operating room. Wall openings for extract air in the vicinity of the floor and immediately below the ceiling then ensure constant dilution of the dust particles and microorganisms carried by the airstream from the operating zone to the outer areas.

A typical operating theater constructed according to this principle is shown in Figure 34.21. The compact dimensions of the ceiling panel and the elegant integration of the operating lamp can be clearly seen. The fluorescent tubes for basic lighting are mounted behind the clean air distributor in the ceiling plenum box. In this way it is possible to achieve uniform background lighting which is pleasant for the eyes, without disturbance to the field of flow.

Operating theaters with such a small ceiling panel are particularly indicated for sterile operations of limited extension, during which not more than four or five persons work in the immediate vicinity of the wound. Such situations apply, for exmaple, to orthopedic operations such as the implantation of artificial joints.

Occasionally, particularly in heart surgery, it is necessary for a fairly large number of people and a considerable amount of equipment to be positioned within the clean air zone. It is then advisable to opt for a clean area of larger dimensions, an exmaple is shown in Figure 34.21. On the other hand, there are applications in otorhinolaryngology, neurosurgery or dentistry for which a ceiling area of less than 1.2 m × 2.4 m is sufficient.

To permit direct access to the fittings for lighting, and to enable to plenum box to be disinfected, the clean air distributing panels can be easily removed. The operating lamp can be neatly integrated into the ceiling panel and the penetration of the ceiling void by its suspension device represents only a negligible obstacle to the airflow. As in all operating theaters with low-turbulence displacement flow, the operating lamps should be of minimum dimensions and shaped aerodynamically, thus presenting the smallest possible obstacle to the airflow.

Concept Validation

What air cleanliness levels can be achieved using this new concept of airflow in operating theatres? The desired germ level of less than 10 colony-forming units (CFU) per m^3 can be achieved and maintained in the operation zone. It was further demonstrated that the low-turbulence displacement airflow effectively screened off the wound region from any induction of air impurities from the outside. The low airflow velocities in the wound area also helped the patient maintain his thermal equilibrium.

Filter Ceiling

A clean environment without micoorganisms is not only important to ensure that the actual operation is performed without complications; it also reduces the risk of post-operative infections.

The filter ceiling consists of 600 mm^2 modules to simplify installation. To prevent contaminated air from flowing into the operating zone, the ceiling is divided into two separate, perforated zones in which air is supplied in a vertical flow at different velocities. Each ceiling consists of three frames: a top frame, a centre frame with 60mm^2 filter modules, and a third frame. Perforated stainless steel screens (550 mm^2) are attached to the frame, to determine the velocity of the supply air flow. To prevent contaminated air from entering the operating area, the perforated screen ceiling is divided into an outer zone, in which air is supplied vertically at a higher velocity in the inner zone and at a lower velocity in the outer zone. The perforated screens are made of stainless steel and can be easily disassembled for cleaning by hospital personnel.

The air is changed 60-70 times an hour in the operating theater. Efficient and cost-effective concepts are now available for meeting the air cleanliness requirements in operating rooms, and to provide the desirable environmental conditions for the surgery.

FURTHER READING

1. Burm AGL *et al:* A central low vacuum pipeline system for disposal of waste anaesthetic gases. *Anesthe* **31**: 200, 1982.
2. Edward R: Operating theaters and ancillary rooms John Sherral and Son, Altrincham, 39, 1964.
3. Golman JW: How to determine optimum number of operation theaters. Modern Hospital, **3**: 1969.'

4. Granning HM: Minimum requirements of construction and equipment for hospitals. US department of Health, Education and walfare. *Health Resource Administration* 74-4000, 1974.
5. Haslam KR: Liminar Airflow airconditioning in the operating room-A review. *Anesthesia and Analgesia* **53**: 194, 1974.
6. Kenset RG: Air conditioning plant design for Operating Theaters Hospital Eng. **28**: 3, 1974.
7. Machenize A: Hazards in the operating theater environmental control. An Royal College Surg Eng. **52**: 36, 1973.
8. Schicht HH: Clean room technology in surgery. Hospital Management International London 301-03, 1997.
9. Turner RS: Laminar Air flow *J Bone and Joint Surgery* **56**: 430, 1974.

CRITICAL CARE UNITS

The Intensive Care Unit (ICU) has sometimes been referred to as the hospital. The obvious meaning of this phrase is that the ICU should concentrate all of the assets as institution can bring to bear on the care of the critically ill patients. ICU not only concentrates the assests but also may concentrate the liabilities associated with medical care.

Intensive care is as old as medicine itself. However, intensive care has evolved to its present status as a form of treatment of patients with serious life-threatening illness or trauma, requiring specialized and intensified human resources, instrumentation and environment.

The quality of care available in an ICU is related first and foremost to the quality of the nursing care and to the clinical acumen of the medical staff. But without the necessary equipment and an appropriate environemntal design, the safety, efficiency, and economy with which the patient care is delivered will be lessened.

The need for special care of critically ill and injured patients is recognised virtually in every medical speciality. This type of care consists of emergency care, resuscitation, and intensive care. Although critical care medicine has evolved into a new speciality, cutting across the boundaries of other medical specialities, most hospitals rely upon specialists in the various branches of medicine to practice critical care within each speciality. As a result, many different types of intensive care units have been established in prominent medical centers and hospitals.

Many countries have registared their hospitals in different catagories. In the United States, the American Medical Association has classified hospitals into the following four catogories, according to the level of intensive care provided.

Catagory I hospitals These are large regional canters, frequently university hospitals, providing comprehensive medical services. These hospitals have at least one ICU of Type I (i.e., for advanced intensive medical care with 24 hour in ICU covarage by critical care medicine doctors).

Catagory II hospitals These are other teaching hospitals, providing major emergancy medical care, with house officers in most specialities and at least one type II ICU (i.e., basic medical intensive care unit with 24 hours in hospital coverage by regular house officers).

Catagory III hospitals These are usually non-teaching community hospitals providing general emergency medical service. They have a type III ICU (i.e., an intensive nursing care unit with 24 hour ICU coverage by registared nurses and at least one doctor on call in the house).

Catagory IV hospitals These are small hospitals which provide only basic emergency medical services with a physician on call at home. They have no ICU.

A catagory I hospital may have ICUs of all different types, but type I ICU will not normally be found in catagory II hospitals. Similary, catagory III hospitals are not expected to have either type I or type II ICUs.

With intensive therapy, it is usually meant the treatment of patients during a period of their critical illness. It requires extraordinary care, qualified staff, strict supervision, and vary often mechanical aids to support vital functions. The patient may require artificial ventilation, treatment for shock, cardiac monitoring, pacemaking, peritonial or hemodialysis, biological correction of severe metabolic disorders and special protection against infection.

Intensive observation is adapted until complications requiring ventilatory or circulatory resuscitation no longer are a threat.

Intensive or critical care is a method of organizing medicine and nursing so that expertise and sophisticated equipment are concentrated where they are most needed and efficiently utilized. Intensive care is considered to be a very constructive therapeutic method.

ICU patients require careful study and accumulation of experience.

Any patient without terminal illness deserves initial admission to an intensive care unit. In each medical speciality and subspeciality, there are patients eligible for intensive treatment. Advanced age is no reason for rejecting a patient from an ICU. The recovering patient should have an active life of some sort to look forward to.

A strong case can be made for intensive care units if their individual guidelines are set within a general ethical framework reverence for life must be tampered by restraint and an equal respect that takes account of human rights, and that such guidelines give careful consideration to the Salvageability of patients and the condition of Salvageability.

Intensive care exposes the seriously ill to an especially high level of risk from the procedures intended to help them. There is also the danger of overenergetic treatment i.e. so-called over treatment of minor cases and unnecessary treatment of hopeless cases. The fact that it is possible to maintain and prolong life, does not inevitably and in all cases mean that to do so is justifiable or even desirable. Reverance for life must be tempered by rastraint and an equal respect for the dignity of death.

Need for Intensive Care

On an average, most large hospitals will need only about two percent of the number of beds in the clinics which make use of the critical care or intensive care and treatment unit. This percentage may rise to six percent.

The need for surgical intensive care may increase from 4.1 percent to 5 to 6 percent of surgical bed capacity, the reason being the increasing share of outpatient surgery.

In the US, about 5 percent of total medical surgical beds are represented by intensive and coronary care units, though it has been recommanded that 10 percent of the total number of beds in a hospital should be allocated for use in the intensive care unit.

Some experts recommend for intensive observation 1.5 to 2 beds per operation room or 5 to 7 percent of surgical beds or 5 percent of acute beds; and for intensive therapy 2.5 to 3 percent of beds in clinics in need of intensive therapy.

In thoracic surgery and neurosurgery the needs are far bigger. If these units are segregated, the ICU bed need is about 15 percent of the clinic beds.

Whether a hospital should have an ICU for a single speciality or for a group of them; or a multi-speciality ICU, depends on the type of hospital and on the regional health care organization.

Organ systems, clinical syndromes, and patient population may be the basis for grouping the patients, as illustrated by cardiac care units, burn units, and pediatric units.

A general intensive care unit, a coronary care unit as far as possible, heart patients should not be nursed with non-coronary patients, a burn unit, and a neonatal and premature unit have represented the physical subdivisions of critical care areas commensurate with efficient staffing, best patient care, and maximum economy.

In hospitals, which have about 1,000 or more beds other types of ICUs could be added, primarily for patients who have been subjected to cardiac surgery, neurosurgery, or thoracic surgery. Although the concept of sroke intensive care unit or neurovascular care unit has been in existence for thirty years, there still is conflict of opinion regarding its advantages.

Some experts favor only interdisciplinary ICUs. Intensive care and therapy wards are for a group of patients an extension of the immediate post-operative care.

The ICU ought to be lined with the post anesthetic recovery area, the emergency area and the delivery section.

Pediatric Beds

The intensive therapy units have been designed predominantly for adults. The optimum care of the child is accomplished in an area specifically designed as pediatric, and by personnel trained in the care of children.

The pediatric skills are the main considerations for the critically ill child. It is decidedly easier to give children nurses training in intensive care a six month a course than ICU nurses training in pediatric care a course of 13 months.

One ICU bed for twenty pediatric beds including sub-specialities, has been recommended. It has also been assumed that the beds in pediatric intensive care units should constitute 6 percent of all beds in the pediatric clinic or 8 percent of the average hospital paediatric census.

Cost of Intensive Care

Intensive care in hospitals uses up a large sector of personnel. It is difficult to evaluate and compare cost wise the results of intensive care. In the USA an intensive care patient is given 16.76 nursing man hours per day which is 2.85 times more than in medical and surgical units.

Although in the intensive care units efficient use of staff is made; the cost of maintaining it, is from 2.5 to up to 20 times higher per bed than in regular bed care.

It has been estimated that the laboratory procedures may account for about 30 percent of the ICU cost.

Benefit from intensive care is currently impossible to assess because patient populations differ, treatment protocols vary widely, and persistance in life support may reflect the ethical climate of the unit.

Intensive care medicine is extraordinarily expensive, yet results in only a small number of patients surviving to a sueful and productive life. Far more likely is death or survival with poor functional recovery.

Patient in the Intensive Care Unit

The critically ill patient in an intensive care unit may be scarcely visible, let alone identifiable as human, among all the paraphernalia of life support. Monitors and ventilatory equipment surround him like sentinels. Charts and flow sheets hang at the end of the bed, chronicling the vicissitudes of a dozen parameters, pain, sadness, loneliness, uncertanity, fear, helplessness, despair. These are not on the flow sheet. These cannot be read off a monitor or determined by cannulation of a vessal. These cannot be measured or computed.

Obviously, the busy intensive care environment is frequently the opposite of peace and quiet required for the recovery from serious illness.

The noise of the unit creates adverse physiological effects and an emotional strain on the patient, disturbing his rest by day and sleep at night.

Sleep may be disturbed in any patient admitted to an intensive care unit. Patients with severely disturbed sleep patterns stand to have significant residual disability compared to those with a similar clinical state but normal sleep records.

Frequant unnecessary awakenings are due to a general lack of awareness by the intensive care unit staff of noise levels, lighting conditions and other factors that would be conducive to sleep.

The phenomena which can occur for the ICU patients in various degrees include confusion, disturbed memory, disorientation in place, time and sometimes in person, and delusions and hallucinations in which the design, colors, sounds and equipment of the ICU may be involved.

Visual obstruction between the patients is desirable. On the other hand, an exterior view is essential. Daylight and clocks perhaps with digital readings and calendars with large type and pull off pages contribute towards the well-being of the patient. In the US, blackboards suitable for mounting get well cards have been recommended. A surface for flowers and plants, should as far as possible be coordinated with the window location and natural light.

The management of the psychological components is of paramount importance for patients in an ICU.

Length of Patient Stay

- The patients stay in the ICU (the variation in the avarage length are considerable) should be kept as short as possible.
- The avarage length of stay in the UK is five days with a range of two to twelve days. An average stay of two to three days has been reported in university hospitals.
- In the German Democratic Republic, the average length of stay in the ICU is four to five days. In Hungery, seven to twelve days. The average duration of treatment of surgical ICU patients is 4.1 days in the Finland.
- In the United States, the average length of stay has been about four days.
- In New Zealand, less than three days avarage duration of stay has been reported. In Australia the mean duration of stay for medical patients has been three days, and for surgical patients six day.
- In neurosurgical ICUs, the average stay is nine days.

As there is a tendancy that the stay in the ICU is being prolonged, as the average length of stay 5 to 6 days could be suggested for planning purposes.

ICU Size

An intensive care unit of less than 6 beds is clearly uneconomical. However, to reduce the risk of nosocomial infection for most highly susceptible patients, the sizing of the ICU to four to six patients has been suggested in the US.

In the Fedaral Republic of Germany, the optimal number of beds per unit is put at 12 with a minimum of 6 and a maximum of 16. The choice of 6 to 16 beds has been recommended also in Denmark. In the United Kingdom, the optimal size of an ICU is considered to be between 8 and 10 beds. In Hungary, the size 8 to 16 beds is considered as recommendable. In Switzerland 12 beds have been felt to be the maximum in an intensive care unit.

Too big ICUs become ineffective. The need for more beds than in one ICU should be met not by fragmentation and multiplication of ICUs, but by grouping several units into a critical care medicine centre, which enhances the utilization of beds.

As optimal ICU occupancy rate 70 to 80 percent have been suggested.

Spatial Requirements

The current average overall spatial need in the ICU is about 50 m^2 per bed. If the ICU is not planned with single occupancy rooms exclusively, the entrance to the ICU should be planned as an antiroom, where staff, visitors or personnel from other sactions of the hospital must, before entering the patient area, be submitted to the growing routines adapted in the ICU.

There should be an emergancy entrance for patients.

Patient Room

The goal should be a patient area, in which the requirements of psychologically pleasent environment and some elements of a scientific laboratory are balanced. Of the two basic design possibilities the open ward and the single bed accommodation the single bed accommodation has gained preference. The provision of privacy without isolation, in which communication is essential, has been recommended not least for the purpose of noise raduction for all intensive care patients. The patient need for an ICU bed in a single bed room is 17 to 21 m^2. The bed is an environemental influence, which the acutely ill patient cannot escape. The patient's bed should provide conditions for his affective existance and his progress toward an improved state of health. A knowledge of the detrimental effects of bed rest must be a part of bed designars, armamentaria. Such pathologies as bedsores, muscle atrophy, thrombophilebitis, constipation, syncope, atalactasis, and osteoporosis could be alleviated with proper bed mattress and bedding design.

The bed should be readily adjustable to various threapeutic positions, easily moved for transport, should have a locking mechanism for a secure stationary position, and where feasible, a removable headboard. For multiple organ support, ample space should be provided around the bed. Bulky equipment may be accommodated. The space around the bed in a single bed accommodation can be used most efficiently when the shape of the floor is close to a square. The length of the room may be the critical dimension. In the ICU clinical policy decisions on individual patients tend mostly to run from hour-to-hour rather than from moment to moment. Close and often invasive monitoring is adapted to allow for early recognition of problems leading to appropriate treatment before a very critical situation occurs. The simplest method of data storage is the clinical chart kept at the bedside, which represants a discontinuous series of observations. Electrocardiographic material and similar electronic data can be stored either on paper or in a computer system with recall. The amount and sophistication of that equipment varies greatly. There should be shelves upon which equipment and instruments can be mounted and a place for patient charts. A dual channel nonfading oscilloscope and a computer terminal can be mounted on the wall behind the head of the bed. Locating the beds permanently away from the wall of the room gives the staff a 360° access to the patient, except for ECG leads if not telemonitored nasogastric suction, and respiratory connections. All tubes and wires could be run through a junction box under the bed. All tubes, pipes, and wiring for the patient could also be organized and contained in a panel or column at the head end of the patients bed. The utility unit may contain an intercommunication system between the patient and the nurse's station and a telephone for the patient's personal use.

One of the panel's important features is that almost everything required for life support can be done for the patient or to the patient from either side of the bed. Under usual conditions no wires or tubing pass over the patient or over his bed. The equipment cannot be seen by the patient, therefore, he is almost unaware of the instruments and machines that are needed to support his life. If and when a patient gets to an ambulatory stage while he is still receiving critical care, a screen can be used to temporarily cover the panel, so that the area does not look so much like a critical care room.. It has been recommended that monitoring equipment should be maintained outside the patient's room. Bedside monitors could be turned on only when needed. This will reduce the monotony of any constant rhythmic signal and diminish anxiety in those patients who are aware of the significant of these devices. A room adapted for maximum care may be needed as well as a room for hyperbaric oxygen and a room for induced hypothermia. Where the ambiant room temparature has to be decreased to 10°C. For each bed in the open ICU which as already indicated should be avoided an average area of about 20 m^2 should be allowed, with about 3.5 m between bed centres. 15 m^2 for one bed is a minimum.

The pediatric intensive care unit (PICU) should be signed to have at least 12 m^2 allotted for each bedspace. This allows room for extensive monitoring equipment, portable X-ray machines, and working space for special diagnostic or resusitative procedures. There must be at least six electrical outlets per bedspace. Ceiling or wall suction as well as oxygen lines must be provided. The two parameters most commonly recorded are the ECG and the arterial blood pressure. A bathroom for shower baths and where the patient could be washed is a considerable advantage. An area of about 12 m^2 is needed.

Nurse's Station

The nurse's station, to be located centrally within the ICU, may, to some extent also serve as a physician's office. The desk should accommodate charts and provide working space for several people. There should be an acoustically shielded telephone and the cantral monitoring recorder.

Units that have a central command area where all data are read out and all records kept are very satisfactory from the point of view of administration but can lead to isolation of the patient from data critical to his care at exactly those times when maximal bedside information and minimal bedside confusion are important. In units with a large number of isolation rooms, two nurse's stations may be needed.

Linked to the nurse's station there should be a preparation area with a supply of drugs and sera, parenteral solutions, blood, sterile sets, emergency equipment, etc. A refrigerator for drug storage is needed.

The nurse requires a separate accommodation, of about 15 m^2 where she or the physician can talk with relatives and members of the staff in privacy.

Utility Room

Utility rooms of about 8 m^2 size, both clean and soiled, are needed, there should be a refrigarator for pathological specimens, e.g. for twenty-four hour urine.

Treatment Room

Frequently there is a treatment room of about 30 m^2 size within the ICU.

Laboratory Services

The intensive care unit should have access to clinical laboratory services on a 24-hour basis, particularly for arterial blood gas and arterial pH analysis. Laboratory apparatus includes equipment for electrolyte and osmolality determinations, gas liquid chromatography, flame spectrophotometry, and auto analysis equipment for assays of serum or plasma components as blood glucose, urea, bilirubin and enzymes as SGOT, troponin, LDH, CPK, etc. within a matter of minutes. An area of about 18 m^2 is required.

X-ray Services

The ICU is dependent on a round-the-clock service from the diagnostic radiology department.

As radiological consultation and reporting is best carried out within the ICU, high-powered mobile equipment capable of taking films should be available.

An X-ray technologist would cover the intensive care unit portable X-ray work. The films should be reviewed by the ICU physician and radiologist at the same time.

Work Room for Technicians

There is a need for a room of about 18 m^2 with working space for technicians responsible for the maintanance of the increasingly elaborate technical equipment.

Bed Cleaning Room

A facility for cleaning and decontaminating ICU beds within the unit or adjacent to it should be available. The recommended area is about 12 m^2.

Store Room

Materials needed in immediate patient care should be available close to where used. A clean supply store should be in the core of the ICU.

A storeroom is required for bulky equipment, such as respirators, defibrillator, oscilloscopes, dialysis machinary, special beds, oxygen tents, bed scales, and patient lifts.

Free and easy passage to the equipment is essential when a defibrillator or a respiratory machine is urgently needed as no time may be wasted.

It has been estimated that there should be about 9 to 10 m^2 storage space per ICU bed.

Staff Changing Room

Changing rooms both for male and female staff should be adjacent to the ICU entrance.

Staff toilets and showers should be provided.

Offices for physicians and secrataries, and a conference room should be available. The systematic teaching of qualified nurses and junior doctors, which is an essantial part of intensive care, requires in the unit a room with standard teaching aids, blackboard, slide tape machine and dummies for resuscitation.

A well-ventilated room about 12 m^2, clearly separated from the ward area, is needed for coffee or tea breaks.

Pantry or vending mechine should be provided. Comfortable non-institutional furnishing is important.

On Call Rooms

There is a need for a sleeping room with a toilet and a shower for the physician on call.

Rooms for Visitors

A visitor's waiting room is needed as the patient's condition often precludes visiting from more than a few minutes at a time. There should be a generous allocation of space, comfortable furnishing, pleasent decor, and if possible, a window to look out.

Relatives and friends who wish to stay for longer periods close to seriously ill-patient, need adjecent to the ICU overnight rooms of about 10 m^2 area with telephone, toilet and shower.

Coronary Intensive Care Unit

Cardiac or coronary care unit is used by the patients who have or are thought to suffer from acute myocardial infarction, arrhythmias or some other cardiac emergency conditions.

A CICU should not be part of a general purpose intensive therapy unit or of a general medical ward. It has to contain an intensive care section (IC) and an intermediate care saction (IMC) as significant patient risk continues beyond 12 days of hospital admission.

In the United Kingdom, the usual length of stay in the CICU for the patients is 2 to 5 days. In Sweden, the length of stay usually is 1 to 3 days in the intensive care section and 8 to 30 days in the intermediate care section.

In Sweden, it has been suggested that between 6 and 8 CICU beds should be available for every 2,00,000 of the population served. In the United Kingdom, between 6 and 8 CICU beds are required for every 250, 000 to 300, 000 of the population.

In the US the optimal number of CICU beds per million population would be 60, assuming that no patient should have a travel time of more than 30 minutes and that he would have a 95 percent chance to find an available bed in the nearest CICU.

Advances in coronary care have led to a substantial reduction in hospital mortality and to an increase of life expectancy, but they also entail in survivors an increase in the number of myocardial infarction hospitalizations for subsequant attacks.

For coronary intensive care units the sizes of 6 to 10 beds have been most frequent.

A separate nursing station is considered feasible when the CICU contains 4 to 8 beds. For the economics of scale the units of at least with 8 beds have been suggested.

Units of less than 4 or more than 10 beds create difficult staffing problems. More than 10 beds in a unit increase the problems in patient supervising.

The CICU should be adjacent to a general emergency admission unit or be situated near a medical ward in which progressive care of the patient with acute myocardial infarction can be undertaken.

The physiological and hemodynamical condition of the cardiac patient is in some way correlated with the patients style of coping with stress, and his history of previous life stress situations.

Prefarably the patients of the intensive care area of the CICU should be for the most part out of sight of each other but within view of the nursing staff and seem to be best accommodated in individual rooms saperate by walls or opaque and sound proof partitions.

The advantage of single-roomed CICU is felt to be that patient cannot compare their progress with that of any other patient and they do not witness the resuscitation procedures or the death of a neighbouring patient.

To maintain the patient's sense of time and place, window items should be provided. This personal space must not infringe on space required in normal and emergency procedures.

In the coronary intensive care unit the patient is also exposed to physical discomfort in the form of thoracic electrodes for ECG telematry can greatly reduce this IV drip, oxygen cathater in the nose, or face mask. There are generally visual or acoustic alarm devices.

Provided the monitoring appartus is silent, unobtrusive, and out of the immediate view of the patient, the monitoring is usually tolerated well by patients if they have been informed that it saves work for nurses and doctors.

Coronary Care Area

According to American Experience about 13 m^2 is workable and parhaps desirable size for a patient room. According to some Swedish experience more space is needed and the size of 18 to 22 m^2 is recommanded. One of the IC rooms should be even bigger about 30 m^2.

In the case of cardic arrest, the attending physician or nurse must have access to the patient's head. It must be possible to insert a board behind the patient's back without difficulty. Therefore, the bed must be away from the wall.

As there are therapeutic advances in having the patient to spend some time seated rather than lying, a comfortable bedside armchair has to be provided. It has to be located in such a way, that a nurse can easily assist the patient to chair. The chair ought to be in position for comfortable supervision.

At the head of each bed there should be notice boards to display vital data. Another feature which should be attached to the headwall is an equipment organizer. It could take some of the equipment, which traditionally is placed on a cart.

There must be a resuscitation panel, both oxygen and suction are essential and a panic button to alert the staff when cardiac arrest occurs. Sometimes medically-pure compressed air is provided to power some types of breathing apparatus. No service should have less than two outlets. Each service connection should be located as close to the point of use as possible. Ther are functional advantages when oxygen vacuum, compressed-air, and the electrical outlets are provided on both sides of the patient's bed.

With the current popularity of prefabricated modular head wall systems in several countries, notably in the US, and the willingness of several manufactures to customize the headwall to the specific requirements of the staff, the architect often believes that all the functional requirements necessary for patient care electricity, oxygen, compressed air, vacuum, nurse call, reading light and physiological monitoring have been solved with the selection of a headwall unit. If the headwall is not properly designed and installed to integrate with the other elements in the room, IV track, examination lights, bed, work space serious operational problems will occur.

Bedside equipment includes oscilloscopes, which need to be simple, large faced, and provide a stable electrocardiogram. Telemetric equipment reducing CICU stresses is gaining greatly in importance. A minimum of 8 adequately earthed electrical outlets per room area needed. In case of power failure emergency electrical supplies must be available. There should be washbasins in all patient rooms.

An enclosed toilet in connection with the patient room in the intensive care area is not needed, as long as the majority of CICU patients are wired to the monitors. The goal should be to develop a patient room which balances the requirements of the scientific laboratory and those of psychologically comfortable environment. A central nurses station should be provided. Laboratory data, medication, nurse's notes, and vital signs are entered manualy via the terminal keyboard. Also most of the automatically monitored parameters can be manually charted.

The need for central multichannel monitors at the nurse's station largely depends on the design and the number of stafff utility rooms and storages are needed.

Intermediate Care Area

In the intermediate care section, which ought to have twice the number of intensive area beds, multibed rooms with 4 to 6 beds are recommended.

The multibed rooms seem to be the provision of more social contact, with associated freedom of expression of hostile feelings, while lack of privacy leads to higher levels of shame and anxiety. In a multibed patient room, the reciprocal assistance among patients can be considerable as viewing each other is easy.

The closed rooms provide privacy at the expense of human interactions resulting to increased loneliness and displacements of hostile feelings.

An enclosed toilet room but the door without locks, should be provided close to each patient room. Access to showers is needed.

The CICU requires ECG apparatus, defibrillator machines which deliver electrical impulses to the heart respirators, ventilators, intravenous infusion units and monitoring systems.

Having within the CICU laboratory equipment that determine e.g. the acid base levels, depends greatly upon the availability of cantralized pathological services.

Outlets for mobile X-ray apparatus a separate 220 volt power source should be located as far as practicable from the patient beds.

If a portable image intensifier is to be used, the part of the bed that supports the patient's chest must be radiotranslucent, which is not always the case.

To avoid the transport of seriously ill patients elsewhere for introduction or placing catheters, ready access to fluoroscope apparatus is important in coronary care units. A cardiac fluoroscope room should be adjacent to the CICU. Alternatively, portable fluoroscopic image intensifiers are used.

For pacing within the CICU a specific area should be set aside. Appropriate radiation protection should be established.

Common Areas

An admission room where early disgnosis is made, is necessary.

A doctors room, a nurse's room, a medicine preparation room, a secratary room, a room for interviewing relatives, a visitor's room with a toilet, and a doctor's overnight facility are needed.

There should be a ward kitchen, storages for equipment, linen and trolleys, a room for record keeping, staff changing facilities and toilets Janitor's closets and an equipment maintenance-room.

The CICU staff should have access to a conferance room equipped with a conference table, chairs, a chalkboard, an X-ray viewing screen and a provision for audio-visual display and to a comfortable, geographically separate lounge for tea or coffee breaks.

Pulmonary Intensive Care Unit

Chronic obstructive lung disease has been increasing at a faster rate than many other major health problems. Acute respiratory failure is a frequent occurrence in a comprehensive pulmonary care programme.A pulmonary intensive care unit PICU is the major key in such a programme.

In order to provide a good environment, sufficient room must be provided to accomodate ventilators, resuscitation equipment, fluoroscope units and rehabilitive efforts. A minimum space is about 1.8 m each side of the bed centre.

Each bed must be equipped with oxygen, suction, compressed air and space for intravascular pressure and electrocardiographic monitoring.

Every effort should be made to provide a bright, chearful environment. Sound absorbing materials such as curtains, acoustical ceilings and carpeting should be used.

The length of stay in a PICU is about seven to ten days. Patient rooms should have a window with a view.

The nursing station must be equipped with remote monitoring having a simultaneous display of each patient's cardiopulmonary data. The monitors should include crisis monitors with a memory loop or delay capacity so that crisis-precipitating events can be recorded.

Utility and supply rooms are needed A laboratory for around the clock determination of artarial blood gases immadiately adjacent to the PICU is required, as these patients are very unstable. A logistic delay due to laboratory remoteness or unavailable technical assistance is not acceptable.

This laboratory can also function as an additional facility for supporting specialized ventilatory studies and sputum examinations.

A closely intermediate care unit would allow the patients to be continuously observed and monitored by telemetry for arrhythmias. This arrangement facilitates increased rhabilitative efforts while the patient convalesces toward self-care.

Stroke Unit

Neurovascular or stroke cases are admitted predominantly from the emergency department, not later than 48 hours after the event has occurred. The great majority is admitted within 10 hours of their stroke.

The patients are prefarably discharged from the unit to a neurology ward when their general and neurological conditions have become stable, and continuous vital sign monitoring no longer is necessary. Continuous observation of vital sign thus is routine. As soon as possible after admission, all patients should have a skull X-ray, sometimes echoencephalogram, ECG, brain scan, serial ECG, cardiac enzymes over three consecutive days and a lumbar puncture.

The use of computarized axial tomography CT and MRI (Magnetic Resonance Imaging) has considerably enhanced the diagnostic accuracy in stroke patients.

Burn Care Unit

Two phases of the burns illness the shock period and the healing period have to be accommodated. Experts have clearly advocated special burn care units.

Special equipment to meet the peculiar needs of burned patients, such as circ O lactirc beds, ropes, weights and pulleys for postitioning and applying traction to extremities, should be available.

Complete reverse isolation can be a significant factor in the prevention of bacterial contamination of individuals incurring major burn injuries.

The recommended number of beds in a burns ward has been between 6 and 15 beds. The total spatial requirements of about 50 m^2 per bed in the smallest unit are reduced to about 30 m^2 per bed when the size of the unit increases to 15 beds.

Patient Rooms

Plenty of space is essential for the treatment of acutely ill patients, who usually will remain in the shock room for two ro three days. The shock room should be of about 26 m^2 in size.

The ordinary patient room should be about 20 m^2 in size. Special beds or cranes and other apparatus for handling heavy patients may require additional space as well as such procedure as application of grafts.

A few double rooms in the burns unit have been accepted.

Supply of oxygen, a suction apparatus and hand-washing facility rooms must be easy.

Each patient must have individual supplies for his exclusive use. Decontamination of equipment before use by another patient is always necessary.

In all patient rooms outlets for portable X-ray apparatus are needed.

In the management of the burned patient, to decrease evaporative cooling and fluid loss, the room temparature should be regulated to 29°C and humidity to about 30 percent. Many burned patients require an air temperature of 30°C at relative humidities of 50 to 60 percent. When there patient has to lie naked light has been used to maintain the patients body temperature.

Air condition with a high number of changes per hour is desirable.

Various types of unidirectional flow units and axenic chambers are among the techniques for regulating the airconditions. Unidirectional flow in treating the 40 to 60 percent burn victims has been suggested.

In a burn room, a multiple organ support system may require a hemodialysis unit, a respirator, an arterial blood pressure catheter and transducer unit, a monitor for ECG and blood pressure, a heater, a IV drip regulator, a pulmonary artery and wedge pressure monitor, and an intra-aortic balloon pump.

The facility must provide an atmosphere of reality and comfort. Windows should be low enough to look out. There should be clocks and calenders. TV has been found to be excellent for preventing boredom and maintaining morale. Lighting should be reduced at night.

A day room is required for burned patients who are ambulant and are considered suitable for mixing with others at a similar stage of their illness. An occupational therapy room is an asset.

As the patient runs a greater risk of being contaminated when he is outside the unit, it would be best to provide all of the direct care services required by the burn patients within the unit itself.

At least one airconditioned dressing room with stainless bath and mechanical hoist should be provided. A disposable sterile polythene liner sheet is recommended to be used for each bath.

Apparatus have been designed to carry the patient on the strectcher between bed and bath.

It is possible to achieve a considerable reduction in the rate of cross infection among burn care unit patients by excluding common treatment areas.

An operation room within the burn unit is frequently favored. A patient with a burn up to 20 percent total body surface will require an average of one to two debridment and/or grafting procedures during his initial hospitalization, patients with a burn of 20 to 40 percent will require an average of four procedures. A burn of over 40 percent requires four to five procedures.

The medication refrigerator would suffice also for storing the daily needs of homograft and heterograft skin. A specially-controlled blood or plasma refrigerators within the burns unit may be necessary.

Many burned patients require high oral fluid and high caloric intake. Unless a complete kitchen is planned, the nourishment area can be combined with a medication room.

Storage spaces should be ample, as many items of bulky equipment in occasional use in burn wards should be readily available, storages for linen burned patients require two or three times as much linen as the average patient and supplies are needed. House-keeping storages are required.

Male and female changing rooms with lavatories and showers are needed. There should be a visitor's gowing room.

The burns team has to be provided with comfortable rooms for breaks, reports, conferances, and classes as it is important that the team members can get away from the many stress for short periods of time.

Adjacent to burns unit there should be a visitor's waiting room with a lavatory, a skin bank, office for the burn care facility chief and possibly a social worker's office.

Obstetric ICU

For patients with diabetes, Rh incompatibility, hypertension, cardiac complications, renal disorders, with a history of reproductive difficulty, for high risk eclampsia patients, and particularly for those in premature labor under 33 to 34 weeks gestation a special ante and intrapartum unit also referred to as an obstetric or labor or maternal intensive care unit should be provided. The antepartum unit could also be regraded as a fetal intensive care unit (FICU) for all high risk pregnancies. The fetal intensive care could be associated with improved neurologic and biochemical status of the neonate. When the high risk patient has reached her term or it appears that labor may have to be induced or operative interferance considered, she is transferred to the intrapartum unit.

Some 5 percent of maternity patients have been considered to need intensive care. Pediatric coverage and obstetric anesthesia should be constantly available. The minimum nurse requirement is one to two patients. Monitoring of physiologic parameters in both the mother and the fetus requires an additional number of staff. For wholly satisfactory care, the nurse-to-patient ratio should be at least 1 to 1.

To motivate an obstetric intensive care unit of about 10 beds 8 antepartum and 2 intrapartum the annual delivery rate of the hospital should be about 3,000.

Neonatal ICU

An intensive care nursery is to provide the best chances of saving life and of improving physical and developmental status for survivors of serious prenatal illness. Infants admitted to the NICU include pre and postsurgical patients, mostly up to one month of life, out-born neonates transferred from hospitals not provided with special skills, and neonate trauma and burn victims. The maximal admission age of one month is an arbitrary determination. All infants of a size the incubators or bassinets can accommodate could be included. Many of the low birth weight neonates will spend only a few hours in this area for immediate postnatal observation. However, very low weight infants about 750 g may remain in the NICU for a month of longer.

Recent advances indicate that parents should be encouaged to visit as often as possible, to touch and handle their babies from the earliest stages, and to feed them in convalescence. The importance of enforcing strict visiting regulations and to keep all personnal with any infectious illness away from the NICU has been emphasized. Neonatal care has to be regionalized. To justify administratively a neonatal intensive care unit the basis of about 4,000 deliveries a year are needed. The number of NICU beds in a hospital can be estimated on basis of the number of high risk neonates in the catchment area of the hospital, the occupancy rate and the length of patient stay.

$$\text{The number of NICU beds} = \frac{L \times (1B + OB)}{OR}$$

L is the average length of patient stay, IB the number of inborn babies requiring the intensive care OB the number of outborn babies requiring intensive care, and OR, the avarage occupancy rate.

Intensive care is provided for the care and observation of all premature and low birth weight infants, infants of high risk mothers, infants with low apgars, suffaring neonatal asphyxia, birth defects, traumatic births, postsurgical patients, trauma, and burn victims. There should be an intensive care area and an intermediate care area. Two percent of live births need 3 percent intermediate care. The intramediate care area provides care for the essantially well infant who though graduate from the intensive care area, still requires some specialized care.

Three level NICUs have been required. A 28-bassinet unit might have three intensive care spaces, 20-intermediate care areas and 5 transitional care places for short-term observation.

A British expert group has recommended that a unit for intensive care of the newborn should contain at least 24 cots. A smaller NICU containing less than 10 to 12 bassinets is not advisable. A washbasin for each three to four bassinets in needed, as value of washing hands must be stressed rigidly. The requirement for open visibility between the wards in neonatal nursaries limits the choice of materials available. Glass is generally an easy surface to keep clean although problems may arise where it is supported at its edge. Smooth surfaces with rounded corners and lack of dust traps are also important. To have an admission room for infants admitted from other hospitals is an advantage. A facility to carry out microchemistry, hematology, blood gas analysis, and bacteriology is needed as well as access to ECG, EEG, and blood bank services. Biochemical determinations must be based on micromethods to limit blood loss. Radiography by usually a mobile X-ray unit is one of the most important diagnostic tools in the initial and follow up evaluation of high risk neonates, virtually, none of the causes of respiratory distress in the newborn can be diagnosed without good quality chest radiography.

A procedure room may be incorporated into the NICU but preferably it is sectioned off to reduce traffic and to allow better control of techniques such as exchange transfusion, umbilical vessel catheterization, and human puncture.

If neonates are to be operated in the NICU, a minor operation room is needed. It should include a special operation table, instrument and anesthetic trolleys, rails for infusion bottles, and a viewing box for X-ray radiographs, Neonates as well as very small children do not need an anesthetic room. There ought to be a sluice room with an incinerator for soiled nappies, dressings, etc. In larger NICUs clean and soiled utility rooms are needed. A chart storage at the working area in the wards and an instrument room for storage and maintenance of respiratory and electronic equipment is needed. The NICU should include a nurse's station with patient data storage for clerical work. A parant's room to allow feeding, bathing, and in select instances breast-feeding, is an essential facility. The corridors should be at least about 1.8 m wide.

Recent Trends

Several recent changes have occurred in fetal and newborn care which should be identified since they have a major bearing on the optimum design of the facilities for delivering this care:

- The fetus and newborn are viewed as a single patient.
- Parents now, allowed unrestricted access to their critically ill infants.
- Change from compartmantalized to open patient care areas.
- Intensive care by a team rather than an individual.
- Development of the regionalisation concept.

Planning for User Needs

Consideration of design are particularly important in an ICU, in order to achieve the best compromise between advanced technology and operating costs and, also to keep the unit "patient oriented" as well as "staff oriented".

There are particular requirements for intensive care which benefit from specialized design, such as the neonatal ICU with proper distributions of necessary facilities for infant isolators. The CCU presents other specialized needs. There, every affort is made to achieve not only adequate privacy but a quiet, restful environment which still allows optimum electrical monitoring of the heart and prompt resuscitation, with all the necessary equipment quickly available to each bed.

A basic philosophical consideration in the design of an ICU has to do with the level of dependence or independence of the unit in regard to the supporting facilities in the hospital.

Design of an ICU requires clear objectives and accurate information regarding the potential demand for intensive care, which includes not only the type of patients to be cared for, but the volume of patient days per year that is expected.

An architect should develop a programme for use in planning a new ICU. The floor space to accomodate a single bed in a large open room is usually 8.1-9.9 m^2 (90-110 sq ft). The appropriate design of each bed area will depend to, some degree, on the type of the patient to be cared for.

The overall dimensions of the ICU depend a great deal upon the relationship of the unit to supporting facilities elsewhere in the hospital. The total space of the ICU will be made up of the nurse's station, adjacent corridors, patient-bed areas, and support areas. The largest variation in the total size of ICU depend upon the amount of space allocated for support functions. The total area of an ICU generally approximates 2.5-3 times the area required for bed space alone. Thus, for a 10-bed ICU with 130 m^2 (1400 sq ft) for the complete unit, is required.

Some of the important architectural factors to be kept in mind during planning and design of critical care unit include adequacy of the number of beds in the area under consideration suitable relationship to other services, adequacy of sound control in the chosen location, the desirability of an exterior view and exposure to sunlight, and practicality of patient, visitor and service access, as well as internal traffic patterns.

Planning Strategies

To ensure the success of designing a critical care unit with a healing environment, two important steps must be taken by the planners early on the project. The first is to involve as many as possible of the participants responsible for the activities of such a unit into the CCU planing team, including top level management: the second is to do as much decision-making up front as possible. It is at this stage that those decisions can have the maximum possible impact on function, budgets and the ultimate success of the project.

The extent of the care taken to select the right in house participants to work with the design professionals on the design team will be reflected in the final product and its success. Team members should be selected not only for their knowledge and experience in CCU design or operations, care giving or special support, but for their ability to share information, to think creatively, to listen positively, to treat other members of the team with respect and to have the

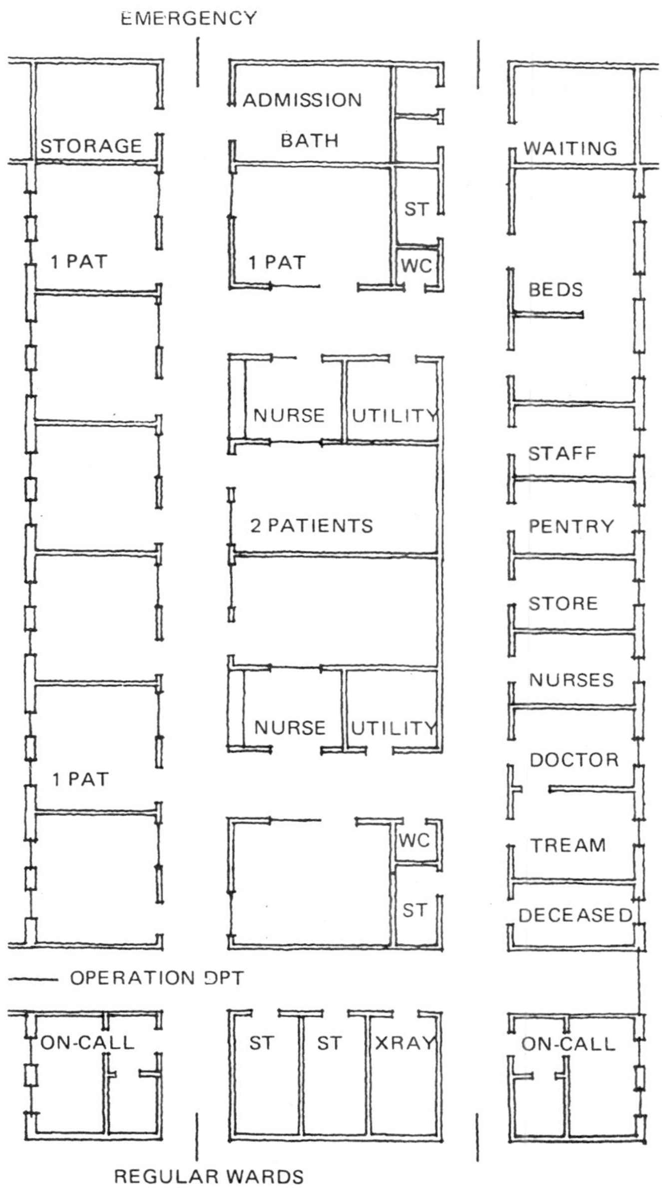

Fig. 34.42: A 12-bed intensive care and treatment unit with two nurses' stations. Pütsep International 1976. Coronary care and burn care patients are not treated in this unit

ability to come to consensus on issues. This involvement will make the team membres feel that their part in the planning is important, and they not only got to have some input on the issues, but become shareholders in success of the project. This design team should include not only physicians and nurses, but also representatives of all of the various management and support staff that have responsibilities affecting the care of the patient and the interaction with their loved ones and visitors. The involvement of a former patients would be ideal.

Team Activities

The first design team meeting should be led by a professional programmer/planner with the skills of a facilitator who can explain exactly what is expected from this early fact finding and programming phase of the project. Team member assignments and responsibilities should be clarified for each participant is understood. This is a good occasion for the facilitator to note that the success of the project and the team will depend upon they carrying out their assignments in a timely manner.

Important events, information receipts and decisions should be drawn up on a schedule or time line diagram for all to keep in their programming manuals. The frequency and location of meetings should also be noted on the schedule, stressing that attendance at the meetings is of paramount concern. Additionally, if a series of special tasks or systems is identified at this time, assignments should be made for task forces to accomplish those issues and chairman appointed to ensure that progress is continuous and above all consistant.

This programming phase should be approached with five well-defined steps, occuring either simultaneously or sequentially:

1. Establish goals
2. Collect and analyse facts
3. Uncover and test concepts
4. Determine needs
5. State the problem.

To assist in gathering the required information, departmental questionnaires should be distributed and discussed at the first design team meeting. There are many facts, concepts and needs that are collected, developed and uncovered that will be important at various phases during the development of the project. Some will seem to be unimportant for the programming phase and obviously, some will be vital to what is being done at the time. The early phase requires that the essance, or distillation of the collected information is sought out and that the other more abstract items should be documented for use in the appropriate phase of the work. If all the information collected is then placed before the design team, a situation will occur which is known as data clog: unable to assimilate all of this data. The forward motion of the design team will slow down or become disorganized. The facilitator should be judicious in the collection and reporting of data and should separate the information into appropriate stacks for use at a later time.

The questionnaires should encompass all of the various aspects of service and support for the CCU, and cover the following issues.

The mission statements of both the institution and the department should, naturally, be mutually supportive and compatible. They will offer guidelines to the design team to focus on the broad aspects, or essance, noted above as well as to define the more specificient delving into the facts greater insights can be gained into the nature of the programme. The CCU mission statement should, of course, detail the level of service sought and the resources that must be genarated to accomplish that mission.

Operational issues Any CCU will operate 24 hours a day, 7 days a week and 365 days a year. A full discussion and documentation on the staffing patterns and the levels of support staff that will be required to operate the unit. This plan of operation will assist in programming the required work space for each individual as well as the spaces required for those support personnel not on a parmanent assignment in the CCU and who will be called to

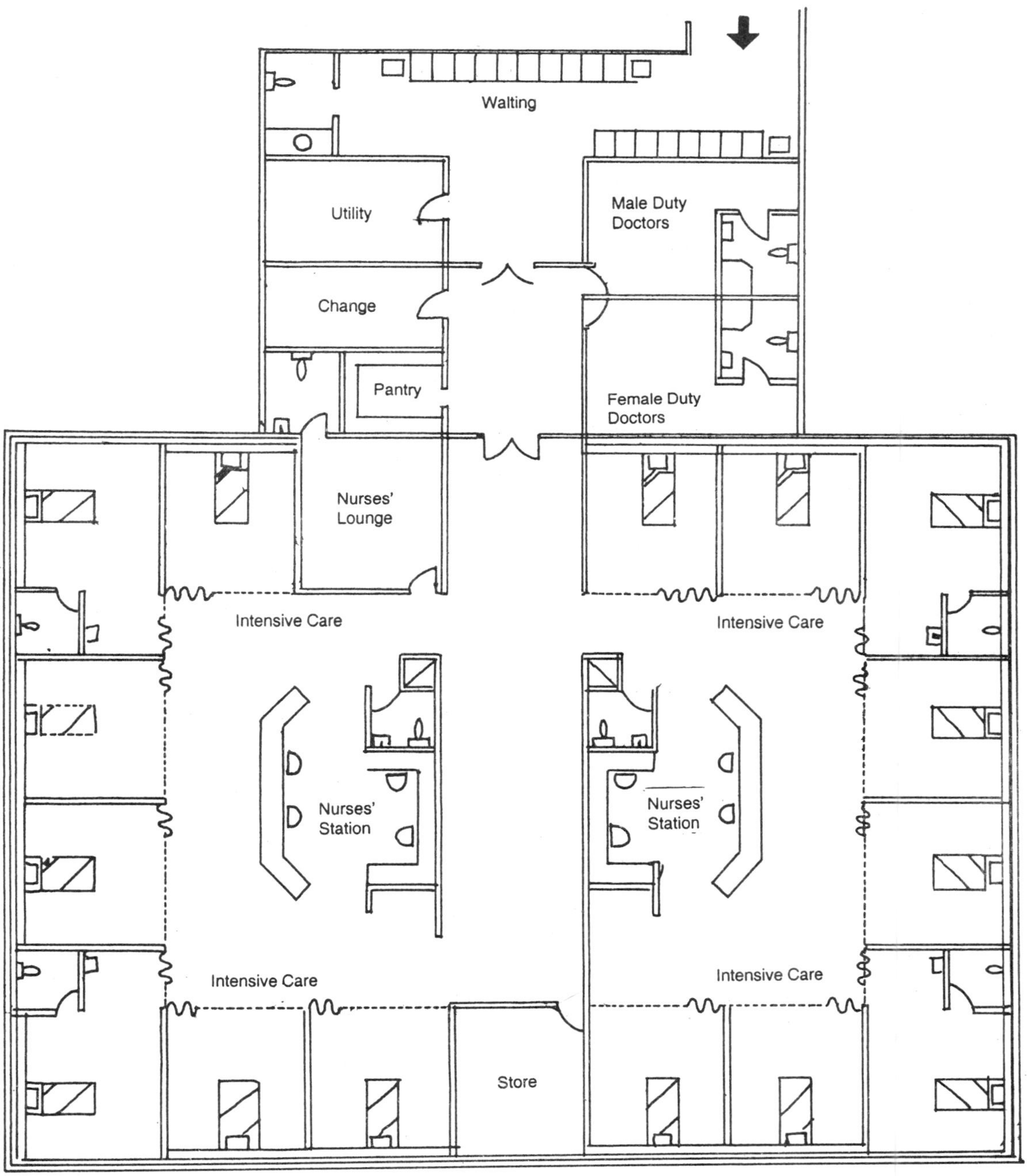

Fig. 34.43: Layout of an intensive care unit

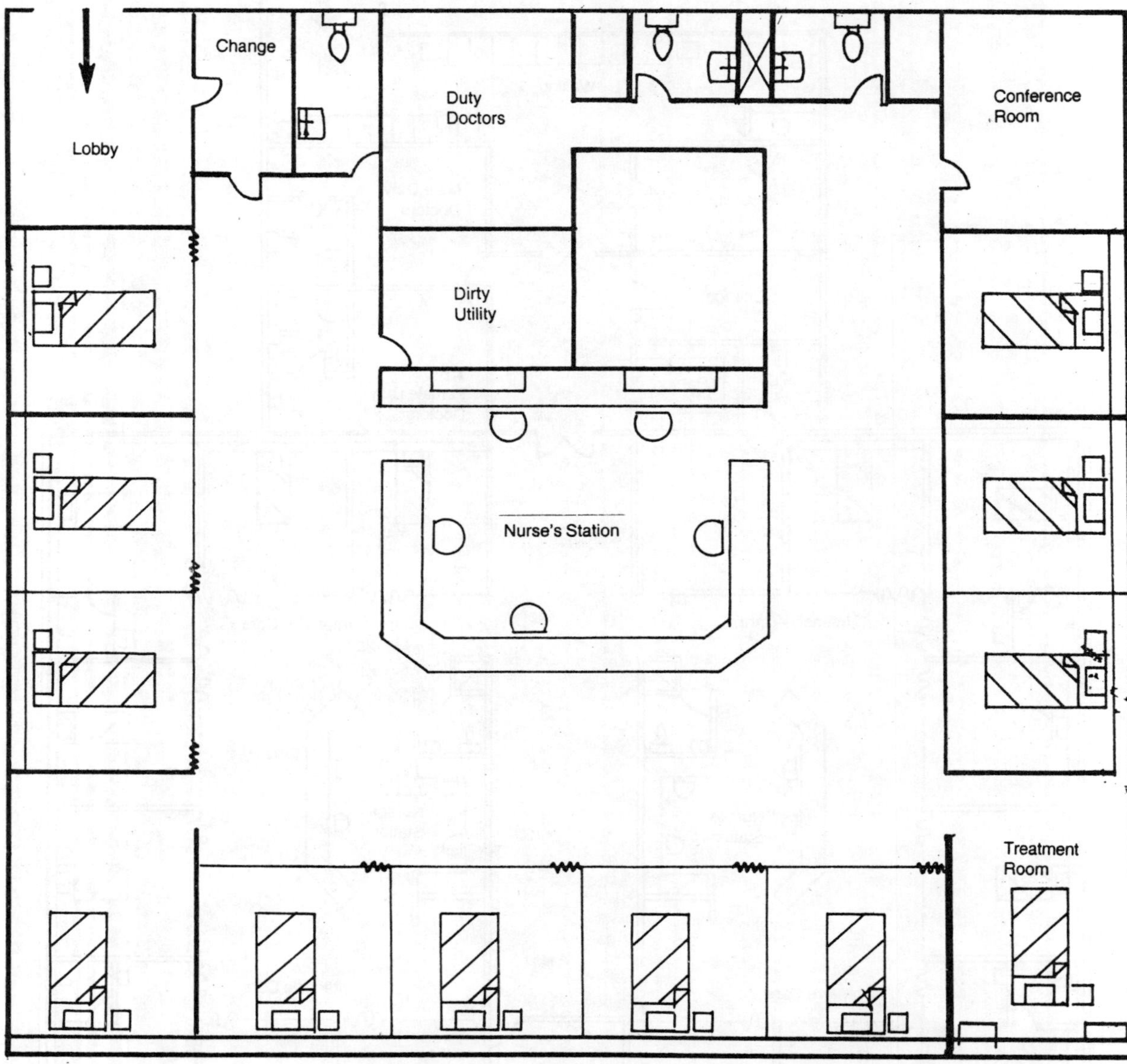

Fig. 34.44: Layout of an intensive care unit

Table 34.1: Space requirements for an average eight-bed CCU (net square feet)

Patient bedroom	175 each
Nurse station	350
Medication area	75
Crash cart	25
Nourishment area	75
Clean utility room	150
Soiled utility room	100
Equipment storage	200
Linen storage	125
Chemistry laboratory	Optional
Catheterization or scanning suite	Optional
Computer room	Optional
Treatment room	Optional
Nurse lounge/lockers/toilet	Convenient to unit
Staff conference room	Convenient to unit
Physician consultation room	Convenient to unit
Office, head nurse	125
Office, unit manager	125
On-call room with toilet/shower	125
Stretcher storage (2)	150
Wheelchair storage (2)	50
Janitor's closet	15

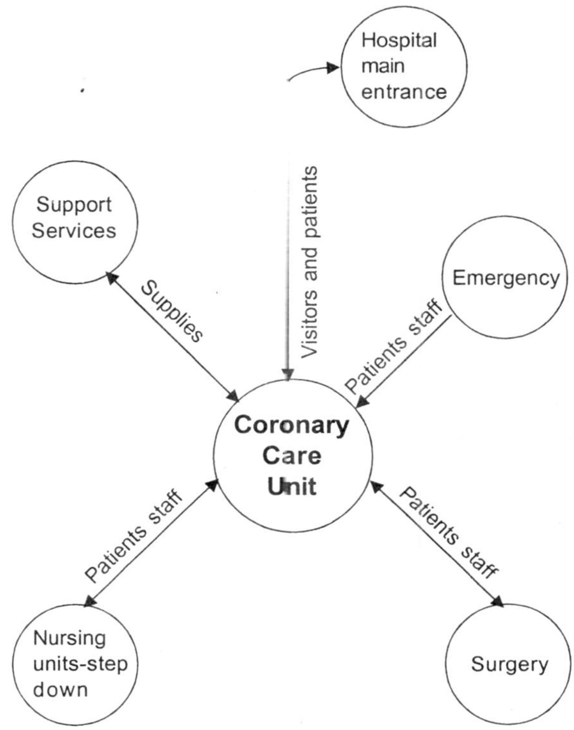

Fig. 34.45: Coronary care unit (CCU) location diagram

active duty either routinaly or in time of crisis. It will also help to determine the proper location and size for supplies and equipment before any hard lines have been drawn on paper.

Uncovering sources of services and supplies. The sources of all services, supplies and equipment can be identified in term of: wehre this service/ supply originates and how it is delivered, and who has the final responsibility for it. Additionally, the design team should evaluate whether this service/ supply is being delivered in a manner that will permit the unit to operate at peek efficiency and effectiveness, or whether alternative means should be part of a work book that follows the projects, progress through to completion.

Development of the systems. The design team must examine the relationships required of all the various departments of services upon which it depends, as well as all the equipment necessary to support its operations and missions. Additionally, the air conditioning, electrics, communications, plumbing and medical gases must be addressed, as should the total environment.

Adjacencies. The design team members should require a study to determine which services and spaces should be located adjacent to which other services or spaces. This study should be concerned not only with the intra-departmental adjacencies, but with inter-departmental adjacencies as well. Support spaces such as supply and ternatively, to decentralize them around the unit for more ready availability to the nursing staff. An example of this decentralized concept might be the use of so-called case carts for specific levels of care that can be nurse servers might also be investigated for inclusion into the planning phase. This concept

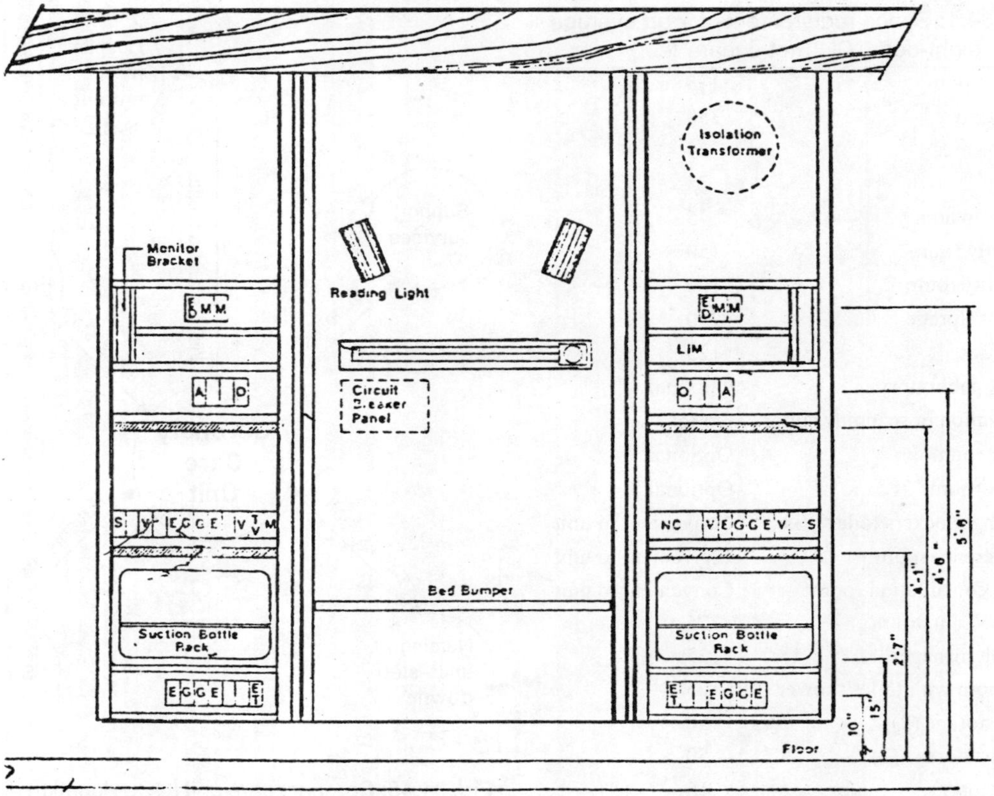

Fig. 34.45: Elevation of headwall for CCU patient room. Hashed lines (/////) = indicate bar rail; A = air; O = oxygen; V = vaccum; E = electrical (single); ED = electrical (duplex); ET = electrical (twist lock); G = ground; M = monitor; NC = nurse call; S = switch (exam light)

permits the replenishment of clean supplies and the retrival of soiled goods by service personnel without the need to enter the patient room.

Conference rooms, the briefing rooms and teaching spaces should be examined to evaluate the concept of shared usage lockers. Toilets and break rooms should be separated from the main area, but still be contained with the department. Given this separation, however, there should be adequate communications to alert the staff of any emergencies within the main CCU.

Environmental issues and needs. The CCU patients needs generally fall into following categories.

- Physical or environmental needs such as windows for views as well as for determining the time of day; clocks and calendars: the ability to gain privacy; the use of soothing colors; shelves for familiar or important objects, and in the case of pediatrics, perhaps toys from home.
- The need for constant observation and professional care
- The need for emotional support and
- The need for communication with staff and loved ones when appropriate.

The CCU staff needs fall into at least six categories:

- The need for space to move around the patient as well as for all the equipment required in a code blue incident
- The need for appropriate lighting levels for patient observation and care

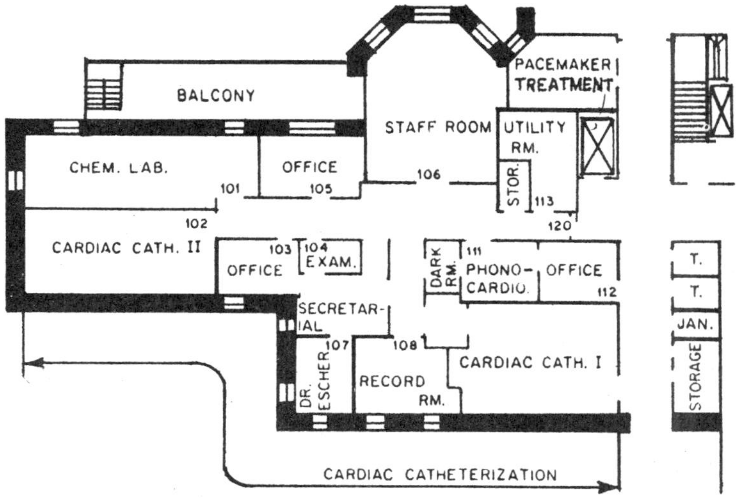

Fig. 34.47a: Reconstruction plans. Catheterization laboratory as of 1971-1974. Originally opened in 1962, housing pulmonary and cardiac physiology, it was revised in 1969-1971 when the catheterization laboratory expanded into the pulmonary physiology work room (102) and office (105), and the pacemaker Center moved its outpatient treatment facility into an outmoded fluoroscopy room and took over room 108 as a minor operating room

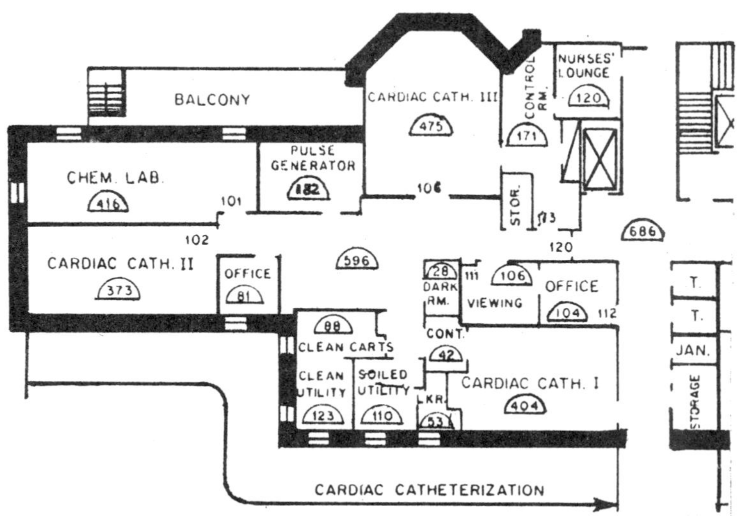

Fig. 34.47b: Revision begun in 1974 with removal of offices, Pacemaker Center, and Phonocardiography to another area and completed 1975-1977 with addition of a new catheterization room together with improved, upgraded, and more specialized facilities for a now primarily operative unit. Section 596 houses nurses' and secretaries' desks and serves as a stretcher and patient holding area

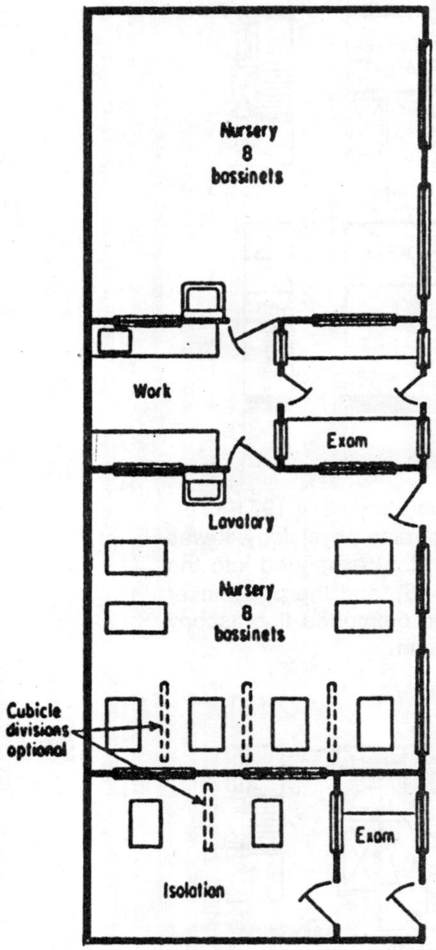

Fig. 34.48: Nursery

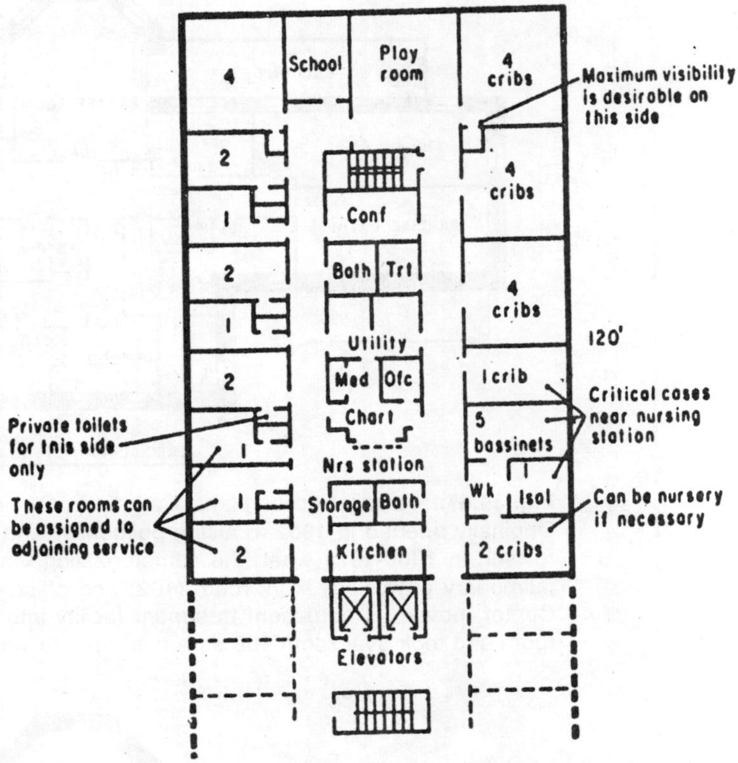

Fig. 34.49: Pediatric unit

- The need to access a myriad of properly functioning equipment in times of great stress.
- The need to have immediate access to support personnel
- The need to have access to family and loved ones when appropriate, and
- The need to get away from the stress of the CCU and still be within easy access of the unit.

The family and loved ones also have needs:

- The need to have the ability to gain vital information about the welfare of the patient
- The need for privacy: with the patient, or by themselves for contamplation or rest, or conferences with the staff to determine patient information
- The need to know that the best is being done for the patient
- The need to gain a sense of control and
- The need to assist in the care of the patient when appropriate.

One of the most serious problems in most CCU designs is the issue of sensory deprivation due to poor lighting: inadequate views; noisy equipment; patients and staff; unfamiliar surrounding and people; anxiety; pain and the separation from family and friends as well as from familiar objects.

Ways of overcoming these problems include providing a variaty of lighting sources and controls

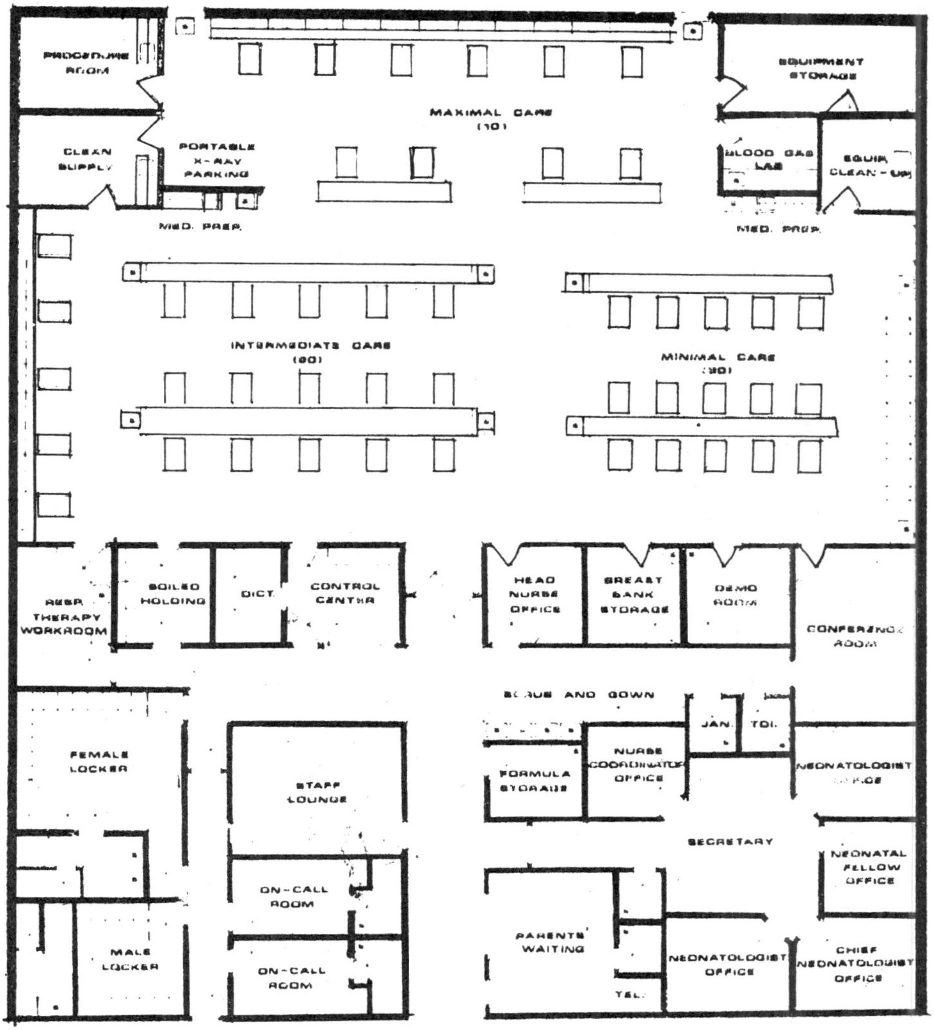

Fig. 34.50: Level III newborn intensive-care unit: open-space concept.

that will fulfill the tasks of the unit. Dimmers for most lighting sources will help provide a soothing environment for the patient and staff alike. Care in locating lighting controls will give the patient some sense of control over their surroundings and allow the staff to have proper lighting when needed. More time and concern should be given to the placement of any lighting in the patient rooms. Early attention to the bed location might permit the patient to enjoy outside views and also observe the entry to the unit as people come and go.

The ability to turn off, or at least reduce, the noise level of the equipment within the patients room or to reduce the amount of equipment in the room, would assist in these and related stresses. Providing separate cubicles for each patient would help in controlling the noise levels from other patients and staff.

The use of sound absorbing materials at the nurse's station, such as carpeting, dropped soffits at the outer perimeter, acoustical tile ceilings and the separation of conferance rooms, debriefing areas and lounges would also be effective in noise reduction.

Permitting 24-hour access by the family or friends, depending on the condition of the patient, would also assist in the well-being of the patients, parents of pediatric patients should be encouraged to help with such chores as changing bed clothes, bathing, hair washing and combing.

There should be provision for chairs and private space around the patients, bedside for the use of spouses and loved ones, which will tend to reduce the stress of this experience for both the patients and the visitors.

The use of colorful curtains and blinds that can be operated by the patient as well as the use of bulletin boards, changeable artwork, and white boards for drawing and writing massages should all be considered to help personalise the room and make for a healing environment.

As far as the staff are concerned, most nursing personnel tend to move the things that make their job easier and more affective closer to the patient to ensure constant observation of the patient, such as using a mobile over bed table for charting. A nurse station be available in each room for charting, medications and other chores. There should be at least one nurse station between two rooms for these purposes. In addition, the traditional nurse station is fairly obsolete these days and more and more CCU designs are incorporating the bedside nurse station concept.

The nurse responsible for direct patient care is always near the patient and the staffing ratios for nurse to patient is usually 1 : 1 or 1 : 2 and the line of sight concept is immediately undone when someone draws the bedside cubicle curtains.

The use of case carts, which contain all of the material and equipment normally used in the specific patient's case could significantly reduce the need for the nurse to leave the immediate area for supplies. These case carts could be sat up prior to the patient's arrival and be tailored to each specific diagnosis.

One very effective tool is full-scale mock-ups. These are very cost-effective in the long run and assist the staff actually to visualise just where everything is to be located, and to make adjustments as required. The mock-ups can be constructed to inexpensive materials or can be built of the material to be used in the actual installation. They can also be constructed in phases, much like the design process itself, with all items roughed in at the beginning and progressing to be more and more precise as the design process continues, culminating in the installation and lasting of actual equipment to be used for the incorporation of the design into final construction documents. This process will educate staff as well as the designer and will, ultimately, reduce the number and cost associated with changed orders during obstruction.

Finally, a determination should be made of the expectation for the CCU of each team member personally and for the CCU design team as a whole and for the ability of mission to be accomplished within its wall, these expectations should be stated in objective terms and, if possible in terms of form function, economy and time. In the long run, these are the criteria on which the success of the CCU will be judged. The design of a successful CCU that encompasses those elements that will ensure a healing environemnt requires a thoughtful, organised approach involving all appropriate personnel. Suggested steps for this are:

- Gain full commitment from the institutional administration.
- Assemble a design team of vital personnel to work on the various tasks outlined above.
- Develop a mission statement for the ICU and gain a copy of the institutional mission statement
- Initiate questionnaires to pull together all of the past, present and future informations on the

various aspects of ICU prior to drawing any diagrams for the unit this will cover the available or required sources of services and supplies, personnel and complete study of the affected systems

- Research existing information and guidelines for ICUs and establish field trips to significant ICUs that are already in operation to gain valuable insights into your own unit, and
- Document all decisions and applicable information for the continued use of the design team throughout the project.

FURTHER READING

1. Axon DC: Planning stratagies for critical care unit design. Hospital management international IHF, London **139**: 142, 1995.
2. Harold Laufman: Hospital special care facilities: Planning for user needs. Academic press, New York, 1981.
3. Porter DR: Hospital architecture guidelines for design and renovation. Health administration press. *Ann Arbor*, Michigan 1982.
4. Putsap E: Modern Hospital: International planning practices. Lloyd Luke Ltd. London 1979.

MULTIDISCIPLINARY INTENSIVE CARE UNIT

Intensive care is one of the important aspects of critical care medicine. It includes resuscitation, emergency care for life-threatening condition and intensive nursing care.

An intensive care unit (ICU) or intensive therapy ward is a nursing unit that is staffed and equipped to look after critically ill patients with potentially reversible lesions who are unable to communicate their needs or who require extensive nursing care and almost constant observation regardless of diagnosis.

Thus, ICU is a special care unit providing the following:

- *A facility* available to all medical staff giving more space, staff and equipment for the care of a patient that cannot be provided in the ordinary wards.
- *A service,* which provides continuous observation of the vital functions and can support these functions more promptly and efficiently than could be done elsewhere in the hospital.

The aim of ICU is to give life support to a patient or prevent threat to life and treat the cause underlying by high standard of nursing care and treatment.

There is a need for concentration of qualified professional staffing and supportive resources into a centre (or unit) where patient admission is by need rather than by diagnosis where patients will be provided extra ordinary care on a concentrated and continuous basis.

The patient will need continuous monitoring of cardiac functions, bed-side system may monitor, temperature, blood pressure, respiration rate and other measurement. More nurses are assigned per patient and they are continuously in the room or within sight of the patient under care.

Type of ICU

a. Single discipline ICU or decentralized ICU, i.e.
   - Cardiac care unit
   - Pediatric ICU
   - Neurosurgery ICU
   - Neonatal nursery
   - Burn Care centre

b. Multidisciplinary or centralized ICU. These usually include medical and surgical intensive care units or combination of all the above.

Physical Facilities

Location It is preferable to locate ICU adjacent to operating suits or recovery room. Easy access from emergency department is also desirable. In a multi storey building, it should be on same floor as operation theatre with facilities like CSSD crystalloid, etc. at easily approachable place.

Beds Number of beds in ICU, will depend upon type of hospital services offered and whether it is centralized or decentralized. In centralized type the requirement may be upto 5 percent of total beds. There should be on an average of 8 and maximum 12 beds. Units of less than 6 are not viable and more than 16 beds unmanageable.

Planning and Design Consideration

The ICU should be organized as a physically and functionally distinct entity within the hospital. Access to it should be controlled in order to regulate traffic including visitors to control hospital acquired infection.

Separate isolation rooms for patients suffering from infectious diseases or those requiring protective isolation should be there.

Direct or indirect visualization of patient from nurses central area is desirable.

Patient care areas should be separate from other areas such as storage staff visitors lounges, etc. Floor space allocated to each bed should be sufficient to accommodate the equipment and personnel necessary to meet any contingency. Usually, it is 140-200 sq. ft. per bed.

A direct intercommunication or alarm system should be provided between nurse's station and patient bedside with connection to other areas and rest room.

Bed should be adjustable to positions required by the patients easily movable. Head boards when present should be adjustable to permit ready access to the patient's head for immediate cardio-pulmonary resuscitation.

If required wall installation of equipment is recommended to facilitate the placement of portable equipment, personnel movement and cleaning procedure.

Adequate lighting should be provided. In active treatment area about 25-30 lux and in nurses/ doctor's room 150-200 lux. There should be floor lights to keep watch on drainage seal suction equipment, etc. Arrangement to make lights diffuse is desirable. Minimum 6 socket outlets 3 each for 5 and 15 amp. and one industrial switch of 9 KV for portable X-ray machines should be there in each cubicle. ICU should have at least two power outlets and alternate supply by stand-by generators.

Adequate ventilation should be ensured with minimum 10-15 air changes per hour. There should be no recirculation of air. Fresh filtered conditioned air should be introduced through suitable filters.

- Temperature 60°-70°
- Humidity: 50-66 per cent

Noise level should be upto 50 decibels. Resilient floor to be provided to deaden sound or moving equipment and staff.

In planning the intensive care Unit (ICU) the architect and the hospital consultant can utilize many of the ideas and schemes that have been developed for the typical patient room of the general hospital. Many aspects of the ICU are unique and must be rethought in planning to meet the special needs of the particular types of patients housed here and of the medical, nursing, and ancillary personnel who care for them.

External and internal relationships of the intensive care unit.

Before detailed plans can be outlined, the external and internal relationship of the ICU must be established. In describing the location of the ICU in relation to other departments. Proximity to good elevator service is the only "must".

Relationships within the unit are at least equally important. In as much as the ICU has been developed to meet the optimal special needs of the seriously or critically ill patient, and of the patient in need of specialized nursing care, it is appropriate to consider the positioning of the patient within the unit.

It is important, first of all, for each patient to be within view of the nurse and, conversely, for each patient to be able to see the nurse. While the comatose patient will be unaware of the nurse's presence, the next patient to occupy this bed may find it most reassuring to see a nurse just few feet away, able to respond immediately to his needs. As reassuring as the patient finds the presence of the nurse, the sight of another patient gasping, struggling, or expiring may prove very distressing. It follows, then that the blocking of vision between patients is desirable.

Variations in Design

To have the largest number of patients within view of a single nurse, it seem logical to place the nurse in the center with patients located on all sides (Fig. 34.50), even though the building may dictate a rectangular form (Fig. 34.51). One possible arrangement, a circular pattern, allows each patient to be placed equidistant from the nurse's station (Fig. 34.52). While there is a practical limit to the number of beds that can be placed along the circumference of the circle without making the central core too large, the ICU bed needs of the average hospital can be met before reaching this limit.

When a portion of an existing hospital is being renovated or the columnar pattern of a multistorey

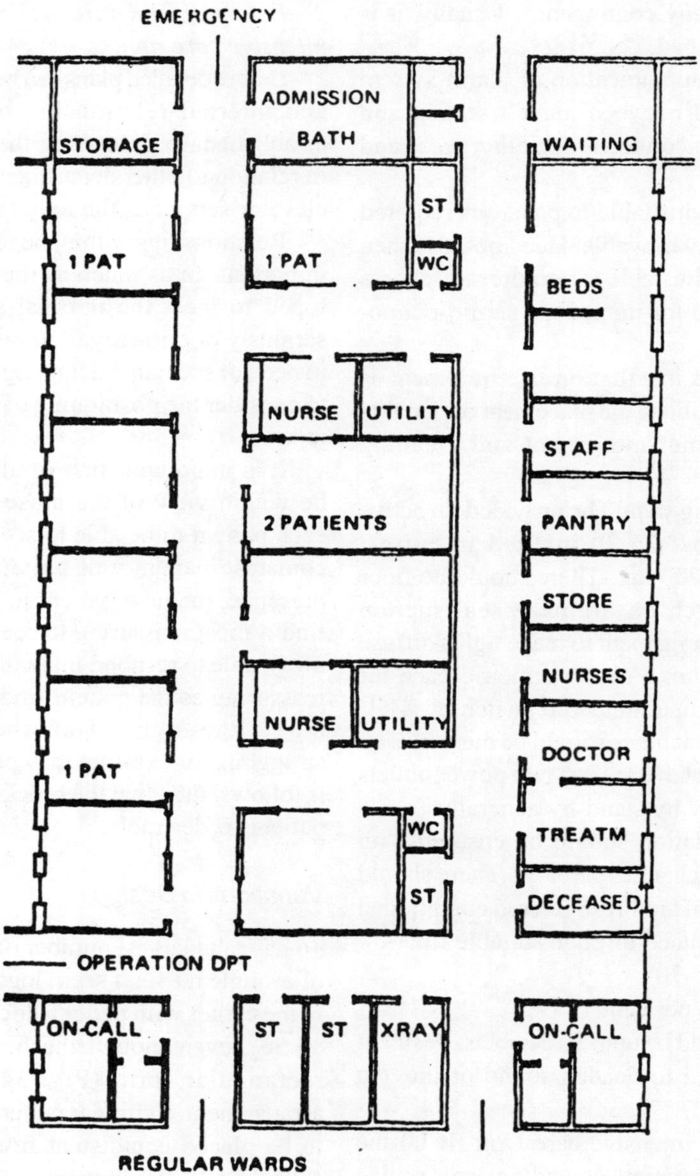

Fig. 34.51: Typical ICU layout

rectangular building is being fitted, difficulties will be encountered. Construction costs for fitting fixtures, casework, etc, to the circular pattern will be greater than the costs for construction utilizating straight lines. Expansion of the unit at a future time when the bed complement of the hospital is increased may prove to be troublesome.

In extending the circular concept, consideration should be given to the semicircle. With a square or rectangular element adjacent to a semicircular

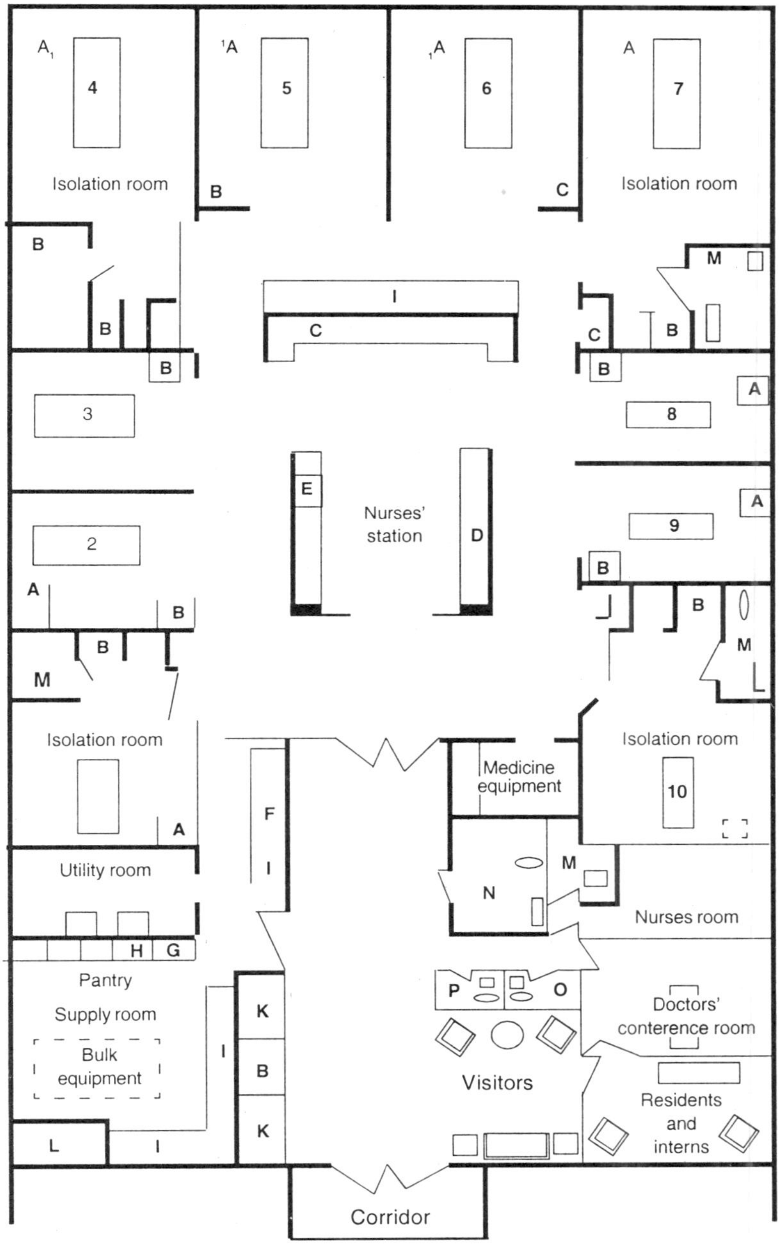

Fig. 34.52: IC ward

element, a unit can be designed with patients accommodated in the circular area, and nurses station and service facilities in the remaining area, utilizing straight walls and traditional cabinet work. A further elaboration of this concept can provide for two semicircular elements connected by a square or rectangular element between them. Again, patients can occupy the circular portions to gain the advant-

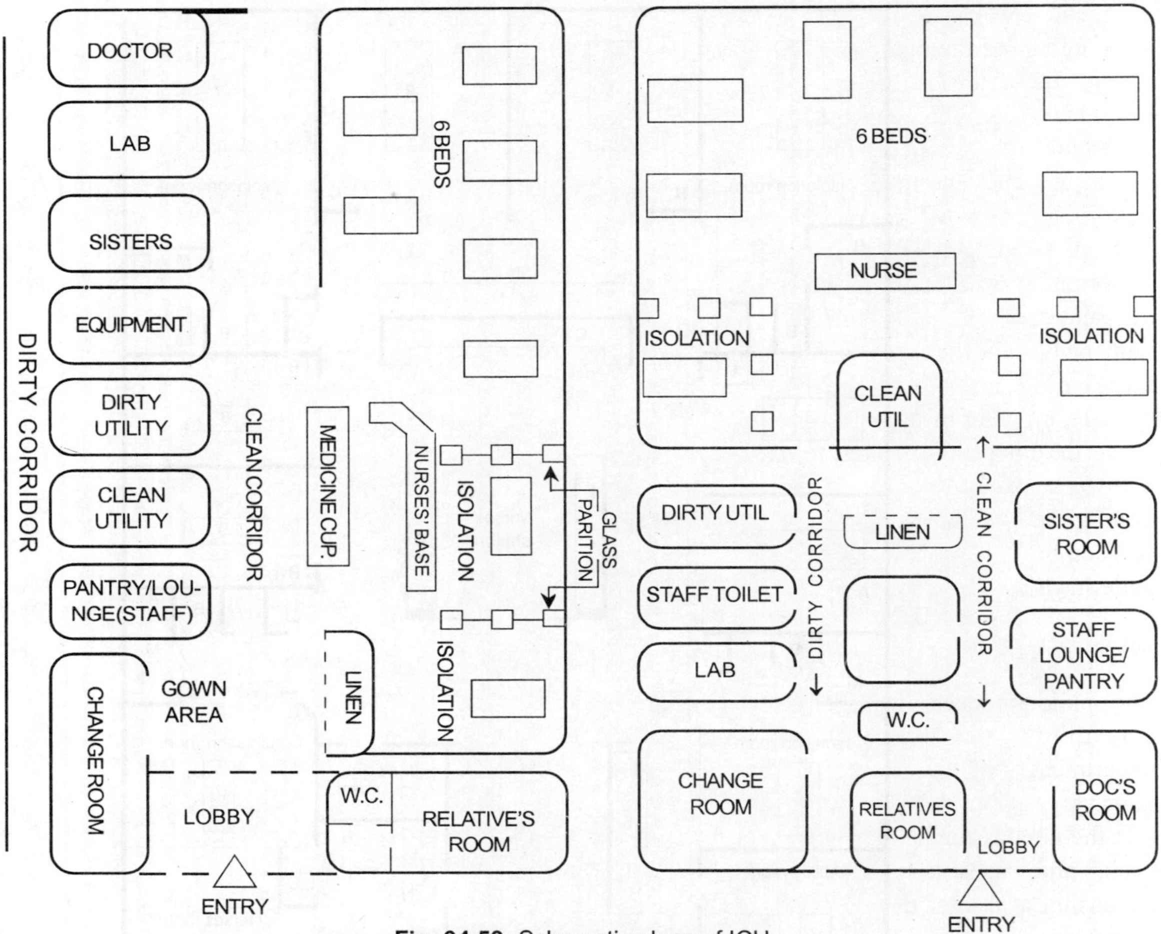

Fig. 34.53: Schematic plans of ICU

ages of the circular design and service functions can be performed within the central linear configuration.

In positioning a semicircular unit, it will frequently be possible to utilize a portion of the floor above the base which usually extends beyond the exterior dimensions of the patient care units above. This will preclude structural problems in designing the upper floors. This concept might be especially helpful when designing an ICU with a double semicircular pattern which takes a minimal amount of area away from the typical patient floor so that the remainder of the area can be utilized as a nursing unit of a practical size. Several other illustrations provide variations of this plan. These schemes, however, may take the ICU too far from the elevator core, making placement nearer the center more feasible. Care must be exercized in designing units of these configurations to ascertain that the area assigned to the nursing care is not disproportionately large for the number of beds provided. It may be possible, if the unit is properly designed, to use the beds at the end of the ICU (and adjacent to another nursing unit) as "swing beds," assigning their use to either intensive care or routine care as the occassion demands.

When structural limitations of the rest of the building are prohibitive but available land is adequate, a circular unit can be designed to extend beyond the confines of the main structure.

No discussion of the layout of a nursing unit would be complete without the mention of a rectangular unit, which existing structures will often dictate in a renovation programme, and relationship to adjoining area will promote in most new construction. Keeping in mind the objective of achieving a workable visual module with enough beds for efficiency of staffing, the central nurse's station with beds on either side is a logical pattern. To increase the number of beds within the visual, module, one end of the unit can also contain bed space, the other end will likely to be needed for entry and work space. A pattern of staggering the positioning of cubicles or rooms around a central station will combine some of the advantages of the circular pattern with the traditional rectangular unit shapes.

Placement by Floor

The opinions concerning placement of the intensive care unit in the base structure with service department or on an upper floor with other patient units vary. Proponents of location in the base argue that the area available here lends to flexibility of design and, particularly, allows greater leeway for expansion at a later date. They indicate, further, that this is not a typical nursing unit in either size or shape and therefore, the upper floor designed for the best—functioning intermediate or routine care unit does not lend itself well to the ICU.

Other opinions maintain that placement in the base poses problems too. If the unit is located near a central elevator core, as it should be, it will not be along an exterior wall. Each room with patient occupancy is required by code to have an outside window. Even if a partitioned ICU with numerous cubicles in classified as one room, it would be desirable to have a window to permit daylight to enter each cubicle. In addition, placement adjacent to such active areas as the operating room, the post-anaesthesia recovery room, or the X-ray suite may make expansion difficult because of the large amounts of space required by these departments when the bed complement is increased.

Proponents of placement of the ICU on an upper floor point out that the function of this area is more analogous to that of the nursing unit than any other department of the hospital, and that the occasional need for emergency, assistance can be satisfied from an adjacent unit. Greater ease of transfer into and out of the ICU is likely to result as well in this location.

How Many Beds Per Cubicle?

There is much advantage in providing each patient with a separate cubicle, it lends to individualized care and generally permits more space for equipment and personnel without encroaching upon another patient's "territory". Of great importance from the patient's point of view is the degree of privacy a cubicle affords from the sights, sound, and smells arising from other patients. Through proper regulation of air flow, with enclosing glass walls and slightly negative pressure within, contaminating interchange between cubicles can be greatly diminished, thereby reducing transmission of infection through the ICU.

Nurses, on the other hand, frequently express preference for at least a few multiple-bed units, pointing out the similarity of needs of certain patients and the unconscious state, which makes privacy less important. The distance between beds can be cut down by elimination of physical barriers, making the nurse's tasks easier when patients of similar diagnosis can be grouped together in one unit. Too many multiple-bed cubicles create lack of flexibility and are to be avoided. The solution seems to be in providing for both single-bed and multiple-bed areas with the unit.

Detailing the Cubicle

The bed can be placed with the head-end at the outside wall. On the partition wall between cubicles, or at an angle. There seems to be little advantage to the last. Utilizing the partition may be the only feasible location with two or more beds in a room, in order to keep the width of the room within reasonable limits. Positioning the bed on the outer wall appears to be the best solution in the single cubicle for greater visibility from the nurse's station and facility of function within the unit. Locating the head toward the nurse's station is excluded from consideration since it defeats these objectives.

Visibility Visual obstruction between patients is desirable. This can be obtained through use of cubicle curtains. Curtains are easily contaminated, however, and must be removed frequently for laundering. The curtains also provide little or no sound barrier and esthetically leave much to be desired. Metal and glass make a more effective barrier possible, although they remove some flexibility. Placement and proportion of glass to metal must be considered. A metal partition at each side, with glass at the foot-end of the room, precludes any lateral vision between rooms. This arrangement may be undesirable, however, because it prevents the doctor or nurse caring for one patient from observating the patient in the next cubicle. A partition, part glass and part metal at each side, can keep the patient from seeing his neighbour but allow personnel near the foot of the bed to see into adjoining areas. Another possibility is glass above the metal below in the lateral partitions so that the patient lying in bed cannot see the next bed, but the doctor or nurse standing at the bedside can see over the metal portion through the glass. A third possibility would utilize glass above and full length at the foot-end so that metal is used only where needed to obscure the patient's vision.

In laying out any floor plan, it is important for the architect to check visual sight lines to determine both placement of the bed and of glass in the partitions to assure that the desired objectives are being met.

Toilets

It is frequently maintained that the patient in the intensive care unit is too ill to use the toilet, therefore it is unnecessary to provide one. While this is undoubtedly true of most patients at some point of their stay in the ICU, a few patients may have bathroom privileges throughout and many more during the final day or two before transfer to another unit. It is widely recognized, for example, that the post-coronary patient undergoes less strain in taking a few steps out of bed to the toilet than in struggling with the bedpan. Therefore, unless ICU policy dictates the retention of only strictly, bedfast patients in the ICU, planning the inclusion of toilets is worthwhile. They provide the added advantage to the nurse of a readily accessible bedpan-flushing facility, if properly fitted, which reduces steps to the soiled utility area and chances for cross-contamination throughout the unit. In view of the somewhat limited use, one toilet per multibed room is undoubtedly sufficient. Where should the toilet be placed? The typical patient room usually has the toilet at the corridor end of the room. This permits more economic use of space, since adjacent area, in providing entry into the room, does not remain unutilized. Further, it allows free use of exterior wall for window space without blocking the patients view.

While this design can be carried over for use in the ICU cubicle, here it does not make as much sense. The patient in intensive care is not very likely to be concerned with the view through the window, if positioning the bed against the external wall is accepted, he cannot look outside, anyhow; and more important still, the toilet room blocks the line of vision between the bed and the nurse's station. By locating the toilet between two rooms, to be shared by both occupants, the width can be reduced so that less visual impairment results. To carry this reasoning a step further, why not place the toilet room along the external wall between two cubicles?

The space adjacent to it can be well utilized as work space for personnel. The question of a lavatory in the toilet room arises, if space permits, it would be welcome. When the frequent use of this facility by nursing personnel for bedpan handling is contrasted to actual patient use, however, the inside lavatory becomes less important. Certainly a handwashing facility (sink) in the work area is of greater importance. Therefore, unless two running water facilities can be provided, a counter-top sink outside the toilet room and in the area most accessible to nurses and doctors is recommended.

Lighting and other Equipment

Lighting of the intensive care cubicle is an important matter, general room illumination, convenience lighting, examination light, and night light should be provided. Color-corrected lighting, combining incandescent and fluorescent light sources, is available and is especially helpful in the ICU where the patients true color must be discernible so that such signs as cyanosis, jaundice, etc. can be recognized. The examination light must be positioned so that any and all parts of the body can be reached with the light. Portable lights attached either to the wall or to the bed can be considered, but they have the disadvantage of requiring one hand to hold, leaving only one hand free to work when no one else is free to assist.

Much equipment is potentially needed for the intensive care patient. It is possible to have much of this equipment mounted on the wall and some of it can be recessed into the wall, certainly consideration should be given to providing through wall piping the services that will be used frequently. This will make life-saving facilities readily available without the delay and personnel time otherwise needed to wheel equipment to the bedside. Some of the newer wall-mounted lighting fixtures have incorporated panels that house outlets of various patient room services. The nurse call system can be located in this console. A geriatric cell button is now available for the incapacitated as well as for the geriatric patient.

Oxygen outlets should be included in the console, no less than one for each patient. Compressed air may also be considered where nebulization, humidification, or other environmental conditioning is required without necessarily utilizing oxygen. It can also be used for spray disinfection of the cubicle upon the patients discharge. If physicians will insist on prescribing oxygen along with treatments, compressed air will probably not be necessary. If used frequently in place of oxygen, compressed air will be more economical. Two or three vacuum outlets per patient's will generally be advisable as a facility to be included in the console, a cabinet can be obtained to provide in a compact assembly the varieties of suction apparatus that may be needed for patients who have undergone complicated surgical procedures. This cabinet can be wall-mounted next to the bed. If it can be recessed, it will still be close at hand without taking up floor space in the room. In either case the necessary drainage bottles are contained within the cabinet instead of protruding in the way of the bed or of personnel. For hospitals in which thoracic surgery patients will be admitted to the ICU, low vacuum for pleural drainage, regulated vacuum for aspiration, and intermittent vacuum for gastrointestinal drainage should be provided through appropriate adaptors.

The patient service console should also include electrical convenience outlets. Enough outlets with proper voltage to meet all needs should be provided to allow the use of any needed equipment without overloading. Two 20-amp circuits should be provided so that two duplex outlets per bed are possible, with one circuit to each. Some equipment, such as a hypothermia unit, will require 20 amps alone. In addition, there should be a second source of current from an emergency generator in the event of a power failure from the primary source. It will be well to provide portable lights that can be plugged into the emergency outlet whenever there is an electrical failure. A wall-mounted sphygmomanometer near each bed will also prove helpful to nursing personnel since it is always handy and need not be carried from bed to bed. IV support brackets should also be readily available. They can be attached to the console or to the bed, or mounted on the ceilling. The most suitable location will be determined by the location of the bed, the console, and other equipment in the room.

The patient service console provides various electric circuits, including emergency power, a sphygmomanometer, IV support brakets, portable X-ray outlets, vacuum outlets, oxygen outlets, lighting, nurse call, and similar facilities.

Despite all the wall-mounted or recessed equipment available, there will always be other items, perhaps less frequently used which will be needed on occassion. If small in size, they will require a place near the bed and off the floor. Accessibility of trays, needles, syringes, and other supply items will require a counter or a shelf. A bedside cabinet, quite useful in the usual patient room, gets in the way in the ICU. The counter containing the sink is a little too far from the bedside. Therefore, shelves behind the bed appear to be a logical solution for placement or storage of the supplies. Recessed shelving offers obvious advantages over well-mounted shelving.

Whether physiologic monitoring equipment is included initially or not, provision should be made for adequate space and wiring. Space requirements will vary with the type of equipment and whether it is placed at the bedside or at a central monitoring station. Portable X-ray outlets should be provided. While they may not be needed in each patient cubicle, a sufficient number, properly spaced, should be planned to serve the entire intensive care unit.

Space Outside the Cubicles

In addition to the nurses charting area, space outside the patient cubicles, but in or near the ICU, must be planned. Clean and soiled utility space is essential. In the interest of good visibility throughout the unit, clean utility might well be in an open area, from which the nurse can see into patient cubicles. A centrally-located counter area with appropriate sink and shelving can be utilized. Because of problems of contamination from infected patients, the soiled utility area should be enclosed. This enclosure can be partly glass, so as not to decrease visibility too markedly. A medication area must be provided within the nurses station. This area can be open so long as appropriate steps are taken to store and safeguard medications. A glass-enclosed cubicle for the head nurse can be most helpful in permitting discussions between nurses or between nurse and doctor, which the patient should not overhear. Metal and glass partitions allow the patient to remain within view of the personnel inside the cubicle. While some of the patients will be fed intravenously, a nourishment station is desirable for the preparation and storage of nourishments for other patients. Linen cart storage or shelving for storing linens (depending upon the linen distribution system in use) cannot be overlooked. Another necessity is Janitor's closet for housekeeping equipment and supplies for this unit. Since some storage of equipment will be neccessary and it is unwise to cluster patient cubicles or corridors with equipment not currently in use, some storage area within the unit is highly desirable. As patient care is becoming increasingly mechanized, the need for storage space for equipment is likely to continue to increase, so planning should be generous in this regard. While it may be used infrequently, due to the nature of patients housed here, one shower or tub shower in the ICU is desirable if space is available. The nursing staff will require toilet, locker room, and lounge facilities within or adjacent to the intensive care unit. A visitors, waiting room outside the unit, but close by, is desirable since visiting regulations will probably preclude visiting for more than a few minutes at a time. The waiting room permits relatives and friends to remain at hand to learn of new developments in the patients condition. The visitor's waiting room should be provided with a rest room, and a public telephone should be available nearby. Finally, a consultation room adjacent to the waiting room will be helpful to the physician in speaking to the patients, family without being overheard by relatives of other patients.

The size and placement of the various cubicles and rooms just mentioned will vary considerably with the size of the intensive care unit, its location within the structure, and the needs and desires of the hospital. Careful consideration and discussion with medical and nursing personnel is of paramount importance, as are other foregoing aspects of the intensive care unit. It is only by considering each item and drawing appropriate conclusions that an efficient, modern ICU can be developed for each hospital.

Equipment

Equipment provided should be suitable for the number of patients being treated. Following should be available.

- Oxygen and compressed air and the means of administration
- Mechanical ventilation assistance equipment including airways, manual breathing bags and ventilators/respirators.
- Cardiac defibrillator
- Respiratory and cardiac monitoring equipment
- Thoracocentasis and thoracostomy sets
- Trachenostomy set
- Tourniquets
- Vascular cut down set—Infusion pump
- Laryngoscopes and gastric suction equipment
- Portable X-ray machine
- An emergency cart within unit should be ready with drugs and equipment as determined by the medical staff.

Staffing

The ICU must be directed by a physician who has received special training, acquired experience, and achieved competence in a speciality related to the care provided in the unit However, traditionally anesthetists have been administering these units because of their expertise in respiratory and resuscitation therapy. They should have the responsibility of implementing policies of the ICU quality, safety and appropriateness of patient care services provided are reviewed and evaluated regularly. Acitivities of a multi-purpose ICU should be guided by a multi-disciplinary committee of the hospital staff. They should be responsible for development and approval of ICU policies, major structural change, major equipment purchases and infection control measures.

Medical Staff

Coverage should meet the intensive care of patient within the unit. The role of house staff should also be defined.

Nursing staff Expert nursing is the most important element in the intensive care of the patient. It is, therefore, essential that the intensive care unit nursing staff should be highly trained and of above average competence. The nursing staff should be knowledgeable about the emotional and rehabilitative aspect of the ICU patient and be capable of applying appropriate therapeutic intervention. The recommended nurse patient ratio, though in practice, it is usually 1:2, the distribution as practical is as follows:

Morning shift	1:1
Evening shift	1:2
Night shift	1:3

A programme for continuing education of nursing staff should be developed and implemented. It should include:

- Recognition, interpretation and recording of signs and symptoms of patients and notification of relevant one to physician
- Initiation of cardiopulmonary resuscitation
- Administration of I/V fluids, blood, etc.

- Administration of emergency drugs as authorized
- Safe use of electrical and electronic equipment
- Control of infection.

Patient and their families, counselling.

Policies and Procedures

Team work based on mutual respect is usually more effective than authority.

However, certain policies and procedures are required to be laid down for avoiding conflicts and confusion in patient care and day-to-day administration. These should be reviewed periodically and should relate to at least the following.

- Admission and discharge of patient
- System of sending consultation and informing physician incharge about his case
- Location of drugs and equipment
- Methods of procurement of drug/equipment and maintenance of essential life-saving drugs, laboratory, X-ray and other diagnostic procedures on pririty basis.
- Checking of expiry dates of drugs
- Infection control
- Procedure to be followed in case of equipment (supplies/services/failure and replacement/repair of equipment)
- Pertinent safety practices (fire orders)
- Visitor control and information to them
- Its role in internal or external disaster planning
- Specification as to who may perform special procedure under what circumstances and under what degree of supervision
- Duties of officer incharge, nursing and paramedical staff working in ICU.

ICUs are cost and labor-intensive area and thus their effective and efficient utilization is most desirable. It is primarily meant for patient in a critical stage of illness and not for all seriously ill patient. The admission and discharge policies should be based on these criteria. Endeavor should be there to keep its occupancy not more than 80 to 85 percent at any time.

Emerging Trends in Intensive Therapy Unit

Intensive therapy usually means the treatment of patients during a period of their critical illness. This unit requires special space and equipment consideration for effective staff functions. In addition, space arrangement shall include provisions for immediate access of emergency equipment from other departments. About 5 percent of the total number of beds in a hospital should be allocated for use in the intensive care. An ICU of less than 6 beds is clearly uneconomical. However, to reduce the risk of nosocomical infection for most hightly susceptible patients the sizing of the ICU to 4-6 beds is recommended. Too big ICU become ineffective. The current overall spatial need in the ICU is about 40 sq. mts. although lower figures of upto 25-30 sq mts have been used.

In a single story hospital, ideal location for intensive care unite will be near to the emergency service, laboratory, surgery, recovery room and other essential services.

In a multi-storey building, locating the intensive care unit on the upper floors helps in keeping it out of the main stream of traffic thus helping to lower cross-infection and providing quite surroundings. Of the two design possibilities for patient rooms the open ward and the single bed—the latter has gained preference. There should be provision for privacy without isolation in which communication is essential.

The spatial need for a ICU bed in a single bed room is 17-21 sq mts. An ICU may assume any shape—square rectangle or circular. For providing privacy, curtains or partitions with glass panels usually at 1.2 m for observation by the nurse but providing visual barrier between patients, should be used. Circular ICU has the advantages of shortest radius of nursing travel distance for a number of beds but is only possible in a new building. In addition to other ceiling lights, lights should be provided on the wall beneath the beds to check drainage bags and bottles under the beds.

Observation of patient color is important hence blue/green lighting is not permitted. Usually 30 lumens/sq ft. at bed level is recommended.

High pressure should be provided in the clean area to prevent inflow of germs and dust from the surrounding dirty areas. Generally 8-10 air changes/hr are provided, There should not be any diffuser directly over the patients's bed to prevent strong air drafts. Thermoneutral zone of 27°-31°C should be the guide for ambient temperature of the ICU, to 25°C for an intermediate care area.

Floors should preferably be of conductive type as most of the equipment in ICU is electrical. Terrazzo in general is used instead of marble or other stones to reduce noise due to walking or falling objects. A terrazzo floor mixed with carbon forms an ideal surface wich can easily be cleaned but is absorbent to some extent which causes stains. in situ mosaic flooring with least possible joints and brass/copper strips 6" apart (both ways) to carry out any static electricity is also used.

For cleaniness and protection of the walls by the movement of the trolleys in situ mosaic finish is recommended for the full height of the wall. All fittings should flush with the wall. Roof should be painted and corners rounded off.

The bed is an environmental influence which the critically ill patient cannot escape. To provide conditions for his effect give existance and improved state of health the ICU bed should.

- be capable of providing a comfortable working height for male 107.5 cm, for female 97.5 cm
- have a mattress at a height of 32.5 cms from the ground for the patient to get in and out of the bed easily
- be readily adjustable to various therapeutic positions, easily moved for transport, have a locking mechanism and a removable head board
- may contain an intercom between the patient and the nurse's station.

Locating the beds permanently away from the wall gives staff a 360° access to the patient.

The head panel gives a neat look to the room

All tubes, pipes and wiring for the patient could also be organized and contained in pannel or column at the head of the patient's beds.

Intensive Coronary Care Units

This term as well as cardiac care unit is used to identify the units restricted to patients who have or are thought to suffer from myocardial infarction, arrhythmias or some other cardiac emergency conditions. They have special needs. They are aware of their surroundings but still need immediate and critical care.

In addition to the requirements of general ICU, the following facilities are also required:

- An ICCU should not be a part of the general purpose intensive care therapy unit and each patient shall have separate enclosure or room for acoustical and visual privacy.
- Each coronary patient shall have access to a toilet.
- Provisions should be made for visual display of cardiac monitoring equipment at each patient's bed location and at the nurse's station.
- All patients should be within view of the nursing staff.
- In case of a cardiac arrest the attending physician or nurse must have access to the patient's head therefore the beds must be kept away from the wall.
- There must be a resuscitation panel with both oxygen and suction.
- Patient's bedside must have a panic button to alert the staff in case of a cardiac arrest.
- There are functional advantages when oxygen, vacuum, compressed air and the electrical outlets are provided on both sides of the patients's bed
- For ICCU the size of 6 to 10 beds is most commonly used. More than 10 beds increase supervising problems. An area of 15-18 sq mtr per bed is required.
- The ICCU should be adjacent to general emergency admission unit or near a medical ward in which progressive care of the patient can be undertaken.
- Since the patients in ICCU are anxious to a greater or lesser extent, they must be kept away from any type of sudden noise or shock. The unit should be located so as to completely avoid any external or internal noise.
- The patients should be preferably out of sight of each other so that they do not witness the resuscitation or death of a neighbouring patient.

Burn Care

There are two phases of burn illness:

- The shock period
- The healing period.

Special equipment is required to meet the peculiar needs of the burn care patients, such as Circ-O-Lectric beds, ropes, weights and pulleys for positioning and applying traction to extremities.

The burn care patient may have to lie on his abdomen or back for lengthy periods. The unit must provide a comfortable atmosphere. Windows should be low enough to look out while lying in bed. TV is an excellent medium to prevent boredom and maintain morale. The recommended number of beds in a burn ward is between 6 to 15 beds. The total spatial requirements of about 50 sq mts per bed in the smallest unit are reduced to about 30 sq mts when the size of the unit is increased to 15 beds. The shock room should be about 26 sq mts in size. Special beds or cranes and other apparatus for handling heavy patients may require additional space. Supply of oxygen, suction and electrical power points for X-ray apparatus are needed. Hand-washing facilities are needed.

To decrease evaporative cooling and fluid loss the room temperature should be regulated to 29°C and the humidity of about 30 percent. When the patient has to lie naked in a shock room, a temperature of 32°C is required. Airconditioning with about 7-10 air change per hour is desirable.

Neonatal Intensive Care Unit (NICU)

NICU is provided for the care and observation of all premature and low birth weight infants, infants of high risk mothers or infants suffering from other chronic diseases.

Three level NICUs have been required. A 28-bassinet unit might have 3 intensive care spaces, 20 intermediate care areas and 5 transitional care places for short-term observation. A unit for NIC should contain at least 24 cots. A NICU would include ward rooms of about 14 to 15 m^2 with 3 incubotors in each.

The number of NICU beds in a hospital can be estimated by the following formula

$$\text{The number of NICU beds} = \frac{L \times (IB + OB)}{OR}$$

(L is the average length of stay OB is the number of outborn babies, IB is the number of inborn babies, OR is the average occupancy rate).

The maximum number of patients which can be properly cared by one nurse is eight.

The minimum space for each bassinet is 2.5 sq mt. It is necessary to place this unit close to, but outside of the delivery suite with a glass partition along the corridor so that friends and relatives can see in without entering the nursery. This unit must be provided with sound insulation.

The nursery unit includes area for:

- Resuscitation:
- Admission and observation
- Routine and extended newborn care (such as general nursery, isolation nursery, premature nursery)
- Nursing station
- Procedures such as circumcision and lumbar puncture

A washbasin for each 3-4 bassinets is needed.

Work space Delivery room and resuscitation area: There should be space for management and resuscitation of the newborn infant after birth. The area should be well-lighted and equipped with:

- Infant bed
- Radiant heat source
- Air, oxygen, and suction points
- Electrical outlets.

Admission and observation area This is for continued observation of the infant during the first 24 hours. This may be a separate room but can be within the nursery. It should have:

- Air, oxygen and suction points
- Six electrical outlets
- Sink
- Trash container

The equipment required is:

- Racks for each clean and used gowns.
- A sink with elbow or foot-operated controls for every 5 bassinets
- One electrical outlet for every bassinet.
- One oxygen, compressed air, and suction outlets for every five to six bassinets.
- A power socket for a portable X-ray unit.
- An area for storage of clean supplies and special equipment such as head hoods, ABG analysers and a panic box
- Separate facilities for temporary storage or disposal of soiled bottles, syringes and diapers.
- Walls and floor should be attractive and be easily cleanable.
- Color schemes—white or off white are recommended because they enhance the observer's ability to detect cyanosia or jaundice.
- Approximate light intensity at 100 lux at the bed level is sufficient.
- Temperature should be maintained between 24° to 26°C (75° to 82°F) for infant comfort and relative humidity should be approximately 50 percent.

Pediatric Ward

The pediatric ward may be an open ward plan. The total room to bed ratio should provide for at least one patient room for every six beds. In addition to other facilities the pediatric ward shall include:

- Space at bedside for visiting parents
- Sleeping space for parents who may be required to spend long hours with the patient
- Separates storage cabinets for toys for use by the pediatric patient
- Space allowance for pediatric beds and cribs equal to those required for adult beds, because of variation in size and potential for change
- Provisions for nutritional needs including infant formula preparation and storage.
- Additional storage for cots, linen and other items need to accomodate parents of the patient overnight.

FURTHER READING

1. The American Association of Hospital Consultants 4, and Functional Design of General Hospitals (Ed. Mills AB) McGraw-Hill Inc. New York, 1974.
2. Ervin Putsep: Modern Hospital: International planning practices Lloyd-Luke Ltd. London.1979.
3. Wheeler ET: Hospital Design and function. McGraw-Hill Inc. New York, 1964.

ACUTE NURSING CARE UNITS

It has been seen that surgical patients change dependency, but sizable majority of medical patients seem to remain in the same dependency category throughout their stay.

Also staying in a regular acute ward unit disrupts an individual's normal mode of operation. He is unable to carry on his regular activities in work, recreation, religion. The loss of contact with family, friends, and co-workers may be felt as much as the physical confinement. The objectives of the hospital system and particularly of the nursing units frequently dictate that the patient be treated as a sick person, not as a person, who is sick. The patient is expected to adjust and adapt. To an ill individual the stress of hospital life may seem unending. Unfortunately, the criterion for patient well-being is rather nebulous. The nursing unit design can contribute towards the patients, coping with the psychological effects of the hospital routines. However, the facility is only one component of a system.

There are ward units also in most unusual shapes and design. In many cases the main aim has been to reduce the walking distances, as in many circles the only argument for nursing economy has been mileage. In the US, the nursing unit design include square units, round units, rectangular unit, pinwheels and clover leaves; single-loaded corridors with patients room on only one side and double-loaded corridors with patient rooms on both sides, schemes for simple circulation and schemes for redundant circulation. Dozens of styles could be shown. Wide variations exist also in other countries. The lowest level nursing unit consists of an open ward, where all the beds are facing the centre of the room. The nurse's station consists of a desk, some storage space, and water supply facilities. At the far end of the ward, there is a serving kitchen, a soiled utility room, toilets and a bath room and a storage. On the next higher level, the nursing unit is divided into units with four or more beds in each and a line of service rooms is added. The added service area contains the nurse's unit with a treatment room, a clean utility room, a nurse's station, a sluice, a soiled linen room, and also administration space, a household unit with kitchen, and wardrobes for the patients. Additional sanitary facilities are arranged. The next step is the adding of a few isolation rooms for critical cases or for contagious diseases.

In the last phase, day spaces are provided, some storages added, and sanitary facilities differentiated.

Single Occupancy Room

As increasing trend towards more privacy in every aspect of life accounts in part for an emphasis on the single occupancy room in hospitals.

It has been found that patients prefer what they are familiar with and tend to preserve the status quo.

However, no strong preference for or against privacy should be stated as an axiom. People, who were alone in their lives, resent being left alone in a hospital. The additional cost for the single occupancy has become a very small part of the very large total cost per day. Nurses like the privacy of the patient, which would give them a closer rapport with the patients, who would be less embarrassed to ask for advice or help. In single occupancy fewer medication errors occur, and there is a superiority in emergency situations. A hospital patient room is a sick bay, but also an individual territory, it is a hotel room, an emergency unit, a family reunion centre. Fulfilling these demands requires more than one specialist. Space restriction can lead to limited freedom of movement, absence of privacy, and lack of personal facilities. All these conditions can have serious psychological and social consequences. It has been suggested that the recovering patients should be given at least the possibility to control the microclimate: light quality, room temperature, air movements, odours humidity. The patient rooms rarely are designed to take into account the psychological influences of proportion and size. Also the windows, open doors and screens affect the patient to perceive the conditions of his socio-physical environemnt.

The configuration of the patient room has to be functionally appropriate. In order to arrive at a suitability, the activities of both patients and staff which are carried out in the room as well as the space requirements of furnishings relevant for the medical treatment and for other convenience of the patient have to be analyzed carefully.

The corner bed constitutes nursing problems. Only the freestanding bed is admissible in hospital practice, when the acutely ill, there is an average of only 2.4 movements of the bed in 24 hours. The ideal room size for etrating different conditions must be known. Figures reflecting dynamic anthropometry and function and the perceptual responses of people should enter the calculations.

All patient's rooms must be as self-contained as possible and directly linked to WC and washing facilities. Washing compartments should separate from WC compartments, self-contained, and doors should be provided. Some of the WC and washing compartments should allow easy access for wheelchairs.

Multipatient Rooms

For reasons of the ease of observability—privacy's very opposite—the single rooms have been opposed. It could be hardly assumed that a patient feels better cared for, if he sees the nurse in the room more often, attending to someone else. Sharing a room in a general hospital is a source of some positive and some negative experiences. It is good to have a roommate to talk to and very important that roommates try to help each other, but it is undesirable to have a very ill roommate and a great difference between the ages of the roommates. The roommates who have too many visitors are quite annoying to other patients. There is no privacy no matter how much it is wanted. Smoking odours, and are noise is an annoying factors.

Although some medical professionals agree in principle with a four-bed maximum requirements, many believe that a larger room configuration has additional therapeutic value in patient care. The bed-landscape reduces the possibilities of good patients-staff contact. Also most of the sheer physical surroundings of large wards are inimical to good communication, because they make private, intimate conversations between doctor and patient very difficult to achieve, and quite impossible if the patient is hard of hearing. Large multi-bed rooms in acute wards for adults represent a significant loss of amenity and of flexibility in the allocation of beds. Their only means to provide some privacy for highly sensitive physical examinations are privacy curtains. They should be provided in any situation in which the patient could be unwittingly exposed.

Single and Multibed Accommodation Mix

Needs which have emerged through development of sub-specialities and changes in the pattern of morbidity, can be effectively met by the provision of single rooms and four-bed rooms in the wards. The optimal mix of single and multibed accommodations in a ward cannot easily be expressed as a single universal percentage, as it depends on a combination of medical, social, and economical factors. The proportion of each type of bed arrangements will vary with the quality level of the clinic, its therapeutic philosophy, the social characteristics of its patients. However, it could be generally stated that at least 33 percent of the ward unit beds should be provided in single bed rooms.

In the size of acute wards, there have been wide variations in basic units 120 to 30 beds as well as in the ward unit combinations 60 to 120 beds. A ward of 24 beds has received broad support, as well as the combinations 2 × 24 and 4 × 24 beds. Larger ward unit combinations, which make the practicing of progressive patient care easier, are being encouraged.

Day Room

Within each multi-bed room, a small sitting should be provided to meet some of the requirements of early ambulation. A central dayroom of domestic character should also be provided for the convenience of ambulant patients.

Most dayroom are lounges and designed for sitting. Whey not have hobby corners, game activity centers, and the like, it has been asked for.

For active pursuits of leisure activities, appropriate settings and equipment have to be provided, while some provision could be made with the patient rooms for activities such as craft-work, it is perhaps more feasible and desirable to locate such activities outside the patient room in special units. Decentralized day spaces seem to be better for debilitated patients and may more effectively contribute to early activation. A separate patient's dining room is invented for ambulant and wheelchair patients to encourage an early return to normal life.

The kind and size of the ward kitchen or pantry depends on the catering policies of the hospital, whatever the catering policy practiced, meals have to be served hot, patient's expectations and dietary demands considered, transportation distances kept reasonable and perfect cleanliness maintained.

Rooms for Nursing Procedures

Analysis of nursing procedures in acute wards shows that all procedures conform to a broad pattern made up of giving and receiving oral or written instructions, preparation or assembly of items for nursing procedures; carring out the procedure in the bed areas, treatment room or bath room, recording results of the procedure, and cleaning or disposal of used items.

These activities require an instructions and recording area, and a preparation area. The instructions and recording area consists of the numbers stations and the doctor's office. The nurse's station should be acoustically closed as it is a source of noise. All clean and sterilized items for nursing and medical procedures should be selected and assembled in one preparation room. Space must be provided for trolley setting. A disposal room is required for the temporary storage of used items awaiting reprocessing and disposal or destruction. Some items are reprocessed in this room and returned to the preparation room, e.g. treatment trolleys. In the US, Gordon Friesen and others have rejected the central nursing station in favor of decentralized nurse servers at each patient room. The combination of inner and peripheral ward corridors is considered to improve the nursing conditions. The inner corridor is mainly the work area for hospital personnel and to a limited extent used by the patients. The peripheral corridor serves the visitors, but it used to some extent also by the patients. When only one circulation space the inner corridor is provided, attention should be paid to the corridor width 2.4 m, which has almost become an international standard, is obviously insufficient and the width of 2.8 m would better meet the operational needs.

Storages

Linen store for bed linen, patients trousers and other clothing and various items used by the staff, but not for storage of mattresses, blankets, pillows and dust generating supplies should be provided. It should be realized that the supply space to the receiving docks of the hospital. If a cart or twin-cart system is to be operated, there are considerable consequences on the ward spacing.

An equipment store has to be provided for spare parts for beds, points, crutches, examination lights, wheelchairs, etc.

Additional Facilities

Office's staff refreshment break-room, interview rooms, laboratory, female and male staff cloaks, domestic service room and some stores are examples of rooms required at ward level but not related to any particular group. They may serve more than one nursing charge. A room for visitor's waiting and relative's overnight stay is considered relatively useful. A centralized overnight accommodation would meet most requirements. Wherever possible, centralized services should be provided with the consequent removal of many avoidable activities at ward level. The range of central services provided will affect the location and size of some of the working areas. The main central services which nowadays provided are sterile and other supplies, catering and housekeeping. Communications and management systems are important elements of the supply and distribution system. A clear statement of an institution's goals, establishing its objectives and categories of inpatients for whom care is to be provided, is needed to determine the character of its ward units.

FURTHER READING

1. Putep E: Modern Hospital. International planning practices. Lloyd-Luke, London, 1979.
2. Laufman H: Hospital special care facilities: Planning for user needs. Academic press, New York, 1981.

MEDICAL MONITORING

Technological advances have revolutionized medical care. Diagnostic tools like magnetic resonance imaging, spiral CT scan, ultrasonography, digital subtraction angiography, positron emission tomography, echocardiography/color Doppler, videoendoscopes multichannel autoanalyser, computerised treatment planning system, linear accelerator, theratron, EEG (electrophysiology), cardiac monitoring, etc. have facilitated prompt diagnosis and accurate treatment. Both invasive and non-invasive diagnostic and therapeutic procedures are being done with high degree of reliability and precision. Non-invasive techniques have become more popular and are replacing traditional interventional procedures. Monitoring is a continuous or semicontinuous visualization of physiological and physical phenomena by means of analog or digital display devices. The data display is presented on a screen or cathode ray oscilloscope. Between data acquisition and data presentation the data are preprocessed, converted, retrieved, processed, and reduced. The information is to draw attention to significant deviations from the accepted or the expected, and to alarm the personnel on duty when some urgent action is necessary. The monitoring devices include thermal recorders, oxygen analyzers, thermistor bridges for multiple site temperatures e.g. patient's skin, rectum, and oesophagus; cathode ray oscilloscopes for displaying electrocardiograms, electroencephalograms, and hemodynamic parameters, blood gas tension recorders; analyzers of drugs and other chemical constituents in blood.

Simultaneous surveillance of several physiological parameters—physiological multi-parameter monitoring (PMPM)—rather than their graphic illustration is the main objective of medical monitoring. This surveillance can easily take place without any graphic registration. The value of PMPM lies primarily in the fact that the simultaneous following of the activities of several organs gives more comprehensive information than the data than the separate registration of the same activities. Impaired activity in one organ may lead to a concurrent functional disturbance in other organs. The time intervals between observations vary according to the monitoring situation and the condition of the patient. Extremely sensitive electronic monitors are now common place. Many of these amplify signals in the region of 1 mV in low-frequency ranges. They cannot be expected to give accurate results, nor can their alarms be reliable in an electrically 'noisy' environment. Measurements of physiological variables alone without further processing may not provide the best guide to patient care. the traditional clinical observation is more complex than simple measurements. The ward chart kept by an experienced nurse contains potentially more information than what a monitor writes out about the same variable.

As the trend in diagnostic examination is going toward more non-invasive technique the risky invasive diagnostic and monitoring techniques will be reduced. e.g. there are already patient, monitoring devices, which do not require insertion, injection or function but utilize a thermistor-transducer which, placed on the skin surface provides accurate reading of the deep body temperature, pCO_2, pO_2, etc.

PMPM by Means of Telemetry

Telemonitoring has positive psychological effect on the patient by removing the wiring to monitoring instruments.

PMPM telemonitoring can be accomplished by using small portable tape recorders or by radio-telemetry (RTM).

Mobility after extended period of confinement would help also to improve the effectiveness of diagnostic monitoring, e.g. by activating cardiac arrhythmias. A cardiac telemonitoring transmitter as an example weighs only about 120 g.

All monitoring units must be interlinked with alarm systems, which operate at predetermined variation extremes of the involved parameters.

Automatic Data Processing

Hospitals are so complex and so specialized in their operation that automatic data processing experience from other fields is often of limited value. The computer by itself is only a piece of machinery, which must be taught everything it does.

Most information systems in hospitals have evolved in a piecemeal fashion rather than through careful planning. The great majority of computer applications to medicine have been excessively modest in scope. Where in other fields, the computer has been utilized to perform tasks previously incomprehensive to mankind, in health care delivery we have been. In medicine the measure of success has often been diagnostic accuracy approaching a skilled clinician.

One of the main tasks of automatic data-processing is to ensure the rational and maximal use of expensive equipment. Several applications such as historical data acquisition, computer-assisted diagnosis, biosignal analysis, etc, appear intuitively to be of great value in improving patient care.

With the support of information systems, the scientific component of clinical decisions will be greatly enhanced. The clinician will no longer have to recall the hard statistical data of past experience. The information system will provide many answers instantaneously, both on a single patient and on similar cases.

A computer-based reliable information system will become a tool in medicine. The physician will be liberated from some chores of memorizing and recall. However, the computer will not reduce the true human task of the clinician to be firmly in charge of the case, to reassure and show empathy, and to develop rational clinical opinions assisted by the computer-produced statistical evidence. The humans role will not decrease. It will only shift. The technology must remain the servant of the clinician. The ultimate responsibility must be human.

The computer has, improved the hospital record keeping, the scheduling of admissions and outpatient sessions. Also storage, retrieval, and analysis of banks of data easily collected and filed has been accomplished.

An electronic picture archieve employs optical disk technology to store the bulk of pictorial data contained in X-ray pictures. Percent storage of electronic picture signals is demanded for the rapidly increasing number of computer tomograms. Efficiency of storage would be improved by data compression techniques, which reduce the data volume of X-ray pictures without loss of diagnostic image quality. the system may be extended to conventional radiographs if state-of-the-art technology such as laser scanning is applied for conversion into electronic signals and re-conversion into photographic hard copies. X-ray, TV system and other electronic imaging systems for infrared, ultrasound, etc. could be directly interfaced.

The visual evaluation process is generally time-consuming and it often makes above average demands on the individuals with respect to concentration and systematic procedure. This is particularly true of light and electron microscope studies and also of the analysis of thermograms. In many problems, the observer is obliged by the criteria employed to make subjective decisions which may compromise the reliability and comparability of the results.

Depending on the type and complexity of pattern recognition requirements and evaluation, image analysis with the aid of the computer would afford many advantages. It also appears likely that similar analysis facilities will be available for images which are variable in time.

Applications have become known on nuclear medicine, blood cell analysis, and X-ray diagnostics.

In an ECG system, interpretation can be assisted by the computer since the average signal has less artifacts and since the computer can perform physical measurements more rapidly, consistently and accurately than the human eye. Computer assisted axial tomography has resulted in a new field of medical expertise. Parallel to this, the computerized methods for ultrasound are rapidly developing.

Where a computerized scheme is to be implemented, great care and preparation are required as well as declared commitment down the head of department and a full discussion with all staff. The installation of a system simply in the hope of general improvement in the service is most unlikely to be successful.

Automatic dataprocessing enables to store, select and combine large volumes of personal information, which has given rise to dangers of international and unintentional invasion of privacy.

Protection of privacy must be guaranteed. The introduction of automatic data-processing systems with insufficient computer security may have a serious effect on the confidence of the general public in the health service.

The value of the computer in monitoring has been mainly in the automation of measurement acquisition, display, storage, retrieval, and charting for the medical record.

New uses for the computer in the laboratory are being developed. They include use of the computer for calculation of hours worked, for workload recording, for individual performance analysis, and for inventory control, all of them administrative tasks whose automation will result in savings. From the patient standpoint, attempts to better assess the effects of drugs on laboratory test results, and either correct the result or alert the attending physician are expected. The computer can be used in microbiology for analysis of organism sensitivity and growth. Storage of coded-diagnostic information can lead to better assessment of the meaning of laboratory results.

Greater value from instrumental monitoring might lie with systems built around small digital computers. They would provide analysis of biosignals, some diagnosis, information storage, retrieval and display. If designed to require only noninvasive, easily applied transducers supported by reliable peripheral instruments for most cases, these systems would provide a significant improvement of medical care.

Minicomputer devices are already being used for ECG and EEG analysis, for evaluation of cardiac catheterization data, patient monitoring, and pacemaker evaluation reporting. Here also cost effectiveness is clearly a very important issue.

Monitoring and Data-processing in Clinical Laboratories

Though automation, which is itself means improvement of the quality of the test data, large numbers of chemical determinations provide a wealth of information. The output also contains a number of previously unavailable determinations.

In all clinical laboratories irrespective of subdiscipline in the field of computerization, the two main tasks are data processing—the clerical work arising from request forms and the generation of reports and data acquisition dealing with the output of a laboratory instrument.

A busy laboratory might handle 500 or more requests daily, and on each occassion the data must be checked to find out if the patient is on files, the data verified or a file created, and the investigations and perhaps diagnosis entered. The data base has to contain the set of identifying data for each patient, the requesting source, and files for result of tests on specimens submitted. The results of the tests done have to be merged into the patient files, and the reports generated and then printed. An efficient system should allow these various procedures to occur concurrently, with on-line acquisition of data from laboratory instrument.

The importance of laboratory data processing is now being recognized. Most obvious is the improved quality of service notably legible reports, a faster turn-round of works, easy inquiry facilities, and fewer errors. The files can be made easily accessible for clinical and epidemiological research.

Computer system have been developed which would help to acutely identify bacteria and thus facilitate proper diagnosis of bacterial infections.

This would be especially useful in identifying organisms seldom encountered.

A computer system has been introduced for use in epidemiologic studies. Biochemical data on bacteria are stored with information on patient identification and hospital location. Each month, the computer puts out information on the distribution of bacteria by patient location. From this and other computer information, it would be possible to more rapidly investigate a local outbreak.

A computer system should not require extra work, be simple to operate and given rapid return-pay off. It also requires a good back-up.

In the first hand computers in diagnostic radiology can be used for data storage and patient identification.

The use of computers is radiotherapy permits the accurate computation of detailed dose distributions in the course of planning and executing the usual sequence of investigative and therapeutic procedures.

Monitoring in the Critically Ill

There are computerized, integrated systems, modular in nature, available for patient monitoring. Automatic sampling of signals from monitors ECGs, pressure, respiration, temperature—is possible as well as plotting trends on a scope e.g. following cardiac output by the dye curve. Monitoring is adapable for pulse waveform analyze; arrhythmia monitoring in conjuctions with a preprocessor; acid base analyze: logging nurse's notes; and generating patient summary reports at the end of each nursing shift.

The electric hazard for patients within the monitoring system the bulk of which is electronic and dependent on main power supply must be reduced by providing isolating transformers and by balanced or positively-grounded electrical equipment.

Electronic monitoring is only an accessory form of patient surveillance. It can never replace direct visual observation of a patient e.g. restlessness in a patient may be a warning sign of cerebral hypoxia even if the cardiac output, electrocardiogram, etc. are within normal limits.

While automated monitoring equipment might increase the technical effectiveness of the nurses by relieving them of some routine functions. Such as charting and checking vital signs, and thus increase the time available to render direct patient care, it cannot substitute human contact and good nursing, especially when dealing with child-patients and patients wakening from anesthesia who are in particular need of human contact and orientating dialogue.

Only the human mind has the capacity to recognize patterns in illness; there are many developments in the course of critical illness that are infrequent or unpredictable, and no transducer or electronic device has been yet devised that will warm of such event. The colour of the patients skin, an increase in his respiratory effort, a change in his pain pattern, impairment of cerebration, development of abdominal distension, or discharge from a wound can only be observed, and their significance assessed, by an experienced nurse or physician.

The computer tends to serve as a partial substitute for nurse performing routine tasks. To capitalize on this substitution the supervisor must make an effort to ensure that the extra available time is channeled into productive activities.

The installation of monitoring systems in the intensive care and treatment units may not be used as an indication or motivation to reduce the number of nurses. Intensive care patients need continuous bedside attendance. Electronic aids can only lighten the work by immediate and objective recording of physiological data. Unduly elaborate monitoring may actually distract from optimal care.

A monitoring period shorter than four hours in intensive care units has been considered to be uneconomical in comparison with manually conducted data registration.

Monitoring devices in coronary intensive care units include automatic electrocardiographic devices without on alarms with printout of the patient bed, time, and data of the alarm, ability to recall or freeze the electrocardiographic pattern; nonfade displays alarms on changes from present parameters of rate, rhythm, and contour; beat to beat rate meters; trend recordings; digital displays; and operational and lead status indicators. In addition, hemodynamic monitoring devices have become part of the CICU.

A significant reduction in mortality has resulted from improved monitoring facilities. The physiological function always monitored in the CICU is the action of the heart by an electrocardiography (ECG). In modern equipment an ECG recorder is a part of the monitoring machine. Frequently monitored are arterial blood pressure, and respiration are monitored occasionally.

Coronary care systems have been oriented more toward the central monitoring station concept, whereas the majority of cardiothoracic surgical units have required bedside monitoring. In most instances these ideas have been carried over in the subsequent design of newer computer-based systems.

In the ICUs and CICUs the monitoring equipment should be of a module system with ready interconvertibility to allow modification of the parameter to be measured as requirements are revised.

Monitoring in Operation Room

In most major surgical procedures, deviations in following physiological phenomena—the oxygen level in the blood; the pH of the blood; the carbon dioxide level in the blood; the pulse rate; the cardiac output and the blood pressure; the blood volume and the body temperature may indicate complications.

Especially in pediatric surgery, patient monitoring is essential to detect the onset of complications. Monitoring of blood pressure, temperature, and blood loss are advocated. Monitoring of internal temperature is considered particularly advisable in all infants and young children undergoing major surgery.

There are technical and practical monitoring problems still to be solved. The electronic instruments must transmit the message from the patient without disturbing the operation area and without being electrically interfered by other equipment in the surgical unit.

Miniaturization of circuits has reduced the size and power equipments of instruments, thus enabling the use of several monitors. Telemetric multiparameter monitoring will very probably be the method of choice for surgery in the future.

Monitoring significantly reduces the risk of general anesthesia, and every patient who undergoes a general anesthetic deserves the extra protection that electrocardiographic monitoring gives him.

An ideal system of medical computerization in the operation room would necessitate a screen which gives continuous visual information of events and trends as the operation proceeds. A minute-to-minute alarm system would indicate when a patient is or will be in trouble.

There has to be a facility to deliver black white paper copies from these display units, so that the essential sequences of the operation could be documented and added to the anesthesia record.

During recent years, some cardiosurgical centres have demonstrated that continuous computer-based monitoring of multiple physiological variables in cardiotomy—open heart surgery may provide the opportunity for prompt and effective reaction to any adverse development in cardiocirculatory function during anesthesia, operation, and the recovery period, which is especially important in cardiotomy patients.

Monitoring in Maternity Units

In maternity units many patients suffer anxiety concerning the welfare of the fetus *in utero* and it seems likely that perinatal monitoring properly explained to the patient, would reduce maternal anxiety concerning the fetus and strengthen the mother's feeling of safety. The benefits of perinatal fetal heart rate monitoring, appear to be a decrease in perinatal stillbirths, a decrease in neonatal mortality particularly of the low birth weight infants, a decrease in neonatal morbidity as measured by neurologic outcome, and assistance in rational labour management.

A labour cannot be monitored more successfully by a computer than by an experienced clinician. Much of the monitor information given to a capable attentive obstrician is at best superfluous and at worst may even seem impertient. However, to the less experienced or the tired clinician such comment could be vital.

Transmitting

The provision of TV cameras in the critical medicine areas has been greatly reduced in the recent years. If they are still used, it has to be notified that the bed area is illuminated at all hours of day and night, causing often disturbance or great annoyance to the patients. This disturbance must be avoided, e.g. by using infrared light monitoring cameras.

Video fluoroscopy-TV-screening calls for closed circuit video installation for X-ray film demonstration and consultations between operation rooms, out-patinet units, and other sections of the hospital on one hand and the radiology department on the other. It can improve collaboration between surgeons and radiologists. A film developed in the radiology department and the commentary by the radiologist can be transmitted to the operation room. In addition, a pneumatic tube for sending exposed films from the operation room to the radiology department is needed.

Closed-circuit TV systems can link surgical teams also to other laboratories. TV camera in the pathology laboratory can be focused over the gross examination area or into a microscope, so that the pathologists will be above to demonstrate the complete specimen or a slide. Prompt delivery of the histological diagnosis, not the televised display of the specimen, is of main importance.

From an EEG laboratory with its own computer, which is linked to monitor high risk patients, the quantitative parameters could be transmitted to the operation room and displayed there parallel to other physiological functions.

Closed TV systems in operation rooms usually have two circuits for vision and two for sound. One sound and one vision circuit terminate within the lighting complex, servicing the permanent, TV camera there. A second pair of circuit terminate in a distribution panel beneath a picture in the operation room and are used in combination with the complementary mobile camera.

Diagnostic and preparatory information as a part of the clinical examination could be obtained by TV, e.g. televised endoscopy.

As TV control room also the operation rooms instrumentation room, if such one is available, could be used.

Recording

For storage of records, also from the X-ray department the computer system has high theoretical possibilities. All departments would be linked to the centre. Information could be scanned, translated to storage numbers, along with its report and the information stored. The radiologist could then dial for requested past information.

For recording operations 16 mm film cameras are in many circumstances preferred to closed circuit TV. A mounted camera should be completed by a mobile camera.

For recording microsurgery a combination of TV monitor and videotape recorder have been used. A tiny microphone plugged into the horizontal arm of the microscope provides the sound during videotape recording. The use of an overhead mirror in spinal, chest and abdominal surgery photography has been recommended. It permits versatility of camera operation, freedom for the operation team and good orientation for the viewer.

ISOLATION OF PATIENTS

Two types of isolation of patients are applied in hospital practice. The more frequent type—source isolation—is used to prevent spread of infection from a patient to other patients and hospital staff. There are four sub-groups of source isolation: strict isolation; respiratory isolation; wound and skin precautions; enteric precautions. Adhesive color-coded labels attached to the isolation room would help to inform the staff of the measures to be taken. Blue would be the colour for standard isolation, red for strict isolation.

The other type—protective isolation—aims at reducing the infection risk for patients whose resistane to infection is markedly lowered. The amount of protection required varies with the type of patient. Maximum protection includes sterilized food, linen, and other supplies. The methods of protective or reversed isolation in which the patient is protected from contamination with strains of hospital bacteria, seem to be in an experimental stage and have to be improved. It is considered inadvisable to mix accommodation for infected patients-source isolation-with that for susceptible patients protective isolation. Physically separate units should be provided for these purposes. Separate nursing and ancillary staff are essential. The requirements for isolation accommodation in a hospital are influenced by the patterns of clinical work and type of specialist units. About 2.5 percent of the beds of a large hospital in a special unit would probably be adequate except during periods of unusually high demand.

Facilities for Isolation

Facilities for isolation and their use vary from country to country and even from institution to institution: there are separate infectious disease units or clinics for patients requiring isolation, special rooms in various hospital ward areas for isolation procedures, and rooms which are used as the situation requires. The transfer of infection by the airborne route e.g. respiratory infections—can be controlled only having the patient in a single room. The control of disease spread by contact depends primarily on barrier nursing, which includes nursing procedures that reduce the risks of transferring infective organisms by direct contact or by way of fomities from person to person.

It is strongly felt that also from the aspect of nosocomial infection, the placing of all beds in single rooms—at least in the intensive care and treatment units—is for the patient the best solution. All patients must be given rooms, not curtained cubicles.

Because isolation may result in a number of additional efforts for physicians, nurses, and patients, sometimes there is reluctance or objection to placing a patient under isolation e.g. for the physician extra time may be required, also nursing care may be more time-consuming, for the patient isolation would decrease social contact.

Psychological Stress of Isolation

Isolation should not resemble solitary confinement. While excessive noise is a frequent cause of complaint in hospital, complete isolation from any audible or visual indications of life outside imposes great psychological stress. Social isolation may affect the patient's welfare. Occasionally elderly patients subjected to prolonged isolation have appeared to suffer from it. Children in isolation wards think that they are being punished, that they have been rejected and are unworthy. They are at risk of withdrawal and regression. Especially for children it is desirable for nurses to spend extra time in the rooms. Mothers may help to look after their babies, if nurses show them the isolation procedures.

Isolation Room

An isolation room has to provide uncluttered space around the bed for equipment and the increased number of personnel involved in emergency care. A room area of about 23m^2 is adequate within an isolation unit and would greatly reduce the need for an operation room. There should be no unnecessary furniture. Critically sick patients should have access to oxygen and compressed air. Distribution pipes from the central gas storage should be provided. The one-patient unit should be self-contained regarding decontamination, toilet, lavatory and sink. An isolation room should be provided with a bedpan-flushing equipment in an adjoining room. In the same space equipment for cleaning the isolation room can be stored, used instruments and other equipment decontaminated, and soiled linen kept in containers prior to disposal.

Disposable crockery and cutlery items as well as paper or plastic cups are recommended.

The sanitation as well as the heating equipment should be easily cleaned and with few possibilities to collect dust. The backs of radiators should be accessible for cleaning; toilets, bidgets, etc, should be fixed to the wall, leaving the floor free. Floor drains and gullytraps should have an enamel finish on the inside.

For effective isolation a separate ventilation system for each room with controlled air pressures to prevent movement of air into other areas has been recommended. Each traditional plenum-ventilated isolation room has between the corridor and the room itself a lock-chamber or ante room for donning the protective gown, mask, cap, shoe, covers and sometimes goggles. A hand-washing facility is included. Adding an ante room or airlock improves the air isolation, possibly by a factor of ten compared with the simple directional ventilation arrangements. With a ventilated airlock the degree of protection may be about 10,000 times that found in an open situation. There should be no cross-circulation or recirculation of air between an isolation unit and other areas of the hospital. The air distribution should be arranged so that all air escaping through door crevices, etc. and excess air flows from the corridors, ante rooms and patient rooms to the toilets to be extracted.

The extracted air should be filtered by means of interchangeable filters before discharge into the open air. The provision of temporary microfilters should be possible.

All ventilation ducts should be provided with cleaning shutters to allow for cleaning the inside of the ducts.

Unidirectional Airflow

High-efficiency air filters can be used to provide particle and microbe-free air as a directed non-turbulent flow in the care of highly susceptible patients. Because it is relatively easy to reduce airborne contamination to a level at which contact and autogenous infection becomes predominant, some of the technical requirements for ventilating patient rooms are less rigorous than for industries. The linear air velocity needed to reduce turbulence sufficiently for unidirectional horizontal flow to be established appears to be no more than 0.1 to 0.25 m/second. Noise control is, however, a major concern.

It is possible to use this form of ventilation to isolate several patients in one room without partitions. Air would enter through the filter bank behind bedheads and is extracted through slot in roof. Only about 10 percent of airflow is to pass into downstream end of the room beyond roof slot. Screens or curtains may be positioned between beds. This arrangement may be advantageous for patients who need much nursing and supervision and for those with claustrophobia in single rooms. Those who come into direct contact with the patients must practice non-contact techniques with regard to clothing, hand preparation, etc. Others who enter the room for activities not needing patient contact need observe only minimal precautions if they remain down stream or to the side of the patients. With this form of ventilation about 90 percent of the air can be recirculated with the addition of fresh air to control smells, carbon dioxide, and other gases. Full air-conditioning is required to control heat gain from the fans. The cost is considerable but convenience and comfort are high and the level of isolation that can be attained is limited only by the measures used to reduce contact transfer. The ease of access itself makes considerable demands on aseptic discipline.

This can be accomplished e.g. in the containment type of plastic isolator.

FURTHER READING

1. Putsep E: Modern Hospital: International planning practices. Lloyd-Luke Ltd. London, 1979.
2. W Paul James, Tatton-Brown W: Hospital: Design and Development. The architectural press. London, 1986.

OBSTETRICS DEPARTMENT

Prenatal care, observation and comfort of patients in labor, delivery room assistance, and care of mother after delivery, as well as nursing care of newborn, are important responsibilities of obstetrics department. Nurses assist doctors in instructing new mothers in postnatal care and care of the newborn.

New type maternity or child-bearing centers demonstrate that low-risk pregnancies and deliveries need not be managed in a traditional hospital setting. The out-of-hospital alternative birth center may include some or all the resources for prenatal care and education, labour and delivery care, immediate post-partum and neonatal care, and follow-up home visiting services. The centre under hospital administration and management may provide some postpartal examinations and health supervision. The centre may be adjacent to a hospital facility or a short distance from a hospital. Clearly understood arrangements for transfer to a hospital in the event of emergencies are important to ensure safety of the mother and infant. The economic feasibility of the out-of-hospital birth centre is dependent on a high volume service.

In the hospital, birth centre usually consists of one or more labour/delivery rooms or a 2-bed postpartum room in the maternity unit, furnished in a home-like decor. Labour and delivery takes place in this room in a bed which may be specially designed to permit use of stirrups if desired or in an ordinary single or double bed. A couch or adjustable chair is provided for the father or family member supporting the mother. Usually the mother and the infant remain in this room until discharge. If a longer hospital stay is necessary, rooming -in care is provided. Sibling visiting and participation, as well as extended family members involvement , is optional. In the UK, a combination of the security of home and safety of hospital is known as 6 hour discharge. Antenatal care is given as for home birth. The midwife is with the mother throughout the first stage of labour, whereafter the mother and her companions are transferred from home to hospital, where birth is given. If there should be difficulties then extra help is available, otherwise after six hours rest the mother goes back home again. According to Swedish experience the distances up to 100 km to the full obstetrical service carry no rate of increased risk of birth during the transport. Experiences from Canada and Sweden indicates that in case of high-risk pregnancies, there is a better prognosis for the baby, if the baby is transported *in utero* to a complete delivery unit instead of being transported to a neonate unit in a incubator.

In the overwhelming majority of cases, birth is a happy event of considerable personal significance, traditionally a time for celebration, it is also crisis period when new behavior patterns, which will influence the family's welfare, are formed.

The birth entails an extensive adjustment process for the mother as it involves and reflects changes in not only her physical state but also in her ability to cope and adapt and in her self-concept as a woman, as a wife, and as a mother. Birth ought to take place in an informal and relaxed atmosphere, not least because almost all obstetric patients are, more or less frightened. Psychiatric disorders are common in connection with Childbirth. The risk of recurrence of puerperal psychosis in a subsequent pregnancy is approximately one in six. Psychiatric morbidity in the puerperium is related to interpersonal and social stresses of various sorts and is not connected with obstetrical stresses. The time of maximum vulnerability in the life of an individual is during the transition from intrauterine to extrauterine life. This critical period and the first few minutes of life commands enlightened acute medical care. Perinatal medicine has abolished the frontiers between the final stage of pregnancy, childbirth and the neonatal period. Obstetrics and pediatrics form one unit. It is important to have a neonatal unit adjacent to the delivery unit. Asepsis in connection with deliveries consists mainly in the preservation of the patient's immunities. This is reached by sustaining her strength, optimizing her general condition, and handling the tissues with utmost gentlness. The transfer of infective material to tissues higher up in the birth passage should be stringently prevented. After delivery, both mother and the newborn babies are susceptible to bacterial infections. The acquisition of organisms of any type by a newborn infant gives rise to changed circumstances but need not be harmful, and in certain situations may be beneficial. This is generally termed colonization and is superficial and confined to surfaces whether external, as on the skin, or internal, as in the gut. The immunological defenses of the newborn against such invading organisms may be incomplete. Where the combination of number of virulence of invading organisms exceeds the infant's ability to limit the spread of those organisms, true infection will take place.

About 2,000 deliveries a year are needed in order to maintain the quality of services in maternity unit. Below this figure, the number of parturitions and the flüctuations in daily census make that the personnel is used in multiple functions, which may lower the standards of patient care.

The number of labour and delivery rooms and obstetrical beds in a hospital depends on the annual number of deliveries in the hospital's catchment area, the ward bed occupancy rate, the time to be spent in the delivery room, and the length of stay in the obstetrical ward.

Because of shorter length of stay of the post partum patient, the tendency is towards an increased number of labor and delivery rooms.

In Poland, three labor beds are recommended per 1000 annual deliveries. One labor bed for each 250 deliveries annually has been a rather general guide in the US.

A simple thumb-rule for determining the size of an obsetrical suite is two labor rooms and one delivery room per 20 post-partum beds, In many countries, a combined labor and delivery room is used. In Sweden, there are three to four such rooms per 28 postpartum beds. In the current medical practice, the labor or first-stage only room, the delivery room and the recovery area are arranged in sequence. There is now a rather general awareness that the normal duration of labor is substantially shorter than the median duration about 13 to 15 hours as quoted in most textbooks. A use of combined labor-delivery rooms would minimize circulation of the patient during labour. However, they may need more space and the furnishing of a combined room is considerably less domestic than the labour room.

After having adapted a queuing theory model for the predication of delivery room utilization, following room figures have been suggested in following chart.

Number of delivery room	*Vaginal delivery service only*	*Complete delivery service 12% cesarean delivery*	*US Public Health Service recommendation delivery service only*
1.	1-90	1-80	1-1220
2.	90-1350	80-1200	1221-1950
3.	1350-4000	1200-3600	2681-3410
4.	4000-7700	3600-7000	3411-4140
5.	7700-9000	7000-9000	4141-5000

The percentage of cesarean deliveries varies in different countries but is generally on increase. There has been a wider indication for it is in discussion, as some feel that cesarean section has changed from an operation of necessity to an operation of choice, with better maternal and fetal results

There is a growing uneasiness among obstetricians as the increasing caesarean section rate is not accompanied by solid evidence that this improves perinatal results. As it still represents a considerable risk for mothers, general cesarean section is not accepted. It would appear that in the future 10 to 15 percent of deliveries would require cesarean section. The section rates will obviously vary with the type of population served.

The delivery suite could take advantage of the administrative and mechanical features of the surgical department by being included in it. Increased staffing efficiency seems to be the principal operating cost saving attributed to this combination.

Spatial Requirements

Family Waiting Room and Early Labor Lounge

This facility should be available in or near the delivery department. In the attractively furnished and decorated room patients in early labor could walk and visit with children, husbands, and others.

Telephone/intercom connections within the labor area and reading materials should be available.

Diagnostic-admitting Room

In the admitting room, which must be easily accessible, the patient is prepared for the labor room. There should be an examination table with a stationary, an adjustable ceiling light fixture, a small laboratory unit for blood tests and urine-analysis and a washbasin. In this room, women could be examined also to ascertain their status in labour without being formally admitted, if they are in early labor.

The admitting room should have an area of about 17 m^2. Facilities to shower the patient and to have an enema performed have to be included. There should be a toilet with a wall-hung-WC-chair and an adjacent washbasin equipment for emergency deliveries should be provided.

Observation Room

It would be optimal to have an observation room, where patients in premature labour—six to eight months pregnant with labor pains-may be treated to slow or to stop the labour.

Labor Room

The sense of isolation, particularly with the first baby, can be overwhelming and the patient in labor can require the company of the husband. Some prefer privacy. Labor or first-stage rooms should be for single occupancy with a floor area of at least 12 m^2. They should be furnished with a homely touch.

A labor-delivery bed could be raised and lowered, it should be adjustable to semi-sitting position. Labor rooms should be equipped with an oxygen source and a suction point for resuscitation. Space is needed for resuscitation of the newborn and for a mobile anesthesia trolley with a device for intermittent positive-pressure respiration, and an emergency cart. A washbasin is needed. Toilet and washroom facilities must be included. They should contain safety bars and emergency call bells. Labor rooms should have temperature and humidity control. Transmission of sound between labor rooms must be prevented.

Patient Lounge

It is important to have a lounge for the first stage of labor patients. The inability of the pregnant women to move about in the labor area is one of the most serious restrictions placed upon her. If the patient can be kept mobile as long as possible, a more normal and easy birth can be made.

In the ambulant group the duration of labor has been shown significantly shorter, the need for analgesia significantly less, and the incidence of fetal heart abnormalities significantly smaller than in the recumbent group. Allowing women in early labor to move around freely and socialize with others will help to minimize problems created by anxiety during labor.

Delivery Room

The second stage of labor can last 1.5 to 2 hours particularly with a first birth. The human female is quite adaptable to many physiological positions and cultural practices, the importance of which have not yet been entirely evaluated. The parturitional posture is not just an arbitrary position assumed by the mother while she is delivering, but instead, is an integral part of the culturally influenced birth process. Rather than have the delivery position dictated by culturally patterned behavior or customs for something as important as the delivery of an infant, it should be chosen from a range of alternatives to suit the individuals physiological processes within the cultural setting.

If the mother chooses to be delivered in a hospital by an obstetrician, her delivery position choices are usually limited: the split delivery bed-table, designed so that one end may be dropped or retracted, allows the woman to be delivered either in the lithotomy position if one end is removed, or in the dorsal recumbent position if the lower end is not altered. For normal deliveries, the usual position of the mother on the delivery table is the lithotomy position, with her buttocks at the edge or projecting over the edge of the table, and with her legs spread apart and in straight leg holders, knee rests, or stirrups. The woman's arms are not to stray into the sterile field. In some cases, the delivery table may have upright handles or hand grips against which the woman may pull in her bearing down efforts. The woman may have to lie flat on the delivery table, but some delivery tables have pillows for her head or for her back to give her a curved spine position. The woman may not have adequate foot support, though, because she has nothing to push against. She is then covered with sterile drapings, exposing only her perineum. A recent innovation has been the adaptation of an adjustable back rest on to a standard delivery table. The adjustable back rest lies under the delivery table mattress and the angle of elevation can be varied from about 5 degrees to about 55 degrees. Women appeared most comfortable with their backs raised at an angle of 30 to 45 degrees,. The delivery table is equipped with stirrups and foot plates, to be used during the second stage of labor in the lowered position so that there is no pressure under the knees, and is also equipped with handgrips thus allowing the mother either to push or to pull while bearing down. Another item is the pillow placed under the mother's head. Using this backrest, the mother assumes a modified sitting position: her back is curved and her head is fixed forward while her legs are bent.

For the mother, this position increases the efficiency of the expulsive effort by directing the force of the voluntary muscles towards the pelvis and by using the force of gravity on the weight of the baby and the abdominal contents. For the obstetrician, this position is compatible with modern methods of obstetric care and asepsis in procedures such as cleansing of the perineum, control of delivery, episiotomy, or the application of forceps. This propped, or semi-sitting, position has also been evaluated in terms of psychological and physical categories of information for both the mother and the baby, The results show no adverse effects while indicating increased comfort to the mother, greater efficiency of the expulsive efforts and considerable advantages in a programme of cooperative childbirth

At each delivery bed, there should be oxygen outlets, also for the babies, suction points, and wall-mounted sphygmomanometers. The access to gas supplies and suction points should be easy.As the importance of mother baby attachment particularly during the first few minutes and hours has been shown and stressed as it facilitates optimal post-partum and extrauterine physiologic adaptation. The opportunity for establishing contact between mother and baby in the delivery room should not be lost. This opportunity should be kept open also for potentially vulnerable preterm babies. The delivery room requires sport light which is directed away from the perineum just before delivery of the infants head all other lights have to be extinguished a radiant heating element to be placed over the delivered baby on the mothers abdomen to prevent heat loss, and a (plastic) bassinet where the baby can be immersed to the face in a 36.5°C water bath until he appears relaxed and comfortable. The vast majority of babies are born normal. However, a significant number will require resuscitation. Even though modern methods have greatly improved, the ability to predict depressed babies, no method is 100 percent accurate. For that reason preparations should be made to resuscitate every baby. The most dramatic changes and so also the most critical changes are related to the transfer from a transplacental gas exchange to a gas exchange via the lungs of new-born infant. The newborn does not tolerate even brief hypoxia episodes, so strict precautions for stabilization of the oxygen environment are mandatory. Oxygen warmed to 32 to 34°C with 60 to 80 percent relative humidity is administered. An incubator prewarned to 35°C should be available in the delivery room. Infants not requiring resuscitation should be placed in this incubator as quickly as possible if a radiant heat source is not available. For care of the depressed newborn infant, a table is needed or a bassinet with non-slippery surface on which to place the baby. The table should be tiltable to provide a head-down position. Radiant heaters will warm the surface on which the infant will be placed, as well as provide a radiant heat source for the infant if resuscitation is required.

Equipment for neonatal resuscitation should be kept as simple as possible. It should include a resuscitator for pulmonary inflation, an oral suction device, oxygen supply, and an overhead radiant heater. When it is dealt with a patient weighing only 900 to 300 g the less equipment there is between the patient and the resuscitator the better the situation will be handwashing facilities.

Storage space must be available. Wall cabinets for resuscitation equipment-measured 65 by 60 by 22 cm have been recommended. A delivery room should have a floor area of about 30 m^2. For obstetrical or surgical lamps a ceiling height of at least 2.8 m is required. A doorwidth of 1.3 m allows the patients to be moved to the delivery room on a labor bed.

It is strongly felt that a delivery room must have a window.

Delivery rooms connected by doorways are believed to make it easier for one nurse/midwife to supervise two concurrent deliveries. Not all find this solution an advantage. Transmission of sound between delivery rooms must be prevented.

Operation Room

If the obstetric suite is a section of the surgical department, the occasional need for immediate surgical intervention is easily met. In an independent delivery suite an operation unit should be included as about 20 percent of deliveries require a surgical intervention. An operation table capable of both head-down and lateral tilt is frequently the first choice for caesarean sections.

Anesthesia Work-room

In obstetric units with more than 3,000 deliveries a year, anesthesia work-rooms should be provided. Basic equipment includes wall shelves, a work counter, a drainboard, and a sink for washing and checking accessories.

Recovery Room

Immediately after delivery procedures are finished, the mother should be assured rest, even if a sedative has been used.

The maternity patient undergoing a cesarean section has had both abdominal surgery and a delivery, and one must consider the unique needs occurring during the puerperal period which are engendered by the individual circumstances surrounding each procedure. As a planned physical assault on the body, the surgical experience becomes an intense event with physiological and psychosocial effects covering a wide range of reactions and behaviors

For rest, observation, and care 12 m^2 recovery rooms are need.

As an infant's first feeding may have an effect on his and his mothers later behavior, breastfeeding in the postpartum recovery room seems to be positive factor and should be encouraged.

The number of postpartum recovery rooms provided ought to be a third of the number of labor rooms.

The recovery room should be placed adjacent to the delivery room and be equipped as a post-anesthetic recovery room. Oxygen and suction should be available. Easy movement of a bed or stretcher and space for attending patients from either side of the bed should be provided for.

The recovery room windows should have shades. Adjacent to the recovery room there should be a toilet.

Nursery for Newborn

All infants to be sent to the normal newborn unit undergo an initial period of intensive observation and visual monitoring. The closer the infant is to term, the better are his adaptive processes. Scales are needed in the examination area of the nursery. About 3 m^2 should be allowed per bassinet. After four to six hours, the newborn has usually made the initial adjustment necessary for extrauterine life and his vital signs and behavior stabilize. Several routine examinations suggests the neonate be unclothed during this postnatal period. An unclothed infant requires supplemental warming. It is of utmost importance to recognize that the normal full-term baby should not require the use of an incubator or other supplementary heating device to maintain his body temperature in an ordinarily adequately heated nursery 25 to 27°C.

Procedure Room for Newborn

A 12 m^2 procedure room is intended for exchange transfusion, not very complex diagnostic and therapeutic procedures and minor surgery of the newborn, as circumcision, or any other elective procedures.

Laboratory equipment, suction, an operation lamp and a washbasin are needed.

Special Examination Room

In teaching hospitals, a room of about 12 m^2 should be provided for maternal and neonatal examination.

Laboratory, X-ray Service

Access to laboratory services, blood bank and X-ray and ultrasonic diagnostic services are necessary.

Sick newborn babies should be examined with minimal disruption of their environment. Equipment designed for pediatric use is available, but not essential. Neonates who are at risk e.g, premature babies, babies born by cesarean section or after a prolonged labor, should have chest X-rays as soon as possible after birth and again at 3,6 and 24 hours, with subsequent films as indicated by the clinical picture.

Film developing facilities must be close at hand. An automatic film processor within the newborn unit may be justified.

Nurses Station

The station should be centrally located within the maternity suite. It should contain desks, a table, shelves, a filing cabinet, bulletin boards, and a couch. The recommendable size of the nurse's station is about 12 m^2.

Generally, at least two nurses per team are required. For 2,000 patients per annum three nurses are required, for 3,000 four, and for 3,500 five nurses.

Obstetrician's Office

The doctors office—about 12 m^2—does not have to be centrally located within the obstetric suite.

Changing Rooms, Retirement Room and Staff Lounge

Changing rooms for both female and male staff should be adjacent to the entrance to the delivery

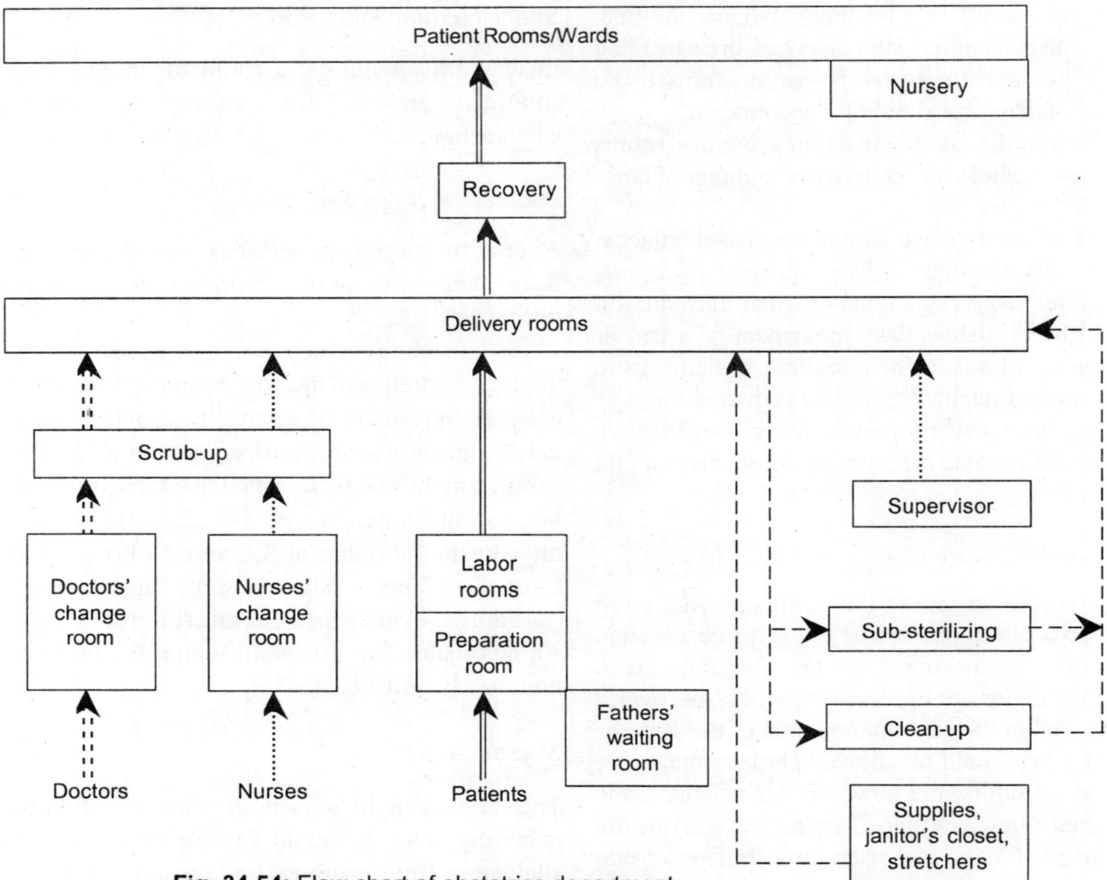

Fig. 34.54: Flow chart of obstetrics department

unit. Toilets and showers should be provided. A small retirement room for every ten female employees is an asset. A washbasin is needed. The needs for a staff lounge have too often been underestimated.

On-Call Rooms

Adjacent to the delivery section, there should be on-call accommodations for obstetricians, nurses and pediatricians.

Nourishment Area, Formula Preparation

A kitchenette for patient catering is needed. It will have to rely on the hospital food distribution system. The required size is about 12 m^2.

An integrated formula preparation room for neonates offers advantages over the dependence on a centralized milk kitchen.

Cleaners' Room

The number of cleaners' rooms–each of about 4 m^2 size–depends on the size of the obstetric department. A bucket sink with hot and cold water, drained, and space for cleaning utensils and mechanical cleaning equipment as well as housekeeping supplies and a cleaners cart is needed.

Utility Rooms Placenta Disposal

Utility rooms, both clean and soiled, with deep double sinks are needed. There should be ample

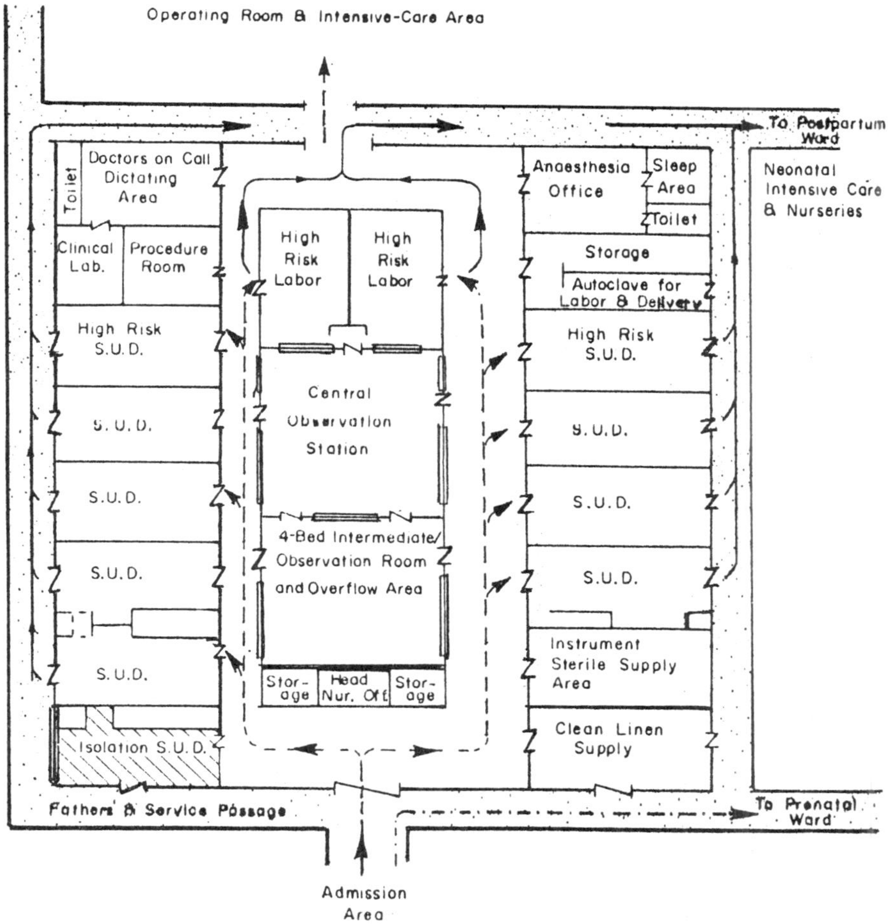

Fig. 34.55: Single unit delivery system—floor plan and patient flow, (Stippling indicates postdelivery; broken arrows indicate predelivery—in labor; alternating dots and dashes indicate predelivery—not in labor)

hampers of soiled linen, because maternity patients often need complete linen changes.

In the obstetric department the typical waste products include soiled dressings, sponges, disposable diapers and underpads, disposable gloves, waste ampules, needles and syringes, disposable masks, disposable catheters, disposable enema units, and disposable blood lancets. There should be provision for disposing placentas.

In large delivery units a room about 8 m^2 area for examination and conservation of some placentas is needed.

A refrigerator, placenta disposal equipment and handwashing facilities are needed. Washbasins should be included.

Storage Facilities

Storage facilities are needed for linen, masks, dressings, underpads, drapes, sanitary napkins, sterilized instrument sets, anesthetic drugs, medicaments, needles and syringes, and disposable gloves. The use of disposable does not require increased storage space. Gas storage rooms with conductive

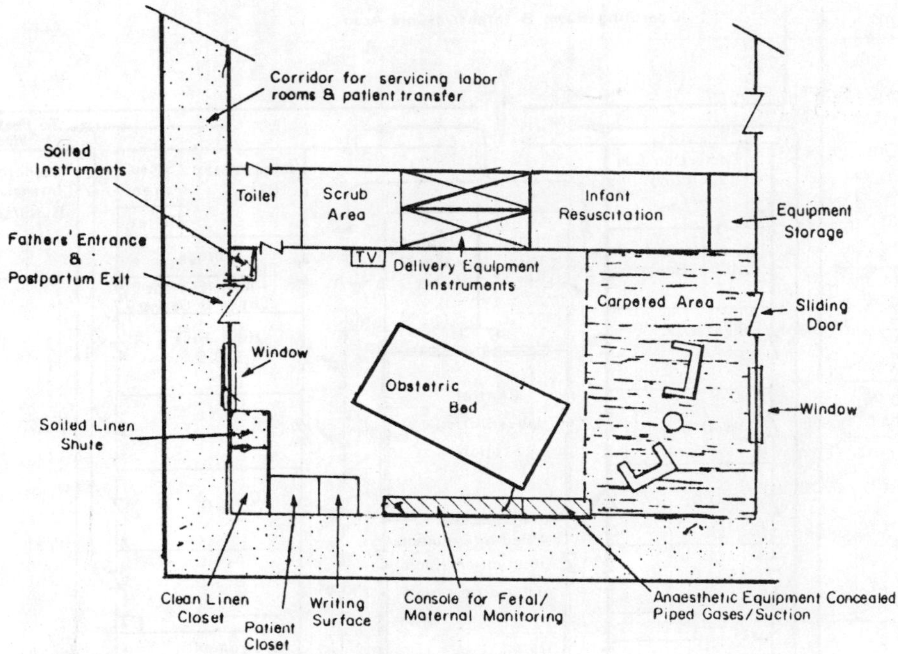

Fig. 34.56: Floor plan of a single-unit labor, delivery, and postpartum room

flooring and gravity ventilation should not be linked directly within the delivery rooms.

A space for a couple of stretchers is needed.

Area for Relatives

A waiting room for relatives and friends near the admitting area should be provided. It should contain comfortable chairs. A public telephone and a toilet should be available. In the cases where husbands are allowed to be present during the delivery, changing rooms in principle like the staff-changing rooms may be needed.

Planning Considerations

Obstetric care and practice has changed dramatically because of technological advances, changes in philosophical and social attitudes. Among the technological advances, constant intensive care facilities equipped with physiologic monitoring and scanning devices, as well as special infection control provisions, are now being built into delivery room design. Also included are facilities to enhance the availability of newborn infant to the mother. The labor and delivery room should be pleasant to the eyes and ears, adequate in size, properly-located, well equipped, and should conform to strict infection control standards.

The number and size of labor and delivery rooms depend upon many factors, only one of which is the number of cases delivered per month. An equally important consideration is the type of cases handled.

$$\text{No. of rooms} = \frac{\text{DLY}}{365 \times \text{DLRD}}$$

DLY = Deliveries per year, excluding cesarean sections done in surgery.

365 = Days per year

DLRD = Deliveries per room per day.

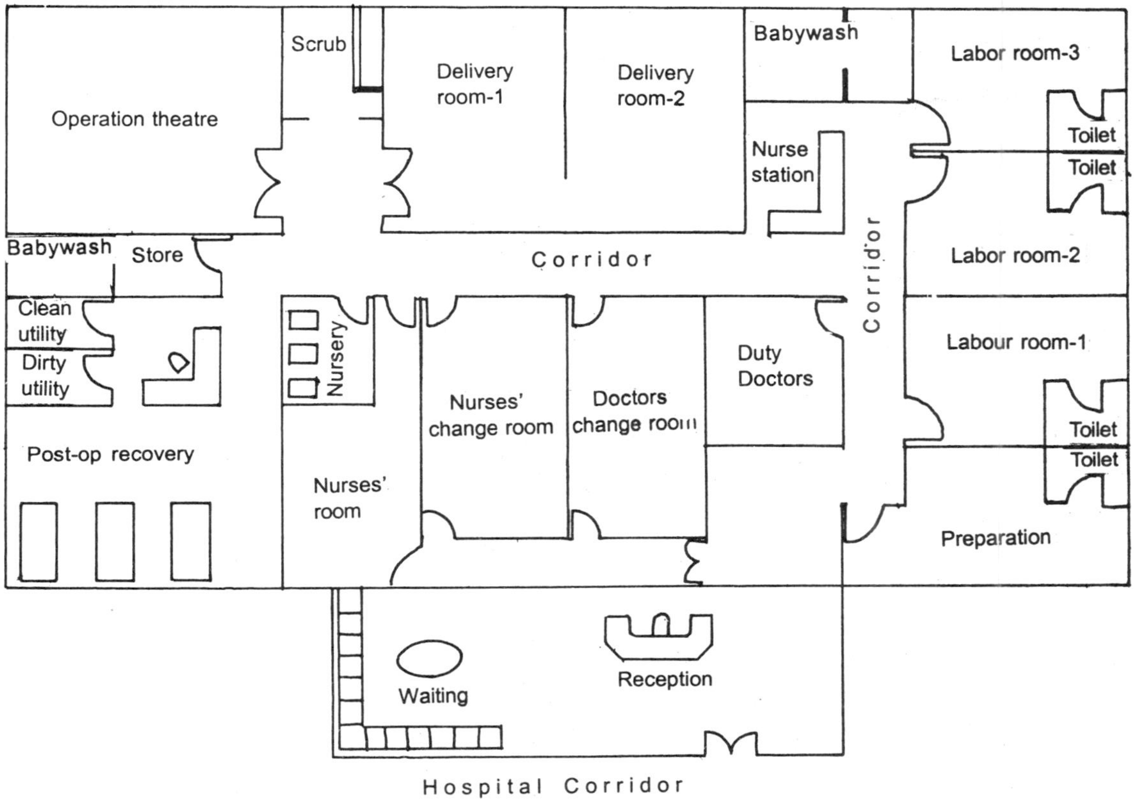

Fig. 34.57: Layout of a labour and delivery suite

This can be 4 to 8 for 24-hour operation.

Here is the sequence of figures:

1. Of the 400 beds in the general hospital, 80 are to be assigned to maternity service, three divisions of 27 beds each plus newborn nurseries.
2. For 80 beds at 100 percent occupancy, the peak delivery load is: 80 beds × 100 percent occupancy =16 deliveries per day (5,840 per year) 5 days average stay.
3. Because deliveries occur at all hours, it is possible to figure an average of five deliveries per room per day, which would call for 3-2 rooms, but because spacing is not wholly controlled, it is wise to allow one additional delivery room.

Labor Rooms

For this number of delivery rooms, the number of labor rooms would range from five to ten, depending upon the number of single rooms in the nursing unit and the admitting practice in the given hospital. If prospective mother are admitted first to their assigned bedrooms in the maternity division and then to labor rooms and if there are as many as 20 percent of the obstetric beds in single rooms, it may be that five labor rooms will suffice, if, however, the practice is to admit the patient directly to a labor bed and only postpartum to her as signed room, perhaps 10 labor rooms should be provided.

SPECIMEN	DATA BANK ACTIVITY UNIT DATA SHEET	Updated 1975.03
ACTIVITY UNIT	Delivery	retrieval index A09 G

ACTIVITIES: Preparation of the mother and carrying out the delivery procedure with assistance of a medical and/ or nursing team.

Minimum space for this Activity Unit : 420 × 480 cm

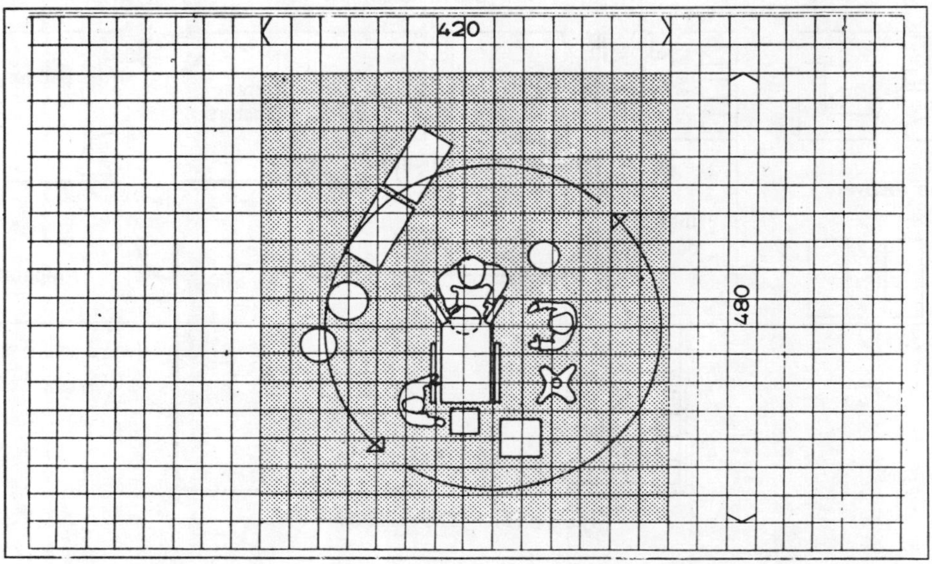

Equipment check-list	Quant.	Specific	Environmental check-list
Shadowless theatre lamp	1		Temperature : 18° C ± 2.
Outlet; medical gas, ceiling mounted, O_2, N_2O, Vac, Med. air	1		Air changes : natural : mechanical : 20/h
Outlet; electrical, ceiling mounted, 240 v, 13 amp, S.O. + low voltage outlet	2		Relative humidity : 55% ± 10
Socket outlet: 13 amp, double, switched	6		Lighting level :
Clock; with sweep, 300 mm dia.	1		480 lux + special lighting.
Table; delivery	1		
Anaesthetic; machine	1		
Stand; drip, mobile	1		
Stand; bowl, double	1		
Trolley; instrument	3		
Stool; Surgean's	3		

Fig. 34.58: Activity unit: delivery

Functional Programme: Delivery Suite

A rule of thumb is to plan one labor room for every 40 patients per month. One labor room should be separated from the others for use in the triage-septic area, for purposes of infection control. In addition, one labor room must be considerably larger than the rest, to be used for high-risk patients. For most labor rooms, dimensions of about 3.6 × 4.2 m (12 × 14 ft) will suffice; for the larger room, dimensions should be about 5.7 × 5.7 m (18 × 18 ft).

The delivery room needs an approximately one room for each 70-80 patients per month.

This includes the separated triage-septic delivery room. Delivery room may be approximately 18 × 18, but here too one delivery room should be considerably larger than the rest; about 6 × 6 m (20 × 20 ft), so it can be used for ceserean section, tubal ligation, and other obstatrical surgical procedures.

It is a good idea to locate delivery rooms near the surgical suite. A busy obstetrical service should have 24- hour anesthesia coverage in the labour-delivery area. A perfect set-up would be a delivery area connected to the main operating room by a door or a flight of stairs.

Proximity to the newborn nursery is also imperative. Pediatricians should always be close to or present in the delivery rooms when high-risk obstetrical patients are in labour.

Labour rooms should measure approximately 13-15 m^2 (140-160 ft^2). The need for larger labour rooms is determined by the necessary equipment and the comfort of the patient. Each room should include monitoring equipment, a Harvard pump for controlled rate of infusion of drugs, outlets for oxygen and vacuum, proper electrical grounding, emergency lighting, and all necessary equipment to conduct a labour. Door size should be adequate and beds should be light enough so that the patient can be moved directly to the delivery room without having to be transferred to a cart. The same requirements hold true for delivery rooms. One room should be larger than the rest but they all have to be rather large. Delivery rooms must accommodate a good-sized delivery table, an instrument table, monitoring equipment, a resuscitation area, a warming crib, anesthesia equipment, overhead lights, emergency lights, mirrors, and walls of cabinets with supplies. Delivery rooms should be a minimum of approximately 27 m^2 (300 ft^2) and about 36 m^2 (400 ft^2) where cesarian sections are done.

Much of the storage space should be in the substerile area. This should also contain instrument sterilization facilities. There should be adequate space set aside for bulky supplies work space for personnel. Packs should be made up by personnel who work in the delivery room complex. There should be a scrub area adjacent to each delivery room and one adjacent to triage-septic area.

Obstetrical recovery area (Constant-care) is required for 24-hour coverage by raised personnel, to check vital signs, vaginal bleeding, height of fungus, etc. The patients are moved out when it is convenient for both the constant-care unit nurse and the floor nursers to do so. The recovery area can also be used for pre-eleclamptic patient following delivery for 12-48 hours, depending on her needs. Other patients who need constant surveillance remain here.

The nursing station must be placed in such a way that nurses are available to the patients and to the admitting section. The lockers' rooms and one-site sleeping facilities have to be carefully designed. There should be enough space for bed, a good-sized lounge chair, and a work-table with a supply lamp.

Clean circulating air and proper maintenance of air handling equipment are mandatory. There is a need for communication facilities in each delivery room.

Single Unit Delivery System

Every fetus has the right to be well-born. To achieve this aim, hospital delivery and the introduction of sophisticated fetal monitoring devices have become the accepted norms.

Three levels of perinatal care are recognized-level I provides largely for the care of uncomplicated maternal and neonatal patients;

Level II has a full range of maternal and neonatal illness; level II centres provide maximum care and are designed to meet the needs of both normal patient and all types of maternal fetal and neonatal illness and abnormalities. It has been estimated that a referral zone of 10,000 annual births is required to support a level III centre; of this number in house births should exceed 2000 per annum. The design of any obstetric single unit delivery system (SUDS) caters to the physical and emotional well-being and rights of the mother. It allows for a natural and personalized child birth experience within the safe confines of a modern obstetric unit.

Two important physical features should be incorporated into the design of the reception area of an obstetric suite: the location should be on the ground level adjacent to the labor-delivery area and, secondly, the decor and atmosphere should be designed and controlled to de-emphasize a hospital or illness-related environment. The lobby leading to the admitting/examination room should be well-lit , carpeted, and wall papered. Comfortable chairs, other furnishings, and piped music will help to achieve this adjective. The reception area can double as a waiting area and should have public telephones, toilets, and some refreshment facilities.

A central station-staffed 24 hours a day a nurse/receptionist should be positioned the entrance to the labour and delivery to receive patients and direct them to appropriate sections of the unit and to control traffic entering labour and delivery area.

It is advisable to have two areas where patients can be prepared for their initial obstetric evaluation and, where indicated, to have procedures such as perennial shaving and enemas. Each admissiontriage

Table 34.2: Functional programme: the delivery suite

	100 beds	*200 beds*	*300 beds*	*400 beds*	*500 beds*
	20	30	40	60	70
Obs beds	1,460	2,200	2,920	4400	5100
Deliveries per year	4	6	8	10	14
Deliveries per room per day	5	5	5	6	6
Delivery rooms	2	2	3	4	4
Combined labour and delivery room	1	1	1	1	1
Single Obs beds	4	4	6	6	6
Labour rooms	4	4	6	8	8
Normal bassinets	23	42	39	56	66
Isolation bassinets	2	4	4	6	6
Premature bassinets	—	—	4	5	6
Total	**25**	**36**	**47**	**67**	**78**
Doctors lockers	6	8	10	15	20
Nurses lockers	6	8	10	15	15
Persons on day shift	11	12	13	19	19
Gross area per user, SFG	120	190	220	210	265
Department area, SFG	1,000-1600	1800-2800	2700-4200	3200-4800	4000-6000
Area per bed, SFG	10-16	9-14	9-14	8-12	8-12

room should be large enough to have an appropriate changing area and examination table with enough space to permit 2-3 attendants to move about freely

The flow of traffic should always be in one direction ; only patients and hospital personnel enter the obstetric suite (labor and delivery) through the main entrance. Many patients now demand privacy when in labor so that they can have a dignified and personal childbirth experience. In SUDS system, each room is designed to care for the patient during her labour, delivery, and for 2-hour postpartum. Depending upon the population being served, 2-4 of these rooms can be designated as high risk; the only difference in the design is the absence of toilets and the provision of more sophisticated monitoring facilities in the latter rooms. It has been estimated that about 10 labor and 3 delivery room beds are required for an obstetric unit catering to 2500 deliveries per annum. A glass-panneled observation station should be centrally situated to facilitate maximum patient supervision and to control traffic. This area looks directly into the 2 maximum high-risk SUDS rooms, into the observation ward and onto the corridor servicing the labor and delivery area. A central console that would admit the obstetrician/nurse on duty to scan patient being monitored would be situated here. A separate room, within the area of maximum obstetrician involvement , should be allocated as doctors' office and dictating area; a clinical laboratory should also be provided for basic blood and urine exams, the assessment of fetal pH and blood gases, and the reading of X-ray pelvimetries. A procedure room for amnioscopy, amniocentesis and ultrasonography should also be provided for. most level III obstetric units require 24-hour staffing by anesthetists suitable office, sleep, and toilet accommodations are needed. These are best situated outside the operating complex.

The area for support facilities should be approximately 7.2 m^2 (80 ft^2), and should contain double sinks and have ample work surface.

The single-unit delivery unit is a combination of labor/delivery and postpartum (2 hours) room which provides for a more specialized delivery. All obstetric procedures, exclusive of cesarean sections, but inclusive of most others that may require anesthesia, one performed in the same room.

The size of a SUDS room will vary according to the space available: 350-400 ft^2 will provide sufficient space to allow for the usual activity associated with a delivery. The room is divided into a carpeted section which should occupy no more than one-third of the floor space and is furnished with two comfortable sofa chairs. The remainder of the floor should be covered in a non-conductive material, an easy-to-clean surface. The walls should be covered with a vinyl textured paper. The roon should have two windows, one opening into the labor and delivery area and the other facing the exterior. Concealed consoles at the head of the bed and along the wall provide electrical, oxygen, and suction outlets, plus piped gases for anesthesia. Provision should be made for a closet to store patient's clothing and personal toiletries. A clean and soiled linen closet with a hatch opening onto the service corridor allows for the restocking of clean and the removal of soiled linen and instruments without disturbing the privacy of the patient. One toilet serves two SUDS rooms.The scrub room should also be shared and have the usual scrub sinks. The infancy resuscitation area is common to 2 SUDS rooms and should be at least 4.5-7.2 m^2 (50-80 ft^2) to allow for adequate space to work. The infant resuscitation unit should be attached to the wall with a special overhead light and adjustable angled table top to facilitate incubation and resuscitation. Shelves should also be provided for necessary equipment. The temperature control should be 2.39-26°C to ensure a proper environmental temperature for the infant. SUDS room is designed to serve as the patients' private "bedroom" for the entire duration of labor and the immediate puerperium. The high-risk labour room should be attractive and more functional. The operating room and intensive care area provide the third component to the SUDS system. It is an area that is devoted strictly to surgical procedures. mainly ceserian section, an intensive-care for seriously ill patients mainly pre—and postpartum and a recovery room. The entire section should be regarded as a sterile area.

A busy obstetric unit should have at least two fully-equipped operating rooms. Ideally, a third should be provided for elective cesarean sections and postpartum tubal ligation.

Postpartum Wards

Every obstetric unit should have prenatal activities -prenatal observation unit and a prenatal clinical laboratory which must be equipped for special procedures such as ultrasound visualization of the fetus and placenta; amniocentesis test for fetal maturity and genetic counselling; intra-uterine transfusion for severely compromised Rh incompatible fetuses, etc.

The prenatal observation unit should be divided into inpatient and outpatient sections. The former or single or two-bedded rooms, each with their own toilets and bathrooms. The purpose is to hospitalize patients with conditions such as pre-eclamptic toxemia, antepartum bleeding, premature rupture of the membranes, multiple pregnancies. The outpatient section provides for the dynamic assessment of fetal well-being and for day-time patient supervision. Each of the above unit will need storage, office, and other staff accommodations together with a suitable waiting/reception area for the patients. The prenatal unit should be separate but adjacent to and in direct communication with both the labor and delivery area and the postpartum wards.

The postpartum unit should be next to the labor and delivery area. The number of postpartum beds vary with the size of the unit, but should be calculated by multiplying the number of annual deliveries by the average length of stay and dividing this by 365 days and the estimated occupancy rate. The number of postpartum beds should be 10 percent less than that of the number of incubators and bassinets due to multiple births and longer stay of infants. Patients should be given the choice of either private or semi-private accommodations. Both should have private bath and toilet facilities. The rooms should be spacious (13.5m^2-150 m^2) and the furnishing and decor-attractive. There should be adequate closet space for clothing and other personal belongings. Concealed consoles behind each bed should be provided with piped oxygen and suction. The ratio of private to semiprivate rooms should be 2 : 1.

A unit delivering 2500 infants per annum would need 20 private and 10 semi-private wards. The postpartum unit should be next to the labor and delivery area. The number of postpartum beds will vary with the size of the unit, but should be calculated by multiplying the number of annual deliveries by the average length of stay and dividing this by 365 days and the estimated occupancy rate. The number of postpartum beds should be 10 percent less than the number of incubators and bassinets due to multiple births and longer stay of infants.

Patients should be given the choice whether private or semi-private accommodations, both should be private bath and toilet facilities. The rooms should be spacious (13.5m^2-150m^2) and the furnishing and decor attractive.

One or two well-baby nurseries should be centrally located within the postpartum unit and be equipped with bassinets that can be easily wheeled into the mothers' room. A procedure room-for doing circumcisions and other minor procedures-should be incorporated into the design of the nursery.

The neonated intensive care should be situated close to the SUDS and operating rooms.

FURTHER READING

1. Cooperman NR: Labour and Delivery Room facilities. In Hospital special-care facilities. Lanfman H (Ed): Academic Press. New York , 1981.
2. E Todd Wheeler: Hospital Design and Function. McGraw-Hill 1964.
3. Notelovitz M: The single unit delivery system: Obstetric unit Design for the 1980s. In Hospital Special-care facilities Lanfman H (Ed): Academic Press, New York, 1981.
4. Putsep E: Modern Hospital. International Planning Practices: Lloyd-Luke Ltd. London, 1979.

DAY CARE FACILITIES

Medical day care has been defined as a setting where lengthy attendance at least two hours—special equipment, rest of recovery, nursing services and the like can be conveniently scheduled for patients and staff.

The types of procedure are mainly time consuming investigations such as those which involve the collection of specimens for analysis over a period, of several hours patients may require some form of preparation.

The procedures may include blood transfusion and transfusion of special blood products, sigmoidoscopy, paracentesis, phlebotomy, taking of serial blood samples, and stimulation and tolerance tests.

In the rest and recovery section, 10 beds could be regarded as a minimum unit and about 20 a maximum. The accommodations would include two examination and treatment rooms, a day and dining space, a utility room, a kitchen, stores a nurses station, a Janitor's closet, a telephone box, a utility room, a kitchen, stores, single or multiple patient rooms, families and patient changing rooms, lavatories. A dermatology day care unit for psoriasis treatment should include a therapeutic bath, whole body ultraviolet irradiation room and a room for application of tar. There may be specialized day care facilities for diabetic, rheumatologic and pulmonary patients.

Surgical Day Care

In surgical day care or minor elective surgical operations and procedures are carried out on patients who are admitted and discharged on the day operation. Required laboratory and X-ray studies with the exception of preanesthetic physical and laboratory evaluation, are performed in the 48 hours prior to admission.

Operative procedures not exceeding 90 minutes in duration are best suited for outpatient anesthesia, provided that they are associated with minimal bleeding and only minor physiological derangement. The bulk of these operations are operations on superficial structures.

It has been roughly estimated that up to 60 per cent of operations now performed in general hospitals could be handled on procedures lend themselves to performance on outpatients. At any rate, the current variety of surgical out-patient procedure is expected to increase. The indications for outpatient surgery must be based on the skill of the surgeon, the complexity of the proposed operation, the conditions of the patient, the facilities available and the needs of the community. The length of surgical procedures should not exceed 90 minutes and they should not require significant sedation or pain relief in the postoperative period. Surgical day-care units have good psychological effects of the patients, as their anxiety is alleviated. The use of general anesthesia for outpatients is much more feasible than ever before. The number of outpatients receiving surgical treatment necessitating general anesthesia has increased dramatically. A programme of anesthesia for outpatient surgery can be conducted without compromising patient safety. Patients are admitted about two hours preoperatively to perform the preanesthetic physical and laboratory evaluation. To obtain these studies on the previous day is considered unnecessary. If there are symptoms of acute upper respiratory way or other infection, the operation is cancelled. A higher incidence of drowsiness, headache, nausea and dizziness occurs when the operation length exceeds 15 minutes. Therefore, before discharge in the afternoon, each patient must be examined by a surgeon or an anesthesiologist. Patients should be accompanied by a responsible adult when they are permitted to leave the surgical day-care unit after sedation.

The fact that the patient leaves the surgical day care unit before being completely recovered and is away from professional observation requires that the patient's condition during and operation be satisfactory before dismissal, monitoring gains importance in that situation as the physiologic state could be assessed to make known physiologic deviations which would prevent or retard dismissals.

Arrangements must be made for about 10 percent of the patients to spend the night after the operation under medical supervision. A collaboration with the admission unit of the hospital seems to be good solution. Concerning infants and children, the principal advantage of out-patient surgery is the elimination of the inconveniences connected with hospitalization. The ratio of pediatric day patients to pediatric inpatient is frequently estimated to 1:1.

It has been found that pediatric out-patient surgery can be safer, more convenient, and more economical than conventional management on inpatient basis. In the day-care units emotional trauma, fear and anxiety of the children is minimal. The children are happier, less frightened, and therefore seem to recover more smoothly. The maximum emotional disturbance occurs in children under five years of age, e.g. the age group accounting for 50 percent of the cases qualifying for day surgery. The parents may be anxious about the care of their child postoperatively, but much of this can be avoided. Most operations in children, especially those in the younger age groups require general anesthesia with its attendant need for thorough preoperative assessments in this respect that day surgery, as it is generally practiced, is most likely to be unsatisfactory.

Although, it has been felt that day-care surgical units should be small and widely dispersed to be of most value to the public and to maintain a friendly and concerned atmosphere, hospital attached units are to be preferred not least because of the curity of the back-up facilities provided by a general hospital. However, the day-care surgical unit should be distinctly segregated from the rest of the hospital. Out-patient surgery has to be provided in facilities, which are designed for that purpose only and not in the operation department, although the latter alternative has been required.

Emergency cases are not to be handled in the surgical day-care units. However, the facilities could be used for acute care in case of a community disaster. The approximate space requirements for an ambulatory surgical unit elements are:

- A receptionist's unit 15 m^2
- A waiting area for the patients 25 m^2
- A waiting area for relatives and friends 25 m^2
- A light refreshments service and patient lavatories 3 m^2
- A nurse's office desk 16 m^2
- A clerical office 13 m^2
- Two changing rooms with lockers and rest cubicles and anesthetic room 16 m^2
- An operation room 28 m^2
- Plaster room 22 m^2
- A scrub-up 6 m^2
- A recovery area with bed bays* 50 m^2
- An instrument room 10 m^2
- Stores 25 m^2
- A utility room 8 m^2
- A disposal room 8 m^2
- A laboratory 10 m^2
- An X-ray apparatus room 12 m^2
- Two staff changing rooms 12 m^2
- A staff lounge 12 m^2
- A doctor's office 12 m^2
- A consultation room 12 m^2
- A cleaners room 4 m^2

At least two operation rooms and one endoscopy room are needed.

The number of operation rooms is

$$\frac{A \times T}{D \times M \times Q}$$

The number of out-patient operation room depends on the number of annual operations A, the time in minutes under which the operation room is disposed per operation, T, the number of annual working days D, the time in minutes during which the operation room is available M, and on the realistic usage quote Q, which varies between 0.55 to 0.8.

The frequency of operations in the main specialities per 100 outpatient is estimated to be in surgery-orthopedics 2-5 in gynecology 4.0 in ENT 2.0 and in ophthalmology 0.8.

The length of ambulatory operation time, which includes preparation and postoperative rearranging of the operation room is about 30 minutes for surgery-orthopaedics, 25 minutes for gynaecology, 40 minutes for ENT, and 25 minutes for ophthalmology. The modern operation room suite is designed for major surgical procedures. The large rooms, conductive flooring and extensive anesthesia equipment for exceed the requirements for same day programmes. Therefore, a simplification and reduction of ambulatory surgery rooms must be achieved.

FURTHER READING

1. Ervin Putsep: Modern Hospital: International Planning and practice. Lloyd-luke: London, 1979.

AMBULATORY SURGERY FACILITY

Rising costs of hospitalization, shortage of hospital beds, and chronic overcrowding of operating room facilities are influencing factors in the search by hospital managements for a less expensive method for providing quality surgical care. Answer is the ambulatory surgery: an innovative method of delivering health care provides a convenient place for ambulant patient/surgeon contact and a workable approach to quality medical care at a reasonable cost to the patient.

Ambulatory surgery facility should meet the following requirements:

- It must be licensed as a health facility.
- It must be inspected regularly by an accredited inspection unit.
- Quality care must be ensured by formal planning and supervised evaluation.
- It must be a part of the health system and not a further fragmentation of this system.
- It should maintain a doctor/patient relationship.
- Cost in time and money to the patient must be less than for a similar service in the formal hospital setting.
- Community must accept such a service as one that is needed and desirable.

Approximately 40 percent of all surgery performed could be performed on an ambulatory basis. Ambulatory surgery is one area in which enhanced qauality of care and cost savings can occur simultaneously. If patients spend a shorter time in the hospital, health care delivery resources are used more effectively, which in turn can help stabilize escalating hospital costs. Few laboratory tests are done and less drugs are prescribed for such patients. Ambulatory surgery can reduce bed congestion in busy hospitals. More beds become available for more seriously ill patients, and this will delay or reduce the need to provide additional inpatient beds in a community.

Ambulatory care does not separate the patient from his family unit as is the case with inpatients, susceptibility to nosocomial infection is negligible, and psychological stress associated with hospitalization is reduced:

Types of Ambulatory Care

- Integrated
- Separated
- Satellite
- Freestanding.

Integrated Facility

The hospital establishes a formal ambulatory surgery programme by incorporating it into its existing, inpatient surgical programme. Construction of more operating rooms is not required, and the ambulatory surgery patients use the same admitting, preoperative, and post-operative areas as do the inpatients.

Separate Facility

A facility within the hospital or on the grounds of the hospital usually connected by some structure to the hospital.

Satelite Facility

A separate ambulatory facility located some distance from the hospital.

Freestanding Facility

Non-hospital model and independently operated.

Freestanding Birthing Centers

Short-stay birthing centers are cropping up in hospital and freestanding centers. About 40 percent of all the births in the United States now take place in these centers. Such centers are attractive because births in these facilities cost significantly less than nursing homes and corporate hospitals.

Cost can be reduced in birthing centers by eliminating un-needed tests that are routinely ordered in hospitals.

Short-stay Surgery

The success of ambulatory surgery in providing safe, cost-effective care to satisfied patients and their surgeons is prompting hospitals to explore variations of the ambulatory model. As hospitals provide increased services to patients and better serve the needs of physicians and all other components of the health care system, their efforts will be directed to:

- Limiting hospital stay
- Lowering hospital charges
- Expanding self care areas
- Increasing consumer satisfaction.

Demand

The changing demand for health care (willingness and the ability of consumers to purchase health services) is shifting preferences towards substitute ambulatory care and away from inpatient care. One more reason for hospital involvement in ambulatory care is competition. Factors that increase demand for ambulatory care include the expansion of coverage by insurance companies and other third party payers.

When considering the development of a formal ambulatory surgery programme, hospital administrators encounter some difficulties. Ambulatory surgery reduces the number of inpatient beds used. This will reduce revenue for the corporate hospitals unless there is a large patient waiting list for admission or unless the number of ambulatory surgical procedures performed can offset the effects of reduced inpatient occupancy. Hospital administrators with a strong philosophic committment to patient needs is reflected not only in the great increases in ambulatory surgery programmers, but also in many other attempts to provide cost-effective quality health care. Hospital administrators have to face this responsibility, meet the challenge, and successfully reach their objectives.

Establishing Ambulatory Programme

The hospital administrator must very carefully ensure that the process is properly managed and that input is obtained from all key areas (surgeons, anesthesiologists, nurses, etc).

The committee for establishing this programme must have medical staff representation (various surgical disciplines—those who are going to use the facility and also anesthesiologists). Many other surgical specialities will eventually be interested in the programme, but their membership on the original committee, though valuable is not necessary. Other representation should include administration, nursing, etc. All hospitals with an active surgery programme whose schedule includes operations that can be done on an outpatient basis should make a formal ambulatory surgery programme available to the surgeons and the potential patient in the community.

Before the programme becomes a reality, the optimum level of ambulatory surgery that could be performed should be determined. This is essential for projecting space requirements. By retrospectively reviewing the operating room schedule for a number of months and comparing each surgical procedure with the patient's admission profile, the hospitals potential ambulatory case-load can be determined with reasonable accuracy. Information to be obtained includes the patients age, the distance he/she lives from the hospital, procedures with the potential to be done on ambulatory basis.

Once the decision is made to establish a formal ambulatory surgery programme, other major issues need to be resolved. A subcommittee can be formed to handle the details of location, construction and finance.

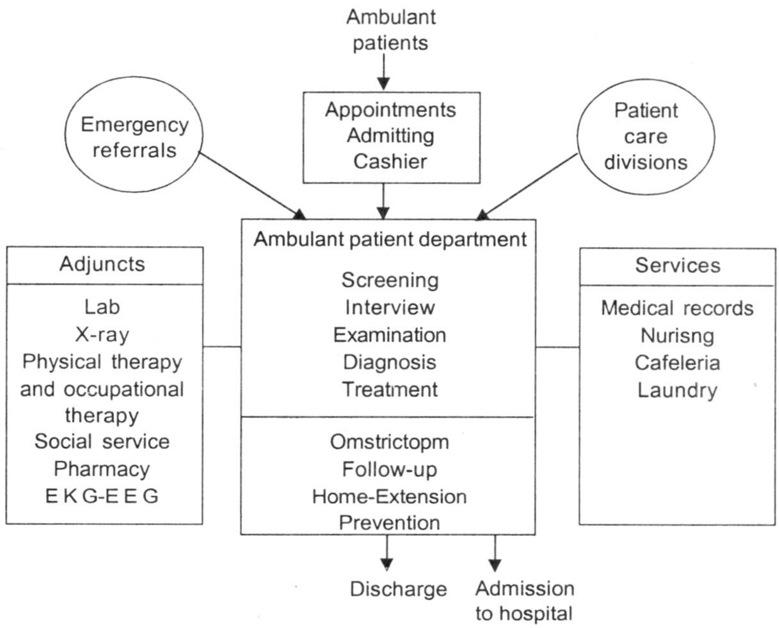

Fig. 34.59: Functional relationships, ambulant patient department

Charges

Hospitals should charge for each service separately, If a patient has had an ambulatory surgery procedure performed, he or she should receive either an itemized bill showing individual charges for each item or alternatively, a single blanket price for the particular procedure that would be an accurate reflection of itemized costs, itemizing significant cost analysis, both in establishing the original charges and maintaining an up-to-date profile.

Selection

Surgical Procedure

Six procedures appropriate to the ambulatory setting are among the ten most frequently performed:

- Biopsy
- Dilatation and curettage
- Excision of skin lesion
- Tubal ligation
- Cataract extraction, and
- Inguinal herneorrhaphy

The common procedure that can be undertaken in ambulatory setting include:

Orodental procedure

- Tonsillectomy and adenoidectomy
- Pelvic laparascopy
- Breast biopsy
- Arthroscopy
- Cataract extraction

Non-surgical Procedures

There are growing pressures to perform a variety of non-surgical procedures, usually on an ambulatory basis:

- Aspiration of breast mass
- Bladder irrigation
- Bone marrow aspiration
- Bronchoscopy
- Cardiac artereography and catheterization
- Chemotherapy (antineoplastic and anti-bacterial)
- Cystoscopy

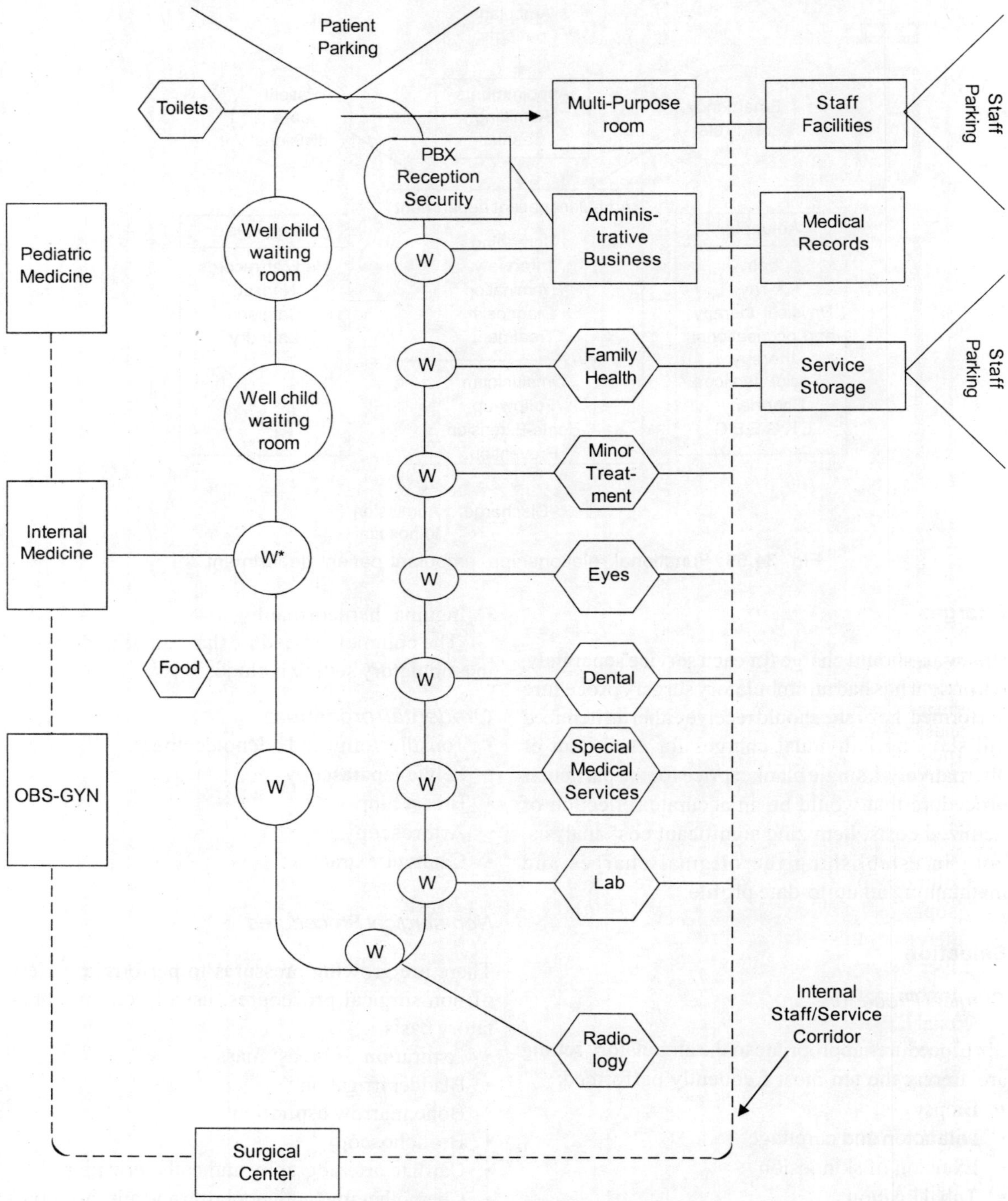

Fig. 34.60: Concourse concept of an ambulatory care facility: smaple flow diagram

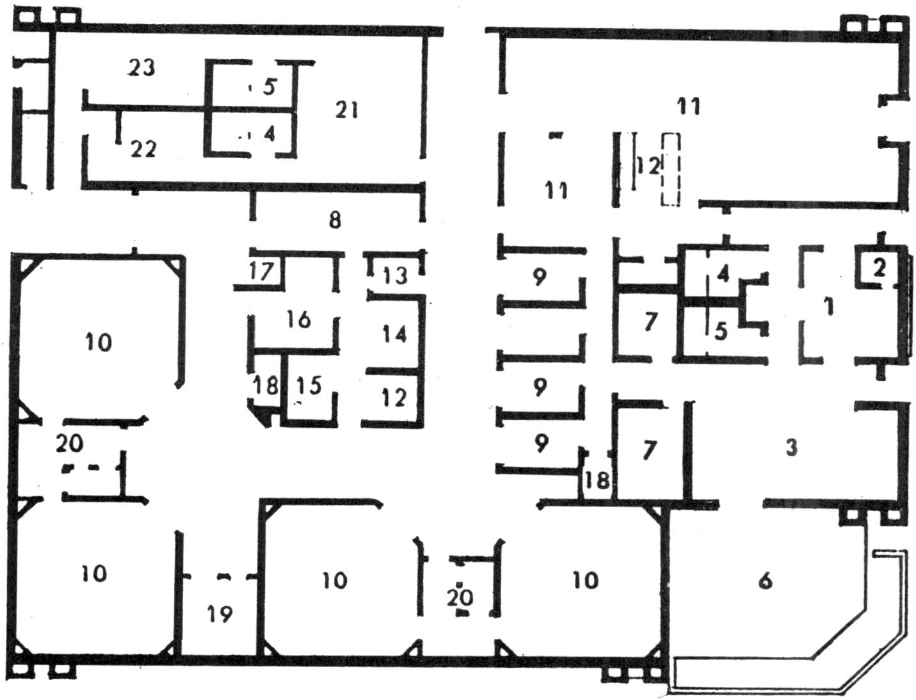

1. Reception room	2. Clerk	3. Waiting room	4. Men's toilet
5. Women's toilet	6. Patio	7. Office	8. Storage
9. Preoperative room	10. Surgery	11. Recovery room	12. Nurses' room
13. anesthesiology	14. Workroom	15. Sterile storage room	16. Cleanup
17. Trash	18. Janitor	19. X-ray dark room	20. Substerile room
21. Lounge	22. Men's locker room	23. Women's locker room	

Fig. 34.61: Floor plan of ambulatory surgery center

- Colonoscopy
- Esophageal varicial sclerotherapy
- Intercostal tube drainage
- Liver biopsy (Percutaneous)
- Lumber puncture (diagnostic)
- Renal Biopsy
- Sigmoidoscopy
- Thoracentesis

Operation Room Equipment

The same high quality of the equipment is required in the ambulatory setting as in the inpatient facility. The equipment includes:

- A reasonably modern anesthesia machine capable of delivering common anesthetic agents
- A full compliment of tracheal tubes and other artificial airways and laryngoscope blades
- Appropriate monitoring devices and resuscitative equipment
- Suction
- Conventional operating table
- Electrocautery machine
- Sterilisers
- Surgical instruments
- Ancillary operating room equipment appropriate to the type of procedures performed (e.g. operating, microscope fluroscopy).

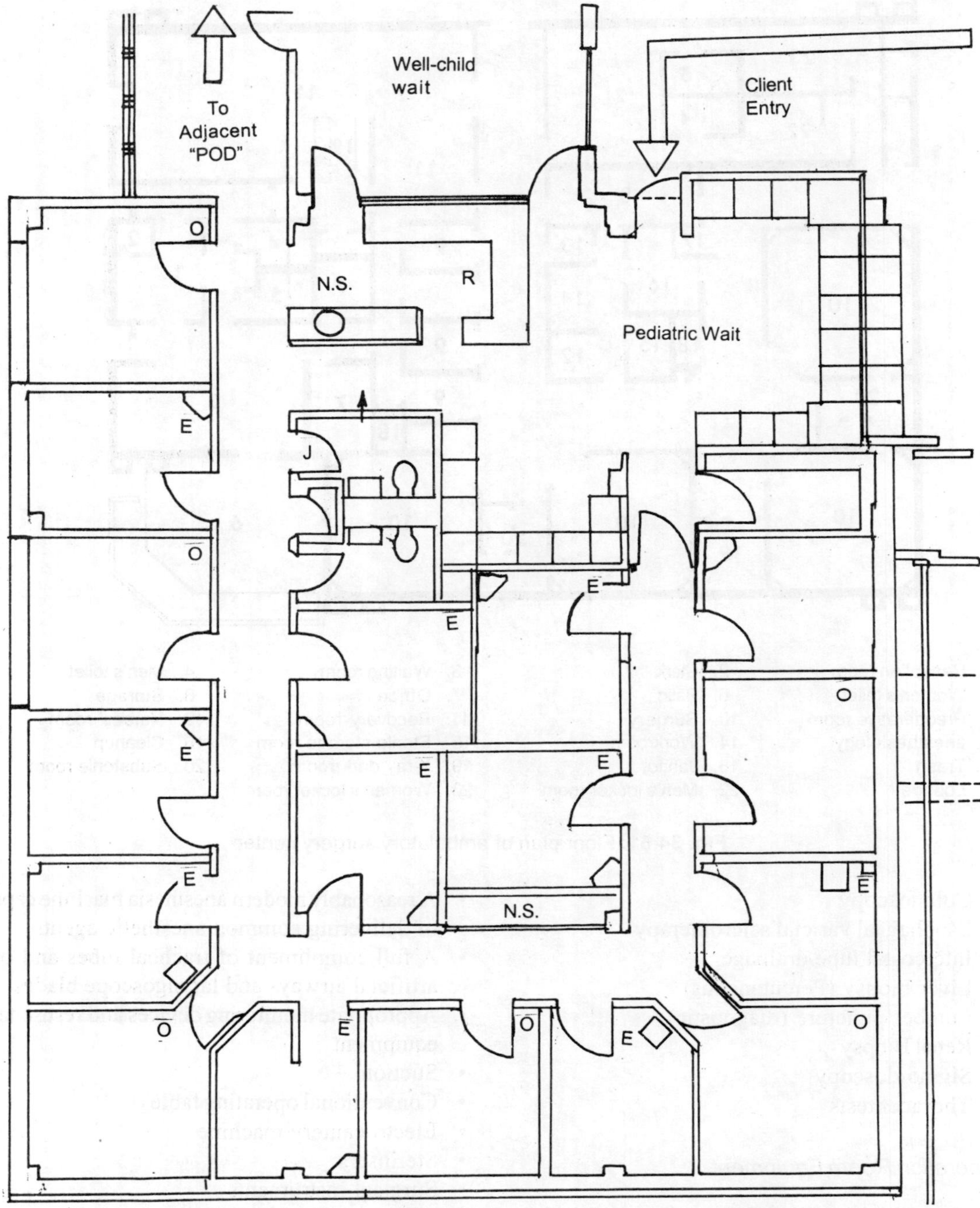

E = Exam room N.S. = Nurses' station O = Office R = Reception J =

Fig. 34.62: Basic layout of a six-provider "pod" ambulatory care facility

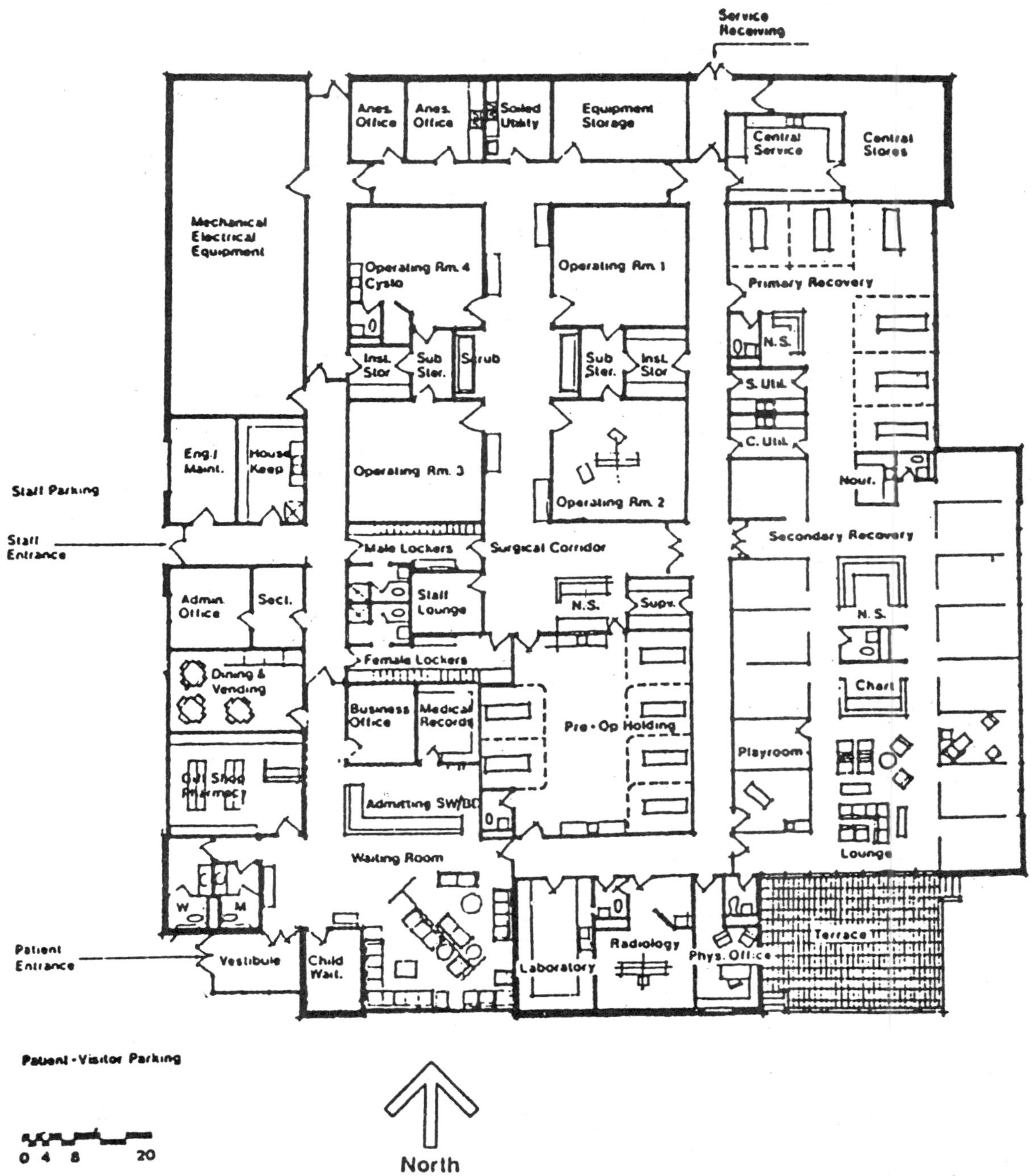

Fig. 34.63: Prototype floor plan of a freestanding ambulatory surgery facility

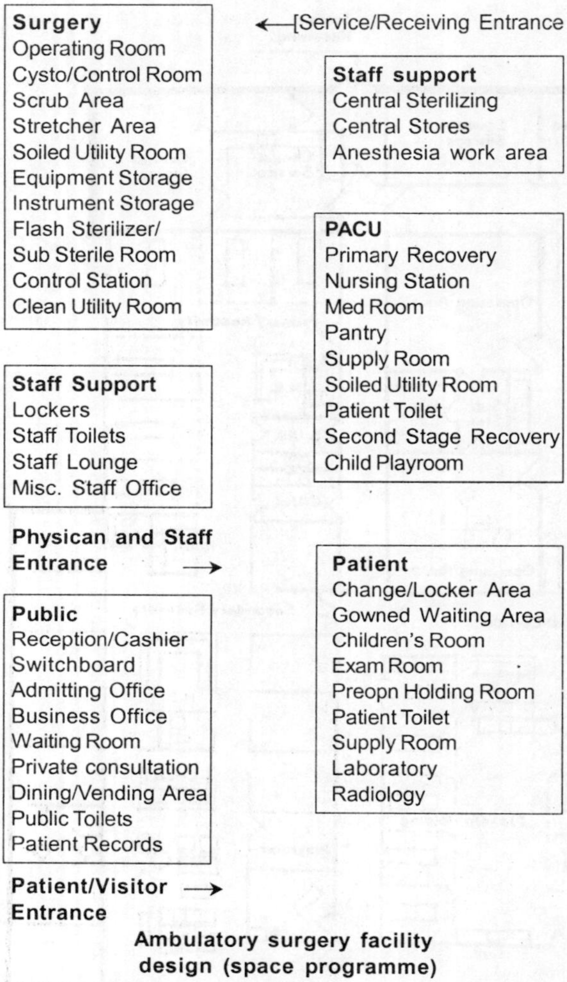

Fig. 34.64: Major zoing and room elements of an ambulatory surgery facility by functional area

Monitoring Equipment

Physiologic monitoring entails the continuous observation and assessment of the patient's condition and response to the anesthesia and surgery:

- Precordial stethoscope
- Sphygmomanometer apparatus
- Electrocardiogram
- Neuromuscular function
- Temperature monitoring
- Oxygen monitoring

Resuscitation Equipment

Even under the best circumstances, medical emergencies will occur. The facility must be trained and equipped to undertake a cardiopulmonary resucitation.

The Emergency cart must contain those items likely to be needed during cardiopulmonary resucitation and other medical emergencies. The cart should also contain electrocardiogram monitor, if one is unlikely to be otherwise available, a defibrillator, and appropriate sizes of the following items:

- Airways
- Endotracheal tubes
- Laryngoscope
- AMBU bag and masks
- Suction catheters
- Syringes and needles
- Intravenous catheters
- Minor surgical tray (for cutdown and tracheostomy)
- Adhesive and gauze sponges

Facility Planning

A well-designed and efficiently-staffed surgical facility greatly contributes to the success of an ambulatory surgery programme. The cardinal rule of facility planing is from following function. It is imperative that the facility be well planned in its early stages, so that its early stages, so that its design conforms to the desired function.

Facility Analysis

Existing building must be analyzed to determine what facilities are necessary to accommodate all of the institution's programmes (including ambulatory surgery). Master site plan should be prepared in such a way as to identify major departmental zones and logical sequencing of construction and renovation.

Functional Programming

Functional/space programming describes the need, function, and facilities required for an ambulatory

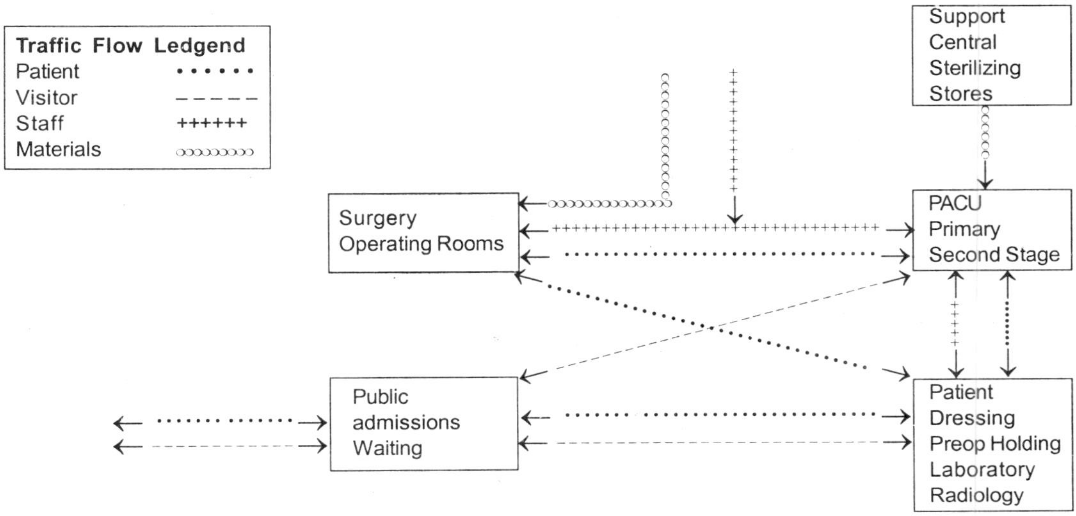

Fig. 34.65: Internal traffic patterns of an ambulatory surgery facility

surgery programme. It contains a departmental description, work load analysis, staffing requirements, department organization, functional considerations, and space allocations. It delineates the number, size, and type of each room together with the appropriate narrative to describe this information. This document (functional programme) after revisions with staff input, should be given to the architect to prepare drawings. It serves as the foundation for all further planing.

Schematic Design

It is the architect's translation of the functional programme into drawings. These drawings show the scheme of the departments.

Feasibility Study

Once the schematic design has been developed, more accurate costing can be done. The cost estimates provide the basis, together with future volumes, to conduct a financial feasibility study.

Design Development

Drawings are prepared in more detail, on a larger scale. Consideration is given to the details of the rooms. Major equipment items are identified (equipment lists,), special mechanical systems (ventilation needs and special lighting, etc) are listed, specific door locations are noted. A room detail summary is prepared, identifying each room, and its detail of equipment, finishes and so forth.

Working, Drawing and Specifications

Very detailed drawings (construction drawings) are the prepared showing minute details in the new facility with a specification to explain the drawings.

Bidding and Construction

Working drawings and specifications are sent to several contractors who prepare bids. The project is awarded to the successful bidder, and the contractor begins to construct the facility.

Planning Process

The following team members may be involved:

1. *Planning or building committee* Represents the owners of the project.
2. *Project director* Directs all the team members responsible for day-to-day activities of the project.

3. *Architect/Engineer* He takes the functional programme and translates it into drawings. Responsible for coordinating the many disciplines (civil, mechanical, electrical), necessary to design the physical structure.
4. Construction manager/General contractor.

Site Selection

Whether the ambulatory surgery unit is located inside or outside a hospital facility, its location must afford convenience, flexibility, and marketability.

After selecting site, there are three major criteria in developing it:

1. *Location of site elements* (identically, the site should be developed by using one-third for buildings, one-third for drives and parking, and one-third for landscaping).
2. *Driving* (to allow for easy and direct access to the site and buildings. Separation service and staff traffic from patient and visitor traffic is desirable).
3. *Parking/Entrances* The key parking-entrance relationship include:
   - Patient and family parking to the main entrance of the building.
   - Doctors parking to the doctor entrance
   - Staff parking to the staff entrance
   - Service-related drives and parking to the receiving dock and service entrance.

Master Planning describes the conceptual process one takes in considering all the potential programmes, services, and facilities to be offered on the site for the next 5 to 10 years.

Once these items are identified, the physical facilities required for them should be estimated (in terms of size) and situated on the site. This provides with a development plan for the future. It allows for orderly development of buildings and facilities.

Equipment Planning

At first, a generic equipment list is prepared on a room-by-room basis. As the design process continues, specific equipment (by manufacturer and model) is selected.

Groupings

Group I Fixed equipment is permanently affixed to the structure. It is not "plugged in". Life expectancy is typically 10 years or more (sterilizers, washers, radiographic systems, etc).

Group II Movable equipment, life expectancy 5 years or more (surgical table, wheelchair, lab equipment, etc).

Group III Consists of small, durable items, easily transported, and having a life expectancy of 3 years or more (surgical instruments, reusable trays).

Steps in Equipment Planning

- Programming
- Inventory and evaluation of existing equipment
- Budget estimates
- Architectural planning and design
- Purchased specifications
- Bid evaluation and purchasing
- Coordination and scheduling of equipment delivery and installation.
- Coordination of staff orientation and training
- Preventive maintenance programming.

Project Cost Components

The project cost budget aids facility planning through identification of capital needs. A well-planned expenditure budget provides assurance that the equipment and facility needed are available at the proper time, helps to define the risk involved, and facilitates the establishment of priorities for asset acquisition.

Functional Programme

Department Description

The ambulatory surgery department will be separate unit located within the hospital but not using inpatient surgical facilities. Existing hospital services will complement the ambulatory surgery department. This programme allows surgical patients to return home the same day as their surgery. No overnight hospital stay is required.

Workload Analysis

Three operating rooms (including a cysto operating room), 5 preoperative holding beds, 5 primary PACU beds and 2 secondary PACU beds will be needed to support projected volumes of service.

There should be 16 parking spaces allocated for patients and their families.

Staffing Organization

- One anesthesiologist will be available and on site during normal hours of operation.
- Three to four anesthesiologist will be available to staff the operating rooms.
- Five nurses will staff the PACU/holding area
- Three to four circulating nurse/surgery technicians.

Functional Considerations

Patients' flow will be as follows:

- Admission/reception waiting/change area/ gowning-preoperative holding—operative room primary PACU—second stage PACU-change area-discharge.
- There will be separate zones for waiting. Preoperative and postoperative, and operating room areas.
- Maximum nurse/patient visibility is desirable, allowing for reasonable patient privacy. The quality of the final ambulatory surgery facility design is directly related to the quality of time and effort given to the facility planning process.

General Guidelines

Ambulatory surgery programme should have atleast two operating rooms. This allows for optimal patient throughput . Each operating room can accommodate 1300 to 2000 procedures per year, depending on average length of procedure, available hours of surgery per day, number of operating days per week, and the efficiency of the operating room turnover.

There should be some minor operating rooms also that can be used for minor and minimally time consuming procedures.

The preoperative holding area is used to prepare the ambulatory patient for surgery. There should be a minimum of 1.5 preoperative holding area for operating room.

The primary recovery area is used for the immediate stage of postanaesthesia recovery. Strethchers are used in this area. Usually, 1.5 primary recovery stretchers to one operating room is sufficient.

The second stage recovery area is for patients who have required consciousness, require less nursing care, are being readied to go home. The area should be comfortably furnished for patients with recliners, chairs, couches, etc. This is a minimal care area where a patients attendant can be allowed. Secondary stage recovery time vary between 1 and 6 hours.

Functional Programming

A successful planning process begins with a concept. That concept is the foundation of the ultimate programme and facility design. To define the concept (ambulatory surgery), a planning team needs to be assembled. Representative from surgical disciplines, anaesthesiology, nursing and management should be included. To successfully define the concept, differing views must be considered and a consensus reached. A functional programme is the planning teams plan to coordinate all the different aspects of providing ambulatory surgery. It is the programme for physical and operational development.

The functional programming comprises of four major sections:

- Description (describes the proposed function of the ambulatory surgery programme).

- Workload analysis (will serve as the basis for projecting staffing requirements and space)
- Staffing levels (staffing by job category are projected)
- Programme for design (specific design criteria to be used for planning the facility).

Quality Assurance

The development of an active quality assurance programme can readily be achieved by organizing a defined committee consisting of a medical director nursing administrator and medical record officer

The committee will:

- Identify problems
- Develop solutions
- Disseminate information
- Reasses at a later date
- Correlate with educational activities
- Report activities to responsible parties.

Quality assurance is an ongoing, cyclic, non-punitive process designed to promote excellence in the health care delivery system.

Looking Ahead

The Philosophy of the ambulatory surgery facility is based on the demonstrated need for surgical services that can be completed safely within a day from admission, through surgery and recovery, to discharge. These services include the responsibility for providing individualized care to maintain or restore physically and emotional stability in the patient. Implementing such philosophy demands cooperative planning of all involved personnel and defined standards, policies and procedures.

Defined standard and established policies and procedures serve as operational guidelines for providing efficient, safe care to surgical patients and their facilities. These standards include maintaining a safe controlled, and consistently monitored environment and keeping accurate records and reports.

FURTHER READING

1. Amin Tabish: Planning Tomorrows Hospital Today. *JAHA* **2(2)**: 714, 1990.

HOSPITAL STANDARDS FOR THE CARE OF HIV INFECTED PERSONS

Most people who have AIDS or who are infected with HIV face emotional and often physical sufferings. It is vital that they receive support, care and compassion from the people around them. Since AIDS is transmitted only through sexual intercourse, blood, and between mother and child, and because the virus is not spread through casual contact, persons with HIV infections should be treated like any other person, whether in the workplace, at school or at home. They should be accorded the same respect, rights and dignity as any one. According to their capacity and the range of medical services which they are able to provide, hospitals are obliged to accept patients who need inpatient care, and to guarantee to those patients the necessary and adequate medical and hospital services appropriate to the type and seriousness of their illness. This requirement also applied to HIV infected and AIDS patients. AIDS patients in state III and IV may, (so that they may receive the best possible care), be sent for further treatment to hospitals, which have specialized experience and adequate equipment and staff to deal, in particular with the after-effects of HIV. Any person employed in a hospital is obliged within the framework of tasks that he is required to perform, to provide the best possible care for AIDS patients, except when social circumstances may justify exceptions. In order to protect hospital staff and patients the hospital authorities must provide general information for hospital personnel concerning the dangers to be faced, in particular the ways in which HIV is transmitted, and must give general training a protective measures against HIV infection. The doctor must inform the patient of the fundamental elements of the proposed examination or treatment, but not of its particular details. In this context, the extent of the explanation to be given will depend on the urgency of the intervention and the intellectual capacity and knowledge of the patient.

Development of Hospital Facilities

The patients may be kept in an area adjacent to, but separate from the main ward. This would minimise the risk of both accidental spread of HIV and hospital acquired infections in AIDS patients. All facilities needed for investigations and management of AIDS patients as well as strict compliance with infection control procedures, should be made available to the hospital centres. Each hospital may identify, among its staff, individuals from various specialities who have shown interest in providing care for the AIDS patients, so that their services can be utilised optimally.

AIDS patients require hospitalization for treatment of acute pathogenic or opportunistic infections and treatment of acute life-threatening emergencies. Many will require emergency or elective surgical intervention. Facilities for all necessary investigations and therapeutic procedures in AIDS patients should be made available in the hospitals. Every effort should be made to provide optimal care for the patients. Special efforts may be made to explore feasibility of involving non-governmental/voluntary agencies for providing home care to chronic and terminal cases so that they can rest their life in comfort and die with dignity. Most HIV-infected persons may remain symptom-free for prolonged period (upto 10 years) and then develop clinical manifestations of AIDS. During the asymptomatic period, they may require health care for problems related or not require health care for problems related or unrelated at HIV infection. All HIV infected persons should receive prophylactic and therapeutic care needed.

It is obvious that the hospital will not only be dealing with clinically developed AIDS but with the patients coming to the hospitals with unrelated illnesses and infected with HIV and capable of transmitting the infection to others. It can be emphasized that health care workers have more danger from this latter category of persons rather than with those patients who are having full-blown AIDS disease. Therefore, different facilities will be required to cater for patient's needs at different stages in the progression of the disease, from testing and diagnosis to outpatient treatment to inpatient care and treatment for periods of acute illness and finally terminal care. There are significant personnel, legal and patient treatment reasons that why the hospital must plan and prepare how it will deal with this particular type of patient population. Unless there is an adequate planning foresight, training and development of work culture and motivation among the health care workers it will not be possible to provide the desired health care to the deprived ones.

Diagnostic Facilities

Planning and design issues here include increased workload, additional space needed (especially for testing and counseling purposes) slow throughput and the need for confidentiality.

Patients are likely to go to a clinic for sexually transmitted disease for antibody testing, creating an increased workload, coupled with slow throughput due to counseling needs, may result in additional clinic sessions leading to increased requirement for consulting and/or examination rooms. The importance of maintaining confidentiality for all discussions with the patients may necessitate additional sound proofing of consulting and/or examination rooms. Depending upon the local demands, it may be appropriate to organize separate clinic sessions for AIDs and STD patients.

Blood samples for testing will generally be taken in a phelebotomy room with the staff following appropriate infection control procedures.

AMBULATORY TREATMENT

For those patients diagnosed as HIV positive and who develop further symptoms, additional tests and treatment may be required. Patient may require a variety of procedures such as lung function tests, bronchial biopsies, endoscopic procedures, CT scan and so on. The time required for cleaning and disinfecting equipment could lead to increased equipment requirements, particularly for items that are frequently used.

It has been estimated that patient diagnosed with AIDS made an average of 102 outpatient visits over a mean of 22.4 weeks duration. Additionally, HIV positive patients may require a 3 monthly follow-up outpatient visits. The effect of this additional diagnostic/treatment workload on these areas call for additional provision of treatment facilities in the OPD.

An attempt should be made to see AIDS patients in groups in given sessions during the working hours of the patient clinic. Efforts should be made to minimise direct contact between patient with AIDS and other patients, especially those who are severely immunocompromised. Contact with their blood and secretions should be avoided. The area of contact should be carefully washed with an effective disinfectant solution. Examining table covers should be cleaned after seeing an AIDS patient or after the group as the case may be.

AIDS patient should be educated about their responsibility to protect others from infection, including other patients, health care workers and friends.

Lack of treatment facilities in OPD may lead to admission as an inpatient—an inappropriate use of scarce resources as most procedures can be carried out on a day-care outpatient basis.

Inpatient Services

For those HIV positive patients who are diagnosed as having developed clinical AIDS (and for some patients with AIDS-related complex), episodic bouts of acute illness or infection may demand admission for treatment as an inpatient. In between these bouts, patients may recover and be sufficiently stabilized to return home. Patients who are less seriously ill but nonetheless require constant nursing care may also be admitted as inpatients, if they do not have anyone to care for them at home.

In the terminal stages of the disease, patients may develop further bouts of acute illness from which they fail to recover and eventually die in hospital, or they may be stabilised but declining.

Arrangements for the Care

Although several models for the care of AIDS patient are available, yet the best way is to establish an AIDS unit. This is managed by a team of dedicated workers including.

- Physicians with expertise in various aspects of AIDS.
- Nurses
- Counsellors
- Infection control officer
- Ward boys

Other professionals who would be willing to look after an HIV-infected person, for consultation of various clinical problems which could arise.

On long-term basis, it is preferable to have postings of residents, nurses and ward boys, etc. on rotation basis. But due to general feeling of fear and resentment, for the time being, it is a practical option to have a group of nurses and supporting staff who are specially earmarked for health care of AIDS patients. Before they start working with the patients, they must be given a short training on the infection-control measures. The personnel of this unit along-with the infection control unit must be made in charge of imparting awareness on infection control and monitoring its effectiveness/success.

Inpatient treatment raises a series of special planning and design issues.

Use of Single Vs Multi-bed Rooms

Precautions such as single room isolation are not generally indicated, if there is a special AIDS unit. But single rooms with integral WC, washbasin and shower may be required for those:

a. Who have secondary infections such as tuberculosis.
b. Patients with uncontrolled bleeding and open wounds.
c. Patients with severe and persistent diarrhea.
d. Who are unconscious or mentally confused.
e. Patients who are immuno-suppressed to avoid secondary infections.
f. Female patients may require privacy.

Disadvantages of single rooms

a. Patients may not be easily observed as in multi-bed areas.
b. Patients feel isolated both physically and psychologically.
c. Additional nursing staff support.
d. No mutual emotional support afforded by the presence of other patients.

Space Requirements

Uncertainty about incidence and prevalence of disease makes it difficult to estimate likely in-patient requirement in a hospital. The scale of provision will also be affected by location (urban Vs rural population served) and by regional and district strategies regarding the concentration or dispersion of hospital facilities for people with AIDS. It has been estimated that from diagnosis to death, AIDS patients occupy an average of 50 bed days, each with an average length of stay for a single inpatient occupancy of 17.2 days AIDS patients are highly dependable and require intensive nursing care, a bedspace of 21 sq metres/bed is indicated.

The actual mix of single Vs multi-bed rooms provided will clearly be a matter for local decisions based on balancing local requirements with facilities available. Ideally multi-bed bays should have their own sanitary provision. This will provide flexibility and make it easier to nurse patient with AIDS in a compartmentalized ward with other patients.

Treatment Facilities

Inpatients may also require access to further tests and treatment procedures. These may be carried out at the bedside, in a treatment room of the ward, or elsewhere in the hospital, depending upon provision already available for outpatient treatment. Provision for blood gas analysis may also be required at ward level.

Privacy and Confidentiality

Confidentiality, especially for patients with AIDS, is an important issue and may require appropriate procedures to control unauthorized access to inpatient areas, and appropriate sound-proofing in those areas used for discussions and counselling between patients, doctors and so on. Control of access as well as good observation of patients may therefore influence the location of the nurse base within the ward.

Counselling Facilities

In addition to medical and nursing care, patients will require counselling and emotional support in order to cope with their anxieties about their illness, with the possibility of death and with breaking the news of their disease, and perhaps their sexual orientation, to their families. Nurses and medical staff also need considerable support and counselling in order to cope, particularly with terminal care of patients. Appropriate facilities for staff and patients therefore need to be provided for counselling purposes at a ward level. Such facilities should be located away from the bed areas and in spaces which are not already used for office purposes as these uses may not be compatible with counselling.

Storage Provision and Disposal

Control of infection procedures, resulting in an increased use of disposable items (such as gloves, aprons) may require increased storage provision at ward level. As patients may be encouraged to wear their own clothes as much as possible while in hospital, it may be necessary to provide wardrobes or increased personal storage space at the bedside.

Overnight Stay

Overnight provision needs to be made for partners, friends and relatives of those patients who are terminally ill. This could vary from a folding bed at the patient's bedside plus access to WC and washing facilities to the provision of separate overnight stay facilities elsewhere in or near the ward.

Staff Changing

Facilities for staff changing will only be required at ward level, if it is a local policy for staff to change into theatre-type gowns to carry out certain procedures. Generally, the use of plastic aprons and gloves is all that is required for carrying out procedures, and for dealing with spillages and so on.

Kitchen Pantry

Severe loss of weight may be a significant problem for some AIDs patients. For those patients who are mobile, use of kitchen/pantry to make snacks may be encouraged by staff. Ideally, this space should be provided within the ward boundaries. Disposable crockery is not generally required except for those patients with bleeding lips or gums, or those requiring isolation due to other infections.

Flooring

As some patients may suffer from severe and persistent diarrhea, it may be more appropriate to provide hard flooring rather than carpets within the bed areas.

Procedures following Death

It may not be possible for partners and relatives to view a body when it reaches the mortuary. Appropriate provision should therefore be made at ward level.

The health care workers should wear masks, gowns, gloves to avoid contact with blood, body secretion of patient. Specimens from patients should be labelled and placed in a special bag or container labelled for transportation.

Operating Room

Disposable gowns and sheets should be used in the operating room. The room should be treated as it would be within a contaminated case. If a glove is torn or a needle stick or other injuries occur, the glove should be changed immediately and instruments involved should also be removed from the sterile field.

Intensive Care Unit (ICU)

Respiratory equipments should be treated according to procedure established. Other procedures are as per operating room precautions.

Labour Room

Same as operation theatre precautions.

Transfusion Rooms and Chemotherapy Unit

Precautions as in inpatient department.

Gastroenterology Laboratory

AIDS patients should be scheduled in the late afternoon so that the endoscopy room toilets used by these patients can be closed to further use until thoroughly cleaned. All personnel in the room should use cap, masks, gowns, gloves and shoe covers. These will be removed on leaving the rooms. Endoscopists should wear eye protection.

Cardio-pulmonary Laboratory and Cystoscopy Room

AIDS patients should be scheduled at the end of the day, so that the room can be cleaned and all the contaminated surfaces washed within 1:5 dilution of 5.25 per cent sodium hypochlorite solution.

Bronchoscopists and assistants should use water-impermeable surgical gowns and gloves, masks and goggles. Separate bronchoscope should be used for AIDS patients. Bronchosocopes should be washed with cidex and then it should be gas sterilized after examining each AIDS patient. All removable pulmonary functioning tubings should be changed after examining each patient, washed with cidex and gas sterilized. Separate disposable mouth pieces and air filters (Pall 1.3 micro filter) should be used for each patient.

Rehabilitation Services

Same as outpatient department.

Radiology and Radiation Therapy Area

Gowns, gloves and masks to be used by health care personnel, masks to be used by patients if coughing. Procedures described for operation theatre and gastroentrology laboratory should be followed.

Dialysis Unit

AIDS patients can be dialysed using infection control precautions. Universal blood and body fluid precautions should be used. The dialyser to be discarded after each use. An individual dialyser must never be used on more than one patient.

Dental Surgery

Personnel should wear gloves, masks protective eye wear when performing dental or oral procedures. The general safety procedures should be followed as in operation theatre. All re-usable instruments should be properly sterilized. The instruments that cannot be sterilized should at least be flushed the outside surface cleaned and wiped with a suitable chemical germicide and then rinsed. Dental equipments and surface that are difficult to disinfect (light handle X-ray unit heads) should be wrapped with impervious backed paper aluminium foil for clear plastic wrap. The covering should be

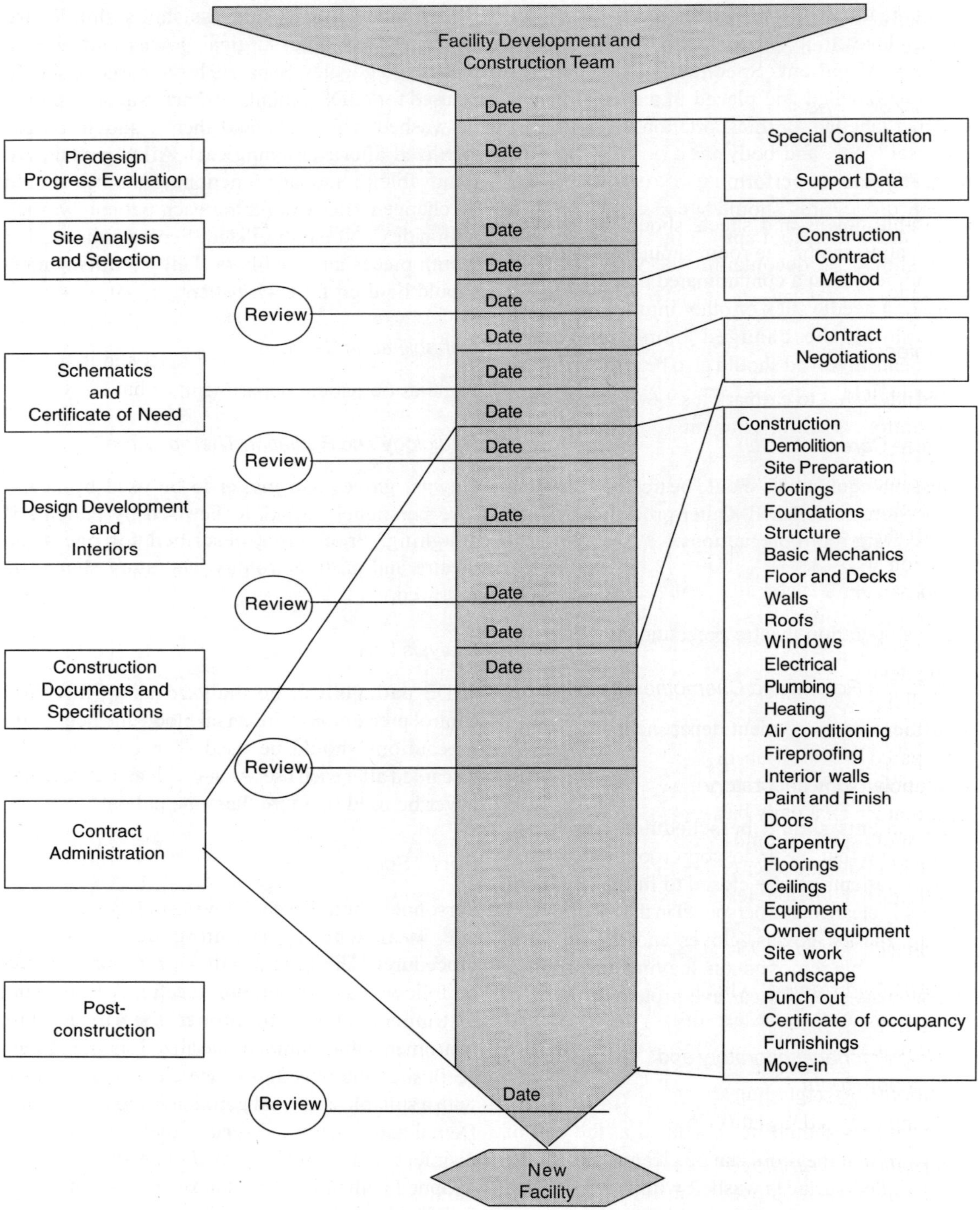

Fig. 34.66: Predesign and program evaluation: Process and schedule

discarded and clean covering should be put in place after use with each patient.

Mortuary Services

Universal blood and body fluid precaution to be taken. All persons performing or assisting in post-mortem procedures should wear gloves, masks, gowns, and waterproof apron. Surface and instruments should be decontaminated with chemical germicide.

Laboratory

1. It is advisable to earmark a separate area in the laboratory dealing with microbial culture, if possible.
2. Specimens should be labelled before submitting to pathology department.
3. Staff should wear gloves, caps, gowns, eye protection device, masks. Gloves to be changed and handed washed after completion of specimen processing.
4. Mouth pipetting is prohibited. Mechanical pipetting device should be used for the manipulation of all liquids in the laboratory. Laboratory work surfaces to be decontaminated with freshly prepared 1:5 dilution of sodium hypochlorite solution. The reagent should be prepared in each laboratory on a daily basis.
5. All individuals should wash their hands with providine-iodine after completion of laboratory activities and before leaving the laboratory.

Person with HIV or AIDS in Employment

HIV/AIDS screening whether direct, indirect or asking questions about test already taken, should not be required.

Confidentiality regarding all medical information, including HIV/AIDS status must be maintained.

Information to employer There should be no obligation for the employee to inform the employer regarding his or her HIV/AIDS status.

Protection of employee Persons in the work place affected by or perceived to be affected by HIV/AIDS must be protected from stigmatisation or discrimination by co-workers, unions, employers or clients. Information and education are essential to maintain the climate of mutual understanding necessary to ensure this protection.

Access to services for employees Employees and their families should have access to information and educational programmes on HIV/AIDS, as well as to relevant counselling and appropriate referral.

Benefits HIV infected-employees should not be discriminated against, and should have access to and receive standard social security benefits and occupationally-related benefits.

Continuation of employment HIV infection is not cause for termination of employment. As with many other illnesses, persons with HIV related illness should be able to work as long as they are medically fit for available, appropriate work.

Policy Development and Implementation

HIV/AIDS workplace policies should be:

a. Communicated to all concerned.
b. Continually reviewed in the light of epidemiological and other scientific information.
c. Monitored for their successful implementation.
d. Evaluated for their effectiveness.

Policy Principles

Protection of human rights and dignity of HIV infected persons, including those with AIDS, is essential to the prevention and control of the infection. Workers with HIV infection who are healthy should be treated in same way as any other worker.

Most people with HIV infection want to continue working, which enhances their physical and mental well-being, and they should be entitled to do so. They should be entitled to contribute their creativity and productivity in a supportive occupational setting. The approach taken to HIV/AIDS and the workplace must take into account the existing social and legal context, as well as national health policies and the global AIDS strategy.

It is also the right of all individuals who seek medical help to be ensured that health care facilities are not a focus of nosocomical HIV infection. All efforts must be made to strengthen infection control measures in all health care delivery systems to prevent HIV and other nosocomial infections. Strengthening of the infection control measures and allaying apprehension in the users as well as providers of health care is essential for ensuring appropriate care for HIV-infected persons. Each hospital should explicitly state its policy on matters related to infection control and containment. It is further recommended that each hospital should have a Hospital Infection Control Agency. This agency should, from time to time, review policies, procedures and practices in order to improve infection control. The hospital infection control agency need to review the present status and define appropriate changes to be made so that infection control becomes a reality. The HIV/AIDS case treatment area may be the first area where these measures will be implemented.

While providing such health/medical care facilities, it is also the right of the health care workers (HCWs) that infrastructure be made available which will be of utmost safety against accidental exposures to HIV while delivering health care.

Once the safety of the health care facilities is ensured, all the hospitals shall ensure that an HIV-infected patient requiring health/medical care is not refused medical help. However, the domiciliary facility for the management of such cases should be used to the fullest extent so that the patient is admitted only for the management of an acute problem. Appropriate prophylactic and curative therapy including elective and emergency curative surgical procedures should be made available to all seropositive individuals. For the time being, (till the clinical load is not enormous) patients with clinical HIV disease requiring inpatient care should be admitted in the general hospital in an area adjacent to but separate from the main ward. This would give a chance to HCWs (healthcare workers) to get used to the stringent infection control measures in the health care setting. This area will thus serve as a model for learning infection control measures in action. It would also reduce the risk of these immuno-suppressed patients acquiring nosocomial infections in the hospital. All facilities needed for investigation and management of these patients as well as strict compliance with infection control procedures may be made available to such a set-up. The hospital should provide the out-patient services for ambulatory care of HIV-infected persons. All the usual infection control measures must be ensured in the OPD setting also. Counselling services must also be available in the OPD. Hospice-type facilities must be developed and provided for the care needed for chronically and terminally ill patients. Assistance of voluntary and private organisations may be sought for provision of the required care.

Providing health care to the HIV-infected persons requires HCWs with knowledge, attitude and skills to deal with the special situation. Therefore, it must be ensured that HCWs are given appropriate professional and educational training both during professional schooling as well as in-service or in-practice through continuing medical education. Reagents necessary for the diagnosis of HIV infection should be manufactured locally as early as possible. In addition to reagents for ELISA test, reagents for simpler tests (such as visual assays or particle agglutination) suitable for use in smaller hospitals must be developed, quality assured and marketed. The necessary Research and Development (R and D) may be entrusted with the department of biotechnology. These principles are equally applicable to hepatitis B virus as well.

Each district hospital in the country should have one STD clinic. This can be achieved in a phased manner. It is also recommended to simultaneously revamp the existing STD clinics according to the norms recommended. To fulfil needs, all these clinics should have an access to nearby laboratory where facilities for testing for HIV is available. It is therefore desirable that more centres for HIV testing should be established. It is also recommended that such centres, in the initial stage, should be established in all the university/teaching hospitals as they already have a basic infrastructure for such a set-up.

All practitioners looking after STD patients should be networked in geographic units (e.g. city/district) for the collection of statistical data. The leadership, may be assigned to district STD centre or medical college hospital in specific geographic units. These centres should establish rapport with all STD practitioners and obtain anonymous information on cases and in return, should provide diagnostic facilities and continuing education.

In order to monitor the functioning of various STD clinics, a monitoring cell should be created both at center and in all the states. This will ensure proper functioning of the clinics, data collections, analysis of epidemiological data should point out the pitfalls in the working of STD clinics.

Vulnerable section of society should be approached through government and non-governmental organizations (NGOs) to educate them about the risk of contracting STDs and about preventive measures (use of condom). This risk group should be motivated to volunteer for periodic check-up (STD and HIV).

Health Education

Reorientation lectures for the doctors and nurses should be arranged periodically. Relevant information regarding the recent developments in the speciality (STD and AIDS) should be circulated amongst doctors from time to time. This will inform them about diagnosis, management and how to coordinate with nearby centres for further management of the patients.

Paramedical workers and technical staff should also be made aware of various facts of STD and AIDS.

Lectures should be arranged through government/NGOs for opinion makers of society (teachers, social workers, politicians, etc.).

In the undergraduate teaching, stress should be laid on teaching of various aspects of AIDS.

The perception of HIV-induced illness is changing. The emphasis in treating AIDS patients should be compassionate, low technology, cost-effective care. Patient care in the community should be encouraged and facilitated as much as possible, to allow them to live as normal a life as possible. It is not only the physical effects of disease that disabled patients, daily life in its many dimensions may also be effected by the impact of AIDS. Though incurable, HIV-induced disease is treatable leading to an overall improvement in the patient's quality of life and survival, provided there is a will, love and compassion.

FURTHER READING

1. Amin Tabish, Safaya AN: Standards for the care of HIV infected persons. *JAHA* **3(2)**: 15-22, 1991.
2. DGHS, Govt of India New Delhi. Proceeding of National AIDS Review communittee Meeting, 26th Dec, 1990.
3. Rawlinson C, Masson G: The design implications of caring people with AIDS. Hospital management international. Year Book of International Hospital Federation. 89, 1989.
4. Singh YN, Amin Tabish: Management of AIDS, a new challenge to hospitals. *Jr of Acad Hosp Admin* **2**: 1990.
5. US Dept of Health and Human Services, Center for Disease Control, Atlanta, Georgia, Guidelines for prevention of transmission of HIV and hepatitis-B virus to health care and public safety workers, morbidity and mortality weekly report. Recommendations and Report, 1989.
6. WHO-AIDS Series 2: Guidelines on Sterilisation and High Level disinfection methods effective against Human Immuno Deficiency.
7. WHO-AIDS Series 5: Guide to planning Health Promotion for AIDS prevention and control, 1989.

Healthcare Facilities for Elderly People

Changes in health care are not simply adding years to life—they are also adding an increased quality of life to those years. Older people make much heavier demands on health and social services than do young adults. The most elderly make the heaviest demands of all. The very elderly also tend to be proportionately highly represented in the most intensive forms of non-home-based care (such as increasingly important. Identifying and assessing need and then organising an appropriate response is essential. Elderly people can benefit from measures to improve their health and well-being. Care of the aged will depend on the effectiveness, the adequacy of provision and the degree of co-ordination of the services. A comprehensive system must be evolved to provide education, leisure activities, health, social services and legal assistance. Investment in research and training to enhance the quality and cost-effectiveness of care is important. Rational planning, supported by research evidence need urgent attention. Emphasis need to be placed on setting and maintaining high standards of community, hospital and residential facility care. The work done in hospitals and the way in which this work interlocks with that carried out by community and volunatry organisations will determine the effectiveness of geriatric services. Old age can be a time of continuing participation in the life of the community and personal fulfillment. A holistic approach is required to respond to the challenges posed by increasing number of elderly population.

Advances in health care are not simply adding years to life they are also adding increased quality of life to those years. Most people can now expect to live to old age in developed economies. In developing countries, average life expectancy is less but their massive populations mean that the old are numbered in millions. The impact of these demographic developments have been reflected in medical sciences by increasing research and knowledge, in society by improved services and among elderly people themselves by increasing expectations in health and social support. As the elderly are far more likely than the young to experience health problems, their use of health care facilities is high, and this of course is one of the reasons why planners are concerned about the economic implications of increases in the size of the very old population. With aging, the need for support for old people becomes increasingly important. Identifying and assessing individual need and then organising an appropriate response is essential. The elderly population is getting bigger. Simultaneously the working population is declining. Estimates suggest that within 50 years, the UK could see 25 percent of the population supporting the rest.[1] More than 60 percent of the people 65+ have long-standing illness, over 70 percent of the people 80+ have some form of disability, 7 percent of people 75+ live in long-stay hospital or care homes and this rises to near 30 percent for 85+, 5 percent of the people 65+ and 20 percent 80+ suffer to some degree from senile dementia, the number of people 80+ will increase by 50 percent over the next 20 years and will double over the next 40 years.[1]

Demographic Revolution

By the year 2000, more than 410 million persons were aged 65 and over, with about 41 percent living in developed countries. Sweden's population has the highest proportion of elderly persons: 17 percent.[2] By the turn of the century developing nations will have 59 percent of the world's population over 65, up from 54 percent in 1985.[3]

In 1985 China, India, the USA and the USSR each had more than 25 million citizens aged 65 and over. China had 80 million in 1985 and expects 240 million by 2040. By 2020, 72 per cent of people over age 60 will be in the developing world.[3] Japan has the highest life expectancy at birth of any nation: 77.1 years (1985). The speed of the aging of Japan's population is remarkable. While it took 45 years for the UK to move 7–14 per cent of its population aged 65 and over, Sweden required 85 years and France 115. It took Japan only 26 years. The USA will reach the 14 per cent in 2010, or 66 years. The USA will reach the 14 per cent. This world-wide demographic revolution is a major success story of 20th century (Table 34.3).

By the beginning of 1990's an estimated 15.7 per cent of population were aged 65 and over and 7 per cent were aged 75 and over in UK. There were 23 people aged 65 years for every 100 people aged between 15 and 64 years, by the year 2030, 31 over 65 year olds will be present in population for every 100 younger adults.[4] By the year 2025, there will be more than 10.7 million people over retirement age compared with 7.7 million in 1995, in England.[5] The number of people over 85 will have grown by over uses its resources. In 1994/95 the NHS (UK) spent £ 2,455 for every person aged over 85 compared with just £ 235 for every person aged 16-44.[5]

Country Experiences

The elderly populations of many developing countries are increasing rapidly. These demographic changes are a direct result of the success of socio-economic development that has led to declines in mortality rates at all ages and reductions in fertility.[6] Adequate disability and life expectancy data are essential for planning health and social policy but are century insufficient.

Japan has put in place a health care financing system that gives essentially free care (only a 5% of copayment is required) for all persons over age 70. The system for delivering health care emphasise hospitalzation a "Golden Plan" was announced in 1990 for expanding home and community-based service particularly rehabilitation and adult day care. Japan is creating a national institute on aging. The

Table 34.3: Population structure and dynamics (1990)

Demographic region	*Population % 60+*	*Population (millions) 60+*	*Deaths (millions) 60+*	*Probability of dying (%) 60+*	*Life expectancy at 60*
Sub-Saharan Africa	5	25	1.3	49.4	15
India	7	59	3.3	48.9	16
China	9	101	5.4	41.5	16
Other Asia and Islands	6	41	2.0	44.9	16
Latin America and Caribbean	7	31	1.2	33.0	19
Middle Eastern Crescent	6	29	1.4	42.0	17
Formerly Socialist economies of Economies	17	57	2.7	36.3	18
Established market economics	18	145	5.9	27.6	20
Demographically developing group	7	286	14.6	43.8	17
World	9	488	23.2	40.1	17

Note: Demographically developing group includes sub-Saharan Africa, India, China, Other Asia, Latin America and Caribbean, and Middle Eastern Creascent region.

Source: *World Development Report 1993.*

government policy for health care financing shaped distinctive Japanese patterns of elderly care provision.[7] The financing system provided a hidden subsidy through national health insurance coverage of long-term hospitalization-that encouraged high institutionalization rates of elderly in medical facilities.[7] Public financing for long-term elderly hospitalization, however, has ot been matched by government attention to quality of care, resulting in serious quality problems and reflecting a social tradeoff between cost and quality.[7]

Sweden has long been acknowledged as in the forefront of systematic development of social service, medical care and geriatric assessment. Social security systems are based on need.

China has a population with one in twenty elderly (80 million). Its village system provides roles for elders. The guiding concept is of generations standing together.

UK has been guided by the "Beveridge Plan" of 1940's in developing a "Cradle to Grave" set of social entitlements. The state currently funds 70 percent of the estimated £ 10 billion cost of the paid care, but this will fall to 50 percent over the next 20 years. Theoretically, this means private provision needs to increase from £ 3 billion to £ 15 billion, calling for a massive growth in funding from the private sector.[1] The demand on the state purse will continue to increase at the same time as it attempts to contain costs. Long-term care will have to be funded, at least in part, by those who require it, which means a carefully planned programme of pension, savings and specialist services.

Approximately 200 billion dollars are spent each year on personal health services for the 29.2 million Americans (12% of the total population) who are over 65. The elderly account for over one-third of health spending. Medicare and medicaid together cover approximately two-thirds of health care expendiutre for older persons and a considerable proportion of these costs is incurred in the last year of life.[8] The proportion of the population over the age of 65 is expected to increase into the next century, heightening concern about health care spending.[9] Life expectancy beyond the age of 65 is also expected to rise. Estimates of the upper limit of average human life expectancy range from 85 to 100 years.[10] The elderly population has been growing at faster rate than the younger population. The USA's population will be 13 per cent elderly by 2000 AD, 17.3 per cent by the year 2020 and 21.2 per cent by 2030 AD. USA is getting a late start on meeting the needs of long-term care in accord with sound principles of geriatric medicine. The health care for elderly is funded in four basic ways: private health insurance, Medicare, Medicaid, and out of pocket expenditures. Old age is a territory populated largely by women. Because women outlive men by an average of seven years, the ration of women to men increases sharply among the elderly.[11] Longer survival brings women greater risk of living alone and in poverty, of having chronic illness, becoming frail, and being hospitalized and institutionalized.[12] According to a recent study,[13] the increase in life expectancy over the over the past 30 years is due in large part to the access to services provided through the medicare programme. Medicare is still a popular programme on which millions of older people, disabled people, and their families depend. Total Medicare payments will be more substantially affected by the expected increase in the absolute number of elderly people.[11] The projected increases in Medicare expenditures will result largely from the increase in the size of birth cohorts and the proportion of each cohort living to the age of 65.[8] It is generally agreed that per capita Medicare costs are rising so rapidly that the costs of current benefits far exceed the contributions that were made bythe beneficiaries who now receive them. The rise in the Medicare costs can be curbed if advance directives and do-not-resuscitate orders are more frequently discussed with younger patients (rather than the last two years of life) and plans are made before crises develop. Substantial cost savings are more likely to be achieved through health care-financing reform in which reimbursement mechanisms are designed to encourage the use of long-term and primary care services aimed at maintaining functional independence and avoiding hospitalisation. Such reform would require integrating Medicare financing for acute care with financing for long-term care. The objective would be to allocate care more appropriately while dominating incentives for cost shifting. Care should focus on preserving function, with careful consideration and discussion of the costs and potential benefits of acute care hospitalization. Such an approach may facilitate limitations on the use of costly procedures that are based on factors other than age, such as effectiveness of outcome.[14] It is felt that Medicare could be imporved by the addition of comprehensive geriatric assessment, coordination of care, and integration of short-term and long-term care. A recent study[15] showed that comprehensive geriatric assessment of older people living in the community has already proved to be clinically effective and less costly than conventional care, since it helps reduce the need for nursing home admissions and other forms of extensive care. There is also scope to offer Medicare beneficiaries more choice in the health care plans available to them and to ensure that the government pay the same amount no matter what plan a beneficiary chooses. Elderly people who want to receive care in more expensive settings or who want to buy more benefits than come with the basic plan may do so, but at their own expense akin to the Federal Employee Benefits Plan (FEHPB). Under FEHPB, the federal government sets its dollar contribution to the premium, offers a large choice of plans to its employees during annual! open-enrollment period, makes information available to its employees to help them choose wisely, and monitors the plans to make sure they are fulfilling their contractual obligations.[16]

Long-term Care Systems

Long-term care is the lifeline for all elderly persons currently in nursing homes and who live in the community.[17] The prevailing bioethical model of decision making, with its emphasis on individual autonomy and life-sustaining medical care at the very end of life, is inadequate. It is inadequate because the chronically ill person who depneds on multiple supports for survival, in a nursing home or at home, cannot function as an isolated person in making decisions any more than in the rest of daily life: that person's intimate involvement with family and professional care givers necessitates their participation.[17]

Most developed countries have publicly supported programmes of social and personal care (e.g. respite care, home helps, adult day care); services are allocated accoridng to need. Among goals commonly found in long-term care services in developed economies is the prevention of impoverishment (a major exception is the USA where the only available public funding is part of public assistance for the poor medicaid).

Expansion of hospital, nursing home and community-based services is recognised as necessary adaptation to population aging in most developed countries.

Sweden has one of the most systematic approaches to long care system. A continuum of services is available to elders, including nursing home care and housing. About one third of GNP goes for health and social security.

In UK, commerialism in long-term care has burgeoned; in 1986, about 168000 of the 426800 beds were in the private, non-voluntary sector.[18]

In Australia, long-term care is mostly in the private sector counting retirement villages, hospitals and nursing homes operated by voluntary agencies and private corporations. State governments provide a smaller portion of aggregate service.[19]

In Japan, the government announced (in 1990) a 10 year "Golden Plan" for the welfare of aged, in preparation for having a population of 16.3 percent elderly in 1000 AD and 23.6 percent in 2020, approximately the proportion expected in Sweden and Germany. The comparable proportions expected in the USA are 12.8 percent and 17.2 percent and in the UK 15.4 percent and 18.7 percent. Japan at present is well below the other countries (at 10.3%). A prominent feature of the plan is support of family care gives in a way that permits them to continue in paid employment away from home during working hours. It also includes systematic development of personnel and faiclities, particularly in the community a tripling of spending in the 1990's compared with the 1980's. Day care services, including functional training will be provided in 10,000 centres in 1999. The programme will innovate "domicilliary care support" centres, offering home visiting, counselling and care co-ordination. The plan examplifies attempts to systematize and balance the institutional and community-based aspects of comprehensive geriatrics, the social and medical components and the housing and family considerations. The plan calls for primary prevention, rehabitation and prosthetic extending, to housing and other environmental modifications to assist mobility and other functioning.

In the Canadian province of Manitoba, a set of well-integrated elements of comprehensive geriatrics can be found. The financial framework is tax-based plan of universal coverage of health. A strong home care programme makes possible the maintenance of patients with their families for as long as feasible.

In the USA, a novel approach to systematizing is the Social Health Maintenance Organisation (SHMO). The key feature is "Case Management" offering framilies' advice and service. The SHMO pool funds from Medicare (primarily an acute care programme for elders) and Medicaid (acute and long-term care programme for the poor). In 1990, a congressional commission advocated a geriatrics-informatic plan for universal coverage of long-term care through social insurance, with a supplementary role for private insurance. The policies offer indemnity payments for individuals determined by physicians to need nursing home care.

Case Management has evolved as a flexible, pragmatic and compassionate strategy for improving client access and care continuity within fragmented systems of health care continuity within fragmented systems of health care and social services. The first generation case management programmes have been designed for various settings that serve different target populations with varying social, medical and psychological needs. This proliferation of categorical case management progrmames is a mixed blessing. While a categorical focus reflects both historical and public financing priorities, it creates a potentially duplicative and an inefficient system in an era of limited resources. Efforts are being made (in USA) to introduce accountability demonstrating value-added benefits and identifying best practices for structuring case management-client focused. The first step is reaching agreement on two critical dimensions of case management-major goals and essential service.[20] The key function of case management is to develop integration of services. the specific interventions of case management include: liaison activities to appropriately integrate clients into the health care system, health promotion, counselling, disease prevention, health education and screening, and community resource linkage. The case management team usually consists of nurses, therapists and social worker. To provide comprehensive services to aged there is need to develop co-operative relationship and mechanisms for information exchange with providers at all system levels that will serve as a bridge across the great divide between all levels of care.

Triage- a non-profit organisation has been able to provide a broader range of comparable services for its population at the same cost as Medicare and Medicaid. Moreover, vulnerable persons were able to remain at home and presumably with greater life satisfaction than in a nursing home.[21]

Triage (the process of establishing criteria for health care prioritisation) permits society to see cases in the context of diverse moral perspectives, limited resourc and competing health care demands. Triage planning offers a useful model for identifying and eliminating wasteful medical care. Prioritising cases require a triage method that is rational, fair and consistent-evaluating prospective cases according to seniority, acuity (severity) and risk.

The Living At Home Programmes fill gaps in the existing social service/medical care system by co-ordinating service for groups of frail elderly at risk for institutionalisation, thereby allowing them to remain at home.

Hospice (which focus on support for dying patient and their families), is not an institution but a service that may be rendered in various settings and the care is covered by a few insures.

There is growing movement to develop Adult Day Care facilities to provide treatment for the patient assist families in making adjustments and finding aid. The cost of care is less than of nursing home.

Health Care Facilities

Older people make much heavier demands on health and social than do young adults. The most elderly make the heaviest demands of all. The very elderly also tend to be proportionately highly represented in the most intensive forms of non-home-based care (such as hospital based inpatient care). In addition to having their highest rate of hospital admissions this group also have a much longer average length of stay in such care when compared to other sections of elderly population. Elderly people with acute illness present a particular challenge for the service seeking to provide the most effective clinical management of their condition and to maximize their level of independence. Elderly people will often have several problems coexisting which require skillful assessment and treatment, but their functional capacity will be equally as influential in determining both recovery and future living status. Older people need support to enable them to enjoy active, fulfilling and independent lives.

Nursing Home

In the USA there are more nursing home beds than acute care hospital beds. There are between 6 and 7 thousand acute care hospitals with a total of approximately one million beds. Three quarters are run for profit and a large proportion of these are run by organisations that own several or chain of nursing homes.[21] The key staff is administrator. Nursing home care in the USA is presently a 30 billion dollers industry.[22] Nursing home care represents about 20 per cent of total spending on health care for the elderly.[14] The quality of medical care provided in most American nursing homes is far from optimal.[22]

Utilising nurse practitioners to provide health care for nursing home patient has been tried at Massachusetts. Nurse Practitioners provide not only a substitutive role to that of medical care but also a complimentary one should be instrumental in enabling policy decisions that encourage the full utilisation on nurse practitioners.[23]

Hospital-Based Service (Acute Care)

Age is an inaccurate means of classifying health cre need, alternative organisational approaches that avoid age-related admission policies need to be rapidly developed to avoid age-rationing of health care. In the use of specialized acute care unit, emphasis should be on rehabilitation, independence in self care, and detailed planning for home discharge.

In-patient Care

Various models that have evolved are:

Age-defined approach (usually 75 years and over) provides a ward environment and care team.

Integrated approach all acutely ill persons are admitted to an acute medical ward, which deals with other groups and are care for by a group and are cared for by a group of physicians.

Need-based approach there are separate elements of geriatrics and general medicine but the decision about which team takes care of patient is governed by his/her care needs.

It is the success in achieving recovery rather than the response to illness per se which is the real test of the quality of hospital services. Integrated multidisciplinary services where access to care is independent of age but is determined by need for care offer the best value.

In Italy an innovative model of health care-acute care orthopedic-geriatric unit offers several advantages over traditional models: decreased patient mortality and length of hospital stay, a lower incidence of complications, and less need for specialist consultations. Cost/benefit ratio is very low. The model has also become a valuable teaching tool and a rich source of pathophysiological and clinical data for geriatric research.[24]

Long-term Care

The aim of long-term care facilities should be to allow the old person to have maximum dignity and self-determination. The elderly person's environment should provide a sense of security and cheerfulness. Emphasis should be on personalized care, retention of personal possessions and own washing and bathing facilities, well-designed modern environment and right to privacy. There is broad range of facilities available for elderly people who require long-term care and support who can not manage within their own homes. The health services in the UK continues to provide "long-stay geriatric beds", which usually care for elderly people who require nursing care. The local authroity social service department provides places in homes for the elderly. The private sector provides places in homes for the elderly. The private sector provides places in private nursing homes as well as in rest or residential homes; the not-for-profit and voluntary organisations also provide some residences. and nursing home care. In UK all patients in NHS long-term care are under the supervision of a consultant in Geriatric Medicine or Psychiatry. Those inhabitents of nursing homes are under the care of individual general practitioners. Nurse staffing tends to be low in most of the long-term care setting. Social interaction with patients in seen as one of the hallmarks of goods quality nursing in long-term care wards. Slowing down of hospital discharge rates, improved facilities for rehabilitation and recovery and hospital based respite and long-term care settings. Social interaction with patients is seen as one of the hallmarks of goods quality nursing in long-term care wards. Slowing down of hospital discharge rates, improved facilities for rehabilitation and recovery and hospital based respite and long-term care need to be encouraged. A comprehensive service requires the provision of acute, rehabilitative and continuing care. Slow-stream rehabilitation is very important. placement in long-term care should only take place after a complete multidisciplinary assessment and the team making the decision should review the long-term outcome on regular basis.

Special Units Within The Service

During last two decades a gradual specialization within rehabilitation has become evident reflected in the development of orthopedic geriatric and rehabilitation units. Their particular advantage is that all staff involved may accept and develop similar techniques and approaches so that whole of the patient's treatment round-the-clock is consistent.

The Day Hospital

Day hospital follows a medical, paramedical and nursing model. The facility is provided by a statutory and voluntary agencies. Day hospitals attempt to dissociate the diagnostic and therapeutic aspect of hospital treatment from the hotel aspect which requires patients to be looked after at night and throughout the weekend when no investigation or treatment is being carried out. The Day Hospital also allows a closed and prolonged supervision of patients suffering from chronic diseases so, if isolated completely from hospital care, would almost certainly deteriorate and require readmission.

In the UK, the department of Health and Social Security allows two geriatric day hospitals and two psychogeriatric day places for every 1000 people aged 65 and over in the catchment area served by these services.[23] Most of the patients attending day hospitals suffer from stroke or disease of locomotor system (arthritis, etc).

Ideally day hospital patients should be transported in well-heated vehicles with comfortable individual seats with safety belts. A vehicle may carry 6 to 10 passengers and requires to be equipped with lift which will take both disabled people and patients in wheelchairs.

Day hospitals provide a reception area, a dining and general activities area, therapy area, consultation and treatment rooms and staff rooms. Efficiency and cost-effectiveness of a day hospital will depend on the care with which appropriate patients are selected. The importance of audit in improving effectiveness of use of day hospitals cannot be overemphasized.

Psychogeriatric Service

The aim of psychogeriatric service is to deploy and enhance the skills of the health profession in meeting the needs of the mentally-ill old people, and in supporting those who care for them. A psychogeriatric service normally accepts any referrals of persons aged 65 and over within a defined geographical area. In UK generally the catchment area is the size of 200,000 people, of whome some 15 per cent will be aged 65 and over. Three basic hospital facilities are essential-an acute assessment or admission unit, a long stay unit, and facilities for day patients.

Wherever possible, admission units should be in general hospital, for elderly patients. If such a unit is to receive all inpatients from a comprehensive district service, then it will need about 1 bed/1000 old people, a 30-bed ward will usually be appropriate for a typical health district.

Educational interventions to improve understanding of mental health for elderly should be considered to address the inadequacies in contemporary mental health care.[26]

Community Care

As older people increase in number and live longer, they are making society aware that old age offers opportunities and challenges as well as problems. The majority of the people will continue to live in community either with their spouse or children or members of the family or alone.

The nature of services provided in community is critical in determining successful outcome of care for old people who do have needs. The multidisciplinary primary health care team is a cornerstone in the care of the elderly which can organize itself in such a way that some of this need is ascertained and problems are recognised early. Community nurses have a major role in caring for elderly. Specialist nursing services, community psychiatric nurses or palliative care nurses are an important adjunct to general community service.

National Health Service and Community Care Act 1990 (the UK) requires a combined approach to the assessment of need led by social service department, in which all agencies and professional disciplines collaborate. On the basis of such assessment a care manager will be appointed to take the lead in ensuring the services identified by the assessment are delivered. This role will include the commissioning of the social care components of the individual's care package. Social workers and some helps deliver such form of service to elderly people in their own homes.

Many old people attend day centres, lunch and recreational clubs. Respite care can be a major importance in allowing dependent older people to remain in their own homes.

Collaboration is crucial for the delivery of effective community care. Discharging an elderly person from the hospital requires careful co-ordination between health services both in the hospital and the community as well as social services, other agencies such as housing departments, and of course, patients, their relavites and carers. For effective collaboration, it is imperative that all players should be clear about their roles and responsibilities.

Home Health Care

In the UK many social services departments have developed their home help services based around a much wider range of tasks being provided in response to individual need than was previously the case. The potential for a joint health and social care approach to domiciliary care for older people is being examined via the provision of domiciliary workers who undertake both the functions of district nurse auxiliaries and local authority home care workers. This model has particular merit in meeting individual need across the health-social care divide.[3]

A problem in the provision of home health care for elderly people is the limited number of family members available for caregiving. Current trends suggest an increasing emphasis on the family as an appropriate caregiver.[27] Patient care provided through outpatient clinics and Home Settings offers such alternatives. In recent years home care become increasingly high-tech, including intravenous infusions, parental nutrition, supplemental oxygen, monitoring devices, chemotherapy and pain management as well as dialysis. These resources can permit the treatment of patients with severe chronic illnesses in their homes, but they can also permit care managers to send patients home from the hospital sooner than the patients and families may wish. Overall, home services may save 30-50 per cent in costs compared to costs for the same service provided in hospital. The major savings come from moving the charge for hospital room. There are opportunities for innovative home care programmes. What people want is the security of care that a medical-nursing team can bring to their homes rather than the power of hospital technology in their houses.[28]

Respite Care

Given the importance of familiar surroundings to many older people (and especially those with dementia) models of respite care involving care workers looking after the person in their own home are becoming more common.

Informal Support

Depending on the need of aged, the type of support provided by families varies enormously. The factors influencing this interaction include: the nature of the housing of the elderly person and of the family, the quality of the family relationships, the attitude of the elderly person towards independent living, and financial considerations.

Rehabilitation

Rehabilitation has to work from consumer's perspective to enhance autonomy. The challenges are the concurrent effects of aging, multiple pathology, different priorities and expectations and the rapid onset of disability during acute illness. Epidemiological information is vital if a rational approach to the price of rehabilitation is vital if a rational approach to the price of rehabilitation is to be built up. There is need to develop cost-effective menas to control the burden of illness caused by chronic degenerative diseases.

The logical place to carry rehabilitation of the old people is in their own homes. A selection of elderly, dependent patients can be cared for in their homes after short-stay hospital discharge and benefit from primary home care intervention programme in terms of improved medical and functional outcome and less long-stay hospitalization.[29] However, rehabilitation facility may be organised within a seperate geriatric unit, provided it is equipped to deal with acute medical emergencies or may be done in an integrated fashion with internal medicine. Rehabilitation patients often need the full range of investigation facilities, require surgical procedures and referral to specialist opinion. Separate rehabilitation units can be made to work, provided that a very structured approach to rehabilitation is maintained using clear objectives, monitoring and discharge planning. Specialist rehabilitation units, orthogeriatric units, stroke units and day hospitals have shown the evidence of effectiveness.[30]

Health Promotion

The promotion of health through education, disease prevention and health protection are beneficial in old age. Programmes include: detection and treatment of hypertension, smoking cessation, exercise, healthy eating weight control, psychological preparation for retirement, and social welfare.

Spurred on by Health of the Nation (the UK) initiative, Age Concern has introduced a national health promotion programme, Ageing Well. The prominent feature of its pilots is the use of its senior health mentors, trained old people who give advice to their peers. Nurse Practitioners in adult health, family practice, and gerontology must expand their repertoire of health promotion and health maintenance strategies to meet the needs of the elderly women.[31]

Role of Traditional Medical Practitioners

Many simple health activities do not require extensive professional training or major facilities and equipment. Health workers based in clinics or in their own communities play an importnat role in delivering these services. The traditional health practitioners have enormous potential as public health workers and providers of essential clinical services, if governments can give them the appropriate training, information and incentives.

Terminal Care

Care of dying must be patient-centered, holistic with due attention paid to physical, emotional, social and spiritual need and to be comprehensive, it must be team care. Terminal care means a commitment to pain and symptom control, the relief of social and emotional problems, a sensitive recognition of spiritual needs and concern for the needs of the relatives. HOSPICE care requires an integrated team who are energetic about rehabilitation. Most Home Care services aim to compliment the work of primary health care teams, with 20 patients per specialist nurse. Palliative care services need to be separately identified and funded.

SUMMARY

In meetings the challenges of health care and productive aging, roles are played by the individual, family, community, employers and government. Care of the aged will depend on the effectiveness, the adequacy of provision and the degree of co-ordination of the services. The work done in hospitals and the way in which this works interlocks with that carried out by community and voluntary organisations will determine the effectiveness of geriatric services. A comprehensive system must be evolved to provide education, lesion activities, health, social services and legal assistance. Investment in research and training to enhance the quality and cost-effectiveness of care is important. Rational planning, supported by research evidence is not an urgent attention.

REFERENCES

1. Patrick Sharp: Chronic care in old age: who will provide? Geriatric Medicine, 25th anniversary issue; 9, 1995.
2. Torrey BB, Kinsella K, Taeuber C: An Ageing World. US Census Bureau International Population Reports Series **95(78)**: Washington DC, 1987.
3. Kinsella K: Ageing in the third world US Census Bureau International International. Population Reports Series **95(75)**: Government Printing Office, Washington DC, 1988.

4. Donaldson RJ, Donaldson LJ: Essential Public Health Medicine. Kluwer Academic Publishers 357-87, 1993.
5. NHS Executive: Annual Report 1994/95. NHSE, Leeds, UK, 1995.
6. Jitapunkul S, Bunnag S, Ebrahim S: Health care for elderly people in developing countires: a case study of Thailand. Age-Ageing: **22(5)**: 377-81, 1993.
7. Kobayashi Y, Reich MR: Health care financing for the elderly in Japan. *Soc Sci Med* **37(3)**: 343-53, 1993.
8. Lubitz JD, Riley GF: Trends in Medicare payments in the last year of life. *N Engl J Med* **328**: 1092-96, 1993.
9. Bureau of Census, Day JC: Population Projections of the United States, by age, sex, race, and Hispanic origin: 1993 to 2050. Current population reports, 25, 1104. Washington DC: Government Printing Office, 1993.
10. Olshansky SJ, Carnes RA, Cassel C: In search of Methuselah; estimating the upper limits to human longevity. *Science* **250**: 634-40, 1990.
11. Butler RN: On behalf of Older Women: Another reason to protect Medicare and Medicaid. *N Eng J Med March* **21**: 794-96, 1996.
12. Davis K: The unfinished agenda. Improving the well-being of elderly people living alone. Final report of The Commonwealth Fund Commission on Elderly People Living Alone. New York: The Commonwealth Fund. 1993.
13. Manton KG, Stallard L, Tolley HD: Limits to human life expectancy: evidence, prospects, and implications. *Popul Dev Rev* **17**: 603-37, 1991.
14. Kramer AM: Health care for elderly person myths and realities. *N Engl J Med* **332**: 15, 1027-29, 1995.
15. Stuck AF, Aronow HU, Steiner A *et al:* A trial of annual in-home comprehensive geriatric assessment for elderly people living in the community. *N Engl J Med* **333**: 1184-89, 1995.
16. Wilensky GR: The score on Medicare reform.minus the hype and hyperbole. *N Engl J Med.* **333(26)**: 1774-77, 1996.
17. Lawrance B, Mc Cullouhgh and Nancy L Wilson: Long-term care Decisions: Ethical and Cenceptual Dimensions. Baltimore, Johns Hopkin University press, 1995.
18. Johnson ML: Long-term Care for the Elderl/in England in Schwab T (Ed): 175, 1989.
19. Moss B: Long-term care for Elderly in Australia in Schwab T (Ed) 242, 1989.
20. Falik M et al: Case Management for special Population-Moving Beyond Categorical Distinctions. *J Case Manag Summer* **2(2)**: 39-45, 74, 1993.
21. Kane RA, Kane RL: Long-term Care Principles, Programmes and Policies Springest-Veriag New York, 1987.
22. Melillo KD: Utilising Nurse Practitioners to provide health care for elderly patients in Nursing Homes. National Academy Press Washington DC, 1986.
23. Melillo KD: Utilising nurse Practitioners to provide health care for elderly patients in Massachusetts nursing homes. *J Am Acad Nurse Pract* **5(1)**: 19-26, 1993.
24. Incalzi RA, Bernabei R, Carbonin P: The orthopaedic-geriatric unit: a new model of hospital care. *Ann Ital Med Int.* **10(1)**: 49-52, 1995.
25. DHSS Geriatric Hospital Service, DHSS London, 1971.
26. Barnes CL, Given BA, Given CW: Caregivers of elderly relatives, spouses and adult children. Health-Soc-Work, **17(4)**: 282-89, 1992.
27. Mein AL, Bygren LO: Efficacy of the rehabilitation of elderly primary health care patients after short-stay hospital treatment. *Med-Care* **30(11)**: 1004-15, 1992.
28. Campion EW: New Hope for Home Care. Editorial. *N Engl J Med* 333 **18**: 1213-14, 1996.
29. Peterson CC: The accuracy of older and younger Australian's understanding of mental health and ageing. *Int J Ageing Hum Dev* **36(2)**: 129-38, 1992-93.
30. Reid J, Kennie DC: Geriatric Rehabilitation Care after fracture of femur: one year follow-up of a randomised clinical trial *BMJ* **299**: 25-26, 1989.
31. Swinson MM: Primary health care of elderly women. *J Am Acad Nurse Pract* **4(4)**: 143-47, 1992.

APPENDIX A

Age dependency ratio in OECD countries

Country	*1990*	*2000*	*2010*	*2020*	*2030*
UK	23.0	22.3	22.3	25.5	31.1
France	20.9	23.3	24.5	30.6	35.8
Germany	22.3	25.4	30.6	35.5	43.6
Italy	20.1	22.6	25.7	29.3	35.3
USA	18.5	18.2	18.8	25.0	31.7
Japan	16.2	22.6	29.5	33.6	31.9
Average for all member countries	19.4	20.8	22.9	27.6	33.3

Source: Organisation for Economic Co-operation and Development-ageing populations: the social policy implications, Paris 1988.

RENAL DIALYSIS UNIT

Renal dialysis is required for patients with the metabolic aberrations of end-stage renal disease and uremia. For the treatment of uremia two dialysis techniques are available : hemodialysis and peritoneal dialysis. Hemodialysis is currently the major treatment modality for patients suffering from the end-stage renal disease. In this procedure, the patient's blood flows through an extracorporeal dialyser, a device which exposes a minimum volume of blood to the maximum possible area of a semipermeable membrane. as the blood flows across one side of the membrane. It tends to come into diffusion equilibrium with a stream of dialysate, a balanced electrolyte solution, flowing across the other. Fluid removal obtained by varying dialyzer blood pressure.

Peritoneal Dialysis

Peritoneal dialysis is used for patients in acute renal failure or in hyperkalemia. The 1- or 2-litre bottles of dialysate are hung so that the fluid flows by gravity into the peritoneal cavity, where diffusion and osmosis take place. Substances thus removed flow by gravity into the drainage bottle or bag. This is called an exchange, and 40 litres of exchange is usually considered one dialysis. Because this method, sometimes called the manual method, uses an open system, the patient is quiet susceptible to infection. However, this technique is extremeley simple, require little or no requirement, and can be performed in even the most remote or tiny hospitals on an emergency basis.

Comparison of Hemodialysis and Peritoneal Dialysis

Hemodialysis	*Peritoneal dialysis*
Advantages	
• Three times as efficient in achieving normalisation of blood chemistries • Rapid treatment in acute renal failure • Long-term chronic intermittent maintenance	• Does not require heparin, circulatory access, of patient or venipuncture • Safe,can be performed overnight without a nurse in attendance • No special equipment or trained staff is required • Patients with unstable cardiovascular conditions tolerate peritoneal dialysis better • Dialysis disequilibrium syndrome is rare.
Disadvantages	
• Requires permanent circulatory access • Requires heparin • Requires special equipment and a highly-trained staff • Dialysis disequilibrium syndrome occurs more frequently than with PD • More expensive than peritoneal dialysis	• Inefficient • Too slow in treating severely catabolic patients • Often not technically feasible • Causes large protein loss • Cannot be used satisfactorily in certain categories of patients on long-term hemodialysis • Risk of peritonitis • Can cause hyperglycemia

Peritoneal dialysis, while popular as the first choice of treatment for patients with acute failure who require dialysis, has not reached the degree of popularity for chronic renal failure that has been attained by hemodialysis. However, peritoneal dialysis is increasingly being chosen as the primary method for long dialytic therapy for a larger expense of the patient population with end-stage renal disease. It takes four to five times a many hours of peritoneal dialysis to achieve the same status clinically as one can with hemodialysis.

In addition to the manual method of peritoneal dialysis, two other techniques are gaining increasing acceptance. One makes use of peritoneal dialysis machines to automatically perform all the exchange required in one dialysis. The other technique, continuous ambulatory peritoneal dialysis (CAPD), is conceptually different from either the manual of automatic cycler methods. Whereas these methods are used intermittently, hence the term intermittent peritoneal dialysis (IPD), CAPD is a new clinically applicable maintenance dialysis technique which utilizes a low dialysate flow rate with a prolonged dwell time.

Hemodialysis Systems

A typical hemodialysis system consists of the following major components: circulatory access, blood pump, dialyzer, method for anticoagulation, dialysate delivery equipment, and monitoring equipment.

Circulatory Access

The external shunt and the internal arteriovenous (AV) fistula are the two major means of access to the circulation. For patients with inadequate vessels, grafts have been interposed internally between an artery and a vein to create a graft AV fistula. Grafts fall into the following classifications: biologic, semibiologic, and prosthetic. A bovine artery is an example of a biologic graft; a mandril-grown graft is an example of a semibiologic graft; and a Teflon graft is an example of a prosthetic graft. The other means of access is though percutaneous of the femoral vein.

Blood Pump

A blood pump is a device used to assist the heart in propelling blood through the tubing and the dialyzer.

Dialyzer

The dialyzer or artifical kidney is available in three designs: the coil,the parallel flow plate, and the capillary (hollow fibre). Each type consists of a semi-permeable membrane. Blood pumped through one channel of dialyzer is contained on one side of the membrane while dialysate, pumped through another channel of the dialyzer, is contained on the other side of the membrane. The dialysis process was previously described.

Anticoagulation

Blood tends to clot when it comes into contact with foreign substances such as dialyzers. In order to prevent clotting, anticoagulation is used. Two methods ofanticoagulation (heparinization) are used, continuous or intermittent. Continous heparinisation is achieved by infusing heparin throughout dialysis via a calibrated infusion pump into the arterial blood line (inlet) of the dialyzer. Intermittent heparinization is done by administering a loading dose of heparin at the beginning of dialysis with a syringe and administering smaller doses through dialysis.

Dialysate Delivery System

The purpose of the dialysate delivery system is to prepare and deliver dialysate of the required chemical compostion to the dialyzers. The dialysate delivery system may be incorporated in a single patient system or may be part of a dialysis system which includes a dialysate central delivery system delivering dialysate to several (up to 20) patient stations. For example, one type of central delivery system continuously makes dialysate from dialysate concentrate and water (1:35 ratio) and delivers the dialysate via gravity or a dialysate delivery pump to various patient sations. The patient station is equipped with its own pump to either deliver the dialysate through the dialyzer under positive pressure (coil-positive pressure system) or deliver the dialysate through the dialyzer under negative pressure (hollow fibre negative pressure). Some patient sations are universal in that they have the capability of using coils or hollow fibre dialyzers.

Another type of delivery system is the batch system. There are central delivery batch systems as well as batch systems incorporated in a single patient system. The difference between a batch system and a proportioning system is that in a batch system a quantity of dialysis is made and stored for use during dialysis. The batch system, like the proportioning system, uses gravity or a delivery pump to send dialysate to the patient stations.

Water Treatment

It may be necessary to treat water before using it to make dialysate. Two processes to treat water are *reverse osmosis* (RO) and *deionization* (DI).RO is the process of forcing water under pressure through a semipermeable membrane. RO purifies the dialysis water of all classes of contamints including more than 99 percent of bacteria, pyrogens, and particles; and more than 95 percent of dissolved organics and dissolved polyvalent inorganics (e.g., heavy metals). DI is the proces of removing dissolved ionized compounds from water by iron exchangers. Water treatment is necessary if trace elements exist in the water supply in harmful amounts. These trace elements, such as copper, fluoride, aluminium, and calcium, can cross the membrane of the dialyzer, enter the patient's bloodstream, and cause complications.

Filters remove suspended particles in the water and should always be used. Ro and DI require expensive equipment and should be used if an analysis of the water shows that race elements exist in harmful amounts.

Dialysis Monitors

A dialysate delivery system should include monitors that indicate variable in the system. Both audible and visual alarms should be present to alert the operator when preset limits are violated. Parameters that are monitored during hemodialysis include variables in the dialysate channel and variables in the blood channel. Factors monitored in the blood channel include arterial pressure, venous pressure, and air in the blood as it is returned to the patient. Factors monitored in the dialysate channel include concentration (conductivity) of dialysate, dialysate flow rate, dialysate temperature, dialysate pressure, and blood in the dialysate.

Design and Construction of a Dialysis Facility

The process of designing and building a dialysis facility is an interesting logistical operation. Assuming that the market and feasibility study have been completed, and government approval and financing have been obtained, the following narrative describes the steps and procedures necessary to develop a typical out-patient facility.

In hospital facilities may be built *de novo,* or more commonly, are developed in renovated space. Some units in hosiptals limit their services to inpatients while others are used for both inpatients and outpatients. Acute dialysis units are usually located in emergency areas of the hospital.

The first step involves selection of an architect. The architect will provide assistance in determining the construction budget and space requirments for the facility and in selecting the site. Criteria for selection of the architect include exellence in design, technical competence, and sound project management.

Because dialysis facility projects usually involve small building, a smaller firm that can give the project closer attention may be better choice than a larger one. Architectural fees will normally be based on an hourly schedule rather than a percentage of the project cost. However, most architects will establish a guaranteed maximum fee.

Following selection of an architect, the next step is to extablish a space and functional programme. A 20-station dialysis facility will usually require between 540 and 756 m^2 (6000 and 8500 ft^2) of gross floor area or about 27 and 38.25 m^2 (300 and 425 ft^2) per patient.

The two choices available in construction facility are building or remodelling. Surprisingly, these is no clear-cut construction cost advantage in remodelling an existing space. Remodelling costs usually approximate new construction costs with the exception of a clean, empty, heated, air-conditioned space such as is found in a new office building.

If remodelling is chosen, the following factors should be considered. Space should not be encumbered by such fixed elements as weight-bearing walls,chimneys, or a large number of columns in locations that would interfere with use of the space. If the unit is not going to occupy a ground floor, the floor structure should be adequate to support the equipment and dialysate loads. Ceiling height should be sufficient to accommodate the maze of piping and ductwork that will be installed.

In choosing a land site, sufficient site area must be available to accommodate the parking required by zoning codes, as well as that actually needed. The site must provide delivery access for trucks as large a tractors trailers. An outside space should be provided for a trash dumpster.

The assistance of an attorney should be obtained in negotiating the lease or purchase of the selected site. After settlement of the lease or purchase, preliminary architectural plans are prepared. An approximate construction budget should be prepared by the architect, as well as budgets for medical equipment and furnishings (the construction costs, depending upon the equipment, degree of remodelling, type of construction, level of finish, and geographical location). The major built-in medical equipment, namely the central delivery system, if any, bedside dialyzers, and water treatment system, should be selected and orders placed for equipment purchase.

Upon approval of the final architectural design, the working drawings and specifications for construction are begun. The time to make changes is before the working drawings nearer completion, a construction contract should be negotiated with a competent general contractor. During this period of negotiations, interior design work should be undertaken.

Development of a multiple-station unit will probably take 4-5 months if remodeling is used and 5-8 months for a new building of approximately 540 m (6000 ft). After completion of construction comes, the check-out phase of the contractor's work, working the equipment and debugging, delivery and installation of furnishings and supplies, and familiarising staff with the facility.

Thus, it can take anywhere from 8 to 14 months from the beginning of architectural design work to the first dialysis treatment for a 20-station facility.

GUIDELINES

Renal Dialysis Unit

When facilities for renal dialysis are provided, these shall be so located as to be available for both inpatient and outpatient use.

a. *Patient areas*
   1. The acute dialysis units; individual cubicles, separated by nonflammable cubicle curtains fixed noncombustible dividing partitions or movable screen units, shall be provided for each patient cubicle.
   2. Bed cubicles or spaces shall have at least 150 square feet per bed and lounge chairs shall have at least 120 square feet per chair. These areas are exclusive of corridors, alcoves, vestibules and circulation areas. The minimum depth of a bed cubicle or space be 13 feet and the minimum depth for a chair cubicle or space shall be 10 feet .

3. The maximum area of any multi-unit dialysis room shall not exceed 5,000 square feet.
4. Surgical-type scrub sinks, fitted with other than hand controls, shall be provided for patient using chronic dialysis units, at a ratio not to exceed one sink for each 10 patients served. The sink shall be located in an alcove or other space directly adjacent to or within the dialysis room. It may not be located in patient toilet. Scrub sinks may be omitted in acute units.
5. A patient toilet room, with water closet and lavatory, shall be provided in each unit.
6. Handwashing facilities, for staff use, with other than hand controls, shall be provided in all units. No lavatory shall be located more than 25 feet from each bed or chair served.
7. Every dialysis unit shall have the capability of providing special emergency services when needed.

b. *Service areas*
   - Nursing station
   - Toilet
   - Clean work room for all the functions of the unit
   - Clean linen storage area
   - Soiled workroom
   - Facilities for sterilizing
   - Nourishment Station
   - Medi-prep area
   - Equipment storage room
   - Office space
   - Refrigerator

c. *Special plumbing requirements*
   - Water supply pipes to dialysis machines shall be sized larger than regular water supply pipes to ensure rapid water supply.
   - At least one floor drain in each dialysis unit.
   - Water used for dialysis should be analysed periodically and treated as necessary to maintain a continous water supply that is chemically and biologically compatible with acceptable dialysis technique.

FURTHER READING

1. Avram MM, Eliot Altman: Renal Dialysis unit. In Hospital Special Care Facilities Laufman H (Ed): Academic Press, London, 1981.

CARDIAC CATHETERISATION LABORATORY

Cardiac catheterization facilities have evolved to include traditional hospital-based laboratories with in-house cardiothoracic surgical programmes, hospital-based laboratories without on-site surgical programmes, freestanding laboratories, and mobil laboratories.

The goals of freestanding and mobile cardiac catheterization facilities are to reduce costs while offering services in a convenient location for low-risk patients.

Because of the cost-containment considerations and the documented safety of diagnostic cardiac catheterization, there has been an increasing pressure to perform catheterization on an ambulatory outpatient basis. In general patients who are not appropriate candidates for ambulatory catheterization include those with severe peripheral vascular disease, mechanical prosthetic valves, severe congestive heart failure, bleeding disorders, severe ischemia during stress testing, ischemia at rest, severe left main or proximal three-vessel disease, critical aortic stenosis and severe co-morbid disease.

The design of a special facility must be carefully considered. There are important questions to be asked, some of which are elaborated here.

1. What is a cardiac catheterization laboratory, for? Is it to be general all-purpose installation? Will it handle high-quality coronary arteriography, cardiac physiology, temporary pacemaker insertion, permanent pacemaker implantation, His buneld diagnostic studies, advances cardiac electrophysiology, radio isotope imaging? Will it be for adult patients, be a pediatric unit, or serve both? Is it for diagnosis, research, or both? What case load will it carry initially and in the future, in each of the categories it serves and in total? What flexibility for shifting direction and load can be preplanned? What limits are set in light of space, budget, engineering problems, and authorization? Keep in mind that with each discipline added and each step-up in sophistication, there are added problem, complications and cost.
2. Why is this facility being built? Is it a new venture, expansion, or upgrading of an existent unit? If it is a new venture or an expansion, does it meet a community or regional need and have requisite planning ranging from federal, state, regional, city, and community levels now have input into need and cost and will veto or curtail readily. Justification must be clear on the basis of community needs, case load, justaposition to a surgical program if the unit is primarily diagnostic, and private or grant support if it is research. Upgrading of an ongoing establishment is more of an internal decision based on need, safety, and available funds.
3. Where is it to be? Where is this facility to be built? Is it wholly new and going into a new building where there may be considerable freedom in planning? Is it new or expanding but more or less constrained by having to be fitted into anixisting building? Is it being upgraded with the limits of old space and the problems of adequacy of supporting structure and utilities?

Is the catheterization laboratory to be housed in a diagnostic X-ray department? Will it be dedicated or shared? Should it be part of a cardiology division's diagnostic aids along with phono and echocardiography, electrocardiography, and stress testing? Should pacemaker implants be done in the catheterization laboratory or in surgery? Should temporary pacemakers be passed in the coronary-care unit, at the bedside, in X-ray, or in the cardiac catheterization laboratory? The choices and answers vary from institution to institution and are greatly dependent on departmental clinical orientary and institutional policies, politics, and jurisdictions.

4. Historically, the cardiac catheterization laboratory began as a subdivision of cardiology, utilizing fluoroscopy to implement physiologic studies. With the advent of contrast radiography and advanced roentgen diagnostic methodology and equipment, radiology departments assumed a vested interest, particularly where case loads were low, facilities shared, and the equipment in the precincts of radiology. Facilities vary widely in situation and structure-ranging from fully equipped units, in and staffed by cardiology, with their own laboratory, developing, viewing, and storage areas, to units in radiology, run by radiologists. concentration, however, in one discipline or anothers is not a guarantee of excellence in either. Of the two extremes, the cardiology facility is more likely to include a greater variety of physiologic and electrophysiologic studies, and the radiology facility to stress anatomic aspects. Many grades of compromise and cooperation have evolved with the laboratory physically in one bailwick or another.

   At Montefiore Hospital and Medical Centre, the laboratory, a maximaly multipurpose unit, is one floor immediately above Radiology with separate and complete facilities. Radiology supplies, maintains, and staffs radiologic equipment, skilled cardiovascular radiologist is on immediate call, attends contrast studies, and contributes materially to technical and interpretive expertise. Patient scheduling, all physiologic studies, all cases done without contrast studies, and the paramedical non-radiological and nursing staff are under Cardiology. Cardiologists do most of the adult studies and pediatric cases, but training can be across the board for both, and radiologists rotate to do coronary angiography. In addition, a sophisticated pacemaker and arrythmia group (cardiac surgeons and cardiologists working across the board) use the unit for their pacemaker implantation and changes, his bundle studies, and arrythmia analysis. The administrative head of the laboratory, a cardiologist, also holds a staff position in radiology. The system functions well, because in the end, the parties concerned at all levels are determined to have it so, and the individuals who work together have evolved an excellent modus vivendi.

5. When will it be built (or altered)? A time schedule must be set on three levels, long-range, short-range, and daily. The long-range plan decides the scope of the project for the foreseeable present, establishes feasibility, location, budget, and basics of equipment and operation. This must include a time table for purchasing. Orders placed at the start of a 2-5 year new building project may result in premature delivery of equipment that is obsolete by the time it is finally installed. Contracts should stipulate later model options when installation times remote and budgets must accommodate. Conversely, orders placed late with firms with long delivery dates may delay projects. Both are particularly true in cardiology and radiology, where the equipment is caught in the current explosion of electronic, computer, and nuclear technology and cost. In new construction of expansion, this timeframe must also include choice of staff. Cardiac catheterization and electrophysiologic activities required extensive speciality training of physicians, nurses, and technicians, even of maids and porters.

Cardiac catheterization facilities have evolved to include traditional hospital-based laboratories with in-house cardiothoracic surgical programmes, free-standing laboratories, and mobile laboratories.

Personnel in the catheterization laboratory should be trained in cardiopulmonary resuscitation and preferrably in advanced cardiac life support.

In order to maintain proficiency, laboratories for adult studies should perform a minimum of 300 procedures per year, and cardiologists performing diagnostic catheterization should perform a minimum of 150 procedures per year.

The necessary equipment for the laboratory includes the radiographic system (high resolution X-ray imaging: a generator, X-ray tube, image intensifier, video system, cinecamesa), Physiological data monitoring (equipment for determining of cardiac output and blood gas determination, as well as a standard 12-lead ECG machine) and acquisition instrumentation, sterile supplies, and an emergency cart. Also included are support equipment consisting of a power injector, cineangiographic film or digital archiving, film processors and viewing equipment.

The hospital staff and the patient must be protected from the harmful effects of sadation.

Space

The space requirement is around 700 square feet which includes 500 square feet for procedure-room area, 100 square feet for control-room area, 100 square feet for clean preparation/store. The procedure-room size and the size of door should depend not only on the type and extent of equipment and staff but allow for patients delivered by coronary unit bed instead of stretcher, attached to respirator at the head, a balloon pump at the feet, attended by extra staff to service these supports, and/or with other physicians, residents in the laboratory as observers.

In determining appropriate space, construction, and cost, considerations may also be given to:

- power (3000 KVA generators) to allow adequate penetration and resolution at cine film exposure of 80-150 frames per second or high speed cut film the laboratory should be powered individually from a separate main feeder line with backup connections
- ventilation (air-conditioned and zoned)
- X-ray protection and structural stress (floor or ceiling bracing may be needed to support heavy equipment)
- cleaning, scrub sinks and cable conduits (washable walls, counters, and base cabinets; wires should be off the floor, in the ceiling or sub-floor)
- gases, suction, (piped-in facilities with wall outlets) anesthesia, emergency drugs, and carts
- X-ray protection (X-ray aprons should be all enveloping to guard backs as well as fronts)
- miscellaneous: exercycles, oxygen collecting or consumption containers, densitometers, oximeters, catheters, syringes, connectors and tubes.

Personnel

Staffing in the cardiac catheterization laboratory include the Chief of service, cardiologists, nurses and radiological technologists. All members should be trained in cardiopulmonary resuscitation and advanced cardiac life support.

Requirements for caseload are based on several considerations. to sustain and sharpen the professional skills and teamwork of the staff and provide maximum data with minimum morbidity, 300-350 adult cases or 150 pediatric cases per year appear to be the least needed.

Equipment

The physical requirements for the catheterization facility includes the radiographic system, physiological data monitoring and acquisition instrumentation, sterile supplies, and an emergency cart besides a power injector, cineangiographic film or digital archiving, film processors and viewing equipment.

High-resolution X-ray imaging is required for optimal performance of catheterization procedures. The necessary equipment includes a generator, X-ray tube, image intensifier, video system and usually a cinecamera. The advantages of digital acquisition and archiving include the ability to have on-line review, quantitative computer analysis of high quality images, image manipulation capabilities, and flicker-free images at very low frame rates thereby minimizing radiation exposure.

Continuous monitoring of blood pressure and the ECG is required during cardiac catheterization. Systemic, pulmonary and intercardiac pressures are generally recorded using fluid-filled catheters connected to strain-gauge pressure transducers and then transmitted to a monitor. Equipment for determination of cardiac output and blood gas determination, as well as standard 12-lead ECG machine, is necessary.

Cine Trace and Television Monitor Display of Physiological Data

A unique feature should display physiologic data directly on the X-ray television monitor instead of a separate slow-fade phyiologic date oscilloscope. This removes extra-overhead bulk and keep all information centered in one easily encompassed visual field. The present system takes the physiologic data of a 12 channel recorder and utilizing a special channel. The 2-channel bank under the large oscilloscope of the Electronics for Medicine VR-12 recorder. These can be postioned or amplified individually and canned by a 2- or 6-econd sweep. This selected data is fed to a small, dedicated non-fade display oscilloscope, scanned by an approximately matched camera, mixed (in the matrix) with the television image and visualized as a non-fade display on the X-ray television monitor. The circuits are designed so that when X-ray into used, the physiologic display is full-screen, usually with a 6-dec sweep. When fluoroscopy or cine are used the physiologic data displaces to the lower left corner of the field as a 2-sec display. Both displays are easily seen on the travelling room monitor in the catheterization room. Closed-circuit television to classrooms and senior staff office display the identical information and, in addition, utilizing a general observation camera mounted over a wall-hung cabinet to the viewer left of the clock, can elect a full view of the room. During videotaping or cine filming the physiologic data is also recorded, obviating the need to recall separate paper or computer recorder information when reviewing the case. In addition, for cine filming or taping, the elaspsed time or elaspsed frame number are recorded digitally. The cine trace and the time references are very helpful in rapid identification of temporally-related events for diagnosis and for research.

Radiation Safety

The patient and laboratory personnel must be protected from the harmful effects of radiation; installing and maintaining optimal X-ray imaging equipment will reduce unnecessary radiation exposure. The amount of radiation exposure to the patient can be reduced by limiting fluoroscopic and image acquisition time, collimation of the beam to the anatomical region of interest, using low-intensity fluoroscopy, acquiring images at lower frame rates, maintaining a minimum distance between the image intensifier and the X-ray tube. Personnel in the laboratory can limit radiation exposure by minimizing acquisition and fluoroscopy timings and 15-frames/second acquisition rates. The most important factors are maximizing distance from the source of X-ray and using appropirate shielding (led aprons, lead thyroid collars, lead eyeglasses, and movable leaded glass barriers).

PULMONARY MEDICINE

The services provided by the Pulmonary medicine department include respiratory therapy, pulmonary function test and arterial blood gas, bronchoscopy, pulmonary rehabilitation and sleep laboratory. Respiratory therapists provide such services as the maintenance of mechanical ventilators, administration of aerosols, oxygen, nebulisers, humidifiers, intermittent positive pressure breathing (IPPB), performing pulmonary function tests, arterial blood gas studies, etc. Respiratory therapists carry out various therapies as per the orders of the pulmonary medicine specialist under whom they work.

Location

Although both inpatients and outpatients receive therapy for a variety of conditions, the inpatients account for 90 per cent of the care given by the department. Besides, almost all the therapeutic work is performed at the beside. Diagnostic functions are undertaken in the department. The department should, therefore, be conveniently located for service to inpatients. Because much of the work is performed away from the department, breakage of small but expensive mobile equipment while transporting is a common problem. The location should not add to this problem.

In addition to the in patient areas, the other major users of pulmonary medicine are intensive care units, post-operative area, and emergency room. The department should have easy access of these areas. Close proximity to vertical transport is necessary.

Design

Pulmonary medicine requires a wide range of expensive but fragile equipment including ventilators, flow meters, humidifiers, nebulisers, etc. These need a fairly large storage area. After use, the equipment must be disassembled, washed, cleaned, reassemble, serviced, packaged, separated and sterilized. Facilities for these activities are essential as also a good distribution system. The services required are oxygen, suction and air. A good communication system is very important.

Organization

The chief of the department is a pulmonary specialist or a physician with an interest and training in pulmonary medicine.

There are no formal training programmes for therapists. In the absence of such a training, the therapists require extensive on-the-job training under a physician specialist in an established department.

It is advisable to cross train therapist staff to rotate between diagnostic and therapeutic sections. In many hsopitals pulmonary medicine units have been combined with cardiology departments to form cardiopulmonary service departments. Cardiology and pulmonary diagnostic testing have been combined to form a cardiopulmonary laboratory unit. This integrated unit has proved beneficial as it has provided improved and integrated cardiopulmonary services and better staff utilization.

Facilities

The space requirements include:

- Physician's office cum examination room
- Chief respiratory therapist office
- Room for bronchoscopy (with cardiac monitor and provision for oxygen and suction).
- A fairly large room for sleep laboratory. The lab must be equipped with many pieces of equipment to monitor heart, EEG, blood pressure, oxygen saturation, carbon dioxide, respiration, etc.
- Space for technicians with charting facilities.

- Treatment room(s)–can be partitioned into cubicles for examination and treatment.
- Clerical area.
- Storage area for movable equipment, small-processed equipment and supplies. To enable the therapist to respond to calls quickly, it is recommended that the processed equipment and supplies and stored in emergency carts, and the movable equipment is stored on the opposite side.
- A small repair room where therapist dismantles, cleans, maintains, and repairs small items of equipment routinely. The room should have utilities, a work bench and small-mounted cabinets.

Respiratory Therapy Department

The objective of Respiratory Department is to provide optimal respiratory care to its inpatient and outpatient population. The services offered should ideally be a continuous process of the efficient daily execution of treatment prescribed by qualified physicians.

Space requirement for inpatient service is 6-5-8.36 square meters (70-90 sft. per 1000 yearly admissions or 800-1200 sft.) for every 100 acute beds. The plans and layout of the area must provide for a sensible pattern of traffic flow. Overall space must be provided for: storage, sterilization, maintenance of equipment, laboratory, administrative work area, conference area, stores and distribution.

The types and quantity of respiratory therapy equipment include ventilators for continuous mechanical ventilation, gas therapy and aerosol equipment, blood gas analysis equipment, monitoring equipment, diagnostic and therapeutic devices, pulmonary function laboratory (blood gas analysis machine, spirograph machine, body-box plethysmograph, EKG machine, calculator, bronchoscope, capnograph, treadmill), manometers; manual resuscitators, sterilization equipment and educational equipment.

The entire unit must be kept maximally versatile. Keep the proximity of the services rational. Review work flow and keep traffic to a minimum in interior areas. To modulate the unit, given the square footage, divide respiratory care into three principal functional modules, the respiratory therapy module, the pulmonary function module, and the office module. Ideally, the department should be placed most proximal to its largest users. If a hospital is large, or made up of individual buildings, it may be necessary to utilize a satellite system. Respiratory care is a key service which is administered throughout any inpatient area.

35 The Support Zone

PHYSICAL MEDICINE AND REHABILITATION

Physical medicine includes both physical and occupational therapy. It is concerned with the diagnosis and treatment of certain musculo-skeletal defects and neuromuscular diseases and problems.

Physical therapy, includes exercise, manipulation, massage, thermal treatment, hydrotherapy, and electrotherapy. The patient may be assigned a routine including any or all of these. The physiatrist (specially trained in this field), or the therapist, assists the patients physician in working out the most beneficial routine. Actual treatment is given by him or under his direction by trained physical therapists. Each treatment may take considerable time, and hence this department, while often a busy one, does not handle large numbers of patients daily as does radiology.

Occupational therapy, also deals with physical handicaps or deficiencies, but its techniques are applied through processes of demonstration and training and not primarily manipulation. Its purpose is not to replace the physical exercise and training of physical therapy, but to supplement it with training in activities. Physical therapy may help a patient regain motor control of a disabled member of his body.

PHYSICAL THERAPY

The major functions of physical therapy include:

- To restore body function
- To hasten convalescence and shorten the patients stay in the hospital
- To prevent and minimise residual physical disabilities
- To return the individual to optimum living.

Location

It should be centrally located to accomodate all categories of patients. It should be close to the elevators with easy access to both outpatients and inpatients. It should be adjacent to other rehabilitative services (Occupational, and Speech therapy) as well as social and outpatient services. The orthopedics department should be as close as possible. The department should be located on the ground floor.

	100 beds	200 beds	300 beds	400 beds	500 beds
Physical therapy					
Massage, plinths	3	4	5	6	7
Hydro, arm and leg whirpool	1	2	2	3	4
Hubbard tank	1	2	2	3	4
Hot pack machine pool	–	–	–	–	–
Waiting seats	–	–	–	–	–
Exercise room	1	1	1	1	1
Helpers	2	3	5	8	9
Secretary	1	2	2	3	3
Occupational therapy					
Therapy room	–	–	1	1	1
Shop	–	–	–	1	1
Therapist	–	–	–	–	–
Helpers	–	–	2	2	3
Total Staff	3	5	10	15	18
Department area, SFG	1000	1800	3150	4000	4800
Area per user, SFG	333	315	267	265	

Design

An assessment of the physical facilities required for the department should be made in the earliest planning and design stage. In designing the department, one has to pay attention to three major functional areas:

- a hydrotherapy area
- a gymnasium
- a cubicles (treatment area)

In addition, there should be designated areas for waiting patients and support services (administration, staff facilities, storage and toilets).

Organizations

The physical therapy department may be part of a comprehensive rehabilitation service or it may be a department by itself where there are no other rehabilitative programmes.

Space and facilities are required for:

- Reception and control station
- Office and clerical area
- Offices for physiotherapists
- Waiting area
- Patients toilets
- Storage
- Janitor's closet
- Staff lounge
- Conference room
- Ramps with handrails at the main entrance
- Individual treatment cubicles
- Hand washing facilities
- Hydrotherapy, area
- Work stations and counters and different areas of work
- Space for paraffin wax bath
- Exercise area with all facilities.

OCCUPATIONAL THERAPY

Occupational therapy evaluates and treats individuals whose abilities to cope with or perform the tasks of daily living area threatened or impaired by physical illness or injury, the aging process, congenital or developmental disability, psychological and social disabilities.

Occupational therapy translates the ability to move into activities that we all do every day—bathing, dressing, hygiene, grooming, eating, transferring, home making and leisure time activities.

The goal of the occupation therapy is to return the patient to his/her optimum level of independence.

The occupation therapy should be located adjacent to the physical therapy department. One of the areas that should have received attention in designing the department is "Activities of daily Living" room which is equipped with cooking range, refrigerator, oven and other gadgets needed for daily living.

Many of the areas needed for the occupational therapy unit are common areas among the various sections of the physical therapy department. Additionally, the occupational therapy should have the following facilities.

- Activities of daily living room
- Work areas and counters suitable for wheelchair access
- Hand washing facilities
- Storage
- Crafts room.

HYDROTHERAPY

The advantages and therapeutic values of hydrotherapy are well known in the rehabilitation of patients with orthopedic, rheumatological, and neurological diseases.

In many cases, the process of rehabilitation should be gradual, without putting too much weight on the body. The ideal situation is to put the patient in water, where the weight of the body is reduced because of the upwards pressure of the water. To achieve this, a pool with adjustable depths is required. There are three ways to achieve different levels in pool.

- A gradually declining floor (one long ramp)
- A floor with various fixed heights (large steps), and
- A height-adjustable floor
- Walking over the 'width' of a gradually declining floor of the only five percent has the effect of walking with a difference of leg length of 1.5 cm. Acceptable would be a maximum length of 3 percent slope, which would require a very large pool.

A pool that is equipped with an adjustable floor is desirable. It is essential to aim for project management solutions rather than just buying products for rehabilitation center.

The pool area should be well-lighted by natural light and designed to give a feeling of spaciousness. The pool should be large enough to allow the patient to progress through his full rehabilitation, i.e. from using the full support of a stretcher, to partial support them on to walking and then to swimming and other recreational activities.

Planning of Hydrotherapy Department

Hydrotherapy department also requires considerable space and should be adequately separated from other parts of the unit.

Hydrotherapy Department normally has a pool for underwater exercise. Owing to the weight of the pool, this section must be placed on the ground or basement floor, regardless of the location of the rest of the physiotherapy department.

Facilities for toilet and showers should be available next to the hydrotherapy rooms

A hydrotherapy department needs tile or terrazo floor. The department should be a self-contained unit having:

1. Registration/Reception area for the patients.
2. Large hall as waiting area for patients and relatives.
3. Clean and dirty utility rooms.
4. Changing rooms.
5. Bathrooms with facility for shower bath.
6. Toilet for males and females.
7. Store room for linen, etc.
8. Store room for equipment.

The following factors must be kept in view while planning:

1. The toilets and showers for patients should be easily accessible from the hydrotherapy rooms.

Both should be planned with due consideration for the difficulties of wheel chair patients and should not be planned in cramped and inaccessible areas.
2. The plumbing must provide for sufficiently hot water at constant pressure.
3. Floor drains must be placed with due regard for possible overflows from tanks and tubes.
4. The flooring should be of daddo-terrazo or mosaic type. But should not be very slippely.
5. It should have as few doors as possible and these including corridors should be wide enough to allow easy transit of a stretchers and wheel chairs and turning around of these equipments if required.
6. A place for parking wheel chairs, trolleys and stretchers, so that communication remains free.

Equipments

Hydrotherapy equipment is used more frequently in institutions for nervous and mental diseases than in general hospitals. Equipment of following nature as used:

1. Continuous (tub) bath.
2. Douches and sprays (providing hot and cold water in jet or spray).
3. Showers.
4. Sitz baths tubs
5. Tables, rubber sheets, blankets (for giving wet packs).
6. Infrared or luminous heaters.
7. Whirl pool baths.
8. Faradic and galvanic apparatus.
9. Exercise apparatus for muscle education.
10. Equipment for an occupational therapy workshop.

Physical Facilities

In smaller hospitals one hydrotherapy room may be utilized for all forms of treatment. It has been recommended that if more rooms are available, one room for men and another room for women should be assigned.

The most important equipment is one of the three types of tanks designed for under water exercises:

1. A large pool where the technician can work in water with patient.
2. A pool with 3½ to 4½ feet (105 to 140 cm) deep and 8 by 15 feet (2.5 by 5 meters) in external dimensions.

As all the staff and patients must take a shower bath before entering the pool, the shower should be sited close to the pool. The shower cubicle should be large enough to take a wheelchair or stretcher. The temperature of water must be thermostatistically controlled. Handrails are fixed on all walls. Floor should have a slope to allow water to drain quickly.

Watever the type of pool, it is surrounded by a handrail made of stainless steel 1½ inch in diameter and fixed 2 to 3 inch from the pool wall.

The steps lending to pool should have 6 in risers and that be 1 foot in depth. The width of steps should be 2 ft. so that both rails can be easily grasped. If pool is of raised type there should be small platform at the top.

Every one entering the pool has to immerse his/her feet in a solution of chlorinated water and this is provided by a foot bath placed near the steps. It is best built into the floor with its own taps and drainage.

The side walks surrounding the pool are at least 4 feet wide on three sides and 8 feet or more on the fourth side where the hoist and steps are placed and there is room for stretchers and chairs. Slips, proof, ridged of studded tiles are used for the flooring which is highly sloped to allow effective drainage of surplus water.

The pool can be cleaned by periodic hosing when empty. It is helpful if the walls and floor join in a curve.

Should be well away from water and should have conduit fittings. All switches and apparatus properly earthed and all leads should be properly insulated and all points should be periodically inspected.

There should be 3 times as many cubicles, as the number of patients treated at time, separate dress for staff—both men and women should be available in clean utility room.

Temperature of dressing room should be 21°-24°C. Comfortable resting room with adequate cushioned chairs for the staff must be provided. The therapist should work for one and half hour in a half day session and take rest after every half an hour session.

Wringer, drier, heated cupboard to keep linen, sheets, dressing gowns, skin suits and clothing of staff to dry up.

Rehabilitation Concepts

A lot of patients with orthopedic (post-surgical and post-traumatic), rheumatic and neurological diseases join an intensive rehabilitation programme. Hydrotherapy should be part of the programme when:

- The disease has a general impact on the body, when restricts functional activities in such a way that the patient has difficulty to increase the physical capacity by just "dry land" activities.
- The disease specifically affects the lower extremities and a progressive weight-bearing

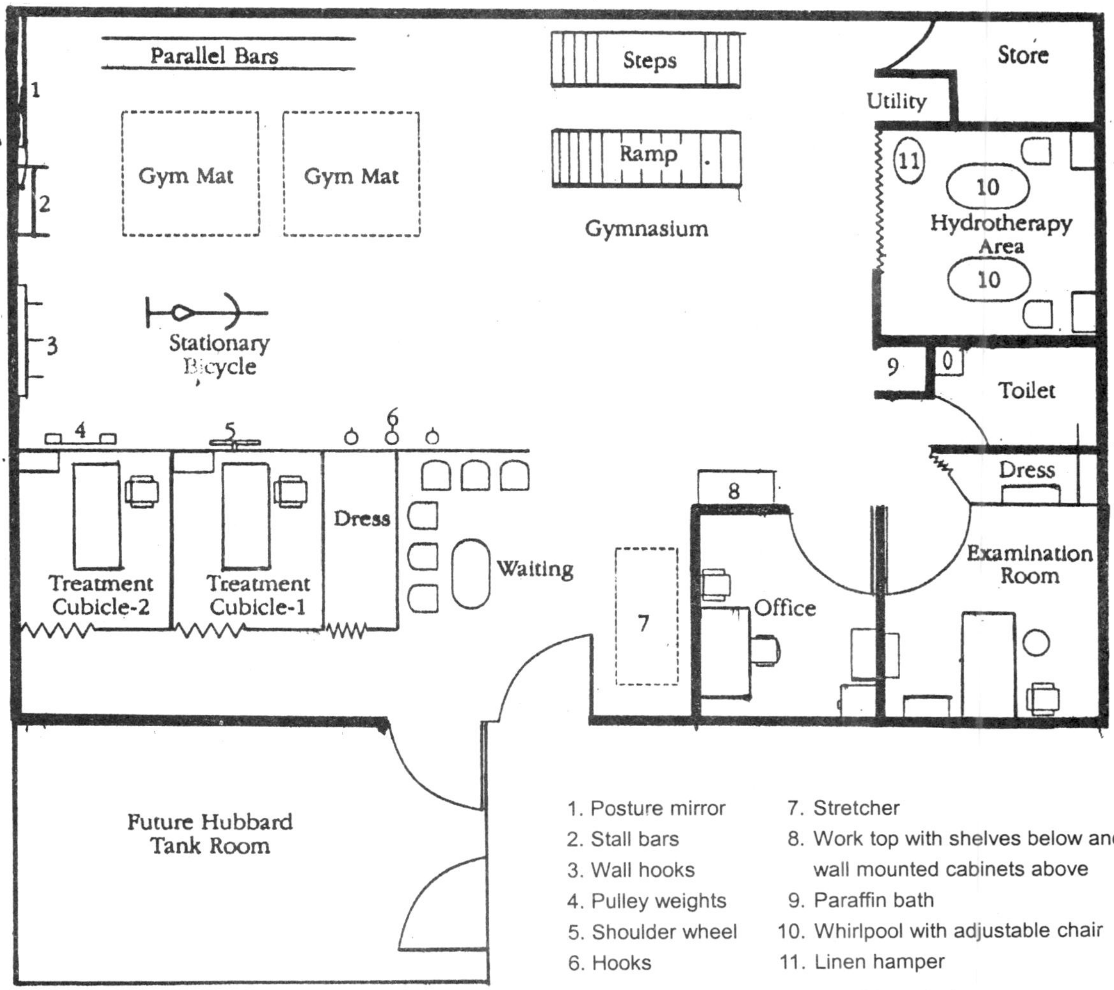

1. Posture mirror
2. Stall bars
3. Wall hooks
4. Pulley weights
5. Shoulder wheel
6. Hooks
7. Stretcher
8. Work top with shelves below and wall mounted cabinets above
9. Paraffin bath
10. Whirlpool with adjustable chair
11. Linen hamper

Fig. 35.1: Layout of physical therapy department in a medium-sized hospital

programme is the key activity in the patients rehabilitation.

In many cases the process, the rehabilitation should go, gradually, without putting to much weight on the body.

What could be better than to put the patient in water where the virtual weight of his body will be reduced becasue of the upward thrust of the water.

Specific advantages of having a therapy pool with height-adjustable depths are given below:

Different Levels in the Pool

In a swimming pool usually there are 2 or 3 standard fixed depths: deep, half deep and shallow.

For rehabilitation the necessary depths vary generally from 0 cm to 180 cm.

Depending on rehabilitation programme being used, the following water-depths are required.

Water depth in cm	*Adult*	*Child*
Walking exercises NWB	140-160	70-80
Walking exercises PWB*	100-130	50-80
Hydrotherapy: General	100-130	
Hydrotherapy: Halliwick method	110-130	110-130
Hydrotherapy: Bad Ragaz Method**	115-125	
Aqua jogging	180	
Swimming	50-140-180	20-120-180

* NWB is non-weight-bearing, shoulders immersed/PWB is partial-weight-bearing, immersion between trochanter and xyphoid.

** The patient floats, this depth is ergonomically advised for the therapist.

There are three ways to achieve different levels in a pool:

a. Gradually declining floor (one long ramp)
b. Floor with various fixed depths
c. Height-adjustable floor

Gradually Declining Floor

A normally a declining percentage of 6 to 7 percent. This seems not to be very much, however if you walk over the "width" of a declining floor of only 5 percent if already has the effect of walking with a difference in leg length of 1.5 cm. Therefore, a declining percentage of maximum 3 percent is acceptable, resulting in a very big pool.

A danger exists, that, specially with group activities. The users will float unnoticed to the deeper water, and get into trouble. This also intensifies the level of attention and responsibility of the physiotherapist.

Floor with Various Fixed Depths

A floor with various fixed depths gives the required differences in water depths. However, steep ramps or steps are necessary to move from one level to other levels.

For patients with impaired locomotive systems this might be very difficult, resulting in the need to use patient-hoist systems.

Ramps and steps reduce the effective therapeutic area of the floor resulting in bigger pools and higher water contents of the basin. This influences negatively the energy needed to keep the basin at the right temperature level.

Differences in levels, realized by ramps or steps, areas dangerous and take extreme attention to avoid casualties. The different levels have to be separated in order to separate the different user groups.

Specially children have to be protected in order not to enter the deeper areas. Fences, lines, and other visual signs can be used in or underwater.

Fences seem effective, however in every day practice they will not be used after a while because of the hassle. Lines are not sure enough and can easily by passed by the users. Visual indications are unclear due to current and waves, and may not be noticed.

The fixed levels however, will give a strongly-reduced space per level, as result of which this therapy will be difficult to perform.

The Pool with A Height-Adjustable Floor

A pool that is equipped with an adjustable base, solves all above mentioned problems.

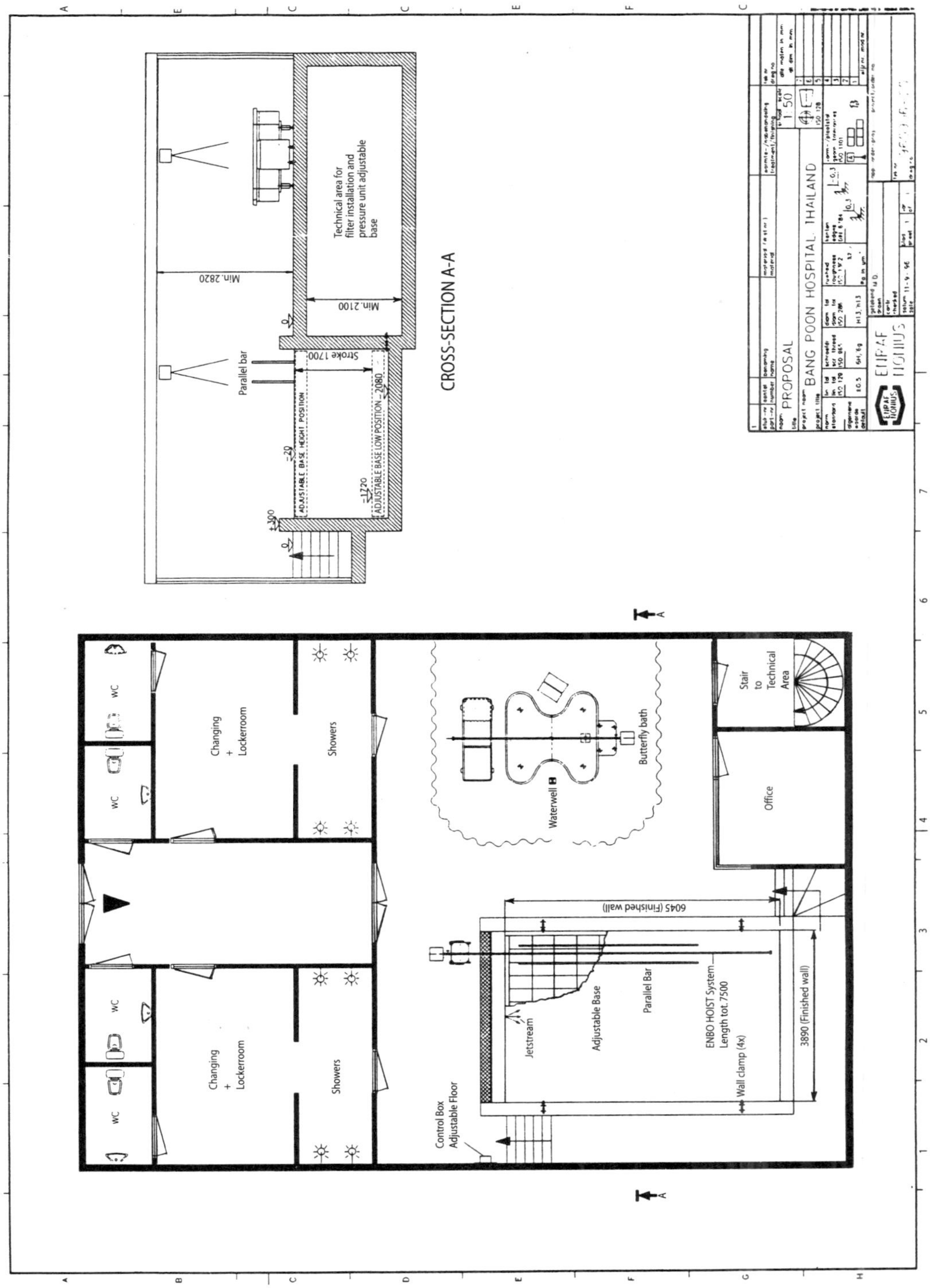

Fig. 35.2: Hydrotherapy-I

a. The physiotherapist can precisely set any desired depth of pool to the needs of the group he wants to treat.
b. He can move the base up and down during treatment.
c. When treating wheelchair-or bed-bound patients, the base can be moved up to the top level of the pool. The wheelchair or stretcher can then be pushed on the base and with a simple push on the button, the base slowly sinks into the pool, allowing patients to stay in their chair or stretcher land slowly getting used to the water.

Further

a. When the base is in the top position it works as an isolation blanket, thus saving energy.
b. No one can fall in the pool accidentally
c. The pool with adjustable base can be smaller due to the effective use of the available space, and thus decreases the amount of investment in the pool.
d. A smaller, but more effective pool, contains less water, therefore energy consumption is reduced.

The pool with an adjustable base is safer and will save the physiotherapist from lot of work.

Required Floor Surfaced Area

The advised required floor surface area can be summarised in the following table:

Floor Surface Area in m^2 exercises(m^2)	*Dynamic exercises (m^2)*	*Static*
Group of 2-5 persons	8-20	2-5
Group of 6-10 persons	24-40	6-10
Hydrotherapy: Halliwick Method	5m^2/patient	3m^2/patient
Hydrotherapy: Bad Ragaz Method	12m^2/patient	

How Does a Height-Adjustable Floor Work?

The adjustable swimming pool base is developed especially for physiotherapy and rehabilitation. The construction is simple but very stable. The base is covered with a non-slip surface of light blue prefab tiles and is provided with a decorative stainless steel frame. The floor is continously adjustable to a maximum of no less 175 cm. The modular system allows the creation.

The operation of floor is very simple. Security for the physiotherapists and the patients is guaranteed since the height adjustment system uses low voltage.

For the adjustable pool base, no expensive contructional provisions are needed. The floor is suspended on stainless steel cables which are attached to wall clamps. The moving parts include a hydraulic cylinder and a number of pulleys. The cylinder is connected with a compression unit installed outside the bathroom.

Only little maintenance is needed and the operational safety is outstanding.

Technical Components

The principal is very simple. In a small to medium size pool (max. 45 m^2) the base hangs on steel cables, and the base is pulled up with a hydraulic device.

With bigger pools (max. 100m^2) floaters are fitted under the base which will push the base up. With steel cables, the base is pulled down.

The water hydraulic device will never lead to the contamination of the pool, as compared with system using oil-hydraulic.

On stainless steel frame, PVC tiles are fitted with special clamps. It is impossible to remove the tiles with base hands.

The spaces between the tiles allows the water to circulate, facilitating the up and downward movement of the floor.

With this open circulation through the floor and an optimal hygienic water-condition is achieved. (No dead water under the height-adjustable floor).

The adjustable floor is made of standard components. The construction includes a stainless steel support frame and impact-resistant hot pressed prefab tiles with dimensions of 300 × 500 mm. The tiles can easily be detached for cleaning and maintenance of the bath on the floor. The maximum area is 45 m^2.

The components of the floor can roughly be divided in four groups:

a. Stainless steel-support-frame and tiles
b. Moving parts
c. Compression unit
d. Operating unit.

Stainless Steel-Support-Frame and Tiles

The frame, which is always under the water surface, is made of stainless steel. It is delivered in separate components and is mounted on site. This means that it is always possible to install the Enraf-nonius adjustable base, even when building is in an advanced stage.

The stainless steel frame is composed of two main girders, which are connected by a number of cross-girders. Four pulleys keep the floor in place. Figure 35.1 shows the composition of the frame.

The hot-pressed prefab tiles are placed on the support frame and attached with special clips. the tiles have dimensions of 300 × 500 mm and are provided with little notches to ensure a space around each tile of 6 mm for the water to pass through which is important for a good water circulation. The total thickness of the base is 30 cm.

Thanks to the application of standard components and tiles, the dimensions of the floor are variable. The maximum surface is 45 m^2.

Moving Parts

The adjustable floor is fixed via cables to wall clamps, which are embedded in concrete in an earlier building stage. The cables are led by guiding pulleys to a water hydraulic cylinder.

In case of elongation of the cables, the cable length can easily be adjusted. The guiding pulleys are made of nylon, quality 6.

Compression Unit

The single-acting hydraulic cylinder of the adjustable base is connected via a high-pressure hose and a wall-or floor duct to a compression unit outside the bath room. The wall of floor duct is always embedded in concrete in an earlier building stage.

Water is used a hydraulic fluid, this means that the bath water cannot be polluted. The compression unit is comprised of a motor, a vane pump and a switch box, which are placed above the water tank.

The tank is provided with a float construction which automatically renews the water.

The motor power depends on the surface area of the floor (minimum power 0.6 KVA, maximum power 2.2 KVA).

The compression unit can be supplied and installed in an early building stage.

Operating Unit

- The operating unit for adjustment of the floor is mounted to the wall.
- The switch box of the compression unit is electrically connected with the operating box. A safe low voltage is used (12 V).
- The operating box includes two buttons (floor up and 'floor down') a pilot light and key switch.
- The adjustment speed of the floor is about 50 cms per minute.
- The operating box can be delivered and mounted in an early building stage. The dimensions of the box are 250 × 160 × 120 mm.

Maintenance

The adjustable floor is very easy to maintain. Emptying the bath and cleaning the floor is required

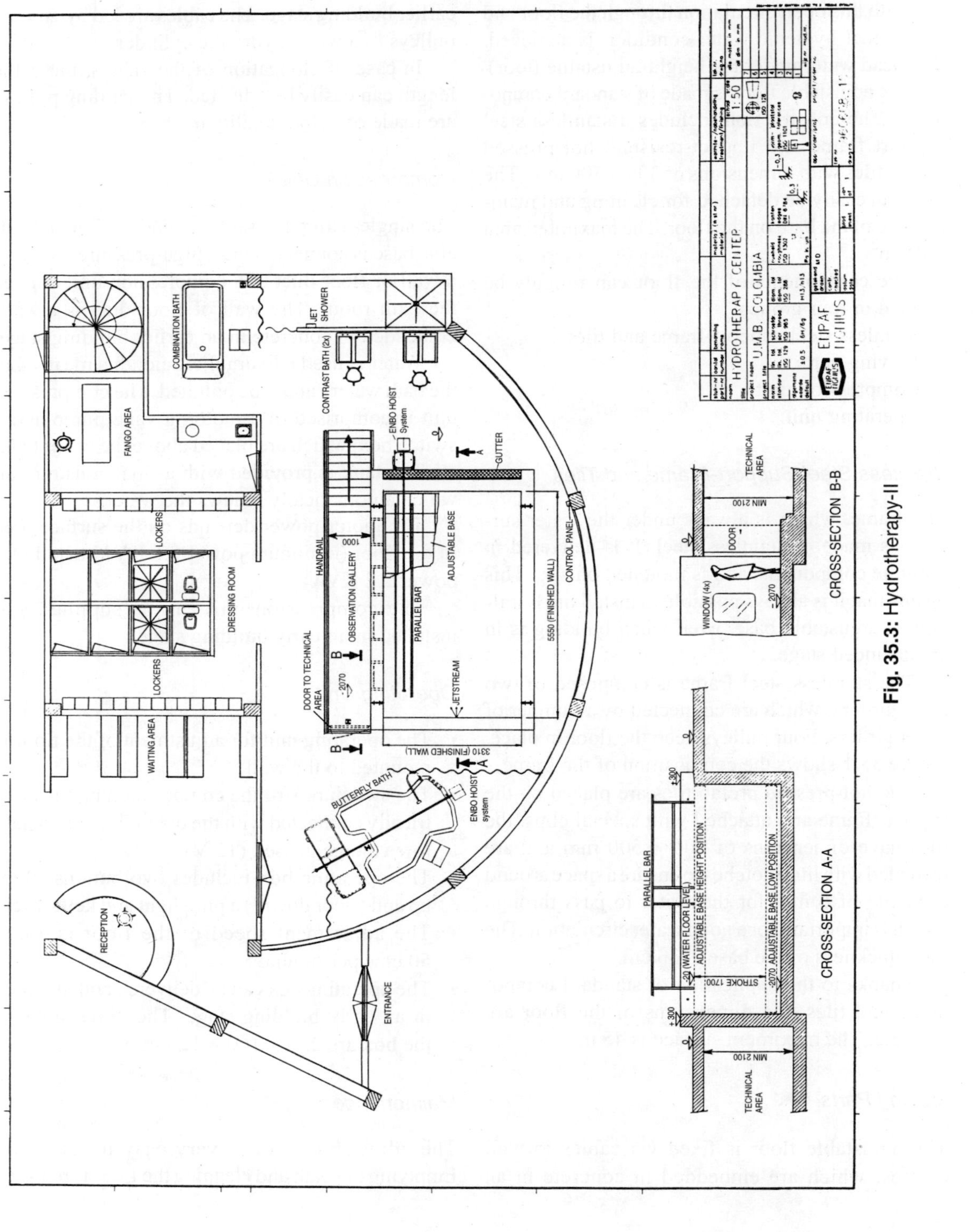

Fig. 35.3: Hydrotherapy-II

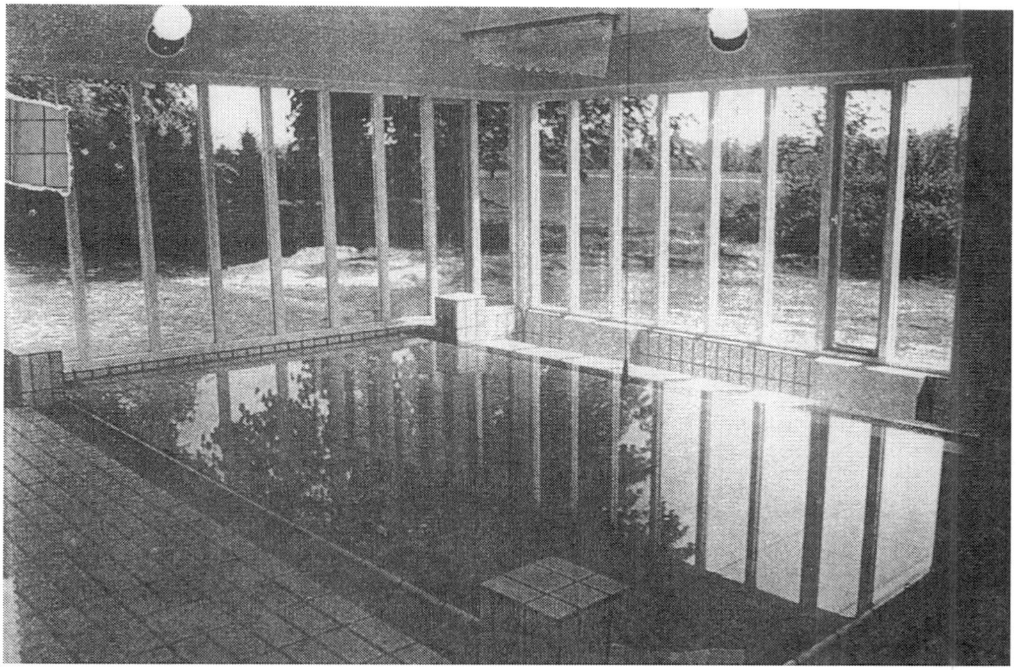

Fig. 35.4

only once in a year. Daily maintenance is restricted to cleaning the prefab tiles with a hard broom.

The water condition, however, should be controlled by a reliable water treatment installation.

Do Not Use Acid Cleaners

Do not use acid cleaners when cleaning the bath room in general. Even the vapour of such a cleaners can corrode the stainless steel parts of the floor.

Annual Maintenance

Once a year the floor should be entirely cleaned and all running parts checked. The floor is supplied with special legs on which the floor has to be placed for the annual maintenance.

Installation

Items of special attention during building include:

1. The dimensions of the bath and the location of the wall clamps
2. The installation of the compression unit
3. The location of hydraulic duct
4. The location of the operating box.

Dimensions of the bath and placement wall clamps.

The user determines the dimensions (length and width) of the bath. A choice can be made from the standard dimensions.

Bath Dimensions

The following dimensions are measured with finished bath walls. Certain tolerances apply to these dimensions, as well as the permitted deviations in parallelism and square.

Special attention has to be paid to following issues:

- If a floor adjustment of 175 cm is desired, a depth of at least 215 cm is required.
- As to the parallelism and square of the walls, the following deviations are allowed:
- Maximum deviation in parallelism, length and width: 15 mm.

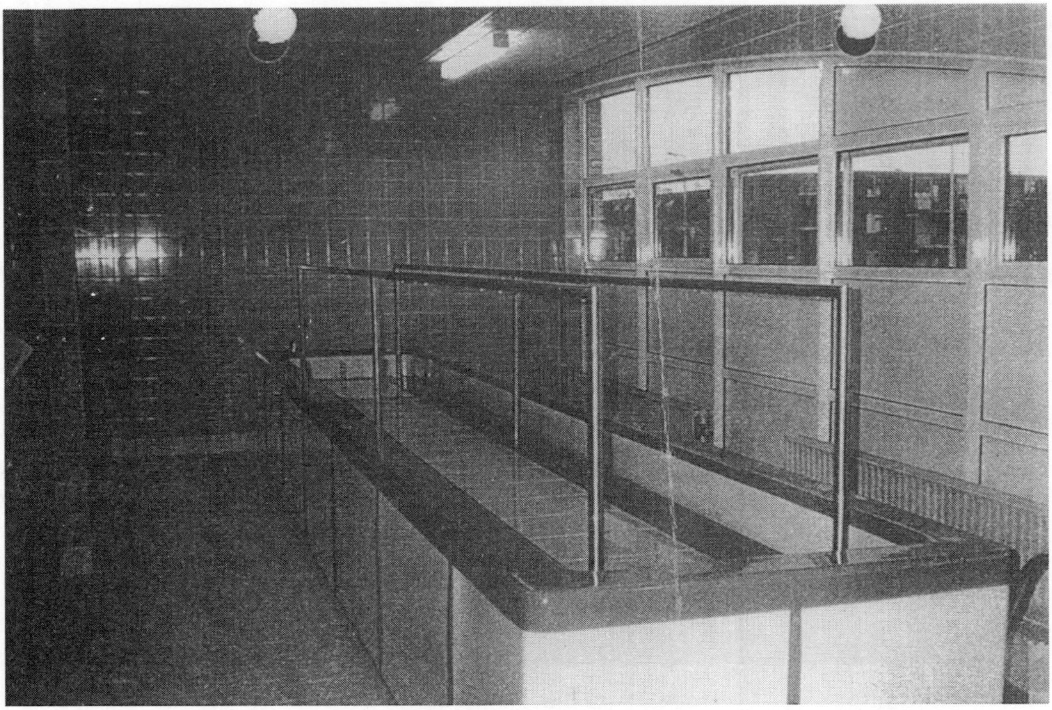

Fig. 35.5

- Maximum deviation in square: 20 mm difference between the diagnosis.
- Maximum deviation is perpendicular: 5 mm.
- The dimensions of the bath are measured at three different heights: at the bottom, at the top and in the middle.

Wall Clamps

The maximum load permitted for the wall clamps varies from 8.600 to 37.000 newtons, depending on the size of the floor.

- As the position of the wall clamps are important, the manufacturer the constructors by drilling the

Lengths in (mm)	*Nominal*	*Minimum*	*Maximum*
	5055	5030	5080
	5550	5525	5575
	6040	6020	6070
	6540	6515	6565
	7035	7010	7060
	7530	7505	7555
	8025	8000	8050

Widths (mm)	*Nominal*	*Minimum*	*Maximum*
	1850	1820	1880
	2150	2155	2175
	2440	2405	2465
	2725	2700	2760
	3025	2990	3050
	3310	3280	3340
	3600	3570	3630
	3890	3860	3920
	4180	4155	4215
	4180	4155	4505
	4475	4445	4505
	5350	5320	5080

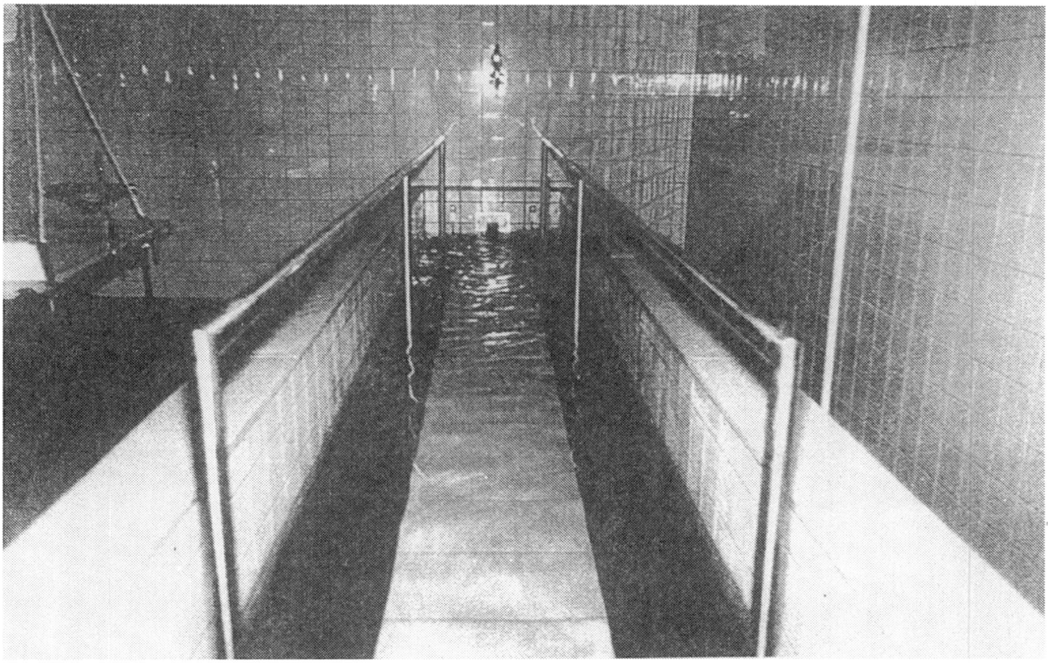

Fig. 35.6

holes for the wall clamps on site during the installation period.

- The wall clamps are mounted in the drilled holes with a special fixation compound. In this way the correct location of the clamps is always assured.
- A drawing with drilling instructions is supplied with the clamps.

Installation of the Compression Unit

The compression unit has 5 connection points:

- Water supply
- Power supply
- Water supply to/from the cylinder
- Overflow from the reservoir
- Connection with operating unit.

Attention should be paid to the following:

- The length of the pipe between the compression unit and the floor-duct should not exceed 5 meters for pressure fall reasons. In many cases the compression unit is installed in the water treatment room next to or under the bath.
- The compression unit must be accessible for service.
- The water supply pipe should be provided with a 5 micron filter. No iron pipes should be located between this filter and the hydraulic conduit.

Location of the Hydraulic Duct

The hydraulic duct is the part of the hydraulic pipe that is embedded in the bath wall or bottom. The duct is composed of a stainless steel pipe with screw thread and a welded anti-leak plate on both ends. The hydraulic duct is embedded in concrete in an early building stage. The location of the duct is chosen in such a way that the distance between the compression unit and the floor/wall-duct is as small as possible.

Location of the Operating Box

The operating unit for adjustment of the floor is mounted to the wall.

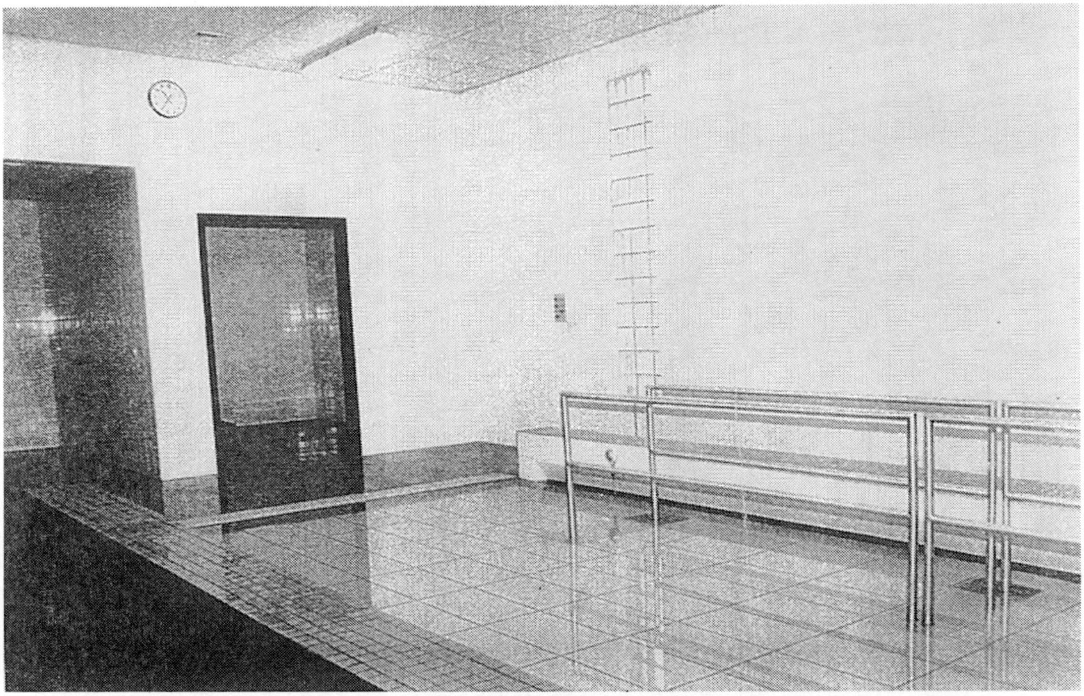

Fig. 35.7

The switch box of the compassion unit is electrically connected with the operating box. A safe low voltage is used (12 V).

The operating box includes two buttons ('floor up' and floor down') a pilot light and key switch.

The adjustment speed of the floor is about 50 cm per minute.

The operating box can be delivered and mounted in an early building stage. The dimensions of the box are: 250 × 160 × 120 mm.

The Filtration Installation

Hygiene is very important in the field of physiotherapy and rehabilitation. Therefore, to prevent the adjustable floor from interfering with the water treatment, spaces are provided around each tile for the water to pass through, allowing optimal filtering.

A special feature of the system is that the hydraulic fluid is simply mains water, so pollution of the bath water is impossible.

A therapy pool is much different from a normal swimming pool. The average temperature of the water is several degrees higher and therefore composes a good environment for bacteria.

Also many patients when put into warm water, become incontinent. Many patient have a weak health and are vulnerable to infections caused by dirty water.

Therefore, a therapy pool ends a special filtration installation.

The filtration installation is specially designed to provide maximum safety to patients and trouble-free operations for the maintenance-staff of the hospital.

The installation filters and monitors the water constantly, 24 hours a day, and adds automatically chemicals and fresh water to the pool depending on the use and pollution of the pool.

A good filtration installation is essential for a health pool.

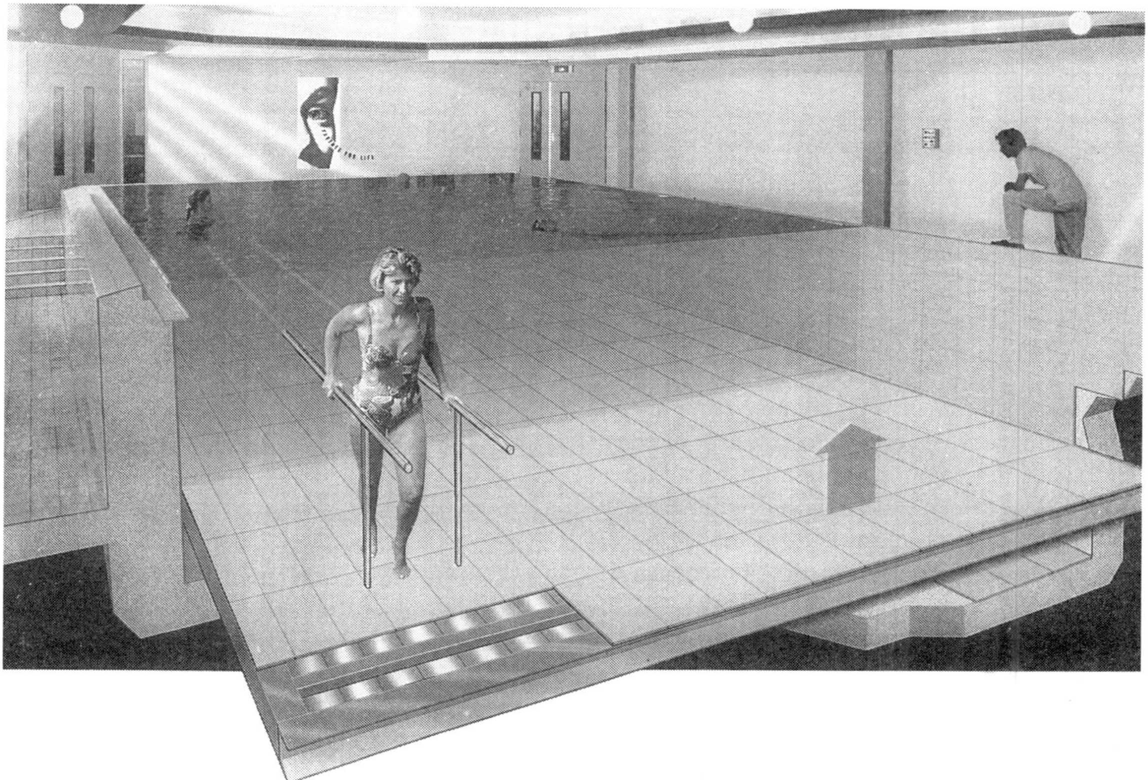

Fig. 35.8

Water Conditions and Environment

The frame and the adjustable floor are made of stainless steel. Unfortunately, even stainless steel can corrode under certain conditions:

- Iron particles in the water can cause galvanic corrosion of the stainless steel.
- Too high an acid and/or salt content attacks the stainless steel.
- Water that is too hard or too soft can cause deposits on the stainless steel.

To avoid corrosion, the following guidelines should be followed:

Rehabilitation

In some hospitals the department of physical medicine expands into a complete rehabilitation service involving other elements besides physical and occupational therapy. These may include speech therapy; functional training for paralytic and paraplegic patients and for others physically handicapped; vocational training for those who can qualify for selected tasks in a general workshop, and a sheltered workshop for those whose capacity prevents their qualifying even for selected work; social service and vocational guidance, including job placement; parent education; special education for the handicapped, and general education for those children who must spend a protracted time in the rehabilitation center. Thus rehabilitation can go well beyond the physical medicine facilities of the normal acute general hospital; yet the elements named do serve needs often encountered in the acute hospital.

FURTHER READING

1. Further N: Rehabilitation in the Netherlands. Ed. Enraf-Nonius 1996.
2. Lamback J: Why Hydrotherapy? Ed. Enraf-Nonius 1997.

LABORATORY PLANNING AND LAYOUT

Design of the clinical laboratory floor plan and work flow pattern contains both quantitative and qualitative elements. Frequently, concerns focus only on the amount of space available and not on how efficiently the space is being used.

Design of Laboratory Space

The question of size in planning a laboratory is always a concern. Several factors need to be considered while determining the space required for an efficient laboratory. These include the scope of procedures to be performed, the intended operational approach for performing the procedure, the anticipated size of the laboratory staff, and the setting (e.g. a teaching versus a non-teaching institution).

Space Allocation

When either relocation or a new facility is planned, the laboratory manager is usually provided information on how much space is allocated for the laboratory. Several terms are essential to convert this information to meaningful figures. The term used to describe the total area based on outside location or building dimensions is the gross area. By contrast, the net (useful) area is the portion between the walls available for laboratory work space excluding building support, mechanics (e.g., ventilation shifts for communiction and transport, storerooms), Another helpful term is use factor, which represents a percentage ratio of net useful area to gross area. The usual use factor for clinical laboratory facilities is 60 percent.

Scope of Services

The scope of procedures provided by the clinical laboratory reflects the type of hospital, facility, or population it serves. Even so, it is inadequate to project laboratory volume on the basis of the number of hospital beds or annual admissions. Such a projection does not include services provided for outpatient department, dispensaries, special clinics, or emergency departments. In light of the skyrocketing hospital costs, the number of procedures performed for patients from some type of ambulatory care facility or department is bound to increase at a faster rate other than growth. By their nature, some types of hospitals, such as teaching medical centers with research programmes, have increased tests over admission number predictions. Even daily census or percentage of occupancy figures are inadequate predictors owing to seasonal variations, competing providers of similar laboratory services, or the economic conditions of the community.

Laboratory Structural Design

Medical laboratories follow two basic structural designs: modular and open. Both of these have advantages and disadvantages, and the choice of design has historically reflected the laboratory director's preference and philosophy of management. The key point is to recognize the positive and negative characteristics of each design to optimize efficiency and productivity, Indeed, it is possible to use a combination of the two designs within the same laboratory.

Modular Laboratory Design

Figure 35.9 shows the floor plan of a modular laboratory. The emphasis is on departmentalization, with a separate room for each laboratory division. This creates a degree of "turfdom". The separation of laboratories by walls has both good and bad effects on interdepartmental communication.

The Williamsport Hospital	
No. of beds	***400***
Total Sq ft net	12,703
Sq ft bed	31.8

Area	*Sq ft net*	*Area*	*Sq ft net*
Blood bank	479	Microscopy	321
Chem-manual	1,831	Miscellaneous	2,747
Chem-special	246	Patient Handling	2,034
Cytology	473	Serology	316
Hematology	866	Storage	330
Histopathology	1,188	Teaching	518
Microbiology	937	Utility	417

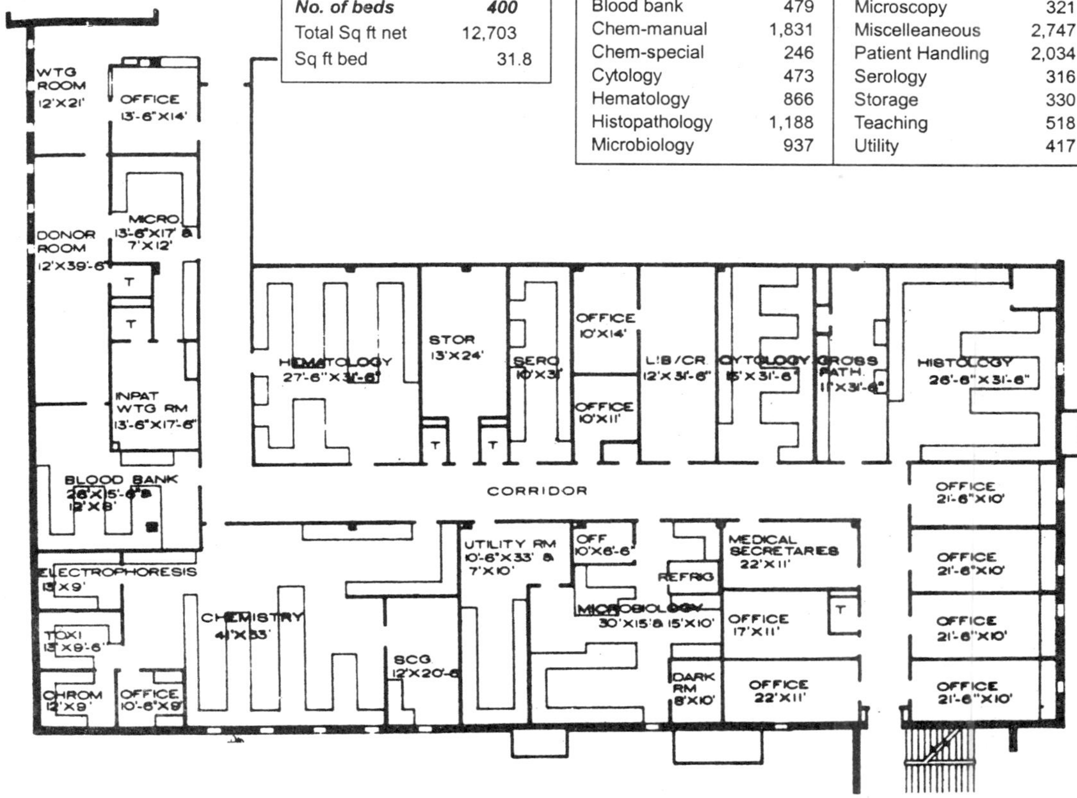

Fig. 35.9: Modular laboratory design

Although discouraging, the walls do not facilitate easy interaction among divisions when it is appropriate. Moreover, there is little sharing of laboratory equipment in a modular design, there is also little encroachment of space. The modular design appears to be less flexible if expansion is needed, although most walls are removable. There is some merit to the separation of areas from a visibility standpoint to discourage interdepartmental checks and criticism during workload peaks and valleys. The noise level is reduced in those laboratories where loud instrumentation is not used. The modular design promotes safety. In that contaminated specimens can be localized, and in case of fire, the modules would contain the burning materials.

Open Laboratory Design

Figure 35.10 is an example of an open laboratory floor,plan with this design, many of the departments interface freely without dividing walls. For some laboratory administrators, this approach is more esthetic pleasing because it gives the feeling of roominess. The open floor plan promotes interaction between departments and fosters the concept of "one big, happy family". This can have a negative effect if interaction between department interrupts the daily routine. Visiting is less controllable, and it becomes obvious to all when a particular department is slow. At the same time, a department that is short of staff will feel unjustly busy if personnel cannot be shared. The open floor plan

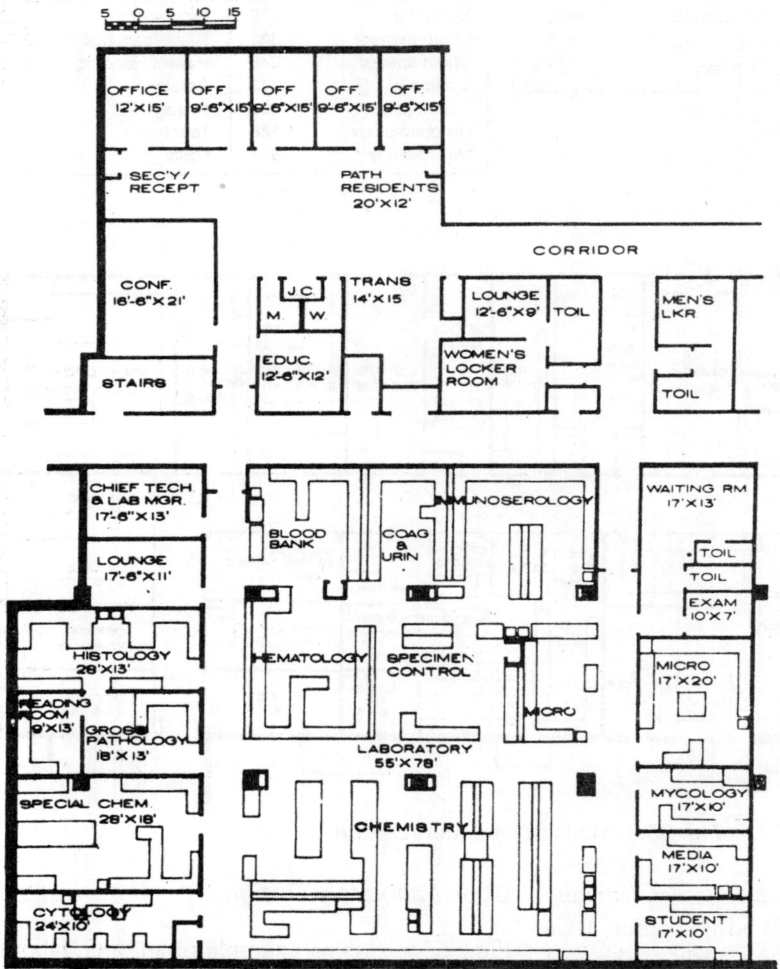

The Williamsport Hospital	
No. of beds	***370***
Total Sq ft net	9,810
Sq ft bed	26.5
Area	*Sq ft net*
Blood bank	300
Chem-manual	1,333
Chem-special	518
Cytology	273
Hematology	950
Histopathology	701
Media prep	170
Microbiology	732
Miscelleaneous	3,483
Patient Handling	451
Serology	460
Teaching	309
Urinalysis	130

Fig. 35.10: Open laboratory design

lends itself well to the sharing of equipment, and expansion is easily accomplished within the confines of the laboratory of simply rearranging several benches of reallocating a bench to the expanding department. There is less control of noise and safety hazards in the open design, and planning for both of these concerns is important if this floor plan is adopted.

Laboratory structural design should be consistent with the level of specialization and automation used. Many laboratories today are collapsing several automated areas (hematology, chemistry, endocrine) history. The open laboratory design for a core laboratory is the more logical approach. In addition, current trends towards total laboratory automation and the use of roboties makes an open design more logical, figure 35.11 to 35.13 shows a conceptual approach to movement of specimens and information in a primarily open design using roboties and total automation.

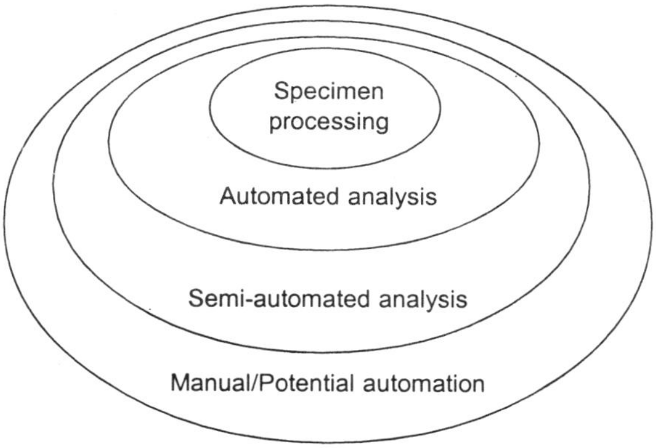

Fig. 35.11: Schematic representation of a laboratory floor plan, organized based on automation levels

Design of Laboratory Work Flow

Several other key planning, organizing, and controlling strategies deal with the flow of specimens into the laboratory and through the department for analysis and the return of the report to the requesting physician.

Layout Flowchart

Physical layout has important effects on the efficiency of work procedures. The layout flow chart allows the laboratory manager to study physical layout to eliminate unnecessary steps. Following is an example of the benefit of studying the layout

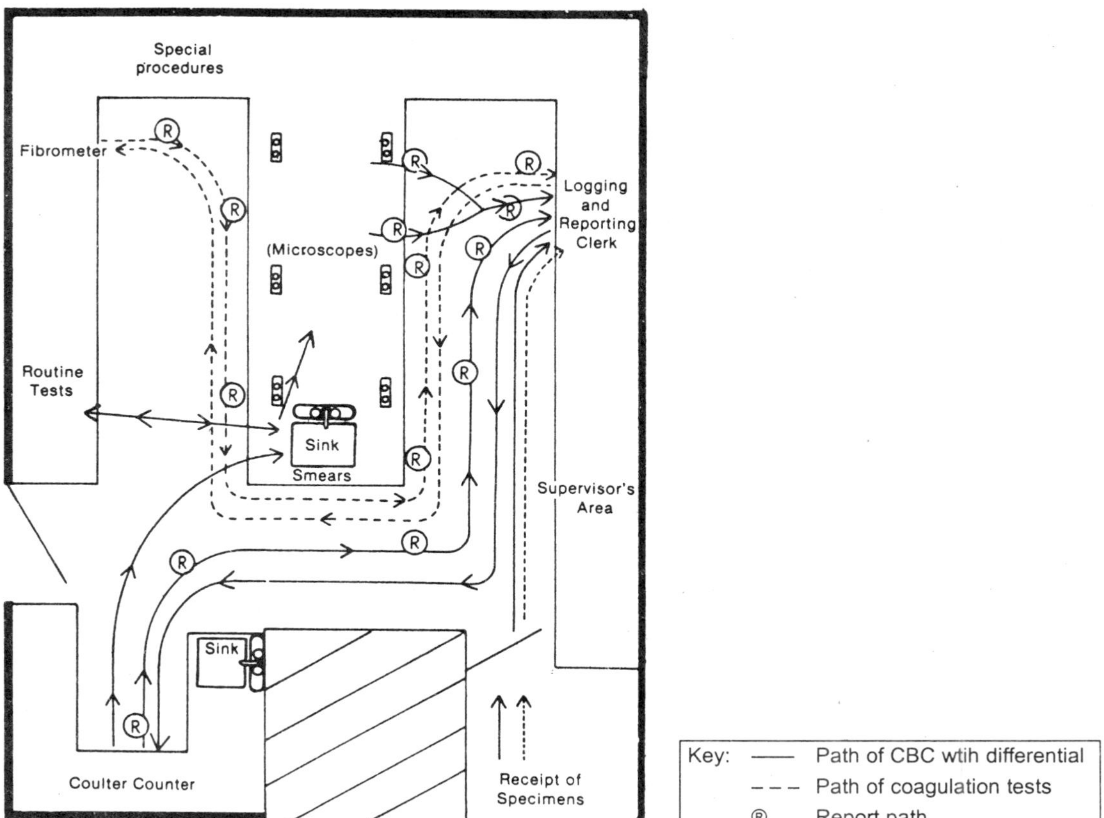

Fig. 35.12: Laboratory layout flowchart before workflow study

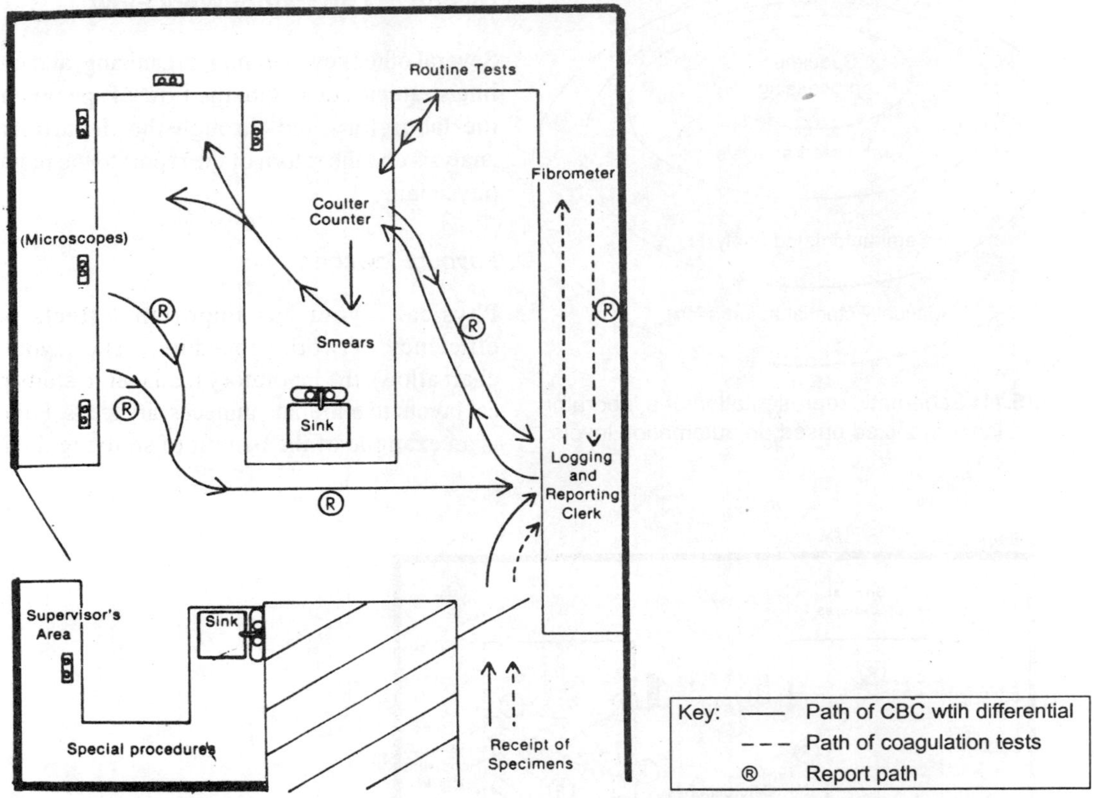

Fig. 35.13: Laboratory layout flowchart after workflow study

work flow of complete blood count (CBC) and coagulation procedures within a hematology department.

Before the study figure 35.14, specimens entered the laboratory by passing the supervisors area to be logged in by the recording clerk. The CBC specimen then was carried to cell counter in the far corner of the laboratory, judiciously placed so that it would be away from excessive traffic. The specimen then travelled back to a sink area so that smears could be made and stained. Sometimes a routine test, such as reticulocyte count or sedimentation rate, would briefly sidetrack the specimen before the differential was performed on the central island bench. The path of the CBC report, once the differential was complete, was relatively short, although the path of reporting immediate (stat) hemogram results from the cell counter followed the same trip across the room as the specimen originally followed. Coagulation procedures were also placed away from traffic, but this necessitated taking the specimen from the clerks area, around the end of the central island bench to the far area of the laboratory, and then returning along the same route with the report.

A rearrangement of analytical equipment, which was done after the layout work flow was studied. The clerk reporting results was moved closer to the specimen point of entry into the department. The supervisor was relocated to the comer alcove, because the routine specimen flow did not require his interaction. The path travelled by the CBC

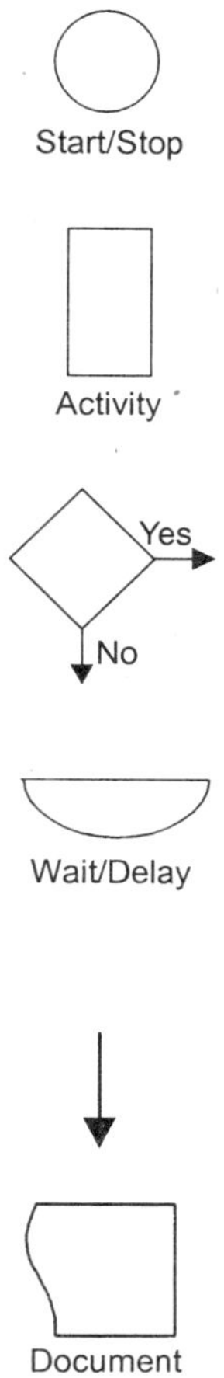

Start/sop to begin or end process.

Ask: Who provides information?
Where does input/process begin?
Which department(s) originate the process?

Single step in the process should be described inside the rectangle.

Ask: What is done with the information?
Who transmits/translates the data?
How does the information get to the next step?

Decision step shows a branch point with alternate paths.

Ask: What happens at each step.
Who makes the next decision?
What factors influence the decision?
What happens if the step is not complete?

Waiting or delaying period.

Ask: How long does each step ?
Where does the process slow down?
What takes the longest? Why?
How long does it take to repeat a step?

Arrows show direction or activity flow.

Ask: Does the same information go to multiple departments?
Is each arrow necessary?

Documentation of reporting is needed.

Ask: Which and how many forms are needed before proceeding?

Fig. 35.14: Flowchart symbols

specimen was shortened considerably by placing the cell counter on the central island bench and relocating the coagulation testing on the same bench as the clerk. Reporting of stat hemogram values CBC results and coagulation procedures was facilitated by these relocations. Technical staffing was improved too. The person operating the cell counter could perform coagulation tests with the instrument located directly behind him. The technologists performing differentials took advantage of the opportunity to stand up and stretch when taking stacks of completed CBCs back to the clerk for reporting.

Operational Flowchart

Another helpful tool in assessing the efficiency of laboratory testing is the operational flow chart. The flowchart is a symbolic representation of a system broken down into its sequential component steps. A process is first reduced to its basic steps, and these steps are then placed in proper sequence, Finally, the steps are graphically displayed in a flow chart emphasizing decision points and alternate pathways. This technique is especially useful if several individuals must share in the operation of a process. It can also be used to emphasize decision-making modes and describe the degree of responsibility and authority the technical staff has in deciding how a specimen is processed. Figure 35.6 shows some of the symbols frequently used in flow charting, and figure 35.15 is a flow chart for the process of uninalysis.

Network Analysis

At time, a laboratory manager may want to add a time and efficiency dimension to the operational flowchart, which is best accomplished by using a network analysis technique. Network analysis is a schematic and mathematical approach to the planning of a project which shows the relationships among different activities and how their timing will affect the overall project. Several components of a project are evaluated, including the shortest possible completion time, activities with delay potential, and extra-effort to cost-benefit analysis.

The two most commonly used network analysis approaches are the programme evaluation review technique (PERT) and critical path method (CPM). PERT is appropriate when one or more of the completion points must be reached at a specific time or in planning a project where a high degree of uncertainty exists a) totally new project, for example). The CPM technique, while similar, does ot require a specific point completion time as in PERT.

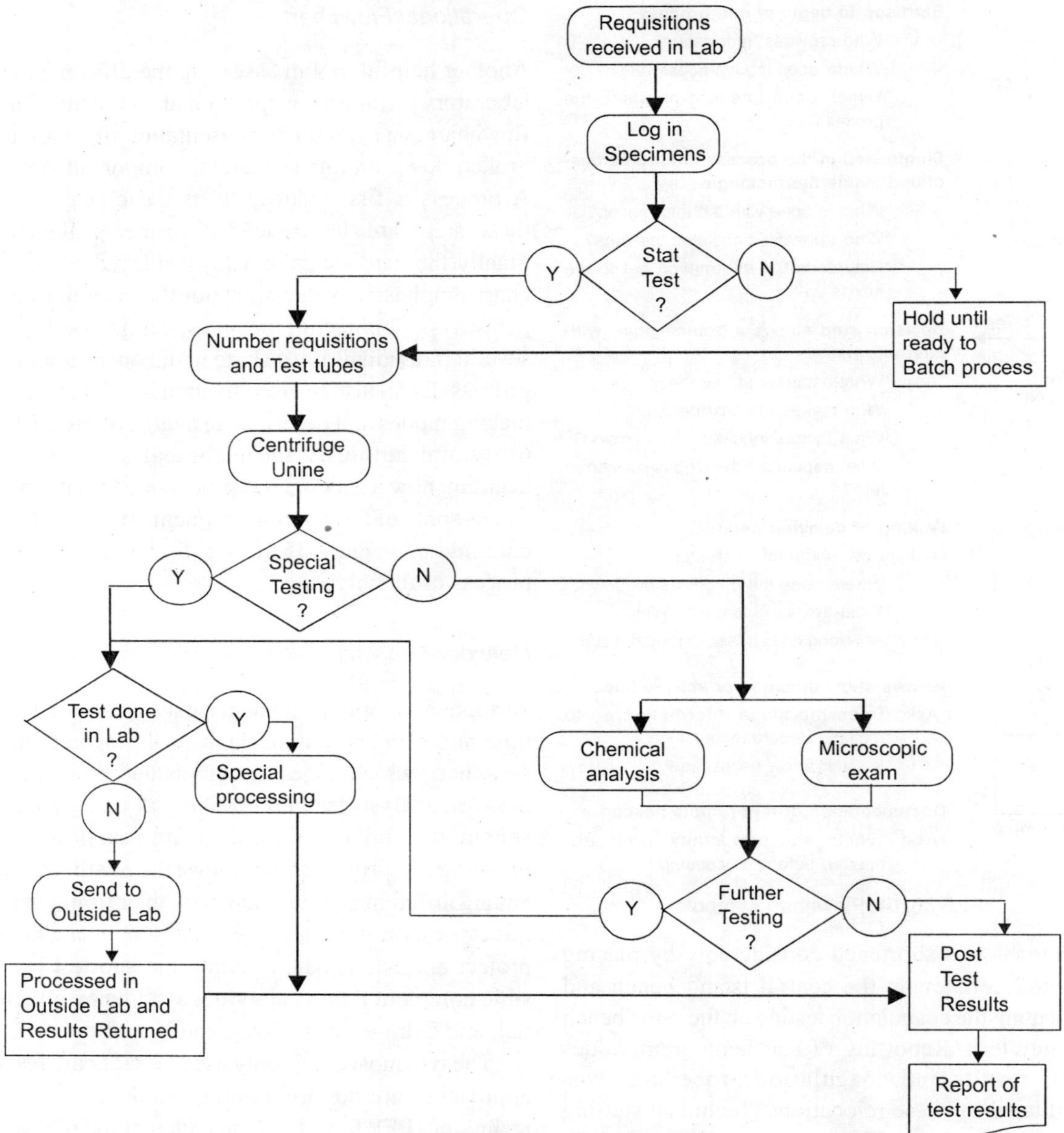

Fig. 35.15: Urinalysis flowchart

The basis of network analysis includes construction of activities and events (Figure 35.16). An activity is an operation requiring time between two events, such as drawing blood. An event is a time when one or more activities commence or are completed. For example, the receipt of the requisition in the laboratory (event) must precede the blood-drawing (activity). The critical path is defined as the chain of events and the total time all of the project but exclusive of some events in the overall project. Float is a term for spare time (slack) resulting from the difference between the time to accomplish the

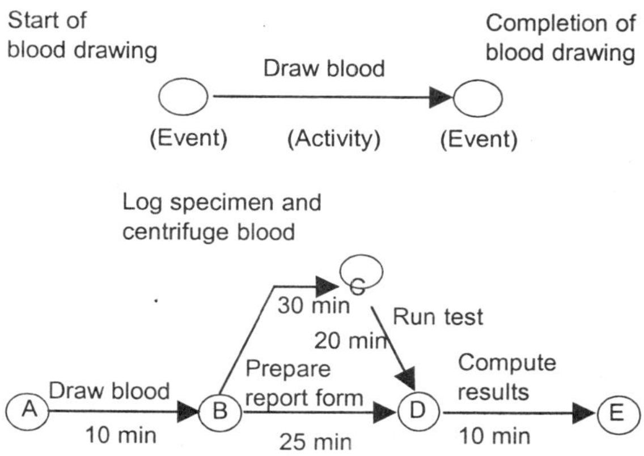

Fig. 35.16: Network analysis—critical path method

critical path and the non-critical path. Two activities can branch from a given event, thus creating concurrent activities within the project.

A laboratory building is costly and is intended to last for many years, during which time the nature of the work is almost certain to change, and hence some degree of flexibility is desirable in order to make updating possible. This may be achieved by the use of demountable partitions or lightweight non-load-bearing walls in some areas so that for example, two small laboratories can fairly easily be made into one large one. Most construction today is in modular form i.e. dimensions are standardized throughout to include room sizes, lengths of bench units, etc. Such dimensions being usually based on a 300 mm unit. Thus, a room may be square e.g. 4.5 m by 4.5 m or rectangular, e.g. 7 mm by 3.5 m and bench units of 1.5 m length would fit into either room (Figure 35.17).

There are advantages to both the square and rectangular layouts. The former makes better use of natural daylight and tends to be more flexible in terms of furniture arrangement. Whilst the latter allows longer runs of bench surface, if doors and windows are on the shorter walls. Some rooms do not require daylight and these can usually be sited in the center of the building.

It is important to remeber that rooms other than laboratories will be required e.g. stores, offices, library, cold storage facilities, etc). and that a considerable floor area is occupied by corridors, staircases, landings, lifts, entrance hall, etc, which may well account for as much as 30 percent of the total space. From a safety aspect, these areas must be adequate to allow rapid escape in the event of an emergency and corridors must be wide enough to allow easy passage of trolleys.

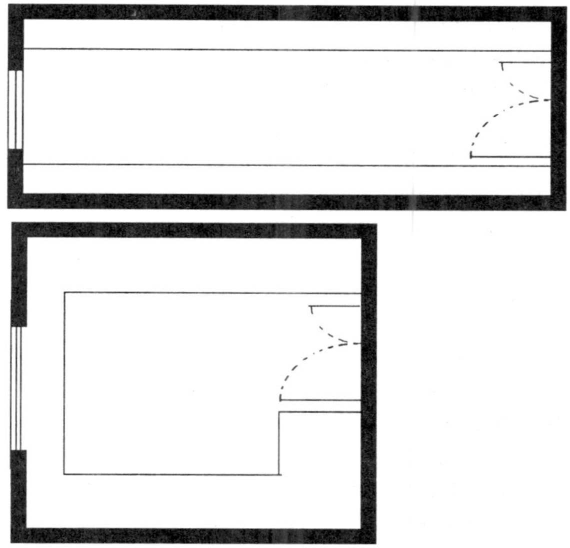

Fig. 35.17: Square and rectangular modular laboratories—each has one window and a 'door and a half'

Staff also have to circulate and a knowledge of the main functions of each department will assist in deciding how they should be accommodated in relation to one another. Some activities will need to be sited close to each other, whilst other may benefit by being separated (e.g. to reduce the hazard of cross-infection).

The architect's attention should be drawn to any unusual hazzard that may not be apparent to him, such as high-level radioactive work or the housing of animals under controlled conditions, and a decision can be made as to whether special areas are set aside for this work or if purpose-designed cabinets or isolators should be installed. The problems of goods delivery, waste disposal, bulk storage, temperature controlled rooms, glassware washing, etc., must also be discussed in detail as they may be of considerable importance in the day-to-day work. Armed with this information, the architect will be in a position to prepare a provisional specification and plan which can then be discussed and modified as necessary.

Space Requirements

These requirements vary with the type of work being done, but the following suggestions form a useful guide:

Research laboratories	20-25 m^2 per worker
Routine diagnostic or clinical	15-20^2 per worker
School teaching laboratories	21/2-3 m bench per student
University teaching laboratories	2-6 m bench per student

Storage space outside the laboratories will also be required to the extent of 8-10 percent of laboratory floor area. In teaching departments, laboratories can often be used as lecture rooms also. But in other establishments this is seldom practicable and an area may have to be set aside for discussion seminars and similar activities.

Laboratory Layout

The basic plan for laboratories has evolved over many years and since the 1920s the development has been based on the concept of rooms arranged on each side of a central corridor. This system has much to commend it, since it is very economical in space, improves communication from one room to another and simplifies the provision of laboratory services. It is based on a structural module, the size and shape of which is designed to meet the requirements of the individual worker. Benches are at right angles to the window wall and provide uninterrupted runs. Daylight is utilized to the maximum and rooms can therefore be deeper than would otherwise be acceptable. The modules can be subdivided by lightweight partitions to provide offices, store rooms, instrument rooms. etc.

If the site is of suitable dimensions, a two-corridor system of similar modules is possible (Fig. 35.18).

The area between the corridors is used for rooms which do not require daylight, such as cold stores, photographic dark rooms, etc. Staircases and lifts, where required, are constructed at the ends of the building. The dividers between laboratories are non-load-bearing partitions which can be removed to provide double or triple-sized rooms if necessary. Intercommunicating doors between laboratories are not only useful in everyday situations but also provide a second exit in the event of a fire. The provision of two staircases, one at each end of the floor, also ensures a means of exit should one be unusable during an emergency (this is usually a statutory requirement). Should this not be possible, an external fire escape must be provided.

In teaching departments, the lecture rooms and laboratories are usually separated by a central staircase. This has the advantage of noise isolation, and in an emergency the laboratory side can be shut off rapidly by fire doors (Fig. 35.19).

In large laboratories, the bench units may be used to divide the room into working bays giving each worker his own area but retaining good communication between staff by not isolating them from one another (Fig. 35.20).

The individual laboratories in teaching establishments will in general be much larger than those in research or industrial organizations, and the actual size is calculated from the number of students expected to work in them and from a study of the syllabuses. Experience has shown that once a building is occupied there is a tendency for the number of students to increase over the years and the resulting overcrowding is both frustrating and hazardous. The corresponding increase in staff will also aggravate the problem. Where possible, allowances should be made for this eventuality at

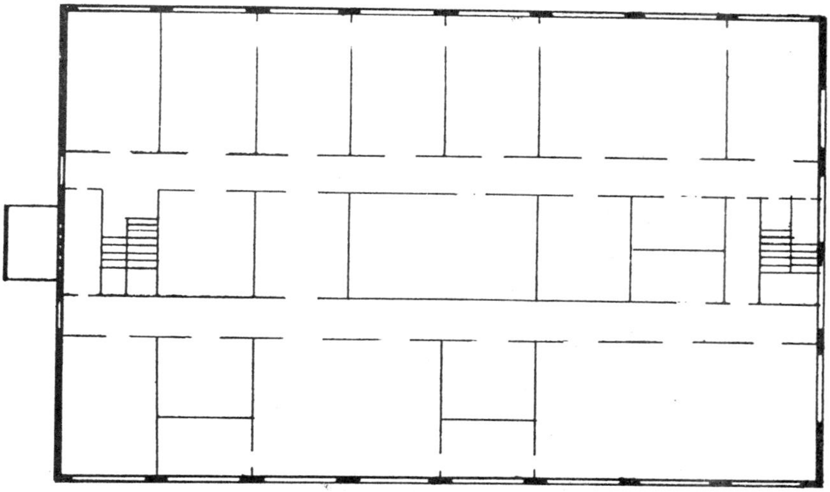

Fig. 35.18: Laboratory arranged on a two corridor system

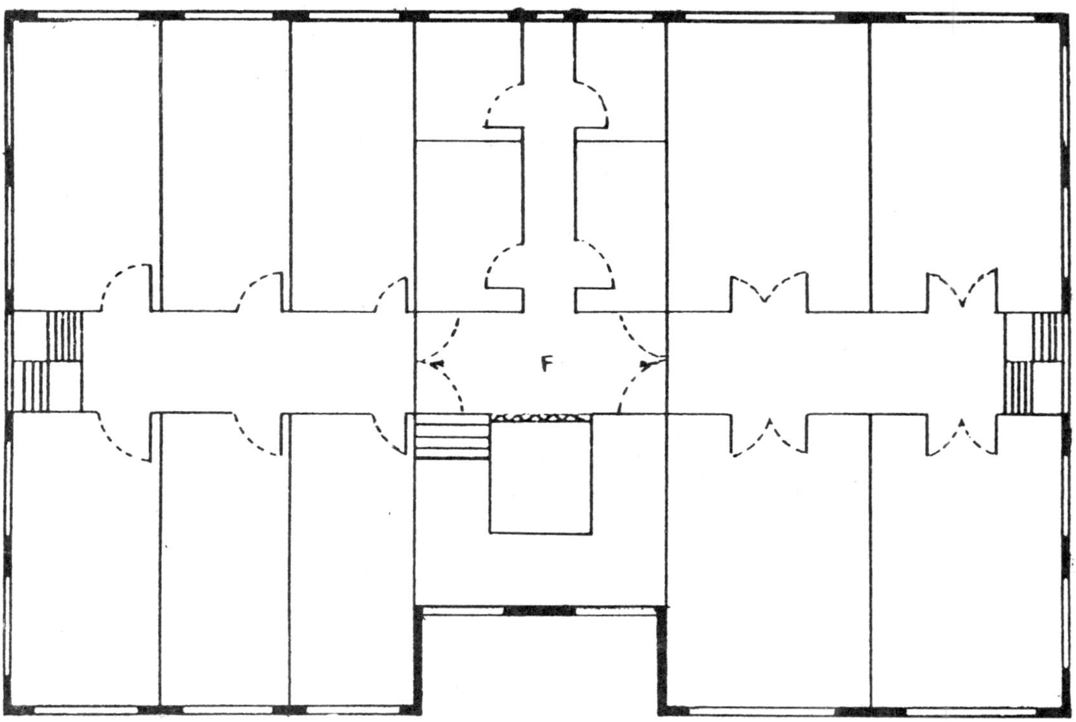

Fig. 35.19: An arrangement suitable for a teaching establishment, in which laboratories and lecture rooms are on either side of a central stair well and lift shaft (F, fire doors)

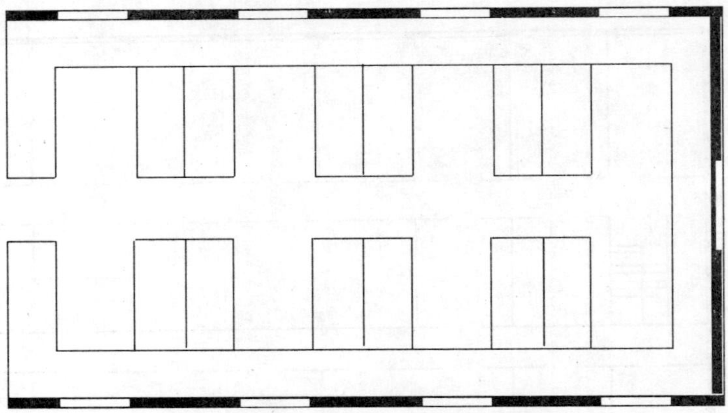

Fig. 35.20: A large laboratory divided into working bays by peninsular bench units

the planning stage, or alternatively provision must be made for extensions to be added in the future. Such extensions could take the form of an additional floor or a lengthening of the building. The latter is preferrable as it can be done with the minimum of disruption.

Provision of Services

The methods used to carry services from the incoming supply to service points at the benches vary enormously and a great deal of thought has been put into this problem over the years by architects, mechanical service engineers and laboratory

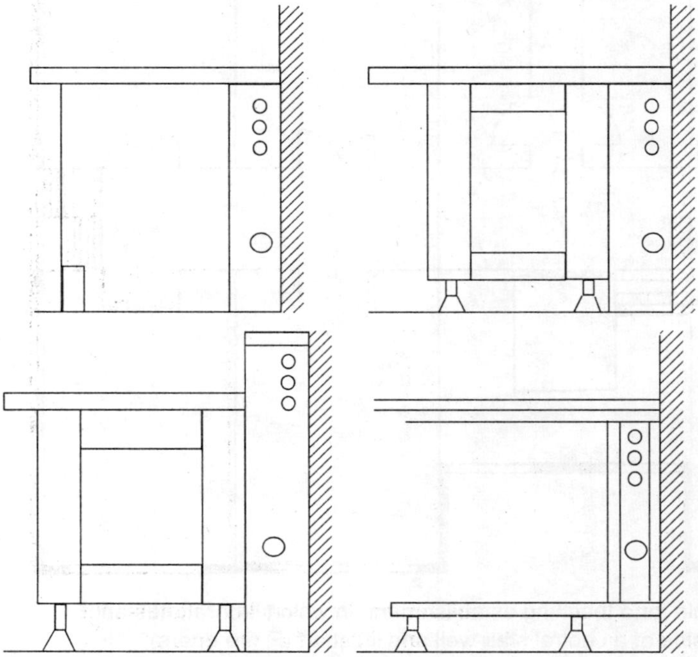

Fig. 35.21: Services fitted behind underbench units: (a) services virtually inaccessible; (b) removable bench unit giving improved access: (c) services run in a spine installed behind a free-standing bench unit: (d) cantilever bench construction showing cupboard unit removed for access

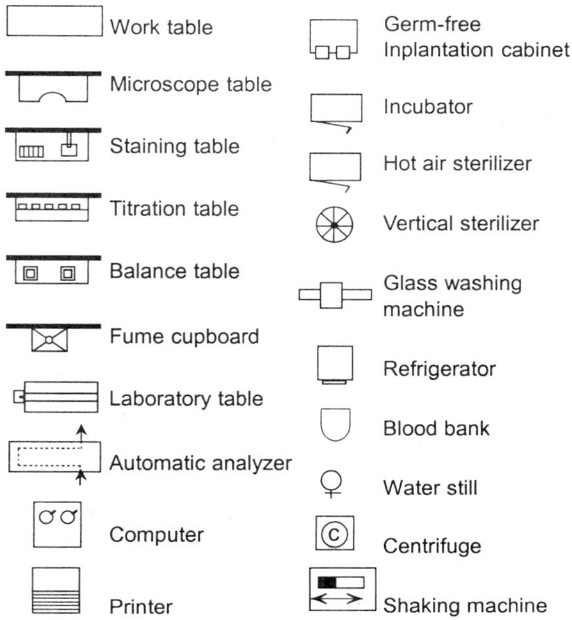

Fig. 35.22: Some symbols of medical chemistry and hematology laboratory equipment

users. Ideally the runs should be kept as short as possible, be readily adapted for alternations and extension, be easily accessible for maintenance, be protected from accidental damage and tampering, should not be in the way of benching, apparatus, etc. and be kept out of sight. It is doubtful if any system has yet been devised which fulfills all these criteria but some at least approach the ideal.

Services should rise upward from the intake level and be distributed horizontally at each floor level in order to feed benches in each laboratory. Current practice is to install service ducts for rising mains and carry branch pipes in the voids between floors or behind bench units. Ducts and voids are provided with access points for servicing. The mass of pipework and cabling in laboratory buildings is so great that space required for them must be designed into the building, and can represent a significant percentage of the total volume. Corridor walls can be utilized for access doors to rising mains at the points where they are connected to horizontal sub-mains feeding the laboratories. The same space may house ducting for fume cupboards or general ventilation.

Service pipes to the bench outlets may be below bench level, above bench level in a service spine or dropped from the ceiling void: waste pipes must, of course, be below bench level.

The service spine is a very statisfactory arrangement but requires the bench to be set away from the wall about 15 cm, with the result that the incorporation of this feature produces, on each side of a room a significant loss of width between benches. The main advantage to dropping services from the ceiling void is that partitions between rooms may be removed without disturbing the pipework. It does, however, require larger ceiling voids to provide access for maintenance together with duct covers in the floors above, and these are difficult to keep watertight.

A building consisting of more than one floor will require at least one lift, which should have a capacity of at least one tonne. It is the common practice to install one lift for passengers and another for goods, although in many cases, a single life will suffice provided it is of adequate capacity.

Floors

The architect will decide on the type of floor construction, having due regard to its load-bearing capacity, it is important to remember that vibrating equipment can represent a load of two or more times its static weight. It may be desirable to have some sections of floor isolated from their surroundings to prevent vibration from one piece of equipment affecting other apparatus. For example, an electron microscope could not be operated satisfactorily if it were not isolated from a nearby heavy-duty freezer compressor.

Floor covering material is important from a number of aspects, e.g. safety, comfort, ease of maintenance, resistance to chemical and solvent attack, life expectancy, cost and appearance. Today there is a wide choice of materials available Traditionally, linoleum has been most commonly used and still has much to recommend it. It is available in wide rolls (which minimized the number of joints) and fulfills all the requirements mentioned above. Vinyl coverings are also popular but tend to be slippery when wet and are attacked by some solvents.

Areas which are frequently wet, such as animal rooms, are usually covered with asphair, but this is easily dented and may give rise to pockets where infected materials may lodge. Quarry tiles are useful in these areas, provided they are well laid and grouted.

Hardwood is a pleasing finish for staircases and corridors but unsatisfactory in laboratories owing to the large number of joints and the high cost of maintenance, offices, libraries and similar areas may be covered with synthetic fibre carpet which is quiet comfortable, hard-wearing and inexpensive.

Workshops and other areas where mains voltage equipment is being used under difficult conditions must be provided with a floor covering which is a good electrical insulator linoleum is generally considered to be satisfactory in these a.eas.

Windows

Most laboratories require large window areas to enable natural lighting to be utilized as much as possible, to provide at least part of the ventilation and, in some instances, to provide a means of escape in emergencies. They should be easily opened by the smallest person likely to occupy the room, be readily cleaned with minimum disturbance to the occupants, be fitted with closures which prevent access by unauthorized persons, and incorporate frames which are resistant to the corrosive atmosphere present in some laboratories. The siting of windows must be chosen carefully as they occupy wall space which could be used for other purposes. Two smaller windows may be less wasteful of space than one large one. Double glazing, although costly, may be an advantage if the normal ambient temperature is particularly low for long periods of the year. It also assists in the reduction of noise from traffic, etc.

Doors

The usual practice is to provide laboratories with a docr and a half, i.e. two leaves, one larger than the other. The large leaf serves as the normal entrance and the small one is also opened when large items need to be taken through the doorway. Suitable widths are 90 cm and 45 cm. Laboratory doors should be fitted with glass panels to enable one to see if it is safe to open the door and to enable a visual check to be made on the room without opening the door. It may be desirable to arrange for all laboratory doors to be lockable and local regulations may require certain doors to be locked when not in use, e.g. flammable solvent stores and dangerous chemical stores. All locks should operate on a 'master key' system.

Benches

The choice of bench units will depend on the degree of flexibility required. Fixed benching is acceptable where the techniques used are unlikely to alter, but if the type of work is likely to change fairly, and rapidly some degree of flexibility is desirable, bearing in mind the increased cost. Modular units are extremely flexible but do not provide an uninterrupted working surface. Floor standing equipment is readily accommodated by removing one or more units.

Whichever units are chosen, rigid construction is essential. Timber frames and worktops are the most commonly used, but metal units are becoming increasingly popular as corrosion-resistant finishes of improved quality become available. Floor-standing frames are usually cheaper but brackets cantilevered from the walls have the advantages of giving an unobstructed floor space and better access to service pipes Figure1.6 Bench units are available in heights suitable for standing or sitting work, e.g. 75 and 90 cm.

A wide variety of benchtop material is in used, hardwood being the most popular. Top grade teak is becoming scarce and very expensive and whilst some of the alternative hardwoods are satisfactory, may be not. Several factory-made timbers, such as blockboard, are well suited as benchtop materials, provided they are covered with an impervious plastic laminate fixed with a good-quality adhesive. These materials wear well, are easy to keep clean and are resistant to most chemicals. They can, however, be damaged by heat or impact but are not difficult to replace. In laboratories where infected materials are handled, the smooth finish of the laminate is readily disinfected.

Linoleum work surfaces are excellent in areas such as instrument rooms and are easily replaced if damaged. Sheet lead may be used where corrosive acids are handled in quantity, but the cost is so great that it is doubtful if such expense can be justified. Quarry tiles are suitable for this type of work but must be fixed and grouted with acid resistant products.

Cupboards and Drawer Units

The bulk of laboratory storage is in under-bench cupboards, although wall-mounted units are used to house small, light items. As with benches, these may be constructed of timber or metal. Under-bench units are usually floor-standing and arranged so that they can be pulled out for cleaning and for access to services. The units may also be suspended from the bench top, in which case they usually slide sideways to gain access to services. Sliding doors are most suitable for wall-mounted cupboards but hinged doors are more satisfactory for under-bench units. Drawer units are useful for small items in frequent use at the bench. Good-quality workmanship is vital, because badly made drawers tend to stick and their contents may be damaged when trying to force them open.

Fire-resistant cabinets for the storage of flammable solvents should be provided in those laboratories where such materials are in use. Units are available with built-in automatic fire extinguishers. These should be large enough to hold one bottle of each solvent required but not so large as to encourage the keeping of large volumes which should be stored in proper solvent store.

Other furniture, such as desks, chairs, filing cabinets and lockers, should be provided wherever necessary. Desks and filing cabinets should be lockable; the latter should be of fire-resistant construction. In some laboratories, a safe may be required for the storage of confidential documents, or for materials which are valuable or dangerous.

Mechanical Services

The main difference between a laboratory building and any other building is in the type of mechanical services required, and the correct provision of these services is of paramount importance.

Heating and Ventilating

It is generally accepted that 20°C is a suitable temperature for most laboratories. A higher temperature tends to be oppressive and a lower temperature is uncomfortable and reduces manual dexterity. Heating is usually provided by hot water radiators fed from a central boiler or by ducted warm air. The latter system may be unsuitable in some laboratories as it introduces a possible hazard where infected or other dangerous material is involved. In instances where the ambient temperatures are likely to be above 20°C for long periods of the year, or where a large amount of heat is produced in the building, full air conditioning will be necessary;

In most laboratories, some form of mechanically-assisted ventilation is desirable to maintain a healthy environment. It may not be necessary to use this continually but it should be installed in areas where noxious or dangerous fumes are likely to be generated. Many volatile materials are dangerous if inhaled for long periods and good ventilation helps to keep these to a minimum concentration. Ventilation is measured in air changes per hour,an average figure for laboratories being 6. If large amounts of noxious fumes or gases are produced, it is usually better to provide efficient fume cupboards rather than to overcome the problem by increasing whole-room ventilation. A ducted warm air supply is provided by one or more fan units working in conjunction with a balanced air extract system. The latter will of course remove heat from the building and this heat loss must be allowed for in the calculations for the heating requirements.

Some rooms may require their air supply to be filtered and this is normally done by installing disposable filter elements in the supply ducts. These should be capable of removing particles of diameters larger than 5 um and will need to be replaced regularly. Electrostatic duct removes are efficient but are expensive to install and require considerable maintenance.

Fume Cupboards

These cupboards will be required in some laboratories, particularly those involved in chemistry of radioactive work. Current models available for specialist manufacturers are extremely efficient and are correctly matched to the ducting and extract fans.

The rate of extract required will vary with the type of work for which the fume cupboards are used. This rate is measured in terms of air velocity over the working surface. For general work, a minimum of 0.4 m/s is recommended and for work with highly toxic or radioactive material, a minimum velocity of 0.5 m/s is required. These velocities are measured with the sash open to height of 600 mm. Too high a velocity can cause light powders to be drawn into the extract system. It is not generally appreciated that the design of a fume cupboard has a marked effect on the rate of air flow; smooth working surfaces, an absence of sharp corners and a profile of sill and jambs which streamline the airflow will increase efficiency considerably, the provision of baffles improves the air flow over the working surface regardless of whether the sash is raised or lowered and some designs permit air from the room to enter the cupboard near the tope to assist with purging.

Most substances handled in fume cupboards are hazardous in one way or another and many be corrosive, it is therefore essential for the units to be constructed of corrosion-resistant materials. Timber is generally unsatisfactory unless it is plastic-coated and various plastic materials such as welded PVC or glass fibre reinforced resins are better. Toughened glass panels have some advantages but it is difficult to seal them effectively, Asbestos working surfaces, even if sealed, are not satisfactory and in view of the health hazard now known to exist, this material should not be used. The sash must be shatter-resistant as it presents a large area of glass at face level. Toughened glass, wire-reinforced glass or plastic such as polycarbonate are suitable materials and can also be used for side panels where these are required. The sash must be well-balanced either with counterweights or spring units, so that it may be opened or closed easily and rapidly in an emergency. Once a fume cupboard is installed and connected to its ducting, it is a major task to move it, and its position must therefore be considered carefully before installation. Siting close to a door should be avoided, because draughts caused by opening and closing the door can cause spillage of fumes; areas where staff circulate should be avoided for the same reason.

Gas, water, drainage lighting and electrical outlets will be required in the fume cupboard and the location of such outlets and their controls is important. A small sink, sufficient for a condenser tube, is adequate and this should be mounted flush with the working surface so that it may then also be used when washing this surface. Controls must be outside so that they may be operated with the sash closed. Electrical outlets must also be external to the fume cupboard and must be switched units preferably of a flashproof design. Adequate lighting units must be installed and sealed against corrosive vapours and provision made for changing tubes easily.

The material used for ducting should be selected with care, as it is usually somewhat inaccessible once installed. PVC or polypropylene are satisfactory materials but in the event of fire they will soften and distort. If the temperature rises greatly, PVC produces dense toxic and corrosive fumes, polypropylene and PVC are perhaps the only available materials suitable for use with perchloric acid.

Fans should be manufactured in such a way that the motor is not situated in the air steam, although for small installations axial fans coated with protective resins are adequate. For larger installation, centrifugal fans are more satisfactory, practicularly as the motor can be removed for service without disturbing the ductwork.

The outlet to atmosphere must be arranged so that fumes cannot re-enter the building. This is best achieved by using an outlet of adequate height above the building. Consideration must also be given to prevailing weather conditions and to the proximity of other buildings which may affect the distribution of fumes in the immediate locality. The design of the actual cupboard is an important consideration and varies considerable from one type to another, although they may look very similar, The main variation is in the arrangement of the extract and baffle. The more advanced systems produce a more uniform air flow over the working surface whether the sash is open or closed. but of course one must accept tha higher cost of a more sophisticated design.

Most fume cupboards have a working surface at normal bench height but for some purposes floor-standing units may be required. These enable workers to walk into them, and large equipment such as gas cylinders may also be wheeled in and out.

Lighting

Modern buildings are usually provided with large window areas in order to take advantage of natural lighting which, in most latitudes, provides sufficient light for much of the working day, However, natural lighting must obviously be supplemented with artificial lighting.

Laboratories require a level of illumination of about 600 lux (1 lux = 11 lumen/m^2). Reception areas, libraries and stores need about 200 lux and offices about 400 lux, these levels being generally provided by means of fluorescent tubes fitted with diffusers. The number and wattage of tubes needed depend on several factors, such as the decor of the room, height of fittings above the bench and on the cleaniness of the fit light output from fluorescent tubes decreases with age and an old tube in a dirty fitting can give as little as 50 percent of its rated output. Measurements are taken at the working surface.

Tubes are manufactured to give various colors of light, the 'daylight' types being the most acceptable for laboratories. In areas where accurate observation of color is necessary, such as in photographic units or paint control laboratories, 'color matching' cubes are necessary. These give an output approximating to north daylight. In offices and circulating areas, 'warm white'tubes give a less harsh illumination. Warm white and daylight tubes are the most efficient, producing about 65 lumen/W, whereas the color matching type produces about 42 lumen/W. Even the lower figure is substantially better than tungsten lamps, which give about 14 lumen/W, it is advisable not to mix different types of tubes in any room as the effect is distracting. Inadequate illumination is not only unpleasant but produces severe eye-strain, especially in older persons, and after long periods may result in permanent damage to the eyes. Fine graduations on equipment are difficult to read with poor illumination, and errors can be made and accidents caused. Similarly, lighting which is too bright gives rise to discomfort due to glare; this may cause severe headaches in many people. Gloss paint and shiny working surfaces increase glare, although this can be greatly reduced by the use of diffusers with the lighting units.

Even illumination overall is most desirable; if a working area is alternately dull and bright as one moves about, the eyes cannot accommend maximum spacing to height ratios for their fittings and these figures should not be exceeded. Illumination reduces with the square of the distance between light source and working surface, and the height of the fittings will therefore influence the number of fittings required. It is important for the ceiling to be well illuminated and fittings should allow a proportion of their light output to be projected in an upward direction. If flush fittings are used this is not possible, but the provision of a light-colored floor covering will overcome this problem to some extent. Fittings for laboratories should be chosen for their performance rather than by their appearance.

For certain types of work involving fine examination or assembly, very high levels of lighting may be necessary—this can be provided by local high-intensity adjustable lamps. There are models available which are fitted with a magnifying lens, the light source being either tungsten filament lamps or fluorescent tubes. The latter are preferable as they produce practically no heat. In premises which are occupied at night, it may be necessary to provide emergency lighting in certain areas such as staircases, corridors and rooms where essential work is being carried out. In the event of a supply failure, the emergency supply can be switched in manually or, preferably, by supply can be switched in manually or, preferably, by automatic means. Generators may be used for this purpose or storage batteries can be utilized. To enable the existing lighting units to be used, batteries are normally coupled to an inverted to provide electric power at the same potential as the normal mains supply, without this facility, low-voltage lamps will be necessary in addition to the normal lighting.

Electrical Supplies

The amount of electrical and electronic equipment in laboratories appears to increase continually and in many departments there is a shortage of mains voltage outlets, making the use of multi-way adaptors an undesirable necessity. The cost of providing adequate outlets at the bench is only marginally greater than purchasing adaptors and far more satisfactory. The maximum load likely to be drawn by bench-standing apparatus is about 1 KVA per metre of bench, e.g. a laboratory having 14 m of bench requires about 14 KVA. i.e. 60 A at 240 V. In addition, equipment such as autoclaves, stills, etc. will require separate supplies of suitable rating. Bench outlets should be fitted with flashproof interlocking switches mounted above the back edge of the bench and distributed along its length in such a way that long-trailing leads are not required. They should be wired as a ring main and each laboratory provided with an easily accessible master switch to enable the supply to be switched off in an emergency, local fuses or overload cut outs should be installed to ensure that a short circuit does not interrupt the supply to other parts of the building.

Three-phase supplies are required for some equipment where large motors or high-power heaters are involved, such as workshop machinery, glass-washing machines and large mixers, and at least one three-phase supply of adequate rating should be available on each floor. There may also be a need for supplies at voltages other than the normal main supply, and if these are fed to benches, special outlets correctly labelled must be used to prevent the accidental connection of the wrong supply to a particular piece of apparatus. Many electronic devices operate from d.c. voltage of 5-80 V and these may be energized from individual power packs in each laboratory or from one central unit. The former system is preferred, because greater stability is achieved and the problem of voltage drop over long cables is avoided.

Emergency Supplies

In the event of a breakdown of the public elctricity supply, equipment which must be kept running may be switched, either manually or automatically, to an emergency supply, usually from a generator. The cost of generators rises rapidly with their power output capability and, with few exception, it is not feasible to supply the entire building. It is good practice to connect selected outlets to the emergency supply is a feed for equipment which must be kept running at all times, Refrigerators and freezers will normally hold their temperature for several hours if not opened, and unless prolonged power failure are anticipated they do not require standby power.

Gas Supplies

In the past, a large amount of gas was used in laboratories for equipment such as ovens, stills and incubators, but today the traditional bunsen burner is probably the only gas appliance in common use. As this does not appear to be a totally statisfactory substitute for this basic service, most laboratories will require a gas supply, except in those areas where a high fire risk exists. In such areas, gas should not be installed, even if it is proposed to blank off the pipes.

All outlets should be of a safe construction with levers wich lock in the 'off position. A very small leak can cause a build-up of gas to an explosive level in a room which is left closed for a long period such as a weekned. If double outlets area spaced along the bench about 2 m apart, the use of long connecting tubes is avoided. Some laboratories have master stopcorks, clearly marked outside the rooms so that they can be turned off in the event of a leak or fire.

Water Supplies

Adequate supplies of cold water must be available in all laboratories, one outlet per 3 m of bench is sufficient for the majority of situations. A teaching laboratory catering for a large number of students will probably require twice this number. Since the supply is normally taken from storage tanks at roof level, the pressure varies with head of water. This problem may be overcome by using a booster pump to raise the pressure to about 3 kgf/cm^2 which is satisfactory if water jet suction pumps are to be used. Some local authorities will not permit the use of these pumps, however, owing to their high water consumption. High-pressure outlets should be color coded for easy recognition. Several types of outlets are available and these should be chosen according to their function. Most will be suitable for connection to flexible tubes for use with condensers or similar apparatus, but at least one tap in each laboratory should be of a larger bore because large volumes of water may be required quickly in an emergency such as an acid spillage.

In general, the demand for hot water in laboratories is fairly small but is useful for warming solution, hand washing, etc. and at least one hot tap should be provided in each laboratory. Mixer taps are well worth the small extra cost. On no account should gas water heaters be installed in laboratories, but if a hot water supply is not available an electric storage-tube, water heater is a satisfactory and an inexpensive alternative.

Drainage

The very large sinks common in laboratories a few years ago are giving way to smaller units or drip cups. One function of sinks in the laboratory is to carry away the cooling water, or the outlets from water jet pumps, and for the disposal of small amounts of waste materials. Large sinks are therefore not necessary for these purposes.

Sinks are made of various materials, glazed fireclay being the most satisfactory for the majority of applications. Stainless steel is also used but some grades are of dubious quality and need to be chosen with care. Polythene, polypropylene and glass fibre sinks are easily scratched and difficult to keep clean. Whichever type is chosen, it is important to ensure that the joint between bench top and sink is water tight and will remain so under all conditions.

Waste pipes and fittings are an important feature, because replacement of an unsatisfactory system is a costly and disruptive exercise. Even with the greatest care, corrosive materials do find their way into the waste pipes and not only damage the system but cause further damage to the building because of eventual leakage which may go undetected for a long period.

Plastic materials, such a polythene, are very satisfactory, provided they are of good quality and correctly fitted. Long horizontal pipe runs tend to sag and must be properly supported. Demountable joints and cleaning eyes are necessary to enable blocked pipes to be cleared. In some laboratories, large catch pots are used to take waste from several sinks but it is better to install individual traps for each sink. The design should be such that the trap can be dismantled without the use of tools to enable blockages to be cleared quickly and small items such as magnetic stirring bars to be retrieved.

In laboratories where highly toxic or radioactive materials are in use, special consideration must be given to the waste system. Glass or glass-lined iron traps and pipelines are recommended when working with highly corrosive liquids. Although costly to install, they have a very long life and require the minimum of attention.

Distilled and De-ionized Water Supplies

Distilled water may be supplied to individual laboratories or to supply points on each floor from a central still. Alternatively, individual stills can be installed in those rooms where a supply is needed. Where demand is very large, the former system may be preferable but it has some disadvantages. Pipework and storage tanks of a suitable nature are expensive and can give rise to contamination of the whole supply if corrosion, leakage or algal growth develop. Water lying in pipes for long periods may leach soluble, materials from the glass or metal or from jointing materials. When the sill is shut down for repairs or maintenance, the entire building is without a supply. The capital outlay for a large still, together with the provision of power supplies, cooling water, etc., is very considerable although the output in terms of l/kVA may be higher depending on the design.

Small stills producing 4-8 1/h are relatively inexpensive, take up little space, can be easily maintained and may be shut down individually for servicing. Whilst gas-heated units are available, electric heating is more satisfactory and produces about 1.3 1/h per kVA. Regular descaling is necessary to achieve this output. Particularly in hard water areas, and it is advisable to select a design which can be descaled with the minimum of dismantling. With some models no dismantling whatever is required. If live steam, free of volatile impurities, is available in the building, strip action stills may be used to advantage. These consist of a condenser into which the steam is passed via a system of baffles to strip out major contaminants which are flushed away with the cooling water. Such units are certainly maintenance free, take up minimum space and have a high output.

Storage of distilled water should be in reservoirs of either glass, PVC, polythene or polypropylene. These may be fitted with float switches which out off the still when full and restart it when water is drawn from the reservoir. High-purity water may be produced by de-ionization with resins formulated for this purpose. Anionic and cationic resins may be used in separate columns, mains water being passed through each in turn; alternatively, a mixed resins may be regenerated by the user, while in the latter a new resin bed is installed when required, the exhausted one being returned to the supplier on an exchange basis. Units are available in various sizes from small bench units up to large installations providing several hundred gallons per day.

In soft water areas, the amount of de-ionized water produced can be very large before the resin becomes exhausted, but in hard water areas the output is considerably reduced. It is often more economical to distill the supply water first and to pass this directly from the still to the delonizer and thence to a storage reservoir. Whichever system is used, it is essential to monitor the quality of the output by measuring its conductivity. Despite the cost of the resin, de-ionizing can be an economical way of producing high purity water because, unlike the still, no heating is required. The actual cost will depend on the concentration of dissolved impurities present in the supply water, which will vary from one area to another.

Steam Supply

Certain laboratories will need a piped steam supply as a service for heating, operating autoclaves, etc., or for conversion to distilled water. It is costly to install, but if a high-pressure boiler is used for space heating, the additional cost is not great. All pipework must be of a high standard and properly lagged to prevent heat loss and to avoid accidental burning. Open-ended steam valves should not be fitted to benches as they are a hazard, and steam should only be used on apparatus to which it can be directly plumbed. Reducing valves must be fitted in the supply lines at the appropriate points, and only apparatus designed to withstand the supply pressure and which are fitted with reliable safety valves may be used.

Piped Gases

Gases which are used routinely may be piped at reduced pressure (e.g. 4 kgf/cm^2) to suitable outlets in the laboratories from a central cylinder store. Only gases which are non-flammable and non-toxic should be supplied in this way, compressed air, nitrogen, argon, etc. may for example be piped to laboratories engaged in gas chromatography, but on no account should such gases as acetylene, hydrogen and chlorine be supplied by this method unless the pipework is installed outside the building,

Outlets at the bench must be fitted with pressure-reducing or flowcontrol regulators, clearly labelled and regularly maintained. Oil or grease must not be allowed to come into contact with them and readily accessible shut-off valves must be installed outside the laboratory for use in emergencies.

Stafety in Design

At all stages of design, safety is of paramount importance, in most countries, building legislation will impose certain design requirements but little if any guidance is given regarding details such as floor coverings and lighting of stairways. Each room should, wherever possible, have more than one exit which, at ground floor level, may be an opening window of sufficient size, in small rooms where two doors would take up valuable space or otherwise be impractical, a 'kick-out' may be incorporated in one of the walls, preferably a corridor wall. This consists of a hole covered with a light panel which is easily broken down and of sufficient size to allow a large adult to pass through. It must, of course, be clearly labelled and unobstructed at all times on both sides. The corridors and staircases must be provided with self-closing doors to contain smoke and reduce draughts which would encourage the spread of fire. Apparatus producing ionizing radiations, such as X-ray equipment, must be housed in rooms which are screened to prevent radiations passing to other areas. Such screening (usually lead panels, lead-loaded concrete or barium-loaded bricks or plaster) is extremely heavy and very costly and allowance should be made for its inclusion where necessary.

Decoration

Decoration serves a number of purposes apart from providing a pleasant environment. It has a marked effect on the level of lighting (particularly daylight utilization) and can reduce the cost of artificial lighting. It preserves the structural materials of the building and provides surfaces which are easily cleaned and disinfected.

For general laboratory use, light colors are preferred for ceilings, walls and floor coverings. Gloss paints tend to produce glare, so that matter or eggshell finishes are more satisfactory. In areas where hazardous materials such as radioisotopes and bacterial cultures are handled, gloss paints may be necessary as decontamination is more easily carried out. Timber apart from bench surfaces, may be gloss painted or treated with varnish.

Plastic laminates make excellent decorative finishes in areas where dirty material is handled, such as in animal houses; although expensive, such laminates require little or no maintenance, Ceramic tiles can also be used to advantage in these areas.

Decoration in offices, common rooms, lecture rooms, etc. is not so restricted and the careful use of colors can be very pleasing, As the decor is not subjected to such harsh treatment as it is in laboratories there is no reason why wall coverings or emulsion paints should not be used. Where an office is occupied by one person, he may be given the choice of colors: if a number of person use the room. However, the scheme should be chosen by mutual agreement. There is no doubt that peoples' temperaments are affected by the decor of their place of work and they can become inefficient and even aggressive in surroundings which they find depressing of otherwise unpleasant.

Allocation of Floors in Multi-storey Buildings

Deciding which rooms should be sited on the various floors of a building is not such a simple exercise as it might at first appear. Incoming goods must be delivered and waste materials disposed of ; hence there is a good case for sitting departments with a large throughout on the ground floor. It can also be argued that laboratories using heavy equipment should be on the ground floor, where flammable materials are handled, the risk of fire spreading is reduced if these laboratories are situated on the top floor. One is soon forced to the conclusion that nearly all departments should be on the ground floor and, indeed, if a large site were available, a single storey building has a great many practical advantages.

There is seldom a good case for using basements as working areas. Boiler plant, ventilation systems, long-term storage facilities and so on can be accommodated below ground level without condemning staff to work in depressing environments. The ground floor forms a natural reception area with offices, meeting rooms, cloakrooms, etc. adjoining. If sufficient space is available stores (with access for delivery vehicles)should also be at ground floor and, indeed, if a large site were available a single-storey building has a great many practical advantages. There is seldom a good case for using basements as working areas. Boiler plant, ventilation system, long-term storage facilities and so on can be accommodated below ground level without condeming staff to work in depressing environments. The ground floor forms a natural reception area with offices, meeting rooms, cloakrooms, etc, adjoining. If sufficient space is available, stores (with access for delivery vehicles) should also be at ground level, perhaps at the rear of the building.

Workshops and laboratories using heavy apparatus are also best placed at ground level, with remaining laboratories on the upper floors. Animal accommodation is usually on the top floor as it is easier to isolate these rooms, although waste disposal can present some difficulties. Service rooms which are shared by all departments, such as glassware washing or photographic facilities, are best positioned near the center of the building to reduce to a minimum the distance between them and their users.

Rooms which are devoid of daylight are occassionally to be found in the central core of large complexes. Such areas are ideal for storage, photographic dark rooms, toilets, etc. but should not be used as normal working areas where staff would be expected to remain for long periods of the day.

Laboratory Organizational Structure

Organization in the clinical laboratory refers to structure and process. Structure examplifies stated relationships of framework. While process deal with interaction. The three key elements of organization are the tasks to be performed, the individuals who are to perform the tasks and the clinical laboratory as a workplace.

Organization of the Pathology Laboratory

Figure 35.17 is an example of an organizational chart for a clinical laboratory. Note that this structure includes a core or central laboratory rather than multiple specialized sections. Although a standard fixture in most organizations, the chart serves only limited functions, one of which is providing visualization who is doing what and the chain of command.

Organization plays an important role in the effectiveness of the clinical laboratory by defining the relationship between tasks, individuals, and the workplace. the basis for this relationship is authority responsibility, and accountability. A laboratory manager possesses authority within the organization if he has the right to issue instructions that others are expected to follow. Authority is generally attached to as position, and its location on the organizational chart implies degree of consent. Responsibility refers to the group of tasks or duties assigned to an individual or position in the organizational structure, and accountability is the obligation to a higher authority for the successful fulfillment of assigned an individual or position in the organizational structure, and accountability is the obligation to a higher authority for the successful fulfillment of assigned tasks. The organizational structure is a visual aid for evaluating each of these basics. For example, when investigating the difficulty a laboratory supervisors is experiencing in maintaining sufficient inventory (responsibility), the laboratory director may realize that the problem is in the purchasing system, which does not accept the supervisors signature on requisition (authority).

The organizational chart also attempts to show relationships between line and staff, in this organizational concept, a line position is one in which a superior exercises direct supervision over a subordinate. A staff position is advisory, supportive, or auxiliary, These terms were defined in industry, and health-care institutions seldom use the same connotation. When a laboratory manager speaks of his staff, he generally is referring to his technical personnel, who are serving in line positions. Individuals involved solely in academic instruction and research would be defined as staff to the functioning anatomic and clinical laboratories. Another component of the structure, more visibly staff, is the administrative section and its role is supportive to the primary laboratory testing function. There are times when line-staff conflicts occur, stemming primarily from a failure to define clearly the operational difference between the two. This may produce a conflict when the rightful prerogative of a line supervisor is usurped by a staff administrator.

Organizational Design and Hierarchy

An organizational hierarchy is a multilevel, vertical structure, signifying who outranks whom it designing or evaluating a laboratory organizational hierarchy, several characteristics should be considered.

Departmentation or Specialization

The design of all organizational structures includes a division of labor. Overall goals are divided into activities. These activities are subsequently separated into departments to achieve a degree of specialization. In the medical laboratory, departments have reflected uniformity of technique (chemical analysis), uniformity of specimen required (whole blood for haematologic analysis, uniformity of function (administrative support). In any large laboratory, it is obvious that specialization has a positive effect on efficiency. Under the supervision and responsibility of the pathologist, services performed by the medical technologists fall into five major sections.

Bacteriology, Immunology and Parasitology Section

i. Cultures and chemical, immunological and animal studies used for identification of bacteria, fungi, spirochaetes and viruses.
ii. Antibiotic sensitivity procedures.
iii. Preparation of vaccines.
iv. Intradermal testing and studies of antigens and antibodies.
v. Procedures for detection and identification.

Biochemistry and Diagnostic Radioisotopes Section

i. Biochemical analysis of blood, body fluids, body excretion and tissues for the determination of nutrition and metabolism functions, acid, base balance, hormones, function tests retention of substances, abnormal moelcular and related procedures.
ii. Diagnostic radioisotopes include blood volume determination, thyroid function studies, fat diagestion and absorption studies, iron absorption and renal and liver function studies.

Blood Bank Section

Responsible for the drawing of blood from donors, the processing of donors blood, the typing and compatibility procedures, the manufacture of blood products and the transfusion service.

Hematology and Hemostasis Section

i. *Studies of blood* Hemoglobin determinations, cell counts and differential counts, hematocrits, sedimentation rates, staining and differential counts on bone marrow aspiration.
ii. Cell count and differential counts of spinal fluid, urine and other body fluids.
iii. Hemostasis studies are concerned with the evaluation of blood coagulation mechanism and vascular factors in the diagnosis and treatment of hemorrhagic diseases.

Tissue Preparation Section

i. Processing of tissues and preparation of microscopic slides from autopsy and surgical specimens.
ii. Preparation of smears for exfoliative cytology study.
iii. Histochemical studies and use of special stains as aids to diagnosis.

The number of departmental personnel, and to a lesser degree: the number of postions, is directly related to the work load and the size of the hospital. The laboratory workload will vary, depending on the census and the quality and kind of medical practice in the hospital. Whether ration of personnel needed are based on beds, patient days, or number of procedures, a basic starting point to complete daily man hours needed will be to obtain an average (median) figure representing tests per patient per day. The average number of tests performed becomes an excellent index for determining average man hours.

The larger the laboratory work load, the greater the need for functional groupings and specia lisation. Mycoy considers that the ratio of pathologists and technicians should be based on the number of procedures, as under:

30,000 examinations/month	One Pathologist and One Addl. Pathologist
Over 15,000 examinations	One Bacteriologist
Over 30,000 examinations	One Biochemist

For each 10.000 examinations one clerk

As regard to the requirement of technologist, data developed by Owen and Finch, from a survey of 350 general hospitals are given below:

Tests performed annually per medical technologist

Laboratory Unit	No of tests
Hematology	13,400
Urinalysis	30,720
Serology	11,520
Biochemistry	9,600
Biochemistry	7,680
Histology	3,840
Parasitology	9,600

Mac Eachern recommends that under the direction of the department or under the head of each sub-department should be one or more technicians, the number depending upon the completeness of the laboratory and the volume of work. The ratio of pathologists and technicians to hospital beds, recommended by him is as:

Beds	Pathologist	Technician	Stenographer
< 50	1 part time	2-3 full time	as needed
50-100	1 part time	3-5 full time	part time
100-200	1 full time	5-8 full time	part time
200-300	1 or more full time	8-10 full time	1 full time
300-500	3 full time	20-30 full time	2-3 full time

Control of Pathology Services

The director has responsibility for all pathology services performed within the hospital. This comprises control of the collection of specimens, performance of procedures, the areas where procedures are performed and the personnel involved.

Work Control Programme

The services offered by the department and to a patient are done only upon the request of physician. The following working principles have been recommended by:

a. In order to avoid misunderstanding and errors in the patient name, location and examination ordered, the request forms shall be made out by the floor nurse or other authorised floor personnel. The department will not consider a procedure to be ordered until the request form is received.
b. The time the report is needed may be indicated by use of terms as routine, today and stay, depending on the urgency.
c. Request form should be delivered to personnel at a central point in the department which makes necessary arrangements with the proper section. This will avoid duplication in collection of specimens.
d. The department will schedule certain procedures for specified days, and may limit the number of other procedures scheduled on any day.
e. The services of the department must be available every hour of every day.

Quality Management

Defined as the periodic systematic surveillance of people, tools, methods, and reagents, quality control guarantees the laboratory's stated limits of precision with some reassurance of accuracy.

Quality assurance requires, laboratory programmes to have three components: monitoring of important aspects of care and outcomes, problem solving to ensure actions were taken to imporve care and outcomes, and documentation and reporting of activities. The quality control programme are measured in terms of accuracy and precision. The common meaning of the term accurate is the true or actual value. In pathology, this term permits an obtained value which may be the true value or slightly above or below the true value. The variation is due to the fact that the clinical condition is a dynamic process, and the results must have a reasonable time relationship to the collection of specimen. Other factors which enter into the decisions are—volume of specimen, viscosity, presence of interfering substances, equipment errors, technologist errors, etc. The term precision indicates the ability to perform repeated determinations on one specimen and obtain results which are closely grouped. This is not a direct measurement of accuracy. If an error or errors are repeated to an equal degree in each of the repeated determinations the result may be very precise but not accurate.

The following quality control measures have been recommended:

a. Preparation of standard solutions consisting of known pure substance dissolved in water, in which the concentration of the substance is known. This can function as accuracy controls when they are included daily with the determination of unknowns.
b. Extensive use of standards, usually obtained commercially, which are prepared with serum as a solvent vehicle. These serum standards are available containing either constitutents in the normal range or constitutents in an abnormal range. This also acts as excellent accuracy control.
c. The use of standard deviation is the third control methods. The standard deviation is obtained by the performing at least ten duplicate analysis, taking the difference between each pairs, squaring each of the differences, adding the squares of the differences and apply the formula:-

$$SD = \pm \frac{\text{sum of (differences}^2)}{2N}$$

N = Number of duplicate analysis. If one performed 100 analysis on the same meterial $\pm$ 1 SD will include 68 percent of results, $\pm$ 2 SD will include 95 percent of results and $\pm$ 3 SD will include 99.7 percent of results.

The procedure method with the lowest standard deviation should be the best.

d. Testing of the equipment and instrument is another quality control measure.

The best control programme is based on the pathologists and department personnel's awareness of the sources of errors and faithful adherence to an organized plan.

Reports and Records

The basic function of the report is to provide promptly and accurately the results of pathology examinations, with the growth in size and complexity of the department, the problem of reports and records has also grown. No pathology report is valid until the medical staff receives the report on it.

Many systems of reports and records are available. There is no one system that is best for all institutions. The system used must satisfy the purposes of many groups whose requirements can be incorporated into the principles on which the reports and records are based. It should meet the following requirements:

a. Request forms should be simple and easy to use. The clinical pathology reports should carry the normal values of the procedures not commonly ordered.
b. The department should have an indexing system whereby records of all procedures performed on a patient are available.
c. The minimum time the record to be kept would be governed by the time period of the statute of litigations. In most cases it is three years.
d. It should meet all legal requirements, particularly in cases of autopsy, notifiable disease, in the event of refusal of procedure by a patient.

A Model Laboratory Quality System

To transition the laboratory quality system framework from a table on paper into an actual working reality, some specific activities are necessary. The activities correspond to those taken in industry to implement the ISO 9000, 9001, 9002 and 2000 series quality standards. They include the formation of the quality system manual, the reorganization of laboratory technical operating procedures, the redesign of the internal assessment programme, and the application of continuous quality improvement programme.

The quality system documentation pyramid is presented in a hierarchy of quality policies, quality processes, standards operating processes, and related forms: Level I—quality manual; Level II—quality system processes; Level III—work instructions (SOPs); Level IV—forms, documents and records.

Appropriate use of laboratory testing by the medical staff is as important to laboratory testing as having an effective quality system.

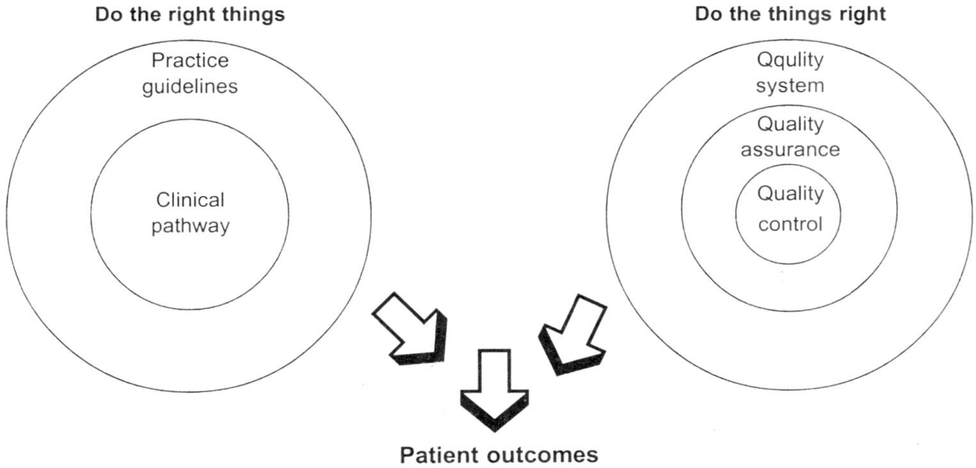

Fig. 35.23: Laboratory quality: The right information at the right place at the right time

Laboratory quality includes: The right information at the right place at the right time. The key to pursue actively two important quality objectives:

- Do the right things
  - practice guidelines
  - clinical pathways

Laboratory participation is vital to answer questions regarding the appropriateness, frequency, and timing of labòratory tests and to assist in developing a cost-effective laboratory test ordering protocol for the clinical pathway's particular diagnosis, treatment, or procedure.

The laboratory quality system provides the means to ensure that the laboratory does things right. Policies and procedures are in place, people are trained and competent, processes are assessed for weaknesses, and corrective action is taken when problems are identified.

SUMMARY

The clinical laboratories should operate within an unified system and the technical control should be exercised by pathologists. The emergency laboratory should be located in close proximity to the intensive care and emergency wards. Central collection room should be properly organised and supervised by a pathologist. A side laboratory should be established for OPD patients.

FURTHER READING

1. Heeb Joseph A: Adminsitration of the Hospital Laboratory Service, Hospital Progress **49 (8-10)**: 1968
2. BS 3202: Recommendations on Laboratory Furniture and fittings. British Standards Institution, London, 1959.
3. Hospital Laboratory Services, WHO Technical Report series 161 (1959).
4. Hughes D, Cullingworth R: Laboratory fittings and waste systems *Chemistry in Bratain* **8**: 470-70, 1974.
5. Lighting in offices, Shopa and Railway Premises. Booklet No 39, Health and safety Executive HMSO, London, 1976.
6. Nuffield Foundation, Divsion for Architectural Studies. The Design of Research Laboratories, Oxford University press 1961.
7. Owen JKMT: Modern Concepts of Hospital Administration, 1962.
8. Report on General Hospitals, Committee on plans and projects, New Delhi 1964.
9. Report on Delhi Hospitals, Hospital Review Committee.
10. Synder JR, Wilkinson DS: Management Functions in clinical Laboratory. In management in laboratory medicne. Synder JR, Willinson DS (Eds): (3rd edn.) Lippincott-Reven Publisher Philadephia, New York 1998.
11. Tabish SA: Textbook of Hospital and Health Services Administration. Oxford University Press. 2000.

PLANNING A MEDICAL LASER PROGRAMME

The advent of laser was the most outstanding breakthrough in surgical techniques in the twentieth century. Laser has resolved so many problems that its use in surgery is limited only by the bounds of surgeon's innovative imagination.

The most widely used laser in surgery is the carbon dioxide laser, introduced in the early 1970's.

Until 1985, the flow-through laser technology prevailed, providing high performance lasers, especially in pulsed and super-pulsed modes of operation. In 1985, the sealed-off technology entered the scene, significantly improving user convenience by eliminating the need for laser gas mixture cylinders, reducing the weight of the system and improving its mobility. Due to the inherent long-term power degradation of the laser tube, a considerable long-term cost burden was added that jeopardized the overall system performance. In 1990, a technological breakthrough as introduced-the Tubo charge technology–which merges the performance of flow through lasers and the convenience of sealed-off tubes into one single CO_2 laser system.

Major trend in the hospital market segment is the development of accessories which will enhance the penetration of the CO_2 laser. The introduction of wave guide delivery system has had a very positive impact in laparoscopy. Micro-spot (another accessory), copies the laser system to an operating microscope and provides burn spots as small as 120 μm at 300 mm working distance thus creating new opportunities in otorhinolaryngeology and neurosurgery. The greatest advantage of CW ND:YAG laser lies in its wave length (1.06 um, near infrared) which is easily transmittable through commercially available silica fibres. Areas like urology, gastroenterology, pulmonary medicine, and hysteroscopy where flexible delivery system (endoscopy) provide substantial clinical advantages is the real arena of this laser.

Bio-Physical Aspects

Laser is an acronym for Light Amplification by Stimulated Emission of Radiation. This is an electromagnetic radiation, not X-radiation and, as such, is not expected to produce a new generation of iatrogenic malignancies. This unique and exciting new form of energy brought to medicine marvellous tool could accomplish new treatments of previously intractable disorders as well as improved treatment of mundane problems. This brilliant form of energy is many times more powerful than the energy of the sun yet can be focussed microscopically to spot sizes as small as 30 microns. Lasers can be directed into seemingly inaccessible areas by mirrors or fibrotic cables or can be directly applied into sensitive areas such as retina without damage to intervening structures.

Basic Components of Laser System

An external power source hyperexcites the atoms in the laser medium so that the number of atoms possessing upper energy levels exceeds the number of atoms in a lower energy level, a condition termed as population inversion. This "pumping system" which imparts additional energy to the atoms may be optical, mechanical, or chemical. These atoms in a hyperexcited state spontaneously emit photons of light. The photons of light bounce back and forth reflected by precisely aligned mirrors located at either end of the laser tube. As they move along the laser chamber, they gain greater momentum and energy and produce more spontaneous emission by striking other atoms. Photons of energy with equal wave length, frequency, and energy eventually escape through the 15 per cent partially transmissive mirror as the laser beam.

Laser light may be delivered in different modes of operation:

- Continuous wave lasers
- Pulsed lasers
- Model locked lasers.

The optical cavity (laser chamber) contains the active lasing medium which usually determines the name of each laser:

- Ruby
- Argon, etc.

There are four types of lasing materials

- Solid state (ruby crystal)
- Gas (helium, argon, CO_2)
- Semiconductor (gallium arsenide)

The laser beam can also be described according to characteristics of the beam, termed modes:

- Gaussian
- Complicated.

The laser light that emanates from the laser chamber is very bright light of the highest luminosity. It is all of the same wavelength (monochromatic). All of the light waves are in phase both spatially and temporarily, or coherent. The energy is highly collimated (all rays are parallel to each other).

Laser systems are an adjunct to standard surgical systems. Laser is a new and different scalpel (optical knife). There is no direct contact with the field of surgery other than by light, accomplishing a desirable "no-touch" technique. Because of sealing of blood vessels and lymphatic, a relatively dry fields of surgery is produced. This reduces post-operative edema. Sealing of nerve ends results in less pain in the wound. The high temperature produced by the laser wound have the ability to sterilize the wound against contaminants such as bacteria, viruses, and fungi.

Laser Effects on Tissue

Laser light interacts with biological tissue in four very specific ways. It may either be absorbed, reflected, transmitted, or scattered. Only absorbed light exerts an effect on tissue. Major results of the above effects may be classified as:

- Coagulation (photocoagulation, hemostasis, necrosis)
- Vapourization (cutting, tissue evaporation)

Cutting with a laser is accomplished by a small well-focused spot size and lymphatics are simultaneously sealed, there is relatively dry surgical field. Incisions made by lasers eventually have the same scars and tensile strength as scalpe incisions. The CO_2 laser is able to be focussed microscopically to 30 mm incisions.

Varporisation or evaporation may be accomplished by a partially or completely defocused beam and is very valuable in debulking tumors, precisely removing individual cell layers, and ablating minor cutaneous lesions such as warts.

Delivery system

- Angioplasty
- Gastroenterology
- Ophthalmology-otolaryngeology
- Bronchology
- Gynecology
- Orthopedics
- Dermatology
- Plastic surgery
- Neurosurgery
- Thoracic surgery
- Dentistry.

There are three elements of delivery system:

- A distal tip, suitable to ensure the required interaction with the tissue.
- A proximal connector
- The interface to allow the link of delivery system to the laser.
- A wave guide transmitting the laser radiation from the connector of the tip.

Lasers that use fibreoptics are very simply focussed and directed by merely aiming the fibres. There is usually a lense for focussing at the end of fibre.

Advantages

The CO_2 laser beam incises the tissue without mechanically cutting it, through evaporation of the tissue. The incision can be made gently and quickly and the incised wound is sterile and free of bleeding because of low divergence, high density and wave length of the laser beam. The infrared light of CO_2 laser is well absorbed by the body tissue, which contains about 90 per cent of water, causing tissue to evaporate to a very small penetration depth (0.23 mm) while blood vessels to 0.5 mm are severed. Besides small penetration depth and precision of incision, lasers have other advantages like:

- Narrow necrotic zone omitting, restricting, or minimizing postoperative edema, resulting in quicker wound healing.
- Elimination or limitation of bleeding, making the operation area more easily seen while the trauma due to hemostasis is decreased.
- Reduction of operative complications with respect to traditional surgical practices.
- Diminishing of post-operative pain.
- Decrease in hospitalization time.

Hazards

The hazards of lasers may be grouped as those to eye, skin, and associated hazards, e.g. fire, X-ray, electrical, fumes, toxic materials, etc.

Effect on tissue are governed by the following factors:

- The energy or power density of the beam
- The absorption in tissues at the laser wavelength
- The time in beam is healed at a given area
- The protective effects of heat removal by thermal conduction and by circulation.

Protection

The most reliable protection system against laser radiation injury are those protective features that are engineered into the laser design or that are designed into a facility i.e. these systems are least subject to human error. When it is not practical to incorporate engineering safeguards in a device, it becomes necessary to rely on procedural safeguards and use of protective equipment to minimize the potential for injury.

Standard operating procedures should be developed.

Medical surveillance of laser using personnel should be included in an overall laser programme. Every employee working with lasers should receive a base line eye and skin examination at the time of employment, along with laser user who are already employed but have not been examined.

Facility Planning

To start a medical laser center:

- Perform a feasibility analysis
- Assess specific laser needs
- Selection and purchases of laser and related equipment
- Maintenance of laser systems
- Facility planning
- Establishment of safety rules and operating policies
- Selection and training of a laser programme coordinator
- Training of hospital personnel
- Training of and issuing of credentials to physicians
- Establishment of laser use charges
- Marketing of laser services
- Maintaining upto date information.

The decision to purchase a laser and implement a laser programme in a hospital requires sound thinking, decision-making and planning.

Providing laser facility to patient carries with it a commitment to quality care as well as concern for safety of both patients and personnel.

Lasers are capital equipment with the potential to enhance revenue. Health care consumers are aware of this new technology and are even demanding laser treatment. An administrator has to determine whether the hospital will benefit from the capital expenditure to provide the services to the community. To determine utilization potential, research (preliminary data gathering about procedures, the community to be served, the clinicians interest) is essential. Appreciating the fiscal impact, of prospective the fiscal impact, of prospective pricing, shopping wisely for the appropriate laser and ancillary equipment and learning to calculate the actual cost per use will assist with the financial decisions.

Preliminary research has to be conducted regarding the community to be served and what laser services are other hospitals providing. Outline the demographics and project a profile that depicts the types of illnesses and health care needs of the target population now and in the future. Analyse the needs of your hospital. What departments are potential users of the laser? What is the volume of the patients having treatments applicable to the laser? Identify the specialities that will be the highest users. Train the surgeons if not trained already and prepare the anaesthesiologists for the use of laser. Nurses should be included in your gathering of perception about lasers.

What types of lasers are to be purchased? If one has determined, e.g. the speciality that will use the laser on the highest volume of patients is otorhinolaryngology, then one needs to look at CO_2 lasers, find out the wattage delivered to tissue by each model. Otolaryngologists usually use 10-15 W with the CO_2 laser. Obstetricians and gynecologists need 25-35 W for infertility procedures, but neurosurgeons may want higher power levels for removing fibrous cranial tumors. Plastic surgeons need lower wattage ranges. Power levels affect cost. Lower-poured lasers cost less money.

The purchase of laser can affect hospitals and revenues in very subtle ways. When you have all of the facts about the cost of the laser or lasers that will best serve your situation, you will need to complete a cost analysis. A formula for determining the cost per procedure might include:

Depreciation of the Laser

Total purchase price: Life expectancy (3-5 years). Divide the cost per year of life by anticipated number of procedures.

Disposable Items used with the Laser

Gases Price per cylinder (if applicable): by average number of procedures per cylinder.

Drapes Cost of sterilizing process or disposable, per item.

Total Cost per Patient

This cost per case can help you decide whether or not a laser will increase revenue for your hospital. If your hospital is one that adds a cost per patient for use of capital equipment, this method can be used for your patient charge.

Before you buy a laser, know what you are getting for your money. That should include all accessories that are additional to the cost of the laser unit. Policies and procedures must be developed prior to use of the laser and ideally should be available for education and inservice sessions. Personnel in the work area need to understand the rational behind the policies, with whom responsibilities rest and the importance of adhering to them.

A laser planning committee can be established to develop policies and procedures for laser use. The function of the committee will be to make certain the needed policies and procedures are developed. Many individuals can be involved in developing the policies. However, once they are developed, someone must ensure it that they are implemented and followed. Adherance and understanding is greater if personnel are directly involved in the development.

Specific laser policies include those on safety of both personnel and patients, credentialing of medical staff; how to operate the laser; maintenance of laser; location and storage, laser safety committee; scheduling for laser procedures; documentation of laser surgery.

Education and training should be considered for all personnel who will be working with the laser surgeons, anestheologists, nurses, and technicians.

Laser Committee

The responsibilities of the committee are:

- Coordinate the detailed formation of a laser programme.
- Evaluate and select the laser system to be purchased.
- Identify, develop, review and approve the policies and procedures.

- Ensure compliance with safety protocols and credentialing criteria.
- Assist in the budget process and development of hospital charges for laser use.
- Provide ongoing monitoring and evaluation of all aspects of laser programme.
- Ensure appropriate documentation.

Membership

Membership of laser committee may include:

- Medical Director or delegate
- Laser safety officer
- Medical staff representative from each speciality using or intending to use laser
- Chief of anesthesia or delegate
- Nursing supervisory personnel or delegates from clinical areas where the laser systems are used.
- Staff members specifically responsible for laser (Co-ordinators).
- Bio-medical engineering representative
- Hospital administration representative
- Nursing administration representative
- Quality assurance representative.

Physical Requirements

Installation requirements vary greatly between laser system and also between lasers manufactured by different companies.

The "argon laser" requires special `hard wiring' for permanent electrical connection. This laser is water-cooled and requires at least 50 psi of dynamic pressure with connection to a water source and drainage system. A constant flow of at least 2.5-5 gallons/min is needed and a capital air tank must be provided if flow transients are likely to occur. Power needed is between 190-240 V supplied from three phase 50/60 Hz, four-wire, WYE connected source. Each phase should rate 40A three phase switch must be in the input line. Normal phase voltage is 208 V. Argon lasers connected to a slit lamp require 100-240 V AC, 40-60 Hz. Argon laser may be placed anywhere in the room.

Carbon dioxide lasers require 11-120 V AC/ 7.5-15 A and may be connected to standard room outlets since they have a self contained power supply. Cooling is accomplished by recirculating water systems, lasers must be conveniently mobile.

Nd:YAG lasers may require connection to both plumbing and electricity depending on the manufacturer. Power required varies from 208 V AC, three phase, 50A, 50 Hz to 380 V AC three-phase, 25A, 50 Hz. The water flow rate varies and some lasers are air cooled. Beam delivery is by quartz fibre. Newer laser systems use 110V-222VC power.

If new operating room facilities are being designed, provisions for window protections, warning signs, power switches and interlocks should be considered. Painted facilities with special finishes—dark blue, flat black—may be used to minimize reflections. Recent interest in the free electron laser technology may rekindle interest in the design of special operating rooms to house these devices which are likely to be inherently larger and may generate associated ionizing radiation.

Remote controls, such as foot switches, are often used, to operate a laser. Foot switches are shrouded to prevent accidental activation of laser beam.

Future Trends

The primary lasers in medical use today are:

- Argon
- Carbon dioxide
- Excimer
- Nd:YAG

Major future trend in laser technology include

- Coronary angioplasty
- Photo-dynamic therapy
- Corneal sculpting, and
- Orthopaedics.

New lasers which are being researched and have potential to expand medical laser application into areas which have only been dreamt about are:

- Helium laser
- Erbium laser

- Alexandrite laser
- Titanium doped saphire laser,
- Smart laser' (broadly tunable laser coupled to a tissue identification system) where the laser wavelength can be tuned to the type of tissue targeted.

Coronary Angioplasty

- *Excimer laser* a VU laser emitting at 308 mm, vaporizes plaques and blood vessel wall is not endangered;
- Pulse dye laser turned into a 'smart laser', which is capable of distinguishing between normal and calcified tissue and able to irradiate selectively.

Photodynamic Therapy (PDT)

Treatment of tumours in conjunction with a drug that concentrates selectively in tumours and when exposed to a specific laser beam a photo-chemical reaction occurs, resulting in a toxic agent which kills the cell.

Corneal Sculpting

The idea is precisely to reshape the cornea to form a contact lens-like contour. The appropriate laser is excimer.

Orthopedics

There is presently no safe and efficient bone cutting laser. The excimer laser seems to be a solution.

The use of lasers in medical and surgical applications is rapidly expanding and impinges upon many disciplines from the clinical laboratory to the operating room.

Health-care providers are in a unique position to make decisions for the future relating to innovative technology for quality patient care. The team approach to decision making about developing, implementing or expanding a multi-speciality laser programme is the wave of the future. Administrators, clinicians nurses, and medical personnel will have to continue their education and increase their skills in laser technology and patient care. Administrator has to play a vital role in the development of a laser programme which requires strategic planning, with careful analysis of the appropriate financial information to determine the feasibility of the development of a laser programme. Appointment of a laser task force to survey the medical staff, determine the laser system appropriate for the facility, develop and approve policies and procedures, and recommend credentialing criteria. Participate in training of laser support personnel, and with a cooperative effort implement the laser programme. Administration will have responsibility to establish a laser programme that meets corporate goals.

FURTHER READING

1. Apfelberg B David: Evaluation and installation of surgical laser system. Springer Verlag: New York, 1987.
2. Burkardt SS: The medical use of lasers. *J Operat Room Res Inst* 1982.
3. Flasher JC: The medical laser: An indispensable tool of physician and surgeon. *Medical Instrument* 1983.
4. Hikether SE: How Lasers Work *AORN J* 1983.
5. Lundergan DK: Developing and maintaining a laser safety program. Honolulu: Hawaii, 1985.
6. Osoff R: ANSI Standards for clinical laser Safety-Clin Laser Monthly, 1984.
7. Rockwell RJ: Laser safety Hazards, Inspection and control. Laser Institute of America, Ohio 1982.
8. Tabish SA: Planning a Medical Laser Programme. *JAHA* **2**: 65-70, 1990.

RADIODIAGNOSIS DEPARTMENT

Programming for better medical and surgical care frequently depends on the availability of prompt, thorough, and skillful diagnostic services. Among the many modern diagnostic techniques, X-ray examinations contribute vitally to facilitating effective medication and treatment. The modern radiologic department frequently services as a centre for daily consutlations in the hospital as a focal point for the provision of teaching or teaching cases (for medical, dental, nursing and allied personnel and as an important link in the research programme of the institution. A carefully planned department assures an efficient flow of service that may be scheduled promptly and expedited with a minimum of movement and distance for the staff and the patient. In modern hospitals, the mission of the radiology department revolves around the acquisition, manipulation, storage, retrieval and analysis of images. Since the early 1960s, significant progress has been made in the conversion of analog images into digital formats. The digital handling of images has had a dramatic impact on the ability of the radiologist to manipulate and to analyse radiographic studies. The shift to digital formats is resulting in the introduction of major computer resources into the department. Areas specially affected include CT, digital subtraction angiography (DSA), MRI nuclear medicine and ultrasound.

The therapy unit includes treatment of varying intensities ranging from superficial therapy to cobalt therapy.

Function

The primary function of radiologic department is the provision of radiologic services of adequate quality and quantity of hospitalized patient; secondary functions include clinic and other outpatient services, teaching and research.

Planning

The primary planning is based on patient traffic, which includes accessibility, promptness of attention, comfort, convenience, privacy, thoroughness of examination or treatment. The main aim is to provide prompt and accurate examination and treatment in pleasant surroundings. This can be achieved by following a strict appointment system. The secondary planning is based on film flow, as the efficiency and speed with which reports are delivered. The tertiary planning is based on technicians' traffic, in order that a minimum of personnel can expedite the exmination and treatment with maximum efficiency and minimum fatigue. The quartan planning is based on achieving most effective traffic pattern for the radiologist and provisions staff so that they may interview, examine and treat patient as quickly and thoroughly as possible.

The planning and design of the radiologic department is guided by the following factors:

a. Daily average number of patient examination. This depends on the type of hospital, community need, proportion and extent of outpatient and inpatient examination and the pattern of facility usage.
b. The quality and extent of diagnostic and therapeutic services to be provided.
c. Number and type of X-ray machines needed.
d. The staff needed for the estimated volume of work.

The department of radiology should be planned and organized according to the estimated patient peak load during the five year period to follow, with due allowance for prospective expansion for teaching, associated research programmes and other developments. One third of this figure is contributed by inpatients and the remaining are outpatients. The staff needed for this volume of work usually includes:

1 Radiologist, 2 or 3 Technicians, 1 Receptionist, 1 File clerk and 1 orderly (as needed).

In planning a cobalt installation, it should be understood that each type of machine and its location within the building will present a different problem which will require an individual solution. Therefore, during preliminary design stages, close co-operation between architect, radiologist and radiation physicist is necessary to develop an efficient and economic layout. The design of the structural system of the building of teletherapy unit depends on (a) the type of machine (b) strength of the source (c) desired location, and (d) the shielding required for floor walls and ceilling.

Physical Facilities

The Radiodiagnosis department should be located on the ground floor, conveniently accessible both the outpatients and inpatients, and to related medical services. When it is planned to include megavoltage radiotherapy equipment it may be advisable to choose a location below the ground surface, if adequate airconditioning is provided. However, it should be borne in mind that high moisture content is dangerous where high voltage apparatus is used. In the average hospital, it is preferable for the diagnostic and tehrapeutic divisions of the departments to be located together.

The fundamental requirements of the department are best satisfied by locating the X-ray rooms at the end of a wing. In this location, the activity within the department will not be disturbed by through traffic to other parts of the hospital, and less shielding will be required because of the exterior walls.

Layout

Every radiologist has specific ideas on the most suitable ways of arranging and operating the administrative functions of the department. Some of the variables involved are assignment of personnel and functions, reception of patients, sequence of patient examination, film distribution, and staff viewing facilities. However, the planning and layout of the department should be free from individual bias. The following items of physical facilities are essential for radiography:

a. *Administrative Spaces*
   - Waiting room 150-300 sq ft
   - Receptionist 80-100 sq ft
   - Clerk
   - Doctors viewing room
   - Radiologists office 200 sq ft
   - Film files.

b. *General facilities*
   - Dressing rooms
   - Patient's toilet room
   - Technician's toilet and workers

c. *Storage facilities*
   - General storage
   - Clean linen and gown storage
   - Janitor's closet

d. *Diagnostic X-ray rooms*
   - X-ray equipment room 100-200 MA=250 sq ft
   - Control booth 500 MA=400 sq ft
   - Storage cabinet and waiting counter

e. *Film processing and distribution areas*
   - Dark room 100 sq ft
   - Film processing area
   - Collection and distribution area

f. *Barium mixing facilities*

g. *Optional facilities*
   - Inter communication system
   - Refrigerator
   - High-speed film dryer

h. *Electrical installations*
   - Voltage
   - Illumination

i. *Radiation protection*

k. *Air-conditioning*

l. *Fire safety*

Waiting Room

The size will depend on the patient load. One hall may be so planned as to serve patients waiting before and after registration. This is located at the entrance of the department. From here the patient is directed to an assigned dressing room. A separate area may be provided for wheelchair and stretcher patients. Sufficient chairs or benches should be provided for waiting cases and their attendants.

Receptionist Counter

The administrative functions and business records of the department, scheduling of appointments, receiving of patients and assigning of patients to dressing rooms are handled by the receptionist. The size of the counter should be sufficient to accommodate a clerk's seat and record chests. It may be 80 to 100 sq ft and juxtaposed to the waiting hall.

Doctor's Viewing Room

It should be located near the office of the chief radiologist so that he may be immediately available for consultation. Its location within the administrative unit provides privacy so that diagnostic comments and discussions will not be overheared by patients.

Radiologist's Office

In large hospitals, the department is placed under a specialist. He needs a spacious room where he engages himself with the study of films and holding discussion with other specialists. Adequate number of viewing boxes are essential.

Film File Storage

Since it is desirable to keep active films for at least five years, sufficient linear feet of filing space should be provided. Bulletin cup boards may be provided in the chiefs room or in the radiology museum if provided.

Dressing Rooms

Three dressing rooms for each X-ray machine should be provided so that equipment and staff can function without delay. Each look mirror. For the purpose of patients; valuables, the doors may be equipped with locks. A dressing room suitable for wheel chiar patient may be provided.

Patient's Toilet Rooms

Toilets should be immediately available for patients undergoing fluoroscope, and other waiting patients. A minimum of two toilets should be provided for each X-ray room. One of the patient's toilet rooms is designed to accommodate a patient in a wheelchair. One toilet should be provided with a bedpan flushing attachment. Each toilet room should be equipped with a grab bar for use of elderly or weak patients.

General Storage

For bulky supplies, a storage cabinet equipped with sliding doors and adjustable shelves may be located in the corridor near the X-ray rooms. Materials such as films, opaque solutions, developing solutions, and office supplies are stored here.

Radiographic Units

Theatres may consist of any one of the following equipment and the number of rooms could be one or more depending on the size of the hospital

a. 50 MA Units
b. 100 MA Units
c. 200 MA Units
d. 500 MA Units

The optimum size of X-ray room is about 252 ft. Ceiling height requirements vary for different X-ray machines, but a minimum of 9 ft. 6 inch is recommended. The machine and transformer should be placed so as to allow adequate space for admittance of a bed or stretcher in the room. Mounting the transformer and the wall is recommended to save floor space.

It is recommended that the control panel be wired to a signal outside each X-ray room to indicate when the machine is one to prevent other personnel from entering the room.

Control Booth

It is essential that the control booth be located to the right of the machine so the machine so that the patient may be observed when the table is inclined, since machine with a end pivoted tables tilt to the right. Under this arrangement additional shielding is not necessary as the primary beam would be directed towards the outside wall.

Dark Room

This room is located between two X-ray rooms to facilitate handling of films. The size of the dark room need not be more than 100 sq ft. The following items may be provided:

a. A hatch window between the X-ray rooms and dark room.
b. A counter for loading and stacking casettes.
c. A partition to separate loading counter from the film processing area.
d. A light lock between the dark room and the light-room, equipped with interlocking doors.
e. A utility tank with a drain board, located opposite the processing tank, for mixing chemical solutions and hand washing.
f. A film processing area consisting of developing tank, fixing tank and washing tank placed in that order.
g. Exhaust fans.

Film Drying

Atmospheric drying is generally resorted to. As this is time consuming, a steel cupboard, filled with a network of heating elements at top and an exhaust fan at the bottom, may be improvised for the purpose. Film dryer units are also available. Barium mixing facilities small rooms of size 100 sq ft to 120 sq ft each may be provided for the preparation of barium meal and for injection in large hospitals.

Cassetteless Radiography

Casseteless radiography is a system in which magazines are loaded with X–ray film. Upon activation of the system, a film of appropriate size is automatically fed into a chamber between a pair of stationary "intensifying" screens where it is tightly sandwiched. A phototimed X–ray exposure is then made, the sandwich is then opened and the film is transported out into a dry–to–dry 990 sec film processor. The magazines can be loaded with about 1–day's supply of films. Once the radiographic system has been initially loaded with film technologist need not be concerned with the film in any way until it appears in the receiving bin of the film processor, 2 min after exposure. The need for a dark room is eliminated and the need for loading, unloading, transporting, and storing cassettes is eliminated.

Cassetteless units are available in either vertical or horizontal configuration. The vertical configuration is used for chest radiography and accepts a standard 14 × 17 in (35 × 42.5 cm) film. The design of the system is such that patients in wheelchairs, as well as ambulatory patients, can be radiographed. When dealing with ambulatory patients, one examination can be completed every 2–min.

The horizontal configuration is for table-type radiography and is used for bone and visceral studies. In this system, four different film sizes are loaded into individual magazines. The X-ray table is in a fixed position in relation to the film exposure chamber. The body part to be radiographed is then moved over to this area on a "floating" tabletop and a phototimed exposure is made. The film is then automatically transported to the 90-sec day-to-day film processor.

To increase the versatility of the room, a separate overhead table and well bulky unit can be intermembered for upright radiography. If the room is made light–tight and if sodium vapour illumination is used, these films can be processed in the same room by hand-feeding the exposed film into the film processor. The system can now do all categories of routine radiographic work.

To handle the increased capacity, an adequate number of dressing rooms and patient waiting areas must be provided. These areas should be located adjacent to the elevations to decrease patient flow problems.

It is reasonable to expect that 80 cases can be done in one room in a normal working day. Conventional radiography systems under the same conditions result in caseload of approximately 25 per day. Approximately 40 percent of the procedures done by the department can be done with this equipment.

Approximately 80 percent of the departments daily volume can be done by these two types of radiographic systems.

The advent of cassetteless radiographic units should result in a dramatic decrease in the number of radiographic rooms and dark rooms, resulting in substantial savings in building costs.

Radiation Protection

Protection against ionizing radiations in excess of tolerable amount is necessary. The barrier design should be checked by a qualified expert before the construction plans are approved and the completed installation should be surveyed with radiation detecting devices before the facility is used.

Primary barriers should be provided on all surfaces of the X-ray rooms which are exposed, or which may be exposed, to the useful beam between the X-ray tube and occupied areas. Secondary barriers should be provided on all other room surfaces where protection is needed. In determining secondary barriers, consideration should be given to direct or leakage radiation or other scattered radiation.

Air Conditioning

Air conditioning with positive ventilation and a well defined pattern of air movement within the department is necessary to provide an acceptable environment. In order to prevent odours from the radiographic and fluoroscopic rooms, darkroom, toilet, and janitors closets, the ventilation system should be designed so that a negative air pressure relative to the adjoining corridors will be maintained in these rooms. This can be done by adjustment of exhaust fan in the rooms and corridors. The following conditions are recommended for the comfort of the patients and personnel.

a. Administrative and waiting area: A temperature of 72°F with a relative humidity of 50 percent and a ventilation rate of 1, 1½ air changes per hr.
b. Patients and technicians corridors A temperature of 75 to 80°F with relative humidity of 50 percent and 2 air changes per hour.
c. Fluoroscopic and x-ray rooms A temperature of 75 to 80°F with RH 50 percent and 6 air changes per hour.
d. Dark-room A temperature of 72°F with RH 50 percent and 10 air changes per hour.

Facilities for radiotherapy may be provided to hospitals, as listed below in order of a capacity for penetration:

a. Infra X-ray therapy (15-2KV)	Small (dermatology, Gynae, ENT, Eye.)
b. Contact therapy (50KV)	
c. Superficial therapy (10-18KV)	Medium
d. Intermediary therapy (80-160 KV)	
e. Convergent therapy (160300 KV)	
f. Rotation deep therapy (160-300 KV)	
g. Cobalt therapy	

Physical facilities for radio therapy will include the following:

a. *Waiting room* One for each sex, of size 100-150 sq ft with toilet facilities.
b. *Pysician's room* The specialist incharge of the department should also be provided with of room of size 150 sq ft. The staff of the department should also be provided with room of size 150 sq ft. A toilet should be provided.

c. *Therapy rooms* Each therapy room should have adequate space for accommodating the therapy apparatus, the high voltage generators control desk and dressing cubicle for patients.
   i. Contact therapy room will include the apparatus, bed and dressing cubicle within size 120 sq ft.
   ii. Superficial and intermediary therapy rooms will include the apparatus and bed. Control desk and dressing cubicle are provided outside the influence of radiation. Size of room may be 150 sq ft in addition 50 sq ft. For control and dressing.
   iii. Deep therapy rooms will be designed functionally similar to superficial and intermediary therapy rooms. To prevent deep penetration, strong protection is required. The size of room may be 200 sq ft.
   iv. Cobalt therapy involves deeper penetration and greater radiation and requires protection of still higher order. The size of the room may be 300 sq ft.

Structure of Radiotherapy rooms: The design of structure should be such as to prevent escape of radiation. The thickness as walls, floors and ceilings has to vary with the intensity of radiation. For superficial and intermediary therapy rooms, 13.½" thick walls and 6" thick RCC roofs will be adequate. They may be painted with lead borne paints. For deep and cobalt therapy rooms the walls and ceiling should be or RCC 12" and 14" thick. Door should be made radiation proof.

Mobile X-ray Unit

In large hospitals, X-ray facilities are required additionally in the emergency, orthopedic, dental and operating departments. The equipment may be of moible type. Stereoscope, and in teaching hospitals sometimes a laminograph for taking pictures at successive layers. There may be a special unit for taking a sequence of exposure, rapidly, almost like a movie, used in angiography and called cineradiography. X-ray units are also often required in one or more of the surgical operating rooms for orthopedic work and for gallbladder operations. Such installations make a ceiling-mounted tube mandatory. The room used for cystoscopy also requires a special X-ray unit which is an integral part of the cystoscopy operating table.

Portable Units

Portable X-ray units, now available up to 500 ma, will require storage space adjacent to the X-ray department for control. A 4-by 5-in. Chest screening unit is sometimes located in admitting, and a separate radiographic unit may be needed in emergency. If radiology can be located close to emergency, it is better to take the emergency patient to the radiology department or to use a portable than to have a separate and little-used unit installed in emergency. Even where economy of investment in equipment is not a prime consideration, better results will for a fluoroscope in the ambulant patient department. Here the consideration is not only cost of equipment but also the desirability of having the radiologist present to assist the internist, the surgeon, the orthopedist, the urologist, and other in interpreting the X-ray shadow picture, whether it be one film or on fluorscopic screen. Having a separate fluoroscope in the clinic for convenience of the internist tends to encourage his independent use of it without counsel from the radiologist and may thus prevent the best and fullest utilization of the professional staff. There is also some danger of excessive use.

FUNCTIONAL PROGRAMME

The functional programme for a 500-bed hospital with an active ambulant patient service may be:
- Five radiographic units-300 ma for general work.
- Six combined radiographic-fluoroscopic—two 500 ma and four 300 ma for GI work
- One special head unit
- One radiographic unit in the orthopedic operating room

- One radiographic unit in a major operating room
- Two portable units-one 25 ma and one 300 ma.

Central service rooms necessary to support these diagnostic units include first a darkroom, desirably located so that films can be passed into it through lightproof boxes directly from the radiographic rooms. The special requirements of this room, including automatic developing, are fully detailed in the literature. Storage space is needed for unexposed film and for developed films and supplies. A film viewing room with banks of shadow boxes should adjoin the film filing room and also departmental offices for the radiologists and technologists.

Planning by formula is dangerous, but programme data can be formulated.

$$\text{No. of radiographic rooms} = \frac{\text{DTY}}{\text{DW} \times \text{WKS} \times \text{HD} \times \text{DTRH}}$$

DTY = determinations per year

Figure radiographic and combination radiographic and fluoroscopic rooms separately if the load figures are available. Also take out determinations for cytoscopy, emergency, cast room, and other operations.

DW = days per week in operation
WKS = weeks per year in operation
HD = hours per day in operation
DRRH = determination per room per hour

DTRH vary from 2 to 6, depending upon the determination. Use 4, or if experience indicates otherwise, use 3 (i.e., 15 to 20 minutes per determination).

The determination of how many diagnostic units can be justified in a given size of hospital is difficult (Fig. 35.24). The factors in this calculation follow:

1. The estimated number of determinations for hospital bed patients each patient visit counts as a determination, regardless of the number of pictures taken.
2. The same for ambulant patients.
3. The days and hours of scheduled service in the X-ray department.
4. The estimated capacity of each diagnostic unit in determination per hour.
5. The extent to which teaching is carried on.
6. The percentage of special cases requiring extra time and attention.
7. The relative limitation of budget upon floor space and equipment.

The point is to estimate the load and to programme the reasonable personnel and facilities to carry it (the rule of three). The load from hospital bed patients for general radiographic and GI work may be calculated thus:

1. Medical patients may be average 1.5 determinations per patient admission, which generates.

$$\frac{1.5 \times 80\% \text{ occupancy}}{8 \text{ days average stay}} = \begin{array}{l}0.15 \text{ determination}\\ \text{per bed per day}\end{array}$$

2. Surgical patients may be average 3.0 determinations per patient admission, including specialities, giving

$$\frac{3.0 \times 85\% \text{ occupancy}}{5 \text{ days average stay}} = \begin{array}{l}0.5 \text{ determination}\\ \text{per bed per day}\end{array}$$

3. Maternity patients may be average 0.4 determination per patient, giving

$$\frac{0.4 \times 70\% \text{ occupancy}}{6 \text{ days average stay}} = \begin{array}{l}0.05 \text{ determination}\\ \text{per bed per day}\end{array}$$

4. Pediatric patients (mostly surgery) average 2.5 determinations per patients, giving

$$\frac{2.5 \times 60\% \text{ occupancy}}{5 \text{ days average stay}} = \begin{array}{l}0.3 \text{ determination}\\ \text{per bed per day}\end{array}$$

5. Mental and other long-term patients are negligible, perhaps 0.1 determination per patient admission, giving.

$$\frac{0.1 \times 95\% \text{ occupancy}}{20 \text{ days average stay}} = \begin{array}{l}0.5 \text{ determination}\\ \text{per bed per day}\end{array}$$

Because most radiographic work can be scheduled at will, it is possible to use average figures rather than to figure peak load requirements. Not many patients must be X-rayed immediately as an emergency.

If actual figures on X-ray determinations are available, it will be more accurate to use them than

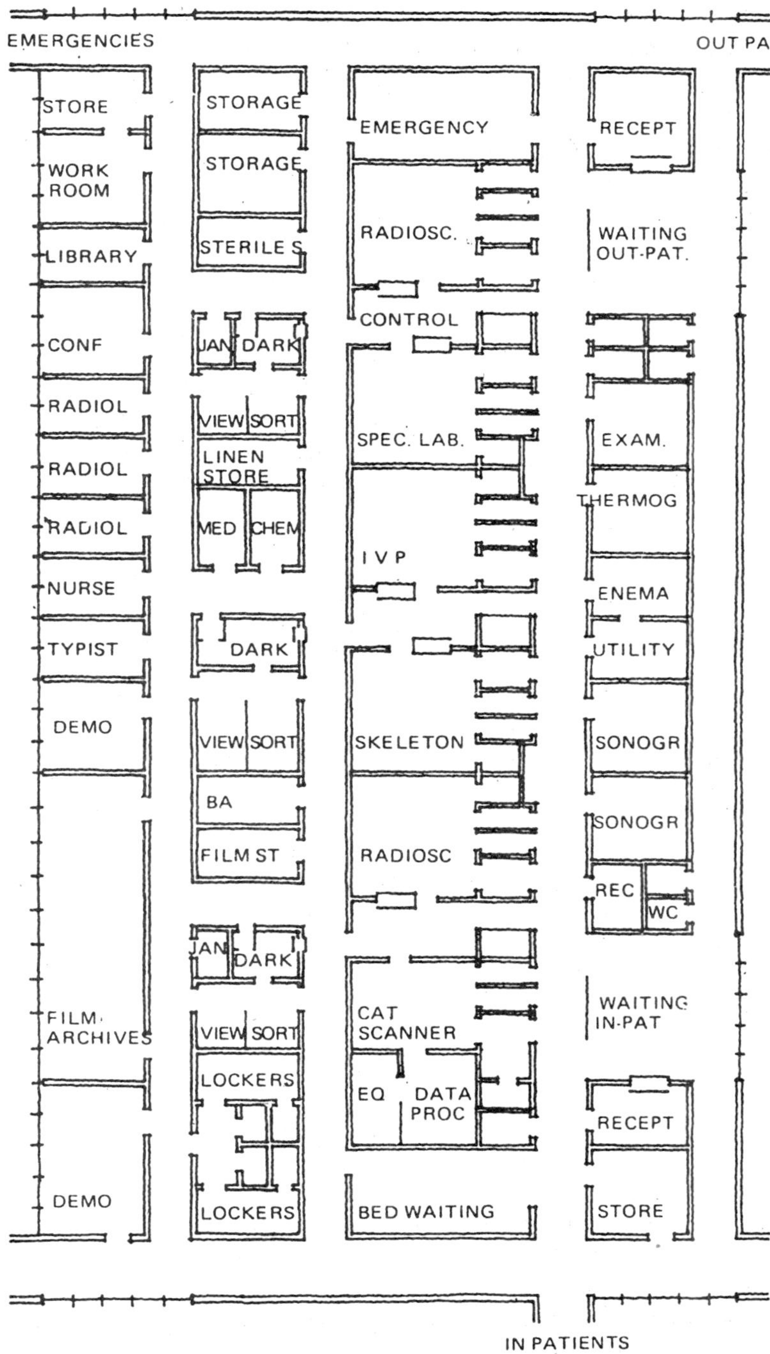

Fig. 35.24: A linear radiodiagnostic department for a 600-bed hospital

to calculate the loads as indicated, but with a new hospital where experience figures are lacking, the estimates should be used. Local conditions, however, can modify the load units suggested.

From these factors can be estimated the load from bed patients for a sample 500 bed hospital.

Type	*Factor*	*No. of beds*	*No of determinations per day*
Medical	0.15	152	23
Surgical	0.5	168	84
Maternity	0.05	70	3.5
Paediatrics	0.30	70	21
Psychiatric	0.005	40	0.5
		500	**132**

Consideration must also be given the kinds of determinations. Again applying empirical factors, we find the following.

Unit	*% of total*	*Determinations per day*
General radiographic	50	68
GI	30	40
Other special	20	26
	100	**132**

The units for cystoscopy, other operating rooms, routine chest stereo, and portable should be excluded, since they are set by factors other than the quantitative load, and the cystoscopic determinations, if known should be deducted from the third category above.

	100 bed	*200 bed*	*300 bed*	*400 bed*	*500 bed*
Determinations/year	6600	13300	20000	29000	36500
Days per week	3	5	5	5½	5½
Hours per day	5	5	7	7	7
Determinations per hour	3	3	2-3	2-4	2-4
Radiographic units	1	2	3	4	4
Combined radiographic fluoroscopic	1	1	2	3	4
Special units	–	–	–	1	1
Orthopedic OR	–	1	1	1	1
Cysto OR	–	–	–	1	1
Portable unit	1	1	1	1	1
Total units	3	5	8	13	15
X-ray therapy	–	1	1	2	2
Radium therapy	–	–	–	1?	1?
Radiologists and researchers	½	1	4	6	9
Technologists, etc	4	10	13	20	22
Department area, SFG	2400-3000	4600-5800	6600-8400-10800	10000	13000
Area per user, SFG	600	475	440	365	370
Area per bed SFG	24-30	23-29	29-28	21-27	20-26

These quantities will support only emergency outpatient loads using the diagnostic room itself, as is sometimes done, is both to free the diagnostic room for capacity use (four determinations, per hour) and to give the patients privacy while undressing and dressing. In a small unit with light load these may not be critical factors and the dressing room may be omitted, but toilets must be provided. The problem is complication.

Construction Recommendation

Ceiling mounted equipment requires properly designed rigid support structures located above the finished ceiling. The bottom of the structure should be flush with the finished ceiling. Through–button or welding of these structures is recommended.

A light-out type ceiling is recommended in most radiological departments for ease of service, installation and remodeling. This may be a 60 × 60 cm or 60 × 120 cm grid system.

Room lighting requirements vary with the examination and equipment involved. Both general ceiling and cove lighting are recommended. Dimmer controls on lights are required in some rooms, particularly special procedure rooms and fluoroscopic rooms.

Trough or trench ducts with removable covers are recommended to facilitate the installation of the required cable connections between the various equipment components.

Trough or trench ducts with removable covers are recommended to facilitate the installation of the required cable connections between the various equipment components.

Trough or trench ducts simplify the equipment installation and permit plugged interconnecting cable type installation. This type of design dramatically reduces installation time and also allows future changes.

The ampacity (for the X–ray diagnostic rooms) of supply branch conductors and overcurrent protective devices shall not be less than 50 percent of the momentary rating or 100 percent of the long-time rating, whichever is the greater.

The rated ampacity of conductors and over-current devices of a feeder for a two or more branch supplying circuits supplying X-ray units shall not be less than 100 percent of the momentary demand rating of the momentary ratings of the X-ray apparatus.

Provisions should be made for emergency electrical power in the event of a power failure.

Specifications should be made 480V, 240V, and 208V three–phase 60Hz power supply, delta and Wye type systems for single-phase equipment. A 480V system is recommended.

Voltage regulation must not exceed full momentary load of a specific KVA at a certain power factor percentage. The phase-to-phase utilization voltage has limited tolerance and daily voltage variation, due to causes other than X–ray equipment, and must not exceed a ± percentage factor (± 5 percent).

The relative humidity in all the examination rooms be maintained at between 35 to 60 percent. Air-charge rate should be received.

Rooms and corridors should be bright, cheerful, and habitable for staff and patients. Murals are often used.

Diagnostic Radiology

Diagnostic X–ray rooms are grouped according to their specialty with the radiograph rooms located nearest the patient waiting areas. The rooms are also situated around the darkrooms in an effort to keep film cassettes carrying to a minimum.

Toilets serving the fluoroscopic rooms are designed so that the patient can enter the toilet directly from the diagnostic rooms and exit from the toilet without re-entering the X–ray room.

Adequate dressing booths must be provided. X–ray control booths should be designed to provide adequate radiation protection for the operator.

LASER IMAGING IN CLINICAL RADIOLOGY

Hospital departments of clinical radiology (X–ray departments) use many different diagnostic-imaging modalities of which plain radiographs (conventional X–ray film exposures) are only one example. Most conventional radiographs are made using a combination of film and screen, the film exposure being predominantly due to light exposure in response to X-rays, by two rare–earth phosphor intensifying screens, between which the dual emulsion–coated radiographic film is sandwiched in an X-ray film cassette. Other imaging modalities in radiology departments not involving direct or indirect exposure to radiographic film include digital radiography, digital subtraction angiography, computed tomography, magnetic resonance imaging, ultrasound scanning including Doppler ultrasound, duplex Doppler ultrasound and colour flow Doppler ultrasound, nuclear medicine scanning and infra-red thermal imaging. All of these result in a video image viewed on a television monitor screen, from which hardcopy must be made; this was traditionally achieved by photographing a TV screen with inevitable deterioration in image quality.

Laser imaging is the modern preferred method of accurately producing such hard copy, which is the superior reproduction of the television image, by converting analog or digital signals from an imaging system into a laser beam which scans a photographic film. The signal from which the image is constructed can be transferred from its source to the laser imager through hard wiring, fibre optical cable, or on digitally recorded disks; each method has advantages and disadvantages in particular situations. This paper describes the application of laser imaging in clinical radiology departments.

Imaging Modalities Producing a Video Output

Digital radiography In digital radiography, an X-ray image produced by an image intensifier is recorded digitally and stored in a computer memory, replacing the conventional X-ray film (an image intensifier is a device for greatly enhancing the faint fluorescence of an input phosphor screen in response to radiation, electron release and capture, causing much brighter fluorescence of an output phosphor screen viewed by a TV camera). The resulting image is viewed on a TV monitor.

Digital subtraction angiography Digital subtraction angiography (DSA) previously known as digital vascular imaging (DVI), is similar to digital radiography but may be included as an "add–on" to older fluoroscopic imaging equipment as well as being built into digital radiographic instrument.

In DSA, summated TV frames early in a sequence of images during a dynamic vascular examination are subtracted pixel by pixel from latter summated TV frames, following intra-vascular injection of a radiographic contrast medium. This results in imaging only those structures in the field of view opacified by the contrast medium, with subtraction of overlying bony structures. This is analogous to a similar technique applied in the past using photographic subtraction of a plain radiograph taken before contrast medium injection from a later one in which the blood vessels were opacified by contrast medium. DSA is very sensitive and can satisfactorily image considerably diluted contrast medium. For example, faintly opacified arteries can be imaged following intravenous injection of contrast medium, which becomes diluted when mixed with blood during the passage through the right heart chambers, the pulmonary vascular system and the left side of heart before entering the systemic arterial circulation. This is a less invasive procedure than conventional arteriography, and can be performed on an outpatient basis. The image data may be recorded digitally, as in digital radiography, or on older systems may be recorded on magnetic recording tape in analog form. The subtraction images can be viewed dynamically on a TV monitor either as a continuous real time image showing the gradual appearance and disappearance of contrast medium in the blood vessels being studied, or as regularly upgraded static images at short time intervals. The optimal images can then be frozen for production of hard copy.

Computed tomography Computed tomography (CT or computer assisted tomography–CAT scanning) uses measurements of X-ray attenuation recorded by an array of detectors from a thin fan–beam of X-rays. The X-ray source and detector array rotate circumferentially around the patient. This results in millions of measurements of X-ray attenuation, which can be used to reconstruct an image of an axial slice through the patient by computer analysis using a back-projection method.

Images can be reformated in other planes, such as coronal and sagittal, by summating information from adjacent axial slices. It is possible to constructed 3-D images of bones and of blood vessels opacified with radiographic contrast medium. The latest generation of CT scanners use helical or spiral scanning instead of planar scanning of individual axial slices, resulted in decreased scanning time and allowing better dynamic imaging of blood vessels following contrast medium injection.

Magnetic resonance imaging Magnetic resonance imaging (MRI) uses the principles of nuclear magnetic resonance (NMR) to produce cross-sectional images without the use of ionising radiation. The patient is placed in a strong magnetic field, typically 0.5–1.5 Tesla (5000–15000 Gauss-where the earth's magnetic field is 0.7 Gauss). Radio-frequency pulses are applied at the same frequency as the precession frequency of the protons (hydrogen atoms) present in the body, causing them to resonate like tuning forks of the same frequency. Some of the protons that are aligned with the applied magnetic field will invert and "flip" as a result and, if the radio–frequency pulse is long enough, the protons will all precess in phase rather than randomly. When the radio frequency pulse is removed the protons will revert to their former state; those which have inverted will return to their earlier alignment, and they will cess randomly. This results in very small magnetic field changes which can be detected by receiving coils, amplified and reconstructed into cross–sectional images in any plane.

Ultrasound scanning Ultrasound scanning uses a probe operating by the piezo–electric effect to emit ultrasound frequency 3.5–10 Mhz into the patient, and receive internal echoes from internal structures, producing real–time, grey scale image displaying the echo–intensity as a 2–D image on a TV monitor. Doppler ultrasound allows flow within the vessels to be displayed, in duplex Doppler, the 2–D image and Doppler waveform are displayed simultaneously, allowing accurate placement of sampling gate over the region of interest. Color flow Doppler allows different colors (usually red and blue) to flow in different directions, so that adjacent arteries and veins are displayed in different colors superimposed on the monochrome ultrasound image.

Nuclear medicine Nuclear medicine imaging, or gamma camera scanning, produces images from gamma rays emitted by a radionuclide injected into the patient. The most common radionuclide used is technelium 99–m (Tc99–m, which is tailored to image different structures or physiology by chelating it with compounds to target specific organs or physiological functions. The emitted gamma rays are detected by a gamma camera consisted of a large lead–sheilded crystal that scintillates when a gamma ray enters it. Groups of phtotmultiplier tubes behind the crystal detect and localize the scintillations, and a computer analyses the resulting electrical signals and reconstructs an image.

Thermal imaging The thermal imaging camera detects infrared (I–R) radiation emitted by the patient, displayed as an image on a TV monitor.

Production of Hard Copy of Video Images

All of the above imaging modalities result in TV images from which hard copy must be made. It is possible to produce hard copy on paper from dry silver copiers or printers, but the preferred medium in hospital practice is a film analogous to a radiograph which is viewed by transmitted light on an X–ray viewing box. In the past, this was achieved using a multi-formal camera, in which a light-sensitive film was used to photograph an image from TV monitor. Essentially, the device consisted of a light–tight black containing a TV monitor screen and a movable lens and/or film, enabling multiple images from the TV screen to be recorded on different parts of the film by photographic means. This had a disadvantage of being a rather large piece of equipment dedicated to one particular imaging modality, with some degradation of hard copy image due to loss of contrast and re resolution plus distortion.

Laser Imaging

The laser imager is a much more sophisticated method of converting an analog or digital signal from an imaging modality into hard copy. The electronic data of image is converted into a digital signal from which a laser beam of corresponding intensity scans across a photographic film exposing it in proportion to the brightness of an image line by line, in exactly the same manner as the electronic beam scans the phosphor screen of a TV monitor. This results in true reproduction with loss of contrast or resolution, free from distortion. The image can be electronically smoothed so that the TV lines are not visible. The photographic film is designed with sensitivity to match the wavelength of the wave output of the laser.

A laser (light amplification by stimulated emission of radiation) is an intense, parallel, coherent beam of light with fixed frequency and phase. The laser beam can be shaped with a collimator lenses or deflected by mirrors. Lasers have many applications in commerce and industry; they are common use in laser printers and CD–players. Laser imagers in clinical radiology use a helium–neon [HeNe] laser or a laser diode.

The HeNe laser is a thermo-emittimng valve, with a warm-up period of 15–20 minutes, emitting a red light of wavelength, 633 nm. It is permanently "on" when the system is operating and has a life-span of 15000–20000 hours. The solid state laser diode has the practical advantage of no warm-up time, and is therefore "on" while printing (about 8 seconds per film), emitting radiation in the infrared range of wavelength 780-820nm. It has a life- span of 80000–100000 hours, sufficient for more than 36000000 films. The laser is self-calibrating using optical feedback to maintain constant output.

The laser optical by which the laser beam is scanned across the film can be galvanometer moving coil system, which can however be prone to interference from vibration or outside electromagnetic fields. A more reliable system uses a rotating multi-faceted mirror which has a faster write speed. The laser spot (pixel) size is 65–85 mm, with a spatial resolution of 11.5–15 line pairs/mm, comparing well with the conventional radiographic film/screen resolution of 4–6 line pairs/mm and mammography non-screen film resolution of 12–16 line pairs/mm.

Laser imagers with a horizontal film transport system can scan a film in eight seconds, with a total film cycle time of 23 seconds allowing a throughput of 156 films an hour. Such rapid throughput is required where multiple imaging modalities require hard copy from the same laser imager. To scan a film in 8 seconds requires imaging of 20000000 pixels, a pixel burst rate of 2500000/second. A single image could have a matrix up to 1024X1024 or more than 1000000 pixels, each of which could be 8, 10, 12 or 16–bits in depth depending on the imaging modality, requiring up to 16000000 bits of information for each image. The image format on a 43 × 35cm film could be 1:1, 2:1, 4:1, 6:1, 9:1, 12:1, 15:1 or 20:1, although for most applications 12:1 is used. Special customer formats can be accommodated with images of different size on the same film and there is also the facility of printing 20 small images on a film which can be cut out for direct mounting into 35mm projector slide mounts.

The first laser images were linked to a single imaging modality (as, for example, the multi–format camera), but the technology quickly progressed to laser imagers with increasing numbers of input channels. The outputs from the various imaging modalities which are served by one laser imager can be in many different TV standards with differing TV line numbers, scan frequencies, interlacing and so on, and may in the form of digital or analog signals. Interfaces are needed between these different inputs and the laser imager computer memory to convert them into the same digital format for the laser to print, this can be quiet difficult technically, but will become easier in future with the adoption of internationally agreed standards for digital communications, DICOM 3 (digital image communications in medicine) and DEFF (data exchange file format).

Linking multiple users to one laser imager can cause difficulties in image data handling due to the large quantities of image data that may be transmitted to the imager in short period of time, or even simultaneously. Early laser imagers used a computer disk as a temporary buffer or permanent means of image storage, but this is relatively slow, can only operate in the read or write mode at any time, and could crash. Thus, while image data is being loaded into the disk, previously loaded data of other images cannot be transmitted to the laser printer. Use of a computer random access memory (RAM) offered a solution, but a multi–modality single RAM can still only handle one input at a time, leading to possible delays if several users attempt to input images simultaneously. The best solution is multiple individual RAM access up to eight inputs, each of which can accommodate two users. Further expansion of the number of users is possible by means of data transmission through digital image stores on computer diskettes which can be loaded into a single input via a digital signal reader. This has particular advantages in ultrasound imaging. For most fixed imaging modalities, such as CT, MRI and so on, a hard link is best, preferably a fibre–optic cable linkage, allowing reliable transmission of images without degradation over distances of up to 1km, thus accommodating imaging modalities which may be sited remote from the main diagnostic imaging department in different parts of the hospital. For shorter distances, hard wiring with copper cable is as alternative.

The digital image manager uses a small recording unit fixed to each ultrasound machine. Images are recorded digitally onto a disk similar to a computer diskette. Each disk automatically encoded with data to instruct the laser imager on the image format to be adopted and on the appropriate contrast and exposure settings related to the particular ultrasound scanner, images stored during scanning can be relayed through the ultrasound video monitor and edited or deleted. Although the disk must be manually removed from the image recorder and physically transferred to the digital disk reader, this is compensated for be significant advantages. First, being mobile, many ultrasound machines are used in more than one location, in particular in intensive care units, and special care baby units, in addition to their usual location in a dedicated scanning room. With a digital imaging system, the recording device is permanently coupled to the ultrasound scanner and thus accompanies the scanner wherever it is used. Second, this system expands the number of ultrasound scanners that can access one laser imager input. The digital disk reader has up to four ports serving any number of ultrasound scanners.

When multiple users input data simultaneously into the laser imager, these are stored individually in the separate multiple RAMs, and then printed in order unless clinical priority has been assigned to an urgent examination which can then jump the queue. Additional handling capacity and versatility can be added to the laser imager by adding a "slave" imager, providing dual printing facilities with the dual printer sited remote from the main unit. Since each imaging modality is programmed to send its images to either the main laser imager or the dual printer, these can each be sited nearer the modalities served in a large department. This arrangement also enables arrangement enables imaging of all modalities to be transferred to one of the laser printers during routine maintenance of the other printer or its film processor.

Input of image data from the linked imaging modalities can be controlled by a linked keypad or through the host imaging modality operating system. This allows choice of format by the user and local storage of image data until the chosen format is filled and transmitted to the laser imager. The exposed laser imager film, after scanning, needs to be developed, fixed, washed and dried.

This is best accomplished by a permanently linked automatic film processor into which the exposed films are directly fed.

A laser imaging system such as that described forms a local area imaging network. This can be upgraded, to a full local area network (LAN) or wider, allowing viewing and manipulating of images on remote terminals in picture archive communication systems (PACS). Available networks include token ring (IBM System), ethernet, fibre distributed data interface (FDDI), Asynchronous Transfer Mode (ATM), Integrated Services Digital Network (ISDN) and Wide Area Network (WAN).

Recent developments in laser imaging include colour laser imagers, allowing printing of colour images from colour flow Doppler Ultrasound and nuclear medicine examinations. The latest development is the dry laser imager. This disposes of wet chemical processing with its associated costs and problems connected with the disposal of spent developer and waste fixer chemicals. The dry laser images produces hard copy indistinguishable in quality and appearance from conventionally processed laser film by photo–thermographic processing with no additional cost.

Furthermore, the unit has a smaller footprint (occupies less floor space) than a conventional laser imager/film processor combination, so it can be fitted into small spaces in existing departments. It is compatible with existing laser imager systems and can provide an upgrade path for existing users.

Laser imaging offers high film quality, high throughput, and versatility to the clinical radiology department. It has revolutionized the production of hard copy both from older and newer imaging technologies with video outputs.

Organization and Staffing

The department should be under the direction of a qualified radiologist. One radiologist is necessary for every 25 patients per day. Busy departments will therefore, need, several qualified radiologists to work in the diagnostic and therapy divisions. The increased use of computer based digital equipment and the arrival of magnetic reasonable imaging (MRI), position Emission Tomography (PET) scanning, cyclotrons, and sophisticated contrast media require a cadre of basic scientists within the department who can provide quality assurance and scientific support for the sophisticated procedures utilizing these new and often prototype technologies.

The number of technicians required for a load of 30-35 patients per day varies from two to three, depending on the type of examinations performed and the amount of non-technical help available. It has been estimated that 2.5 films are required per examination of each patients. At least two clerks or secretaries are required per 30 patients to interview patients, make appointments, type and transmit reports and maintain accurate records.

Patient traffic flow pattern within the department should be evolved by the radiologist in consultation with the chief technician, the representatives of the administrative, medical and nursing staff. It should be ensured that unnecessary waiting and cross patients flow are avoided by adopting a suitable systems.

Records

Policy for reporting: All diagnostic and therapeutic procedures should be reported by the radiologist. Diagnostic reports should be reported as rapidly as possible. Reports for therapeutic procedures are usually provided at the end of the course.

Film identification Every X-ray film should permit identification of the patient, the date of examination and the orientation. Identification may be by means of a direct radiographic method (lead letters and numbers), a photographic method or adhesive labels affixed after processing.

Film filing As a general rule, only a portion of the current films can be available in the X-ray department it self. There is no perfect numbering system. One method is to prefix every X-ray number by

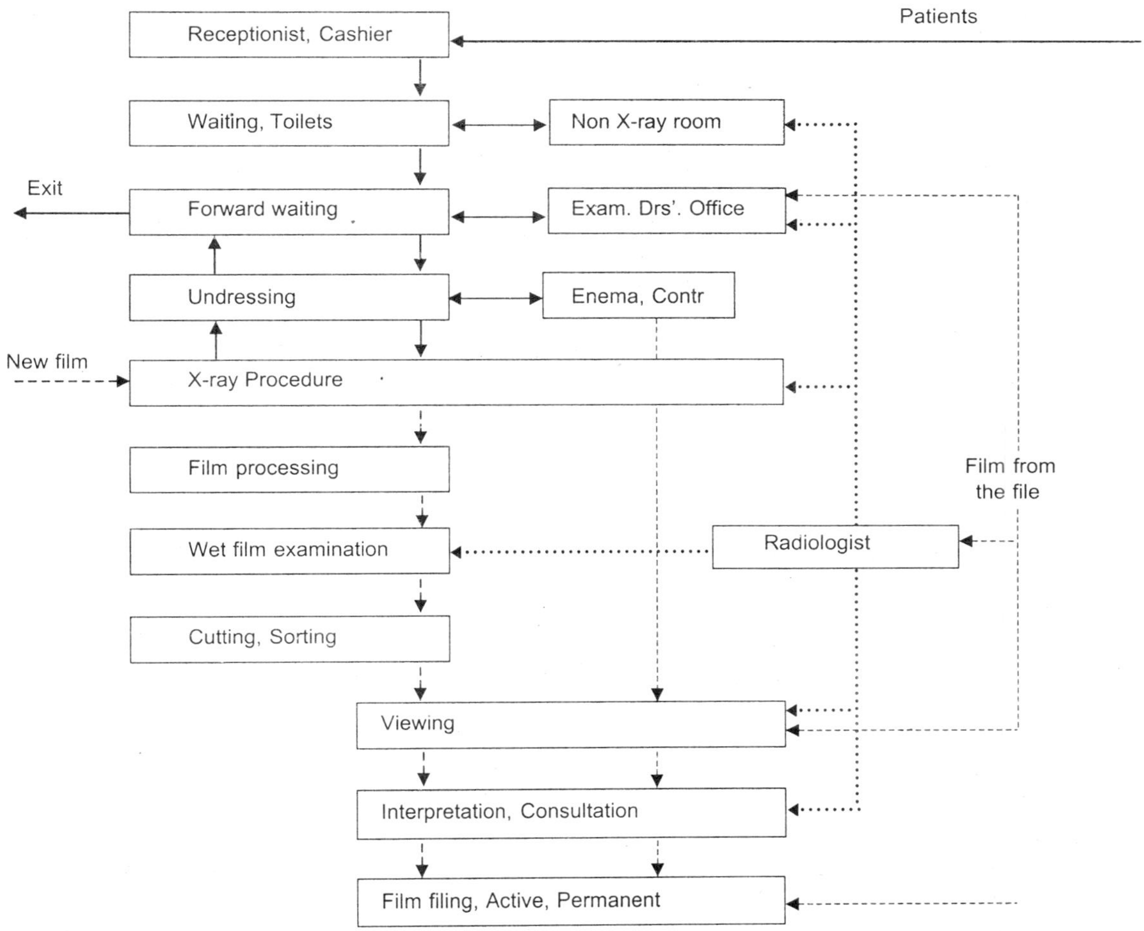

Fig. 35.25: Patient, radiologist and film flow in radiodiagnostic departments

the year. Another method is to have a permanent inactive file number. As regards shelf space, it has been estimated (Scott) that 2½" running inches are required for each 25 diagnostic X-ray examination.

All records are indexed in such a manner as to make them readily available for subsequent references. No better system has been devised than a card index similar to that used in the medical record office. X-ray diagnosis index should be used to enable a study of groups of films pertaining to the same radiological condition.

Film storage has always been a major problem in the hospital. At present Nitrocellulose films have been replaced by acetate X-ray films. Standards have been determined for filing acetate films. The following precautions may be noted:

Both exposed and unexposed films should be stored in metal or other fire resisting container.

Exposed films not of recent date and surplus stock of unexposed films should be stored in a vault as under:

1. It should be located outside the building.
2. Ventilation should confirm to approved standards.
3. Light should be provided by ceiling fixtures protected by vapor proof globes; no portable light being allowed.

4. Automatic sprinklers should be sufficient in number.
5. Automatic fire door with the fusible link inside the vault is essential.

Radiation Protection

The need of the radiological department shall be responsible for observance of any regulations or codes of practice (International Commission on Radiological Protection 1955) on radiation protection, and for the instruction of all personal regarding radiation hazards and methods of control. The following measures are recommended:

Personnel Tests

All new personnel in radiological work shall have a pre-employment blood examination. Blood count, haemoglobin and total and differential white cell count.

Protection

1. When new equipment is installed or when new X-ray departments are opened the site is monitored by a recognised specialist. Modern equipment is shock-proof provided insulation/earthing is serviceable.
2. Personnel monitoring is carried out either by photographic or by ionizing methods. Where the quantum of work is considerable, it is advisable of X-ray workers to carry photographic devices (film badge). In other cases where isotopes are used for diagnosis, treatment and research it is absolutely essential of roll personnel involved to carry ionization devices (Decimator) for protection.
3. The lead aprons and gloves should be worn by technicians.

Experience has proved that the best precaution in the case of total irradiation of the body with X-ray or gamma rays, is not to exceed a 'tolerance zone' generally accepted as 0.3 per week. For local irradiation, 4.5 per week is assumed to be the limit.

CONCLUSION

Because hospitals vary widely in size and scope, no uniform design and facility can be made applicable to all types of hospitals. However, most of the principles for planning, and smaller institutions. There is no doubt that in larger hospitals there will be sub-divisions of diagnostic radiology into subspecialities, such as, angiocardiography, neuro-radiology and paediatric and radiology; use of automation in radiographic exposures, in processing, in recording diagnosis and in transmission of records will occupy the present methods; there will be increasing use of televised roentgenograms permitting immediate consultation for smaller affiliated hospitals located at a distance. Despite all these dramatic developments, a majority of patients will still be interested in personalised medical care provided with competence and kindness and at a reasonable fee. There will continue to be need for personal efficiency, tact promptness and gentleness.

FURTHER READING

1. Amin Tabish: Textbook of Hospital and Health Services Administration. Oxford University Press, 2000.
2. Lawrence F, Wolper and Jesus J Pena: Health Care Administration, Principles and Practices, 1987.
3. Vincent, DC: Administrative and X-ray service. Hospital Management, **108**: 6-67.

MEDICAL RESONANCE IMAGING

The basic function of a radiodiagnostic department is to provide a broad spectrum of diagnostic procedures by directing electromagnetic waves through areas of clinical interest and recording them in a manner that can be interpreted. These studies can include fluoroscopy, radiography, computerized scanning, ultrasound, and other image-forming techniques. The department is responsible for conducting and interpreting the procedures.

Medicine is essentially a search for reduction of uncertainty. The diagnostic process traditionally has relied in combination of educated observation, experience and logical induction. Quantification is relatively recent.

In medicine, and radiology in particular, the opportunities for detailed and scaled observations and diagnostic features or statistically designed trials and laterally for computerized handling of data have offered some solutions to the problems of numeration and proportionality. The shift of radiological paradigm in 1972 with the advent of computed tomography (CT) and the subsequent explosion of microtechnology have provided an opportunity to express and to quantify in detail the content of an image and in particular the ability of biological tissue to interact with various forms of radiation.

Access to a quantitative data, sophisticated interactive display systems and powerful image processing facilities have further facilitated approaches to both tissue characterisation and cellular metabolism.

The newer innovations of CT after that have resulted in significant reduction in radiation.

- Faster imaging time
- More comfort to patient
- Volume acquisition
- Reduced contrast usage
- 3–Dimensional reconstruction of bone, soft tissues and vessels.

The CT Scan Imaging has reduced its peak with the introduction of various spiral/helical CT Scans and sub-second scanners and millisecond scanners. They are able to scan whole body in single or two breath folds, cardiae and other organs in real time and three-dimensional imaging.

Magnetic resonance (MR) proton imaging with its high contrast multiplanar facilities and absence of ionising radiation is currently without doubt the most sensitive and least invasive modality of structural change in CNS. It seems likely in the developed and the developing world to become the primary investigative tool for intracranial disease and many musculo-skeletal disorders.

Since the introduction of clinical imaging in 1972 the techniques of MRI are changing to give better results to help the patient care.

The newer innovations of MRI are :

- MR Angiography to rule out vascular abnormality non-invasively
- Magnetic transfer contrast.
- Chemical shift imaging.
- Magnetic resonance spectroscopy diffusion and perfusion image.

The advantages of MRI are:

1. Excellent tissue characterisation
2. Good spatial resolution of tissue
3. Non-ionising radiation involvement.

Disadvantages are: no metals, implants prosthesis, pacemaker, arterial clips, etc. should be found in patient's body.

All the grandest discoveries of science have been but rewards of accurate measurement and patient, long and continual labour in the minute shifting of numerical results.

The early investigation into the nature of the effect about 150 years age by Christian Andreas Doppler is an interesting story. Because of his work, the effect is named after him. The Doppler effect was used by bats, dolphins and other animals long before humans applied it to their needs.

Doppler ultrasound has been in use in diagnostic medicine for many years. Fetal heart rate monitoring was the first. Application that developed largely in 1980's extended its use to virtually all medicine specialties.

The newer applications of 1990's are:

1. Doppler power imaging
2. Colour Angio
3. 3–D Angio and organ reconstruction, etc.
4. Trans–cranial color duplex Doppler
5. Contrast enhanced color imaging.

Colour duplex image is an elegant technological advancement that superimposes a two-dimension colour flow image on the standard B mode image.

Spiral CT Scan: Trauma

Old Patients—to see exquisite contrast enhancement to detect abnormalities in various organs of human body.

a. Normal organ vascularity with subtle lesion enhancement.
b. Tumor vascularity.
c. Staging of malignancies.

CT Angiography (MIP and surface shaded 3D Angio) of cerebral vessels and other vessels.

Three dimensional reconstruction of various parts of body in;

a. Trauma,
b. Facial reconstruction,
c. Oncological planning.

All these procedures are very easy to do on spiral because we can cover 40 cm in 41 seconds supported by high computer capacity.

The concept of nuclear magnetic resonance (NMR) originated in 1936 by the Dutch-physicist CJ Goter. However, more than 40 years elapsed between the first description of NMR principle and the production of first clinically relevant image. The first successful NMR experiments were described by Bloch and Purcell independently in 1946, paving the way for the development of NMR spectroscopy as a powerful analytical tool in chemistry and biology. Damadian (1971) and Lauterbur (1973) indicated the potential of NMR to obtain images of the intact human body. During the 1980's–advances in engineering and computer technology were combined with newly developed scientific and clinical understanding to produce a completely new addition to the medical diagnostic armamentarium. Continuos research in this field is widening the role of MR in clinical practice.

MR Physics

The hydrogen nucleus is universally used for imaging because of its great natural abundance in biologic tissue. In the presence of an external magnetic field, the hydrogen nuclei precess. After addition of radiofrequency energy, there is deflection of the net magnetization vector by 90 degrees. These deflected spins are temporarily in phase and the excited nuclei are precessing in synchrony. They return to equilibrium after the excitation pulse and this is termed magnetic relaxation. There are two types; longitudinal (T1) and transverse (T2). Most of the pulse sequences commonly employed are designed to exploit the differences in relaxation times to optimize visualization of structures. On MR, the same tissue can be show to be dark, bright or other shades of grey, depending on the pulse sequence used. Various pulse sequences can be used to produce T1 (TR) and short echo times–TE. T2 weighted images (long repetition times and long echo times). Conventional T2-weighted images take a longer time as compared to T1-weighted sequences. In general, T1 and T2-weighted images represent anatomy and pathology respectively. On routine spin echo T1-weighted images water, CSF, urine I are dark (hypointense) while fat and all paramagnetic substances like melanin, intra and extracellular hemoglobin, proteinaeceous fluid are bright (hyperintense). On T2 weighted images, CSF or water is bright and fat becomes grey. Gadolinium DTPA, which is the most commonly used paramagnetic contrast agent enhances tissues on T1-weighted images by shortening their T1 relaxation times.

Types of MR Systems

There are basically two types of magnets used in MR machines–permanent and superconducting. Permanent magnets are usually of low field strengths, in the range of 0.2 to 0.3 Tesla (T). These systems are comparatively cheaper and have a very low maintenance cost. MRI using superconducting magnets are in the midfield to high field strength ranging from 0.5 to 1.5 T. The higher the field strength, the better is the image resolution and shorter is the time taken to do the study. However they are more expensive. High field strength magnets incorporate newer software like MR angiography, fast spin echo and 3D imaging, etc. for routine clinical use.

Magnetic Response imaging, or MRI, is one of the most remarkable diagnostic technologies available today.

This new diagnostic imaging modality provides pictures of the inside of the human body as never seen before, utilizing magnetic properties of the human body, exeternal magnetic systems, and radio frequency waves. Excellent sectional images of the body are obtained in any desired plane giving minute anatomical details. The MR system consists of a large, sophisticated magnet weighing about 5 to 7 tons and having specially designed electronics, computers, consoles display television monitors and documenting devices.

It is so precise that physicians can often get as much information from MRI as they would from looking directly at the human body.

The MRI is superior to other systems in being relatively non-invasive. It potrays the morphological details of the human system with excellent resolution and without loss of definition. It does not require hospitalization usually. To date, no harmful effects have been observed from magnetic influences.

MRI can help diagnose a variety of conditions faster and safer than ever before. It is especially invaluable in:

Brain

The unique contrast resolution of MRI, is the fact that it can present images in multiple planes without loss of definition, and the very important aspect that calcium does not interfere makes the head the most important structure of the human body that benefits from MRI. The advantages of MRI over any other modality are in the following conditions:

MRI

Brain	–	Where CT is equivocal
	–	Tumors, infections.
	–	Pituitary.
Spine	–	Cord abnormalities.
Musculo skeletal	–	Muscle/soft tissue abnormalities. Marrow abnormalities.

Colour duplex Doppler finds its applications in:

- Almost all the vascular structures in the human body like carotid, vertebral, femoral, arterial, venous, renal arteries, etc.
- Pregnancy, cord abnormalities.
- Thyroid eye balls, testes, breast.
- Ultrasound soft tissue and joints.
- Ovarian and uterine abnormalities.
- Transplant kidney.
- Transcranial Doppler
- Middle cerebral artery, posterior cerebral artery, Basilar arteries, etc.
    - Intracranial neoplasms; for slaging and pre–operative surgical and/or radiation management.
    - Early detection of cerebral metastasis
    - Medical diseases of the brain (i.e. multiple, demyelinating diseases, transient ischemic attacks, and brain infarcts)
    - Posterior fossa and temporal fossa–lesions in particular
    - Cerebello-pontine angle tumors
    - Pathology of the cranio-verbal junction
    - Pituitary lesions (i.e. pituitary adenoma, suprasellar masses etc.)
    - Orbital pathology.

Spine

The spine and spinal cord with surface coils constitute the second most important area of the human body for MR investigation, because of the ability to see the spinal cord in sagittal, coronal, and axial planes without injecting contrast medium.

- Primary lesions of the spinal cord (syringomyelia, cord tumors, etc).
- Extramedullary lesion (i.e. metalais, meningiomas neurofibromas)
- Disc diseases (degenerative disc disease)
- Postoperative evaluations of the spine
- Destructive lesions of the vertebrae.

Cardiovascular

The ability to study the cardiovascular system with cardiac gating and in multiple projections without contrast medium makes MR a unique modality. Indications for MR studies of this systems include:

- Morphology of the cardiac chambers (i.e. congenital heart diseases, ventricular aneurysms cardiomyopathies, intracardiac thrombi and tumors)
- Diseases of the aorta (i.e. aneurysm, dissecting aneurysms)
- Diseases of the pericardium

Chest

The MRI is useful for:

- Hilar masses (i.e. differentiate vascular vs. nonvascular)
- Some mediastinal tumours
- Staging of broncogenic carcinoma
- Diseases of the chest wall.

Abdomen, Retroperitoneum and Pelvis

Indications

- *Liver* diffuse liver diseases, e.g; hemochromatiosis, evaluation of solitary and multiple space occupying lesions.
- *Kidney* masses (diagnosis and staging); perirenal pathology; transplant viability; renal vein thrombosis.
- *Aorta* aneurysms, dissection and occlusion.
- *Interior vena cava* thrombosis, tumour thrombi
- *Adernal* Masses (diagnosis and staging)
- *Pelvis* diseases of the uterus, staging of carcinoma of the uterine cervix, benign prostrate hypertrophy, prostatic soft tissue neoplasms. Diagnosis and staging of the bladder tumours.
- *Retroperitoneum* tumours, nodal enlargements, abscess etc.

Musculoskeletal

Indications

- *Bone* tumours, infections infections, avscular necrosis.
- *Joints* almost all joint diseases, cartilage injuries, tears etc.
- *Soft tissues* tumours, inflammation, hematomas.
- *Cartilaginous* epiphysis before ossification.
- *Congenital* hip dislocation.

Breast

As non-ionising radiation is utilized in MR, it represents no biological hazard to women. The best indication is in the study of dense breasts as an adjunct modality to mammography and ultrasonography.

Advances in MRI

MR Angiography

MRI is inherently sensitive to the detection of flow. Development of multiplanar data acquisitions, sophisticated RF pulse sequences and post-processing of data into 2 and 3 dimensional display format has resulted into acquisition of not only morphological but functional information non-invasively. The two techniques most widely studied are time–of–flight (TOF) and phase shift. The TOFMRA technique is best suited for studies of defined regions containing tortuous vessels with fast flowing blood, such as carotid arteries and the circle of willis. Phase shift (gradient refocused) methods rely on velocity induced phase differences to discriminate flowing blood from surrounding stationary tissue. These techniques are sensitive to the detection of slow flow in small vessels. Further advantage of this method is that a precise measurement of blood flow velocity can be done. These techniques are used successfully in the evaluation of aortic aneurysms dissections and coarctation, of aorta made pulmonary artery in the pulmonary atresia and carotid bifurcations. On MRA aneurysm, and AVM can be visualized well in the brain. The relationship and effect of tumours on adjacent vascular structures, e.g. meningioma invading dural sinuses are more easily appreciated than conventional spin echo imaging. Recent developments in abdominal imaging allow use of MRA in detection of renal artery sterósis and portal vein thrombosis.

Inversion Recovery and Fat Suppression Techniques

These techniques are another method of spin echo imaging that may be performed to enhance TI contrast. Short TI inversion recovery (STIR) is useful in reducing unwanted signal from fat and for enhancing contrast for lesion detection. This is particularly true in retro-orbital region, liver and bone marrow.

Fast Spin Echo (FSE) or Turbo Spin Echoimaging

This new method using complex physics helps to reduce patient study time by up to 30 to 50 percent without compromising image quality. With this techniques high quality T2 weighted images are obtained in a fraction of time required for conventional imaging. Development of fast spin echo techniques allow visualization of intrahepatic biliary radicles and extrahepatic bile duct without use of contrast medium. High signal from bile can be extracted and post-processed to produce 'MR cholangiography' images.

Cine MR

It allows images to be seen in realtime allowing study of CSF flow, joint kinetics and cardiac movements in systole and diastole.

Newer Coils

New coil designs have not only improved resolution, but also allow larger areas to be covered in one image. For example the new phased array spine coils can image the dorsal and lumbar spine together with high resolution images.

Gradient Echo Techniques

In these techniques, scan time is reduced by use of gradient and short TR. They are very susceptible to magnetic susceptibility. This can be useful in identifying soft tissue calcifications and iron in hemosidern deposits surrounding hematomas. They are used to obtain MR angiography sequences. In view of good TI contrast available and speed of acquisition. Gradient echoimaging is well suited to obtain dynamic Gd DTPA images of liver.

MR Control Media

Clinical investigations have demonstrated the potential of new RF pulse sequences combined with MR contrast agents. Paramagnetic Gd–DTPA, combined with dynamic scanning, can provide functional information on tissue and organ perfusion where as superparamagnetic iron oxides have a role in the tumor screening. Intravenous superparamagnetic iron oxide particles are targeted to hepatic reticuloendothelial system where the particles are promptly sequestrated by phagocytosis, giving rise to a profound reduction in signal intensity of healthy liver. Because tumor nodules are devoid of phygocytic koffer cells, there signal is not affected. Early studies have shown that lesions as small as 2 to 3 mm/in diameter can be visualized and the technique looks promising for tumor screening.

MR Spectroscopy (MRS)

MRS is the only noninvasive technique capable of measuring chemicals in the body. Current research shows that MRS show difference metabolism in brain tumors, reduction of PCr/Pi ratio in acute stroke, changes in the phospholipid metabolism in Alzheimer's disease and other dementais. MRS can also be useful in evaluation of patients of ischemic heart disease and cancers. At present multivoxel MRS is essentially a research tool. The unique ability of MRS is noninvasively measure a variety of metabolites in human body guarantees this technology a permanent place in biochemical research and diagnosis of human disease. Newer machines have at present single voxel MRS which is very easy for routine clinical use. This is essentially a pushbutton technique which takes only 5 to 15 minutes of additional time. Early results show that it is very useful for differential diagnosis and measurement of response to therapy for ischemia, infraction and malignancy.

Diffusion/Performance Imaging

The advent of echoplanar MR imaging has led to development of these new techniques. These can be used for very early diagnosis of acute ischemic stroke much before conventional MR techniques can show them. The earliest change to occur with reduced blood supply is reduced diffusion coefficient of water molecules into the extracellular space, this can be detected by diffusion imaging within minutes of a stroke. A difference between diffusion and perfusion images helps identify the ischemic penumbra or the ischemic tissue at risk in an acute stroke unit, this could then be effectively treated with thrombolysis similar to the way in which acute heart attacks are treated.

Functional MRI

Functional MRI, an existing new MRI technique noninvasively combines functional localization with high resolution anatomic information. Functional MRI uses principle of echoplanar imaging to obtain images of the entire brain within few minutes. These MR techniques detect signal changes coincident with the activation of sensory motor of visual cortical regions. In activated areas of the brain there is increased neuronal activity with changes in regional cerebral blood flow with a slight increase in concentration of deoxyhemoglobin. Deoxyhemoglobin is paramagnetic and slightly distorts magnetic field around it oxygenated hemoglobin is not paramagnetic. The difference can be measured using sequence specifically designed to enhance this effect. The clinical application of functional MRI include:

1. Accurate mapping of sensory, motor or visual coritical regions helps to delinate exact relation of tumor from the functionally sensitive area to plan surgery.
2. For early detection of ischemic lesions or infarcts.
3. Information about hemodynamic changes of brain. Future research in functional MR scan even allow analysis of "mind" in human being.

Rapidly advancing MRI techniques having made a phenominal impact on not only the neuro sciences but also on musculoskeletal and body cavity (cardiac pelvis) imaging.

Advantage like precise anatomical delineation and multiplanar capabilities of the MRI have made neurosurgery invasive the "viewing wand" technique using MRI has added to the accuracy and curtailed the invasiveness of neurosurgery. MRI provides the cystal clear rode map for gamma knife surgeries. The measure advantage of MRI is ability to pick up lesions when they are very small for example the average size of acoustic tumors at diagnosis has been reduced by almost 50 per cent to an average of 2.5 cm since the advent of MRI.

Thus the advent of MRI and the rapid strides which have been made in the precision of imaging has set the stage for a revolution in the concept of diagnostics.

COMPARISON OF VARIOUS IMAGING TECHNIQUES

Radiographic Techniques

Radiographic imaging techniques gain their imaging advantage from the availability of a high photon flux. Whether detection is done with a screen-film combination (X-ray) or scintillation detectors (CT), an abundance of photons produces a minimum of statistical fluctuation. X-ray techniques rely on a single physical property of the imaged part, that is, electron density, which corresponds to physical density in grams per cubic millimeter.

Plain radiographs are two-dimensional projection images in which a fine pixel format (film grain size) is used to produce a time-honored, proved, high resolution study. The theoretical limits of radiographic detail are determined by the film screen grain size and radiation scatter. Despite the advantage of good spatial resolution the projected superimposition of objects in plain radiographs obscures individual objet detail. Although CT uses a less efficient detector system and a considerably larger pixel size than that used in plain film radiography, a greater conspicuity and diagnostic accuracy is achieved through the two important features of tomographic display and post–processing. Computed tomographic scans now can achieve slice thickness down to 1 mm. Image windowing and centering can separate high-density (bone) and low-density (tissue) structures without re-examination. Computed tomographic scanning provides a sufficient dynamic range of quality imaging with adequate density definition to enable the identification of small droplets of air and fine bone trabecular detail in the same study.

The advent of CT in the mid 1970s allowed visualization of the brain that was not available with previous imaging techniques. The skull, cerebrospinal fluid, and grey and white matter are identified in submillimeter detail. Acute hemorrhage is easily differentiated from normal tissue because of its higher density, which is attributed to spilled blood proteins.

The general availability of radiographic instruments and short examination times have made radiographic methods the keystone of the standard imaging department. Sub-second exposures (in plain radiography) and exposure times of 1to2 seconds (with CT) have permitted studies in patients who are unable to cooperate fully. Precise anatomic detail has been the basis of radiographic diagnosis. Major deficiencies of film-screen radiographic methods are the short dynamic range and lack of diagnostic specificity, and the absence of a quantitative response to therapeutic measures. Diagnosis with these methods relies solely on anatomic changes based on the size and location of abnormalities. The use of contrast agents further enhances the identification of abnormalities as the result of tissue perfusion, but gives inconsistent results about histology, metabolism, or response to therapy. A further deficiency of plain radiograph methods is the limited control they provide for scatter, and the radiation hazard they create. Artifacts produced by bone shielding and beam hardening are particularly prominent in CT examinations of the posterior fossa of the head.

MAGNETIC RESONANCE IMAGING

With the discovery of nuclear magnetic resonance in the 1940s, the development of CT techniques in the 1970s, and the perfection of greater signal detection in the early 1980s, MRI was born. A truly volume/pictorial method with hazard and with greatly improved contrast was achieved by entirely different maneuvers than had been used in earlier imaging methods. Multiplanar projection was achieved through volume imaging.

The mechanism of imaging display in MRI is based on the individual electromagnetic properties of the atoms within tissues. Conversion of this information into high contrast scan is done by perturbing the individual magnetic fields of various tissues with radiofrequency waves while atoms are used the influence of the high magnetic field of the scanner.

Plots of spin-lattice relaxation times (T1) and the spin-relaxation (T2) after releasing of the radio frequency energy applied by the scanner have yielded images of the body with challenging anatomic detail. Relaxation times have provided to correlate with the concentration and mobility of tissue hydrogen nuclei in the field of view. Tissues with relatively high quantities of free water yield prolonged T1 and T2 times. By conventional agreement, prolonged T1 gives a decreased signal (dark) on T1–generated images, while prolonged T2 is plotted as a bright signal (white) on T2 scan. The MRI can accurately depicts the quantity and thermodynamic state of hydrogen ions which identifies the relative quantity of water and fat in tissues. The gray and white matter of the brain are clearly distinguished. Operator–controled maneuvers produce images with either enhanced T1 and T2 plots.

The vastly expanded contrast sensitivity of MRI has significantly improved the diagnosis of neurologic abnormalities without radiation hazard or the need for contrast-enhancing agents.

Despite the increased sensitivity in detecting white matter abnormalities afforded by MRI, the technique suffers from non-specificity of tissue response. Because MRI essentially depicts the number of mobile hydrogen ions in an area of tissue, edema, tissue devitalized by a stroke, demiyelinization, and neoplasm all produce similar findings T1 and T2 values have not yet been effectively used to differentiate various clinical disorders, nor have they been adequate identified changes in tissue response to therapeutic interventions.

Neoplasms contain increased free water (mobile hydrogen), and are revealed by prolongation T1 and T2 times on MRI scans. However, necrosis secondary to stroke, or primary delimitating diseases, give the same signal characteristics as seen with tumors once these abnormalities occur, the MRI signal pattern changes the little therapeutic response.

The advent and acceptance of contrast agents in MRI has resulted in a greater sensitivity in detecting perfusion abnormalities and alterations in the blood-brain-barrier. The diagnosis of brain neoplasms, and particularly of matastic tumors, has been improved immensely with prior intravenous administration of gadolinium. The mechanism of enhancement by MRI contrast agents is blood pool visualization (i.e. blood flow and tissue perfusion).

A summary of the advantages of MRI includes; (1) high contrast and high sensitivity, (2) absence of known hazards, (3) easy manipulation of images by varying pulsing techniques to enhance T1, T2, or hydrogen ion concentration, (4) elimination of artifacts produced by bone shielding (absence of hydrogen ion in cortical bone), and (5) ability of MRI to characterize vascular flow. Third-party reimbursement for MRI has led to the rapid proliferation and availability of the technology.

Disadvantages of MRI include; (1) high cost of the equipment and installation, (2) low signal output, which results in slow image acquisition and therefore, the extreme sensitivity of MRI images to motion, with the need for patient cooperation, (3) claustrophobia, which prevents up to 10 percent of patient examinations, (4) absence of a signal from calcium, (5) low specificity of T1 and T2 findings (poor tissue characterization by MRI is no achieved. Further disadvantages of MRI include the absence of an accepted orally-administrated contrast medium to delineate the gastrointestinal tract in abdominal imaging, and the absence of contrast agents specifically targeted to different organs and diseases.

Magnetic resonance imaging of other elements, such as sodium has not succeeded in increasing the specificity of diagnosis with this technique. Magnetic resonance spectroscopy (MRS) has yet to become a significant clinical tool in differentiating tissue viability, and has achieved no place in clinical practice. It remains entrenched in sophisticated chemistry laboratories, using instruments with ultra-high-energy magnetic fields. Major problems of spectroscopy include its low signal output and difficulty in discriminating selected volumes. The abundance of phosphorus 31 in normal muscle makes the analysis of deeper organs difficult. The individual phosphorus peaks are poorly resolved, and quantitative analysis is virtually impossible. Even with high-quality phosphorus spectra, quantitative evaluation of tissue viability is difficult because of the abrupt changes in adnosine triphosphate (ATP) concentration with tissue death, producing an all-or-more response.

POSITRON EMISSION TOMOGRAPHY

Although radiographic and medical resonance imaging produce highly sensitive and detailed scans, it remains difficult to identify metabolic activity of the tissue and to quantify the response to treatment with these techniques. Positron emission tomography is based on characterizing the response of tissue to the introduction of tracer-tagged, metabolically active agents. The goal of PET scanning is to differentiate normal tissue with enhanced or arrested metabolism. The objectives of PET imaging are identification of tissue-specific essential nutrients, appropriate labeling of these nutrients with positron emitters (without changing the chemical properties), and the development of sensitive and precise detector systems for quantifying the accumulation and clearing of specific agents by individual tissues. But without inexpensive, user-friendly instrumentation, PET will have difficulty getting out of the research laboratories.

The ultimate end of PET imaging is the development of automatically produced organ- and tissue-specific targeted agents. It is predicted that this, combined with the relative quantification of radiopharmaceutical uptake, will achieve the discrimination of disease from normal metabolic processes.

Two major deficiencies of PET are its low photon signal response and the basic principle of annihilation, which establishes fundamental limits to spatial resolution (i.e., 15 percent of positrons emitted from carbon 11 are annihilated at 1.05 mm from the carbon nuclei). Large voxels are needed to capture sufficient numbers of photons over prolonged periods of producing reasonable, statistically valid data, in diseases of cerebral white matter, such as multiple sclerosis, in which MRI excels as a diagnostic method, PET fails to identify any characteristic signal patterns. Hence, the utility of PET in the brain is predominantly in the study of metabolically active regions of the cerebral contex and basal ganglia. In comparison, MRI holds its greatest advantage in displaying anatomic changes of white matter and abnormalities in the posterior fossa. Computed tomography is unsurpassed for determining bone and calcium abnormalities and the identification of acute hemorrhage.

Positron emission tomography has achieved no place in the delineation of intracranial hemorrhage. Whereas MRI maintains advantages over CT in determining the age of subacute and chronic hemorrhages, CT remains the clinical tool of choice for identifying acute bleeding. Magnetic resonance imaging is unexcelled in the diagnosis of the accumulation of methemoglobin, which produces a strong signal on T1 and T2 weighted scans. In the diagnosis and identification of the extent of cerebral changes secondary to stroke. MRI is superior to either CT or PET. An immediate demonstration of cerebral changes secondary to cerebral vascular insufficiency is possible with MRI because of the high-intensity signals generated in the region of ischemia on T2 weighted scans. With the use of CT, cerebral changes secondary to infarction require hours to days before they can be diagnosed by decreased signals in the region of infarction.

Limited experience exists in the diagnosis of acute and chronic cerebrovascular disease by PET. Collections of individual studies lead to the belief that the place of PET in cerebrovascular disorders will be in the relative quantitation of flow and cerebral perfusion. The major value of PET is cerebrovascular disease may be in the differentiation of depression. Alzheimer's disease, and multiple infarct dementias. Further methods are being investigated for identifying those patients with cerebrovascular disease who will benefit most from interventive therapeutic proedures (i.e., endarterectomy). The redistribution of perfusion after acetazolamide challenge may become an effective selector of those patients who will benefit from surgical therapy.

Positron emission tomography has received increased attention for the grading of tissue viability in patients with neoplasms, particularly in the differentiation of viable tumor from necrosis secondary to radiation or inflammatory disease. When combined with clinical findings and anatomic CT and MRI, PET provides new information that influences medical therapy. PET accurately predicted the diagnosis and tumor grading. Unique advantages of PET scanning occur in several settings, aprticularly in brain tumors. Hypometabolic tumors are generally low-grade neoplasms and are less responsive to radiation and chemotherapy. It has been argued that therapy is inadvisable for these lesions. The differentiation of primary neoplasm from surrounding edema also is more accurately assessed by PET.

Positron emission tomography is particularly indispensable and probably the only imaging technique capable of distinguishing radiation necrosis from viable tumor. The sensitivity of CT and MRI for identifying gross anatomic changes is unquestioned; however, anatomic changes associated with either regression or progression of tumor are ambiguous. Occasionally, tumors may loose their viability during successful therapy, giving a false impression of tumor progression. In such cases, PET scans give a classic appearance of decreased or absent tracer uptake. Similar signal deficits are recorded with cerebritis.

Comparable conclusions also are possible with abdominal tumors. A nonspecific defect of low attenuation is identified in the right lobe of the liver in the CT scan, which proved to be hepatocellular carcinoma on histologic examination. A PET scan reveals a high concentration of activity from accumulated FDG. In a series of seven patients with primary neoplasms, PET scanning was effective in differentiating primary hepatic malignancies from benign tumors. The diagnosis and differentiation of tumors metastatic to the liver has been less reliable because of the variable signal responses that occur with different tumors.

A relative value scale for the image quality provided by PET, CT, MRI is presented in Table 35.1.

Table 35.1

Relative Value Scale (1–4*)

	PET	*CT*	*MRI*
Spatial resolution (detail)	1	4	3
Contrast/sensitivity	1	3	4
Tissue charcterization	4	1	2
Quantitaion	4	1	2
Cost/Time	1(HCFA)	3	2

*Highest value is 4, lowest 1

Although PET suffers in spatial resolution, its specific tissue contrast sensitivity and tissue characterization make it a valuable primary diagnostic method as well as an adjunct to CT and MRI.

The future development of PET scanning is likely to follow two courses: (1) development of specific chemical agents that identify individual metabolic and disease processes, and (2) development of less expensive, automated, and user-friendly radiopharmaceutical production units. The expense of PET without reimbursement has shifted its progress. There appears to be a renewed commitment by industry to achieve lower costs and a more efficient output from PET. Clinical trials and the validation of protocols are needed to define the cost effectiveness of the technique. The success of PET depends on its ability to provide specific information techniques and unnecessary therapy.

With the commercial availability of PET scanning devices, progress toward defining the role of this new imaging technology in community medicine is accelerating. The contribution of PET to ideal imaging, to complement conventional methods will be clarified within the nect few years.

Magnetic resonance imaging (MRI) and radiographic computed tomography (CT) were accepted within 5 years of their introduction. Each of these diagnostic methods was enhanced by industry, funded by third-party payers, and readily established in clinical protocols. For the past two decades PET has been ensconced in university laboratories as a research tool. The emergence of smaller, less expensive automated radiophramaceuticals give purpose to the following analysis.

To permit the discussion and comparison of conventional and PET techniues, the following standards for an "ideal imaging system" are adopted. The ideal system must be capable of producing high photon flux, must produce no hazards, and must contain a precise and efficient detector to allow total capture and the discrimination of true from artificial events. Pre and post-processing of the generated signal must be available to establish patterns that create repeatable, unique, and quantitative formats for a particular clinical entry. To be of ultimate clinical value, the technique must be; (1) capable of diagnosis and the quantitation of tissue response before and after interventional maneuvers, (2) readily available to health care professionals, and (3) affordable to the general public through pooled public insurance funds. Only techniques that allow high patient throughput are acceptable for general medical use.

To assist in analyzing and comparing various imaging systems, image quality is characterized by four criteria: spatial resolution, contrast discrimination, signal characterization, and signal quantitation.

Spatial resolution is a measure of the capacity to define fine detail when an excess of photons is available, whereas contrast discrimination represents overall sensitivity signal detection at low photon flux. Signal characterization implies that the properties of the processed signal are unique to a particular entity; this permits the retrieval of truly new information that could not be gained with current conventional imaging techniques.

In the past three decades, CT and MRI have been accepted as routine clinical tools for resolving particular problems. Despite certain shortcomings, these imaging methods have become invaluable in clinical practice and have come to represent "gold standards" of medical diagnostic imaging. The individuals who discovered them were awarded Nobel prizes within one decade of publishing the first scientific papers on their works. Their general use has spawned a large industrial production and research activity. Yearly advances in the technology of the two methods have accelerated patient throughput and enhanced imaging quality. Yet CT and MRI fall short of the goals and objectives of an ideal imaging system, because they produce little direct metabolic information, are inconsistent in tissue characterization, and have offered no reliable means of accurately determining tissue response to therapy. Neither the Hounsfield units in CT nor the TI and T2 values used in MRI have yielded adequate tissue determinants, and both modalities are inconsistent in differentiating benign from malignant disorders.

Neurological Disorders

The first applications of PET to have reached clinical use are in neurological disorders and brain tumors. The parameters that can be studied are energy, glucose utilization, oxygen metabolism, cerebral blood flow, and amino acid transport, and possible also the rate of protein synthesis.

Brain disorders that so far have lent themselves to study by clinical PET include epilepsy, brain tumors, cerebrovascular disease, dementia and degenerative brain disease. The most common types of tracers for PET imaging in neurology are F_2-deoxyglucose, ^{15}O (as CO, O_2 or CO_2, and H_2O), ^{11}C-labeled glucose, and amino acids, and ligands for neuroreceptor studies (dopamine, opiate, serotonin, and benzodiazapine receptors). Several tracer-kinetic models have been or are being developed and validated for neurological applications of PET, and are now being used in a research environment. They are time-consuming and not practical for daily clinical work, but are needed for research and for validating any diagnostic method that may evolve from the research laboratory into the clinical area.

Cerebrovascular disease is another application of PET with PET one can measure cerebral blood flow and oxygen and glucose metabolism in areas that are detected by the ischemic process. Positron emission tomography is potentially valuable for monitoring the treatment of cerebrovascular disease and for evaluating stroke patients for rehabilitation purposes. If decreased cerebral blood flow and glucose utilization are coupled with an increase in the oxygen extraction fraction in the affected region, viable tissue is expected to exist, and the patient may benefit from the technique such as interventional endarterectomy. Instead of measuring cerebral blood flow, metabolism/and oxygen extraction, we have adapted the acetazolamide challenge method (originally demonstrated with stable xenon gas and CT) to PET using ^{15}O-labeled water to evaluate cerebral blood flow reserve in patients with significant lesions of the carotid or intracerebral arteries. Because of the short half-life of ^{15}O, pre- and post-Diamox cerebral blood flow studies can be done within 1 hour. In normal subjects, acetazolamide increases cerebral blood flow through vasodilation.

The direct costs of a clinical PET center include equipment, facilities, personnel, and maintenance. A "classic" PET center requires three types of equipment: a cyclotron, a PET scanner, and laboratory equipment for radiochemistry and blood analysis. It is best to resist the temptation to buy a larger cyclotron (higher energy, more particles) than necessary, because its higher complexity and operational costs may actually limit its utility. A 16 MeV cyclotron is adequate for most clinical PET centers.

When starting a clinical PET center, a whole body unit should be purchased, to reach as broad a patient population as possible. Consider the number of slices and axial coverage provided by particular scanners. We believe the scanner should obtain as many slices and provide axial coverage as large as possible, to cover the organ of interest. Another consideration is the great range of necessary ancillary equipment for PET. The laboratory equipment for PET varies from mundane items such as radiation monitoring to exotic items such as high-pressure liquid chromatography (HPLC) devices or "hot cells" with remote manipulators, which are necessary for quality control and the production of certain radiotracers.

Most of the PET centers now in operation are impressive, extensive facilities. To understand this, one should recognize that the majority of these centers developed from research orientations. Many started in a national laboratory. The amounts of money and the facilities required were probably larger than what is necessary for clinical PET. Both a cyclotron and a PET scanner should easily be housed in a 1,000 to 1,500 sq. ft space, with some ancillary space in addition. Cyclotron shielding must alternate both gamma radiation neutrons, for which the shielding materials are typically different. Gamma radiation requires lead; neutrons require materials such as borated water. We prefer self-shielding for a cyclotron. A regulatory advantage of this approach is that the shield itself, rather than the room that contains the cyclotron, becomes the containment. If the shielding is adequate, a non-radiation worker can actually stand at the shield during cyclotron operation. Inner locks or restricted access to the cyclotron room are unnecessary. Depending on the size of the cyclotron, it can be less expensive to have self-shielded cyclotron that to manufacture a thick-walled concrete vault to house an unshielded cyclotron.

A modest amount of shielding is required for the PET scanner. Most manufacturers incorporate lead into their scanners to shield against activity originating in other areas of the scanner room and areas of the patient's body that are not in the direct field of view. When installing a PET facility in a nuclear medicine operation, one may want to consider the effect of a patient emitting 511 KeV photons on Anger cameras in adjacent imaging rooms. We have had to pay particular attention to this problem at Johns Hopkins because we use rotating anger camera SPECT systems in rooms adjacent to our PET scanner. When the camera is rotating, there is point at which it faces directly into the PET room. We did studies to ensure that the additional count rate that the Anger camera receives from the 511 KeV photons generated in the PET scanning process did not produce artifacts in our SPECT studies. The PET scanner, and particularly the cyclotron, consume a lot of electricity (about 150 kw when operating). Most of this electricity becomes heat, requiring some cooling (obout 250,000 BTU per hour).

A big advantage of having the PET operation in the heart of the nuclear medicine clinic is that it minimizes new problems in managing radioactivity in patients. It also permits the integration of PET into the routine clinical process of scheduling patients, archiving data, presenting data in morning conferences, and other activities.

Having a cyclotron and a PET scanner close to each other (approximately 40 feet at Johns Hopkins) facilitates communication between the chemistry team and the PET scanning team. If problems develop in positioning a patient or putting in an intravenous line, for example, the cyclotron team can continue bombarding the target and delay any required chemical synthesis. Once the synthesis begins, the activity decays and the millicurie dose decreases. In some of our studies in which specific activity is a consideration, it decreases, raising the possibility that we may not be able to use the dose for the study for which it was intended. On the other hand, if the cyclotron teams having trouble with radiotracer production, they can inform the scanner crew, who may delay preparing the patient. This type of close physical proximity between the chemistry operation and the scanning operation is very important. One cyclotron (either an 11 MeV or certainly 16 to 17 MeV machine) can support three of four PET scanners with ease, depending on the types of studies being done. A typical run of [^{18}F]2-flouro-2-deoxyglucose (FDG) provides enough doses for four or five studies, enabling the simultaneously provision of radiotracer for several scanners.

There is much discussion about the personal requirements of a clinical PET center. The minimum staff required includes a doctoral-level technical director either a chemist or physicist. This individual must know about the chemistry and the physics of radionuclides and PET scanning, oversee the quality control of radiopharmaceutical production, and oversee the quality of the images and numbers produced by the PET scanning team. One chemistry technologist is still necessary at this point, even with automated synthesis devices, the "black boxes" used to produce radiopharmaceuticals, two certified nuclear medicine technologists are required to perform the scanning, including data acquisition, processing, archiving, and any required blood sampling during acquisition. Free standing PET centers and administrator for financial operations maintenance of supplies, and management of accounts.

Although it has been assumed that the equipment for the center will be amortized over an 8-year period at a 10 percent annual rate, the PET scanner should probably be amortized over a 5-year period and the cyclotron over a 10-year period. Many established PET centers have cyclotrons that are 20-25 years old and still useful. Scanners are more quickly outdated with 5-year-old scanners lacking contemporary technology and performance. I think we will continue to see a more rapid evolution of PET scanners than of cyclotrons.

Maintenance costs are a significant fraction of the yearly operating budget for a PET center. They can be estimated to be seven and a half percent per year of the direct equipment costs, although this is probably a conservative figure. Some analysts offer figure as high as 10 percent, frighteningly high number. Given the complexity of the cyclotron and the PET scanner, I strongly believe, having had to fix our PET scanner on a number of occasions, that a maintenance or service contract is well worth its cost. For the sake of simplicity, all indirect costs may be combined and calculated as 50 percent of direct costs. These indirect costs include electricity, cooling, facilities, maintenance, and insurance.

It is tempting to think that a PET center with only a scanner and rubidium 82 generator would be less expensive. This is not likely to be true. Without a cyclotron the costs of the equipment loan and maintenance decrease, and the personnel requirement are reduced. Except in a few unusual situations, a clinical PET center should include a cyclotron as well as the PET scanner. In the future it is hoped that the regional distribution of PET radiopharmaceuticals will be practical. Because of the short half-lives of the radionuclides employed, notionwide coverage from a single distribution site, which is frequently possible with other radionuclides and radiopharmaceuticals, will never be possible in PET. Large metropolitan areas could potentially be served by a single cyclotron, radiopharmaceutical, and distribution center. PET must adopt this approach in order to become a widespread clinical reality.

Given the number of PET studies one must conduct in a year in order to break even, one must consider study throughput. Study throughput depends on three issue: the properties of radionuclides, the speed of the PET scanner, and the number of patients available for particular studies. The most uncertain element in this is the patient population on which the clinical demand for scanning is based, including the numbers and types of patients, because this affects the radionuclides, the tracers, and PET scanner requirement for a particular center. The properties of radionuclides and the configuration of the PET center affect throughput in important ways. For example, carbon 11 has a 20-minute half-life. If four scanners were available, four doses of a particular radiopharmaceutical could be simultaneously made and four patients scanned. In PET centers with only one scanner, one cannot make four carbon 11 doses and have three of them sitting in syringes while scanning the first patient, and then two sitting in syringes while scanning the second patient, and and so.

DESIGNING A CT SCAN ROOM

CT scanner rooms could be described as a cross between X–ray room, operation theatre and computer room. Elements common to all three types of facility usually feature in the design of a scan room.

As with all installations, it is better to build CT scan room in a vacant clear area or on a Greenfield site. Many hospitals have compromised and built CT rooms in areas stolen from other departments. This often leads to scanning in a room the size of the broom cupboard with the control room reduced to the size of a shoe box.

Components of a CT Scanner

The components of the CT scanner can be broadly divided into the following:

The scanner This is subdivided into a couch, on which the patient lies, and the gantry, which houses an X-ray tube and bank of X-ray detectors. The gantry and table are sited within the scan room.

The control console This controls the scanner and allows the radiographer and radiologist to send and receive data. This is sited in a room directly adjacent to the CT scanner. A clear lead glass window and lead lined door separate the two areas. In some smaller scanners the control desk may contain all the computer hardware necessary to control the scanner and process the data. In these cases, the demands on air-condtioning are less stringent.

The generator This devices the scanner and powers the X-ray tube. Generators have become progressively smaller as technology has improved. They are usually accommodated in a separate room, sometimes with the controlling computer (where electrical interference is not a problem). However, if space, or constraints on running cables are a problem, the generator can be sited inside the scanner room.

The computer In more advanced scanners, the computers required to process the data from the detectors and display it are enormous. These types of computers need separate rooms with carefully controlled temperatures.

Air-conditioning is one of the most fundamental considerations when designing a CT scan room. It can be the most costly element in the design of the room and often causes the greatest design problems. Frequently, air-conditioning plants are installed with a much larger capacity than is actually required. This is often the result of an over–zealous works department, or designs being implemented before selection and purchase of the scanner. Turnkey, if available, is the best option.

Pre-Installation

Temperature control is exacting. In the scan room it is important to maintain a constant temperature because fluctuations cause the performance of the X-ray detectors to change. This leads to the production of artifacts on the completed scans, upsets the calibration and affects uniformity in detector performance. Extremes of temperature are not too good for the patient either. Air-conditioning is also required in the computer room, if present, and in the control room (depending on the manufacturer).

Preparation of the area in which the scanner is to be installed is similar to conventional X-ray rooms. Level flooring are correct positioning of the floor trunking are important. CT has the advantage of not requiring are reinforced ceiling to support heavy cables and monitors. It is cost-effective to site the scanner in an existing X-ray room, because lead protection will already in position. In some cases it is useful to install computer flooring in the computer room, which helps to reduce maintenance time. As with air-conditioning, it is better to opt for turnkey in pre-installation.

Location of Scanner

The position of the scanner within the scan room is critical. It is important to consider the type of patients being scanned, their specific needs, and their mobility. Patients on trolleys and beds will require large access doors. With very sick patients, it is often important to have rapid access to the patient's head. The gantry should, therefore, not be squeezed into the corner of the room so that the anesthetist and associated equipment cannot get behind it. Provision of piped gases and suction at the head end of the scanner is ideal.

The best position for the scanner is usually at a 45° angle to the long axis of the room. This allows access to the both sides of the couch. Table and gantry controls are usually duplicated on each side of the scanner.

It is also helpful to provide the following within the scan room:

CCTV This is often provided by the manufacturer and positioned the wall behind the gantry so that it shows the patient's head after the X-rays have passed through the gantry. The picture from the CCTV is transmitted to a monitor in the control room.

Intercom A two-way intercom is usually provided in the gantry allowing communication with the control room.

Panic button This is useful for isolated departments and a bell and a light should be situated outside the room to the nursing station or corridor.

Telephone If required, it may be useful to have simple ring-out only telephone.

Blinds any windows or lead glass viewing panels should have blinds attached. This prevents embarrassment if the patient has to undergo any internal preparation while on the table.

The medical physics department using the CT scanner specifications will calculate radiation doses and provide a complete description of shielding requirements. These will be similar to a conventional X-ray room. All doorways to the scan room require warning lamps and radiation signs.

Space Communications

Generally, three separate but adjacent rooms are desirable: the gantry room 22.5-27 net m^2 (250-300 net ft^2); the room continuing computers, operator's console, and possibly the power equipment (13.5-18 net m^2 or 150 to 200 net ft^2); and a room permitting independent viewing, reading, interpretation, and possibly filling functions (9-13.5 net m^2 or 100-150 net ft^2). Consideration should be given to measures which permit effective resuscitative efforts. Such measures include sufficient space for the activities of the resuscitative team; immediately accessibility to oxygen and suction equipment, perhaps ideally piped in from a centralized source; immediately availability of an emergency cart for resuscitative.

Air Conditioning

Dedicated, autonomous climate control systems for the CT facility should be seriously considered in many hospital environments. Backup window units may constitute an economic alternative. The gantry room and computer room should have independent temperature control.

The CT scan rooms tend to be cold, with the temperature under 21°C, and control of patient temperature may become difficult. The neonate or infant is especially prone to develop hypothemia, and facilities to add or conserve heat, especially during anesthesia, should be established.

The induction facilities-to eliminate delays in the CT schedules-should be in an adjoining room with storage space for anesthetic equipment and defibrillator. When not employed for anesthetic purposes, the induction room would be available as a holding room for patient preparation.

Piped anesthetic gases and vacuum with connectors for anesthesia machines should be provided in both CT and induction rooms. To accommodate ventilators an appropriate electrical power source oxygen connection are required.

Provisions have to be made for waiting with toilet facilities and dressing rooms.

For postanesthetic observation there should be a nearby recovery unit.

The computers, generally situated adjacent to the scan room, are so temperature critical that frequently the room must be air-conditioned. A temperature of about 21°C is required.

The difficulty of working in a limited space in an environment not conductive to intensive-care support of potentially high-risk patients-head injuries, etc. is often not appreciated. A complete CT unit would require an area of about 70 to 90 m^2.

Protecting the Equipment

It is important to fire-protect the massive investment that is made in a CT facility, particularly if the money for the scanner has been raised by public appeal or on a leasing agreement. The best fire protection for the computer and the generator room, although not the cheapest, is halon gas. This causes the least possible damage to the equipment. Protecting larger areas such as the scan room is usually left to the hospital smoke detector system.

A CT scanner area must be provided with changing facilities and a WC. Preparation for body scans requires the patient to drink contrast media. This outlines the bowel and allows differentiation of normal tissue and lesions. Thus there is the need for WC and washing facilities. A waiting area with a drinking machine is not a good idea.

It is important to consider all aspects of the project before purchasing and installing the scanner. This includes both the need for the scanner and its possible position within the unit.

EXTRACORPOREAL SHOCKWAVE LITHOTRIPSY

The introduction and success of extracorporeal shockwave lithotripsy (ESWL) parallels the era of minimally invasive therapy, for some of mankinds oldest recorded maladies. Overnight the major trauma of a large flank incision approach to a minute kidney stone was replaced with extra corporeal generated and focussed energy by ESWL devices. This success of ESWL has led to the search of other less invasive alternative to traditional methods of surgical management. The future of medicine will further demand the amalgamation of physicians and technology. ESWL is only the beginning.

Today, since ESWL is well established worldwide, the medical and economical environment has changed in so far as cost-effective use of lithotripsy device becomes more and more a mandatory condition. Purchase price, installation expenditure and running costs are to be taken into account as well as performance, indication range, re-treatment rates and multi-functional use of the device. These features determine the overall profitablity calculation. Are there significant differences in this respect between modern lithotripters? There are! It is important whether kidney, ureteral, common bile duct and gallbladder stones can be treated or whether ureteral stones cannot be localised. It counts, whether the re-treatment rate is close to one, or two or more treatments for every stone are required. It is cost effective to use the costly X-ray and ultrasound components of a lithotripter, for diagnostic and therapeutic procedure other than lithotripsy, as long as extra corporeal lithotripsy has been finished for the day. These and other aspects make a difference between different lithotripters.

Modern lithotripters have been significantly changed, due to more than 20 years of clinical experience. The following basic features are of major importance and shall be available at every up-to-date lithotripsy system.

Acoustic power and fragmentation efficacy: as the key component of a lithotripter, a pressure wave source first of all has to deliver a sufficient amount of acoustic energy for fragmentation of all kinds of stones. Most of the available sources today have less energy reserves than needed for single treatment fragmentation of large or persistant stones. Some do not feature the dynamic range for gentle treatment with low power whenever sufficient and increased energy when necessary.

A wide dynamic range–starting with low power and significant energy reserves for difficult stones–is the first and mandatory requirement for a modern lithotripter source.

Energy distribution and pain sensation to minimise tissue damage, the acoustic energy is most favorably coupled to the patient's body via a large coupling area with low energy density. Only a small focal zone should contain enough energy for fragmentation, whereas all other areas to be passed by the pressure wave should not be affected. Precise focussing by large aperture system is the technical answer to this problem. Pressure wave sources using large aperture angles of 80-90° enables a gentle energy propagation throughout layers of tissue and organs, and provide the highest energy concentration in a restricted focal area simultaneously.

In order not to exclude obese patients from extracorporeal lithotripsy treatment, a focal depth of at least 15 cm is required, so that a source diameter of about 30 cm is appropriate. Due to the low energy density on the skin level of the patient, pain sensation is reduced to the lowest possible value, offering the capability of anesthesia-free and potentially ambulatory treatment in many cases.

Incorporation of ultrasound and accuracy of localisation Ultrasound localisation, as one of the two common targeting modalities, has the advantage of featuring no radiation hazard and providing real-time monitoring of the fragmentation procedure, as well as targeting control.

Ultrasound, however, is of limited accuracy compared with X-ray localisation. The principle of ultrasound imaging is based on pulse echo techniques, evaluating the flight time of ultrasound pulses from the transducer crystalto reflecting target and back to the crystal, now acting as a receiver. Mapping the flight times of echo pulses for different spatial directions results in a two dimensional image of the interfaces of organs and tissue in homogeneities. The actual spatial distances are precisely reflected by the ultrasound image only if the propagation velocity of the ultrasound pulse within the body is precisely known and constant. Individual variations of about 5 per cent, however, have to be taken into account. The deviation of the geometrical focus position and the ultrasound display may thus come up to 10-20 mm as proven by our own measurements. But 10-20 mm deviation is not acceptable, since a target concernment may be completely missed by the pressure wave focus.

Nevertheless, ultrasound is a valuable localisation modality when incorporated in a coaxial alignment with the pressure wave path. Ultrasound and pressure waves, while propagating in a similar fashion through living tissue, behave similarly with respect to deviations and, therefore, targeting inaccuracies are minimised by in line ultrasound configurations. In line ultrasound targeting is another key feature which fits well with the requirement of smooth energy coupling of large aperture source as described above.

In line ultrasound increase fragmentation of efficiency by minimising the number of shots passing the stone, due to inaccurate targeting, and helps to keep potential tissue damage at the lowest possible level.

Lifetime and running costs The lifetime of a therapeutic source and accordingly the running costs have a direct impact on the economic situation. Evidently, reduced running cost have to be achieved by avoiding costly spare parts, like park plug, and providing the highest possible lifetime of critical components.

Interdisciplinary use There was a time when it was necessary to decide what type of lithotripter to invest in urinary or biliary. Still, today, there are systems being claimed to be especially matched to the needs of biliary or urinary lithotripsy. The reasons are historical. Today, there is no logical reason to built dedicated lithotripters. The interdisciplinary use is limited only by the localisation modality. Therefore, modern lithotripter should be suitable without compromise of interdisciplinary use.

Multifunctionality

Lithotripters are, by their nature, large machines and incur a large capital outlay. To justify such a cost, the hospital will naturally wish to ensure good use of such a machine, especially considering the most advanced machines incorporate sophisticated X-ray technology. Hence the new generation of machines have the ability to incorporate leg holders and urological basins, enabling the following procedures to be performed on the machine:

Urology Transurethal resection, endoscopic and percutaneous lithotripsy (mechanicla, hydraulic, with ultrasound or laser), endoscopic calculus extraction, percutaneous nephrotomy.

Cystoscopy, antigrade and retrograde uretemoscopy, crystography and urethocystography, antigrade and retrograde pyelography, plain radiographs of the renal tract and angiography.

Gastroenterology endoscopic retrograde papillotomy (EPT), endoscopic calculus extraction, endoscopic retrograde lithotripsy in the biliary tract (mechanical, electrohydraulic, with ultrasound or laser), percutaneous transhepatic puncture of the gall-bladder and bile ducts; gastroscopy, choledochoscopy, retrograde cholangiography (ERC).

Current Machines

Present day machines are generally smaller, more sleek and more mobile than their first generation relatives. Most are dual purpose, capable of fragmenting both renal and biliary stones. In some models the large water tank has been replaced by either shallow water coupled or a 'dry' liquid filled cylinder. Most modern machines have both X-ray and ultrasound imaging capability. The user has a variety of energy to choose from, including the venerable, reliable and efficient spark-gap generator, as well as lithotripters that are electromagnetic, piezo-electric and even micro-explosive energy sources.

In spite of vast differences in appearance, size, accessories, efficiency and cost, all ESWL machines are designed around the same basic principle of operation. An energy source creates a short duration accoustical wave that can be focused from outside the body to a precise internal location. A combination of direct energy transfer and cavitation effects result in stone fragmentation. All lithotripsy machines must incorporate four main features to function:

- An energy source
- A shock wave focusing method
- A stone localisation system, and
- A machine-to-patient coupling device.

The energy source (generator) creates an external shock wave that is focussed by a hemiellipsoidal reflector or electronic lens. This focal point (F_2) is positioned by an imaging device fluoroscopy, plain film X-ray or ultrasound so that it coincide with the spatial co-ordinates of the urinary or biliary tract tone.

The shock wave is coupled to the patient's skin by water bath or liquid/membrane arrangement (cushion), and a series of shocks are administreted until the stone is fregmented.

The need for anaesthesia or analgesia will vary with the machine type and power setting. For the first generation water bath lithotripters this usually means general endotracheal anaesthesia, but most current machines have modified the body surface area over which the shock wave enters (and/or reduced the peak power of the shock wave) such that intravenous sedation is usually satisfactory anaesthesia.

Depending on machine type, one or more treatment sessions may be required to eachieve maximum fragmentation efficacy.

Subsequent improvement in lithotripter design have led to significant changs in generator type and configuration, patient handling methods and stone localisation systems. Each change is attempting to enhance one or more of the basic four features that all ESWL machines share.

The shock wave created by an lithotripter follows the basic physical low of acoustic energy. The shock wave bring about destruction of a stone when the delivered energy at F_2 exceeds the intrinsic tensile strength of the calculus. Both cavitation effects and direct acoustic energy absorption appear to play major roles in the actual breakdown and fragmentation of the stone. Numerous factors related to a given machine's design attempt to optimise these acoustical events. The energy delivered, the configuration and duration of the hock waves, the volume and shape of the second focus and the accentuation of the shock wave by intervening tissue, affect the ability of a machine to fragment stones.

There are several methods of generating shock waves, as presented in the commercially available lithotripters of today. The first is spark-gap consisting of an electrode-ellipsoid system in which high voltage is discharged underwater and results in an expanding plasma that generates a shock wave. Spark-gap technology is found in some devices. Some manufacturers employ an electromagnetic source for shockwave generation. Piezo-electric crystal arrans are found in lithotripters made by Diasonics, EDAP, and Wolf. Even microexplosive energy has been utilized in some systems.

Technique of Pressure Wave Generation

Commercial lithotripsy devicies presently make use of three different physical principles of pressure- or shock wave generation. Electro-hydraulic spark plus systems are powerful but noisy, costly and inconvenient due to frequent change of worn out electrodes; piezo-electric systems lack at least in clinical praxis the necessary power. A high re-treatment rate is reported of all today's piezo-electric systems. Electromagnetic principles are used based on flat coil generators with acoustic lenses for pressure wave focusing. Although power and lifetime make the electromagnetic system most favourable for extracorporeal lithotripsy, restrictions of the acoustic lens limit their efficacy due to a limited aperture and local depth. This drawback has been overcome by an innovative source design, making use of a highly efficient reflectror geometry instead of an unfavourable acoustic lens.

The innovative pressure wave soruce the new source design is based upon a cylindrical acoustic impulse generator which is coaxially aligned with the parabolic reflector. Acoustic pressure waves are generally on the surface of a hollow cylinder and radiated radially perpendicular to the cylinder exis. Focusing of the primary cylindrical wave is accomplished by a rotational symmetric reflector with a parabolic surface contour.Since the pressure wave generator is designed as a hollow cylinder, space is available to incorporate an in-line or coaxially aligned ultrasound localisation system. Ideally, the axial area is a low pressure zone, protecting the inline ultrasoundtransducer from the potentially destructive effects of high power pressure waves. Storz Medical, Switzerland developed a pressure wave source with an aperture of 30 cm . Due to the large aperture, the pressure field exhibits a favourable distribution with respect to gentle and pain-free coupling.

The focal depth-distance from reflector rim to focus-is 165 mm, long enough for even very obese patient and any stone locality.

The focal size is 6 mm in lateral and 28 mm in axial direction which is well matched to the whole range of stone sizes. With an 84.5°, the aperture angle is within the favourable range.

Cylindrical pressure wave generation is based on electromagnetic principles, working similar to a loud speaker with a comparatively large cylindrical membrane. The amount of acoustic energy generated for every square area of the membrane is lower than in a system with smaller membranes, resulting in an increased lifetime of the pressure wave source.

The acoustic output is adjusted in nine steps from 10-100 MPa-100-1000 bar, measured with transmission type PVDF-probes-covering the whole range, from gentle low energy fragmentation of brittle salivary gland stones up to powerful high energy treatment of bulky and resistant gallbladder and staghorn stones.

Lithotripsy Applications

ESWL has applications in the treatment of calculi of the kidney, ureter, gallbladder and common bile duct. Regardless of the application, ESWL has generally been contraindicated in those patients with untreated bleeding disorders, pregnancy, gross obesity, uncontrolled sepsis and where the store cannot be targeted and treated through safe acoustic window.

Occasional reports have demonstrated the potential usefulness of ESWL in pancreatic and salivary gland caluli. Although ESWL has gained and maintained a major role in the management of renal and ureteral stones, it remains at the investigational stage for biliary calculi (at least in the United States). Although gallstones can be readily targeted and fragmented by ESWL, the ability of the gallbladder and common duct to clear these fragments is very different from the kidney and ureter. Ancillary measures, common to the success of urinary ESWL, are not readily applicable to the biliary tree and the success of concomitantoral dissolution therapy plus ESWL for gallstones, has been less efficacious than originally hoped.

In spite of these difficulties, gallstones can be successfully fragmented and cleared from the gallbladder with ESWL. When ESWL and oral bile salts are used together for patients with solitary stones, 20 mm or less in size, 76 per cent of patients are stone free 9 to 12 months following lithotripsy with high energy, sparkgap lithotripsy.

In both renal and gallstone patients, the direct side effects of ESWL appear to be minimal. Serious complications are rare, especially when care in patient selection, stone localisationand proper selection of athe acoustical treatment window are attended to.

FURTHER READING

1. Chanssy C, Schmiedt E, Jocham D, Brendel W *et al*: First clinical experience with extracorporeally induced destruction of kidney stones by shock waves. *J Urol* **127**, 417-20 1982.
2. Hill CR: Physical principles of medical ultrasonics. Series in Applied Physics, Ellis Horwood Limited, 1986.

RADIATION ONCOLOGY DEPARTMENT

Radiation oncology deals with the treatment of patients with cancer and other tissue growths. The treatment is basically a tissue destroying procedure. Cancer is treated by ioninsing radiation either alone or in combination with chemotherapy, etc.

Electromagnetic waves can be generated by X-ray equipment, linear accelerators, isotopes and betatrons.

The department varies in size depending on the types of services and programmes offered and the sophistication of the equipment it has. Cobalt unit is used for deep radiation therapy, and the linear accelerator uses recent technology to treat a wide range of oncology cases. A simulator is used to set the teletherapy fields to plan the treatment with accuracy so that the cancerous area receives the maximum radiation dose while the vital structures.

There are three steps in the treatment:

- Initial evaluation of the patient and development of a treatment plan
- Determination of the workload related to the type of treatment plan.
- The application of radiotherapy or chemotherapy or combination of both.

Initial evaluation of the patient and development of treatment plan is done using treatment planning system (TPS).

The location of the department should be preferably be on grade level. The radiation protection required dictates the use of high-density materials in thick walls, ceiling and floor. The department requires floor loading of such magnitude that any other level will raise costs intolerably. It should be ideal on the ground floor in close proximity to the outpatient department. Since about 50 percent patients are outpatients and are ambulatory, proximity to or easy accessibility from the outpatient department is important. It is desirable to locate the department adjacent to radiodiagnosis department.

The department,should be designed to present a cheerful and pleasant atmosphere which concentrates on the patient comfort.

Facilities and space requirement include:

- Reception control.
- Waiting area (Close to reception).
- Dressing rooms near treatment area.
- Consultants chamber.
- Chemotherapy room.
- Nurses station.
- Therapy rooms and control rooms.
- Radiation physicist room with treatment computer.
- Staff facilities.
- Patient toilets.
- Storage for supplies.

Radiation therapy can be divided into four categories:

Brachytherapy Ionizing radiation using radium or the equivalent, or radioactive cobalt, caesium, or iridium. These isotopes are used in the form of needles for implantation of tumours, or in applicators to be placed against the tumour or inserted into a cavity containing a tumour.

Superficial therapy Ionizing radiation with energies from 8 to 140 kilovolts. Relatively, soft X-rays are used for non-infiltrating cancers, such as skin cancers.

Orthovoltage therapy Ionizing radiation with energies from 150 to 400 kilovolts. this equipment has been replaced largely by megavoltage units. It is used in the treatment of infiltrating surface malignancies and often as a supplement to megavoltage therapy such as intraoral and intervaginal treatment.

Megavoltage therapy Ionizing radiation of greater than one million volts. This includes cobalt 60 and a variety of accelerators using high-energy

Table 35.2

Facilities	New patients per year	Personal		Equipment	
		Patient Care	***Planning***	***Radiation Sources***	***Support***
Complete Radio-therapy Center	1000	6 Therapists 3 Physicists 8 Techs 2 Nurses 6 Residents	3 Dosimetry/Mold room techs 2 Simulator techs 2 Electronic and Machine shop techs	Two 1–8 MV X-ray or cobalt One 10–25 MV X–ray and electron beam One 100–400 KVP X–ray Radium sources on hand	2 Simulators 1 Computer
Clinical Radio-therapy Center	1000	4 Therapists 2 Physicists 2 Techs 2 Nurses 4 Residents	3 Dosimetry/Mold room techs 2 Simulator Techs 1 Electronic and Machine shop techs	Two 1–8 MV X–ray or cobalt One 10–25 MV X–ray and electron beam One 100–400 KVP X–ray Radium sources on hand	2 Simulators 1 Computer
	500	2 Therapists 1 Physicist 4 Techs 1 Nurse	1 Dosimetery/Mold room tech	One 1–8 MV X–ray or cobalt One 10–25 MV X–ray One 100–400 KVP X–ray radium source	2 Simulators 1 Computer
Affiliated Radio-therapy Center	200	½ Therapist 2 Techs ½ Nurse	—	One 1–8 MV X–ray or cobalt One 100–400 KVP X–ray radium	—

X-rays. The term cobalt therapy enjoys the reputation as being synonymous with all mega-voltage therapy. This, of course, is not true. In addition to cobalt, most of the radiation therapy centers have more sophisticated accelerators which deliver radiation at 4 to 12 million volts. A few of the large centers have accelerators and betatrons which produce X-ray at 25 to 35 million volts.

In the linacs of linear accelerators, electrons are accelerated in a linear tube by high frequency power generators. Electrons are emitted for a gun, travel down the tube gaining energy all the way to hit a target and produce X-rays at the end of the tube or to be let out. The main advantages over the cheaper cobalt machines are the higher quantum energy of the radiation, better depth dose curves and better collimation and the much higher radiation intensities of the X-ray. The maintenance of a linac is more complicated and costly than that of a cobalt unit.

In the betatron, electrons are accelerated by induction and guided by magnetic fields. The betatron is basically a very simple and reliable, though expensive machine for producing very high energy electrons. Unlike radiation from other common sources, the dose it delivers drops off very sharply after a certain depth and, in general, a lower amount passes through the patient on the side away from the point at which the radiation enters. These advantages are countered to some extent by the fact that an electron beam is not particularly well focused and radiation is scattered to tissues around the cancer.

A betatron and a linac are complementary and can serve most of the needs. It has been stated that the ideal combination is a matched pair of super

Table 35.3: Checklists of Basic Information in Planning a Radiation Therapy facility

	Initial	*5 Year Projection*		*Initial*	*5 Year Projection*
1. Number and type of patients to be accommodated daily			4. Other integral space		
Average number			Waiting rooms		
Peak number			Inpatient		
Impatient workload			Outpatient		
Number ambulatory			Dressing rooms		
Number in wheel chair or stretcher			Examination rooms		
2. Staff			Head and neck		
Radiotherapists			Female gynecology		
Residents (Trainees)			General		
Radiation physicist			Treatment rooms		
Physics and dosimetry personnel			Record rooms		
Technologists			Communications		
Secretarial and computer personnel			Chemotherapy facilities		
Maintenance and janitorial personnel			Diagnostic radiation facilities		
3. Therapy equipment (Number and types of Units required)			Patient photography facilities		
Simulator			Nurses and technicians spaces		
Superficial			5. Architectural points		
Orthovoltage			Heating, Air–conditioning, Noise control		
Megavoltage			Electrical conduct requirements		
Cobalt–60			Treatment room, lighting control		
Linear Accelerator(s)			Shielding (Safety requirements)		
Betratron			6. Treatment Planning rooms		
Other			Dosimetery		
Radium and other sealed source of for interstitial or intracavitory therapy			Mold room		
			Machine shop		
			Electronic and maintenance shop		
			7. Computer Facilities		
			8. Other ancillary facilities and space		

voltage machines either cobalt or preferably linear accelerators.

Where both machines are readily available, a clinical preference for linac treatment leads to a higher linac/cobalt ratio. This element seems usually to outweigh the factors which might otherwise tends to increase the observed cobalt unit case-load. Among them the slightly longer down time required for maintenance and repair of accelerators. Where choice exists, cobalt is used for a higher population of the simpler palliative treatments requiring fewer, less accurately defined fields than the conditions treated by linear acceleration.

Evaluating and comparing the patient benefits of the different types of radiotherapy is a complex matter. Whatever the medical benefits of the radiation, they must also be weighted against its side-effects, which range from the almost immediate skin reactions and radiation sickness to possible longer-term complications involving the heart, the lungs, and deep tissue reactions.

On account of the high-dose rates, the irradiation times have become so short that the setting up times for the full utilization of these expensive units have become extremely significant.

Radiation therapy, for optimal use of professional staff and equipment, and economy consistent with high quality care would still be best performed in a limited number of medical centres.

According to the UK estimates, a population of one million requires in a radiotherapy department, two cobalt machines or one cobalt machine and one linear accelerator or betatron machine. In addition there is a need for a superficial X-ray machine and a deep X-ray machine—200 or 250 KV—for palliative therapy or for use when one of the supervoltage machines is not working.

All machines should be replaced in 12 to 15 years.

The assumption as a bread guide for planning has been that a cobalt machine can treat 300 to 400 patients annually, and the linear acceleratory 600 to 800, Raison suggests on the basis of 400 cobalt patients per annum 560 linear accelerator patients and on the basis of 800 patients taken on an accelerator 500 patients for a cobalt machine.

A cobalt unit, can treat 30 to 40 patients in a day of seven hours with two radiographers to each machine and a linear accelerator treats 60 to 70 patients in the sametime. Because of the very short treatment, times the number of radiographers has to be doubled.

To establish a radiotherapy unit 7,000 to 10,238 medical treatments and/or examinations per annum are requested.

A regular 700-bed hospital for example, requires in addition 12 to 24 beds when radiation therapy is introduced in the hospital, a 1,000 bed hospital 40 to 60 beds and a hospital of the highest medico-technical standard about 50 to 80 beds. In these ward units, special precautions against radiation have to be taken.

Elements of Radiotherapy Unit

The clinical examinations section of a radiotherapeutic clinic includes a reception area including a registration room, examination and consultation rooms, rooms for medical staff and social workers, waiting areas including bed or trolley bays, storages, toilets and telephones.

The consultation rooms should be separated from the treatment area. The ration of examination and treatment rooms has to be high as many patients are old and slow to undress. The inevitable number of follow up examinations often produce large clinics. Insufficient rooms may result in insufficient use of medical staff. A darkened cubicle or room should be provided for examining otolaryngological patients.

An acceptable clinic room design from the functional point of view does not necessarily become acceptable when a mirror image of this is produced.

The treatment section comprises the treatment planning room for time-consuming dosimetric planning which requires access to a computer assisted scanner, simulator, mould room, medical staff-medical officers, physicists and technicians and secretarial and record facilities, rooms for the unit stands, spaces for machinery including the power supply components and the control room. The planning procedure may require the taking of check X-rays and the use of simulator.

This simulator is an essential piece of equipment and mandatory for all megavoltage units. The accommodation will comprise the main simulator room and control area, an X-ray processing room, and a clinical room for the preparation of the patient for minor surgical procedures.

A computer assisted tomography coupled with computerized treatment planning and dosimetry offers a great potential for improving radiation therapy through accurate localization of tumour and critical normal structures within the host and by utilizing the tissue density and X-ray attenuation coefficients to increase the accuracy of dose computations. Such a system will utilize measurements from the actual patient for corrections necessary for dose perturbations resulting from tissue heterogeneity. A special CT scanning unit is needed in larger radiotherapy units. A treatment room needs 45 m^2 to 56 m^2 has been preferred for its irradiation area including the 1.75 m wide maze, about 15 m^2 for the stand, and 35 m^2 for the machine room.

Various methods are used for providing access to the treatment or radiation room. The most convenient is achieved by means of a door leading directly into the room. In the case of megavoltage installations, however, such a door requires heavy shielding even when located in a wall exposed only to leakage and scattered radiation. It may be very heavy and require an expensive motor drive as well as means for emergency manual operation. A maze arrangement is generally the most economical, as shielding of the door can be greatly reduced, usually to less than 6 mm of lead, if it is exposed to multiple scattered radiation only. The required lead equivalence of the door will depend upon radiation energy, maze design, weekly workload and beam orientations. The principal objections to the use of a maze are increased space requirements and sometimes less convenient access to the treatment room, particularly for stretcher patients.

Direct window viewing is used in most superficial and orthovoltage installations. For megavoltage installations the cost of the high-density glass and its lead frame may be significant. Indirect viewing by means of mirrors is more economical but may be less satisfactory.

Closed circuit TV provides considerable flexibility, as both camera and display can be located for maximum convenience. Therapy equipment control panels and TV displays for several facilities may be placed in close proximity to each other; several cameras may be used to view the patient from different angles; a pan-tilt mechanism for the camera may be operated from the control panel to view any portion of the treatment room; and additional displays may be located elsewhere. Disadvantages of such a system include the need for auxiliary viewing in case of TV equipment failure, and the cost of maintenance.

In therapy installations, means of oral communication between the patient and control room shall be provided.

The people outside the treatment room must be protected from accidental radiation. The walls of the treatment room likely to be hit by the direct radiation must be made of baryt concrete, the other walls may consist of normal concrete. In treatment rooms, there is a hazard due to high concentrations of ozone and the oxide of nitrogen. An air flow across the room to reduce rapidly the gas concentrations and about 12 air changes per hour should be provided.

The machine control room or station needs not border on the treatment room. It should allow adequate space for the radiographer team and some students, altogether approximately six people.

The radiotherapy mould room suite is a key supporting facility, its activities are diversified over a range of technical skills. The prime function of this suite is to produce skills and applicator for tumour sites. Here, patient impressions are taken, appliances constructed, plaster of paris technique applied as well as cold setting resion formulations, epoxy/polyester techniques, etc. practiced.

The main work laboratory should have benching, cupboards, and drawers. Work cubicles should be provdied for construction and fitting procedures to afford privacy to patients.

The plaster room of about 11 m^2 size should have tilted surfaces and floor drainage.

A vaccum forming and injection molding bay is required as well as store for materials. As the mould room uses inflammable materials, good ventilation is essential.

To reduce the hazard of transporting radioactive sources, the insertion of radioactive materials is undertaken in the operation room. A single-operation-room operation unit is needed. Extra space must be allowed for radiation protection equipment.

The place of chemotherapy in radiotherapy oncology department is increasing steadily-palliative at first but sometimes curative when combined with other disciplines.

As many patients may attend for multi-agent injections, there must be adequate waiting space, rooms for injection therapy and a recovery unit containing at least three couches is needed for outpatients awaiting transport after treatment.

The radioisotope laboratory has for its solid sources a general service area where applicators and accessories are stored together with shielded containers and appliances for transporting radioactive materials. Records of radioactive materials. Records of radioactive material in stock and in transit use must be kept.

A radiopharmaceutical room is needed to produce under aseptic conditions substances which are injected intravenously into the patient.

Rooms for general *in vivo* and *in vivo* counting are needed, where gamma cameras and rectilinear scanner are used. Additional rooms will be required for imaging equipment.

A sub-waiting area will enable to separate patients who have received radioisotopes from other waiting patients.

Officers for registration, consulting rooms, and rooms for secretarial staff and data recording equipment are needed as well as a xeroxing bay. Any large radiotherapy unit has to allow a seminar room for daily meetings to review case reports, notes and films and to keep staff generally informed.

A staff library with a section for medical slides is needed as well as offices for photography, and documentation and statistics, as well as accommodation for research.

Provision for ample storage space is essential. Equipment not in regular use should not be left around in treatment rooms as it can bee unsightly in departments and worrying for ill patients. There should be mechanical engineering and electronic worship facilities. Hospitals where radiotherapeutical experimental studies are conducted, require and animal quarters. Wherever possible, rooms with no outside windows should be avoided.

Radioactive Waste

Radioactive waste from telecurie and brachycurie treatment in the kilocurie or 100 millicurie range with a half-life of about five years. These preparations, as well as cobalt 60, regarded as no longer useable after a few years. These wastes are not bulky but are highly active and need to be fully screened at all stages.

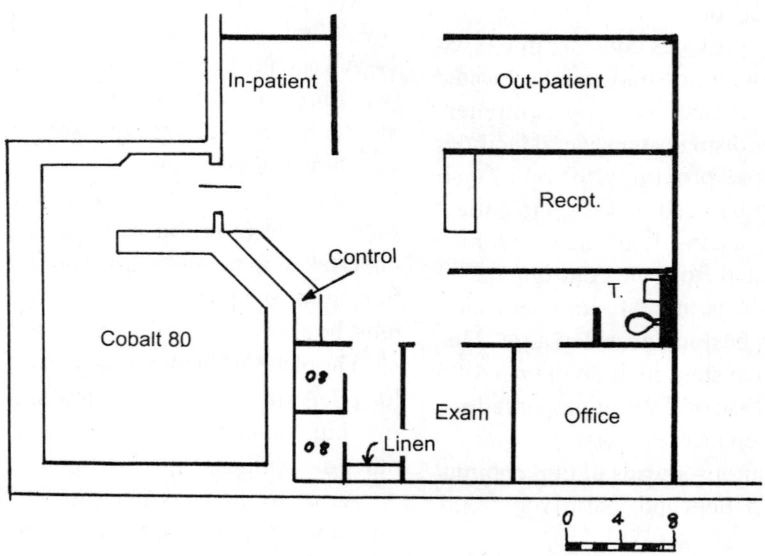

Fig. 35.26: Affiliated radiotherapy center. The single cobalt suite might be located in a community hospital remote from a radiotherapy treatment center. But a suite of this size could be associated with a medical center. The layout shown contains minimal facilities. Patient waiting areas and reception, dressing, and examination rooms have been provided

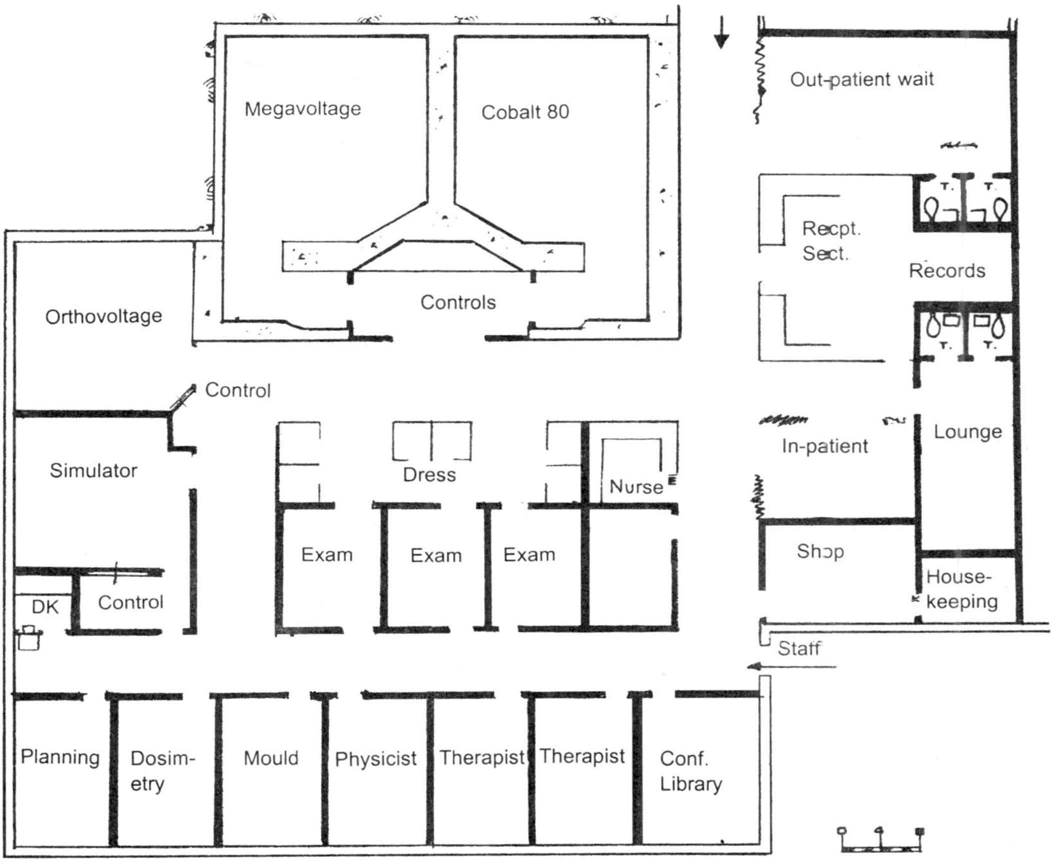

Fig. 35.27: The clinical radiotherapy center might be considered a moderate-sized department. The receptionist has visual contact with all waiting patients. A nurses' station is located central to the various functions. Individual patinet dressing booths are shown directly outside the examination rooms and across the corridor from the treatment rooms. The staff corridor is separate from patient traffic. A darkroom has been provided close to the simulator room

Waste from nuclear medicine and other applications are bulky but with a half-life of less than 14 days can be treated as inactive waste after 24 half-life periods. Iodine 125, with a half-life of 60 days, needs special storage. When providing facilities for storing of these wastes, the national regulations have to be observed strictly.

3–D Treatment Planning System

In the past few years, the dawn of the new perspective in how radiation therapies administered, using three dimensional treatment planning systems, has influenced the approach and outcome of cancer cases.

Randolph Hemingway,
Precision Therapy International

Three dimensional (3–D) treatment planning systems have allowed the radiation oncologist and the physicist to treat patients with ports outside the typical co-plannar fashion defined by convention. The result is an escalated those to the tumor and a

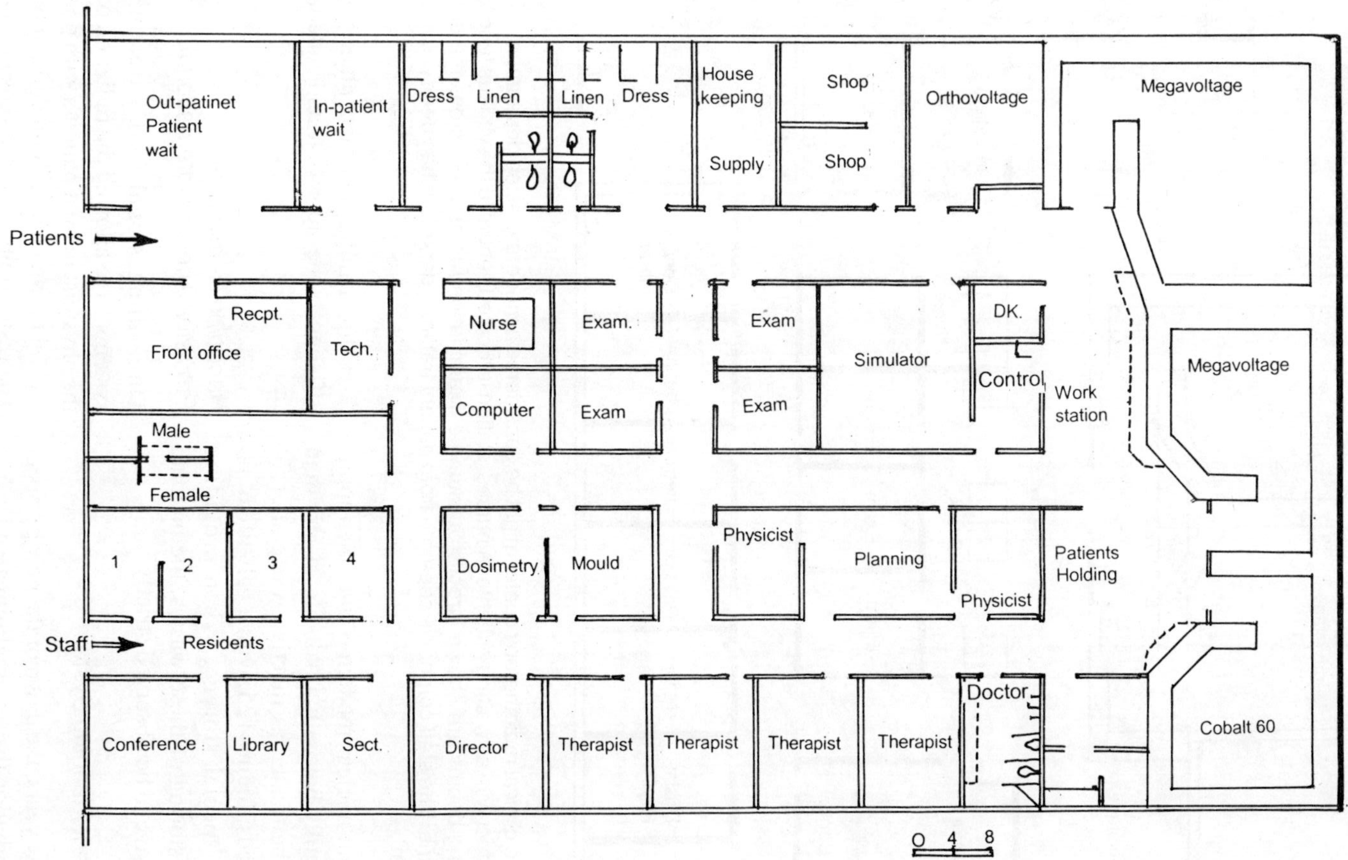

Fig. 35.28: A complete radiotherapy center with resident training program requires larger treatment and staff facilities. The receptionist and nurses' station are convenient to the patient waiting areas. A waiting area for gowned patients is separate from the main waiting area and is divided into separate areas for male and female ptients. The examination rooms are convenient to the gowned waiting areas. The inner staff functions are away from patient traffic. A treatment planning room is located central to physicist, therapist, and simulation. Residents' offices have been included. Facilities are shown for radium storage preparation

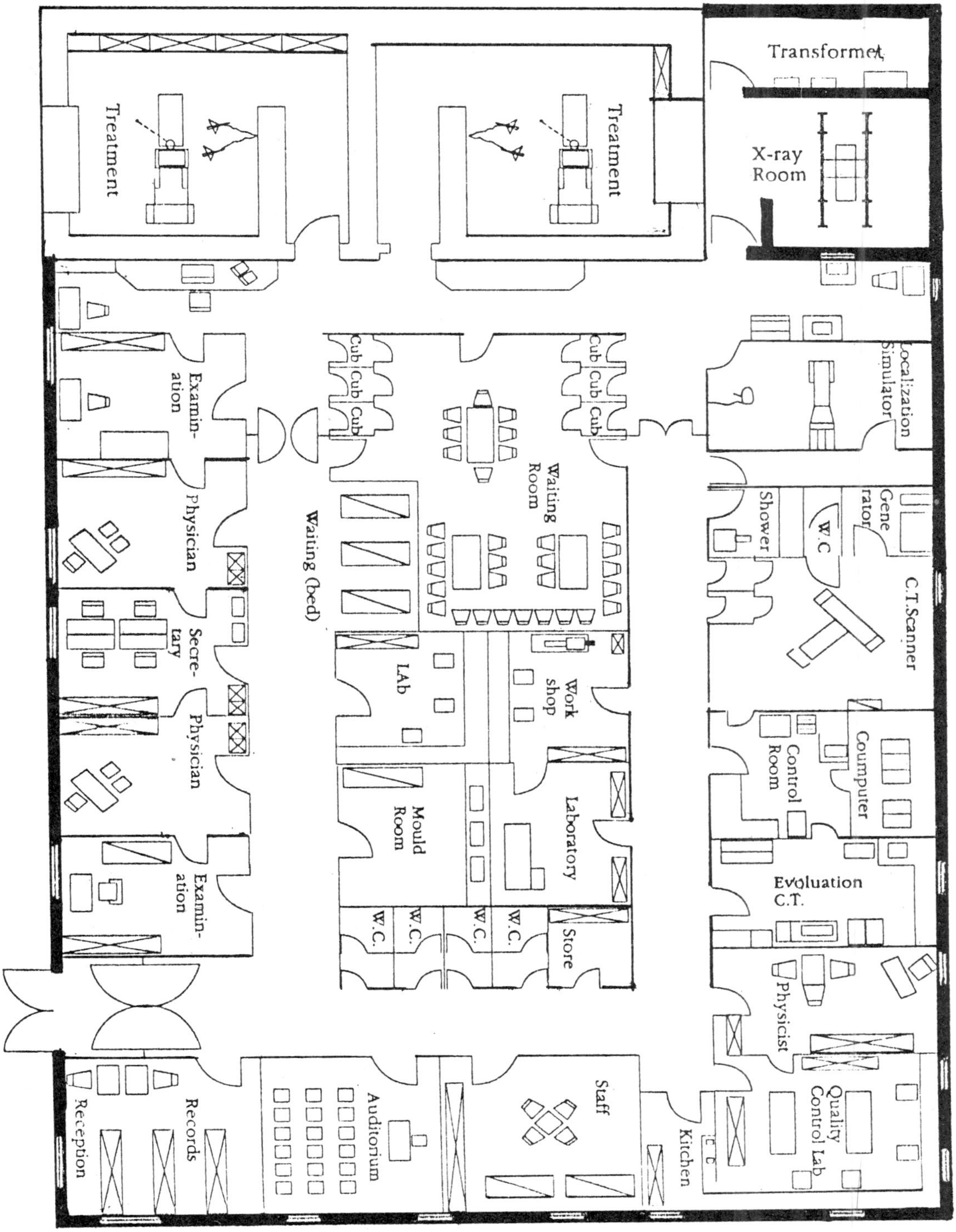

Fig. 35.29: Layout of radiation therapy department

minimized dose to sensitive structures, yielding better tumor response and less morbidity. Inevitably, the outcome is improved quality of life for the patient.

Ultimately, the objective in radiotherapy treatment of malignancies is to deliver a tumorcidal dose to the lesion while minimizing exposure to the surrounding tissues. This is often accomplished through creative strategies aided by a treatment planning system. Until recently this process was limited to delivering radiation through co-plannar portals. The ability to venture simple plane of radiation required great inside and faith today with the aid of computerized 3-D treatment planning it is possible to reconstruct, visualize, plan, calculate and evaluate sophisticated dosimetery with a verifiable means.

The essential difference between 2-D and 3-D computerized treatments planning systems are graphical presentations and dose calculations. 3-D systems require true user interface tools for field determination verification. Dose optimizing through beam modifications with tools such as true colour compensations and other forms of dose intensity modulation are highly desirable. Dose calculations using volumetric reconstruction of 2-D computerized tomography (CT) scans and interpretation of tissue densities should model a close depiction of actual measured dose.

Hardware Equipment in 3–D Image Reconstruction

With the aid of accelerated central processing systems and graphics processors in high performance workstations, reconstruction of 2-D to 3-D images by surface rendering is a reality. Mega-floating point operations (FLOP) ratings exceed 300 on many workstations. Million instructions per second (MIPS) exceed 180. The result of such a configuration is true interactive rotation in real time, a virtual reality is in planning a 3-D, volumetric subject. Complex routines of redundant mathematical calculations that used to take days are now accomplished in minutes. Even peripherals such as printers are far superior, with the ability graphically to duplicate image like that displayed on a high-resolution monitor. All the basic hardware tools are available to accomplish optimal 3-D planning.

Dose Calculation Algorithms

One of the major significant dilemas in calculating true doses is the algorithms ability to predict the actual dose measure. The Monte Carlo formula for dose calculation is the most accurate. Unfortunately, the workstations are not prepared to handle such a laborious task in a reasonable time frame. Most of the alternatives have been modifications of 2-D photon algorithms. One of the most popular approaches has been modifications of Clerkson or scatter integration. The beauty of the approach is the manner which scatter is handled. The data comparison with the measure dose in most cases is within a 2 percent deviation. The use of a more controversial approach is the convolution method. Some developers tout a higher accuracy rate, yet the approach has not been approved by the US Food and Drug Administration. Variation from these two methods may vary by 1 percent. Electrons are being adequately calculated with a 3-D derivation of the Hogstroms Pencil beam. In summary, the approach to dose calculations has evolved so that they have become more predictable and more reliably generated.

The determination of pixel by pixel electron density calculation by CT number (Hounsfield) has allowed for more sophisticated dose prediction with modeled 3-D images. Higher quality CT scanners have enabled the calculation of accurate tissue densities throughout the study series. Such methods are equivalent path length (EPL) can be used in predicting perturbation of electron transport.

With the aid of these more sophisticated calculation methods, interest in optimizing tumor doses in a volumetric manner recedes. True dose compensation method examines the calculated dose for the scatter integration and attempts to optimize beam profiles. From this calculation there is an output to the milling machine for shaping. This device is then used in the linear acceleratory tray, much like a wedge.

Other works in progress include true intensity modulation with aid of internal interactive veins, or leaves, that after the dose distribution in a dynamic form. Multileaf collimation and dynamic wedges play a significant role in dose distribution and therefore should be an integral part of the ideal planning system.

Graphical Interface and Interactives

No less important than the calculation approaches are true tools for planning. Virtual or 3-D simulation may best describe the process of a 3-D planning computer system. There will be a significant decrease in the use of simulators and CT scanners will appreciate in the near future.

Some of the essential tools are as follows:

Beam's eye view (BEV) should be interactive in space with the true functions of the accelerator; i.e., collimator, gantry, field size and couch angle.

Room's eye view (REV) much like BEV, should be interactive.

Non-coplannar beam allows for placement in an orientation not parallel to the cross section.

Digital reconstructed radiographs (DRR) are as close depiction of how the actual port film should look.

Dose volume histogram (DVH) are as graphical plot defining dose versus volume of a known structure.

Surface rendering is an aid for outlining 2-D structures in a 3-D manner with coloured wire frame, transparencies and opaques. Autocountering of structures and volumetric display of dose distribution are critical.

Sagital and coronal reconstruction of transverse slices for 2-D visual interpretation of beam placement and dose evaluation.

Icons illustrates interactively the teletherapy unit's physical orientation.

Design of treatment aids, such as Bolas, custom blocking, compensation and wedges. Another consideration for a planning system would be the ability to correlate with other imaging modalities. In many cases, magnetic resonance imaging (MRI) may host valuable information in tumor volume determination. Since MRI does not yield density correction, a fusion of this information to CT is invaluable.

CT interfaces are of the essence to properly facilitate efficient image acquisition. Many sites are opting to choose a dedicated CT to ensure patient position. Immobalisation of the patient has become critical to precise field placement.

Future Needs

Automation of radiotherapy centers is becoming more critical as treatment plans become more complex. Linear accelerators are now digitally controlled with options such as dynamic wedges and multileaf collimators. Record and verify computer interfaces confirm necessary parameters of machine positioning. Block cutters and compensator machines are automatically designed devices for beam shaping. Dosimetery measuring tools are linked to a management package for routine data collection. Picture archiving computer systems (PACS) transport and manipulate portal images, treatment plans and diagnostic studies.

More developers are running in parallel, and are not adequately addressing the open architecture requirements to integrate these tools. Conformity in software and hardware development is needed with room to grow. Closed architecture operating systems force use either to emulate functionality thereby slowing it, or to run operations independently causing poor efficiency. All systems should be planned for compatibility.

The evolution of 3-D treatment planning has resulted in the use of better defined target volumes and allows for more accurate dose evaluation. The initiation of more protocols relating to non-coplannar treatments are planned three dimensionally.

The data link protocol started by the radiation therapy oncology group will facilitate such information. Ultimately higher, more homogenous dose distributions will be delivered to the tumor and will be minimised to the normal tissue. The result yields an escalation of doses by as much as 10 percent. It is hoped that future studies will show improved local tumor control and an improved quality of life for the patient.

THE BRACHYTHERAPY

Brachytherapy is a specialised method of delivering a bniologically significant dose of ionising radiation to a critical target volume using radioactive sources placed in or near the target volume. HDR (high dose rate) Brachytherapy by virtue of its dose rate and fractionation has radiological effects similary to fractionated external therapy. LDR (low dose rate) has the potential for superior delivery of ionising radiation to the target, but has the advantage, and disadvantage of delivering the dose over a longer time. Because LDR is basically infinitely fractionated radiation, one would expect the long-term side effects to be decreased, compared to HDR. Pulsed dose rate (PDR) brachytherapy aims to maintain the repair advantage of LDR while utilising the radiation protection advantages and planning flexibility of a stepping source.

Applications of Brachytherapy

- Intravascular
  - to prevent restenosis
- Treatment of
  - Head and neck carcinoma
  - Nasophysingeal cancer
  - Endobronchial carcinoma
  - Lung cancer
  - Carcinoma of the esophagus (intraluminal brachytherapy, external beam radiotherapy: EBRT, associated with HDR brachytherapy)
  - Prostate cancer (HDR combined with external beam radiotherapy)
  - Carcinoma of the cervix
  - Retroperintoneal sarcomas
  - Breast cancer
- The concept of IORT is essentially based on achieving a maximal local dose escalation by actually visualising the target volume at the time of surgery and as direct irradiation of the target volume as possible, while minimising the radiation to any interventing or underlying normal tissue. The techniques (to extend the boundaries of surgical resection) allow for both, organ/function preservation in less advanced cases by substituting radiation for more extensive and mutilating surgery, while they can actually improve local control (and possibly overall survival (in cases when local relapses are a major problem despite maximum surgical resection.

Intravascular brachytherapy (both by beta and gamma emitters) has been shown to prevent neointimal proliferation (restenosis) after balloon or stent injury. The introduction of radiation therapy to the cardiac catheterisation laboratory is a new concept. The use of vascular brachytherapy for peripheral arteries require the patient to be transported to the radiation oncology suite for treatment with a closed-end lumen delivery catheter positioned in his peripheral arteries. There are two classes of device for coronary use: catheter based systems, and radioactive implants. Currently there seems to be accumulating a preponderence of evidence supporting the notion that endovascular radiation can alter the natural history of coronary interventional procedures.

In contrast to external beam radiotherapy treatment planning, brachytherapy treatment planning covers only the reconstruction of applicators with the aid of radiographs and a few anatomically defined reference points. The dose calculation is performed on the basis of predefined arbitrary planes.

The radiation oncologist must be thoroughly familiar with the basic principles of physics and dosimetry of irradiation, skilled in the performance of interstitial or intracavitary brachytherapy, and knowledgeable in the clinocopathological features of tumors to optimally use radiation therapy in the management of patients with cancer.

The New Brachytherapy

The radiation oncologist must be thoroughly familiar with the basic principles of physics and dosimetry of irradiation, skilled in the performance of interstitial or intracavitary brachytherapy, and knowledgeable in the clinocopathological features of tumors to optimally use radiation therapy in the management of patients with cancers. Empty catheters are placed through the tumor in the operating room, and then after loaded with iridium-192.

The radiation exposure to staff, and the person loading the radiation sources into the implant, can be reduced using remote afterloading. This is achieved because every time a nurse enters the patient's room, the radiation sources are withdrawn into the shielded safe of the remote after loader.

The most important factor in the rapid growith of remote after loading brachytherapy is the added treatment control which is offered by this technology, the trend towards outpatient also encouraged the use of HDR remote afterloading system that enable the doctor to deliver a fractionated treatment in only a few minutes, rather than 30 to 70 hours of a conventional LDR treatment.

Modern afterload also enable the radiation isodose distribution to the optimised to treat a particular tumor geometry, or patient anatomy. Treatment optimisation can be achieved by using the stepping source with its variable dwell position and times. The techniques including singular value decomposition optimisation and geometry based Iterative optimisation.

The use of optimised brachytherapy using a small stepping source, controlled by a remote after loading system is a technique that will expand rapidly, making manual implants obsolete.

Brachytherapy has been used since the early 1900's to achieve local control of cancerous tumors. Originally, radium rubes were placed in corks to treat cervical cancer, and radium was also used interstitially in glass or metallic tubes. Surface tumors were treated by using individualised wax or plaster moulds, in which rasium tubes or needles were embedded.

By the 1960's and 1970's cessium-137 sources had often become the radionuclide of choice for intracavitary therapy. The cesium-137 was encapsulated in 2 cm long, platinum/iridium tubes, with an active length of 1.5 cm (Amersham type G-tubes). There were different source activities commercially available such as 5 mg, 10 mg, 20 mg and 25 mg radium equivalent. However, very little control could be exerted over the positioning of, for example, sources within ovoids (colpostats). This often resulted in a policy of 'standard' loadings for vaginal ovoids and uterine tandems as in the Manchester system. The results obtained were consistent, but relied considerably on the skill of the doctor placing applicators in position and in using gauze packing to avoid high rectal and bladder doses.

Iridium-192 and Manual Afterloading

The introduction of iridium-192 wire and seeds has resulted in an increase in the use of interstitial therapy for treatment of breast and head and neck cancers. Empty catheters are placed through the tumor in the operating róom, and then afterloaded with iridium-192.

In Europe, the standard practice for interstitial therapy is to use iridium-192 wire cut-out length and inserted into a flexible nylon carrier. This is then introduced into the patient's implant catheters. In the United States, worries about possible radioactive contamination when cutting the wire, resulted in the development of iridium-192 seeds, usually encased in nylon carrier with a 10 mm spacing between seeds. The length of the implant can be altered, but normally all the seeds are of the same activity. A few hospitals order 'dumbell' loading of the seeds in the carrier activities higher at each end, and even fewer hospitals arrange for the seed ribbons to be removed at different times. With such non-standard practices, it is difficult to guarantee the quality control needed to prevent mistakes.

Radiation Exposure and Manual Afterloading

Although the use of manual afterloading procedure removed the radiation exposure to the doctor implanting or inserting the catheters, there was still radiation exposure to the person loading the radiation sources and to the nursing staff in the ward or room containing the patient. The ALARA principle states that radiation exposure must be as low as reasonably achievable. The normal working practices or reducting the radiation exposure by using time + Distance + shielding do not always achieve Alara since major surgery results in an increase in the required nursing, and too much shielding increases the time that the nurse must spend near the patient. radiation exposure of radiation therapy personnel results primarily from brachytherapy procedures. Even when conventional after-loading procedures are followed, radiation exposure of nursing personnel, implant technologists, and medical resident staff may be of concern. Since many hospital employees are young, consideration of radiation exposure in the medical profession is important.

The New Brachytherapy: Ratiation Production and Remote Afterloading

However, the radiation exposure to nursing staff, and to the person loading the radiation sources into the implant, can be reduced using remote afterloading. This is achieved because every time a nurse enters the patient's room, the radiation sources are withdrawn into the shielded safe of the remote afterloader. In the mid 1980's the majority of remote afterloading systems were used to match conventional low dose rate treatments supplying radiation protection and a better degree of treatment control than could be achieved using manual afterloading or pre-loaded techniques.

Control of Radiation Removal

An interesting side effect of the introduction of remote afterloading is the control of radiation sources. Nobody has to remove radiation sources in the middle of the night, since the remote afterloading system automatically achieves this task. Also, it is not possible to lose radiation sources or as has been reported to the author from more than one hospital, accidentally remove the radiation sources from the wrong patient.

Treatment Control

The most important factor in the rapid growth of remote afterloading brachytherapy is the added treatment control which is offered by this technology. The trend towards outpatient treatment also encouraged the use of HDR remote afterloading systems that enable the doctor to deliver a fractionated treatment in only a few minutes, rather than the 30 to 70 hours of a conventional LDR treatment.

Optimisation

Modern remote afterloaders also enable the radiation isodose distribition to be optimised to treat a particular tumor geometry, or patient anatomy. The use of conventional brachytherapy resulted in a relatively fixed treatment isodose distribution, with very limited ability to optimise any treatment. The most common HDR remote afterloading system, the micro-selectron-HDR supplied by Nucletron, uses a small 1.1 m diameter by 6 mm length stepping source of Iridium-192. The position of the source within each catheter can be programmed in 1 to 28 possible dwell positions. Depending on the step size selected, 2.5 mm or 5 mm, this gives a treatment window of 12 cm or 24 cm. This treatment window can then be moved anywhere within the last 30 cm of the applicator.

In each of the dwell positions the treatment time for the source can be programmed to be in the range 0 to 999.9 seconds. This effectively gives an infinite variable source activity in each position. The variable dwell time also enables the isodoses to be shaped in each catheter for this system which has 18 catheters (channels). An example of this optimisation capability is where the single source has been programmed to give a linear, a dumbell and a pear-shaped isodose distribution.

Obviously it is still possible to give a standard source loading and standard dosimetry, however, to take full advantage of the extra degrees of freedom for treatment control presented by the moder remote afterloading systems, sophisticated brachytherapy treatment planning is required.

Treatment optimisation has been an unattained goal for many years, but this ideal can only be fully realised using the stepping source with its variable dwell positions and times. Two optimisation techniques are of particular use if we wish to take advantage of this new degree of control

- Singular value decomposition optimization (SVD)
- Geometry based iterative optimization (GBI)

Singular Value Decomposition

Optimization was developed for the special requirements of a multiple catheter bronchial implant, where the catheters are placed through and around a bronchial tumor. The catheters can take virtually any angle or curve and this type of implant is totally different from the conventional parallel needles of a breast or template implant. SVD enables the physicist to obtain a uniform isodose distribution with the diverging or converging catheters avoiding hot spots. The prescription is usually at 1 cm from the catheter envelope.

Geometry Based Iterative

Optimization was developed to optimise a large interstitial implant, such as prostate template, where it may be required to have a uniform isodose distribution throughout a multiple needle implant, or to have different dose regions within the same implant. The tumor volume is defined by the needle placement and apart from defining the needle or catheter length, it is not necessary to define specific dose optimisation points. The technique enables the physicist to correct for a certain amount of misplacement, or curvature of the needles.

Is the use of remote afterloading brachytherapy, particularly HDR brachytherapy, a viable treatment technique? The remote afterloading LDR treatments match clinically the conventionall LDR brachytherapy dose rates, but with complete radiation protection and a degree of added control. HDR brachytherapy is not new and has been in use for over 3 years for treatment of cancer of the cervix and endometrium.

The new factor is the small controllable iridium-192 stepping source which enables any body site to be treated. Palliative treatments of the bronchus and oesophagus are an excellent appliction for this outpatient treatment technique. The convenience of outpatient treatment for the cancer of the cervex, prove to be advantagesis.

The use of optimised branchtherapy using a small stepping source, controlled by a remote afterloading system is a technique that will expand rapidly. Within the next 10 years, most radiotherapy departments will be using this form of brachytherapy and it will become ethically necessary to use the added treatment control. Manual implants will then become as obsolate as the use of radium sources, which is already obsolete. This is the result of the inevitable march of technological progress.

The new treatment methods illustrate the tremendous degree of control now possible with brachytherapy.

FURTHER READING

1. International Conference of Canere Nursing, London, September.
2. van der Lssrse: New developments in computerized brachytherapy treatment planning. Clinical aspects of brachtherapy, 1989, 57-71.

NUCLEAR MEDICINE DEPARTMENT

When the Hungarian chemist George von Hevesy, used radioisotopes to study phosphorus metabolism in human bone in 1935, he could have had little idea that his research would lead to a radically new way to diagnose heart, kidney, lung and many other disorders.

A little over 66 years have elapsed since Hevesy collected his Nobel prize for chemistry and his legacy–nuclear medicine–is now available in about half of US and Japanese hospitals and one in three European hospitals. Today, nuclear medicine is used mainly in diagnosis and to a lesser extent, in treatment. It relies on the fact that radioisotope are unstable elements whose atomic nuclei 'decay' into more stable forms while, at the same time emitting small amount of beta and gamma radiation.

When these small amounts of radioisotopes are injected into the blood stream, swallowed or inhaled, they selectively deposit in particular tissues or fluids of the body and decay, generally over a period of a few days. The radiation which they emit can be analysed by special cameras outside the body which produce quantitative pictorial images and measurements.

Unlike other forms of scanning, such as X-rays and computerized axial tomography which primarily provides structural information, nuclear medicine provides valuable information about the function of various data.

For example, it is used to determine the functional defects in the heart and blood vessels. Doctors can see the effects of injury on the movement of the walls of the heart, they can measure efficiency of heart contraction and they can locate areas of the heart with insufficient blood supply due to blocked vessels.

Similarly, when radioisotopes are inhaled they can be used to evaluate blood flow to the lungs and the distribution of air in the airways. Obstructions in the air sacs or blood clots in the tiny blood vessels of the lungs can be picked up. In the spleen and liver, nuclear imaging can show tumours and abscesses and, in the gall bladder, blockages and inflammation. Bone imaging with radioisotopes is more sensitive than X-rays in detecting both stress fractures and the spread of cancer to the skeleton. Staging tumours in this way is important in deciding what treatment should be given–and when–to either slow the spread of the disease or to provide pain relief from bone metastases.

For imaging, radioisotopes which emit gamma particles are used because they can be detected by the cameras used in nuclear medicine. Beta particle producing isotopes which are often used for therapy have shorter wavelengths. They cannot be used for imaging. The first radioisotopes to be used in medicine were those of hydrogen (deuterium or heavy water), phosphorus (phosphorus-32), sodium (sodium-24) and potassium (potassium-42). Before long, researchers were using radioiodine (iodine-131) to measure thyroid function and, later, to suppress thyroid function.

The mid-1970s dramatically changed the field of nuclear medicine with the development of radioactive nuclides. Prior to the 1970s, hospitals were forced to use radiopharmaceuticals (tracers) sourced directly from the reactor. These tracers had to be used quickly or else their usefulness would diminish. The newly developed "inactive" pharmaceuticals could be stored at the hospital and conveniently "activated", as needed using a generator.

The 1980s saw the development of computers which allowed sensitive measurement and quantitation of emitted radioactivity. By 1990, the development of high performance SPECT (Single Photon Emission Computer Tomography) cameras provided functional imaging of superb quality and detail. These SPECT cameras used in conjunction with computers can construct three-dimensional images of the body's organs.

Today, nuclear medicine has developed into an important tool with enormous potential in the world market, saving countless lives.

Swallowing, inhaling or being injected with something radioactive–however, low the level–sounds pretty scary. But patients can be reassured that they will be exposed to less radiation than for many X-ray procedures. For example, bone imaging by nuclear medicine techniques given one-tenth the radiation of a bone X-ray. Air travellers on international flights are exposed to a much radiation as compared to certain nuclear medical scans.

Anyone working with radioactive substances wears a device to measure radiation and ensure that their exposure does not exceed allowable limits. Most of the waste generated by a typical nuclear medicine department of hospital contains very short-lived radioactive materials which can be stored on site until the radiation disappears and it can be disposed off with the rest of the hospital refuse. Only small amounts waste have to be sent to licensed disposal facilities. There is little doubt of the usefulness and safety of nuclear medicine for imaging and therapy. But what about the cost? As financial constraints bite into health budgets all over the world, there is growing pressure on health care providers to show that they are getting value for money.

In 1993, the British Nuclear Medicine Society commissioned an evaluation of the cost effectiveness of nuclear medicine. A review of over three hundred papers in the world, literature was carried out to provide evidence of the cost effectiveness of the nuclear medicine in a variety of clinical areas. At the end of 1994,the conclusion from the review were published and a number of diagnostic applications were considered to be of proven cost effectiveness or warranting further study. These are summarized in Table 35.4.

Of particular interest, bearing in mind the growing use on nuclear medicine in cardiology, were comparisons of the costs of a range of heart investigations (Table 35.5). These showed that myocardial perfusion imaging using radioisotope costs considerably less than a conventional angiographic investigation and it is also much less invasive for the patient.

Table 35.4: Cost-effectiveness of nuclear medicine

Disease	*Cost-effectiveness score*
Coronary artery disease	
• diagnosis	Medium
• management	High
Kidney	
• hypertension, transplant, urinary tract infection	Medium-high
Lung	
• pulmonary embolism	High
• brain (still in research phase)	Low
Bone metastases	
• primary diagnosis	High
• follow-up	Low
Bowel	
• inflammatory bowel disease	High
Thyroid	
• nodule	Low
• follow-up	High^{+}

High	– Nuclear medicine technique accepted as cost-effective
High	– Literature provides enough information to warrant further studies of cost-effectiveness
Medium	– Literature provides some evidence to suggest that further studies of cost-effectiveness may be warranted
Low	– Nuclear medicine techniques accepted as not being cost-effective or still in the research phase

For the future, nuclear medicine holds promise in the diagnosis of conditions which have evaded other scanning techniques. For example, over the last decade, radioisotopes have been developed which can cross the blood-brain barrier and have the potential for use in routine evaluation of cerebrovascular disease by assessing regional blood flow in the brain. There is growing interest in the use of nuclear medicine to differentiate between forms of dementia, such as those associated with

Table 35.5: Relative cost nuclear cardiological imaging techniques

Technique	*From the literature*	*From 3 key London hospitals*
Stress ECG	1.0	1.0
Rest echocardiogram	1.0	1.3
Stress echocardiogram	1.2-7.4	1.8
Myocardial perfusion imaging	1.3-7.4	2.8-3.7
Magnetic resonance imaging	–	4.6-11.6
Coronary angiography	5.3-18.5	9.6-11.6

Alzheimer's disease and AIDS. Nuclear medicine will continue to be a significant tool in proving safe, effective and painless means of gathering useful information necessary for diagnostic purpose. Its future will be guaranteed as new diagnostic and therapeutic applications are developed.

A value of 1.0 has been given to stress ECG and the other values and ranges are order of magnitude greater.

Nuclear Medicine Department

Nuclear medicine includes all aspects of radionuclide use medicine, including radioimmunoassay methods (purely *in vitro*); wet studies such as absorption tests, excretion tests and hematology test, partially *in vivo* and partially *in vitro*; imaging studies *in vivo*; and therapeutic applications (thyroid and blood diseases).

In the radioisotope unit of the nuclear medical services short-lived isotopes are used diagnostically as tracers to locate lesions tumours. The more long-lived isotopes are used therapeutically.

Through scanning the distribution of radioactive material in the human body is mapped. If a particular organ accumulates radioactive material selectively, an image may be produced which shows the position, size, and shape of the organ. The degree of radioactive material concentration may supply information about its function and lesions.

The trend of new instrumentation and efforts of radiopharmacists indicate that nuclear medicine is returning to an analysis of body functions and metabolism. The safety and relative simplicity of the nuclear examination methods suggest a considerable increase application on different organ systems than heretofore.

Moving Detector Instruments–rectilinear scanners or scintillation cameras–and stationary detector instruments, the so-called gamma cameras are used. Emission CT scanners do the same thing as gamma cameras. The difference is that the emission CTs can provide either cross section slices or slices the entire length of the body, whereas gamma cameras do not. The image of the emission is reconstructed by a computer on a video screen; data can be stored in the computer for later analysis and manipulation.

Emission CT scanners come in two types. The low-energy type, also known as single photon, uses commonly available radioisotopes that are routinely used by nuclear medicine departments. These low-energy radioisotopes can be active in the body for up to an hour, in some cases, and can be stored. High-energy emission CT scanners, also known as positron ECTs. Positron cameras or annihilation coincidence detection device, use high-energy radioisotopes that have a short half-life and cannot be stored. Most often used isotopes are the radioactive forms of carbon, oxygen and nitrogen. These must be manufactured in a readily accessible cyclotron, one that is usually no further away from the treatment area than in the adjacent building.

Radioactive wastes are clearly defined. Methods of their management are established. No reason for variance exists. Adequate installations must be provided to deal safely with radioactive wastes in liquid or solid form, whether from the laboratory or excreted by patients, and for the storage of unsealed sources in accordance with safety requirements. Storage tank for radioactive waste in an advantage when isotopes with short half-life are used. The patient who have died briefly after an injection of a significant dose of radioactive isotopes require the margue to be equipped with a radiation protected refrigerated chamber.

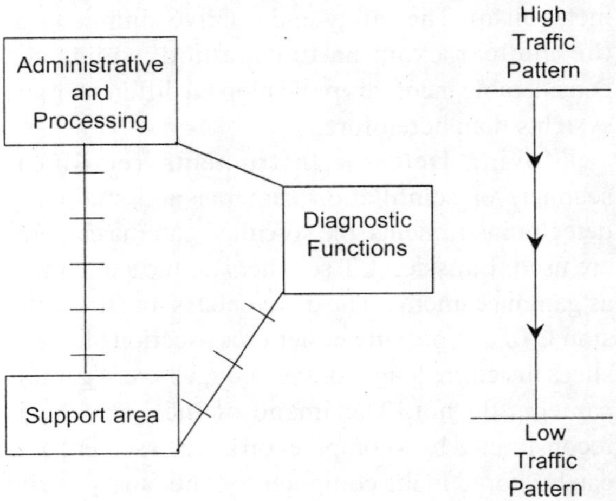

Fig. 35.30: Interrelationship of the three major functional units. The hatched connecting lines indicate lesser physical and proximity requirements

It is estimated that in many countries about 1 percent of the population is annually exposed to nuclear medical examinations. About 50–60 per cent of the nuclear medical services are conducted on the outpatient basis.

In the US teaching hospitals about 30 percent of the patients are diagnosed using radionuclides.

Nuclear medicine is a field in which technology advances are rapid and the demand for procedures is expanding, making planning difficult.

Internationally, the nuclear medical services have not a uniform organizational position. There are complete, independent units, but also units, where some of the activities are spread to X-ray diagnostic units, to radiotherapy, clinical chemistry, clinical psychology, and medical physics.

It has been stressed that there is an ever-growing association between nuclear medicine and

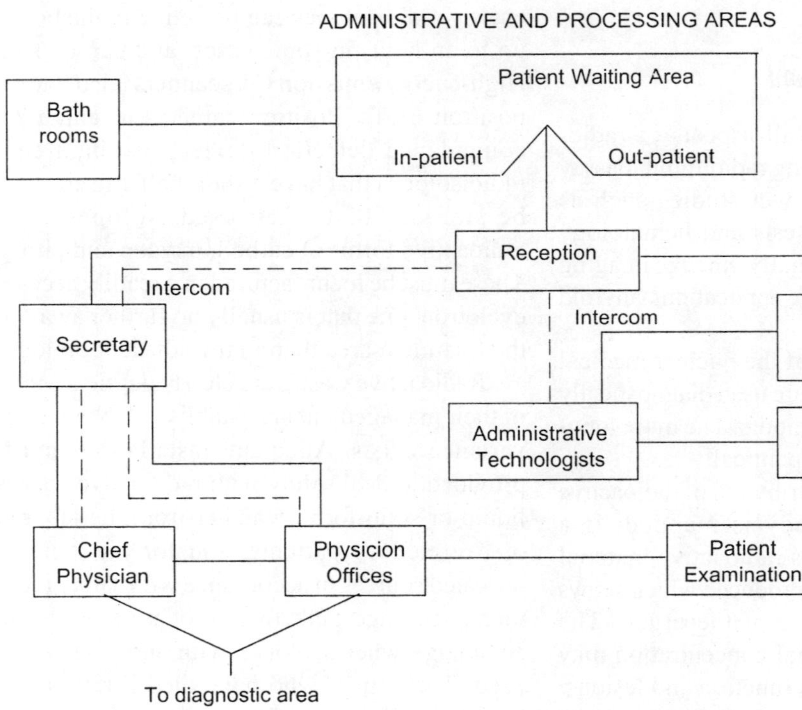

Fig. 38.31: The solid interunit connecting lines indicate the important proximity relationships, the dotted lines the intercommunication requirements

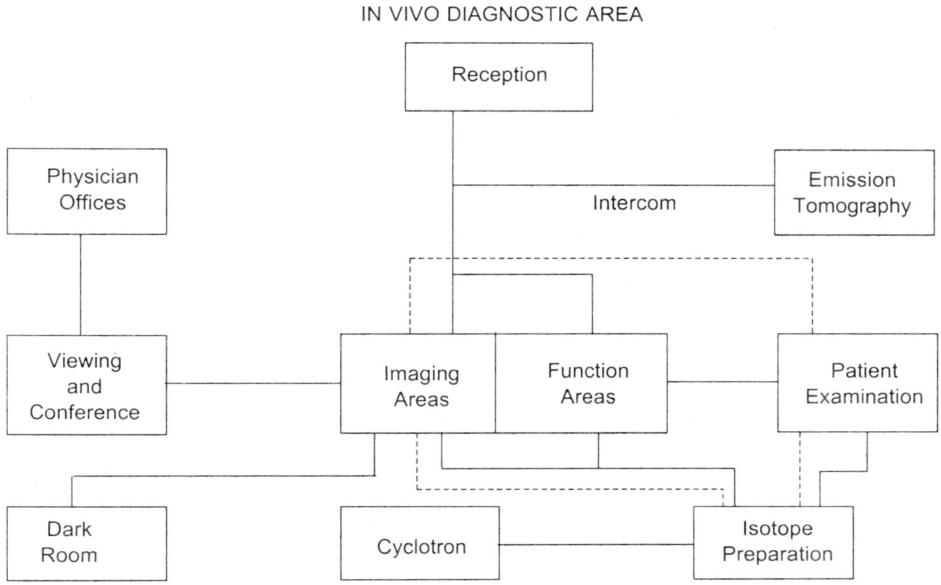

Fig. 35.32: The relationships of reception area to carious patient function units is shown. The dotted lines indicate the intercommunication system

diagnostic radiology, e.g. when isotopic techniques are compared with the standard chest radiograph, it is evident that the two are complementary. Their combination provides a powerful tool.

The office or control center located at point of patient arrival, would be the hub of the department. The size of procedure room or laboratory should be about 27 m^2 and of a scanning room about 15m^2. In the procedure room there is a patient examination table, work counters, a disposal sink, scintillation well counter, wall cabinets, a ventilated cabinet, a desk, a refrigerator, and a wash basin.

Electronic devices for locating the size of the tumour within the body is placed in the scanning room. Instead of a separate procedure room for each measure instrument, larger rooms or bays in which two or more instruments can be operated simultaneously can be used.

Administrative Area

The receptionist is the dynamic code of a nuclear medicine unit and usually has a number of responsibilities. For efficiency and work control there should be an intercommunication system between the receptionist and the technologist in the patient procedure area. Ideally there should be two types of communication systems between the receptionist and the technologists, a voice intercom and a telephone system to route calls to the imaging area. The receptionist must also have communication with the departmental secretary, usually by means of telephone, and advantageously should be in the physical proximity of the secretary. The receptionist should have easy access to the patient medical record files for quick retrieval when a patient arrives for examination. The secretary to the attending physician should be interposed between the receptionist and the physicians' offices.

Patient examination rooms should be adjacent to the physicians' offices. This is very important since many patients require interviewing and examining either before or after the studies. In addition, physicians must have satisfactory access to the diagnostic area.

A frequently forgotten facility is the technologists' lounge. Nuclear medicine procedures often

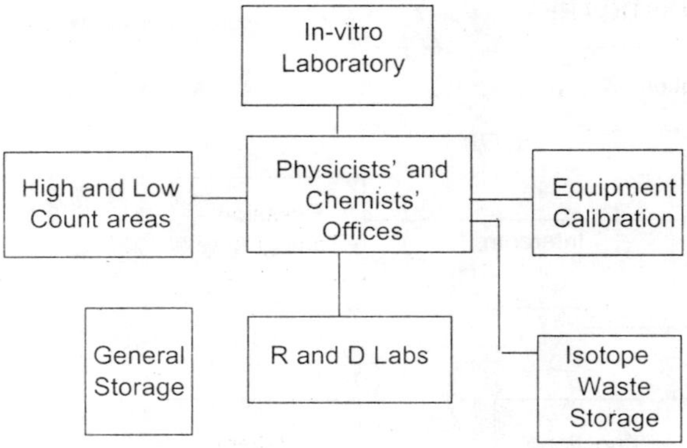

Fig. 35.33: In non-patient area, relationship of these units in *in vivo* and administrative areas is not critical

entail rather complicated logistics that require a number of sequential steps. For a number of reasons there may be extended periods of time when the technologists must be inactive. A readily available lounge is not only appreciated by the personnel but improves efficiency of operation. For example, it provides source for coffee breaks, rest, lunch, and so on, with minimal loss of time. Another advantage is the immediate availability of personnel is in cases of emergency or just to help in difficult situations that may develop.

In Vivo Diagnostic Area

A direct interface between the reception area and the imaging/function areas is mandatory for efficient patient care. The imaging area must be adjacent to the function area where procedures such as thyroid uptakes or dynamic renal studies are performed and the dark room should be close by for film processing. There should be direct access from patient examination rooms since patients will frequently go directly from the examination rooms to an imaging/function unit, particularly for thyroid studies. Periodically technologists will observe an abnormality that requires an immediate attention of the nuclear medicine physician. To avoid tying up the diagnostic area, the patient can return to an examination for further evaluation by the attending.

The film viewing and conference room should be directly accessible to the patient procedure area and the physicians' offices. Question on studies by the technologists and censoring studies are continuous physician responsibilities. These areas must be convenient for the physician or efficient utilization of time will not be attained. To decrease needless traffic in the reception are and the diagnostic area, there should be direct access to the viewing and conference room for the house and attending staff.

The isotope preparation section should be very convenient to the function area and the imaging area. In most hospitals radiopharmaceutical preparation is performed by the technologist who do the imaging. To conserve personnel time proximity

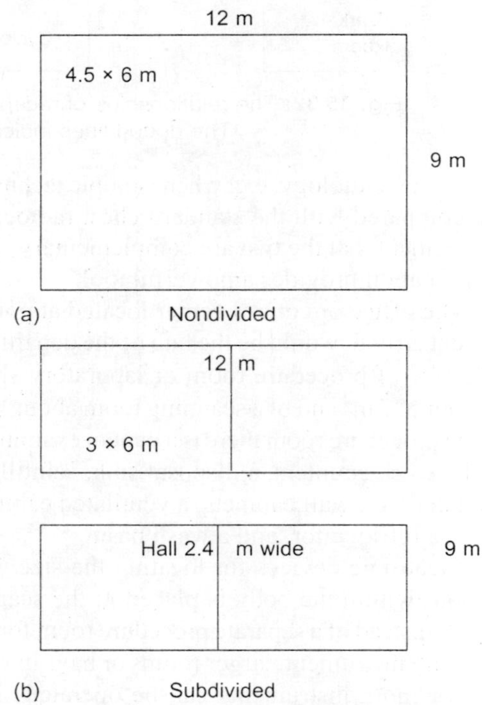

Fig. 35.34: (a) Design of 111.4 m^2 (1200 ft^2) imaging area (multiprocedure room) without partitions, providing space for four examining areas, (b) Design of 111.4 m^2 (1200 ft^2) imaging area (individual rooms) with partitions. Each examining area measures only 3 × 6 m (11 × 20 ft) and 22.3 m^2 (240 ft^2) must be devoted to hall access

is needed not only to the imaging studies but also to the patient examination areas. Since many patients are examined first by the physician, it is convenient to administer the radiopharmaceutical in the examining room.

In larger hospitals and medical centers positron emission tomography will probably be fairly common. This type of imaging requires an on site cyclotron and consideration must be given to these in future.

Non-patient Area

In a 500 bed hospital there may be need for physicists and chemists who require research and development laboratories, special counting rooms for high and low quantities of radioactivity, and space for equipment calibration. The *in vitro* laboratories should be located in the general area of non-patient function. Two storage areas for radioactive materials are required, one for current inventory and one for waste.

Space Requirements

The administrative and processing areas require approximately 180 m^2 (2000 ft^2) for a 500-bed hospital (Table 35.6) and about 108 m^2 (1200 ft^2) for 250-bed hospital. This includes patient-waiting areas, physicians' offices, reception areas, administrative technologist office, technologist lounge and patient-record files.

Table 35.6: Administrative and processing areas

Space Requirements	
Area	*Square Feet*
Waiting–outpatient	300
Waiting–inpatient	100
Reception and filling	75
Bathrooms (2)	150
Secretary office	200
Physicians offices (2)	280
Patient examination	120
Administrative tech. offices	120
Technologists' lounge	225
Patient studies file	300
	2070

The *in vivo* diagnostic area also requires about 180 m^2 (2000 ft^2), not counting the emission tomography and the cyclotron requirements of 72 m^2 (800 ft^2) (Table 38.7). A 200-bed hospital would require 108–117 m^2 (1200-1300 ft^2). Since only the imaging area can be appreciably reduced in size.

Table 35.7: In vivo Diagnostic Area

Area	*Square Feet*
Imaging area (4) with computer	1200
Function area	240
Isotope preparation	180
Darkroom	75
Viewing	300
	1995
Examination tomography	400
Cyclotron	400
	800

The space requirements for the non-patient function are variable (Table 35.8) depending on the size of the hospital and the sophistication of the service. For example in a hospital of 250 beds, high and low high and low counting areas, research and development laboratories, basic science professional offices, and equipment calibration facilities are not needed. On the other hand, an in vitro laboratory and isotope waste storage and general storage are required in all nuclear medicine units. In summary, a total area of 603 m^2 (6700 ft^2) is needed in a 500-bed hospital with research and development activities (Table 35.9). In a 250-bed hospital with only diagnostic service, 225 m^2 (2500 ft^2) should be adequate.

Table 35.8: Nonpatient areas

Area	*Square Feet*
Professional offices	240
In vitro laboratory	400
High and low counting areas	240
Equipment calibration	180
R and D laboratories	300
Isotope waste storage	75
General storage	75
	1510

There are two approaches to the design of the imaging suite for a nuclear medicine service, one is the *open area* concept and the other is the *individual area* concept. In the multi-procedure room concept, the area for the patient and instrumentation is really greater than 4.5 × 6 m (15 × 20 ft) because the space between instruments can be used for patient maneuverability.

General Construction Features

Several of these are very important (Tables 35.10 and 35.11). Exclusive power supplies to the hospital transformer should be available for the imaging instrumentation, as should an adequate exhaust system for radioactive gases. Usually, ventilation requirements are fulfilled by good air conditioning and heating systems that are capable of moving about 100 linear feet of air per minute. Specific requirements can be obtained from the Nuclear Regulatory Commission. The local telephone Company can usually provide excellent help on the design of the intercom and telephone system.

Equipment

For a 500-bed hospital the imaging instruments needed are two Anger type cameras, an emission tomographic scanner, and a third camera devoted entirely to cardiology. A treadmill, electrocardiograph, and a cardiac resuscitation unit with a defibrillator are required for nuclear cardiology. Other pieces of equipment needed are listed in Table 35.12.

The information presented in this report is based on the requirements for an active nuclear medicine unit in a community hospital of 500 beds, or a similar sized academic institution; however, specific needs will vary according to the type of

Table 35.9

Area	*Square Feet*
Administrative and processing	2070
In-vivo diagnostic area	1995
Nonpatient areas	1510
	5575
20% for halls, closets, etc.	1115
	6690
Emission tomography and cyclotron	800

Table 35.10: General construction features

1. Adequate floor loading
2. Adequate width halls and doors
3. Adequate candle power
4. Dimmer or selective light control in imaging areas–sans windows
5. Vinyl type tile floor with very smooth concrete undersurface
6. Shielding–FM and AM signals
7. Well spaced from heavy electric equipment such as elevators
8. Movable walls
9. Planned for orderly expansion

Table 35.11: Utilities and special features

1. Exclusive power supplies to hospitals transformers for imaging and counting equipment
2. Usually only 120 V electric lines required. Exceptions are electrical heating units in laboratories and emission tomographic instruments.
3. Interoffice and laboratory communication is best served by telephone system. Local telephone company best source of advice
4. General ventilation requirements are prescribed by NRC or equivalent state agencies
5. Special exhaust system for radioactive gases
6. Oxygen and suction in patient areas
7. Wash facilities in imaging areas, patient examination areas, and all laboratories
8. Standard utilities in laboratories

Table 35.12: Equipment–patient areas

Stationary Cameras—general purpose (2)
Tomographic scanner
Camera—cardiology
General purpose computer
Radioactive gas recovery system
Probe type detector
Tread mill
Cardiac resuscitation unit
Film processor

institution. For example, a cancer-oriented or neurological.

As patients are fully clothed during nuclear medicine procedures, there is no need for privacy in conventional sense. On the contrary, the area's open atmosphere seem to help patients to feel less fearful during the diagnostic process, and the surrounding activity helps to provide with them some interest. However, use of these open spaces does require that the staff members have considerable insight into patient anxiety.

The large scan area approach seems to provide staff efficiency improvement, good visual contact among staff members, easier modification to accommodate new techniques and equipment. A folding, sound-absorbing wall is recommended to be used to close one bay of the scanning area when a seriously ill or particularly noisy patient is treated.

For radioactive-therapy, a limited number of radiation protected single patient rooms is needed.

The well-protected radiopharmaceutical preparation room or hot laboratory is to provide radioactive compounds to the patient scan areas. In this room these materials are stored and dispensed. A shower for use in case of radiation contamination should be located near the radiopharmaceutical preparation room.

No office should be located near a source of high radiation, such as the hot lab. The high radiation levels in the hot laboratory may interfere with procedures in adjoining rooms, so the hot lab should be isolated, adjoining areas such as the storage area.

In the handling and storage area the departmental layout has to be compact. Sophisticated remote handling equipment is used to reduce personal exposure. Lead is used in shielded areas. The weight of shielding may cause construction problems.

Liquid radioisotopes may present problems relating to vaporization, contamination, ingestion, and waste disposal. The shielding arrangements, however, are considerably simpler in comparison with solid source shielding.

The room temperature in the storage area should ensure that stored liquids do not freeze. As stores may be visited frequently, attention shall be paid to fire risks. Advice should be sought from fire authorities, also concerning an automatic fire detection and warning system. Outside each store there must be a clear warning sign, including the standard radiation symbol and the name of the person responsible for the store. Rooms are needed for film viewing areas, files, patient waiting, and staff lounges and lockers. In all rooms where radioactive nuclides are stored, dispensed, or manipulated chemically, exposed surfaces require appropriate treatment to prevent contamination. Adequate shielding and security of such rooms must be ensured. These rooms should be separated from rooms where highly sensitive counting of low activities takes place.

Safety precautions are much more important in *in vivo* studies than in *in vitro* studies.

Laboratories and clinical rooms where large amounts of nuclides or highly radioactive patients are handled should be as far as possible from counting rooms where low activities are being measured. In multistoryed buildings this may be a three dimensional problem and permissible floor loadings for heavy equipment and shielding have to be considered.

All surfaces in the procedure rooms should be for ease of documentation and cleaning of non-porous, continuous and smooth material.

Plastic laminate covered benches are excellent, although joints and sinks present problems. Stainless steel benches easily incorporate formed sinks, but can be corroded by chemicals. Taps of the sinks for washing of contaminated glassware and other articles should be operatable without using the hands. The drain should be connected directly to a main sewer. The taps should be accessible for periodic monitoring. Floors can be covered with sealed PVC except where hot objects or some organic chemicals may fall on them. Then linoleum may be preferable if cut so that joints do not occur where spills are most likely.

A floor drain is sometimes justified. The drains could be of any material except polyethylen which tends to absorb radioiodine.

Hand washing facilities should be provided and sited conveniently by each working area.

Washing facilities ought to be elbow or foot operated.

Where large quantities of radionuclides are handled, a shower should be available for use in an emergency.

About 10 changes of air per hour should be provided.

Ventilation should be designed so that air from rooms where radionuclides are used and which could under accident conditions be contaminated will not be recirculated or taken into inactive areas. In a suite of rooms used for work at different levels of activity, ventilation should ensure that the air flow is from low to high activity areas.

In adverse climatic conditions it is important that the entire department be air-conditioned to guarantee good working conditions for the staff and to protect the measuring equipment.

The crystals in the gamma camera heads can tolerate temperature variations only from 10°C to 40°C, but cannot adjust to rapid fluctuations. The camera also requires a non-condensing relative humidity between 35 and 60 per cent.

The primary purpose of *electrical design* in a nuclear medicine suite is to provide an uninterrupted and constantly even source of power. Noise on the electrical lines, pure circuit noise on the electrical input panels, sudden voltage surges that occur as other large equipment is turned on or off, and similar problems necessitate the use of isolation transformers to filter the electrical flow.

At the present time a complete radioisotope service is possible only in hospitals of the highest standard.

A complete nuclear medical service would include the following sections and rooms:

Diagnostics Radiopharmaceutical preparation–hot laboratory, application room; area for diagnosis including two scanners and two gamma-cameras; room for radiochromatography etc; data room; two examination rooms; dark room; physical laboratory; electronic shop; radiation protected store for isotopes; laboratory; waiting room for non-ambulant patients; waiting room for ambulant patients; two patient lavatories; room for physicist and chemist; two biochemical laboratories; sample preparation; room for liquid scintillation-counter; rooms for autoradiography; film viewing room; film filing room; staff changing rooms; staff lounge and radioactive waste room.

Counting room room for electronics; two dressing cubicles; patient lavatory; patient shower and staff room.

Therapy Two operation rooms; preparation room; room for dosiometric planning and radiation protected isotope store.

Nuclear medical ward Twelve single rooms with shower and lavatory; two four patient rooms with shower and lavatory; day room; nurse's station; doctor's room; pantry; utility room; two changing rooms for staff and staff lounge.

Experimental animal unit Two animal rooms; preparation room; operation room; staff room and feed supply room.

Central administration Major nuclear medicine equipment in an university medical center covering about 5,000 nuclear medicine procedures per annum may include two scintillation cameras, two 3-inch crystal rectilinear scanners, one thyroid uptake system, two dual-probe 5-inch crystal rectilinear scanners, two gamma cameras, one multi-channel analyzer and scaler, one liquid scintillation counter, two ceiling-mounted X-ray units, one dose calibrator, one automatic well scintillation counter, one stationary *in vivo* multiprobe counting system, and equipment for radiopharmaceutical preparation.

FURTHER READING

1. Deland FH: In Laufman H (Ed): *Nuclear Medicine Service in Hospital Special Care Facilities.* London, Academic Press: 1981.
2. Putsep E: Modern Hospital: International Planning Practices. London, Lloyd-Luke Ltd. 1979.

BLOOD TRANSFUSION CENTRE

Blood transfusion is an increasingly important element of medical treatment. This is a vital but often neglected part of the health service, although blood and blood products have become indispensable in medical treatment. Blood transfusion is a broadly-based discipline that overlaps and intersects many other medical, scientific and managerial fields, including hematology, immunology, genetics, histocompatibility, cellular function and metabolism, protein structure and function, cryobiology, disposable equipment, statistics, bio-engineering, data processing, logistics, standardization, and public relations.

Co-ordinated long range planning is needed for the development and integration of such diverse activities, together with careful consideration of priorities and optimal use of resources.

National Blood Policy

The organization of blood transfusion services should be an integral part of any national health policy. Such a policy should include:

- Any established and relevant legislation, plus applicable government rules and regulations
- Delegation of some or all activities to institutions, hospitals and organizations, with a clear division of responsibilities if several institutions or organization are involved.
- The role of a national blood transfusion committee.
- Blood collection, storage, processing and distribution can be arranged by different organizations.
- Red Cross, Red Crescent blood programme, government blood transfusion services, hospital blood banks, non-profit organization, etc.

Hospital blood banks have the advantage of dealing with both donors and patients and can undertake investigations of both in the same laboratory. They are closer to clinical development trends and thus able to respond quickly to changing needs.

National Blood Programme

A national blood programme is an administrative entity that covers the national needs for blood and blood components. If only one organization is involved, the blood programme is often called a blood transfusion service. The national blood programme may or may not be involved in the preparation of plasma derivatives.

The transfusion service has following responsibilities:

- To take the best possible case of the donor before, during , and after donation;
- To ensure that the best possible use is made of the donor's gift;
- To ensure that the components required are made available promptly and with a guarantee of both quality and safety.

In order to carry out such a programme, the organization responsible for these activities must:

- Employ appropriately qualified professionals to direct the centers making up the total service;
- Provide premises, plant and technical infrastructure;
- Organize donor recruitment, call up donors, and maintain a donor record;
- Encourage training, development and research in blood-related fields.

A blood transfusion centre can meet the demands made on it only if adequate premises are made available.

The premises must be of a suitable size, construction and location to facilitate their proper operation, cleaning and maintenance in accordance with accepted rules of hygiene. They must comply with the requirements for Biological Substance No.1 (General Requirements for Manufacturing Estab lishments and Control Requirements for Manufacturing Establishment and Control Laboratories) and provide adequate space, lighting and ventilation for the following activities:

- Medical Examination of individual to determine their fitness as donors of blood and/or blood components
- Taking blood from donors with minimum risk of contamination or error
- Care of donors, including those who suffer adverse reactions
- Storage of whole blood and blood components pending completion of pressing and testing
- Separate storage of whole blood and blood components, after testing and before distribution
- Laboratory testing of blood and blood components
- Processing and distribution of whole blood and blood components in a manner that minimizes the risk of error
- Performance of all steps in apheresis procedure, where applicable
- Labeling, packaging and other additional operations
- Storage of equipment, reagents and disposable material
- Documentation and recording of data on the donor, the donated blood and, where possible, the recipient.

General Considerations

The blood transfusion centre should be located where it provides easy access for donors and staff, and allows quick and safe transportation of blood and components to hospitals.

Tasks of the Transfusion Centre

In planning a new transfusion centre, due consideration should be given to the following:

- The total amount of blood to be taken; and
- The level at which the centre will operate (national, regional or district), which will determine the different tasks requiring different premises, working conditions, equipment and personnel.

The centre must make special provision for space if it is to:

- Have an outpatient department for activities such as sampling for antenatal serology or treating patients with haematological disease;
- Produce stenile containers (bags or bottles) blood taking and giving sets and other sterile equipment;
- Produce blood grouping reagents.

Hygienic Conditions

The best hygienic conditions must be ensured throughout the premises of a transfusion centre since there is a continuous movement of donors, staff, materials, and blood and blood samples. Blood and blood components taken from the centre are used in hospitals, and external contamination of containers should therefore be avoided. All rooms must be easy to clean with washable floors and walls. The collection and disposal of waste must take place separately from the distribution of clean material, to avoid the spread of infection; provision for the expedient disposal of potentially infective materials by autoclaving and/or incineration must be made. There must be compliance with local by-laws in the disposal of these materials. It is particularly important that special arrangements be made for the disposal of blood samples and, occasionally, of outdated blood: they should not be directly discharged into the public sewerage system.

Air-conditioning is desirable for the greater comfort of donors and staff. Moreover, special conditions, including a supply of filtered or sterile air, or low temperature and humidity, may be required for some types of equipment procedures.

Infrastructure Within the Transfusion Centre

Water Supply

The water supply should never be contaminated with any material potentially dangerous to health;

it must be suitable for production of pyrogen-free water. Installation of filter is often necessary.

Electricity Supply

A reliable electrical supply is essential for lighting and for operation of equipment. A power failure to refrigerators may damage stored blood and blood components, and a transfusion centre must therefore have its own stand-by generator. The cost of damage abused by a power cut will almost certainly exceed the cost of the generator. Special attention should be paid to the possible need for a nonstandard electrical supply and for voltage stabilization, especially when considering the suitability of particular equipment.

Sewerage

Sewerage disposal must comply with the sanitary requirements of the local health authority. It should be noted that highly nitrogenous sewage has a high biochemical oxygen demand rating and should therefore never be discharged in an untreated condition.

Storage

Whole blood and blood components must be stored separately in a refrigerator, refrigerated room or freezer, as appropriate, which is used only for this purpose. Refrigerated room are more economical for larger transfusion centers, where large qualities of blood and components must be accommodated.

Steam

If large-scale production of solutions is undertaken, there should be an adequate supply of steam for cleaning of equipment and operation of sterilizers. The steam itself should not cause or leave a contaminating deposit on the equipment or containers to be cleaned or sterilized.

Distilled Water

A supply of freshly distilled (and usually deionized) water should be available in every blood transfusion centre.

Gas, High-pressure Air and Vacuum

Depending on the tasks undertaken by the transfusion centre, there may be a need for a gas supply for high-pressure air and for vacuum facilities.

Communications

The transfusion centre require telephones and/or fax facilities to maintain communication with hospitals and other transfusion centers, and to call in donors in special circumstances.

Factors Determining Adequate Floor Space

If a transfusion centre is not located within a hospital, the following supporting facilities must be provided with:

- Sterilizing room;
- Laundry;
- Garage;
- Store rooms;
- Changing rooms, toilet facilities and canteen for the staff of the centre
- Workshop for maintenance of the building and equipment.

It is important to plan suitable rooms for all operations; for instance a room containing a laminar air-flow cabinet should be of adequate size for the convenient running and maintenance of the equipment. Where air-conditioning is planned, rooms must be designed with sufficient space to accommodate the equipment.

In the case of multistoryed buildings, the floors should have large loading capacity; where floor space is limited, weight distribution must be carefully considered. The provision of a basement depends on the climatic conditions and the type of ground, and may prove impossible in tropical areas.

It is suggested that a separate room be available for sterilizing equipment and stills (to ensure intensive ventilation and other climatic control).

Functional Plan

The functional plan of a blood transfusion centre is based on the paths taken by the donors, the blood, samples and materials.

Path of the Donor

The path of the donor, refers to the rooms in the transfusion centre through which the donors need to pass. The first of these is centre through which donors enter and then pass through to the donor-record room, where their cards are filed. From here they proced to the donor laboratory and then to the consulting room for examination. If they are accepted as donors, they continue to a second waiting room and await their turns to enter the bleeding room. After donation they go from the bleeding room to the resting room, then to the donors cafeteria where food and liquid refreshment are served by staff who also supervise this post-donation period. Finally, the donors leave the building. These areas should be so arranged that donors can easily find their way (Figs 35.35a and b).

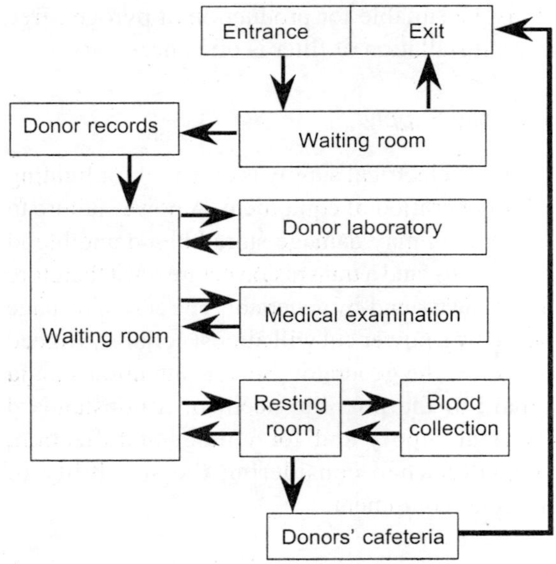

Fig. 35.35a: The path of the donor

Path of the Blood

After withdrawal, the blood can take one of two different paths. If it is not being separated into components immediately, it is put into a refrigerator and stored until the results of laboratory test are available, after which it is transferred to another refrigerator and made available for clinical use. If components are to be prepared immediately however the blood is taken to the appropriate preparation room. The components are then stored in refrigerators or freezers at prescribed temperatures. If the centre has plasma fractionation facilities, the plasma is delivered to that area. Following fractionation, plasma derivatives are stored at the appropriate temperatures.

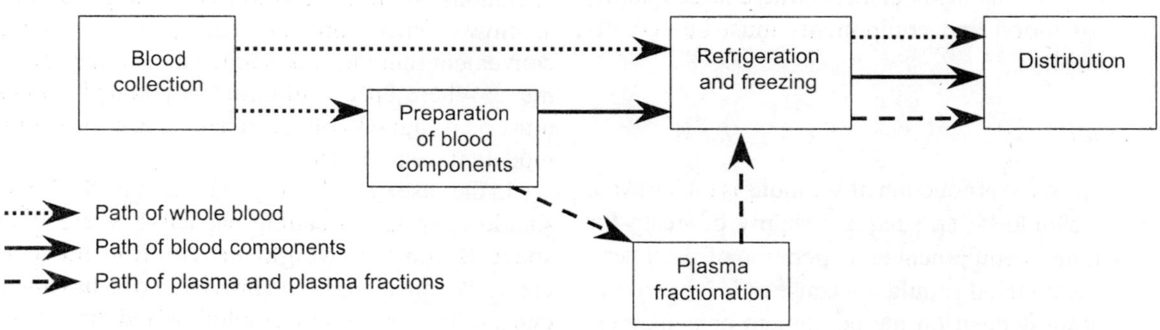

Fig. 35.35b: The path of the donor

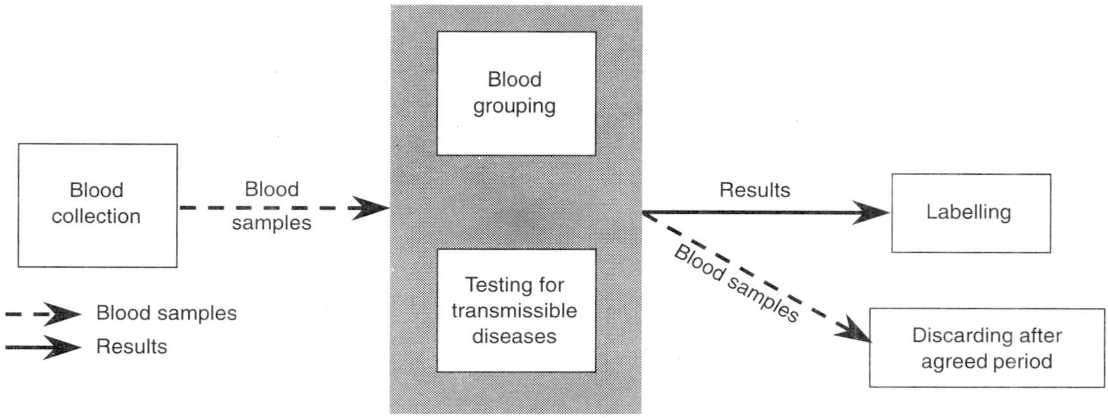

Fig. 35.36: The path of blood samples

The refrigerators, or refrigerated rooms, should be close to the distribution area. The blood and components must be stored in the refrigerator or freezer until issued for use.

Path of Blood Samples

Blood samples are taken in the withdrawal room and delivered to the laboratory for testing, When testing is completed the samples are discarded, preferably after incineration (Fig. 35.36).

Path of Meterials

There is continuous movement of material in a blood transfusion centre, and the arrangement of rooms should be such as to allow this flow to be economical and rational (Fig. 35.37). The material can be divided into four groups:

- Material purchased sterile, or sterilized in the centre before use
- Clean but non-sterile material
- Material to be cleaned
- Waste.

To avoid contamination, the paths of these different materials must be separate from each other.

Before planning the premises, a choice must be made between a central store-room or individual stores maintained by each functional unit of the centre. In the latter case a separate store-room must be attached to each unit. However, even when there is a central store-room, space must be provided in each unit to store material that must be available at all times. Within the store-room, sterile and non-sterile material must be treated separately. A choice must also be made between a central wash-up area for each functional unit. Where a central store-room and central wash-up area are chosen, they must be within easy reach of all functional units.

Waste must be stored in closed containers and collected daily. Its removal from the building must follow the shortest possible path avoiding all aseptic areas. Used needles should never be carried in containers that can be punctured.

Designing a Blood Transfusion Centre

The level (national, regional or district) of a transfusion centre determines its design, although certain principles are valid at all levels.

The building must be designed so that closed working areas (e.g. aseptic rooms) are not exposed to strong sunshine. Climatic conditions such as prevailing winds should always be taken into consideration. If the wind carries dust, ventilation by filtered air may be required in certain working areas to

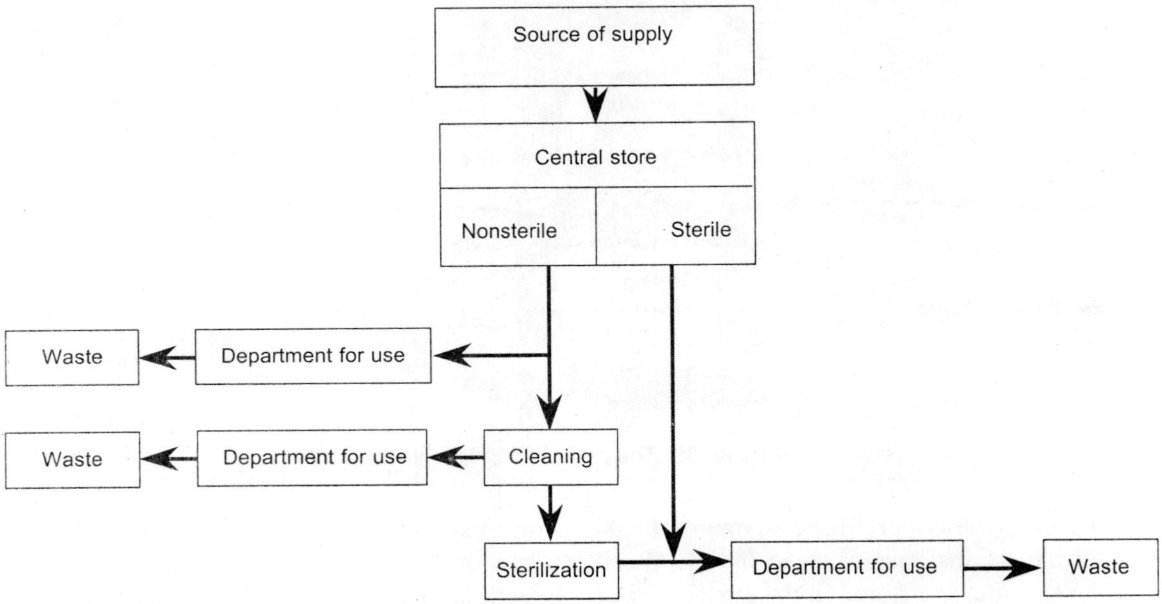

Fig. 35.37: The path of materials

ensure sterility and to protect the equipment from dust.

The building material and style should comply with the general construction guidelines of the country.

Donors, blood and outpatients, where applicable, should follow separate paths in their movements through the building. They should use separate entrances on different sides of the building. In multistory buildings, separate elevators should be available for people and goods.

The design of doors and windows should ensure natural lighting of rooms where possible, and protection against dust and insects. A septic or air-conditioned rooms should have non-opening windows. Loading and unloading facilities and areas should be covered for protection against rain and snow. Access to an adequate stand-by generator must be ensured

Figures 35.38 to 35.46 show the arrangement of units (departments) in various transfusion centers which are in separate buildings on hospital grounds.

Regional Centre

Figure 35.38 illustrates a two-storeyed building in which the following functions can be performed: registration, examination and bleeding of donors, plasmapheresis, testing of blood, production of blood components, quality control and storage and distribution of blood and blood products. The centre also has storage, central wash-up, sterilizing and distilling rooms, an outpatient department, training centre, staff rooms and offices. This is just one example of the layout of a regional centre. Other designs, based on single or multistoreyed concepts, may produce a building that is just as efficient. Where appropriate, however, allowance should be made for sufficient expansion to permit a regional centre to assume the role of a national centre.

District Centre

A district centre will usually be a part of, or closely associated with, a hospital. Its design will depend on the closeness of this association, particularly

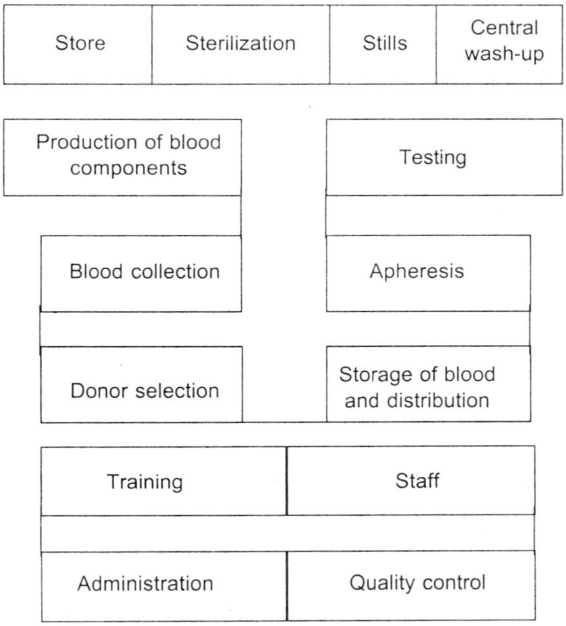

Fig. 35.38: Regional centre-1

with respect to support facilities and infrastructure. The functions of the centre will determine its structure.

Preliminary and Detailed Planning

Figure 35.39, shows the design and arrangement of units within a regional centre, which comply with those shown in Figure 35.38 but are shown in more detail. The arrangement of rooms within the functional units allows for appropriate paths to be taken by donors, blood, blood samples and materials.

Standard Floor Space Requirements

The standard floor space of a transfusion centre depends on the number and type of tasks to be performed. Following standard floor spaces for centres of different sizes performing all laboratory tests, including screening for transmissible diseases, independently of hospital laboratories are recommended. The arrangement and size of rooms within the functional units are based on:

- A district transfusion centre, not attached to a hospital and serving a limited number of medical units in the close vicinity, taking 50 donations per day (all within the centre) and with limited facilities for blood component preparation;
- A regional centre, not attached to a hospital and serving medical units at varying distances, taking 200 donations per day (more than half by mobile teams) and with facilities for processing 80 percent of donations to blood components.

District Centre

The functions of a district transfusion centre are:

- Examination of donors and copllection of blood
- Standard floor space depends on the number of donors to be examined and bled daily. Floor space of 120 m^2 is adequate for 50 donors per day and includes the donors waiting room (which should be cheerfully decorated to help donors feel at ease).

Storage of Blood

If the amount of blood stored by the district centre does not exceed 50 units at any one time, a floor space of 40 m^2 should suffice for blood storage, distribution and administration.

Testing of Blood

If the district centre collects 50 units per day it will require a floor space of 30 m^2 for testing and quality control.

Storeroom and Offices

Another 30 m^2 of space are required for these purposes.

The additional facilities needed in a district centre performing the functions outlined above and preparing a limited number of blood components, will require the following areas:

Cleaning and sterilization	30 m^2
Laundry	16 m^2

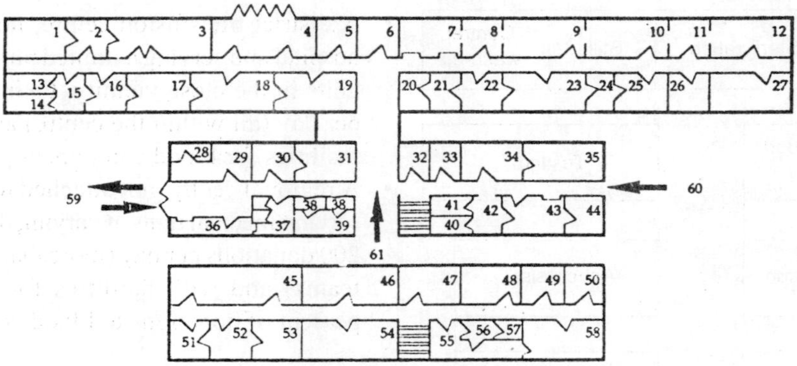

1 S terile storeroom
2 Reception of material
3 Storeroom
4 Garage with ramp
5,6 Toilets
7 Sterilization
8 Preparatory room
8 Stills
10 Central wash-up
11 Store-room for detergents
12 Reception for washing
13 +4°C refrigerated room
14 -30°C refrigerated room
15 Airlock
16 Labelling
17 Aseptic room (for blood derivatives)
18 Centrifuges
19 Chemical laboratory
20-21 Laboratory for testing for transmissible diseases
22 Reception of blood samples
23 Laboratory for donors' blood samples
24 Cross-matching
25 Laboratory for patients' samples
26 Detection of antibodies
27 Preparation of sera
28 Food store-room
29 Donors' cafeteria/snack bar
30 Resting room
31 Blood taking
32-33 Toilets
34 Plasmapheresis
35 Sterile room
36 Donor recording
37 Examination laboratory (including urine samples)
38 Changing room
39 Consulting room
40 + 4°C refrigerated room
41 +30°C refrigerated room
42 Air-lock
43 Delivery of blood and derivatives
44 Duty room, telex
45 Meeting room (lecture room)
46 Staff restroom
47-50 Changing rooms and shower
51 Organization department
52 Secretariat
53 Director's office
54 Library
55 Microbiology
56 Room for thermostats
57 Sterile box
58 Culture medic preparation
59 Entrance for donors
60 Entrance for deliveries
61 Main entrance

Fig. 35.39: Regional centre 2

Garage	20 m^2
Storerooms	20 m^2
Changing and rest room	2 × 20 m^2
Maintenance workshop	20 m^2
Administrators' office	12 m^2
Donor Organizer's office	12 m^2

REGIONAL CENTRE

The tasks of regional transfusion centre are:

- Examination of donors and collection of blood
- If daily bleedings number 200, the donor department should have a floor space of 300 m^2. This assumes that more than half of the total donations are taken by mobile teams (Figure 35.40).

Testing of Blood

This involves the testing of donor, blood samples (grouping and detection of transmissible disease), blood-grouping and cross-matching for hospital

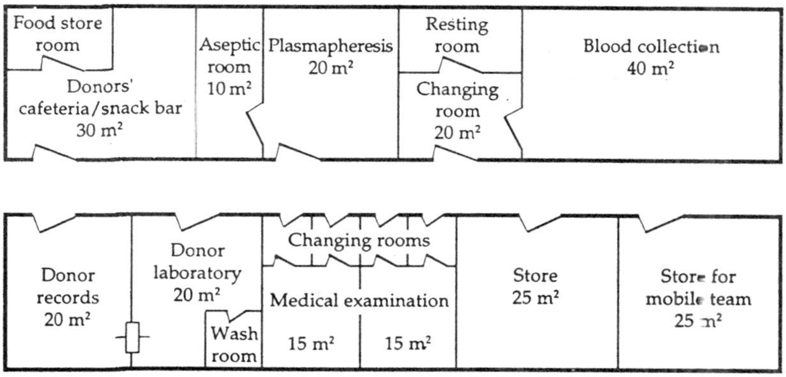

Fig. 35.40: Donor department—240 m^2

patients if it is not performed by a hospital laboratory), as well as preparation of some diagnostic reagent. At least 150 m^2 of floor space are needed to perform these tasks (Fig. 35.41).

Production of Blood Components

The plan and size of this unit are determined by the quality and quality of blood components produced. The following types of blood components may be produced at the regional centre level:

- Red blood cell concentrate
- Red blood cell concentrate, washed
- Platelet concentrate
- Leukocyte concentrate
- Fresh frozen plasma
- Cryoprecipitate.

The unit depicted in Figure 35.42 can process 80 percent of the 200 units of blood taken daily, and occupies a space of 230 m^2.

Quality Control

Microbiological and chemical control of blood, blood components, solutions and reagents is performed here. Floor space should be at least 100 m^2

Storage and Distribution of Blood

The regional centre featured in this example requires a sufficient area to store a maximum 1000 units of blood at 4°C, and an additional 2000 units of blood components at -30°C. the unit has fax facilities, offices and a duty-room, the total useful area is 100 m^2 (Fig. 35.44).

Cleaning

This unit contains the central wash-up room (for cleaning laboratory requirement), stills and sterilizing equipment, and requires an area of 150m^2 (Fig. 35.45).

The regional centre should also have a storeroom of 3 or 2, a garage of 100 m^2 and additional rooms (changing room, toilets) occupying about 70 m^2.

The total useful area of the regional centre is 1500 m^2. It could be valuably enlarged however to

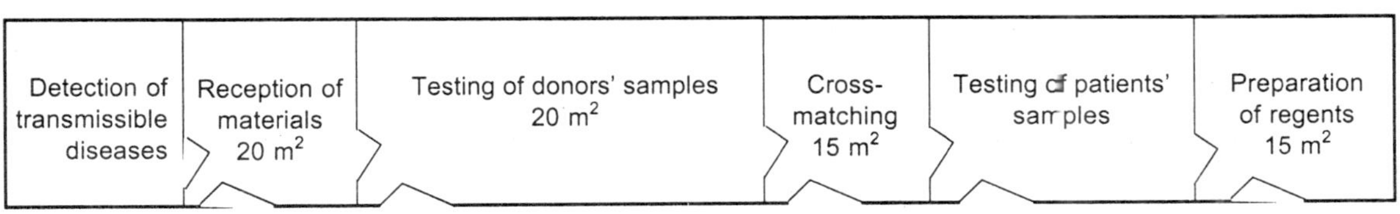

Fig. 35.41: Testing of blood—150 m^2

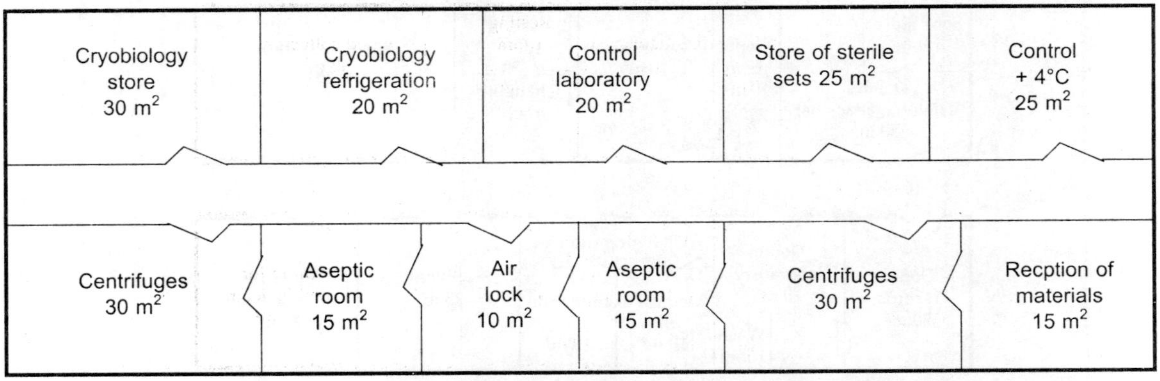

Fig. 35.42: Preparation of blood components—230 m^2

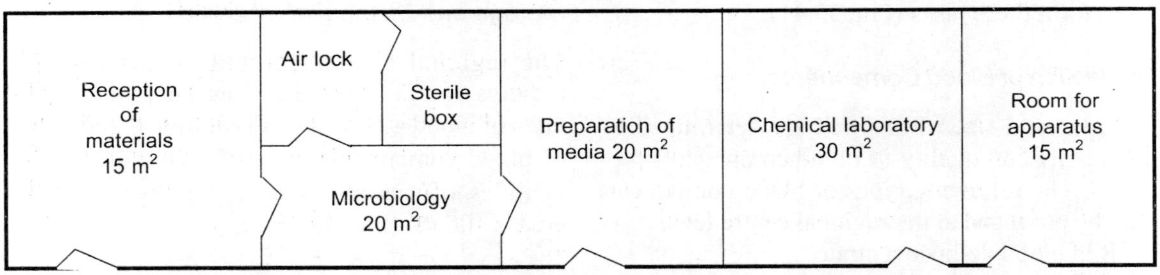

Fig. 35.43: Quality control—100 m^2

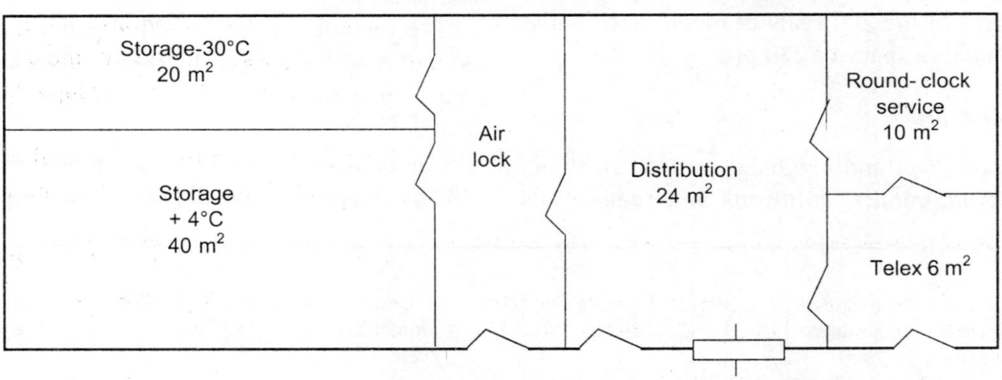

Fig. 35.44: Storage and distribution of blood components—100 m^2

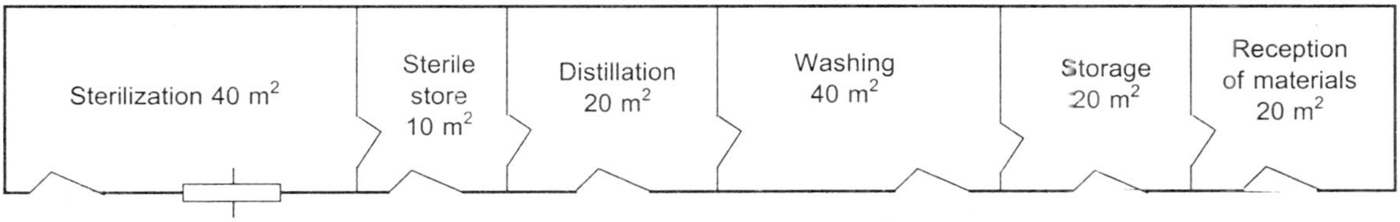

Fig. 35.45: Cleaning—150 m^2

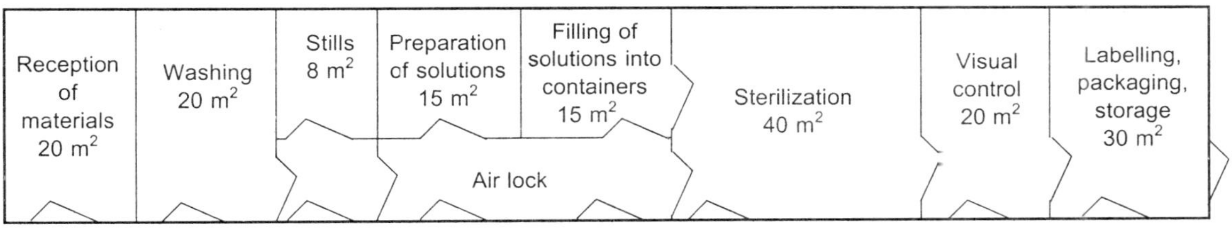

Fig. 35.46: Preparation of sterile containers and solutions

include a training centre (at least 200 m^2), management offices (100 m^2), staff rooms (150 m^2) and an outpatient department (50 m^2), thus increasing the total useful area to 2000m^2.

If the regional transfusion centre is not attached to a hospital, it will need the following additional facilities:

Laundry	30 m^2
Staff canteen	30 m^2
Maintenance workshop	30 m^2

These can be attached as an additional wing to the regional centre illustrated in Figure 35.39.

NATIONAL CENTRE

The design of a national transfusion centre will differ from that of a regional centre if it undertakes a larger volume of work or performs additional tasks. More management tasks and laboratories (e.g. if the centre acts as a national reference laboratory) demand more floor space. If plasma fractionation is to be undertaken eventually, the national centre will then have to be enlarged accordingly; a further separate unit may also be required for production of sterile blood container (Fig. 35.46).

HOSPITAL BLOOD BANK

The most important step in the organization of a blood transfusion service is to appoint a person qualified and experienced in transfusion medicine to head it.

Blood banks at premier institutions or large metropolitan medical colleges have undergraduate and postgraduate teaching programme and super-specialities should have separate departments of transfusions medicine.

The major functions of blood transfusion service are:

- Recruitment of donors and maintenance of donors records
- Collection, preservation and distribution of blood and blood and blood components
- Laboratory procedures
- Teaching, training and research
- Clinical/therapeutic functions.

Location and Space

The blood bank should ideally be located at ground level, closely associated with the hospital it serves or with a major hospital if it serves more than one hospital. It should be close to the emergency services of the hospital and preferably close to the operating theaters.

The areas of the blood bank can be broadly divided into:

- Donor recruitment offices
- Bleeding complex
- Therapeutic area
- Laboratories
- Administrative and clerical offices
- Teaching facilities.

The donor recruitment offices should have:

- Adequate space for the donor organizer and clerical staff and for equipment such as computers and photocopy machines.
- Good telephone facilities manned atleast 12 hours each day.
- Adequate recording and retrieval facilities (Computerized or manual) to store and update data on voluntary donors.
- Access to printing facilities for preparing donor publicity materials.

Bleeding Complex

The bleeding complex should be located close to the front entrance to the hospital, so as to ensure a high visibility and easy accessibility to the donating public. Donors should be able to go to the donor complex without having to go through hospital corridors or hospital security areas.

The bleeding complex should consist of the following rooms:

- Reception room
- Medical examination room
- Bleeding room and apheresis room
- Rest room
- Kitchen/pantry

Rooms should be interconnected and located in such a manner, that traffic is in unidiretional only and a donor who is going in to donate should not clash with a donor who has already donated blood.

Therapeutic Area

Would be used by patients who require transfusions of blood or clotting factors at frequent intervals such as patients of thalassemia.

Laboratories

The layout of the laboratories should be such that there is minimum movement of persons in the corridors and laboratories and limited entry of outsiders to the laboratories.

Laboratories of the blood bank include:

a. Laboratories for processing donor blood
b. Component laboratories:

Basic will prepare:

- Fresh frozen plasma
- Cryoprecipitate
- Platelets
- Packed RBC
- Leucocyte poor RBC etc.
- Relevant coagulation work

Advanced will prepare:

- Freeze dried and heated
- Coagulation factors
- Plasma fractionation

The component laboratories should be adjacent to the bleeding complex so that blood, as it is collected, can be processed without undue delay and without encountering problems in transporting it to the component laboratory.

c. Donor serological laboratory
   - ABO + Rh grouping
   - Antibody screening
   - Identification of antibody in positive screening
   - Labelling donor blood and stocking tested blood
d. Infectious diseases laboratory
   - AIDS
   - Malaria
   - Syphilis
e. Quality control
f. Laboratories for processing patient blood
g. Issue counter/room: will
   - Issue blood and blood components to patients.
   - Receive patient samples for testing.
   - Store crossmatched blood and basic components.

   The issue counter/room should be located at the entrance to the blood bank so that patient samples can be received and blood and blood components issued without disturbance to the laboratories.
h. Patient serological laboratory: will do:
   - Emergency
   - Nonemergency
   - ABO + Rh grouping
   - Antibody screening
   - Identification of antibody in positive screen
   - Crossmatch blood
   - Antenatal work-up

   The emergency section of the patient serological laboratory should be adjacent to the counter room followed by the routine laboratory.
j. Special laboratory will do
   - Platelet and granulocyte serology
   - HLA work

Administrative and Office Area

- Consultants office
- Departmental, administrative and clerical offices
- Staff common room
- Service area:
  - Store
  - Wash room and distillation plant
  - Toilets
  - Housekeeping

Teaching, Training and Research

- Conference Room
- Department library.

Bleeding Complex

• Reception room	25	25	40
• Medical examination room		15	25
• Bleeding room	40	55	100
• Refreshment room	15	25	30
• Kitchen/Pantry	5	5	10
• Apheresis area			40
Day care/therapeutic area		30	50

Laboratory Area

• Laboratory for routine donor work	25	50
• Laboratory for routine patient and antenatal work	35	50
• Laboratory for specialized work: platelets HLA granulocyte serology		50

- Issue counter
- Emergency laboratory 18 20 20
- Hepatitis HIV/VDRL 20 25 30
- Malaria
- Wash room distillation plants etc. 20 25 30
- Component basic and coagulation work 25 30
- Component advanced freeze drying 50

General Areas

- Doctor's office 15 15 × 3 20 × 1, 15 × 1
- Donor recruiter/social worker/clerical staff 25 30 50 × 3
- Blood bank office 15 20 25
- Stores 20 25 35
- Technician's common room 15 20 25
- Toilets 5 × 2 5 × 2 5 × 3
- Trainee-doctor's room 25
- Library/conference room 30

  Total **248** **460** **895**

Special Considerations

Bleeding room and refreshment area and laboratories will be airconditions if ambient temperature is above 28°C.

Laboratories will have emergency power.

- Minimum space for blood bank in category I- 100 m^2
- Minimum space for blood bank in category II- 300 m^2
- Minimum space for blood bank in category III- 895 m^2

Bleeding Complex

- House officer 1 1-2 2
- Nurses 2 3 4
- Social workers 1 2 3
- Lab. attendants 1 1 2

Apheresis Room

- Nurses 2
- Lab. Attendant 1

Laboratory

- Technical supervisor 1-2 4
- Technical assistant 2 4 8
- Lab. assistant 4 11 13 (4 for shift work)
- Lab. asstt. 1 2 4
- Lab. attendant 2 4 5
- Donor organiser
- Associated/clerical part time staff 1 2
- Social worker 2 5 10 (for mobile teams)
- Vehicle driver–part time 1 3
- Service staff, clerical staff
  - Clerk (Typist) part time 1 2
  - Store keeper part time 1 1
  - Sanitary attendent part time (Sweeper) 1 2

Consultants in Blood Transfusion

- Professor 1
- Lecturer 2 3
- Pathologist (part time) 1 Resident

Equipment

Routine work

- Blood Bank Refrigerator: 3 Numbers
- Capable of maintaining temperature of 1-4°C, having
- Audio-visual alarm system and temperature display
  - untested blood 1

Table 35.13: Spatial Requirements for Blood Bank (in m^2)

	• 3-7 UOB/Hospital bed 1000-6000 UOB consumed per year	8-15 UOB/Hospital bed 6000-15000 UOB consumed per year	16 UOB or more per Hospital bed over 15000 UOB consumed per year
UOB (Units of Blood)	100-800 bed Hospital District Hospital Health Service Coorporation Hospital No. super-specialities non-teaching	Per year 400-1000 bed Hospital State Medical College Hospital Specialised Hospital Teaching Hospital	Consumed per year 800-1000 bedded Hospital Premier Institute Metropolitian Medical College Hospital All Superspecialities teaching Hospital and Blood Bank

Table 35.14: Standards for staff for blood bank

UOB (Units of Blood)	3-7 UOB/Hospital bed 1000 = 6000 UOB consumed per year 100-800 beded Hospital District Hospital Health service hospital No superspecialities Hospital non teaching	8-15 UOB/Hospital bed 6000-15000 UOB consumed per year 400-1000 bedded Hospital State Medical Collages Hospital specialized Hospital Blood Bank functions 24 hrs/ day. Teaching Hospital	16 UOB or more per bed Over 15000 UOB consumed per year 800-1000 bedded Hospital Premier Institute Metropolitan Medical College Hospital All superspecialities Hospital Blood Bank.

- tested blood 1
- tested and crossmatched blood 1

Centrifuge table top Capable of 3500 × g with accurate timer in 1 min increments upto 30 minutes. Accurate tachometer. Acceleration to desired speed in approx 30 sec rapid decellaration. Rotor for swing head capable of taking minimum of 16-20, 12 × 100 mm tubes and microplate carrier. Number depends on size of blood bank but approximately equal to number of day technicans on duty.

- *Water bath* (37°C with temperature control) fibreglass.
- *Incubator* 37°C with temperature control of ± 10°C
- *Hot air Oven* for drying glass ware
- *Microscope* binocular
- *1 Kg balance* for weighing blood bags during blood collection.
- *Tube stripper cutter and aluminimum clips* to seal blood bags.
- *BP Apparatus*
- *Domestic refrigerator* without freezer compartment.
- *PH Meter* Not essential for category one blood bank.
- *DRL Agitator*
- *Weighing Machine* for donor

Distillation and Double Distillation Plant

Analytical balance–Not essential for category one blood bank.

Additional equipment for blood bank collecting 10,000 units or more.

- Dielectric tube sealer 2 numbers
- Vortex mixer
- Magnetic stirrer
- Analytical balance
- Plasma separation stand: 3 Numbers

Clean Air Station (Laminar Flow)

- Microplate agitator
- Blood component work
- Basic equipment

Blood bank refrigerated centrifuge for 450 ml blood bags. Swing head 5000 g with wind shield.

Temperature of 0-25°C. Timer at 1 min. Interval upto 60 min.

Accurate Tachometer

Freezer 70°C with alarm system temperature display, and recording thermometer. 24 hours power supply and stand by power.

Dielectric Tube Sealer

- Plasma separation stand
- Tube stripper, cutter, an aluminimum rings
- Platelet agitator rum incubator for platelet storage
- Clean air station.
- Weighing scale of 2 kg with sensitivity of 100 mg.
- 1 kg balance in 5 mg increments for weighting plasma bags.

Equipment (Small Items Blood Bank)

- Blood bag stand stainless for keeping bag upright.
- Test tube racks.
- Flexible table lamps with concave mirror
- Micropipettes-2 ml upto 1000 ml.

Flexible Construction for Expansion of Centre Activities

The national blood transfusion service must always keep abreast of scientific advances (new techniques, new blood components, etc.) and be actively involved in the planning and development of the various blood centres. In the early stages of a national service the transfusion centres carry out only the basic functions–examination of donors, bleeding, testing, storage and distribution of blood. The scope of activities can then be enlarged by adding the following:

- Production of blood components (or increasing production and variety of blood components)
- Improvement of quality control
- Care of patients suffering from haematological disorders
- Independent functioning (e.g. local production of blood containers)
- Production of diagnostic reagents
- Production of sterile solutions for processing blood components
- Fractionation of plasma
- Automation and data processing.

An existing building can be enlarged by construction of a new wing, by adding a new floor (if the foundations of the building permit) or by making use of spare rooms. It is recommended that more floor space be planned for a transfusion centre than is required initially, perhaps 10 percent of the total useful area. These extra rooms can first be used as storerooms but be fitted out later to serve other purposes.

Any enlargement that is expected to take place in the near future should be embodied in the original plans. For example, if the national blood programmer provides for a national centre to start plasma fractionation, the original plan should include a separate department for this purpose.

FURTHER READING

1. Marshall M, Bird T: Blood loss and replacement. Edward Arnold (Publisher) Ltd. Preface, 21, 1983.
2. Masouredis SP: Preservation and clinical use of blood and blood components. In Hematology, Williams WJ, Beutler E, Erslev AJ, Lichtman MA (Eds): Mc graw Hill Book Co, 1983.
3. Pinter J, Szilassy C, Polner G: Design of Premises of a blood transfusion centre. In Hollan Sr.Wagstaff W, Leikola J, Loth F (Eds): *Management of Blood Transfusion Services* World Health Organisation, Geneva 1990.

MEDICAL INFORMATICS

Medical informatics will touch the lives of all those working in health care. Its major concern is with information and the use of new and appropriate technological tools to access accurate and relevant information for clinical purposes. Medical informatics can help to manage information explosion.

Health informatics is a muttidisciplinary endeavour across all health professions. It seeks to advance understanding of the science and technology of information management in medicine. It seeks to develop and apply this science and technology in support of improvement in quality, cost and effectiveness of health care education.

It is quite commonplace to observe nowadays how patients records are reduced to a large mass of poorly structured information, that is to say a mixture of texts, images and numbers. Within medical institutions, particularly inpatient hospitals with related highly specialised outpatient consultations., the situation becomes worse, when there is the least attempt to retrieve specific, relevant information is from medical literature thanks to powerful tools like MEDLINE, Exerpta Medica or Pergamon and Cochrane Collaboration.

Indeed, today, the key question for a health institution is the integrity and the management of data in growing health organizations.

Distributed systems offer the potential for applications and information to be integrated across diverse and physically separated systems, possible bridging heterogeneous hardware and software environments. Distributed systems promise to revolutionize the use of networked resources, services and database, again leading to a minimization of cost. These types of system are particularly relevant now that there is greatly increased computing power on the desktop coupled with modern communication technology.

The technological scenario in an organisation consists of a set of already existing heterogeneous applications and the market is offering quite a number of cheap but isolated applications to support the specific needs of the users in the autonomous units of an enterprise.

Communications

The arrival of computers has permitted a new step with, at the begining, the communication between two computers then between two users of one application. With the increase in the complexity of dialogue between two applications appeared the notion of distributed application: there is not only the exchange of information but the co-operation between similar applications. All this means obviously the putting into place of communication networks which must constantly evolve to reply better to the growing needs of the users and especially of the software which serves to introduce the functions required.

The increasing demand to interconnect equipment of different makes and models, *a priori* incompatible, has in this way led to the definition of standards of communication, independent of the equipment on which they have been introduced. Two series of standards predominate at present in heteroclite environments on one side the series of protocols-TCP/IP (Transmission Control Protocol/ Internet Protocol) defined by DARPA (Defence Advanced Research Projects Agency) for the American Department of Defence and, on the other side, the series of OSI (Open System Interconnection) protocols defined together by two organisation for standardisation, the CCITT (Comite Consultatif International Telegraphique et Telephonique) and ISO (International Organisation for Standardisation). It is, nonetheless, to be noted that, contrary to the Osi series of protocols that are formulated most of the time, the protocols of TCP/ IP are *de facto* standards, in view of their process of normalisation, that is to say fully implemented with come built-in performance characteristics. The approach according to the OSI model lends itself to taking into consideration the heterogeneous application systems in accordance with open distributed architecture.

At a time of the increasing use of cellular telephones, of high resolution digitised television, remote bank transactions, a scientist or even a doctor can carry out a bibliographic research from a distance, as well as consulting a database, e.g. relative to a sequence of nucleotides of human genes based upon a diagnosis of magnetic resonance by specialists from a distance using tele-radiology facilities from a satellite hospital far from a specialised university hospital. These developments linked to communication imply a co-operation more and more extensive between university, researcher, industry and governmental research laboratories. Medical informatics will touch the lives of all those working in health care. Its major concern is with information and the use of new and appropriate technological to access accurate and relevant information for clinical purposes. Medical informatics can help to manage the information explosion that has occurred in medicine and health care generally over the past three decades. Health informatics is a multidisciplinary endeavour across all health professions. It seeks to advance understanding of the science and technology of information and information management in medicine. It seeks to develop and apply the science and technology in support of improvements in quality, cost and effectiveness of health care.

High speed data networks will enable health professionals to share information. Electronic health records are an essential components in providing timely and co-ordinated patient care. Access to other colleagues and experts for consultation purposes will be quicker and easier. Similar speedy access to medically related knowledge basis will be supported through the emerging field of telemedicine. Developments in communication technology should improve the speed and efficiecy of health care administration procedures. The use of new technology and relevant information for the purposes of clinical audit and the development of protocols and guidelines for the care and management of patients which will facilitate the assessment of clinical outcomes. This will provide a foundation for monitoring the efficiency and cost-effectiveness of health care services.

Telematics requires the integration of three fields-(1) those of the intelligent terminals connected to (2) a telecommunication network with a view to assure (3) the support of public or private primary function, relative to buisness administration and to all health fields. The fields (1) and (2) benefit from rapid technical developments, nevertheless, the critical point of telematics stays linked to (3) the capacity to integrate and to make accessible applications in a coherent fashion and compatible to a very large and heterogeneous community of users whose means of communication stay more or less linked to the use of public telephone ("public switched telephone network" PSTN) and to its extensions, also to the eventual interconnection to LANs (Local Area Networks) then to WANs (Wide Area Networks) assuring the bridges between islands of informatics, public, semi-public or even private. The objectives alluded to by telemedicine emphasise the following facilities that previously partly belonged to centralised access to the distant databanks (being regional, international or like MEDLINE, UMLS, or other databanks designed for technology transfer in all sorts of medical specialities and fields). These are medical information exchange relative to patients; requests of laboratories; various data and images; internal or external electronic mail facilities to one or two institutions; and general telematic services.

In concrete terms such facilities allow especially a new sharing experts relative to a greater range of specialities of their technologies. The availability of telemedicine, and also of teleradiology, assures one of the participation of the most appropriate experts for any one question and to take an inventory by way of data bank of technology transfer. The mixed medical information exchanges of images and interpretative reports combined with facilities for video conferences have already made their appearance some time ago as an illustration of this present state of art!

A patient's medical records are nothing more than a poorly structured association of texts, images, numerical data and laboratory results. These texts have, however titles and sub-titles defining a total network of indexable paragraphs of sub-titles more or less comparable. This description gives evidence of a potential administrative use with, at the sametime, the implication of local limitation of PC microcomputers, limited disk space, weak security and confidentiality, and limited accessibility if the number of files continually increases. On reflection, the expansion of communication networks and open/distributed architectures of the client-server type, permits the resolving of this problem by the marriage of technologies notable of the world of MS-DOS and Windows with that of the UNIX world of microcomputer client-server having available database managers of the SQL type accessible in the network model.

In the DIOGENE hospital information system integrating the distributed client-server model, "UNIDOC" takes into account the patient dischrage letter, which needs to be sent to their local doctor, the surgery reports and all the radiology and specialist consultant reports. The word processing system adopted is win word for Windows. The documents are structured by paragraph pre-numbered for each document category. Apart from this, each document category has at its disposition a predefined selection of key words conditioning the filing and querying method of the archives. The identities and socio-administrative aspect of patients are obtained diretly from the this server of patients' identity without having to be recaptured. The documents can be found patient by patient, by doctors and be secretaries. The documents archived on UNIX and Data Base Management server of SQL type can be made accessible to any of the PCs in the network, but under reserve of the right of access control.

The availability of discharge letters and other documents becomes particularly precious in the emergency room, at the patient's reception, if the patient, after a period of time, returns to hospital in a critical state, and where it appears advantageous to verify if the new events/symptoms are not in close relationship with one or more previous hospital stays or with one or other of the external specialist consultations. This same document base constitutes the chosen tool of the epidemiological clinic and the evaluation of the quality of internal documentation as a means of evaluation of the quantity of wasteful care and treatment. The collection of patient's records and their observations in terms of "findings" of positive or negative symptoms and signs can be compared to their equivalent formula in terms of medical knowledge from QMR (Quick Medical Reference) which gives an estimation on the basis of the evaluation of the acoustic signal against noise. These approaches can be combined in matters of medical education with services associated to attitude files or to "knowledge interfaced". Clinical medicine consolidates itself by the support of authentic scientific methodology, that means reproducible and objective, lending itself in this way to decisional, analytical techniques.

The new distributed open architectures of the client-server type which involves the use of multiple and interconnected networks, conditioning on a new manner of co-operation between experts which can be accessible even if they are geographically very far away. These facilities combine a progressively systematic method of remote bibliographic research as a new means of comparison vis-a-vis similar cases detected from patient's files completed by networked computer readable electronic supports. Decisional analysis and evaluation of medical language utilised in referring to the knowledge base will allow clinical medicine to soon become a science rather than an art.

Apart from this, if on the other hand the HIS (Hospital Information System) continues its indisputable service on the so-called transactional activity plans, for example, laboratory examination requests up to the result report, the new architecture and network facilities, notable those of picture archiving communication system (PACS) and of image manipulation, have opened the door of teleradiology already as a specialised branch of telemedicine. Whatever the case, either one or the other, complete, will induce a new distribution of investigative clinical forces in the general apparatus of the distribution of health care.

Knowledge based medical records can facilitate:

- Rule-based care
- Patient-centered communication
- An Intelligent information gathering
- Focused information resources

Practice based on rukes and guidelines generated by kowledge bases can improve patient care and lead to a more patient centered communication structure. This, in turn, leads to informed information gathering and the ability to focus informatrion resources.

ESTABLISHING A FULLY NETWORKED IMAGING PROGRAM

The basic principles of medical imaging changed very little from Roentgen's discovery of X-rays in the 1890s to the early 1970s. It has been said that Roentgen himself probably would have felt quite comfortable with the technology in an X-ray room built as recently as late 1960s. But then things began to change, and change very quickly. Three entirely new technologies burst on the scene. First came computed tomography (CT), thanks to the Nobel Prize-winning work of Godfrey Hounsfield and Allan Cormack.

Computed tomography was rapidly followed by nuclear magnetic resonance, or MRI as it is often now abbreviated, and positron emission tomography, or PET. The revolution was made possible by many events. Of particular significance was the creation of appropriate mathematical techniques such as the fast fourier transform, or FFT.

Then came the computers and computing equipment that used these techniques to create images from attenuation measurements at a fast enough speed and low enough cost to permit the use of the techniques in a clinical setting.

In the 1980s, four fundamental changes occurred in computing as it applied to the medicine. At the beginning of the decade, the personal computer (PC) was introduced by IBM, and changed the face of computing forever. The PC put power and creativity into the hands of millions of people. It and its successors are still a powerful force for change. They have given birth to the modern workstation that is beginning to find its way into mainstream medical imaging products.

The advance in display capabilities is vividly shown in the appearances of various PET systems. The first illustration is of the PET system of the late 1970s. Note the very tiny image monitor and separate monitor for text and commands, housed in a confining box. The next illustration is the representative of a PET system of the mid-1980s. The image monitor has gotten bigger, and a pointing or tracing device known as a trackbal is utilised the 1989 scanner has a single monitor, which is larger than that of the mid-1980s device, and a tiny mouse, much like the one that would now be found on a home computer, has replaced the trackball.

At the beginning of the 1980s, image monitors displayed 256 or 320 pixels on a side, and were 9 to 12 inches in their diagonal dimension. These were replaced in the mid-1980s by the "standard" of today, the 512 × 512 display on a 15-inch monitor. If one looks closely at most of these monitors, it is evident that the information most often is found in the center 13 inches, because of the distortion at the edges of the monitor caused by "bottle curvature". There also may be a very annoying flicker when graphics are put on the screen. Over the past few years, however, it has become practical to have a 16- or even a 19-inch display, with very little curvature and a thousand or more pixels on a side. As the monitors have gotten larger and the pixel density has increased, it has become practical to combine the textual command and control information with the imagery, thereby focusing the user's attention on a single device, reducing head movement, and simplifying the user interface. Studies have shown that clinicians are reluctant to diagnose from an image monitor, preferring to view a sheet film on a lightbox. Clinicians want to see the multiple images in a size comparable to that available on film, and at a very high speed. Today's display technology allows equipment manufacturers to fulfill these requirements. The filmless radiology department has been a dream since the silver shortage of the early 1980s. Emerging technologies now make it possible.

Another area of dramatic change in the computerisation of medical imaging is data storage. Some time ago, the typical medical imaging computer had fewer than 256 kilobytes memory. One or perhaps two costly, noisy, and physically enormous disk drives were attached to the system, each holding, at best, 200 megabytes of data. Today, 8 MB or more of memory is found in a workstation processor, revolutionising the way in which computers are programmed. Gigabytes of disk storage are possible, and most medical imaging systems have atleast 500 MB, with far more on the horizon. Optical storage using lasers to store the data, offers the potential of 600 MB or more of storage on a single 5¼ in. Compact disk—like platter, or more than 2 GB on a laser platter. Think of this as a worlds largest floppy disk, but also think of it as having read speeds equivalent to the Small Computer Systems Interface (SCSI) hard disks. For massive amount of on-line storage, optical "jukeboxes" are a very real, though at the moment relatively expensive option.

The user interface also has changed dramatically. Coming into the 1980s, and fuelled in part by the PC, it was thought that the menu and function keys were the only way communicating with a computer. These protocols tended to be rigid, unforgiving, and single-task oriented. In short, they were machine like rather than human-like. While "user friendly" was an advertising buzzword, many systems were actually user hostile. But marvellous developments were in the works at the Xerox Corporation and the Stanford University in the 1970s for the use of windows, and for a pointing device known as a mouse, to create a desktop environment with which far more people could identify. The Apple Corporation then popularised this with its Macintosh computer. Now it is spilling over to medical imaging. All of the major equipment makers have demonstrated these modern interfaces at medical equipment tradeshows, and the first products in this area are making their way into the field. Ninety-six function keys, lots of typing, separate control and image monitors, and a vast array of knobs and controls, way to use mouse-driven, Macintosh-like approaches.

The computing revolution is now being played out in six areas:

1. The power of the processor
2. The architectural concept of the system as a network
3. Convergence on standardisation
4. Product differentiation dominated software
5. Specialised processing capabilities for digital signal processing and three-dimensional graphics
6. Computer-literate children whose minds are unencumbered by methods of the past.

The advance in processing power closely parallels the popularisation of reduced-instruction set computer (RISC) technology. Reduced instruction set computer technology has been available for several years, but with limited application. It is built on the premise that a processor spends 80 percent or more of its time executing only 20 percent of its total set of instructions. Given that assumption, the processor is optimised to permit those most frequently used instructions to be executed in a single clock cycle.

The first RISC workstation to enjoy any popularity was the IBM PC-RT, which was introduced in the mid 1980s. In 1987 Sun Microsystems introduced its Sun-4 family of products, using a new chipset known as scaleable processor architecture, or SPARC. This new chipset offered with 7 million instructions per second (MIPS) or 10 MIPS performance. A MIP is approximately the computing power of a VAX 11/780 or a MicroVAX II computer. When the Sun-4 was introduced, the processor performance in the range of 2 to 3 MIPS was considered outstanding in that price range. Since Sun's announcement, others have entered this marketplace. Hewlett-Packard and its partner Apollo, as well as DEC, Motorola, Intel, IBM, and others, all have RISC architectures available. Both DEC and Sun have processors with more than 10 MIPS of power.

Accompanying RISC is a most usual vendor strategy. The RISC architectures are licensed to many other vendors, virtually putting to the public domain what was once a most closely guarded proprietary secret. This is being done to promote proliferation of these architectures, thereby encouraging software developers, who have until now concentrated on the Apple Macintosh and IBM PC, to write for these new platforms.

The impact of 10 MIP performance has been dramatic. In the realm of medical imaging, three-dimensional volume packages such as the Mayo Clinic Analyse became real-time and thus practical in a clinical setting. Similar impact is being felt in development groups. Whereas CTI's software group once had seven engineers sharing a single MicroVAX, for example, each engineer now has a 12.5 MIPS desktop workstation at a total cost that is approximately the same as that for the VAX. Productivity gains can be substantial when appropriate development tools are in place. From a product perspective, it is reasonable and affordable to offer individual workstations for clinicians.

The result of RISC technology is that an unprecedented computer computing power will be placed in the hands of everyone. Just where that power will be applied remains to be seen.

It is essential to view medical imaging equipment as a part of a network rather than as a single entity or island. The movement of data will be the paramount key to success. Medical imaging is, or should be, viewed as just another networking challenge. Data must be taken off an acquisition device, value must be added along the way, resources must be shared, and information must be exchanged between specialists and generalists.

Today most data are passed via Ethernet or token rings at less than 10 Mbits per second. Coming soon is a new standard, known as Fibre Distributed Data Interface (FDDI), that will make possible 100 Mbit/sec transfers. This means faster transfers, more data on the network without collisions or delays, or both. This in turn will fuel demand for faster processors and faster peripherals to collect and store the information from those spigots. Most readers are probably familiar with modems and phone-line data transfers at speeds of 2400 bits per second (baud). Really good phone-lines for general uses can attain 9600 baud. At extra cost, 56.6 KB of transfer is attainable. Fibre optic cable offers the opportunity to again raise this by an order of magnitude or even two, while keeping it affordable. Imagine being able to transfer images and other information at those kinds of speeds between outlying clinics and a central hospital facility or researchers at widely distanced locations. If information is power, a fantastic power surge is about to be unleashed as unprecedented amounts of information are put into the hands of vast number of people.

Table 35.15 puts these bits and baud's into perspective as measured by their impact on PET image transfers. A single PET image consists of approximately 260,000 bits of information (128 × 128 × 16), assuming that data compression techniques are not applied. Given this information, the various transfer rates can be compared.

Table 35.15: PET image transfer rate

Date Rate (bits/sec)	*Transfer Time (sec)*
2,400	108.0
9,600	27.0
6.6	4.5
1M	0.26
10M	0.026
100M	0.0026

As networks become capable of operating at these faster rates, enormous pressure will be put on processors and disk drives to accept more data more quickly. Networks are important to a medical imaging environment for a variety of reasons. Correlative diagnostic work using more than one imaging technique is becoming significant. There is a natural relationship between the functional image provided by PET and the structural image provided by MRI. The correlation of imagery with laboratory data is important in many modalities, but especially so in PET. Often records can be updated when examinations are performed, clinicians can get the information more quickly, and billing can occur in a more timely and complete manner.

In medical imaging there is an ACR-NEMA (American College of Radiology-National Electrical Manufacturer's Association) standard for information exchange. The standard defines a protocol for communication between imaging devices, an image data format, and the physical requirements needed to attach a device to a network.

In computing, UNIX is emerging as the operating system of choice in the workstation environment. Although there is some variation between vendor implementations of the UNIX system, the differences are not overwhelming, and two gigantic efforts are underway to achieve a single universal standard. Among languages, C has emerged as the standard choice. Windowing standards will soon achieve consensus. As these standards, and similar ones for graphics emerge, the possibility of software portability stops being a fantasy and becomes real. These changes will be difficult for some people to accept. There are staunch adherents to operating systems like VMS, MS-DOS, and the general IBM environment. There are strong believers in FORTRAN and PASCAL. However, it is believed that UNIX and C will emerge as winners in this millennium and will fuel the computer hardware revolution.

In hardware there are open interfaces such as SCSI and SMD, and buses, such as VME and Multibus. The days of proprietary systems, which served to lock-in buyers, seem to be numbered. With standards, a network perspective, and modern software development practices, the hardware revolution becomes all the more welcome.

As interesting by-product of the hardware revolution is that product differentiation, particularly in mature imaging modalities, will increasingly be defined by the capabilities of the software. While hardware platforms may vary between vendors, their capabilities and costs will be similar. Portability will assure that no one will hold a hardware performance advantage for very long. The leading edge of this effect can already be observed. Most high-technology companies have more software engineers than hardware engineers, sometimes in a ratio of as many as three to one. Project development costs are now more heavily weighted towards software. Further evidence is given by the decision of RISC architecture developers to license their hardware to other companies to create interest in writing software for their platforms.

Specialised chips and processors promise to further unleash creative thinking and the creative use of medical imaging. Three-dimensional graphic and imaging engines are very close to hand. Digital signal processing promises a degree of image enhancement and the quantitative analysis of acquired data that might once have been possible only on multimillion dollar supercomputers.

Clinicians have made diagnoses from film for decades. Digital modalities introduced imagery on monitors driven by computers. Few clinicians today use these devices for primary diagnosis. If it is assumed that modern hardware and software can make it possible to navigate quickly through large volumes of data, and to display large numbers of images quickly, will clinicians accept electronic imaging as the format of choice for primary diagnosis? If the answer is "Yes", radiology and nuclear medicine departments will change dramatically. The tape room and film library may in time give way to the optical jukebox. The film reading station may share space with or even be replaced by the electronic workstation.

Looking ahead, further many "exotic" experimental imaging techniques are being evaluated today. Adaptive histogram equalisation, volumetric three-dimensional imaging, and automated delineation of blood vessels are but a few of them. Will these techniques be used frequently enough by enough physicians to affect the practice of medicine? If they become accepted, they will substantially effect the performance requirements for computer architecture and workstations.

Will digital imaging modalities ever be more than a niche in the total medical imaging world? Digital techniques such as CT, MRI, PET, and digital subtraction analysis (DSA) are responsible for far less than half of all the images taken in a hospital or clinic. Will conventional radiography go digital? If it does, the impact on networks and data storage will be tremendous, since each chest X-ray contains as much as 64 Mbits of information.

NETWORKING

Networking is usually viewed as a method for transferring data from one system to another. Picture archiving and communication systems (PACS) have reinforced this concept by providing means of this moving data from multiple remote instruments to local consoles for display and storage. However, networking potentially provides far more than data transfer alone. In its most advanced form, networking enables users to access executable programmes and data located on remote computers for display or storage elsewhere. For example, in our center, physicians at four separate computers are able to execute an image analysis programme, located on a file server in our imaging laboratory, using image data located on any disk on the network, and to display the results on the local console. New technology will allow the development of programmes that search the network for idle processors (computers) in order to enhance speed in complicated image analysis tasks. The "distributed computing" concept promises to be one of the most active areas in future computer development, reducing the need for data and programme file replication at multiple sites, ensuring common resources (e.g., a common database file), and optimising computing power for all participants in the network.

Radiology equipment is commonly purchased from competitive vendors, each with different computers or microprocessors [usually referred to as central processing units (CPUs)] that control specific functions of the system.

Because each CPU has a unique method of arranging pieces of data, images that are compatible with one machine may not be recognised by another. This CPU incompatibility traditionally required programmers in the research institution to develop utility software for reformatting data when it is transferred from one system to another. As new systems were added additional software was necessary. Today, operating systems and networking software are designed to recognise data structures from other computers and correct for differences in them, minimising the cumbersome and expensive generation of translation software.

The incompatibility of different CPUs is only part of the problem of data transfer. No standard of image display or storage has yet been adopted by various vendors of radiologic imaging equipment, making the transfer of image data from one device to another difficult. To illustrate this problem, consider how an image is displayed on a monitor. One method of display might require the computer to read data from a disk, and begin "painting" the picture from left to right, starting at the upper left corner of the screen. If the data rate arranged on the disk in an order that starts from the lower right corner and progresses to the upper left, the resulting image will be inverted. Various image compression techniques, which reduce disk space requirements, further complicate this. While CPU translation has been integrated into networking software, image display formatting is still accomplished through utility programmes written within an institution.

Compounding these problems is the need for "user friendly" systems for clinicians and technologists, a description that to the researcher often implies "user-hostile." Systems developed to run exclusively from a preset list of functions (as from a menu) commonly prohibit the installation of functions not specifically built into the system by the manufacturer, such as networking capability. Medical imaging companies are understandably reluctant to allow users to modify their systems to access data files, primarily because of patient security and safety interests.

Networking Basics

To fully appreciate the computational potential of a networked environment, it is necessary to understand a few basic concepts of networking hardware, software and physical connections. The following section describe in general terms the components necessary to build a network.

Hardware

Routine clinical services and rapid image transfer to allied departments for research require high-speed data networks. Table 35.16 outlines several options for data transfer rates that can be expected from each modality. The hardware needed for network implementation includes modems on the low end and dedicated fibreoptic cables on the high end.

Table 35.16: Data communication hardware

Link	*Transfer rate (bps)*	*Relative transfer factor*	*Image transfer time (sec)**
Modem	1,200	1	109
	2,400	2	55
Serial Port	9,600	8	13.6
	56,000	47	2.3
Ethernet	10 M	8,333	0.013
Pronet	100 M	83,333	0.0013
Fiber Optics	1G	833,333	0.00013

*Assuming an image of 128 × 128 pixels × 8 bits

A modem (*modulator/demodulator*) converts digital electronic signals from a computer into voice frequency analog signals (modulation) that can be transmitted over a standard telephone line. Another modem then converts the analog data back into a form that is recognisable to the receiving computer (demodulation). As shown in Table 35.16, a typical modem transfers data at a rate of 1200 bits of data per second (bps). High-speed modems are now available for data-transfer rates up to 4800 or 9600 bps, and can be made switchable to automatically select the remote modem bps rate. Nevertheless, these rates are far too slow for routine image data transfer. For example, at typical modem rates it requires 1 hour to send a single CAT scan image (without data compression) to a remote computer. However, several companies have successfully utilised modems to transfer compressed images.

Serial interfaces offer advantages of increased transmission speed and reduced transmission error due to their use of dedicated cables between computers. Serial interfaces are now standard components of most computers, and because they require only that a simple cable be installed, the cost of the resulting networks is low. The major disadvantage is the need to have a dedicated cable between the computers in the network, which limits the physical distance between systems. A further problem is that electrostatic noise can easily contaminate the cables. Serial links are commonly used to connect processors to electronic equipment. In radiology departments, serial ports are used to connect computers to the gamma cameras used in nuclear medicine and to digital X-ray equipment. Typical serial interface data rates range from 96000 to 56000 bps. This is adequate for most text files, short data files and continuos data streams, but too slow for image transfer.

Data transmission over ethernet is controlled by a set of rules defined by the US Department of Defence and known as the Transmission Control Protocol/Internet Protocol (TCP/IP). These rules define physical mechanisms by which computers with different processors and operating systems can communicate. TCP/IP has been adopted as an industry standard for open computing (e.g., for systems designed for networking). Ethernet transmits data at maximum rates of about 10 million bps (Mbps). At this rate, a typical CT scan image can be transferred in less than 1 second. Because the TCP/IP is recognised as an industry standard, Ethernet components are readily available for most computers. The data transmission rates listed in Table 35.16 are maximum rates; actual data transmission rates on the electronic interfaces between the Ethernet Cable and various individual computers. Ethernet coupled with advanced fiberoptic interfaces, holds the greatest promise for routine data transfer in medical imaging.

Software

All computer networks require software to implement the physical transfer of data. Inexpensive commercial software is available for all of the standard networking protocols.

Topology

Various topologies are utilised in computer networks, including point-to-point, star, bus, and ring formats. Topology refers not only to the arrangement of the wires that connect computers on the networks, but also to the logical connections between computer systems. For example, in nuclear medicine network, the mVAX-II series as a hub on a star network for data transfer between five gamma cameras, but physically is linked as a node on a bus network. In this case, a bus-wire configuration operates as a star network simply because the software controlling the network requires all data transmission between cameras to be routed through the mVAX-II. Point-to-point transmission utilises a single communication channel to connect two computers. This can be part of a larger network, or can be a simple system designed for data transfer between two host computers. Star topologies rely on a central host computer connecting multiple outlying systems. The central system acts to control the network. This topology has the advantage of allowing many computers to communicate, but is limited by the reliability of the hub. Bus topology consists of a single "backbone" transmission cable with various devices attached to it by transceiver cables. The devices can be computers, printers, disks, or other peripherals necessary for the function of each system. A ring topology connects devices in a loop, which can optimise the speed of data transmission on a single cable. Internet networks—links consisting of multiple single networks—often are composed of multiple parallel buses or a core ring with multiple bus "spokes". The ethernet protocol utilises a bus or ring architecture to link all systems along a single line. This has the advantage of allowing each system to send the data to all others. Because signals are passed between systems on a first-come, first-serve basis, the speed of high volume data transfer are limited. We have implemented a bus topology for the PET center network. The CT network effectively runs as a point-to-point system with each scanner sending images directly to a common, remote viewing console. Topology is important when planning a computerised facility that is likely to expand. Ring networks must be planned carefully to optimise the line distance. Bus network permits the easy addition of new nodes, but cable placement must be planned in advance to allow access from multiple areas within a building.

FURTHER READING

1. Hoffman J: Changing Face of Computerisation in Medical Imaging. In Hubner KF *et al* (eds): *Clinical PET* Mosby-Year Book. St. Luis, 1992 .
2. Smith GT: Establishing a Fully Networked Imaging Programme. In Hubner KF, Collmann J, Buonocore E and Kabaa G (Eds): *Clinical PET* Mosby Year Book St. Louis, 1992.

MEDICAL RECORDS DEPARTMENT

Medical records are defined as an orderly written document encompassing the patient's identification data, health history, physical examination findings, the surgical procedures, and hospital course. When complete, the second should contain sufficient data to justify the investigation, diagnosis, treatment, length of hospital stay, result of care, and future course of action.

A good quality medical record is one which is accurate complete and timely. The medical record is the principal document by which the performance of healthcare professionals is measured.

The medical records benefits the patient, the doctor, the hospital and public health authorities and contribute to education and research.

To The Patient

It helps the patient in the following ways:

1. It serves to document the story of the patient.
2. It serves to avoid omission and unnecessary repetition of diagnosis and treatment measures.
3. It assists in the continuity of care in the event that future illness requires attention in or out of the hospital.
4. It serves as an evidence to support or to refute the legal questions that arise.
5. It assists the patient and the authorities concerned in fixing the disability entitlements under the workman's compensation act.

To The Hospital

The medical records form the basis of many phases of administrative efficiency.

1. It provides the management with statistical information necessary for decision action in regards to utilisation of resources, planning for administrative control and future references.
2. It also furnishs documentary evidence for purposes of evaluation of hospital care in terms of quality, quantity and adequacy (medical audit).
3. It protects the hospital in the event of legal questions (torts suits).

To The Doctors

1. It assures the doctor of the quality and adequacy of the diagnostic and therapeutic measures under taken by him.
2. It assures the doctor of the continuity of medical care.
3. It helps the doctor in his self-evaluation of medical practice.
4. It protects the doctor in case of legal suits.

To The Public Health Authorities

It gives a reliable mortality and morbidity statistics and thus helps the public health authorities to plan the prevention and social measures to meet the needs of the community Early warning of the incidence of communicable disease is often obtained from the hospital records.

To Medical Education and Research

Since recorded observations and case-studies are the basis of all clinical research, medical records become invaluable in all research, and teaching programmes.

Characteristics of Good Medical Records

1. Complete	Sufficient data to identify the patient, justify diagnosis and warrant treatment and outcome.
2. Adequate	All necessary forms and all relevent clinical information.
3. Accurate	Capable of quantitative analysis.

Functions of Medical Records Department

The functions of the medical record department are broadly classified into the following categories:

- Outpatient
- Accident and emergency
- Inpatient
  – medical record library

Central Admission and Enquiry Office

It initiates documentation of the patients, maintains records of admission and discharges, collects documentation after discharge and forward the same to the central record office. It keeps an upto date information of bed-state of each and every ward. In fact, this is the hub of all administrative activities in connection with admission, discharges documentation and supply of information regarding inpatient of the hospital. Since this office operates round the clock, it also serves as a general enquiry/ information centre for the hospital and may be entrusted with any other activities depending upon resources.

The central admission and enquiry office performs the following functions:

- Registration of admissions and discharges
- Maintenance of waiting list of patients
- Maintenance of bed occupancy board (account of bed position)
- Scheduling of appointments
- Ward's daily census reports
- To see that the hospitalisation charges and the advance money for paying/private wards patients are paid by the patients.
- To file the exemption orders slips if the patient is declared indiligent.
- To prepare the Alpha Index Card of every patient admitted and to arrange them alphabetically to know the location of patients in the wards.
- To receive death information proforma with two copies of certificates from the concerned wards and make entry in the death register. To obtain signature of the relatives in the death register of the time of disposal of dead bodies.
- To send phonograms if no relative of the deceased is available and make entry in the phonogram register.
- To receive the police documents from different police stations for postmortem, make entry in the register and directed to mortuary.

Outpatient Section

In the outpatient department, every patient is given a registration number in the form of a card/ticket and all his OPD records are kept in a folder bearing the same number. The folders are kept arranged in serial order in rows of shelves and are taken out as soon as the patient presents his registration number. The folder is deposited back at the end of the visit and stored in appropriate place.

Central Record Department

Assembling

The order of arranging the medical records in the wards differs from that used in assembling for permanent filing. There need not be any hard and fast rules for the arrangement of various forms and papers of medical record. Each hospital will decide depending upon its special requirement, the order in which the various forms are to be filed.

The general, order of assembling used in the wards observes the following sequence.

1. Graphic chart TPR (temperature, pulse, respiration)
2. Physician's order
3. Nurses bed side record
4. Special reports, lab, X-ray, anaesthesia operation reports.
5. History and physical examination
6. Progress report
7. Records of admissions
8. Summary sheets

The order of assembling followed in the wards may be reversed in the medical record department for convenience in making later demands. While most of the hospitals use the above method of assembling the medical records, some large teaching hospitals prefer to have their medical records arranged in strict chronological order. This arrangement of medical records is known as integrated record.

Quantitative Analysis

The quantitative analysis and re-assembling of medical records are usually done concurrently. It is the responsibility of the medical record officer to check the component parts of the records and analyse the contents for completeness, accuracy, and adequacy. It is done with the help of a 'deficiency check-list'.

Basic records

i. *Summary sheet or face sheet* It is the top sheet of the medical record and contains the patient's identification data, social data, provisional diagnosis, final diagnosis, name of the physician, date and time of admission and discharge, signature of the physician.

ii. *Admission record card* This should show:
   - The full name, address, nationality, age, marital status, religion, occupation of the patient.
   - Name, address, phone number of the nearest relative or friend and of the attending physician.
   - Name of the father/guardian and address
   - Name, address phone number of the employer

iii. Authorisation of medical/surgical treatment
iv. Discharge-summary
v. History
vi. Physical examination
vii. Laboratory reports
viii. Progress notes
ix. Physician's order
x. Graphic chart
xi. Nurses' bedside record

Special records Such as reports of consultation, transfusion, anaesthesia, tissue reports, ECG, X-ray, short-stay reports obstetrical records, New-born records, records of progressive care units, autopsy records, consent forms for surgical interference, abortions, operation. Other special records such as death certificates correspondences, birth certificate, etc.

Deficiency Check

While assembling and analysing the record, a note should be made of all the deficiencies by entering into the deficiency check list or on the top of the medical audit sheet or on the use of a rubber stamp form.

If there are any deficiencies the medical record should be labelled as "Incomplete file" until completed.

Completion of Incomplete Records

This is done by the concerned physician/nurse/unit/department.

Coding

This is done according to the "international classification of diseases".

Indexing

a. Patient-index (alphabetical index)
b. Disease-index
c. Doctor-index
d. Unit-index
e. Operation-index

Analysis and Statistics

Preparation of monthly hospital abstracts and annual statistics.

Reporting

Reporting of the communicable diseases, births and deaths, should be furnished to the hospital, municipal and health authorities.

Numbering

The system of filing patients records in universal use is that of filing records under admission-numbers. This may be done in the following ways:

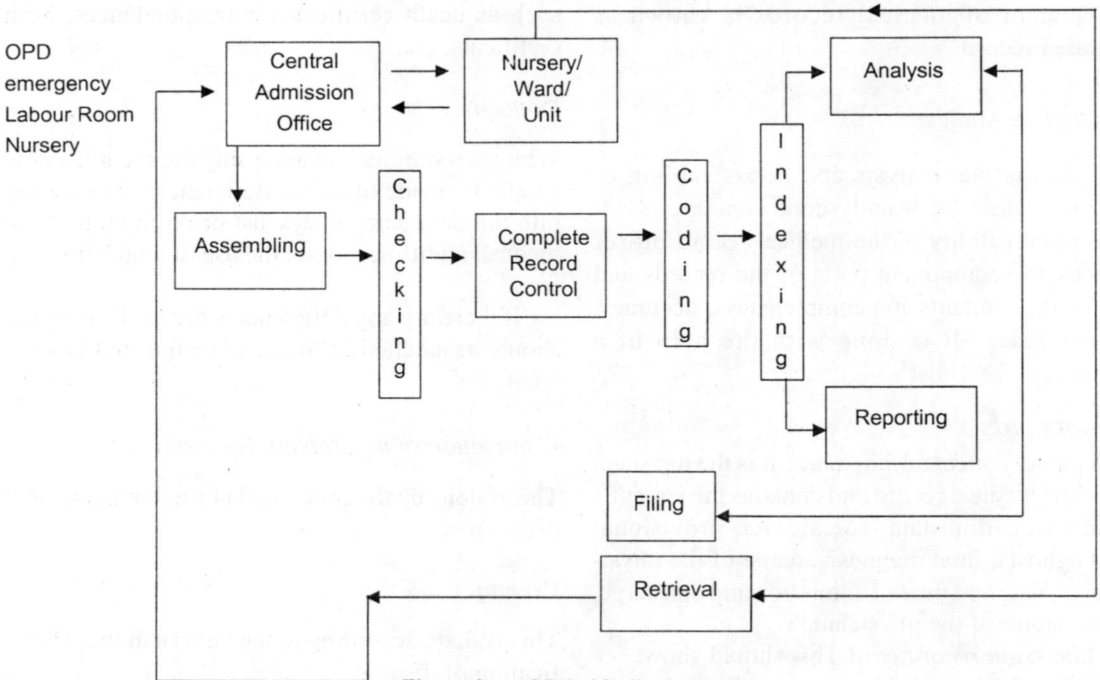

Flow chart 35.1: Medical records

Serial numbering In this method, the patient receives a new number on each admission regardless of the number of re-admissions the number always being the next unusual number either in the patient's register or the number-index.

Unit-number system In this method, the patient is given a number on his first admission to the in patient or outpatient department of the hospital. He retains that number on all subsequent admissions to any department of the hospital. All admissions are filed together in one folder and under one number.

Serial-unit numbering This method is a modification of the serial and unit numbering methods. This assignment of numbers is the same as with the serial numbering but the records are brought forward and filed under the latest number.

Filing System

Decentralised system Under this system, the inpatient and outpatient department have their own individual records and file them independently within the department. There is no connection between the two sets of files, if a patient is transferred from one department to another the records can be seen only through a loan. This duplication of records increases the amount of labour and operating cost. For these reasons, this system is being rapidly replaced by the centralised system.

Centralised system This is an arrangement in which all the case records of a patient whether inpatient or outpatient are filed together within a central department. Under this system, both inpatient and outpatient records are filed together under one unit number.

Methods of Filling

The modern methods of filing can be classified into two categories:

Horizontal filing Under this method, the papers are inserted in files or folders and the folders are

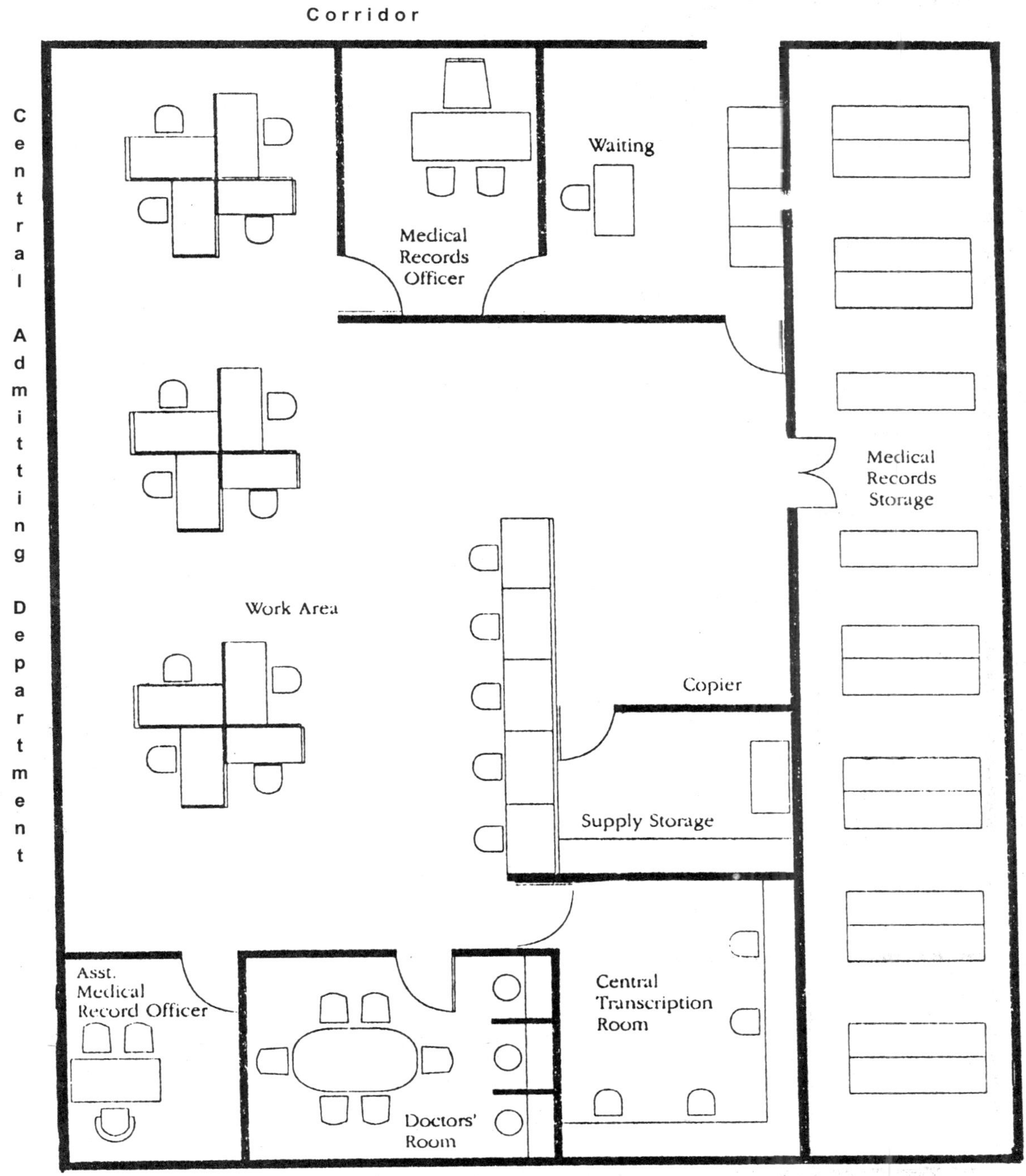

Fig. 35.47: Layout of central admitting department

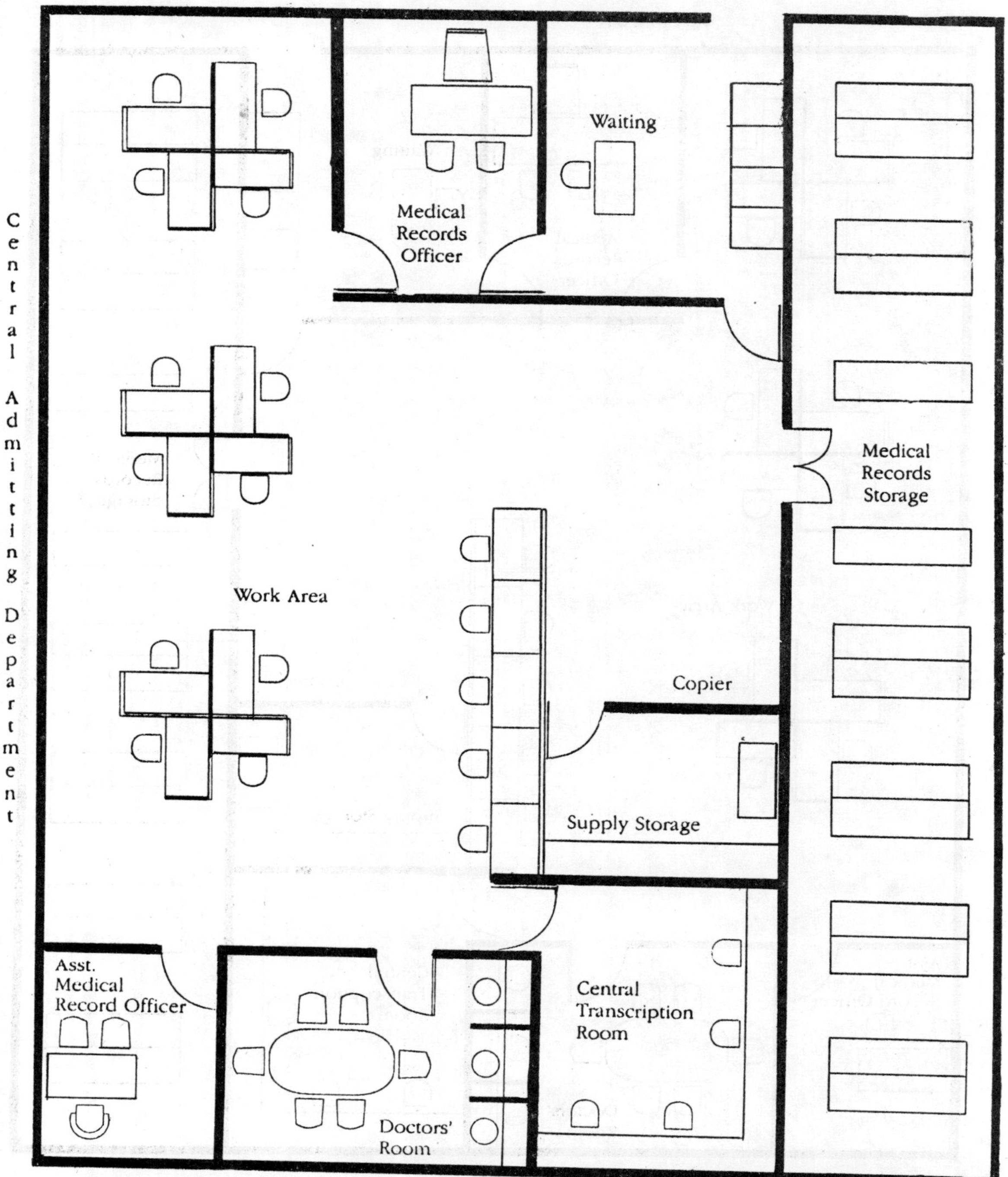

Fig. 35.48: Layout of a medical records department

kept in horizontal position one upon the other and these are maintained in chronological order.

Vertial filing This is the most modern method of filing, in which the files are placed vertically or in a standing upright position.

This method has the following advantages:

i. Facility for ready reference
ii. Economy
iii. Scope for expansion
iv. Adaptability
v. Safety of papers
vi. Wide applicability

Forms

a. Use of files of different colours for different years is useful for easy identification and retrieval.
b. Size should be uniform standard so that these can be easily filed (8 × 11).

Space

a. Outpatient registration
   Average space is 2-3 sq. ft./bed
   for 50 bed 150 sq. ft.
   for 500 bed 1200 sq. ft.
b. Admitting office 125-175 sq. ft.
c. Medical record office

50 bed	175 sq. ft.
100 bed	240 sq. ft.
200 bed	500 sq. ft.
> 500 bed	1200 sq. ft.

d. Storage
   120 to 500 sq. ft. with shelving for vertical storage.
   125 inpatient or 300 outpatient records in one standard 36" shelve.

Storage (Retention)

The length of time for how long the medical records will be preserved, depends upon the hospital or the government policy.

Clinicians want the records to be kept for indefinite periods. One senior medical record officer considers desirable to retain these as follows:

a. Need of the patient upto-10 years
b. Medico-legal: Inpatient-10 years
   outpatient-5 years
c. Teaching/Research-5-10 years

The records older than 10 years seldom required to be retrieved.

The means for decreasing space for storage is to adopt one of the following methods:

a. Microfilming
b. Comprehensive summary

Functions of the three sub-divisions of the medical record department.

a. Admission office	Reception Reservation of beds Initiation Identification Social data Assignment (to OPD or Wards) Notification
b. Ward/Nursing unit	History Examination Diagnosis Investigations Consultations Treatment Progress notes Education Evaluation Discharge
c. Record office	Assembling Checking Incomplete record control Coding Indexing Analysing (Medical Audit Committee) Reporting (Hospital Statistical Abstracts) Filing/Storage Retrieval

Ownership and Uses

The medical record is the property of the hospital and not of the patient, the clinical department or the attending doctor. Therefore, if the medical record is to be adequately protected and yet serve maximum usefulness, it must be considered from two points of view as a personal document and as an impersonal document.

As a Personal Document

The medical record is a confidential and privileged communication and must not be released without patient's consent. Even though, it is confidential personal document and the property of the hospital, the following might be interested in the information contained in it and some information has to be divulged under certain circumstances:

Patient Although the patient has got no legal right to the custody or persual of his record, he may be given a brief summary of his condition, the results of various tests and types of treatment carried out in broad terms.

Relatives and friends No written information should be divulged to friends or relatives who may be informed in the following lines:

a. Condition of the patient serious/very ill/satisfactory/progressing.
b. Date of admission/discharge/death/birth of child.

Press No member of the hospital staff should give information to the press except the administrator himself, and that too should be confined to only date of admission/discharge/death.

In case higher authorities feel that a press hand out is necessary for public information, the ministry or the appropriate authorities usually ask for a brief condition of the patient from the hospital. The official spokesman may then issue suitable handout on the basis of the brief.

LIC The LIC frequently request for details of hospitalisation and cause of death of the patient to dispose claims that arise out of the insurance policy. This information can be given to LIC without the consent of the patient because he has waived his claim to this privilege by a signed declaration in the insurance policy.

Police As soon as a case is declared medico-legal, the medical officer is required by law to give a report about the injuries to the police in case of patients whether treated outdoor or indoor.

However, police should not be allowed to record the patient's statement without prior certification by the medical officer in charge that the patient is in a medically fit condition to do so.

In all the above cases, the hospital cannot be forced to produce or hand over the original record to the patient's above listed except by a subpoena by a court of law.

Court of law According to the Indian Evidence Act, the hospital documents including medical records are admissible as documents of evidence because the entries in the documents are made by persons in the ordinary course of business or in the discharge of their normal professional duty.

The court can therefore, subpoena any document or record or summon the doctor for purpose of evidence in the court under law of torts (liability for negligence).

The types of cases are:

- Patients *vs* doctor suits.

As an Impersonal Document

The contents of the medical records can be used for education, research, public health and so on, where no reference is made to any particular individual and the patient's identification data is not revealed.

However, in supplying information to municipal or public health authorities regarding communicable and notifiable diseases, some personal information has to be divulged in public interest so that the authorities concerned can undertake appropriate public health measures. Normally, public health authorities are interested in impersonal information regarding the number of cases, deaths, births and so on.

SUMMARY

A well-organized medical records department should have clearly laid down written medical record standards, that should be developed in accordance with the institutional mission, objectives and resources and to meet the standards proper comprehensive medical record policies and procedures have to be introduced.

FURTHER READING

1. Huffman EK: Medical Record Management Physicians Record Company, 1972.
2. Tabish SA: Textbook of Hospital and Health Services Administration. Oxford University Press, 2000.

ELECTRONIC HEALTHCARE RECORD

Major benefits of the electronic sharing of health information are that it may:

- Decrease paper work
- Save time and effort
- Reduce costs
- Increase accuracy and completeness, and improve quality
- Improve timeliness
- Improve management of care.

Tension exists, however, between the sharing of health information, where the benefits seem to be clear, and the need to keep a secret, to maintain traditional doctor-patient relationship.

The main problems in "keeping a secret", with regard to the electronic sharing of information, are as follows:

- It can be accessed remotely
- It can be accessed unknowingly
- Copies cannot be differentiated from originals.
- It can be widely distributed
- Data can be easily linked
- Manual systems are difficult to access and thereby perversely secure.

Dangers arise with information association. An address, not normally considered confidential as an isolated piece of data, may acquire confidentiality restrictions by being associated with a diagnosis. The date of attendance at a clinic may be innocuous until linked with the name or nature of the clinic or even that it occurs on the second Wednesday in a month. Information is valuable.

The need is to enable sharing whilst preserving security, privacy and confidentiality.

To first define these concepts:

Secure "safe against attack; intentional or accidental"
"reliable; certain not to fail"
"fixed or fastened so as not to give way"

Private "belonging to an individual"
"not to be disclosed to others"
"kept or removed from public knowledge or observation"

Confidential "spoken or written in confidence"
"entrusted with secrets"

The Electronic Health Care Record

- Is stored in digital format and cannot be read without appropriate technology.
- Can be seen and used at more than one location at one time.
- Can be replicated, where the replica created cannot be differentiated from the orginal.
- Can be processed automatically.

The boundary of the electronic health care record should be that all recordings regarding the care of that patient are made by a responsible clinician. Also, that information does not form a part of the record until a clinician has taken resposibility for that information entering the record (laboratory results etc.).

The purpose of the electronic health care record is to be a record of care that supports the provision of care by the same or another clinician in future; a medico-legal record of the care provided should there be any reason to investigate the competence of clinicians providing the care; and a source of health care statistics.

Security and privacy are particularly crucial issues now because:

- Lack of technical standards currently inhibits passing between institutions and individuals, this enables operation without clear security and confidentiality controls.
- Information technology is being introduced, internationally, to health care records in a climate of clinical, political, economic, and managerial pressure to speed development.

- The next generation will redress technical difficulties and lead to dramatically increased information exchange.

The information explosion is in the centre of:

- A shift from institution based to patient based care.
- Increased ageing population.
- Increased capability of medicine.
- Increased specialisation.
- Shorter hospital stays.
- More information flowing.
- More co-ordination amongst carers.
- More people need to share information.

The risks of communicating information are that:

- There is a risk of serious harm to patients or clinicians.
- The risk involves the health care record and its processes.
- The risk needs to be minimsed without compromising the usefulness of the record.

The attendant consequences are that:

- Minimising these risks will require moral and legal regulation.
- Regulation is both technically feasible and morally appropriate.
- There is at present no European harmonization of legal frameworks.
- For the present, we have to rely on trust and recognition of each others' work practices.

Confidentiality is complex, involving:

- *Access by other clinicians* Health visitors, involved in the care of the under 5s, might be given unrestricted access to the records of children under 5 but what of the records of their patients?
- *Access by non-clinicians* They have no duty to make entries except in the administrative section. They require no access on the grounds of accountability. Patients usually happy with this as it gives them immediate access to information. Non-clinicians may look up a result when a patient telephones, check spellings or details in the record when writing letters.
- *Access by technologists* Technologists have no duty of care and access should be with the consent of the clinician involved.
- *Access by students* Access should involve personal consent of the patient or be via a clinician involved in the care of the patient.
- Access by legal professions and other third parties should involve written consent from the patient.

The commission of European Communities Directive (CEC, 1992, 86) gives guidance on when disclosure of personal information may be made without consent; where disclosure is necessary to safeguard the subject's vital interest; where the data subject has already been informed that the date are to be disclosed; where disclosure is required by legislation making an exception to obligation to inform; where the data are disclosed for one of reasons listed in Article14(1).

Article 14(1) lists

- National security
- Defence
- Criminal proceedings
- Public safety
- Paramount economic reason
- Monitoring procedure
- The equivalent right of others.

Access may be restricted by

- Certain professional groups, e.g. doctors, nurses
- Certain institutions, practice, hospital—certain problems, such as AIDS, termination, malignancy.

It may also be

- Regionally/nationally defined
- Practice defined
- Patient defined
- Carer defined.

The necessity to authenticate a recording by a clinician is real but this has not yet been resolved technically, still less universally implemented e.g. via a health professional user card or screen activated device.

Possible authentication devices for patients include:

- A patient card

  A patient card is dependent on the patient having the card with them when care is required. Patients who are not competent may suffer.
- A patient PIN.

Problems here are that patients in no means always attend themselves concerning aspects of their care e.g. repeat prescriptions. Clinicians frequently access records when the patient is not present. What if the patient is unconscious?

Control of the contents of the record exercised through a responsible clinician has its own problems:

- Conflict of interest between accountability and the rights of patients to control the contents
- Indelible records are a requirement of accountability
- Once entered, data should remian, and amendments effected by creating a new version of a transaction
- Copying to third parties should involve the written consent of the patient and a clear undertaking by that party to use for specified purposes
- Should these permissions be recorded in the electronic record?

In terms of inaccurate data, control of the contents should reside with the patient. If accuracy is disputed by the clinician the data should be annotated with the patient's opinion.

The major threat to systems is from people *within the organisation* in terms of:

- *Altering records* The nature of information stored on digital media makes detection very difficult. Systems can be built so that storage is sequential with complex checks on completeness so that it may be "impossible" to change data retrospectively without detection.

- *Falsifying records* A false date/time may be added by altering system clock. The DOS operating system actually invites you to do this.

- *Indelible records* Even if records stored on indelible media, such records may be copied on to magnetic media where they may be altered then copied back on to a replacement indelible media.

- *Inaccurate recording* A clinician may defensively omit recording important details or falsify them. Continuing access to the record by patients is the only way to establish accuracy.

- *Falsifying identity* By users using another's access code.

The durability of digital storage is not proven. Digital data may be encrypted and require "keys" to unlock it. Software or hardware required may no longer be availabe and keys may be lost or forgotten.

Future IM and T strategies should highlight and/or focus on:

- Information derived from operational systems.
- Little need for separate systems for management purposes.
- The idea that clinical information should be centre stage.
- The idea that primary responsibility rests with clinicians.

The issue finally should not be either to share or keep secret. Patients and clinicians need both. There must be a balance.

FURTHER READING

1. Barnett GO: The Application of Computer Based Medical Record Systems in Ambulatory Practice; *New* England Journal of Medicine, **310**: 1643-50, 1984.
2. Campbell JR, Stoupa R: The patient, the Provider, The Processor: Information Management in Ambulatory Care. In: L SCAMC Proceedings (RA Miller Ed.); IEEE Computer Society Press, 939-40, 1990.
3. Colien MF: Hospital Computer Systems; New York, John Wiley and Sons, 303-06, 1974.
4. Lindberg DAB, Humphreys BL: The UMLS Knowledge Sources: Tools for building better user interfaces.

In: Proceedings of the 14th Annual Symposium in Medical Care; RA Miller (Ed), New York, IEEE Comp. Soc. Press, 121-25, 1990.

5. Scherrer JR: Information and Computers in Secondary Health Care. Paper Presented at international conference on medical informatics. London, BMA and BMIS. 1994.
6. Shephered S: Caring. Sharing and Keeping a Secret. Paper presented at International Conference on Medical Informatics. London, BMA and BMIS. 1994.

CENTRAL STERILE SERVICE DEPARTMENT

Aware of the serious world wide problem of nosocomial infection the World Health Organization conducted studies (1986), in 47 hospitals of 14 countries and recommended that each hospital should follow:

- Aseptic techniques
- Disinfection and sterilization techniques
- Antibiotic policies
- Surveillance of present routines.
- Evaluation of prevention and control measures.

Sterilization (a total destruction of all microorganisms including spores) is usually achieved by heat treatment, that is steam under pressure in an autoclave, and is the safest and most economical method. The objects will become sterile within 15 minutes at 120°C. It should be noted that an item is either sterile or not sterile. It can never be nearly sterile. Fundamental to successful patient care is a reliable sterile preparation of all supplies that are used in daily hospital operation. As a result of technical progress, more and more dedicated and complicated medical instruments and equipment are being used, not only in surgery but also in other specialities. In hospitals today this equipment is prepared in the central sterile supplies department (CSSD) by trained personnel. The discoveries in the field of microorganism, role of asepsis and significance of bacteria in the pathogenesis of disease stimulated Charles Chamberland (1851-1908) who developed first pressure steam sterilizer (autoclave). Schimmel Bush (1860-1895) a German Surgeon, was the first to use the steam sterilizer for the sterilization of surgical dressings. Another eminent worker Von Esmark (1855-1915) proved efficiency of saturated steam in all methods of sterilization. The idea of centralizing the sterile supply was first conceived in American College of Surgeons in 1928 and the same was later adopted by the British Military Hospital during second world war. Nuffield Hospital Trusts pioneering and extensive research on planning and organization of CSSD resulted in concept as a standard hospital practice.

In India, the first ever CSSD was established at Safdarjung Hospital, New Delhi, in 1962. It was later acquired by All India Institute of Medical Sciences (AIIMS) in 1965 and thereafter by Christian Medical College, Vellore, Postgraduate Institute of Medical Education, Chandigarh, etc. At present, many hospitals have either acquired or are in the process of setting up CSSD.

The objective of CSSD is to provide sterilized materials from a central department where sterilizing practice is conducted under conditions which can be properly controlled, thereby contributing to a reduction in the incidence of hospital acquired infection. It also helps in reduction of work load of nurses in sterilization activities.

The other objectives of CSSD include:

- Pooling of materials, equipment and manpower to achieve effective and economical resources utilization.
- to ensure quality control of services rendered
- training of nursing and ancillary personnel in sterilization practice.

Advantages of CSSD

- Need for fewer supervisory staff
- Greater care in overcoming staff deployment problems in case of absenteeism
- Optimum equipment utilization
- Smaller capital and power costs
- Greater flexibility in production planning
- Overall economy.

In the modern hospital, sterilization and asepsis are in the forefront of the continuing battle against hospital acquired infection. The concept of CSSD has been revolutionized by the knowledge of thermal destruction of microorganism, ethylene oxide gas and use of ionizing radiation. As a result of these developments, the process of sterilization has become more complex and sophisticated.

The knowledge explosion in the field of surgery and medical practice and technological advances have resulted in the growth of sophisticated services such as coronary care units, cardiac catheterization, renal dialysis, open heart surgeries, transplantation of organs, etc. The success of these services necessarily depend upon efficient CSSD. The ever-increasing instrumentation in medical practice and enlarged scope of surgery and types of procedures undertaken inevitably carries the risk of infection, therefore, extensive development of CSSD to meet the challenge of increasing risk of infection.

For economic reasons, efficiency of operations and maintenance of high standard, hospitals have found it preferable for all reusable supplies and equipment requiring special cleaning, disinfection or sterilization to be handled centrally whenever possible. The centralization of sterile services resulted in greater uniformity, lower cost, improved performance and better supervision.

Function

The CSSD in a modern hospital processes, stores and dispenses the supplies and equipment required for all aspects of patient care including diagnosis and treatment. In carrying out these functions, a CSSD removes or destroys infectious contamination on reusable items and redistributes them. The role of the CSSD in the prevention of nosocomial infection is very important. The scope of the CSSD varies from hospital to hospital, type of hospital, ownership of hospital, availability of finances, type of services provided but the common items processed are needles, syringes, rubber goods, treatment trays, special sets and dressings, etc. The department is also responsible for the operation of the sterilizers for autoclaving the entire hospital requirements such as theatre linen and instruments packed for all wards and other user departments.

The CSSD is a major service support in the hospital and has direct relationship with the efficient and effective functioning of the key areas of the hospital. CSSD represent a sizeable service cost centre in a hospital.

Essential Pre-requisites

There are a number of essential pre-requisites that should be observed before attempting to sterilise. (a) All items should be cleaned and dried which will ensure that the minimum number of organisms are present on the item prior to processing (b) The packaging must be appropriate for the process and not obstruct the passage of the steriliant While undergoing the sterilisation process (c) The machinery must be able to perform its task within well defined parameters and (d) The maintenance and logging of the process and engineering work on the machinery is essential.

Sterilization processes can be classified as under:

- Heat sterilization
- Gas sterilization
- Liquid sterilization
- Sterilization using ionizing radiation
- Other experimental technologies
- Heat sterilization

Steam Sterilization

Steam sterilization is the most common of all the sterilization procedures used in the health care facility, because steam under pressure has been found to effectively destroy even the most resistant bacterial spores and viruses during a brief exposure. Steam Sterilization is universally used except where the heat and moisture damage may occur to the material being sterilized. In the simplest steam sterilization cycle, air is removed by displacement with steam. This limits the use of such machines to sterilization of unwrapped, nonporous items only. Porous load sterilizers have an operating cycle which incorporates a vacuum assisted air removal

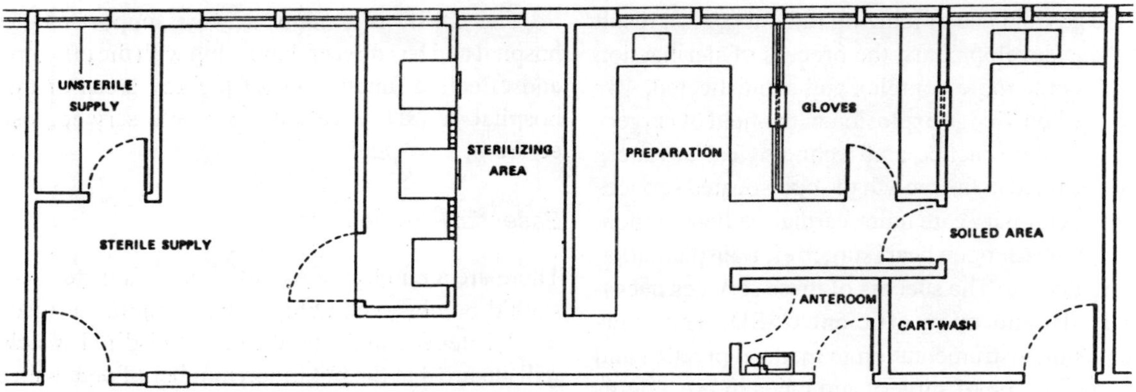

Fig. 35.49: Generic lay-out for central sterile supply

stage prior to steam admission for sterilization and can therefore be used for wrapped goods. The combinations of time, temperature and pressure vary from sterilizer to sterilizer and were published by the British Medical Research Council working party in 1959. Such time/temperature relationship has been recommended as

- 3 minutes at 30 psi at 134°C
- 10 minutes at 20 psi at 126°C
- 15 minutes at 15 psi at 121°C

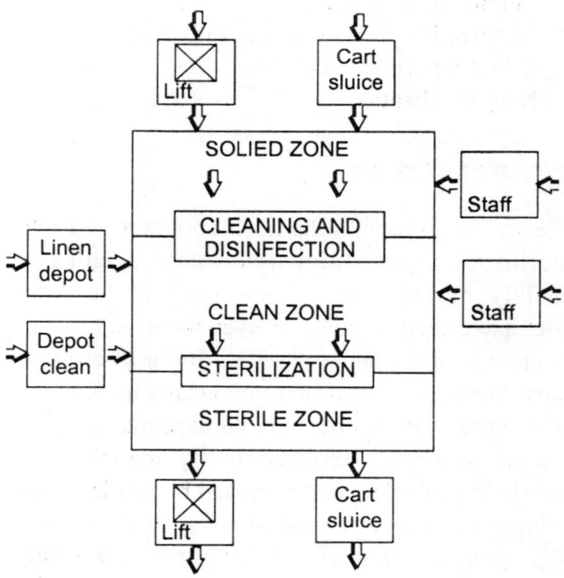

Fig. 35.50: Diagram for central sterile supply departments

The advantage of the process is that steam is a non-toxic, non-corrosive and highly effective sterilizing agent. The process can be easily controlled. Exclusions to the process are items comprising any material which will not withstand exposure to temperatures of 121 to 138°C for the appropriate period at pressures greater than atmospheric, e.g. thermolabile plastics and fiberostic endoscopes. It is also not suitable for waxes/oils, steam-impermeable powders and non-fluid items in sealed containers.

Sterilization with hot-air In this process, articles to be sterilized undergo exposure at 160°C for 2 hours, 170°C for 1 hour or exposure at 180°C for 30 minutes. The efficacy of this process also depends on the initial moisture of the microbial cells. Compared with moist heat sterilization, dry heat sterilization is inefficient. The main advantage of dry heat sterilization is its ability to treat solids, non-aqueous liquids, grease/ointments, closed containers and items which could be damaged by steam or moist heat.

Gas Sterilization

Several gaseous agents have been used successfully to sterilize medical devices, instruments and equipment, especially with the advent of plastics, electronics disposable, and other heat-labile

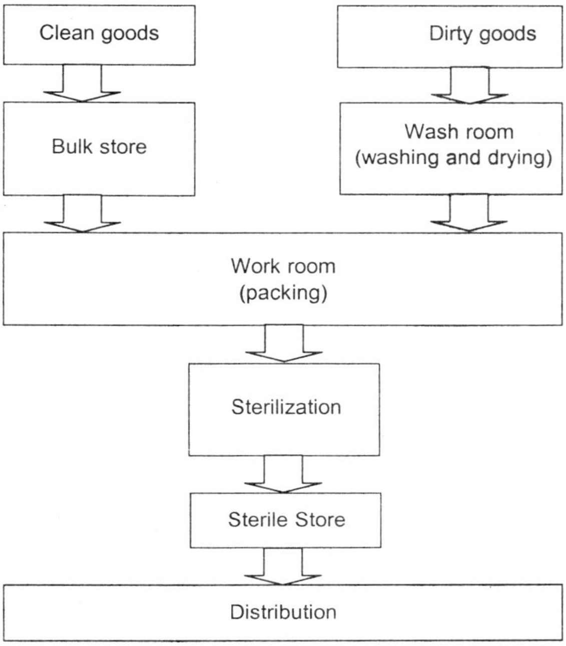

Fig. 35.51: Organisation of work flow in CSSD

components into the medical field. The main methods in use are:

- Ethylene oxide
- Formaldehyde

Formaldehyde has been shown, under appropriate conditions of temperature and humidity, to be both sporicidal and bactericidal. It is still used as a fumigant for rooms and buildings in which massive contamination has occurred. It is the sterilizing gas of choice for decontamination of biological safety cabinets and high-efficiency particulate air (HEPA) filter units. However, it has been demonstrated to be toxic to human being and has been classified as a potential carcinogen.

Low-temperature steam formaldehyde This combination of dry saturated steam and formaldehyde kills vegetative bacteria, bacterial spores and most viruses. All objects exposed to this process are placed in the chamber of an automatically controlled sterilizer in such a way as to ensure the removal of air followed by exposure at sub-atmospheric pressure to the action of dry saturated steam at 73°C in which formaldehyde is entrained. All surfaces must be exposed to the action of this steam/formaldehyde mixture. A variety of cycles are described in which there are variations in the combination of steam pulses, formaldehyde injection, holding stages, and the amounts of formaldehyde employed. Preferred uses are items and materials, including appropriately wrapped goods, not damaged by this process but unsuitable for stream or dry heat sterilization. Plastics (electromedical) qualify for this process. Exclusions are sealed, oily or greasy items such items where chemical reaction may occur between steam/formaldehyde and the article, items contaminated with body fluids, e.g. dirty returns from operating theaters, clinics, etc.

Vapour phase hydrogen peroxide With increasing knowledge of the toxicity of ethylene oxide, this has emerged as a new alternative method of

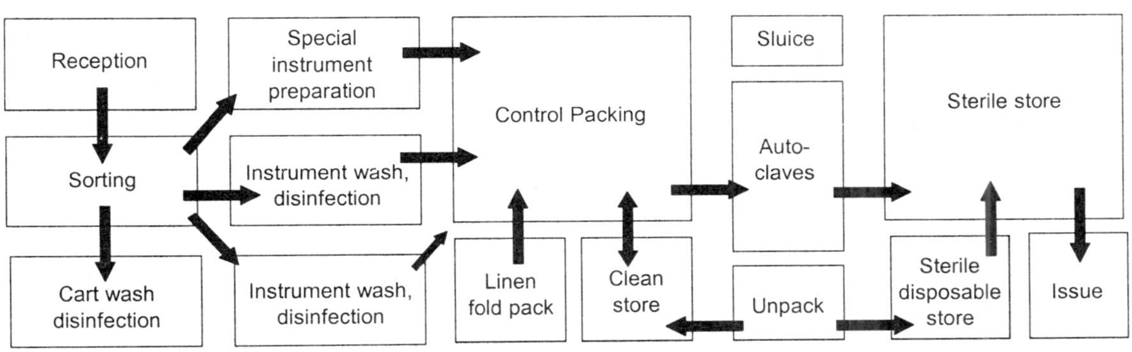

Fig. 35.52: Principal drawing

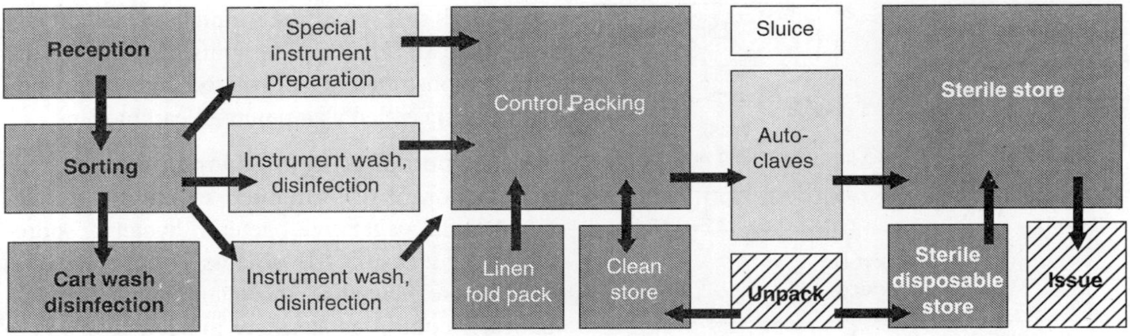

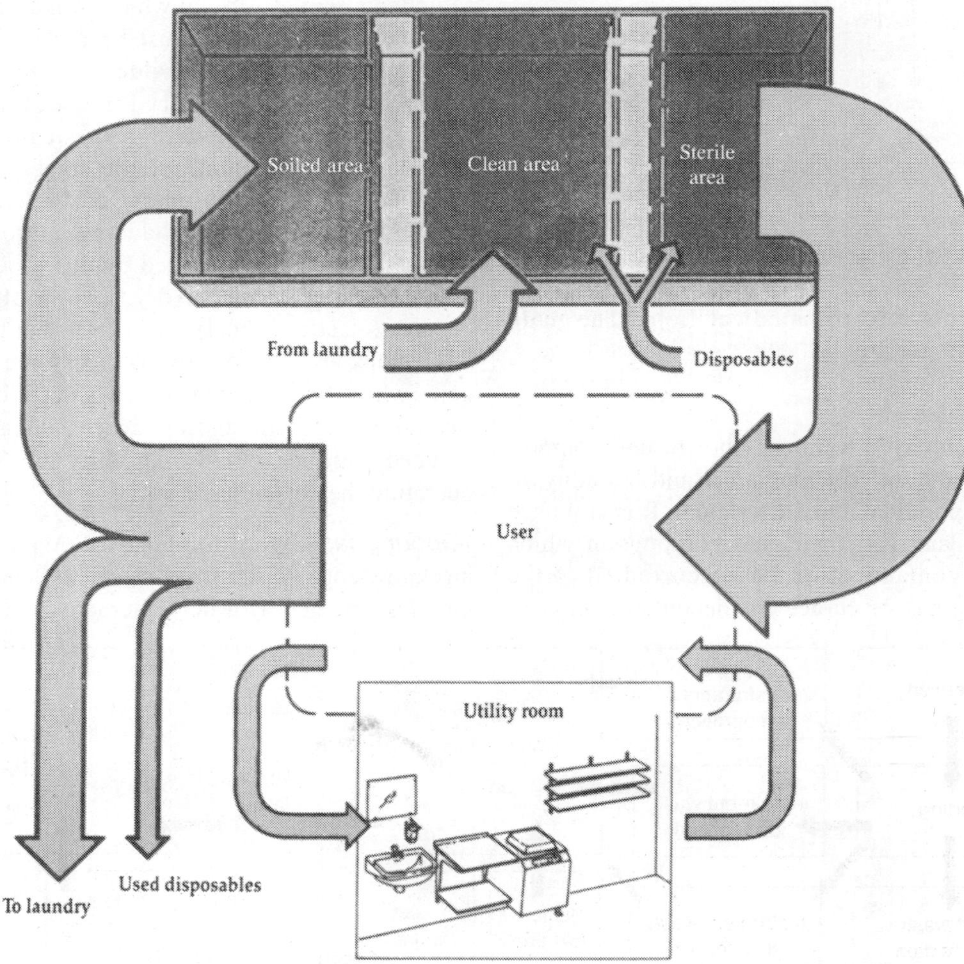

Fig. 35.53: Principal drawing of a CSSD

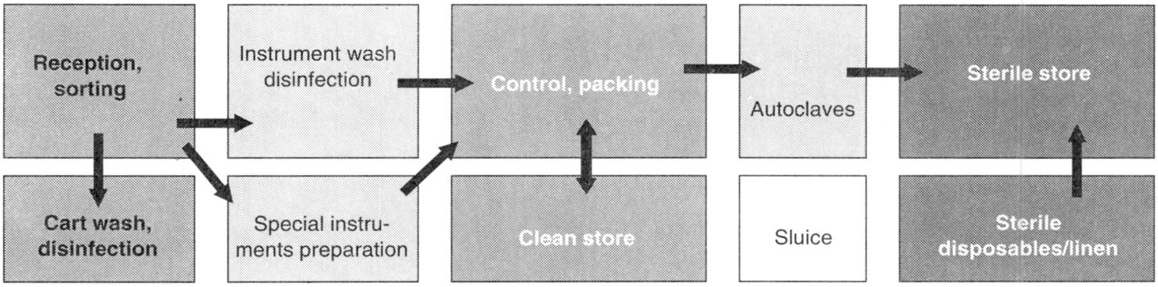

Fig. 35.54: Principal drawing of a TSSU

sterilization for heat labile devices and instruments. This technology is currently under evaluation. Vapour phase hydrogen peroxide generators have shown sporicidal activity, the process shows promise as an effective and self alternative method of sterilization.

- *Gas Plasma Sterilization* is a dry, low-temperature process combining a chemical vapour phase with a gas plasma phase repeated multiple times under vacuum to ensure sterility. Plasma sterilization may become available on an industrial scale in the near future, spurred by increased interest on behalf of medical manufacturers.

Liquid Sterilization

Glutaraldehyde sterilization Inspite of having been used for over a decade doubts remain about its efficacy. Many authors have maintained that liquid chemicals could not be used as an effective sterilization technique and the process is again being evaluated in the UK.

Sterilization by Ionizing Radiation

While ionizing radiation is not commonly used in the hospital for the sterilisation of equipment and medical devices, it is an important process in the manufacture and packaging of devices used in the health care facility. Many of the devices that are supplied "sterile" to the hospital, such as plastic hypodermic syringes and catheters, are formulated to be sterilized by gamma radiation and may be damaged or may not properly function when sterilized in any other manner. These items are considered to be"single use" items and are not expected to be recycled. Radiation causes little or no damage to the materials treated and leaves no residual radioactivity. Radiation of drugs, pharmaceuticals, and tissues for transplantation has also been successful.

Two accepted methods of sterilization with ionizing radiation are in use. These are:

i. Gamma radiation
ii. Electron beam (E-beam)

Gamma radiation has been the traditional method used in this field and reportedly exhibits better penetrative capability than E-beam sterilisation However, of late E-beam irradiation has become as efficient as gamma irradiation in neutralizing microorganisms. Both gamma and E-beam irradiation sterilize through the use of ionizing energy; in the case of E-beam sterilization, the source of this energy is an electrical machine, whereas gamma irradiation uses a radioactive isotope. Beyond this the dynamics of the techniques in terms of how they achieve neutralization of microorganisms are essentially the same, namely through transference of energy from the energy source to the products.

Ionizing energy can have a deleterious effect on polymers, and this is often cited as one of the main disadvantages of both E-beam and gamma irradiation processes. These negative effects range from colour changes to mechanical degradation such as increased birthlessness. However, this effect is much lower in case of E-beam sterilization as compared to gamma irradiation.

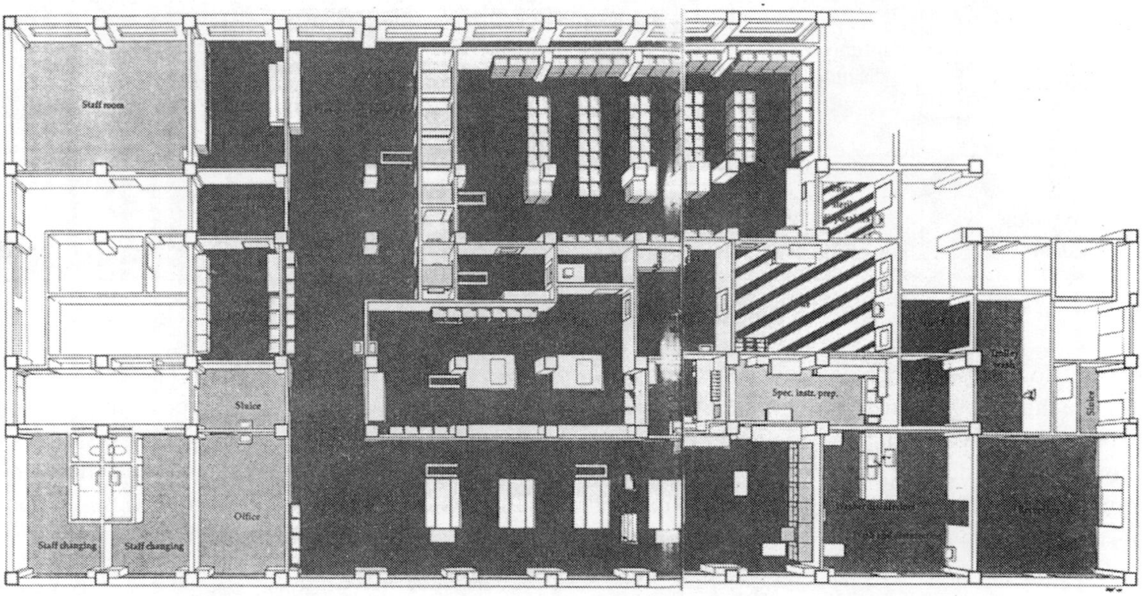

Fig. 35.55a: Large CSSD: This example depicts a large CSSD at the new Beijing Hospital in the People's Republic of China. the 800 bed hospital has a daily flow rate of 430 sterile baskets or 11 cu.m. combined volume

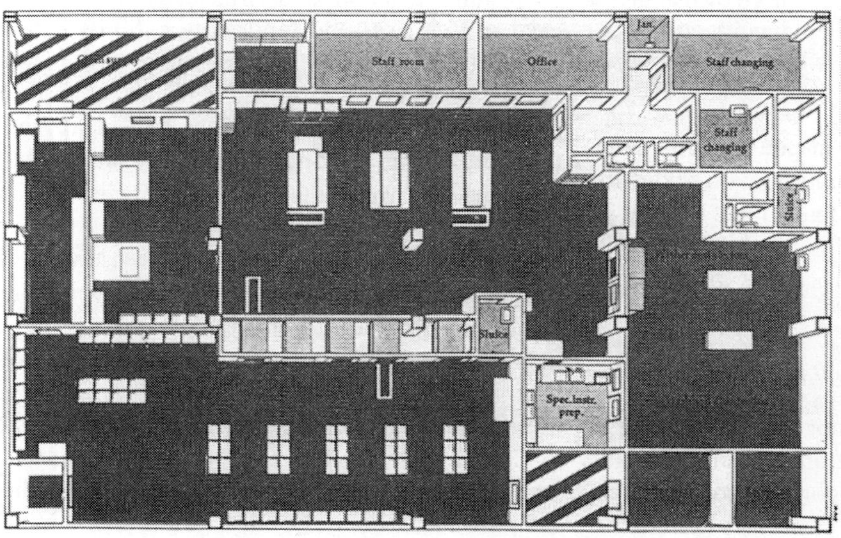

Fig. 35.55b: Medium: This CSSD was designed for a Gulf Hospital in Dammam, Saudi Arabia. The flow of goods for this 500 bed hospital was estimated at 250 sterile baskets or 6.5 cu.m. per day

Other Experimental Technologies

A US company, Pure Pulse Technologies Inc. (San Diego, CA) is marketing a sterilization technique based on high intensity pulses of white light. The method is reportedly simple and effective, providing rapid and continuous on-line sterilization while being easily monitored for process validation and parametric control.

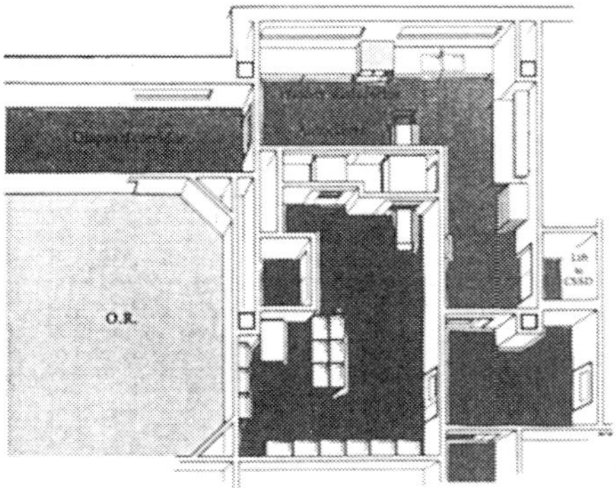

Fig. 35.56: As previously mentioned it is a common practice to combine a CSSD with a small substerile department adjacent to the operating theatre.This TSSU is from the Miners Hospital in Lubin, Poland

Sterilization Using Ethylene Oxide

The use of ethylene oxide (ETO) and its efficacy as a steriliant was first documented by Philip and Kaye in 1949. They proposed an alkylation reaction as the mechanism of action of this material and established the basic conditions under which ETO was effective as a sterilizing agent. This was the beginning of a new era in the field of medical device sterilization. The development of ETO sterilization methods and procedures, pioneered by Philip and Kaye and continued by numerous other investigators, has led to the widespread use of disposable equipment and supplies in the hospital industry. This trend has done much to decrease the possibility of

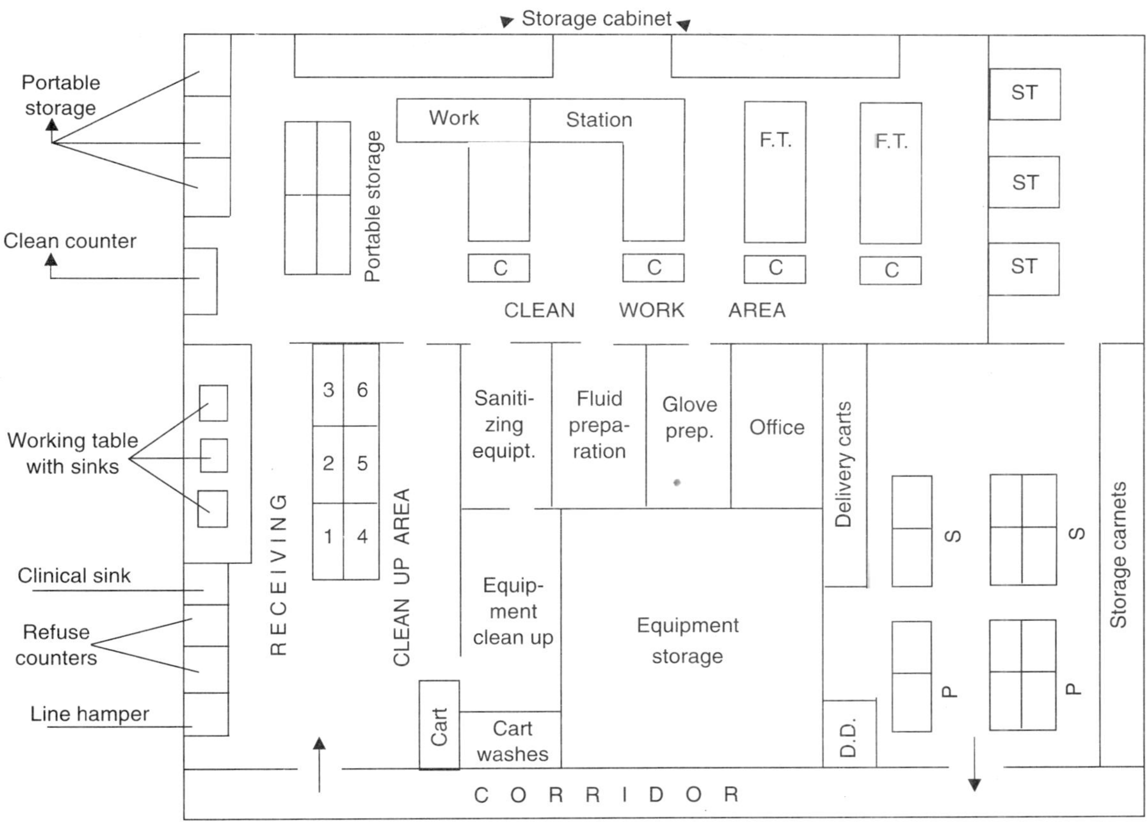

ST—sterilizers; D.D.—despatching Desk; F.T.—flat top table; C—cart; P.S.—Portable storages; 1—work table; 2—utensil washer; 3—worktable; 4—sonic cleaner; 5—glove washer; 6—glove dryer

Fig. 35.57: Conventional central sterile service department

cross contamination and has aided in the battle against hospital acquired infections. It has, however, also led to the discovery of the toxic effects of ETO, and the safety procedures for the use of this material must be carefully considered to avoid personnel, patient, and environmental exposure.

Guidelines for Sterile Supplies

The quality requirements for hospital operations are rising rapidly, partially due to technical progress with new possibilities and knowledge, but also due to higher expectations of the patients.

Fundamental to successful patient care is a reliable sterile preparation of all supplies that are used in daily hospital operation. As a result of technical progress, more and more delicate and complicated medical instruments and equipment are being used, not only in surgery with its special instruments and anesthetic equipment, but also in other departments. In hospitals today, this equipment is prepared in the central Sterile supply department (CSSD) by trained personnel. Only adequate design of a CSSD provides the basis for meeting the higher standards of sterile supply needs for the daily hospital operations in an economical and germ-proof fashion. The functional relationships in the CSSD are clearly outlined by the respective tasks and existing code requirements. The diagram shows the functional relationships of a central sterile supply department.

All possible floor plan solutions are guided by such a functional diagram. Before beginning a design, the volume of sterile supply needs should be established. In order to size the various washing and disinfection machines, packing machines and sterilizers, statistical information in the form of numbers of surgical procedures and so on, must be known as well as the sterile supply need of different ambulatory departments and patient care units.

Epidemiological Procedure

An accurate listing of instruments, meaning the number of instrument-sets for the various procedures has to be put together and the number of anaesthesia procedures in the hospital should be listed. The proper sterile preparation of anaesthesia supplies require adequate machines and installation. Guided by the statistical information, the size of the machines and the preparation cycle can be developed. The so-called use of one-time materials influence the lay-out of a CSSD. Naturally, as more one-time materials are being used, less material has to be prepared through sterilisation. This is only partially a question of economy. It is more a question of epidemiological standards. The results are easily recognisable. For example, the use of one-time covers will eliminate the sterile preparation of the surgery pack wrapping drape. This in turn, means less volume in the laundry, sewing room, and in the sterilizer. Waste-materials removal, of course, becomes an additionally critical factor with the use of one-time material. Setting the cost factor aside, the standard of industrially-fabricated materials is usually higher than that of normal cloth. Also to be considered in this context are the waterproof and limit-free qualities of the industrial products. More details and advantages can be pointed out by material experts. Self-adhesive-cover drapes, because of their many advantages, are being used in more and more areas. All industrially-produced sterile goods are subject to the standards of good manufacturing practice (GMP). This high-quality standard should be reached in the sterile preparation of hospital supplies. All functional and organizational efforts, the interior of the rooms, and the selection of equipment and machines should serve this goal. In some hospitals this goal is reached. Yet, there are areas where many improvements can be made.

Part of the design of a CSSD is the organizational planning of material's handling, meaning the location of cart lifts and the selection of carts and containers. The materials movement itself is done by the materials handling department which makes scheduled runs between supply and receiving stations. The staff of the materials handling department does not enter the surgery department nor the CSSD for safety reasons.

Also here the old rule holds: "Every conceivable chance for bacteria transmittance must be interrupted as often as possible "Enter-rooms" are the basis for a consequent implementation of that rule, A hospital equipped with an automatic materials transport system will use the system in the same manner.

The central sterile supply department is divided in different work areas:

The Soiled Zone

This zone is meant for receiving of used and soiled materials, loading of materials in washing and disinfection machines. Manual cleaning is not being done because of hazards to the staff. In this area all personnel wear special safety uniforms, materials reach the clean zone only after washing and disinfection.

The Clean Zone

It is the largest work area within the CSSD. Here all equipment is checked after the washing and disinfection cycle, then packed as complete instrument sets and prepared for sterilisation (clean-packs). Indicator labels verify the correct preparation, the work process is documented so that, in case it is necessary, it can be proven with which instrument set a patient was treated. This documentation has recently become more and more important.

Working Practice

Responsibility for the department should be given to a specialist who has sufficient knowledge of the surgery department and surgery instruments. A good working relationship with the out patient staff and the anaesthesia staff is important. All personnel of the CSSD should have the chance to familiarize themselves with the surgery department, so that they can understand the goals and importance of their own work in the CSSD.

Rotating work positions-meaning everybody works consecutively at every work position-supports morale and helps make up for lost time during times of sickness or vacation. The instrument sets must be checked twice. The check-lists must be signed and dated by the staff and only then can they be cleared. In the clean area the rule stands " Access only through personnel ante-rooms. Safety gowning and no coffee back corners". The CSSD staff should take its breaks outside the work areas, for example in the cafeteria.

Another problem is the holding of clean supply, for example linen. Basically all linen, gowns and sheets should be folded as instructed by the CSSD and the OP department and delivered in laundry carts. In other words, there should be no handling in the clean area to avoid producing unnecessary and undesirable dust.

The transport cart serves as a storge shelf and is also sterilized. For longer journeys within the hospital, the cart is covered with a hood. This hood can be double layered, outer layer white, and inner layer green. In the receiving areas, these hoods are taken off, this is an additional protection against undesirable influences during transport. Through the sterilization process, the sterile supply reaches the sterile area.

The storage volume of sterile supply should only be as large as necessary to ensure fast enough exchanged of supplies while still holding enough reserves for emergencies. Hospitals with emergency departments have to plan accordingly.

Choice of Equipment

Industry offers a great number of proven machines. It is important to select the right machines for performance capacity and volume reserves. It is also important to choose machines from manufacturers who offer a reliable maintenance service.

When choosing equipment it is necessary to think of the energy requirements, installation preconditions, and the space requirements. An advantageous machine capital cost can quickly turn to a high total cost through additional construction and installation work. Before signing the order, construction and installation costs as well as the energy requirements must be known. Consider the necessary transport into the building, the clear door widths, also the lift doors, the weight of the equipment and so on. Most equipment produces considerable heat during operation. The resulting cooling demands of the air-conditioning system will be very expensive in installation and service. Consider the air supply and air exhaust needs of the equipment.

Electrically-driven steam generators for the sterilizers are expensive to use (50 to 100 KW power demand quickly add up, and will push up the year's maximum needs).

Not much can be done through limiting demand since the sterilisation temperatures and pressures have to be met exactly. The cheapest heat media is still, in the long run, in house generated steam, but it has some problems concerning its purity, hydrazin, and so on. Electrically driven steam generators, therefore, should only be used in emergencies and limited for uses in the kitchen.

If the outpatient department of the hospital is rather large, and the amount of anaesthesia equipment and material sizable, a special department for the preparation of this equipment can be considered.

More and more parts of anaesthesia equipment are made of heat-resistant and pressure-resistant materials and, therefore, can be put in an autoclave. Those parts however, can also be sterilized in the CSSD. In order to make all these decisions, capacity calculations must be made. The complete design of a CSSD should comply with the following criteria:

- Clarification of the epidemiological requirements for the sterile preparation of equipment and materials.
- Quick, economical and safe sterile preparation of all supplies.
- Correct material handling of all supplies in the soiled, clean,and sterile zones.
- Three months after starting operation of the CSSD the work training phase should be finished. An operation analysis can then be made, and the entire materials handling situation can be adjusted after that test.

Planning and Physical Facilities

Location of CSSD varies considerably in different institutions and each location has its advantages and disadvantages. A common consideration which is borne in mind is that the major users like the emergency , ward units, labour room and operation theatre should be near or have direct and easy access to it. At the sametime it should be isolated from other functions of the hospital. It should have adequate supply of water (both hot and cold), steam, compressed air and electricity.

All functional areas should be provided consistently with the basic principle of keeping contaminated and sterile material separate. The minimum area in square feet required per bed is as follows:

- 75-99 beds — 10 sq.ft per bed
- 100-149 beds — 9 sq.ft per bed
- 150-100 beds — 8½ sq.ft per bed
- 250-229 beds — 7½ sq ft per bed
- 300-above — 5 sq.ft per bed.

This space is divided into six basic divisions:

- Clean work area including sterilisation — 40 percent
- Sterile storage — 15 percent
- Equipment storage — 14 percent
- Fluids, needles and syringes — 12 percent
- Receiving and clean-up area• — 12 percent
- Gloves processing area — 7 percent

The department should be so designed that there is no back tracking of sterile goods. There should be a continuous flow of equipment from the receiving door straight through the department to the dispensing door with every possible care taken to eliminate chances of contamination of sterile goods.

In a report on general hospital, the committee on plan projects has recommended the floor space requirement as under:

Facility	Bed Strength					
• General	50	100	200	500	750	1000
– Administration office	—	—	120	120	120	120
– Stotre Room (unsterile)	120	240	160	240	240	240
– Sterilisation Unit						
• Reception and Wash-up area	120	120	180	180	240	240
• Check up and assembly	180	180	240	240	320	320
• Autoclave room	80	80	120	120	160	160
• Storage and issue	120	120	180	180	240	240
	620	740	1000	1080	1320	1320

Areawise space allocation as suggested is given below (Table 35.17).

Table 35.17: Areawise space allocation

Area	*Nature of work*	*Proportion of space %*
• Wash Room		10
• Work room (in which all assembly and packing is done	Clean	26
• Syringe and Instrument (processing is done)	Clean	9
• Unsterile pack store	Clean	4
• Bulk store	Clean	11
• Sterile store	Sterile	16
• Miscellaneous rooms (including gloves room, office, rest room, lavatories)	Clean	19
• Autoclaves	Clean	100

Efficiency of services of CSSD in a hospital depends upon the staff employed in the department and on the personal relationship between the CSSD superintendent and his staff with the medical staff and sister incharge of wards/ departments of the hospital, which will ensure not only smooth flow of supplies but also prevent wastage and loss of instruments.

Systems of Distribution

The "One for One" or basket system Wards send their requisition to CSSD from which deliveries are made in accordance with the demand.

The "milk round"system Daily topping up of each wards stock to an agreed level

The "grocery system A load of standard composition is delivered daily to each ward and unused stock from the previous days issue is returned.

The "Clean for dirty" exchange system One clean article is issued for each dirty article returned to CSSD under arrangements by the user.

Procedure

- One and a half times an average days "usage" is allowed in the wards for use to-day.
- One average days "usage" is held in sterile store for issue to-day and use tomorrow.
- One days"usage" is processed in the CSSD
- A small reserve is kept to meet the peak demands

CSSD is a major service support in the hospital and has direct relationship with the effective and efficient functioning of key areas of hospital- to process, maintain and dispense supplies required by nursing, medical or para-medical personnel in designated departments for the care, diagnosis or treatment of patients.

Working Principles

Some basic working principles, as are:

- All materials must be subjected to procedures of guaranteeing sterility. The sterilisation procedure should be done at a place other than that where the item is used.

- The staff should be trained with knowledge of bacteriological problems.
- System of packing sterile materials should be simple, easily understood by all users, clearly indicating what is sterile and what is not, yet flexible and easy to change if experience dictates.
- The same pack should carry sterile materials to the place of use and non-sterile material back to CSSD as far as possible.
- The packs should be economic and available in simple number.
- The service should be available round the clock.
- The CSSD must provide products in a form which will achieve the greatest saving of nurse's time, which is one of its chief justification.

Staffing

The type of personnel required, besides the supervisor would be mostly technicians and aides, messengers and a clerk. The number of persons required will depend on:

a. Scope of functions
b. Scheduled hours of service
c. Methods of distribution and collection
d. Physical facilities and processing equipment

Cleaning, Drying and Packaging

Cleaning is said to be one of the most important, time and labour consuming procedures in any CSSD. Without efficient cleaning, sterilisation is difficult, and without fool proof packaging, sterilization is a waste of time.

Methods of cleaning range from manual cleaning, machine cleaning, and cleaning, with ultrasonic energy.

Modern CSSDs, use machines with high pressure water jets for cleaning everything other than rubber goods and needles. It can wash bottles and other large items which cannot be accommodated economically in ultrasonic washing machines. After washing the articles are dried in conventional drying oven or in an infrared moving belt drier but the latter does not provide flexibility of exposure for different type of articles. As regards the rubber goods, catheters and tubing should be soaked in warm-water for four hours before washing. After soaking, each catheter should be flushed with a jet of water under pressure.

Gloves are usually washed in glove washing machine, manually or in the high pressure water jet machine. Testing of gloves for puncture and tear is a very important step in their processing. This may be done either with water or compressed air. Ultrasonic cleaner uses sonic energy for cleaning of instruments. The Ultrasonics create cavitation.The implosion (opposite of explosion) generates minute vacuum areas which are responsible for cleaning process. It will be seen from above that most of the articles glassware, bowls, instruments, etc. can be washed and cleaned manually or by means of machines with the help of water and mild detergents. But rubber tubing, catheters, gloves and needles requires special procedures.

Most of the articles, glassware, bowls, instruments, etc. can be washed and cleaned manually or by machines with the help of water and mild detergents. But rubber tubing, catheters, gloves and needles requires special procedures.

Packing material to be used depends on the procedure of sterilisation. Articles to be sterilized by steam require a different material than those sterilized by hot air. Selection of wrapping material also depends on its ability to offer resistance to bacterial penetration. For steam sterilisation, the wrapping materials commonly used are linen or paper. For sterilizing articles by hot air, the items are put in suitable containers made up of glass, aluminum or stainless steel.

In the USA, it is a usual practice to pack all goods in two layers of linen and to sterilize them in an autoclave as a composite pack. The Nuffield Trust recommends use of a reasonable number of basic dressing packs and a large number of supplementary packs to supplement the basic dressing packs. The Trust also recommends use of paper as a wrapping material, which should be easy to open out, economical and can provide bacterial resistance. If the inner barrier is paper, then the out barrier should be sufficiently robust, to protect the contents of the pack against puncturing in transit and moisture. For this purpose, the Trust recommends the use of sterilizable cardboard boxes.

Gloves require detailed attention of skilled and reliable workers. A number of processes are involved before they are packed-washing and rinsing, testing, drying, repairing, powdering, sorting into sizes, turning and pairing. Disposable paper wallets are used and gloves are packed into these together with a commercially prepared powder sachet.

The choice of the method adopted for sterilization usually depends upon:

a. The type of material to be sterilized
b. Possible damage to the material
c. Method of packing
d. Availability of equipment
e. Work load and cost involved.

Dressing packs can best be sterilized by sterilized by steam under pressure. The equipment commonly used is an autoclave and the modern ones are the high vacuum, high pressure type. The time taken for one load is about 30 minutes, and the sterilisation is very effective.

The use of gamma-ray sterilisation for dressings enable the dressings to be compressed, thus reducing the bulk, and wrapped in sealed plastic envelops. This development will be particularly useful when the sterilized dressings are to be transport long distances and overseas.

Instruments are preferably sterilized as under:

- Instruments are part of dressing packs by steam.
- Instruments packed separately in metallic containers and sterilised by dry heat (160°C maintained for one hour). Cutting edge instruments are sterilized by dry heat, as they are likely to be damaged by moist heat.
- Delicate surgical instruments, such as, cystoscopes, heart lung machine or other electrical equipment, which are likely to be damaged by heat or steam can be effectively sterilized by Ethylene oxide gas. These sterilizers are safe, automatic, easy to operate and effective, not only for above mentioned instruments but also for any other types of sterilisation.

Rubber Goods

Rubber goods include catheters, tubing, drainage material etc. Gloves can be sterilised by steam under pressure but certain amount of damage occurs due to high temperature. Manufacturers use gamma radiation and gas for sterilizing disposable rubber goods. The best method for sterilizing glass syringes is dry heat. In the conventional hot air oven, the sterilization is carried out at 160°C for one hour. The other two method used for sterilization of syringes are gamma radiation and Ethylene oxide gas. Both these methods are highly effective and are used commercially for sterilizing plastic disposable syringes.

Shelf life of sterilized items depends on the following:

- Porosity of the wrapper and the method of raping,
- Storage condition.

Under ideal deal conditions, the shelf life may be upto 4 weeks. In any case there is no need to restrilize supplies at the end of one or even two weeks of storage. Beyond this period, most articles will have been issued for use in any case.

Financial Considerations

The cost of establishing a CSSD depends upon capital cost and running cost. The capital cost consists of premises, which may be existing or new, processing and other equipment. The running cost will include labour for processing and packaging, dressings distribution and collection.

The total cost will depend upon the size of the hospital, scope of the services, availability of space, location, type of equipment and various policies and procedures.

Disposable

In recent years, disposable sterile articles are being used in hospitals for patient care. Disposables are those ready to use articles which are discarded after single use, and are more economicaly replaced rather than reprocessed and used. Disposables have gradually been replacing reusables, as these items are convenient to use at any place and at anytime. Disposables provide a high degree of patient safety, comfort and satisfaction.

This development is having an effect on the scope and functions of CSSD. It is felt that hospitals may switch over to disposable items which are difficult to clean, such as, gloves, needles, syringes and catheters. As large number and variety of disposable are produced, the CSSDs will only be required to process those articles which are not or cannot be made in disposable form.

The advantages of using disposable area claimed to be as under:

- Elimination of cross infection: It indirectly reduces the cost of hospitalization.
- Better patient care (comfort, convenience and quality)
- Elimination of labour and considerable nursing time have been saved
- Reduction in cost where these articles are cheaper than reusables
- Convenient, readily available for use and higher efficacy

The problems that are likely to arise in greater use of disposable are those of storage space at hospital and ward level, and the problem of disposal of disposables. Several possible techniques are available for sterilisation and subsequent disposal of waste. Pressurised steam, dry heat, and gases would appear to offer greatest potential for versatality and low cost. As waste is collected, it could be transfered to a large autoclave and subjected to steam sterilisation. It could then be safely compacted and hauked to a sanitary landfill or ground for disposal through sewage lines. The hospital is responsible for the ultimate disposition either by prompt incineration or by destruction and concurrent burrial.

Fundamental to quality patient care is a reliable sterile preparation of all supplies that are used in daily, hospital operations. In future planning of CSSD, serious consideration should be given to the types and members of sterilisers and other major mechanical equipment to be installed.

FURTHER READING

1. Darmady EM *et al:* Central sterilize supply. The scope, function and organiza tion of central sterile supply department in the Potsmouth Group Hospital, 1966. Guidelines for the reuse of disposable medical devices. The American society for Hospital control service personnel. Infec. Control **7(11)**: 561-63, 1986.
2. Mc Gibony JR: Principles of Hospital Administration, 1969.
3. Manton JS: Dressing Packs: A concern for CSSDs for Psychiatric Hospitals. Hospital International, 1967.
4. Tabish SA: Planning, design and management of Central Sterile Supplies Department. *JAHA* **2(2)**: 1990.

DIETARY SERVICES

Dietary service has been considered as one of the major departments of the hospital and incurs expenditure of about 35 percent of the operating cost of hospitals.

The importance of hospital dietary department is not only to give clean, safe, therapeutic and timely supply of food, but to demonstrate to the patient the value of balanced diet and train others to follow it. The hospital food service is combination of two aspects that is nutrition and dietetics. Nutrition is the combination of process by which the living organism receives and utilizes the material necessary for the maintenance of its functions and for the growth and renewal of its components. Dietetics has been defined as the application of the science and art of human nutrition in helping people select and obtain food for the primary purpose of nourishing their bodies in health or disease throughout the life cycle. It includes consideration of the planning of meals for the healthy and sick, together with the selection, storage, preparation and serving of food with due emphasis on economic social and psychological factors.

The function of the department of dietetics can be broadly divided into following three categories:

1. Food service: system management
2. Dietary counselling and
3. Dietary education/Training programme

Food Service System

The dietary service is responsible for prepration and distribution of food to the patients and to run the cafeteria for staff and visitors, and includes:

- Procurement of physical plant and equipment for the use in the department.
- Procurement, storage and accounting of food materials in all its forms.
- Issue of rations and other materials for daily cooking.
- Menu planning and receipt standarisation.
- Preparation and cooking of food.
- Planning and preparation of modified diets for patients with specific diseases.
- Supervision of formula room in paediatric unit.
- General cleanliness

Dietary Counselling

It includes the following activities:

- Dietary counselling to patients including diet history assessing food habits and formulating nutritional care plan according to medical and social needs.
- To take ward round alongwith clinician for dietary counselling and also to know about type of food to be supplied to the patients.
- To organize dietary out-patient counselling and render nutritional advice to patient.

Dietary Education

Organizing formal and informal education and training programme is one of the important function of the, department. It envisages:

- Teaching and training undergraduates
- To arrange courses for in-service and on-the-job-service programmes
- To arrange health education programme for in-patients and outpatient
- To conduct research on various aspects of patient diet, i.e. menu planning, nutritional values of foods, storage of items, modes of cooking, etc.

Planning the Service

The design and physical facilities of the food service department has an important bearing on the standard of food service, labour costs and the morale of the empolyees.

Systematic planning starts from the planning of flow process of the department which will determine the needs and various facilities required for smooth functioning of dietary services such as;

- Physical facilities (location, space, machinery equipment, etc)
- Organizational plan (staff required to run various services
- Financial involvement (budgeting, accounting, costing, use of computer, etc.)

Physical Facilities

The success of the food service programme depends upon an effective combination of facilities, equipment and operational practices.

In the general layout, the most important factor to be borne in mind is the logical workflow, that is, receiving supplies storing and refrigerating them, preparing and serving food, returning trays and washing dishes. There should be adequate space and facilities for performing the work in each of these functional areas.The location on ground floor has the advantage and more convenient for delivery of supplies. With special lifts food is supplied to ward and thus odour and noise can also be avoided. The size of the central dietary department, is influenced by many factors such as number of beds in the hospital, type variety of diet to be served, policy regarding supply of food to employee and staff. However, for smaller hospitals, 2.5 sq. mt. per bed space is required. Bigger the hosptial, smaller is the spatial requirement per bed. Following guidelines are recommended.

Bed	*Sq.mtrs.*	*Per Bed Sq.mts.*
25-50	58.5	1.57
51-100	123.5	1.81
101-300	175.5	0.88
301-500	230.8	0.57
501-750	263.0	0.41
751-1000	278.7	0.37

Lay-out

Work flow in the preparation and service of food should proceed in a direct line. This may be either straight or circular (Figure 35.53).

The equipment in the preparation,cooking and serving areas should be also arranged that personnel can perform task efficiently and effectively. Equipment positioned to achieve single direction work flow will increase work efficiency. Mobile food holding unit offer flexibility in serving areas.

Ventilation, lighting, heating, the type of floors, walls, ceiling, plumbing, steam and water supply- all require careful judgement.

Ventilation

Proper ventilation reduces bacterial concentration in the air, odour, condensation upon interior surface which may drop into food or utensils, smudging of walls and ceiling, excessive heat, and the concentration of toxic gases produced as a by-product of combustion or otherwise. Moisture develops and promotes more. Preference should be given to artificial rather than natural ventilation. Dependence on window area or on natural ventilation is not adequate. Mechanical ventilation will be needfed for promoting the efficiency of employees and for preventing odours from permeating the building. Proper size exhaust fan and stove hoods are a necessity. Face velocity for exhaust canopies should be 75-100 CFM 25 to 30 air changes per hour should be provided in the main kitchen and dishwashing area. Discharges of the exhaust system should be well above the building.

Lighting

Dependence on nature for adequate lighting is not possible. Thus artificial lighting of kitchen is necessary. Ceiling lights that diffuse the rays, if sufficiently powerful, are best. 10 feet candles at a

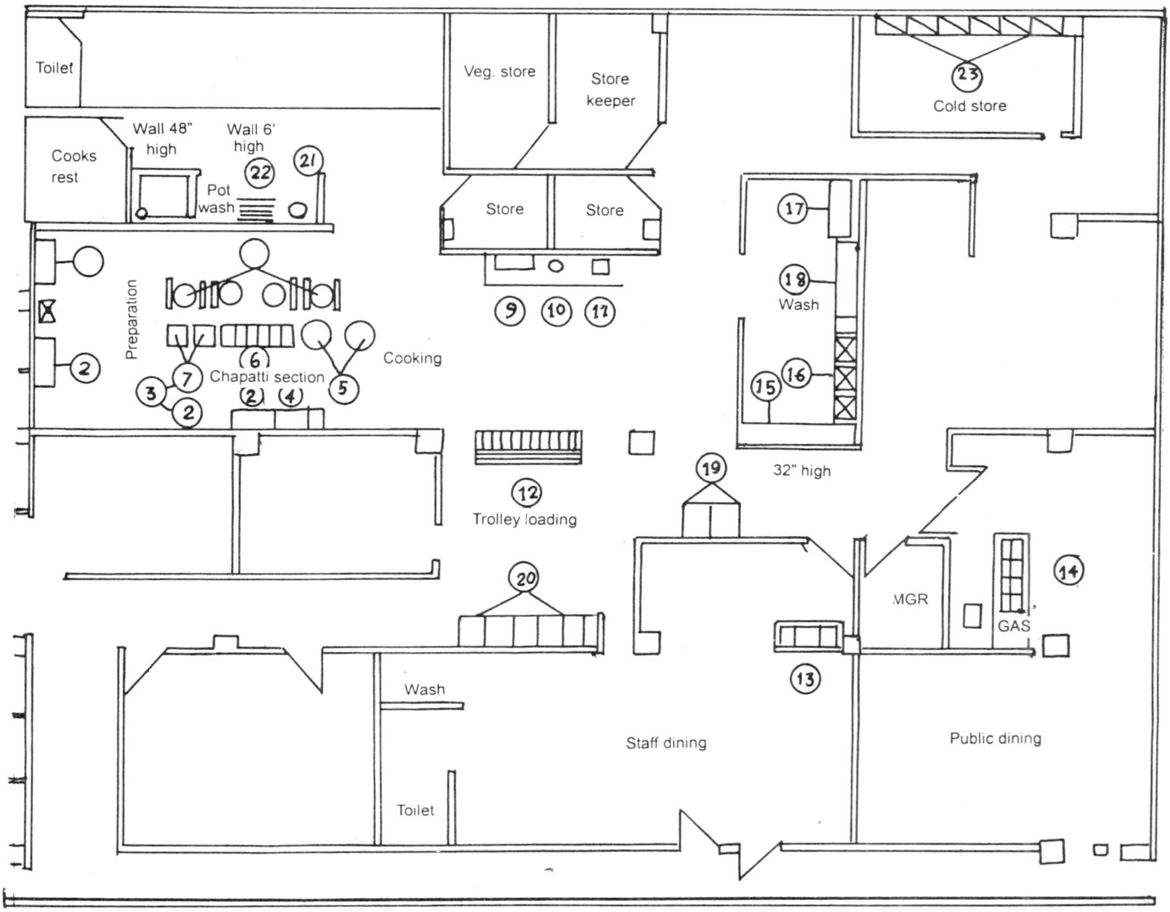

Fig. 35.58: Layout of a hospital kitchen

distance of 30 inches from the floor on all working surface should be provided.

Flooring

The floors of all rooms in which food or drinks are stored, prepared, or served or in which utensils are washed shall be smooth and kept clean. Cement flooring is not recommended, because it gets roughened quickly and hence cannot be cleaned throughly. Floors may be of concrete, terrazzo or tile. Large squares of tile make one of the best kinds of flooring as they are durable, impervious to liquids, and form a level surface. When the tiles are used, it is better to cover the walls also to eliminate all angles where dirt might collect. Floor should be freely supplied with drains to allow cleaning by flushing. If floor drains are used they shall be provided with proper traps and should be constructed so as to minimize clogging, and the floor should be graded to drain.

Steam Supply

Hospital kitchen needs sufficient hot water for various jobs such as washing of dishes, sterilization of dishes and garbage receptacles and cooking, etc and various temperatures ranging for 80-120°C. Thus steam supply with a pressure of 30 to 40 psi. is desirable. Steam pipes are to be carefully insulated to prevent loss of heat. Steam lines should be placed below the floor in a crawl space. This permits a better layout and reduces heat in the kitchen.

Water Supply

Running hot and cold water under pressure should be easily accessible to all rooms in which food is prepared or utensils are washed and the water supply shall be adequate and of a safe, potable quality. Provision of running water under pressure will encourage its use in cleaning operation. To make it safe for drinking, the reverse cycle osmosis process may be used.

Funcational Areas

The major functional areas of the food services department, following the sequence in the workflow, include:

- Receiving area and control station
- Storage and refrigeration rooms
- Preparation and production areas
- Serving room
- Food delivery
- Special diet kitchen
- Dish washing area
- Pot washing area.

Dietitian's Office

The office should be conveniently located so that it should offer un-obstructed observation of all areas of the department. It should be soundproof and well ventilated. Therapeutic dieticians should be on the patient floor, so that these dietitians are readily available to the medical staff and the patients.

Receiving and Storing Food and Supplies

The receiving department in small and medium sized hospital is often combined with the storage areas. It should have easy access from the outside and proximity to the food service department is most important. The receiving entrance should be located where the noise of trucks and unloading will not disturb patients.

Unloading space is usually provided in the form of a delivery dock or platform as high as the floor of the average truck body 1 mt to 1.2 mt. The outside door of the receiving area should be preferably of the double door type with a width of 1.5 mt. Whenever possible, actual checking of supplies should be done as close to the point of storage as possible so that there is less chance of mislaying or losing merchandise after the receipt is signed. A platform scale is the one essential piece of equipment in the receiving area.

Storage

A dry, well-ventilated store-room should be provided for non-perishable supplies such as canned food, bottled beverages, dry ration (staple food), china, silver, glassware, linen, etc. A temperature of 15-20°C should be maintained. Doorways and corridors wide enough for hand trucks are essential, and doors with secure locks should be planned. The most desirable height for the ceiling is store room is 5 mtrs. To support the heavy lead of stacked cases, the floor must be well built.

Metal shelving is desirable, if the budget allows, and should be placed in the centre of the room or at least 0.75 mt from the walls. Aisle space should be wide enough so that the shelves are accessible on both sides. Adjustable shelving often allows a more efficient storage space for all types of supplies. A slotted platform raised about 14 cms above the floor is advantageous for bags of staple food and case lots of canned products. In large hospitals a well ventilated, day store room for one or two days supplies should be located near the area of food preparation. It should have adequate space to store a limited amount of food in cases and sacks. About 46.5 sq.mt of space has been suggested for this store room.

Refrigeration Storage

Perishable foods, such as meat, poultry, dairy products, eggs, fruits and vegetables need refrigerated storage space. Refrigeration storage needs of different hospital vary greatly as a result of frequency of deliveries, type of menu, type of institutional service, budget consideration, etc. Refrigeration space of .04 cu mt per person served including storage facilities for frozen foods is recommended

Refrigeration storage is of three types:

1. *Walk-in* it is convenient for bigger utilization as it is easier for handling large supplies. Accessibility is easier and sanitation is better.
2. *Reach-in* for small hospitals reach in boxes may serve the purpose.
3. *Under the counter* If stores can be received daily under the counter refrigerator can also serve the purpose. Optimum temperature for refrigeration should be between 0 to –4°C.

Food Prepration Room

The preliminary preparation of food involves peeling, washing, soaking, cutting, and sorting of foods before being sent to the cooking unit or the salad unit. This area should be located between the storage area and the cooking unit.

In the large hopsital the preparation area is divided into a meat cutting unit and vegetable unit. In many small hospitals the cut meat is bought, thus obviating the need for a separate meat cutting unit. The minimum equipment's required for the preparation unit is:

- A saw to cut meat/vegetables.
- Double sink with drain boards.
- Table area 1.2 linear meter per worker.

Food Prepration Unit

The cooking unit should be located near preparation unit to facilitate a straight line flow of food from one processing point to another. The provision for institution size pressure cookers, steam kettle will be very advantageous. There should be baking arrangements alongwith cooking range, if not provided separately.

Special Diets Area

Special attention is required to be given in planning to supply special/therapeutic diet menu. Separate diet for each patient is to be supplied from kitchen. This area should be equipped with mixer-grinder measuring balance and good working table.

Those hospitals which admit infants, should have formula room. The formula room draws supplies almost exclusively from refrigerator and prepare food to supply to various paediatrics sections.

Every precaution required is to be taken for sterilization of containers in which food is prepared and the container in which it is supplied.

Food Service Area

Food services may be centralized, decentralized or a combination of both. In a centralized service, all food is prepared and cooked in the main kitchen and the food trays are set up, served, then conveyed to various patient areas by trolley. In a decentralized service, food is cooked in the main kitchen and transported in the bulk to patient areas where the trays are served, either in a floor pantry or at the patient's bed side, both have its merits and demerits. Either system can work satisfactorily, if administration so desires. If hospital has paying wards then food has to be supplied from decentralised kitchen, because it assures hot food supply and short-orders can be attended.

In most of the hospitals kitchen supplies food to all wards in trolleys. Even main food for paying ward kitchen is cooked in this kitchen and supplied in trolleys where separate trays are prepared and only soup and bread are cooked as and when required.

Ample floor area for movement of trolleys and personnel must be allowed and parking area for trolleys, between meals, must be provided.

Dish Washing Area

Although decentralized food service is common, dishwashing should, be centralized so that proper standards of sanitation can be maintained.

The dishwashing room requires almost 0.1 sq. mt for each person served. Floor space must be sufficient for emptying and cleaning of tray trucks. Space is also needed for storing of dish baskets or racks when not in use and for storing of soaps, detergents and other cleaning supplies.

Provision must be made for collection of garbage near the soiled dish counter and for transporting it outside without carrying it through the kitchen or other clean areas. Mechanical dishwashing is desirable for manual diswashing proper facilities must be provided which consists of:

Counter for stocking and scraping of dirty dishes. This should be of non-porous material such as stainless steel, anodised aluminum, etc. sloping slightly towards the pre-rise sink. There should be a 15 cms opening through which rejected food can be scrapped into a garbage can below (or a mechanical garbage grinder). This counter should be 2-3 mts long, 0.65 mts wide, 1 meter high.

Pre-rinse sink with running water at 50 to 60°C to remove remaining excess food which has dried on dishes. This sink should be 1.25 mts long, 0.65 mts wide, 0.4 mts deep, 1 mt. above ground, and connected to the stacking counter on one hand.

Wash sink adjourning to the pre-rinse sink, with same specifications.

After-rinse-clean dish storage: This can be of two types. Either another sink, as described above, into which dishes are dipped, with water at 80°C after which they are stacked on the clean dish counter to dry, or preferably, a clean dish counter adjoining the wash sink, on which are racks or baskets, into which the dishes are placed then the dishes are rinsed by a spray of water at 80°C temperature. Dishes are left to dry in the clean racks which should be pushed into the clean dish storage area. If this drying clean dish counter can extend through an opening in the wall to a separate clean dish storage room that will be better.

Pot and Pan washing

This area (a minimum of 4.6 sq.mt) should be out of the main traffic line near the cooking unit. Rack, table, or movable cart is needed for holding solid pots and pans.

The washing area requires a three compartment sink, one for pre-rinse and soaking, one for washing, both with water at 50-60°C and one for rinsing with water at 80°C. Sinks should have splash back and grease traps. A low concrete basin, with running water and drain, approximately 1.5 × 2.5 mts will be necessary for washing larger pots. Provision of racks for storage of clean pots and pans is to be made near the cooking units.

Table 35.18: Functional programme

	100 beds	*200 beds*	*300 beds*	*400 beds*	*500 beds*
• Patient meals per day					
peak per meal	225	510	765	1020	1275
• Cafeteria meals per day	95	190	285	380	475
peak per meal	147	247	383	536	727
• Cafteria seats (2½	96	163	257	368	506
sitting)	40	60	95	120	160
• Staff dinning seats	—	10	15	25	40
• Other meals	10	20	30	40	50
• Peak total meals	412	777	1178	1596	2052
kitchen peak per meal	201	373	572	788	1031
• Dieticians (including	1	2	3	4	5
assistants) Kitchen	10	20	30	40	50
employees	4	4	6	8	10
• Secretary	—	1	1	1	2
• Others	2	4	6	8	10
Total staff	**17**	**31**	**46**	**61**	**77**

FUNCTIONAL PROGRAMME

Central tray service, hot and cold divided in 20 tray carts to patient divisions for final assembly and serving. Trays returned to central dishwashing.

Nourshment pantry on floors. Nursing staff will serve trays to patients. Cafeteria for visitors. ambulant patients, and hospital personel on pay basis. Auxiliary runs coffee shop.

House-keeping

It is very essenital to maintain high degree of cleanliness in hospital kitchen. Cleanliness is dependent upon good quality of floor, provision of sufficient running water at desired pressure, good drainage system, ventilation and trained manpower to follow the laid down procedure of sanitation. some of the important elements of high degree of house-keeping sanitation are as follows

Garbage Disposal

An area of at least 5.6 sq.mts should be available for this purpose. It should be in an area away from patient units, easily accessible from the service drive way. Garbage cans should be washed with hot water (80°C) after each emptying.

Toilet and Lavatory Facilities

Hospital kitchens shall be provided with adequate and conveniently located toilet facilities for its employees. The doors of all toilet room shall be self-closing. It is required to be kept clean so that flies and other insects may not be present. Provision of liquid soap and soap near hand washing sink is very essential. There must be provision for exhaust fan.

Organization of Dietary Department

Right person, in right number at required time is must to cook required amount of diet according to menu and to serve to the patient, staff and attendants, Staff is also required for therapeutic advice and training/research. It is essential that function of different categories of staff be known. Proper job description is required to compute the workload and number of persons of various categories. The quality of worker and the productivity depend upon the staff working in the organization. The qualification and experience of each staff is needed to be specified. It will further help in calculating the wages/ salary of various staff.

Chief Dietician

Chief dietician will be responsible for :

1. *Administrative function*
    - Purchasing or collaborating in purchase of food and equipment
    - Preparing duty roster
    - Co-ordination with other department
    - Supervision
    - Accounting, control and office work.
2. *Dietary and clinical counselling*
    - Planning and specifying quantity and quality of food to be cooked
    - Menu planning
    - Therapeutic counselling.
3. *Education/Research*
    - Arranging educational programmer for interns, nurses, staff, etc.
    - Conduct research programmes
    - Organise seminar/workshop.

Similarly, description and job specification of all staff need to be written and advertised before appointing them in position.

Staffing Pattern

It is difficult to generalise on the size of staff required in hospital dietary department. Guiding factors will be individual circumstances and policies adopted by the particular hospital and type of services to be envisaged. One kitchen staff for every 20 is recommended.

a. *Administrative and Supervisory Staff*

1. Chief Dietician	
2. Dietician	Administrative
3. Dieticians	Therapeutic
4. Dietician	Technical
5. Steward and Food Supervisor	

b. *Other staff*
1. Head Cook
2. Head Bearer (Food Services Supervisor)
3. Store Clerk
4. Cook
5. Baker
6. Cook helper (Masalchi).

	100 bed	*200 bed*	*300 bed*	*400 bed*	*500 bed*	*750 bed*
Head Dietician	—	—	—	1	1	1
Asstt.Dietitician	—	1	1	—	—	1
Tech.Dietitian	—	—	—	1	1	1
Clerk	—	1	1	—	1	2
Steward	1	—	—	1	1	1
Head cook/	—	—	1	1	2	2
Bearer	—	2	3	4	5	7
Cook	2	2	4	5	6	7
Baker	—	—	—	—	1	1
Cook helper	2	4	5	6	7	7
Reserve plus 10% leave	5	10	15	19	25	30

The working hours of staff needed for preparation of number of meals can be calculated by following formula:

$$H = MR + 12\tfrac{1}{2} \text{ of } \frac{MR}{100} \text{ or } \frac{BMR}{800}$$

H = Total hours of staff time required.

M = Average meals provided per week.

R = Hours of of staff time per 100 meals.

(This does not include 10% leave /sick reserve.)

Job Specification

It is desirable to describe the jobe of all employees of kitchen to make them responsible for specific jobs. To get desired results each operation needs to be studied and best method to do so developed.

Before employing practical interview or on the job, performance needs to be taken into consideration. The job to be performed by kitchen staff are:

- Orientation and training of new employees
- Supervision of work according to schedule (cooking, dishwashing, machine handling, housekeeping)
- Receipt and checking of stores
- Observing safety measures.

Implementation of Dietary Function

The work of the dietary department must be so organised and supervised that food service can be carried out on a fixed schedule. During meal hours the staff are under exacting pressure to meet this schedule and therefore should have a working condition which promotes efficiency. Good working relationship must be maintained also with service departments like house-keeping, engineering and laundry, etc.

Hospital diet must fulfill minimum two criteria; (i) to meet physiological needs and (ii) patients satisfaction. While planning for menu, individual food preference and local food habit should be kept in mind.

Scheduling of menu can provide variety in cooking, flavour, and taste.

Hospital Diets

Generally four types of standard hospital diets are supplied
1. Full/normal/regular diet.
2. Soft diet (light diet)
3. Liquid diet.
4. Therapeutic or modified diet.

Normal/regular diet comprises 80 percent of the total patient food in any hospital, as this group is allowed to eat without restriction. Generally, 1800 to 2500 calories of diet is supplied.

Soft diet is ordered by the physician for limited use in feeding patient unable to tolerate a regular hospital diet. The food used on the soft diet are moderately low in fibre and connective tissue. The soft diet should be an adequate one and may include tender, meat, vegetables low in fibres and some fruits. Liquid diet is served to post-operative patients or to those who are unable to eat solid for good nutrition and thus it is prescribed for a limited time. Therapeutic or modified diet is served on the order of attending physician, details being left to the dietitian.

Indenting and Supply of Diets

Nursing staff keep the dietary department advised as to the number of patients on each type of diet. This is done by the use of a diet order form, which is sent to the dieticiation and at a specified time each day. Since the requisitions stand for 24 hours the best time is usually late in the afternoon when the nursing personnel have an accurate idea of discharge/admission of patients.

Time schedules should be made from both patients and employees to obviate and delay as much as possible. While planning the hospital, it must be assured that one elevator is earmarked exclusively for food service.

Direction and Control

The main job of manager is to direct the activities and to enforce control on it so that work should progress as per plan and if there is any need to change it, it should be based on realistic approach. All managerial functions are inter-departmental. Any control function must be performed in conjunction with planning, organizing and directing. The common goal in supply of food in hospital is to provide quality food at minimum cost. Food cost can be controlled by wise planning, economic purchase method, control in wastage/pilferage. Excess ordering need to be checked by evaluating left over food. Thus, over production can be checked. As far as possible automatic equipment should be used to reduce man-power employed. Wages cost need to be kept low. Periodic check by chief dietician will help in cutting down excess order.

Evaluation of Diet Service

Any of the following procedure or combination can be used for evaluation.

- Audit of account by external agencies. Every organization should arrange audit of account by its own accounts department and then, a registered charted accountant should be required to conduct audit of accounts. This should be the regular feature.
- Constant monitoring and checking according to laid down procedure is vital for proper performance. Any of the following procedure of combination can be used for evaluation:
- Quantitative method
- Sample Survey
- Consumer satisfaction.

Quantitative method For every process, data needs to be maintained, so that periodic check can be exercised and comparison can be made. If it can be properly arranged,performance can be checked by other institutions which will bring cost control and efficiency can be maintained for effective control.

Sample survey Samples can be taken at various points for check on quality control, it is desirable to collect sample from (a) assembling line (b) ward, and (c) left over food. If check can be made, it will clearly show at what stage food deteriorates.

Consumer satisfaction Patient satisfaction is very good index of performance. It is better to distribute questionnaires and collect information through it for assessment of quality of food served.

Equipping Hospital Kitchens

In modern hospitals, the preparation and distribution of meals is very important and because there are many different specializations required, and integrated system is best suited to deal with the problems involved. A correct diet forms an integral part on any therapy and is now considered fundamental to catering planning in hospitals.

On this basis, planning must take into account. The organization of catering services to include food purchasing, its preparation and cooking, the serving of the meal onto trays or in suitable

Table 35.19: Area chedule for hospital of different bed strength

Description	No. of beds	
	750	250
Staff Accommodation		
• Dietitians room with laboratory	180	120
• Steward room with storage space	180	120
• Work man rest and change room	320	180
• Bath and WC	180	120
Total	**860**	**540**
Stores		
• Provision	320	160
• Vegetable store	60	40
• Meat Store	60	40
• Milk Store	60	40
• Day store	60	40
• Equipment store	160	120
• Fuel store	180	150
• Supplies Store	120	120
• Janitor's store	60	60
Total	**1060**	**770**
Kitchen		
• General Kitchen	500	320
• Diet Kitchen	180	120
• Pantry	120	100
• Washing	150	150
• Trolley bay	100	80
Total	**1050**	**780**
Grand Total	**2970**	**2090**
• Circulation 1/3		
Total Floor Area	**4000**	**2700**

containers, their distribution among the patients and the collection and washing of crockery and cutlery.

To implement a catering service in a hospital there are four main alternatives:

- A traditional hotline whereby meals are taken on personalized trays (DP system)
- A refrigerated lines whereby meals are made up in the kitchen on personalized trays (DP system)
- A refrigerated line whereby meals are made up on personalized trays in the kitchen then reheated and served on the wards (DPR system).
- A frozen line whereby meals are made up in a centralized operation then defrosted, reheated and served on the wards.

The traditional hot line is used only in 400 to 500-bed units. The others are planned following certain basic criteria:

- The hospital catering service must be self-sufficient and independent.
- Preparation, cooking and distribution must be carried out independently co-ordinated by efficient planning.
- The operations mentioned above must be as fully automated as possible.
- Transport and distribution times must be kept to a minimum.

Particular attention must be paid to hygiene and cleanliness, both in the planning and proeration stages, and the actual carrying out of the catering programme.

Figure 35.59 illustrate a typical structure, planned and carried out on the basis of the above-

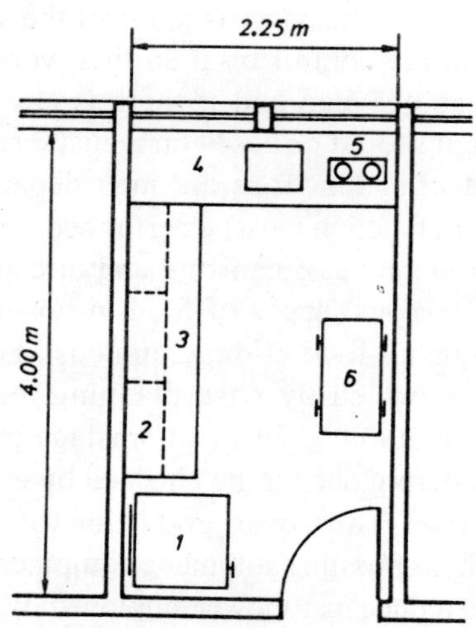

1. refrigerator	2. storage cabinets
3. work counter	4. counter with sink
5. portable stove	6. cart

Fig. 35.59: Room data sheet for floor pantry of centralized food system

mentioned points, At the heart of the system is a computer which uses specific softward packages in order to co-ordinate all the main operatations. The computer works on two fronts: it collects and analyses individual orders for each patient and at the sametime uses the model menus in its memory to programme the necessary operations of preparation, cooking and making up. The computer also automatically controls stocks, food purchase orders and all accounting and administrative operations is general.

The kitchen must be placed as centrally as possible in relation to the wards and at the same time be easily accessible for deliveries of foodstuffs. The avoidance of typical disturbance factors for the patients in the wards must also be a prime consideration. A second important factor to be considered is that of a rational division of the space available. Not only is it important to study a functional lay-out which requires minimum labour and personnel, but also to pay attention to hygienc and statutory standards, correct positioning and building specifications for certain critical areas with regard to hygiene are essential in order to avoid creating second source of contaimination (Fig. 35.60).

At this point, kitchen planning and the catering service programme must develop along the lines of the selected system. On of the most up-to-date systems with potential for future development is the refrigerated line (DPR system). It is useful to consider some of them more closely. Whichever organizing system is adopted, a precise goal to achieve, if the service is to be effectively managed, is that of keeping to minimum overall standing time between making up meals, transporting and distributing them, the total time which these operations require should be one of the parameters which most influence the standard of service. One reason why the refrigerated line is particularly attractive is that it gives the full saturation of the equipment in the kitichen. In fact, the cooking programme for the refrigerated line (DPR) takes a working day for the preparation of various meals, and makes it possible to utilize the same machine more full than the hotline.

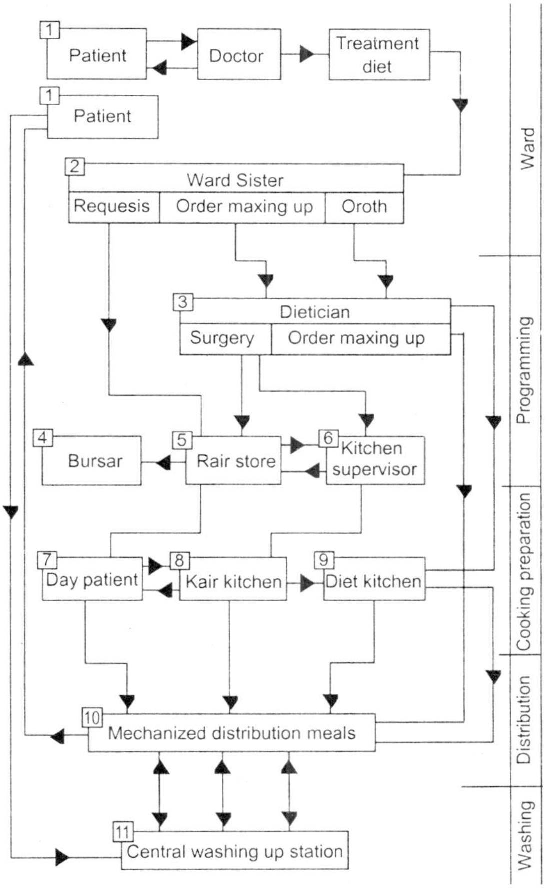

Fig. 35.60: The connections between hospital catering services

It is obvious that with this system the cooking programme must be closely linked to the time necessary for the special chilling equipment to lower the food temperature.

Choice of Equipment

One of the most important points in hospital kitchen planning is the choice of the equipment. This choice has a direct influence on the quality of the meal as well as its cost and management.

In the, recent past there has been a change for traditional equipment, pans and large-size monoblock kitchen units, to more sophisticated and flexible appliances having a much more specialized function.

For instance on the market today, there are food preparation machines such as vegetable washer tanks with production per cycle from 5 to 35 kg. each cycle taking only two to three minutes.

For larger scale users, there are continuous belt vegetable washers from 150 to 800 kg/h. There are also specialized machines for mincing, dicing, slicing and so on.

For boiling in water or for steam cooking there is now à wide choice of continuous or batch cooking machines, with various functions and sizes, and these machines have time and temperature controls that allow for automatic operation.

In particular, this steam cooking equipment ensures improved nutritional quality of the food, as mineral salt and vitamin loss is reduced to a minimum and the colour and appearance of the food is maintained. In addition to these advantages, steam oven, which are being used more and more frequently in hospital kitchens, notably reduce cooking and reconditioning times as well as saving energy. Convection ovens and mixed type ovens for both steaming and convection cooling have also become very popular and are widely used for both cooking and reconditioning. The most complete and rational system of distribution is the DP systems. This system overcomes the typical drawbacks of traditional methods and is based principally on the overall coordination of all the operations involved in providing meals for patients.

To this end, all the various stages of planning, production, inspection and distribution are centralized. This gives a new functional layout (Fig. 35.56) which allows suitable meals to be served to the patients in the right conditions, at the right moment and at minimum cost.

In brief, the result of this process is a personalized tray which is made up on a special line. The line is essentially a conveyor belt flanked by specially designed trolleys. These trolleys each have a specific purpose, from containing and maintaining the Bastronorm containers at the ideal temperature, to the transport of the trays and the crockery. The

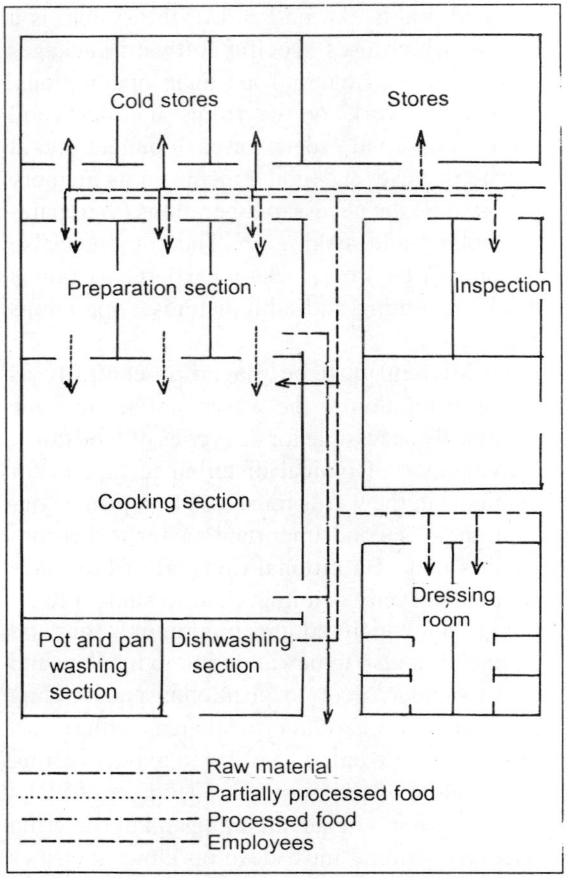

Fig. 35.61: Schematic diagram of the hospital kitchen

system is complete with are all made to Gastronorm dimensions.

For dishwashing, there is a wide range of machines on the market, roughly divided as follows:

- Fixed basket machines for 320 to 960 platesh/h (particularly suitable for ward kitchenetts),
- Moving basket machines for 1800 to 4000 plates/hr.
- Conveyor belt machines for 2650-900 plates/hr.

The machines described in (b) and (c) are used when all the dishwashing is done in the central kitchen.

Below, in order to co-relate effectiveness to cost, is a summary of the organizing and administrative advantages to be gained by the use of the methods

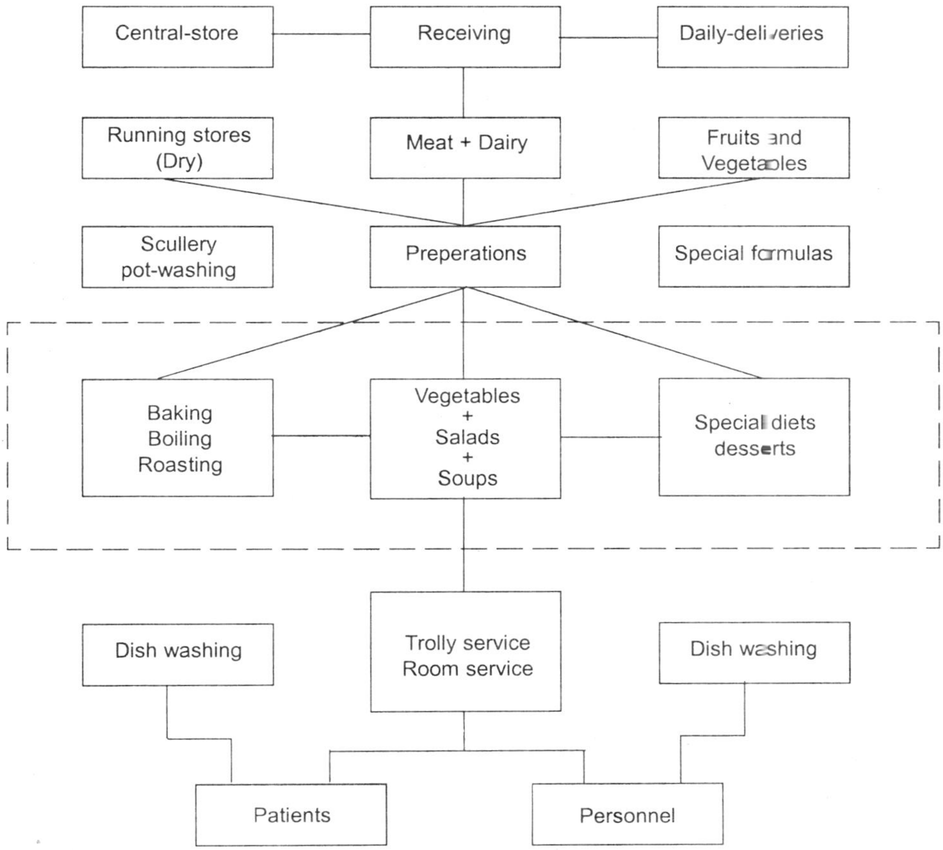

Flow chart 35.2: Dietary department

described, immediately reflected in the overall cost of catering services:

- Large savings on basic ingredients and the advantage of savings due to computerized programming of purchases and control of stocks.
- Simplified, centralised operrations for dividing the food into portions and making up meals, resulting in obvious savings and allowing staff to be fully occupied.
- Reduction in costs due to rationalised handling and transport systems for the food at all the various stages of its transformation.

Purchasing equipment has to be based on scientific methods. There is a need for a professional approach to integrated system

FURTHER READING

1. Amin Tabish: Costing of Dietary Services as part of an operational management-budgeting system.Jr. *Health and Population: Perspective and Issues* **16(1and2)**: 31-36.
2. Clean catering-Deptt: of Health and Social Security, Ministry of Health, Northern Ireland-1985, London, Her Majesty's Stationary Office.
3. Food service manual, American Hospital Association, Chicago-10, Illinois, USA, 1954.
4. Rose JC: Handbook of Health care Food Services Management. Aspen Publications Inc. Rockville, USA, 1984.
5. Rawland and Rawland Hospital Management and Guide to Department. Aspen Publication Inc.Rockville, Maryland, USA, 1984.

THE HOSPITAL PHARMACY

The pharmacy be located in an area which is convenient for providing service to the many departments and personnel who make daily use of such service. Therefore, this is primary consideration. It is irrelevant where the pharmacy is located in the hospital so long as it meets the test of convenience.

In hospitals of less than 200 beds the pharmacy should be located on the first floor, in the center of the activities it is called upon to service frequently, easily accessible to the elevator, and near or adjoining the out-patient department. This will provide the most efficient service and conserve main-hours of work.

Though it is recommended that the pharmacy be all located on one floor, it may be varied in larger hospitals when first floor space is at a premium. Basement is not desirable for pharmacy.

Pharmacy facilities should preferably be located either in or immediately adjacent to the out-patient department. It is not suitable for a cashier, nurse or other hospital personnel to accept the prescription from the patient and send it by pneumatic tube or by other means to the pharmacy located in some other section of the hospital and return the medication to this person for delivery to the patient. Although main-hours be conserved by combining in-patient dispensing unit. This advantage should not take precedence over locating the out-patient pharmacy facility in the immediate area serving out-patients. If a low volume of work does not justify such a location, then it would seem best either to not offer out-patient pharmacy service or to have the patient carry his prescription to the in-patient pharmacy.

In general, the in-patient pharmacy appears to be reasonably well situated to render the services required of it. Where possible, all sections of the in-patient pharmacy–storage, dispensing, manufacturing, parenteral solutions, etc. should be contiguous. When these functions are separated from the main pharmacy, it is recommended that they be in a direct vertical relationship of being able to respond to the clinical needs of the patient on a current basis. In addition, such a system makes available to the patient, physician, and nurse the services of a pharmacist in a clinical capacity rather than as just a dispenser of medications. By being on the nursing floor, the pharmacist is available for the taking of patient drug histories, maintaining patient drug policies, observing the patient for drug reactions and toxicity and dispensing unit-doses and intravenous products with additives.

Floor Space

The following floor space and its distribution is recommended.

Area distribution for general hospital pharmacies

Areas in Square feet		*Beds*	
• Compounding and Dispensing	50	100	200
• Laboratory	205	320	495
Parenteral Solutions Laboratory		185	200
• Active Store room		125	200
• Manufacturing Laboratory			120
• Office and Library			105
• Circulation			60
Total	**205**	**630**	**1180**

The areas shown in the above chart are net areas and do not include walls and partitions. Additional storage space of approximately 170 square feet per 100 beds is provided for bulk storage in an area directly beneath the pharmacy and separate from the main hospital store room.

Translating the above figures into a square foot per bed ratio, the following is noted:

Areas distribution square feet per bed

	Beds		
• Areas in Square feet	50	100	200
Compounding and Dispensing Laboratory	4.1	3.20	2.40
• Parenteral solutions Laboratory		1.85	1.00
• Active Store Room		1.25	1.00
• Office and Library			0.53
• Circulation			0.30
Total	**4.1**	**6.30**	**5.91**

The number of additional square feet of space to give the type of service the pharmacy should provide is given below:

Beds	*Space*
100	8.12 sq.ft/bed
200	6.62 sq.ft./bed
300	5.39 sq.ft/bed
400	5.00 sq.ft/bed

It is important to recognize the fact that pharmaceutical services in the hospital have expended considerably therapy suggesting that, until more up-to-date information is developed, the recommendations for floor space in hospital pharmacies should be considered minimal for the construction of today's hospital pharmacy.

Furthermore, it is important to note that today's practice of pharmacy provides its practitioners the opportunity to perform variable functions ranging from standard type dispensing methods to unit dose dispensing methodologies. Involvement with intravenous additive programmes, drug information centers and clinical pharmacy endeavours simply means that pharmacy floor space requirements must be determined by factors other than bed capacity and ambulatory clinic patient load. Also, no two hospitals should be compared for the purpose of determining the square footage requirements of the other.

Equipment Planning

The pharmacist, administrators, purchasing agent and architect, as a group, assume the responsibility for the planning and the subsequent purchase of the major equipment items to be located in the pharmacy. The less expensive items commonly used in the daily practice of the profession, are usually purchased by the purchasing agent after he has consulted with the pharmacist.

In selecting the equipment, all parties must exercise extreme care in choosing those items which will provide good service, with minimal maintenance, at a price within the hospitals equipment budget.

The cost of equipment should not be estimated nor should a percentage of the building construction cost be used. Whenever such short cuts are taken, experience has demonstrated that insufficient funds are available for the purchase of the desired equipment. Clearly then, once the equipment list is prepared, it behaves the pharmacist to consult freely with the purchasing agent, manufacturers representatives and vendors as well as to peruse through the latest editions of the catalogues.

Equipment is segregated into two groups: fixed and movable.

Fixed Equipment

Fixed equipment is defined as that which requires installation and becomes attached to the building. The single connection of electric power lines into the building's electric system or temporary attachment to a utility system does not qualify the item as fixed equipment. Fixed equipment is usually included in construction contracts and must be purchased and installed in accord with the requirements of the contract. Examples of fixed equipment are cabinets, counters, sinks, dumbwaiters and elevators.

Movable Equipment

Movable equipment is defined as that equipment which is capable of being moved and is not intended to permanently affixed to the building. This group includes large items of furniture and equipment having a reasonable fixed position in the building

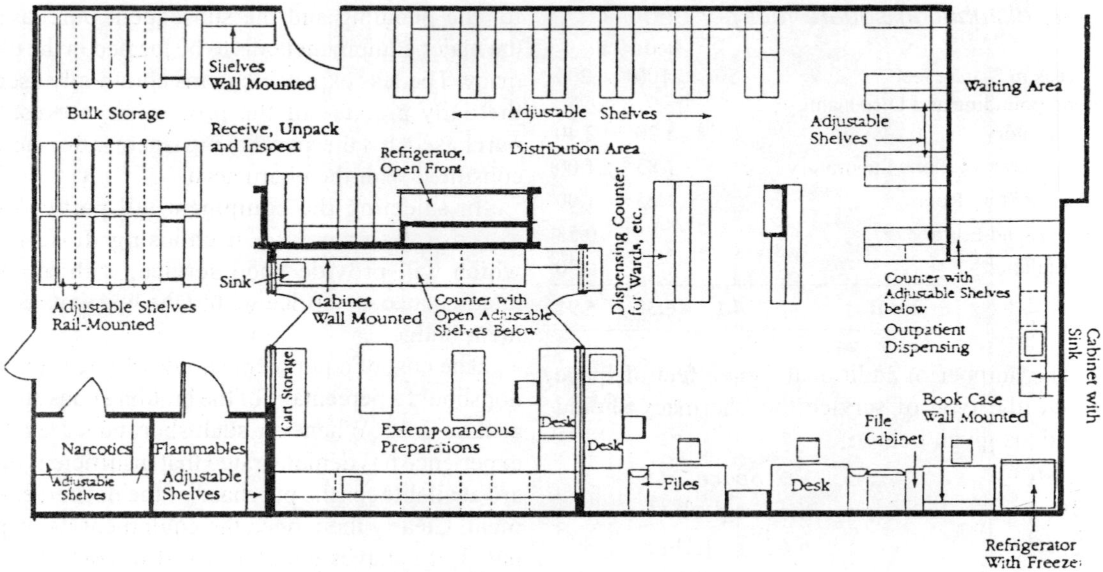

Fig. 35.62: Layout of a pharmacy

but which can be moved. Examples of movable equipment are carts, desks balances, mixers, etc.

Suggested Equipment List

Because the scope of service rendered by each hospital pharmacy will very from one section of the country to the other or for that matter, from hospital to hospital. It is an impossible task to attempt to prepare a standard list of equipment which will meet every need.

Drugs distribution	*Suggested quantity number of beds*		
• Order Review	100	200	300
Fiexed			
• Bookshelves, adjustable			1
• Pneumatic tube station	1	1	4
• Utility pole, phone, electric.			
Movable			
• Cabinet filing	2	2	2
• Letter size 3 drawer	2	2	4
• Card size two-level, revolving	1	1	2
• Visible index type	1	1	2
• Cart, for photocopier, storage	1	1	
• Chair, swivel with arms desk	2	5	2
• Office, double predestal	2	3	6
• Editing special.		2	4
• File, swinging panel,strip	2	2	3
• Photocopier		1	1
• Table, writing 2'×2'	2		
• Time date stamp. electric	1	1	2
• Typewriter electric	2	3	6
• Waste receptacle	2	2	4
Inpatient Dispensing			
• Fixed cabinets, wall-mounted counter, prescription, cabinets bins and drawers below	1	3	6
Dumbwaiter			
• Pneumatic tube station	1	1	1
• Shelving adjustable 12" starting 18"above	0	1	1
• Counter	1	2	3
• Ledge, fixed	0	1	1
Movable			
• Cabinet, filling 5-drawer,	1	1	0
• Cart, delivery,	0	1	2
• Refrigerator	0	1	2
• Biological type, with freezer	1	0	2
• Pass-through, caffeteria type for IV solutions	0	1	1
• Open front. refrigerated case type	0	1	1
• Typewriters. Electric, nonmovable			
• Carriage	1	2	4
Stool,Operators adjustable	1	2	4
Receiving and Storage			

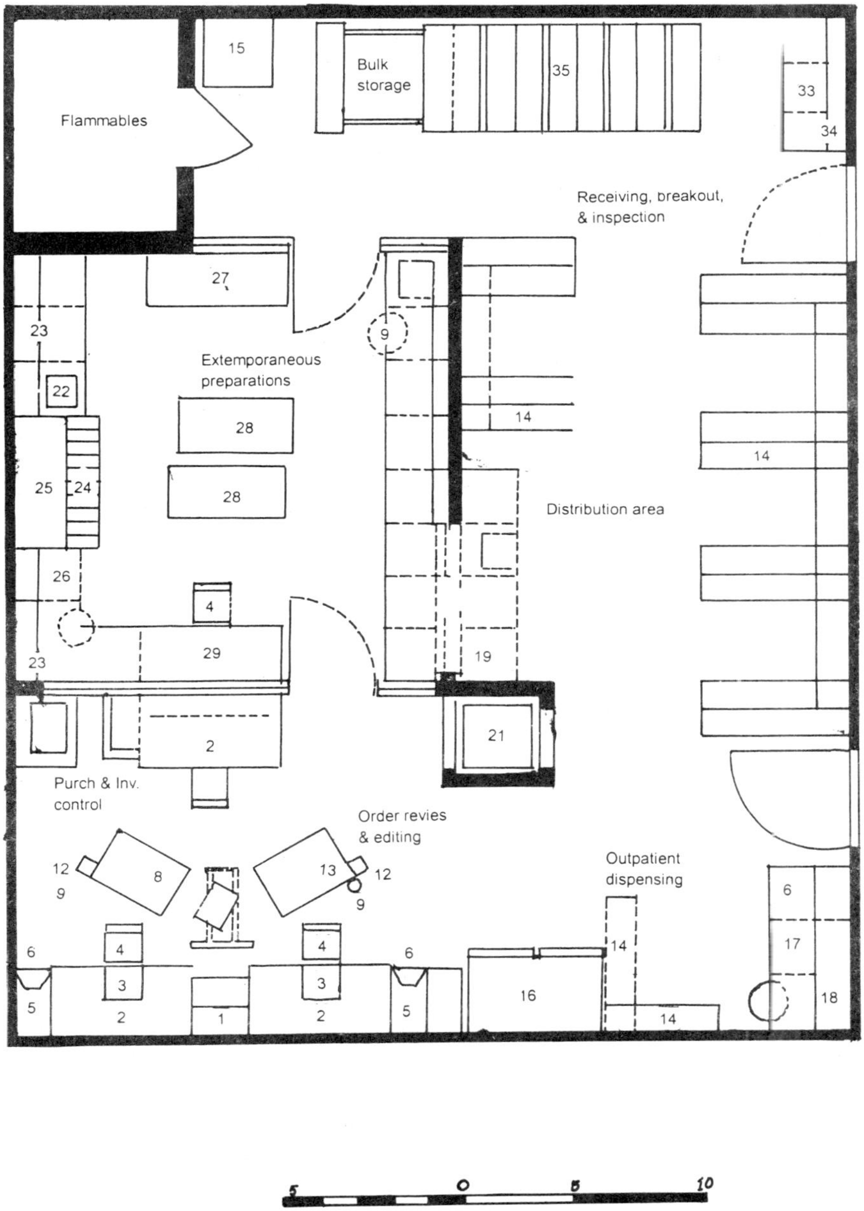

Fig. 35.63: Pharmacy department in a 100-bed hospital. This plan is to be considered as one example of a modern pharmacy design. (From Planning for Hospital Pharmacy, US Dept. HEW Health Services and Mental Health Administration. Health Care Facilities Services, Washington, DC)

Fixed			
• Counter, with adjustable shelving beneath	1	1	1
• Shelving, adjustable wall-mounted 9" Rail-mounted in narcotic vault back 24", room 12"		1	1
• Vent, inlet and outlet, in flammables room	1	1	1
Movable			
• Cradle, drum, Waste receptacle	1	1	1
Purchasing and inventory control			
Fixed			
Bookshelves wall-mounted above desk	1	1	
Movable			
• Cabinet, filing, visible		1	1
• Index type	1		
• One section		1	
• Three section		1	
• Letter size, 5-drawer	1	1	
• Chair, swivel, with arms		1	
• Desk, office, double pedstali		1	
• File, swinging, strip insert		1	
• Waste receptacle		1	
Extemporaneous Preparations			
Fixed			
• Cabinet, wall-mounted. counter with sink, drainboard,	2	2	2
• Adjustable shelves beneath			
• Counter, with open adjustable shelving beneath	1	2	5
• Shelving fixed ledge	0	1	1
Movable			
• Bins, autoclavable	10	10	20
• Cart, flask transport	1	1	2
• Cart, utility flat tope Locking wheels	2	2	2
• Chair, Swivel	1	1	1
• Desk, office, single	1	1	1
• Pedestal, file drawer	1	1	1
• Hood, laminar airlow,	1	1	2
• Waste receptlac	2	2	4
Receiving and Storage			
Fixed			
• Counter, with adjustable shelving beneath	1	1	1
• Shelving, adjustable, wall-mounted, g" Rail-mounted in narcotic	1	1	1
vault. Back 24"-sides 12", inflam-		1	1
mable room 12".		1	1

• Vent, inlet and outlet, inflammable room	1	1	1
Movable			
• Cradle, drum,	1	1	1
waste receptacle	1	1	1
Purchasing and Inventory Control			
Fixed			
• Bookshelve wall-mounted above desk	1	1	
Movable			
Cabinet, filling, vesible index type			
• One section		1	
• Three section			
• Letter size, 5-drawer	1	1	
• Chair, swivel, with arms		1	
• Desk, office, double pedstall	1	1	
• File, swinging, strip insert		1	
• Waste receptacle		1	
Extemporaneous Preparations			
Fixed			
• Cabinet, wall-mounted Counter with sink, drain board adjustable shelves beneath.			
• Counter, with open adjustable shelves beneath	2	2	2
• Counter, with open adjustablel shelving beneath	2	5	
• Shelving fixed ledge	0	1	1
Movable			
• Bins, autoclavable Cart, flask transport	10	10	20
• Cart, flask transport	1	1	2
Cart, utility, flat top, locking wheels	2	2	2
• Chair, swivel	1	1	1
• Desk, office, single	1	1	1
• Pedestal, file drawer	1	1	1
• Hood, laminar airlow	1	1	1
• Waste receptacle	2	2	4
Outpatient Dispensing			
Fixed			
• Cabinet, wall-mounted		1	
• Counter, with sink, drain board, file drawer		1	
• Counter, with file drawer bins, and shelf beneath.	1	1	
• Door, flexible, pulldown type for outpatient dispensing counter window		1	
• Panels acoustical			

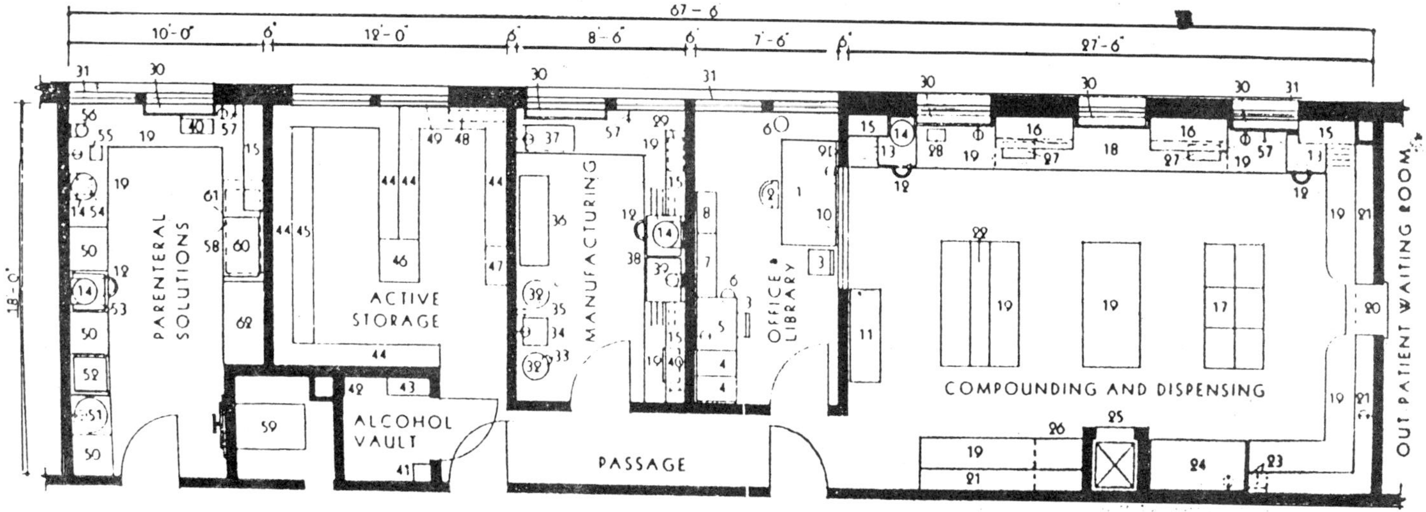

1. Desk excutive
2. Chair executive
3. Chair staight
4. File and drawer
5. Table, writing
6. Receptacle, waste paper
7. Case, book
8. Rack, carboy
9. Outlet, telephone
10. Glass panel
11. Rack, carboy
12. Can, sanitary waste
13. Sink, with goose neck spout and drainboard, graduate rack above, cabinets below
14. Tank, glass, distilled water, 12 gallon
15. Cabinets, adjustable shelves
16. Cabinet, drug, sectional type, with shelf above counter
17. Cabinets, drug, sectional type
18. Counter, prescription and drawers below
19. Counter, cabinets and .... below
20. Window, dispensing
21. Shelves, adjustable, open starting 18 inches above counter
22. Shelf, above counter
23. File, prescription
24. Refrigerator, with biological drawers 32 cubic feet
25. Dumbwaiter
26. Safe, narcotic, under counter
27. Scale, prescription class A
28. Scale, prescription, heavy duty
29. Scale, counter
30. Heat outlet grill, inlet grill in base of cabinet
31. Cuards, at all windows
32. Tank, mixing or storing, 20 gallons, mounted on stand with casters
33. ....
34. Filter ....
35. Outlets hot and cold water
36. Rack, filter
37. Mill, colloidal
38. Sink, two compartment, with dramboard, goose neck spout, cabinets below
39. Still, 2 gallon per hour
40. Hot plate, double element
41. Vent, outlet, 8 inches above floor to atmosphere
42. Vent. inlet, near floor to atmosphere
43. Shelves, starting 42 inches above, floor
44. Shelves, 12 inches wide, adjustable, open
45. Shelves, 24 inches wide, 36 inches high adjustable
46. ____________________
47. ____________________
48. ____________________
49. High windows
50. Rack, bottle
51. Cleaner, bottle pressure
52. Sink with goose neck spout
53. Sink, with distiled water .... omit hot and colt warer supply
54. Drip pan with waste connection in counter top
55. Pump, suction and pressure
56. Still 10 gallon per hour
57. Outlet gas
58. Carriage, sterilizer, under cunter
59. Sterilizer 21 × 36 × 48 inches
60. Oven, hot air, 21 × 14 × 14 inches
61. Counter open below
62. Cabinet, storage; open adjustable shelves

Fig. 35.64: The above plan for a pharmacy for a 200-bed general hospital with slight modification is adaptable to modern day dispensing practices

- Shelving, adjustable, wall-mounted 12"
- Movable Cabinet filling, rotary mechanical 1
- Chairs, guest, for waiting area file, swinging panel, strip insert 1 1
- Refrigrator, biological,with freezer waste receptacle 1

Outpatient Pharmacy (separate)

Fixed

- Cabinet, with drawers and adjustable shelving beneath counter, with drawer and knee space
- Panel, acoustical 1
- Pneumatic tube stations
- Shelving, adjustable wall mounted 12" table
- Cabinet steel double locks plus alarm buzzer
- Cabinet filling letter size drawer 5
- Cabinet filing rotary, mechanical
- File swinging panel strip insert
- Refrigerator, biological with adjustable
- Typewriter, electric 2

Waste receptacle 3

Extemporaneous Preparationing (Outpatient)

Bed

- Cabinet, wall-mounted
- Counter, with drawers and open adjustable shelving
- Sink unit, with drainboard.

Pharmacy Substation

Order Review

Fixed

- Counter, desk height, with drawers and adjustable shelves beneath. shelving, wall-mounted 12"

Movable

- Chair, swivel, with arms
- Waste receptacle

Distribution

Fixed

- Counter, with open adjustable shelving
- Counter, hinged
- Shelving, adjustable, wall-mounted 12"
- Sink unit, with drainboard

Movable

- Cart, with cassette storage- 1
- Hood, laminor airflow, vertical or horizontal 1
- Refrigerator, with freezer beneath counter 1
- Waste receptacle 1

Manufacturing and Packaging

Cleanup Room

Fixed

- Counter, stainless steel, with adjustable shelves and doors beneath double sink 1
- Shelving adjustable 12" wash area 6" high curb with 1" Sill. 1
- Window pass-through into infections filling room 1

Movable

- Cart, utility; stainless steel 23" × 46" with locking Wheels for solution flasks 1
- Table, utility, stainless steel 23" × 46" with locking wheels
- Washer, automatic, laboratory pass-through on rails into injections filling room, to accommodate 25 I flasks per batch, plus two headers for I flasks and one for small glass ware, tubes, and pipetters 1

Injections Filling Room and Still Room

Fixed

- Autoclave, steam, fast
- Exhaust, pass-through into central service autoclave area size suited to solution workload 1
- Counter, stainless with open adjustable shelving beath.
- Still. Capacity 25 gallon per hour (mounted in still room).
- Storage tank 150 gallon capacity, ceiling suspected 1

Movable

- Carriage, autoclave
- Cart, autoclave
- Cart, solution flask drain type 2
- Conductivity meter, recording
- Filling machine, automatic dual nozzle type 2
- foot operated for amps and vials 1
- Hood lamininar airflow, stool, operators 1
- Table, utility, stainless, stainless

- Table, utility, stainless, stainless steel. 35" × 70' with locking whels
- Tank, premix 50 gall capicity with pump agitator unit and hand-operated filler 1
- Mechanism type. Filter membrance 1

Sterile Preparation

Fixed

- Counter, with storage cabinets
- Kettle, steam, jacketed 5-gall capcity
- Shelving wall-mounted 12"
- Sink unit, laboratory type corner 1
- Window pass-through, to Injections
- Filling room and Aseptic filling room 2

Movable

- Balance, prescription, type A 1
- Balance, single beam capacity 4.5 kg
- Chair, Swivel
- Cabinet, filing, letter size 5 drawer 1
- Cart, utility, laboratory type with railed top 1
- Desk, office, single pedestal 1
- Filter, membrance type
- Hot plate, electricit, double element, heavy duty, variable heart

Lockers

- pH meter 1
- Pump, suction and pressure
- Stirrer, small volume counter tope 1
- Waste receptacle 2

Sterile area Storage

- Fixed counter, 1' × 2' for writing 1

Movable

- Stool, 2 steps 1

Aseptic Filling

Fixed

- Counter, stainless stell, open beneath, 3
- Shelving, wall-mounted 12" 3
- Window pass through to labeling and Inspection room 1

Movable

- Hood,laminar airflow, horizontal or vertical.
- Pipetting machine automatic, 2
- Stool, operators adjustable
- Syring, e.g. Corwall type with 4
- Swinnery adopter

Labelling and Inspection

Fixed 1

- Cabinet, floor 1
- Counter drawer units 1
- Counter top units 3
- Cupboard drawer units 1
  - Corner unit 3
  - Desk height 1
  - Small drawer 1
  - Sink unit, corner 1
  - Sink unit, corner 1
  - Shelving, well-mounted 12" 1

Movable

- Labelling machine automatic, with foot operated 1
- Clutch. Plain worktable and offset pad, plus attachments for pressure sensitive labels
- Labeling machine hand operated
- Light-dark inspection box 1
- Stool, operators adjustable 1
  Plate imprinting machine capacity, making imprinting plates for use with labelling machines 1 1
- Typewriter, manual ½ line 16 characters per inch 1

Prepackaging

- Cabinet, e.g. schwartz tpe 3
- Counter, wall-drawer , ope 1

Movable 1

- Filing machine automatic duct type capacity 0.25 to 100ml with sack back device foot operated. 1
- Heat sealer electric stickrstant 2
- Covered shoe packager 1
- Table utility, stainless steel, plat surface 25" × 70" with locking wheels 1

Nonsterile Mixing and Filling

Fixed

- Cabinet, e.g. Schwarz type 3
- Counter, with drawers and storage
- Cabinets beneath jacketed, 20 gall
- Rack, filter: heavy duty, installed flush with counter 2 1
- Shelving, adjustable 18" 1
- Shelving, adjustable wall mounted 2
- Sink unit, laboratory type

- Wash area
- Balance single beam capacity 4.5 kg 1
- Balance prescription
- Blender, electric 1
- Chair, swivel. 1
- Desk, office single pedestal, with file drawer
- Filter press suction pressure type 10 gallon 1
  per minimum capacity on casters 1
- Homogenizer
- Mixer large, taken-mounted
- Mixer-blender for semisolids 1
- Ointment mill, three roller 1
- Rheostat, variable for 110 volt line 1
- Tank, mixing and storage 50 gallon 2
  capacity, with spigot, filter attachement
  on wheels 1
- Filter attachment on wheels 1
- Timer electric
- Washer, laboratory type, automatics, for small glassware and control laboratory items, distilled water rinse
- Waste receptacle, large 1

Administration

Movable 1

- Bookcase, 1
- Chairs Swivel arms
- Credenza Desk, double pedestal
- Dictating machine, recorder 1

Secretary/Receptionist

- Cabinet, filing 5 drawer 1 4
- Cabinet, storage 1 1
- Chair, guest 3 3
- Chair swivel, typists 1 2
- Desk single pedestal secretarial 1
- Dictating machine transcriber 1
- Table corner 1 2
- Typewriter, electric 1 2
- Waste receptacle
- Conference Room

Fixed

- Blackboard wall-mounted 1

Movable

- Cabinet, storage
- Chair conference folding 8
- Projection screen 1
  - Table, conference 2
  - Table corner 1
- Waste receptacle 1

Assistant for Business Affairs

Movable

- Welding machine, electric printing 1
- Bookcase
- Chair,Guest
- Chair, swivel, arms 2
- Table, desk type 1
- Waste receptacle 1

Control

Control Laboratory

Fixed 300-500 beds

- Cunter, with drawers and storage cabinet beneath
- Fume hood, with sink distilled water and electric gas outlets 1
- Shelving wall-mounted 12" 1
  sink unit, corner

Movable

- Balance, analytical, one-pan, substitution weighting reading to 0.1 mg unit 1
- Battery jar, cylindrical 1
- Burrets, micro,class A,3-way stopcock,
- Burner e.g. Fisher, high temperature 5
- Bwets automatic (Class 4) 2
- Burner e.g. Terrill,natural gas 2
- Cabinet, e.g. schwartz type 1
- Centrifuge, clinical 15-and 40 ml tubes 1
- Chromatography apparatus, thin layer type for 8" × 8" plates 1
- Chromotography cabinet, bench type 1
- Constant temperature unit e.g. Tecam
- Electrode, silver billet 1
- Freezer, upright, to include capacity for storing frozen unit-dose injectables 1
- Heating mantle hemispherical for 125-ml flask 1

Extraction apparatus 1

- Hotplate, electric thermostatic. 1
  pH meter, line operated, direct reading
- Incubator, gravity convection large size 1
- Melting point apparatus e.g. fisher-Johns or equivalent for determing melting point of paraffix wax 1
- Microscope, polarizing e.g. Uniton type 1
- Nitrogen distillation apparatus, micro. 1
- Power supply for hydrogen lamp. 1
- Refrigerator, home type 1
- Silica cells for spectrophotometer, set of two 1

- Spectrophotometer, for use in visible and ultraviolet ranges 1 1
- Stirring apparatus, magnetic, variable speed 1
- Stool, laboratory type with back 1
- Support stands, various sizes 1
- Table, for balances, adjusting level 1
- Table utility 1
- Transformer variable e.g. Powerstat type 1
- Waste receptacle.

Control office

Movable

- Bookcase 1
- Cabinet, filing, 5-drawer 4
- Chair, swivel, with arms 2
- Costumer 1
- Dictating machine, transcriber 1
- Waste receptacle 2
- Table, desk type 1

Drug Information

Drug information/ conference Area 100 beds

Fixed

- Bookshelves, wall-mounted 12" 1
- Blackboard, wall-mounted 1

Movable

- Cabinet, filing, side opening 5 drawer 4
- Calculator, electronic, statistical, 1 printing chair, library 4
- Shelving adjustable 12" 4
- Table,reading conference 1
- Table, desk type 1

300-500 beds

- Typewriter, electric, wide carriage ½ line advance, changeable type 1
- Waste receptacle 1

Reception 300-500 beds

- Chair, guest 2
- Chair, swivel 1
- Costumer 1
- Table corner 1
- Typewriter, electric, wide carriage 1 ½ line advance
- Waste receptacle 1

Drug Information officer 1

- Blackboard, wall-mounted. 1
- Bookshelves, wall-mounted 2
- Counter, desk-height, open beneath
- Cabinet, filing, under counter 2-drawer 1
- Calculator, electronic, statistical, printing 1
- Chair, library 2
- Chair, swivel, with arms 1
- Waste receptacle 1

Library

Movable

- Cabinet, filing, side oepning 5-drawer 4
- Chairs, library 3
- Microfilm reder 1
- Shelving, adjustable 12" 1
- Table, reading 1

Propcessing and Records

Fixed

- Counter, with storage cabinets, beneath1
- Pneumatic tube station 1

Movable

- Cabinet, filing, tab card, 8-drawer 2
- Chair, swivel, operator 1
- Collator, punchcard 1
- Keypunch, printing 1
- Photocopier, capable of copying from bund volumes 1 1
- Photographic equipment slidmaking 1
- Sorter, electronic, punchcards 1
- Waste receptacle 1

Teaching

Student Work Area

- Desk-height counter, built-in open 2
- Beneath, with book shelves above, one desk drawer below
- Bulletin board, wall-mounted 1
- Blackboard 1
- Cabinet, filling, 5 drawer 2
- Chair, swivel, with arms 2
  Lacker Lamp, desk type, fluorescent, 2-bulb 2
- Typewriter, electric wide carriage ½ line advance 1
- Waste receptacle 1

Instructor Work Area

- Bulletin board, wall-mounted 1
- Blackboard, wall-mounted 1
- Cabinet, filing 5-drawer 2
- Chair, swivel, with arms 1
- Chair, guest 2
- Costumer 1
- Desk,double predestal, office 1
- Dictating machine transcriber 1
- Table, desk type 1
- Waste receptacle 1

Electrical safety in the hospital pharmacy could be improved if consideration is given to the following guideline principles:

1. Keep electrical power cords as short as possible in order to eliminate electrical leakage.
2. Use equipment with proper ground lines (three-prong plugs).
3. Purchase equipment with power on-off switches which have clearly visible indication of power status (on or off).
4. Eliminate slow blow fusing whenever possible since this type of fusing increases the exposure time of the operator to the electrical hazards.
5. Before permitting personnel to operate new equipment, be sure that they are properly trained in its use. In addition, it is important that they read the instructional manual-particulary the section dealing with safe use and possible hazard.
6. Train operators to disconnect the power receptacle from the power source by pulling on the connector, not on the cable.
7. Avoid the use of extension cords.
8. Do not attempt to make repairs to the equipment
9. Cooperate with in-house maintenance programmes.

Cleanup Area

A pharmacy that is involved in a reasonable volume of extemporaneous compounding or manufacturing should have a cleanup room. A cleanup room designed for joint use by CSSD and pharmacy is the most efficient and economical. Appropriately located, pass-through windows and a curbed floor area with floor drain are the desirable features.

Nonsterile Mixing and Filling Room

The area for mixing and filling ointments should be separate from that for liquids, although both may be in the same room. Provision to hold be made for weighting and measuring, mixing and stirring (sometimes overheat, blending, homogenization, filtration and filling adequate storage space must be provided.

Prepackaging Area

The prepackaging room is for the packaging of oral solid dosage forms into container. In hospitals of 300 beds or less without a manufacturing programme and without unit dose dispensing, it may be possible to pre-package oral solids in the extemporaneous preparations area.

Injection Reconstitution Area

The area for the reconstitution of injection should be equipped with two or more class 100 laminar airflow hoods. Such units are available with horizontal, vertical, covering 90-degree and converging 180-degree flow patterns.

Labelling and Inspection Room

The labelling and inspection room should be adjacent to the filling areas so that the unlabelled drug products can be transferred directly through a pass-through window to eliminate the chance of their being used prematurely. Adequate storage space for levels, printing machine accessories, form etc, must be provided.

Quarantine Storage

Products manufactured and filled in the pharmacy are subject to quarantine until appropriate chemical and bacterial testing is complete. Finished products should be transferred directly to the quarantine storage area.

Refrigeration Facilities

Most hospital pharmacists and architects when developing plans for a new pharmacy are quite cognizant of the desirability and the need for air conditioning and large biological refrigerators in the hospital pharmacy: More often than not, little thought is given to the need of freezer and a cold room. The thermal storage requirements vary from "cold place" to "store in refrigerator" or avoid excessive heat or excessive temperature. The complete list of storage temperature terms and the definitions are as follows.

- *Cold Place* A cold place is one having a temperature, not exceeding 8° (45°F).
- *Refrigerator* A refrigerator is a cold place in which the temperature is held between 2° and 8° (36° and 46° F).
- *Cool place* A Cool is one having temperature between 8° and 15° (46° and 59°F).
- *Room temperature* Room temperature is between 15° and 30° (59° and 86°F).
- *Excessive heat* The expression "excessive heat" designates temperature above 40° (104°F).

Since many of the drugs, so described, are in common use in the hospital, the pharmacist should make every effort to see that proper storage facilities are made available. This is easily done in most hospitals by the purchase of a large biological refrigerator and a freezer. In the small hospital, these two units or, as is usually the case, the refrigerator with a built-in-freezer compartment, provide adequate facilities. The problem which usually arises in the larger hospital is that the refrigerator is too small to accommodate the inventory requiring reaching additional refrigerators.

Although both of these arrangements are workable, it would seem that a less expensive and a less inconvenient method of cold storage within the pharmacy could be had by the construction of a cold room.

A cold room is defined as an artificially cooled room with a regulated temperature range of 12° to 15°C (53.6° to 59°F).

Constructing a Cold Room

In existing facilities, a cold room may be inexpensively constructed if the parties involved will use a little imagination. A little-used corner of the basement storage area should be selected and the necessary area marked off. If windows are present they should be bricked-up or atleast double-panned and sealed against the outside atmosphere with caulking compound.

An electric light fixture and the required number of electrical outlets should be installed with the switch controlling the light fixture being on the outside wall nearest the entrance to the room.

The necessary additional walls of the room may be constructed of concrete, blocks or brick. Where the use of the above building materials is not feasible, a similar result may be had by the use of wood studs with aluminium foil insulation. The inner side of this type of wall should be cement plastered and the outer side "finished-off" by covering with masonite or other inexpensive material. The door should be fit tightly, be no larger than necessary, and be provided with a good automatic door closer.

An electric motor-driven air cooled freon compressor unit with a remote blower-type cooling coil will provide the necessary refrigeration. This unit should be installed with the necessary thermostat and expansion valve required to maintain the desired temperature range.

The blower is mounted in the cold room. To it, a small waste line is installed to drain away the condensate which collects on the refrigerator coil. The compressor may be installed outside of the cold room in order to conserve space within.

Obviously the size of the cold room to be constructed will determine the capacity of the refrigeration unit to be installed. In general, a room approximately 10' × 10' would require one tone of refrigeration to maintain a temperature range of 50° to 60° F

Once constructed, the room may be equipped with the necessary shelving, storage binds, cabinets, and work bench.

Built-in Equipment

One of the most important aspects of a pharmacy modernization of construction programme is that which involves the planning and selection of the built-in cabinets, counters and other types of casework. Due consideration must be given to such details as the height of the bench or cabinet, the size of the shelving or drawers, the types of handles on drawer and cabinet doors, whether or not the shelving is to be fixed or adjustable as well as the type of material which will be installed on counter top.

The materials used in the construction of built-in equipment must be reviewed by the hospital pharmacist in the light of the activity to which the equipment will be subjected. Thus, it is not sufficient to specify that the equipment will be constructed of stainless steel. One should specify whether it is expected to be constructed of mild, cold rolled, annealed furniture steel, the gauges of the metal to be used, the gauges of the inetal to be used in the shelving and whether or not the face of the shelf should be turned back up under the shelf and brought into contact with it in order to provide additional support; and details relative to the doors, adjustability of the shelving, etc.

Special attention should be given to the counter tops. All too often, excellent base cabinets, are provided but the counter tops do not offer resistance to corrosion and abrasion. Accordingly it is of importance for the pharmacist to enquire about the physical properties of the counter finishes, some guidelines are the following:

1. To what degree can it be bent without cracking or breaking down?
2. How much of an impact will it withstand without flaking or peeling ?
3. What effect will a high relative humidity have upon it ?
4. Is it sufficiently hard to resist erosion?
5. If the material is coloured. Is the color retention quality sufficient to resist appreciable discolouration?
6. Is the finish coat abrasion resistant ? Bear in mind that it must resist acids, alkalies oils and solvent.

Many of these units are available from the several manufacturers who specialize in the development and construction of such components.

Electric Lighting and Service

The availability of good electrical lighting and a sufficient number of grounded electrical outlets is mandatory for a smoothy functioning pharmacy.

Accordingly, sufficient lighting must be provided for the various work areas as well as the library and the offices. Although the present literature indicates that 30 feet candles are adequate for general illumination, and 50 feet candles for special areas such as the prescription dispensing area, it is recommended that in any new construction, the services of a lighting engineer be utilized. This is important because each hospital, or unit within the hospital, has particular needs based upon many factors some of which are characteristic of the operation, whereas others may be due to location and environment.

In selecting the type of lighting and light fixture, care should be given to the selection of a unit which will not become a house keeping problem. That is to say that, when possible, a fixture which can be mounted in the ceiling is highly desirable since it will not gather dust and dirt. Fluorescent light is recommended, however, a combination of fluorescent tube and standard bulb in the same fixture provides a better light.

Grounded electrical outlets should be provided in all areas in which the use of electric equipment may be indicated. In addition, thought must be given to the requirements of voltage in the range 220 volts for some of the ovens or mixers in the manufacturing area. If volatile solvents are used in the manufacturing areas or are stored in the pharmacy, consideration must be given to the installation of explosion proof fixtures and outlets.

Ventilation

Air conditioning of the pharmacy is desirable for a number of reasons. First, it obviates the need for the opening of windows and doors through which dirt, dust and other environmental contaminants may enter the pharmacy. Secondly, the use of the various autoclaves, ovens and steam jacketed kettless may render the working environment too hot. Maintenance of a temperature, which is compatible with the official storage requirements for drugs on a year round basis irrespective of the climatic conditions. Fourth, adequate ventilation is essential for the removal of the storage odours which are characteristic of the chemicals used in the manufacture of the various galenicals, preservative fluids and reagents. Fifth, because doors and windows can be kept closed, there can be a saving in the cost of housekeeping service in the pharmacy.

Conveyor and Pneumatic Tube System

Modern engineering technology has made available a means of transporting nearly every item from the pharmacy to its hospital destination. Accordingly, in order to conserve pharmaceutical manpower, thought should be given to the installation of dumbwaiters, pneumatic tube systems and other like devices for the movement of supplies from the pharmacy to their desired hospital destination. The type of combination of equipment necessary will vary with each hospital, therefore, it is recommended that the advice be sought from the hospitals architect and or the various manufacturers and distributors of such devices.

Finishes

Work Counters

Although many of the work counters will be constructed of stainless steel, others will not require such construction. For those units, formica or a similar material is suggested as an efficient and durable surface.

Floors

The floors of the pharmacy proper should be resilient, smooth but not slippery, stain resistant and yet complimentary to the existing or proposed decor of the department. Many flooring materials are currently available which are highly satisfactory and economical. Some of the floor coverings currently in use are asphalt tile, vinyl title, rubber tile and heavy duty linoleum.

In recent years, many architects and designers have introduced carpeting into the hospital pharmacy with aesthetic results. On the other hand, some of the installations have not been complementary to the operation of a hospital pharmacy. Carpeting has proven to be acceptable in the office, library, waiting room areas but has not been acceptable in the various work areas. Much of the complaint centers around the excessive generation of static electricity and the flammability of the carpet material.

Low relative humidity has always been the major problem in controlling static generation in carpets. The lower the relative humidity, the greater the problem. Thus it is important to ascertain the kilo volts of static electricity that a carpet will generate at the normal building temperature and with a relative humidity of 10 to 20 percent Clearly, the lower the kilovolts generated, the more acceptable the carpet will be for pharmacy installation. A high humidity will also produce low kilo volt readings of static electricity. Obviously, a high humidity does not lend itself to the pharmacy comfort.

Walls

The walls of the pharmacy should be painted with a material which permits periodic washing without the danger of losing its original colour. The selection of the appropriate color scheme is here left to the taste and discretion of the parties involved.

In the manufacturing and parenteral products rooms, painted wall surfaces do not usually withstand the constant washing necessary for the maintenance of the desired degree of espouses. Accordingly, it is suggested that a ceramic tile, or other comparable material, be utilized in these areas.

FURTHER READING

1. Barker, Kenneth N: Planning a Hospital Pharmacy Facility, *Am J Hosp Pharm* **28**: **6**: 423, 1971.
2. Brown Thomas R, Barker Kenneth N, Rowland F *et al:* A National Survey of Planning for Hospital Pharmacy facilities *Am J Hosp Pharm* **28**: 532, 1971.
3. Francke DE, Latiolais CJ, Francke GN, HO NFH: *Mirror to Hospital Pharmacists*, Washington DC.
4. Minimum Standard for Pharmacies in Hospitals with Guide to Application *Am J Hosp Pharm* **15**: **11**: 992, 1958.
5. Minilne AM, Taylor WR: Suggested plans for Hospital Pharmacies 50, 100 and 200-Bed General Hospital, *Bull Am Sec Hosp Pharm* **23**: 112, 1950.
6. Milne AM, Burgoon DF, Sim M, Donovan AC: Hospital Equipment and Planning Guide. Public Health Service publication No. 930-D-4 (Reevised 1964), US Government Printing Office, Washington DC.
7. Osterberger, David J: Layout and Design for Mechanized Centralized unit dose Dispensing *Am J Hosp Pharm* **28**: **6**: 447, 1971.
8. Planning for Hospital Pharmacies, Dept HEW publication No (HRA) 77-4003, August, Superintendent of Documents, US Government printing office, Washington DC 20402 p.i., 1997.
9. Swenson Earl S: An innovative Design in Hospital Pharmacy facilities. *Am J Hosp Pharm* **28**: **6**: 440, 1971.

PLANNING OF LAUNDRY SERVICES

Laundry services form an integral part of the hospital. The need of laundry services has been realized with the growth and development of the hospital itself. In India during 1968, Jain Committee on 'Study Group of Hospitals' suggested mechanization of laundry in teaching hospitals where one has to cope-up with huge quantity of linen. Such measures may also be preferred for smaller hospitals where the resources permit. However, hospitals with bed capacity of less than 200 may employ small washing machine.

In India, the contract Dhobi System is prevalent in most of the hospitals. Only few large hospitals in big cities have mechanized laundries. It has been observed that the hand washing system is uneconomical because of increased incidence of infection in operated cases. Thus, small mechanized laundry is the only sensible answer to combat the problem of hospital acquired infection.

Organization of Linen Services

With the establishment of mechanized laundries in hospitals, the laundry managers are delegated the responsibility for the delivery, repair and inventory of linen and they are responsible to the administrator of the hospital. Two different types of systems are adopted for the circulation of linen in the hospitals:

Centralized system which establishes a central supply of linen under the overall charge of laundry manager.

Decentralized system which makes assignment of linen responsibility to various areas and hold these areas responsible for the same.

Types of Linen Services Systems.

- Contract System
- On Premises Laundry Systems (OPLS)
- Co-operative System
- Linen Rental System

Contract System

In India, most of the hospitals own their linen. Majority of the hospitals get the linen washed by contract *dhobies* (washermen). The advantage of this system is the saving of the capital outlay for a modern laundry. The disadvantages of contract system are; the need for a higher linen inventory, higher costs compared to hospital's own laundry, no control over the washing techniques, the services are not dependable, excessive damages to linen due to use of raw chemicals.

On Premises Laundry Systems (OPLS)

Hospital owns its linen and the laundry. All the activities of the hospital laundry is done in the hospital premises. A hospital of more than 100 beds can run an OPLS efficiently and economically. The advantages are; safe handling of infective linen, better linen control, control over washing techniques and chemicals, control over quality of finished linen, control over the cost from direct internal controls in the laundry, and capability to render a higher level of patient care and comfort. An OPLS with modern equipment, disciplined and dedicated laundry workers can emerge on the top as compared to other systems.

Co-operative System

Centralized laundry tends to be more beneficial for smaller hospitals. Many small hospitals can share the services of the highly qualified laundry managers and utilize the modern automatic plant. The centralized laundry organization would include standardization of linen for all the hospitals served, and the establishment of a central purchase committee for linen. An efficient and effective system of pickup and delivery schedules is essential for the success of this system.

Rental System

- The linen supplier takes the entire responsibility and supplies clean linen to the hospitals and is also responsible for replacement, condemnation, and laundering the linen
- The trend today for organizing the linen service is in the following preferential order
- Hospital operated laundry having its own inventory of linen is considered the best.

Co-operative System

- Commercial laundry with hospital purchase linen.
- Linen supply with both purchase as well as laundering on rental basis.

Planning of Laundry Services

Hospital laundry has the following distinct advantages:

- Rapid and dependable service
- Longer life for the textile because the process of washing is controlled (resulting in long-term financial gains).

Minimum Capital Investment in Linen

The overall broad objective of the laundry is to maintain adequate supplies of clean and serviceable linen to the user departments at the minimum cost. This can only be achieved by close co-ordination of laundry operation at each stage and effective linen distribution system.

Whether the laundry is located in the main building of the hospital, in a separate room or with one or more of the hospital operation services, it should be located convenient to the user departments to save time for transportation of linen. The soiled and infected linen received, and clean linen distribution areas should always be physically separated with separate entrances.

The route of the soiled linen from the using points to the laundry and the flow of clean linen from laundry to the using units should be so planned as to minimize the possibility of contamination of clean linen. The arrangements of the equipment should be as per the work flow so that criss cross and backward movement is avoided to conserve the labour.

The laundry should be grouped into specific separate areas as:

- Soiled linen receiving
- Sorting and washer loading
- Clean linen processing
- Clean linen disbursing
- Offices, supply, storage, toilets.

The workload and workflow and dimension of each area should be a major consideration in good laundry planning.

The Indian Standards Institution has recommended the following areas against the bed compliment:

No. of beds	*Area in SFT*
25-50	315
51-100	441
101-300	2520
301-500	3245
501-750	4505

A final assessment of plant and machinery required for a particular laundry can be made only by a professional consultant.

Laundry manager's office should be located as centrally as possible to properly supervise the entire laundry operations. The walls should have large vision panels to allow full view for each area. Two-way communication system is considered between this office and each laundry area.

A toilet, locker and shower facilities should be provided in the soiled linen receiving, sorting and washer loading room and the clean linen processing room. Supply storage room should be adjacent and connected to the soiled linen receiving, sorting and washer loading room. Sufficient space should be provided for the storage of one week's supply of detergents, bleaches and others.

The floor for the laundry should have a smooth, slip resistant and water proof surface, the walls should have a smooth washable surface free from all corners, edges, or projections which normally create extra maintenance problems. Walls and ceiling should be high enough to allow for the installation and repair of all the equipment with a minimum height of 11 feet. Utility services like piping, electrical wiring, should be designed and sized with appropriate consideration for future expansion. The steam supply system should be so designed to deliver steam to the equipment in right quantity and at the desired temperature. Return piping system must ensure removal of condensation from the equipment. Approximately 3 gallons of hot water is required for one Kg of linen processed. It is possible to supply hot water by the pipeline to the laundry at the required temperature directly from the boiler room. Hot water should be available at 180°F.

The Power supply to the laundry is usually 440 volts, in three phase, four-wire alternative current system. The distribution channel must be easily accessible and it should be located near to the load counter and away from the direct path of escaping steam.

Power requirement for determining feeder sizes is:

- For operation of motorized equipment: 3 KW/hr/50 Kg of dry linen. For lighting: 3 W/Sq. ft. of floor space.
- Power supply should preferably be prompt three grid system.
- Good light is important for the laundry. Lighting should be free of glare and shadows. Daylight should be used whereever possible.

Fan blades, ducts, and lint collector should always be cleaned to reduce the fire hazards. Fire extinguishers should be located in the laundry near the clean linen and the processing areas and also near to the electrical components.

There is absolute need for flow of drains in the sorting and washing area. The drain should be equipped with proper sediment and lint trays.

Ventilation system must be able to provide a comfortable environment for the workers. This may require cooling of the area in summer and heating in winter. It must provide safety for personnel and contribute to the quantity of the finished product by the air-borne contamination. Separate mechanically operated supply and exhaust systems are required.

All the equipment should receive the manufactures recommended routine maintenance at the recommended intervals. A plant register should be maintained to give comprehensive detail of the equipment.

Layout and Work Flow

Various types of layouts are:

- Straight through flow (most common)
- To U-FLOW
- Gravity flow (very useful in sloping sites)
- Laundry is divided into two distinct areas: clean and dirty.

Dirty area comprises

- Reception of solid linen
- Sorting (classification) of soiled linen into suitable quantities for processing.

Clean area comprises

- Drying
- Finishing
- Discharge
- A barrier wall between the clean and dirty area is desirable

Dirty Areas

All the linen is delivered to the reception area. Foul and infected linen is treated with special care.

The double-ended washing machine (which themselves form the cross-infection barrier between the dirty and clean areas) have also been recommended. In case of conventional machines, the linen after washing is passed on to the clean side through the physical barrier.

Clean Area

Here, the drying tumblers, calendering machines and garment presses are located. Hydro-extractor removes about 50 percent of the moisture from the wet wash. Drying tumblers using hot air, dry or partially dry the damp linen. Calenders are used for ironing flat articles such as sheets. Garment presses are used for items like overalls and uniform. In addition, various types of folders and drying chambers are also used in large laundries.

Mending Room

The most suitable place for sorting out this linen in the laundry is the finishing section. Some suggest that mending room should be in the laundry.

Economy in the Laundry

Adequate use of automation and labour saving devices help to achieve efficiency as well as economy. Sheet folders, self-dumping washers and the use of conveyor-belts are the important labour saving devices in practice.

Accurate knowledge of cost of production records takes the guess work out of operation. The margin between the production standard and the time paid for, may leave several opportunities for improvements. A uniform work load, well designed work flow method and scientifically formulated wash formulas save the wastage of materials as well as the wear on the linen. A water softening plant can save at least 40 percent of supplies of the wash formula.

Provision of adequate work area, proper light, ventilation, temperature, and humidity adds to the efficiency of the work staff.

Laundry Management

Laundry contributes to good patient care in two ways:

Contribution to the morale of the staff and patients with fresh laundered linen.

Control of hospital infection Comprehensive programme for improving efficiency should include:

- *Production design* Can any operation be eliminated, combined or simplified?
- *Workshops layout and equipment* Can workflow be improved and handling be reduced by repositioning equipment or using mechanical conveyors.
- *Staff training* Can the operators work be expedited and made less laborious by appropriate training, based on motion study principles?

Standardization of linen A review of various types of articles processed is fundamental to any investigation of laundry efficiency, since the design of each article affects the choice of the laundry process and therefore the cost incurred.

Sequence of operation Appraisal of method: It is necessary to establish correct laundry methods for each class of article to ensure that the simplest methods are employed strictly consistent with the standard of the 'finish' strictly required for each type of article.

The main laundering process in a mechanized scientifically managed laundry are:

- Sorting
- Washing-extraction
- Tumbling
- Preparation (for finishing process)
- Flat work ironing
- Pressing
- Hand ironing
- Packing, folding
- Work shop layout and equipment

Laundry can function effectively and efficiently if the building is planned in strict accordance with the production sequence involved through receipt, processing, and dispatch.

Staff training Proper selection and assignment of personnel to a pleasant working area will help in maintenance of satisfied staff. Training scheme for the workers can be devised on the basis of job specification sheets.

Laundry procedures Soiled linen is received in the reception area of the laundry either direct from the wards or via the central linen room. The soiled linen is sorted in the laundry before being fed to the washing machine.

Foul and infected linen are the most potent sources of cross infection in patient care areas as well as in the laundry. Such linen should be packed in strong washable or disposable bags and transported to the sluice plant near the laundry, either in trolleys or in vans. The infected linen should not be mixed with ordinary soiled linen.

The woolen blankets are normally processed in the laundry at a temprature of 90°F with neutral soaps alone, without the use of any chlorine bleach. Laundry process itself is considered quite adequate to kill the pathogenic organisms. Soap and alkali detergents, hot water, chlorination, sudden change of PH and ironing temperature have been known to kill all types of bacteria and spores.

Temperature for washing Usual temperature for washing in laundry is 71°C. The use of 60-65°C water for normal wash periods is sufficient to ensure the elimination of bacteria associated with nosocomial infection.

Table 35.20: Suggested minimum machinery, equipment needs for hospitals of 500 beds

Washing Machines	5
Extractor containers	3 sets
Electric Hoist	1
Extractor	3
Drying tumblers	4
Flat work ironer	1
Garment press air driven	1
Multipurpose Utility press	1
Form Finisher	1
Spotting Board	2
Marking machine-power driven	1
Hand driven	1
Floor Scale	2
Air compressor	1
Soap Tank	2
Starch cooker	1
Metal truck	4

Radioactive linen Such linen should be put through a special washer reserved for this purpose in the washing area.

Human Resource

The key to successful and efficient operation of the laundry is the selection of a technically trained, experienced laundry manager. The suggested norms of personnel are:

Bed strength	*Number of employees*
50	2
100	6
200	11
300	20
400	27
500	32
600	37
700	40

An average worker may be expected to process linen at the rate of 75-115 Kg in course of each 8 hours duty with improved equipment and automated process, this is increasing, so that average number of personnel is declining.

The cost of operating the hospital laundry will be determined largely by:

- The initial expenditure for equipment and space requirements.

Personnel requirement

- A satisfactory location considering economy of operation, transportation, and possibilities for expansion,
- Cost of supplies and maintenance
- Efficiency of operation as checked against attainable standards.

Other Considerations

Attention should be given to the personal needs and comfort of the patient.

Adequate supply of clean linen sufficient for the comfort and safety of the patient and the personal appearance and dress of hospital personnel attending on patients is required.

- Intelligent planning for linen and laundry services is essential to good hospital care which depends on:
  - Total bed capacity
  - Allotment of beds to various services
  - The extent of service facilities

Average amount of circulating patient linen has been found to be a minimum of four times the complete complement of that in use at one time. This allows one set to be in use, one set at the laundry, one available for immediate use, and one for stand by and emergency purposes. To this must be added load from other sources, operation theatre, outpatient, emergency, clinics and employee uniforms.

The total load is usually expressed in Kilograms of soiled linen per day. The average figure for general hospitals is 6-9 Kg of soiled linen/patient/ day plus 12 Kg for each operation or delivery. For hospitals with more than 50 beds, it is usually more economical and more satisfactory for the hospital to operate its own laundry.

Space and Equipment

The average requirement for laundry purposes alone, excluding central linen room, sewing room, and soiled linen room will range from 12-18 SFT/bed.

Saving Labour

In the ironing line

a. *Folding* Hand folding of hot linen coming out of the ironer is very labour intensive and tiresome for operators.

   Folders have now reached a very high level of automation and reliability.

   New feature The folders can now fold in a way that saves the nurse's time when they make up the hospital beds. The sheets and draw sheets are folded like an M instead of the usual two half folds. The sheets with an M fold are much easier to unfold by one nurse.

b. *In the area of Tumble dried articles (uniform)* The choice of textiles number and size of articles greatly influence the productivity in the total linen service system of the hospital.

	100 beds	*200 beds*	*300 beds*	*400 beds*	*500 beds*
Estimated patient days per year	5200	10400	15600	20800	2600
Pounds per year at 20 Ib per patient per day	10400	20800	31200	41600	52000
Pounds per ambulant patient	9000	18000	27000	36000	45000
Pounds per resident	8000	15000	22000	29000	36000
Total pounds per year	121000	241000	361000	481000	601000
Pounds pear day (total × 1.3/260 days)	610	1220	1830	2440	3050
Flatwork	300	600	900	1200	1500
Rough dray	200	400	600	800	1000
Hand press work	110	220	330	440	550
Working shifts per week	5	5	5	5	5
Total laundry personnel	5	8	12	17	22
Manager (and assitants)	—	1	1	2	3
Washer	2	2	4	5	6
Ironers	2	4	5	6	7
Others	1	1	2	4	6

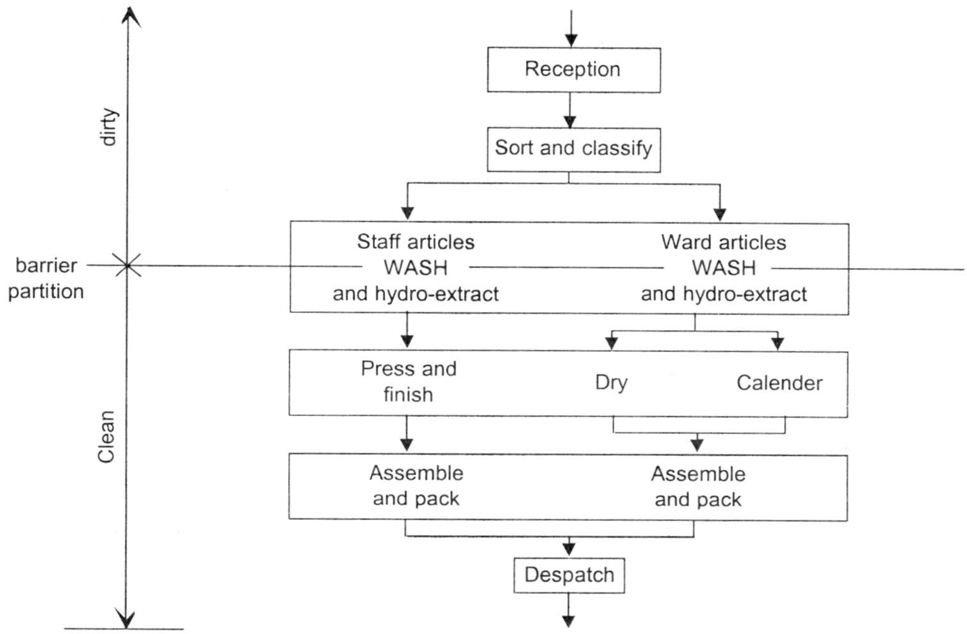

Fig. 35.65: Work-flow diagram for hospital laundary

Quality Control of Laundry Operation

New Technologies are Helpful

Electronic cameras have replaced the eye because the speed at which the linen passes through an ironer, makes it impossible and tiresome for the human eye to detect stains and holes in the linen. The programmable logical controllers (PLC) are used to control the operation of the equipments, can collect and transmit information to a central computer about the actual production, quality and other disturbances that occur. The card controllers are used to control the entire operation of the machine with precise controls over all variables like time, temperature, injection of detergents, etc. They are simple to maintain and most of the components are indigenously available.

Cost Reduction

Pre-sorting of Items (Use of Computers)

Wet section (optimization of water consumption, i.e. requirement and the detergent used):

- Recycling can lead to 60-70 percent savings in consumption of fresh water.
- Double drum progressive laundry systems are more economical
- Reduction in residual moisture (from 55 to 48 percent), energy costs for dryers and calenders can be considerably reduced.

The laundry should, as a part of linen service system, maximize the quality of linen service and minimize the total amount of man-hours involved in the system.

Patients and staff are becoming quality oriented about their linen service. This will lead to a more differentiated linen in terms of textiles, finishing quality, and price/cost. Differentiation demands specialized operation and efficient staff. The system and equipment be made available to ensure that the users (patients and staff) in the hospital receive a good quality linen service, that the laundry can

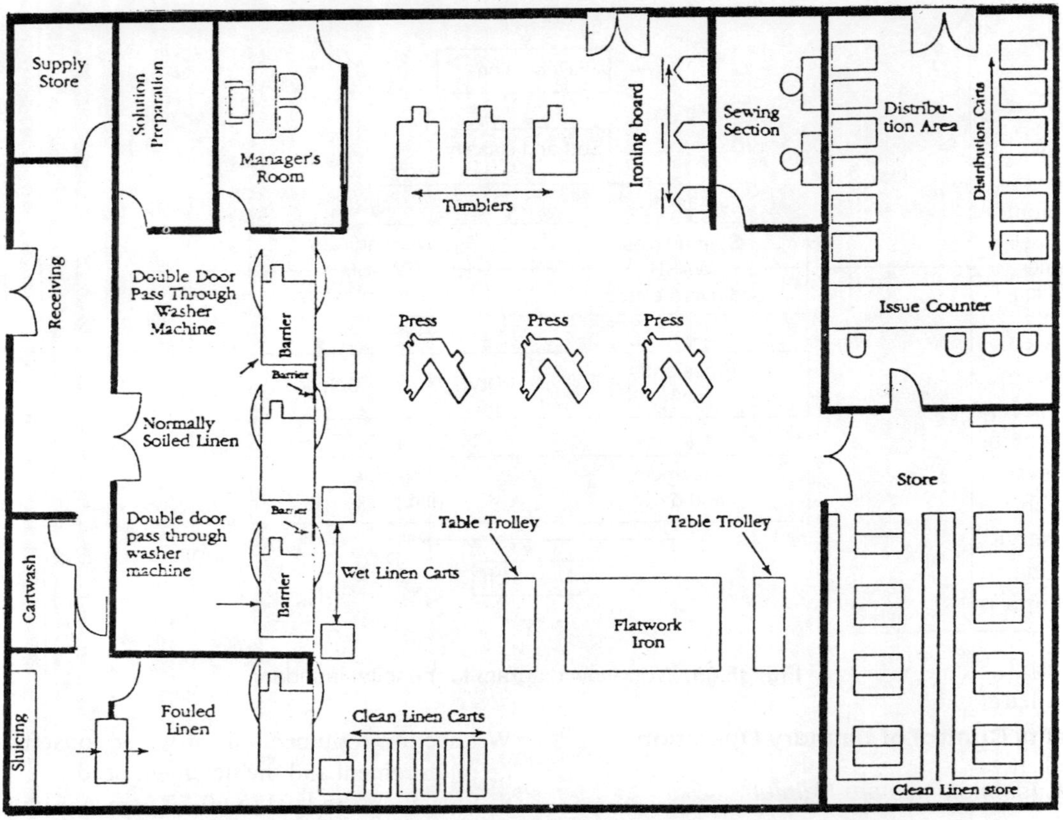

Fig. 35.66: Layout of a typical laundry

supply through automated systems with high production per operator hour, that operators in the laundry have good working conditions and that management has completed control of quality and costs.

FURTHER READING

1. Amin Tabish: Planning of Laundry Service in a Hospital. Laundry World 3(1): 16-27, 1993.

MEDICAL-SURGICAL GASES AND VACUUM

Medical gas system is a necessity in all hospitals. The centralized medical gas system provides an efficient, economical and dependable life support network that supplies medical gases, vacuum and compressed air to the operating department, ICUs and other special procedure rooms.

Medical gas service includes: oxygen, nitrous oxide, medical air 400 KPA (4 bar) and 700 KPA (7 bar), medical vacuum and anesthetic gas scavenging disposal (active) system. piped medical gas systems are fixed pipe installation built into the fabric of the building that transmits a medical gas service from source to the terminal unit. The terminal unit may be wall-mounted or contained within a pre-fabricated assembly, such as ceiling pendent. A minimum pipe size of 12 mm should be used. Wall mounted terminal units should be installed at approximately 1500 mm above finished floor level especially where more than one gas is used at any one location. Pipelines should be installed recessed within the fabric of the building (concealed installation) in all patient care areas. Surface mounted pipes in these areas can be concealed within a vertically mounted headwall assembly if required. Pipes can run in corridors, plant rooms, and other general areas may be surface mounted. Pipe run should ideally follow the shortest possible route and should be installed in horizontal and vertical planes only. Pipelines should be adequately supported along their length by Munsen rings or other approved brass or plastic supports/ brackets at intervals. All exhaust pipes from pressure relief valves, compressed air or vacuum plants and especially gas scavenging exhaust must be routed to discharge outside the building into a safe area. Exhaust outlets must be clearly labeled. Vacuum exhausts should be locate clear of air intakes, and air intakes should be positioned in such a manner that fumes from traffic or other sources can not be drawn into the system.

Medical gas line ball valves should be fitted to each medical gas pipeline system at source and at the point of entry into each building. Each pipeline entering a patient care area should be controlled by area service valve units. The valve should be positioned to enable positive control of the area and should be quickly isolated in case of fire. Pipeline installations should be jointed on-site by a flux less brazing technique with an inert gas purge to prevent oxidation. The technique is only suitable for copper joints and avoids internal contamination of pipelines by flux residues and oxides.

Each pipeline should be clearly identified by the type of medical gas or vacuum system carried by the particular pipe and the direction of flow. Recognized banded colour coded tape is recommended with 9 mm black lettering, to clearly identify the gas service. The identification should be applied periodically along each pipe run especially near valves or other components. Identification should be applied at the point of entry and exit through dividing wall, bulkheads, and ceiling. Colour code yellow for oxygen, navy blue for nitrous oxide, sky blue for compressed air and sky blue for vacuum.

The size of the branch or riser distributor to the recovery ward may be calculated on the basis of 20 litres/minute per bed. Each oxygen terminal unit in an intensive therapy unit should be capable of passing 40 litres/minute if it is intended to use the oxygen to provide the mechanical power for driving them as well as to supply the patient or 20 litres/ minute of the ventilators are electrically driven or driven by the medical compressed air supply. Nitrous oxide terminal unit should be capable of passing 15 litres/minute.

Therapeutic gases are a vital life supporting measures and an indispensable part of the critical care and extensively used for advanced anesthesiology. The supply of medical gases in any hospital should be based on the workload in relation to bed strength of the hospital and the type of hospital. In intermediate care unit, the number of outlets should be around 20 per cent of the bed strength whereas in the intensive care unit (high dependency), it should be 90 to 100 per cent of the bed strength.

Piping system for oxygen, nitrous oxide, air and vacuum are found in all health facilities. Medical gas pipelines should be constructed with suitably sized copper pipes and copper fittings. All pipes and fittings should be delivered to and the site protected in suitable polythene bags and the pipe ends should be fitted with appropriate caps to prevent particulate matter contamination. Pipe joints and fittings must from a permanent joint to ensure system integrity. Pipes should be supplied in a half hard state to enable manual cold formed bends to be manufactured on site. All components and fittings with brass, should be terminated in copper stub pipe to enable the site brazing, should be fitted during manufacturing and the joints chemically cleansed to remove all traces of flux and oxidation especially from internal surfaces.

The design of each medical gas pipeline should be the most economical system that achieves the correct design performance figures required for that gas service. The pipes should be of the smallest possible diameter and frequent step down in their size is recommended. Pressure drops through the pipelines and fittings should be calculated and system designed. The flow rates of terminal units for all installations are started in times of flow at standard temperature and pressure. The rate of flow actually occurring in the pipe lines serving the terminal units will therefore be lower than the stated figures in the case of pressure gases and higher in the case of vacuum, and will depend upon the pipeline operating pressure.

Particulate matter purging is carried out on all pipelines and installations to ensure that the gas flow from a completed installation is clean. Medical quality air is used for the purging process to remove all possible particulate matter and nitrogen is used in the brazing process. Purging should be planned to systematically remove particulate matter contamination with the pressure and flow rates specifically selected for that installation. On completion, the distribution system gas outlets should be tested and the gas flow passed through fibres to ensure that a satisfactory standard is achieved. On completion of all pipeline tests, each gas service is connected to its source and purged with the working gas to remove all traces of air and nitrogen. All line ball valves should be closed with the inlet pressure remaining at 690 kpa (6.9 bar) and downstream pressure released. The pressure should be held for 24 hours without leakage, but for systems with more than approximately 50 terminal units, a pressure loss of up to 15 kpa (0.15 bar) may be acceptable. The system should be exhausted to a vacuum of 210 mm Hg absolute. This vacuum shall be held for 24 hours. A rise of more than 10 mm Hg per hour indicates either that the pipeline has not dried u or that there are leaks.

Pipeline should be seamless type, of high quality copper tubing. Embedded piping should be protected against physical damage. The gas content of the pipeline should be cleaned thoroughly and washed with tetrachloride.

Other less common systems include those for carbon dioxide, helium and certain mixed gases.

The important components of the system include:

- source of supply (central supply room with control equipment)
- distribution system (piping that extends to the points in the user areas)
- point-of-use delivery connections (station outlet valves and pendants at the use points)
- monitoring and control equipment and alarms.

To improve safety and performance of central piping system, greater care in their design, installation, use, and maintenance is needed and greater communication between all of the principals must be stressed.

Controls are intended to prevent tragic incidents. The best system design must go beyond the minimum requirements, and sometimes can be done at lower cost. Safer and more functional systems design cannot be achieved by depending only on national standards and codes. All alternative types of equipment should be compared, product claims verified, experience and problems of other users sought, and finally, tight specifications written accordingly–including performance and design criteria.

Manifold Room

The manifold room usually consists of a cylinder manifold and a control panel. The control panel consists of primary and secondary pressure regulators to ensure delivery of gas to the pipeline at the required pressure provided there is gas in the cylinders. When the cylinders become empty a warning lamp on the control panel illuminates. The control panel also has the pressure gauges to indicate pressure in the cylinders.

The vacuum unit comprises of a vacuum pump with an electric motor. A cylindrical reservoir tank stabilizes the pressure of the pipeline system at all the outlet points. The motor has a negative pressure switch for automatic start and stop. Vacuum pumps are duplexed.

The compressed air unit consists of a compressor with an electric motor, after cooler, air receiver and air dryer. The system instantly provides compressed air through the pipeline wherever it is required. The compressors are duplexed.

The primary supply is that part of the equipment which actually supplies the system. A secondary source automatically suuplies the system when the primary system becomes exhausted. The primary and secondary equipment provide the normal operating supply. When the operating supply fails or is exhausted, a reserve supply automatically takes over.

Usually half of the daily consumption of oxygen and nitrous oxide is kept in the manifold room as reserve supply. In the case of vacuum and air, there is always a reserve capacity in the system itself which lasts for a while.

Oxygen and nitrous oxide are stored separately from flammable gases and liquids. The storage location should be free of combustible materials.

The size of central supply room depends on the system it houses.

Oxygen and Nitrous Oxide

Oxygen for hospital use may be supplied from a bulk tank or from cylinders. It may be stored as a gas or a liquid; the oxygen containers may be stationary or movable. The bulk oxygen system includes oxygen storage containers, pressure regulators, safety devices, vaporizers, manifolds and interconnecting piping with a storage capacity of more than 20,000 cubic feet of oxygen including reserves. The system terminates at the point where oxygen first enters the supply line at service pressure.

Vacuum

Vacuum suction is distributed through a network of pipes. There is a central vacuum supply system with control equipment, an alarm signaling system and a network of piping extending to areas in the hospital where patient suction is required. The piping terminates with outlet valves at each user point. The central vacuum system consists of two or more vacuum pumps which operate either simultaneously or alternately, depending on demand. Each pump should be capable of maintaining 75 per cent of the peak calculated demand. The pump should in normal course alternate automatically. The pumps should be equipped with motor starting device and overload protection.

Vacuum pumps should be of proven reliability and driven by electric motors with good insulation and noise level tested to satisfaction. The receiver vessel should be constructed and tested. The control panels and electric installation should also conform to the latest standards. The bacterial filter element should guarantee 100 per cent bacteria removal.

The medical vacuum plant must be capable of maintaining a vacuum of at least 300 mm Hg at the connection point of each terminal unit with flow of minimum 40 litre/minute within a designed system.

Compressed Air

In the compressed air system, the standard items of equipment and accessories include compressors, shutoff valves on tank outlets, valves on drains, pressure gauges, safety valves, check valves, pressure switches, inlet filter-mufflers, and automatic electric controls.

The compressed air plant should be provided with directly driven electric motor and an incorporating air inlet filter and silencer. Each compressor should be provided with air blast after cooler and auto drains. The compressor air motors should be of squirrel cage type suitable for three phase supply.

Alarm System

System that monitors the pressure of various gases at different areas of the distribution system should be incorporated in the centralized medical gas system. Alarms should be located in working areas of those who use and maintain the system. The other alarm, called the remote signal lamp provides a warning signal can also be used.

Medical Trunking System

The medical trunking system provides a safe and efficient means of delivery services to patients/staff. The trunking system should have modular design of aluminum extrusion, comply with ISO standards, have ability to house medical gas terminals and electric sockets, full range of medical accessories, and available pipe wired and pre-piped.

The system includes: Theatre Suction Trolley, Multimovement Pendent for Operating Room and Modular Wall Panel for ICU.

Oxygen Concentrator

Oxygen concentrators work on the principle of enrichment of air compressed from the atmosphere by elimination of nitrogen. This is done by absorption of nitrogen by chemical granules called zeolite that have the property of absorption of nitrogen. The advantage of an oxygen concentrator is that it reduces the total number of cylinders in circulation and in good condition can deliver oxygen at 90 per cent purity and is cost-effective. It uses atmospheric air and purifies it up to 96 per cent medical grade oxygen continuously. It should be able to produce 350 litres per minute of oxygen and oxygen should be through central pipeline available in hospital at 4.20 kg/sq. cm.

Liquid Oxygen Supply System

A liquid oxygen supply system provides a centralized, convenient and reliable method of storing liquid medical oxygen to supply gaseous oxygen to a hospital distribution system. Liquid oxygen vessels should be located in the open and the surrounding area should be controlled so that no combustible materials or naked lights are allowed within a distance of 20 feet, from the containers and associated controls. Cabin liquid oxygen supply system is usually considered economical if the expected usage exceeds 100,000 gaseous litres of oxygen per week. The installation is specifically designed as an external plant releasing valuable internal hospital space normally used for manifolds. The system consists of a Vacuum Insulated Evaporator with integral control panel and pressure raising coil, Matched Vaporizer System, Oxygen Delivery Control Panel Assembly and Remote Alarm System.

LIBRARIES IN HOSPITALS

Today's hospital library is an active, service-oriented special library. Like other departments within the hospital, the library contributes to the hospitals primary mission of providing patients with the best possible care. The library supports the delivery of patient care by providing physicians, nurses, and other health care professionals with library services to meet their informational educational, and in many cases, research-related needs. Although it is tempting and often expedient to talk about hospital libraries as a homogeneous group, in reality they differ in many ways. This tremendous variety is important for hospital librarians to recognize as they assess the patterns of library service most appropriate for their institutions.

Staffing

The first and most obvious difference among hospital libraries is in staffing. While many hospital libraries are staffed by one person, other have three or more full-time staff members. The educational background of library employees also varies. In the past more frequently than today, hospital personnel with training and responsibilities in other areas, such as medical records, were placed in charge of the library. Today the trend is to provide qualified medical librarians in hospital libraries, whenever possible.

Library Users

Almost all hospital libraries today provide services primarily to physicians and nurses. Residents, post-doctoral fellows, and medical students form part of the libraries clientele in hospitals affiliated with medical schools. Students in other professional programmes affiliated with the hospital, or sponsored by it, may also have access to the library. In addition, many hospital libraries provide services to the hospital administration, professionals in other departments, and other hospital employees.

Some hospitals have also opened the doors of their libraries to people not on their staffs, such as patients and their families, attorneys, and physicians in the local area. Due to increased consumer advocacy and interest in promoting healthful living habits, some hospitals have recently begun to provide health information to the community at large.

Services

The range and variety of services that hospital libraries provide reveal the individuality of hospital libraries most dramatically. Although the broad categories of services are similar, the number of creative variations practiced in hospital libraries can be appreciated by attending a" sharing session" among hospital librarians.

Hospital libraries provide standard library services, primarily in the area of the health sciences. These services include the provision of journal collection, a reference collection, and often a circulating book collection; inter-library loan services; reference services, including both answers to factual questions and literature searches; and awareness services of various kinds, including routines, table-of-contents scans, newsletters, and notification of recently published materials on specific topics. In addition to providing these services to walk-in users or to clients via the telephone, some librarians function as clinical medical librarians, participate on committees as information experts, assess formal information needs, and support other outreach efforts.

Hospital libraries also provide a variety of information services needed by the hospital in all aspects of its organizational operation. Providing total information services, however, means extending the standard library services beyond the subject matter of the health sciences to include any information needed by hospital personnel in the performance of their jobs. Such an expanded mission requires a collection that covers basic references in selected fields outside the health sciences. While hospital operations touch on almost every conceivable discipline, library funcing is usually limited, making extensive interdisciplinary book and journal collections not feasible. Therefore, librarians have taken other approaches to provide total information services in hospitals. Hospital librarians are using local information sources, both formally and informally. Much needed information can be obtained from nearby public and academic libraries, local agencies, institutions, and businesses. When use of other libraries or information agencies is extensive, formal agreements may often evolve. In these formal, cooperative efforts, hospital libraries contribute to and benefit from the agreement. Consortia of hospital libraries constitute the most popular approach to expanding services, and one that fits in well with the overall hospital thrust toward shared services. Finally, initiating total information services is often made more manageable by focusing on one particular need at a time. Limiting the scope of a programme to one area, such as social services, can result in a highly visible, successful programme within an initially limited context.

Many hospital libraries are expanding their services to include various audiovisual services. In some, audiovisual involvement means extending the standard services to non-print media: providing a software collection, a viewing area, interlibrary loan and rental of software, and basic media reference service. Other libraries have expanded the concept of media services to include equipment distribution, projectionist services, and production of such audiovisual materials as slides, transparencies, graphics of various types, videotapes, and slide tape programmes.

Providing library and information service to hospital and clinic patients, and even to the community at large, is another area in which hospital libraries are expanding. Today, many libraries are discovering additional ways to provide health science information to patients. Hospital library services may now included identifying and acquiring pamphlets, books, articles, and audiovisual materials on both general health topics and on specific diseases. These services are provided to health care professionals who use the material with patients in a variety of teaching situations. Some hospital libraries provide the resources directly to the patients or public who have been referred by practitioners or who walk into the library and request help.

Information Needs

Obviously, hospital library roles, staffs and services can vary from extremely limited to comprehensive. Even though some hospital libraries offer limited services because of a variety of circumstances, most librarians feel that the unique hospital environment creates enormous information needs. These needs challenge librarians to provide better and better library and information services, no matter on what level the library currently finds itself. Many factors contribute to these expanded information needs in hospitals.

Expansion of Educational Programmes

Educational programmes in hospitals are continuing to expand to meet the needs of health sciences students, medical students, and residents who are often located in hospitals distant from the libraries of their academic institution. Hospitals are also expanding their continuing and in-service education programmes for employees on all levels, both to respond to increasing certification and regulatory requirements and to improve the quality of professional performance. Patient education programmes of many types are blossoming. Some hospitals are initiating educational programmes directed to the general needs of their employees: physical fitness programs, stop-smoking clinics, parenting classes, and seminars on topics such as rape prevention, stress, and relxation.

Increasing Professionalism in Health Occupations

Increased professionalism in areas that used to be called health occupations is resulting in broader-based educational preparation, a greater variety of specialized education programmes, more stringent credentialing or licensing requirements, and a greater use and production of professional literature. All these developments may increase the need for information by a greater number of health care professionals.

Interdisciplinary Nature of Hospitals

Closely allied to the increased professionalism of hospital personnel is the multidisciplinary nature of the modern hospital. Over 50 autonomous disciplines may practice in today's modern institution with relative independence. They may have separate professional structures, including tools and channels for information. Yet coexisting with this comparative freedom are the demands of the hospital for centralization of certain services and functions, dictated by the need for uniformity, efficiency, regulation, and cost containment. Library and information services can be received as one of many services that are more cost-effective when provided centrally.

Increasing Regulation of Hospitals

Regulatory forces increasingly influence the hospital environment. In addition to the trend of many health care disciplines toward self-regulation, hospitals are continually establishing policies and procedures that conform to external guidelines. Government regulations come from many sources and are directed towards many goals. The issue of cost containment also continues to exert regulatory influence on the programs of the hospital. In view of the complex and rapidly changing nature of regulations and their tremendous impact on hospital operations, effective monitoring becomes essential. Hospitals are coping with the need to manage this large and complex body of new information by hiring administrative assistants, subscribing to newsletters and information services, and sending employees to seminars. However, no effective system of monitoring regulations has become dominant as yet. Thus libraries have the opportunity to demonstrate that they can meet this critical information need effectively.

Library Development

Given both the wide range of possible services and the expanding library and information needs of hospitals, the library program for an individual institution must be tailored to match the needs of the institution, its current resources, and its potential for expansion and development. In designing this tailor-made blend of information services, hospital libraries face a number of common situations that deserve consideration.

To deal with the problems of limited time, hospital librarians need to consider new technologies and alternate methods for performing necessary procedures. They must also become aware of opportunities to share projects, services, and even such products as forms, proposals, or searches. Adapting another library's needs assessment form may take fifteen minutes; designing an original may take several hours. More importantly, librarians need to take a hard look at the real needs of their users and direct library efforts toward services that are needed and used.

Centralized Library Services

In hospitals where several libraries serve different user groups, the trend today is to move toward centralizing library management and resources into one hospital library. This trend, occurring at varying rates in different institutions, make sense for a number of reasons.

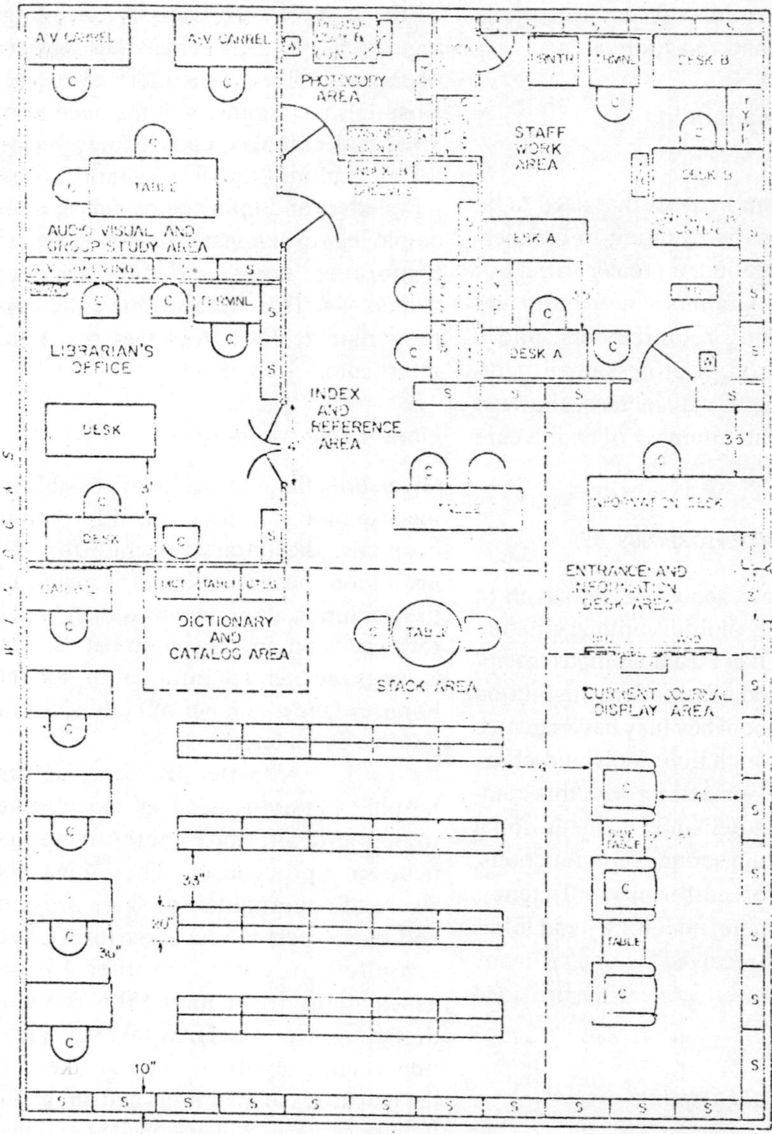

(Area 34'× 53' = 1802 sq.ft.)

Scale:
1/4 inch = 1 foot

Key:
I = Index
TR = Truck
C = Chair
W = Waste-basket
S = Shelf

Fig. 35.67: Sample floor layout for library in 200-bed community hospital

Cost effective use of Library Resource and Staff

Many of the same key resources are required by physicians, nurses, administrators, and personnel in support services. Consolidation of these materials minimizes duplication of these costly resources. It also improves hospital control over purchases by ensuring that materials are stamped as hospital property and kept in a secure environment.

Promotion of the Team Concept

Maintaining separate medical, nursing, and administrative collections supports an older structural model in which the physician was the sole health care decision maker. The consolidation of disparate collections and diverse clientele, however, fosters the health care team concept and recognizes the contributions, interrelationship and needs of all those involved in providing health care services.

Establishment of an Information Focal point

Centralized library services for all members of the health care team identifies the library as a focal point for information gathering. This reduces the time spent by team members in tracking elusive information, increases communication effectiveness, and ultimately facilitates all health care decision making.

The Hospital Librarian

The hospital librarian is the key to effective library service. He or she is responsible for planning library services, for securing administrative approval for those services, for providing them effectively and efficiently, and for modifying them as institutional needs change. In many hospitals, the librarian works also at the task necessary for the operation of a successful library. When the library staff expands, however, the librarian assumes an additional supervisory role. These varied responsibilities require a variety of skills and abilities.

Although most hospitals have similar information needs, each institution's response to these needs is somewhat different. Hospitals differ widely in size, in scope of programmes in governing process in educational affiliation, and in financial support.

To be effective, hospital librarians must understand the operational and organizational structure of hospitals in general and must be able to analyze the specific process, including the political dynamics, in their own institutions. If the hospital is involved in educational programsme, the librarian needs to understand the structure of education for medicine, nursing, and other health professions, particularly in a clinical setting. Only a librarian who thoroughly understands the goals, functions, procedures and organizational dynamics of the institution can provide context-oriented library services.

The Planning Process

Planning is essential to the management of any complex activity, including running a library. Faced with pressures to provide services, librarians are sometimes tempted to neglect planning in favour of immediate action. Planning, however, ensures organized and effective activity. It takes time, but that time is recouped in more efficient operations after implementation.

Planning not only helps a librarian to organize the activity of the library, but it also provides the means by which a librarian can obtain approval to expand that activity. A detailed plan for a projected new service or for the expansion of an existing service shows the administration what is suggested; why it is suggested; how much it will cost; and what impact it will have. The same plans, once approved, can then direct the new activity. By developing plans that identify worthwhile activities, determining the steps needed to accomplish those activities, identifying necessary resources, and establishing policy and procedures, librarians can make the library operate more smoothly.

The planning process can be divided into a series of separate activities that provide an organized adn logical framework. The following activities provide a step-by-step approach to the planning process.

Although the activities involved in all types of planing remain essentially the same, three types are useful in hospital libraries: (1) programme planning (2) project planning, and (3) long-range planning.

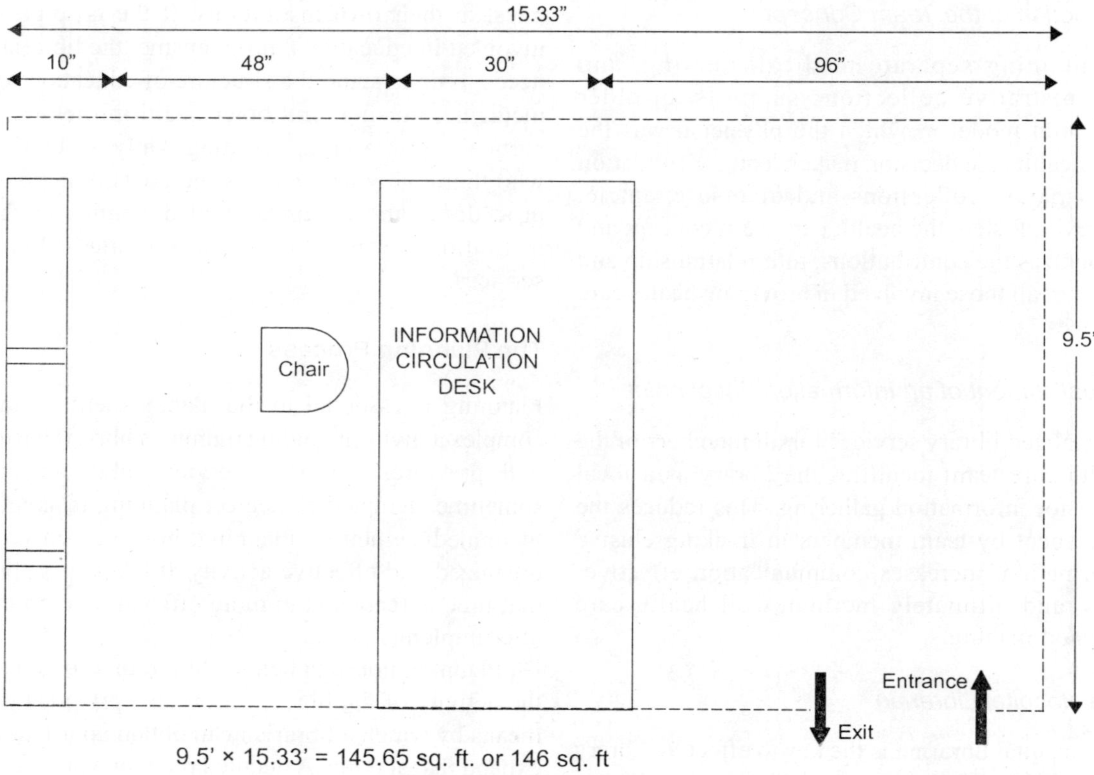

Fig. 35.68: Entrance and information-circulation desk area

Programme Planning

Programme planning involves library activities as a whole. During this type of planning, a librarian decides what services the library will provide, gives a philosophical basis for the library services, and describes how the services will be provided. At this time the librarian has a chance to list goals, determine how much time and money are necessary to accomplish the goals, and establish the guidelines or rules that govern the activity. Programme planning organizes library activity and demonstrates the logic of that activity.

Ideally librarians should develop a programme plan when first establishing library services in a hospital. After library services have been established, librarians can use the planning process to rethink the priorities of their programmes and record the decisions for the hospital administration. Librarian undertake the development of formal planning documents, including goals, objectives, policies, and procedures at various times. They may develop these documents after assuming a new position, before adding a new programme, or when studying, changing, or expanding an existing service. After planning documents have been prepared or revised, they should be submitted to the hospital administration for approval. When planning programmes, librarians should follow the steps described below.

Determining Goals

Determining goals is the first step in the planning process. It involves identifying institutional goals

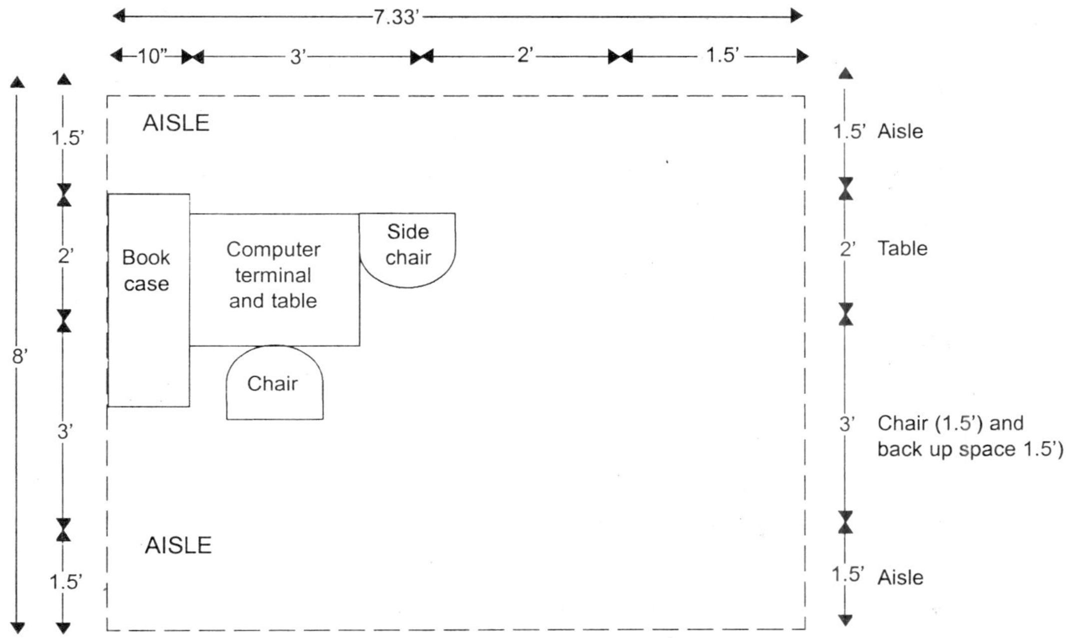

7.33' × 8' = 58.64 sq. ft. or 59 sq. ft.

Fig. 35.69: Computer terminal area

and then formulating library goals to support the goals of the institution. Hospitals may have a variety of formal documents expressing their philosophy. Some hospitals are guided by a mission statement and then develop annual goals from that statement. In most hospital, the philosophical statements emphasize patient care first and then may include education and research.

Mission Statement of a Health Sciences Library

The library will support the work of all hospital employees involved in patient care, research, teaching,and administration by providing a dynamic information service. The library collects and organizes information for this purpose in the form of books, journals, and audiovisuals. The library is dedicated to finding answers to all requests for health care information and can identify and deliver published materials from the worldwide library community. Specific goal statements describe each of the library's major services. The identification of specific service goals will help define the components of library service.

Assessing Needs

An accurate needs assessment is the foundation of any planning process. It provides planning data for librarians and solid evidence of the need for library services. The needs assessment should be carefully planned, based on what the librarian wants to know and how that information will be used. A librarian might need to know what information the hospital staff needs, what sources they already use, how often and how quickly they need material, and whether they would use particular services and sources if they were available.

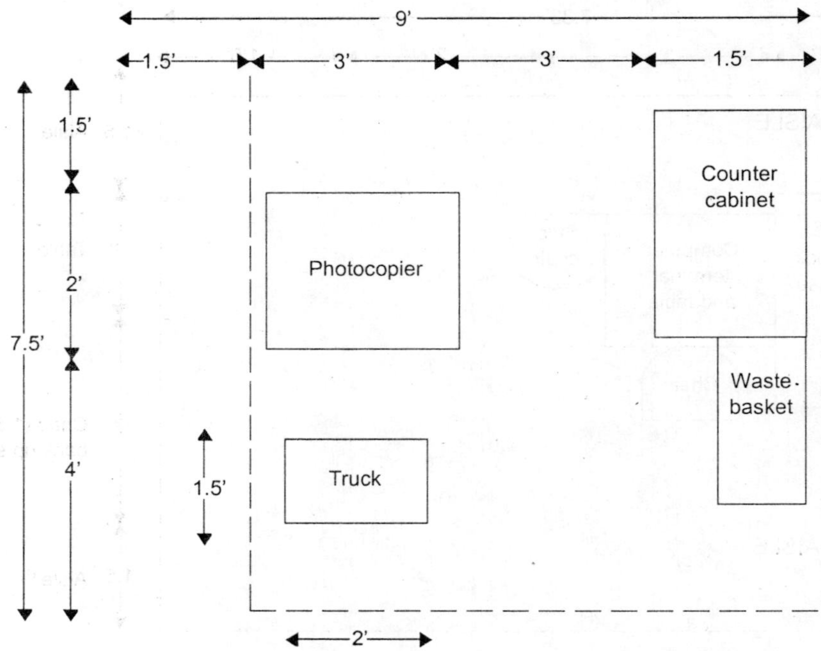

7.5' × 9' = 67.5 sq. ft. or 68 sq. ft.

Fig. 35.70: Photocopy area

Programme Objectives of a Health Sciences Library

1. *Informational and Educational Resources* The health sciences library provides book, journal, and audiovisual collections to meet the informational and educational needs of the medical and nursing staff and all other departments and programs of the institution.
2. *Information* The health sciences library provides information services, including answering factual questions, and compiling bibliographies in a timely manner and in a usable format.
3. *Document Delivery (interlibrary loan)* The health sciences library will attempt to obtain any needed document through interlibrary loan or other appropriate means. Photocopying services are available in the library.
4. *Cooperative Library Services* The health sciences library maintains active, cooperative relationships with local, and where possible, nonlocal libraries. Such cooperation may include interlibrary loans, collection development, reference referrals, technical processes, and other project areas.

Since objectives represent specific actions, more than one objective is necessary to achieve a programme goal. If a librarian wants to be specific, several objectives can be written. Although broad objectives are easier to write, they are less easy to measure and reveal less about the library activities. Specific objectives take more thought, but they are also more useful in organizing activities and showing personnel outside the library what the library does. Objectives not only show the administration what the librarian plans to do, they also provide the librarian with a guide. Objectives can be used to establish the overall activities of the library programme and also accommodate yearly changes. For example a librarian can use the same programme

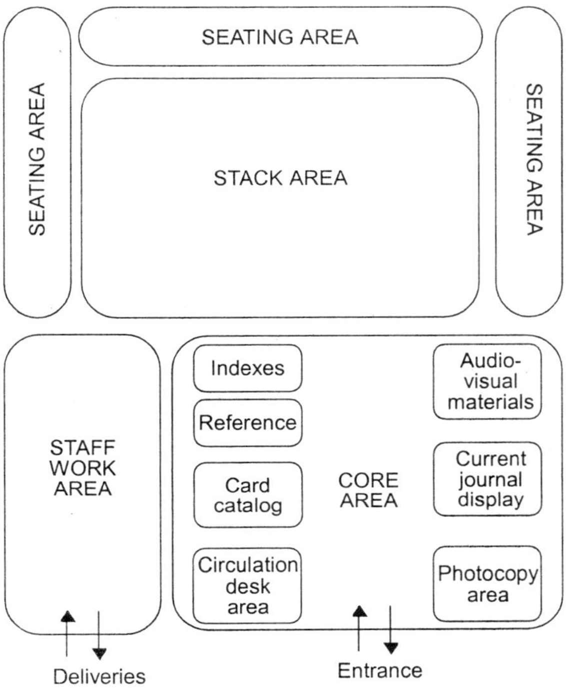

Fig. 35.71: Sample library diagram illustrating spatial relationships

objectives from year to year but modify. Operational objectives for each year's activity. Operational objectives can include a mix of objectives that reflect on going activities and special projects for a particular year.

Information and Educational Resources

Objectives Select, with the input of appropriate departments, 50 new books, 15 new audiovisual programmes, and 12 new journals each year. Subject areas to be considered are internal medicine, nursing, dermatology, pathology, paediatrics, obstetrics and gynaecology.

- Identify, evaluate, and acquire the most receptions of books currently in the collection.
- Acquire selected material.
- Evaluate and withdraw dated material.
- Produce and distribute a list of new books four times a year
- Produce and distribute once a year a list of journals owned by title and subject.
- Update the audiovisual catalogue annually.

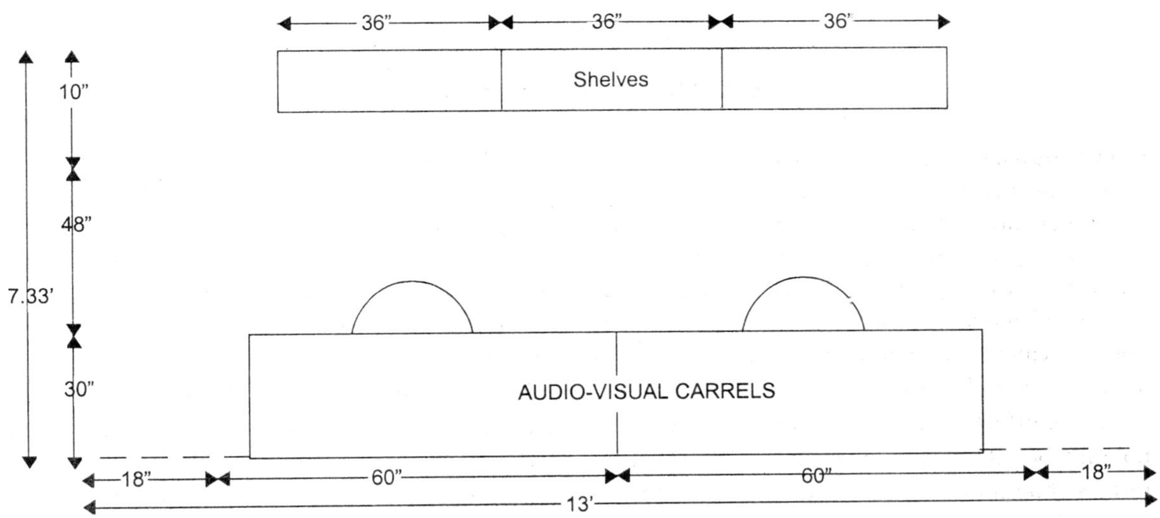

7.33' × 13' = 95.3 sq. ft. or 96 sq. ft.

Fig. 35.72: Audiovisual area (Sample was developed for the requirements of an active library in a 200-bed community hospital

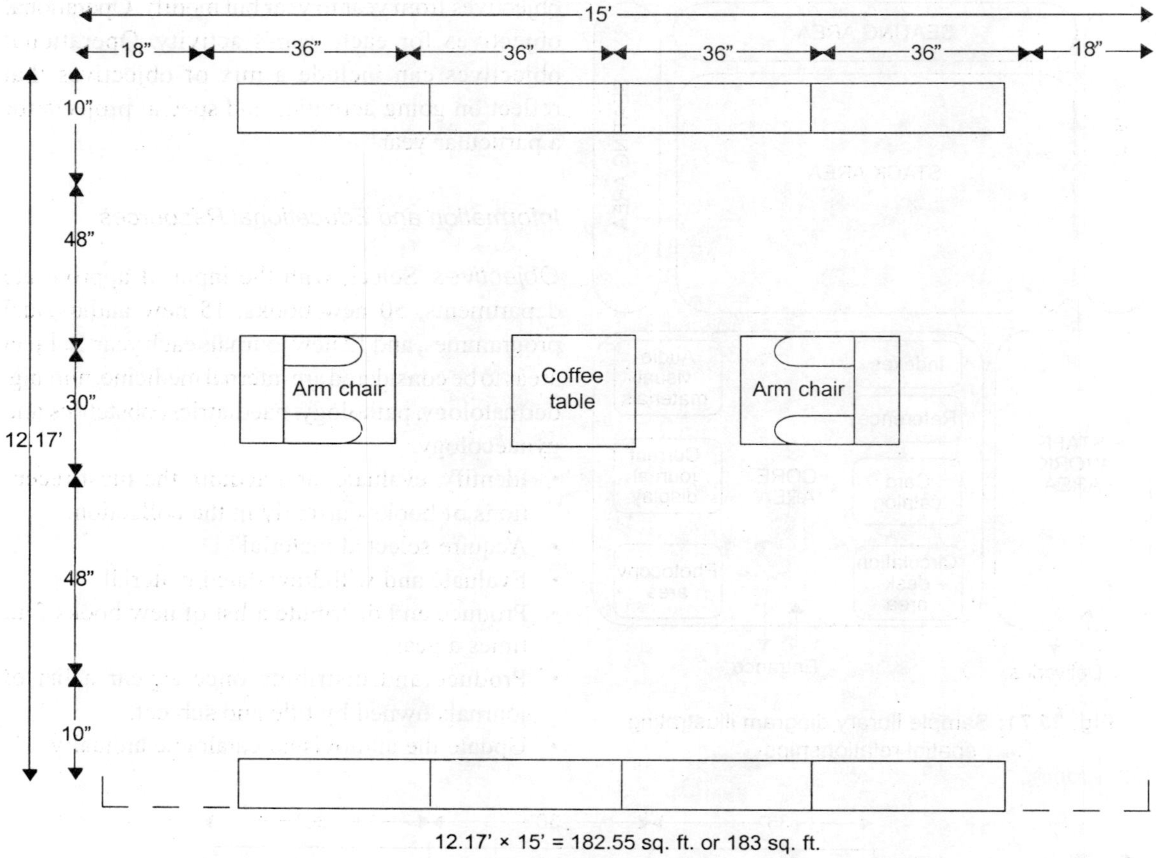

Fig. 35.73: Current journal display area

- Provide a mechanism for staff to request specific titles in specific subject areas.
- Design and maintain systems for the circulation of appropriate of non-circulating materials.

Objectives can be listed in order of importance or grouped under specific categories of priority. The librarian can then assign realistic completion dates to operational objectives.

To be effective, objectives and priorities must not only be set but should also be adhered to. Librarians should incorporate objectives into scheduling, task, assignments, and policies; post them in a visible place; or schedule a specific time during the week to review their status.

Establishing Policies

Policies are the general guidelines or rules that govern the way an objective will be accomplished. By establishing these rules in advance, the librarian can anticipate operational problems, design solutions, obtain administrative approval, and publicize the ground rules to both library staff and users. If a library committee exists, its endorsement and support of library policy is invaluable. In many institutions, policies that affect the entire hospital must be reviewed by the administrtaion and filed in the hospital policy manual. They facilitate the smooth operation of library activity and provide a

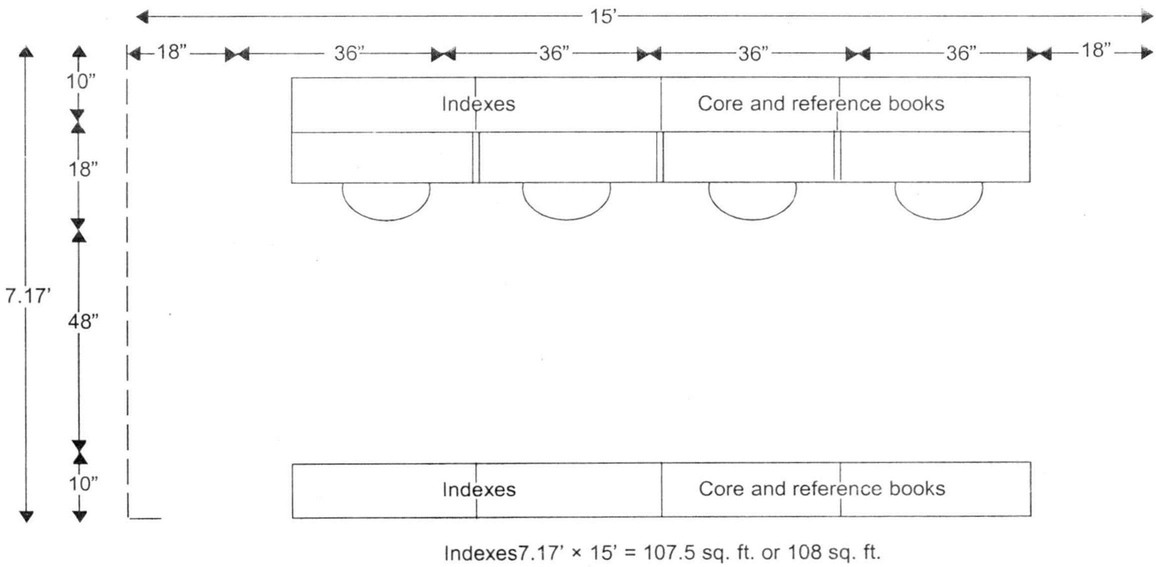

Fig. 35.74: Reference books and index area

vehicle for obtaining the approval and support of the library committee and the administration.

Developing Procedures

Writing procedures is an essential part of planning. During this step, a librarian decides how each objective will be implemented. Once the procedures are used, librarians can modify them, if necessary. Procedures require the logical analysis of a task, provide a written record of the standard practice, and can be used to estimate the amount of time necessary to complete a task.

Scheduling

When planning a new service, librarians should schedule a specific amount of time for each objective in order to integrate the new service into the existing service.

Project Planning

Project planning involves systematizing and documenting decisions that must be made in any case. The dividends gained through increased efficiency and administrative awareness of library activity outweigh the few additional hours involved.

Long-Range Planning

A third type of a planning, often the most neglected type, is long-range planning. This process anticipates institutional changes and analyzes how these changes may affect library services. The long-range planning process often results in a written five-year plan that the librarian presents to the administration and the library committee for approval and support.

Long-range planning prepares the library for future contingencies. New residency programmes, additional outpatient clinics, and new allied health training programmes all have an impact on information needs. Budget increases take time to justify and also must be planned.

Long-range planning is essential in today's dynamic library environment. The effects of automation alone have a dramatic impact. Librarians need to anticipate developments in electronic publishing, telecommunications, and information

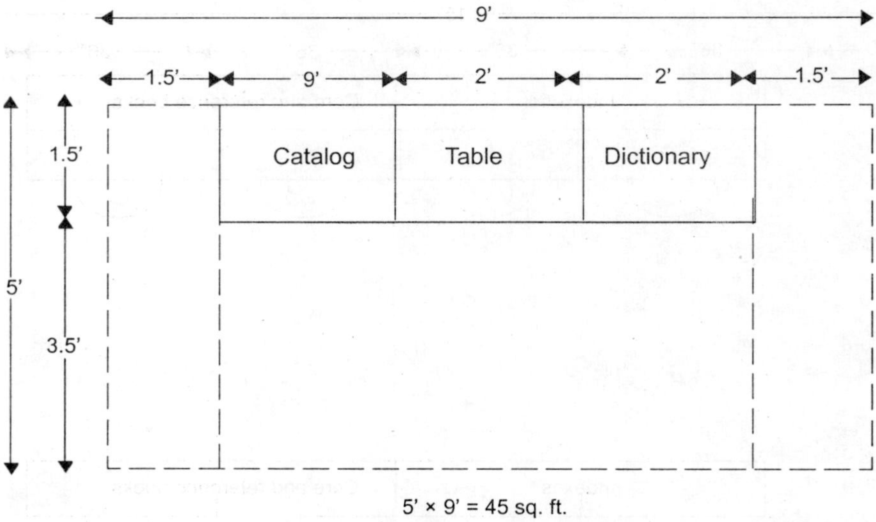

Fig. 35.75: Card catalog and dictionary area

handling, and integrate these changes into regular library policies and procedures when useful. Increased networking among libraries continues to make a variety of new servicers available, Libraries should keep informed about these service and anticipate how they can effect their own Institutions.

The third element in long-range planning is the five year service plan, which starts with the needs assessment, when needs have been documented the new services are planned. With a five -year lead time for planning, however thorough needs assessments may be conducted and major budget requests or grant proposals initiated. As long-range service planning progresses, librarians should document each stage in the annual report and in the annual review and update of the library five year plan.

Evaluation

Evaluation is essential to the entire planning process. A librarian cannot formally plan unless programmes, services, and procedures are analyzed to determine their function, effectiveness and need for improvement or change. The purpose of evaluation is threefold: (1) to determine the effectiveness of existing programmes (2) to determine specific changes that will improve existing programmes, and (3) to justify continuing budget support. Evaluations of individual programmes or services are more helpful in making improvements than evaluation of an entire programme of services.

In order to understand the evaluation process, librarians should examine the four classes of evaluation, effort evaluation, process evaluation, effectiveness evaluation and impact evaluation.

Effort evaluation Librarians can compare the resources used with the results achieved.

Process evaluation Librarians can evaluate processes to determine whether the procedures used in the performance of a service are efficient and appropriate.

Effectiveness evaluation Evaluating programme effectiveness determines whether a service accomplishes its objectives.

Impact evaluation The most powerful form of evaluation is impact evaluation. It assesses the extent to which accomplished objectives actually meet the needs of the parent Institution.

The Physical Facilities

The physical environment of the library significantly influences both library use and library service. Inconvenient space discourages use; poor arrangement of the stocks and furniture makes the user overly dependent on library staff; and inadequate working space for staff results in inefficiency. Conversely, adequate space, easy access to materials, and an organized and clearly marked arrangement of materials contribute to effective library service.

In order to make sure that there is adequate space for the library, librarians must convince hospital management that library services are essential and that adequate space is vital for providing good service. The process of obtaining library space takes a great deal of time and involves many people in addition to the librarian. Because procedures vary for planning and developing space, librarians should learn what the appropriate channels are for their own institutions.

The hospital librarian should be the central figure throughout the planning process. Because librarians are responsible for the effective use of the space given to the library, they must become experts in planning library space. The librarians role includes initiating the study of space requirements, planning a solution to space problems, acquiring administrative approval for plans, and working with the building team to translate plans into a functional library.

Planning new space for a hospital department is rarely done by one individual alone. The library committee, usually representing various user groups, is often very effective in this role because it is familiar with library problems. The purpose of the planning team or committee is to explore and express user needs and desires, react to all aspects of planning, and apply pressure to bring about an effective outcome. The librarian should involve the administrator in assessing space needs. Through this process the administrator can gain a clear understanding of how the library functions and how it contributes to the quality of patient care.

An architect, engineer, hospital space planner, or hospital draftsman provides assistance in space planning by preparing schematic drawings, floor plans, construction documents, and specification. The architect, hospital engineer or planner will also check state and local code requirements and confer with mechanical, electrical, and structural engineers. This person can also assist in selecting furniture, colour schemes, carpeting, wood finishes, and stack materials. Sometimes a hospital will employ an interior designer or ask the advice of a designer on the staff of a large furniture supply firm. This specialist can prepare a layout for library areas, select furniture, decor, colours, carpeting, wood finishes, and so forth. Commercial shelving companies can also be a useful source for advice on placement of shelving.

The range of services provided by these professionals and the overlapping of abilities make it essential that librarians have some knowledge, of every aspect of design. With such knowledge, librarians can make more informed decisions on design, furniture, and aesthetics.

Planning for Additional Space

Responsibility for initiating the planning process usually rests with the librarian. He/she should begin the planning process by evaluating the existing library space.

Evaluating Existing Library Space

New space in a hospital is both expensive and scarce. Before a request for new space is made, the librarian should evaluate the existing space to determine its limitations and identify specific needs for new space.

Data should be gathered on the use of existing space, user populations, and standard or typical library space needs. The analysis of the use of the existing space includes the size of the total space in square feet, the collection size, annual growth rate, seating capacity, and staff size. The librarian should also determine both present and potential user populations by job category: staff physician, resident, nurse, pharmacist, and so forth. The projections of library use should be based on actual hospital programmes or projected new ones.

Considering Alternatives to New Space

By evaluating existing library space. The librarian can identify areas that are overcrowded or no longer functional. They should examine these areas thoroughly and look for solutions that may alleviate the problem without requiring additional space. The size of the collection should be reviewed first. The following methods of reducing its size should be assessed: (1) studying the use of materials to determine the most cost-effective size, (2) withdrawing or storing infrequently used items (3) exploring the use of microforms (4) in cooperative collection sharing arrangements with other libraries.

After reviewing the collection size, the librarian should analyze the use of floor space to determine if any additional space can be gained by any of the following methods: (1) reducing the width of the aisles between stacks, tables, or carrels (2) replacing bulky furniture with smaller pieces, or (3) rearranging the entire layout to make optimum use of tight space. Finally, space outside the library can be considered.

Once all reasonable avenues for alleviating space shortage have been explored and documented, the librarian can begin plans for creating additional space. Additional space can include space in a new building, space in an area vacated by other or renovation of the existing space.

Estimating General Space Requirements

Obtaining additional space is expensive. Therefore, when requesting space, the librarian should project future needs as well as the present needs of the library. To plan for a flexible facility, the space needed to accommodate future growth must be estimated. Rapid technological change has made it impractical to attempt to project growth for more than ten years. Using the completed evaluation of the existing space, the librarian can estimate space requirements by their function and their relationship to one another. The librarian can identify the areas to be accommodated and determine the numbers and types of materials furniture, equipment and people to be placed in each area.

After existing space has been evaluated and alternatives have been considered, a general estimate of required space should be calculated. The librarian should realize target figure, based on projected growth to cite early in the process of selling the need for larger space.

The librarian can make a general estimate of the total amount of space needed for all library activities by calculating the number of seats needed to accommodate users during peak periods. This number is based on 10 percent to 25 percent of the number of potential users. The percentage of potential users may divide into primary users (those who use seats regularly) and secondary users provides adequate seating. For hospitals with extensive teaching commitments, seating 15 percent of heavy users such as students, 10 percent to 25 percent of heavy users such as students, 10 percent of moderate users such as residents, and 1 percent of light users such as social workers or dieticians, may be more realistic.

After the number of seats have been determined. The total is multiplied by 100 to 120 square feet. This estimate usually provides an adequate amount of space for all the furniture, equipment, and materials needed for the entire facility. The formulas for determining the general estimate of total library space follow:

Number of seats	= 10 to 25 percent Potential Primary Users	+1 percent potential secondary Users
Total space for library in sq ft	= No. of seats × 100 to 120 sq ft	

Another type of space estimation involves calculating space needed for broad functions, such as the stack area, seating area, staff area, and core areas. This type of estimate can be prepared fairly quickly using standard formulas. It provides backup for journal estimate, documentation of actual space required and guidance for the architect or space planner.

Stack Area

On the average, 8½ medical periodical volumes can be housed in 1 Square foot of floor space in 7½ foot high stacks, acounting for both stack and aisle space. From 9 to 9½ monographs may be shelved in 1 square foot of floor space. It is a good idea to use the smaller figure (8½ volumes) when calculating space for books and journals to compensate for unestimated growth.

The number of volumes should be calculated based on ten years growth. There are several methods for determining this figure. The simplest is to multiply the number of volumes added during the present year by ten and add this figure to the current volume count. Space needed for the collection is then estimated as follows:

$$\text{Stack area in sq ft} = \frac{\text{Collection size (ten-year projection)}}{8\frac{1}{2}\text{ volumes}}$$

Seating Area

On the average, 30 sq feet per user-seat will provide adequate space for various types of seating, including aisle space around each chair. the librarian should use the number of seats calculated in the general estimate and figure the amount of space needed for seating users as follows:

Seating area in sq ft = No. of seat × 30 sq ft

Staff Area

The formula of 175 sq. feet for the librarian and 150 Sq.feet for other staff members includes space for desks, aisles, equipment, storage and work counters. Space for the staff is then estimated as follows:

Staff area in sq ft = No. of Staff × 150 to 175 sqft

Central Core Areas

Calculating the amount of space needed for central core areas such as the information desk, the card catalog, and the reference section is more involved. For each of these areas, the librarian should make a list of the furniture, materials, and equipment that must be accommodated, omitting seating and working surface for users that may be provided in the reference and index area or the journal display area. Then a drawing should be made of each area. Areas should be drawn independently of each other. Two drawings should be made of each area. Areas should be drawn independently of each other. To draw to scale, the librarian should use graph paper and a scale of 1 : 48 (¼ inch = 1 ft) or 1:24 (½ inch = 1 ft). To accommodate a walkway, one half of a three-foot aisle space should be allowed on at least two sides of each area. The space needed for core areas can be estimated as follows:

Core areas in sq ft = Sum of sq ft for each core area

Trade-offs and space saving may occur later when the librarian makes a detailed estimate of allocated space.

Entrance and Information Circulation Desk Area

The librarian can include entrance space or "traffic" space for users in the estimate of space needed in front of the information desk, Usually six to eight feet is allowed for this "milling room." The size of the information desk, space for staff seating behind the desk, as well as shelving should also be included.

Current Journal Display Area

If the librarian is using standard 90-inch high steel stacks with 36-inch wide sections 10-inches deep, 25 issues can be displayed on 5 slanted display shelves. A maximum of five shelves is recommended for easier reach. The librarian should also allow for one-half of a 4 foot aisle, or 2 feet in front of each display, for standing and passing.

Card Catalog and Dictionary Area

The number of books projected for the collection, and therefore the number of cards to be filed determines the size of the catalog case needed. A standard 17 inch tray will provide 14 inches of net filing space. If filled to 72 percent capacity, such a drawer will hold 1,000 cards averaging 1/100 inch in thickness. The librarian should figure an average of five cards per title. A collection of 1,000 books would require five drawers. Addtional space can be added for a consulting table, a large dictionary on a stand, and space for standing and passing

Audiovisual Area

Audiovisuals should be kept in an area near the circulation desk. Many librarians standard stack sections comprised of shelves 10 to 12 inches dep the most flexible space for softward. Since library holdings of these materials are so varied, as in the format and the method of storing them. No standard measures have yet been developed. Growth projections can be based on present growth rates. Seating estimates are included in the previous estimate for seating.

Photocopy Area

When estimating space for the photocopy area, the librarian should include the following items: the photocopy machine, additional work space on either side of the machine, a book truck, a counter for stapling and cutting copies, a supply cabinet, and space for a large wastebasket.

Computer Terminals

Space for a computer terminal, a chair, and shelves also needs to be estimated. The drawing, should represent "ideal space". Later one, the librarian should locate this function in the most convenient place for staff and users, such as at the information desk or in the librarians office.

Book Trucks

Finally, estimate the number of book trucks needed and calculate the space required to park them when not in use. Small trucks are about 1½ feet wide by 2½ feet long. Large trucks ar 3 feet long by 1½ feet wide.

Totaling Area Estimates

After space requirements have been estimated for the stack area, the seating area, the staff area, and core areas, the estimates should be totalled and compared with the general estimate of space. The results should be fairly similar. If not, the librarian should examine both estimates to make sure that the projected requirements have been analyzed thoroughly. To compensate for wasted space that may be caused by the idiosyncracies or the configuration of the actual assigned space, the librarian can add a 6 percent configuration loss to the estimate. If the general estimate remains much larger than the estimate by area function, the formula chosen for the general estimate may be more generous than is appropriate for this facility.

Making a Detailed Space Estimate

When approval of new space becomes certain, the librarian will want to make detailed calculations of the space needed for materials, furniture, equipment, and people. This estimate should include space for each activity and each item to be accommodated in the new space. Specific space allocations for types of seats, such as lounge chairs or a chair at a carrel, should also be included.

The librarian must be very precise when making a detailed space estimate, since an architect or space planner will be using it to design a floor plan. When the floor plan is completed, the architect will check it against the detailed space estimate for errors or overlooked items.

Central Core Areas

For each of the central core areas. First describe the function and list all materials, furniture, seats, and equipment that will be needed. Then specific measurements should be determined for each item and the total calculated. At this point, possible placement and spatial relationships should be considered.

Stack Area

The function of the stack area should be described in the detailed estimate. The librarian should also list the number of materials, furniture, and equipment needed, such as bound journals and number of carrels for users. If audiovisuals are to be stored in the stacks, they need to be included, as well as the special carrels to accommodate equipment. The area required to house the stacks, aisles, and carrels should be drawn to scale and also estimated in number of square feet.

Shelving

The number of linear feet of shelving required must be determined. Since many journal volumes measure as high as 12 inches, only 6 of the 7 shelves in a 90-inch shelves, this provides 18 linear feet per stack section. In order to allow space for shifting, shelf space is considered at full capacity when it is 86 percent filled. Therefore, in a section for journals with 18 linear feet, 86 percent reduces the space to 15 linear feet and accommodates about 75 volumes at 5 per linear feet and accommodates about 75 volumes at 5 per linear foot. If 84-inch high stacks with six shelves are used, then only 5 may be usable. At 13 linear feet, 65 journal volumes can be accommodated at 5 per linear foot.

When calculating the linear feet of shelving required, use the standard of five volumes per linear foot for books and bound journal volumes. This provides a flexible estimate to accommodate unforeseen changes in the growth of the collection. Stacks usually measure 12 inches in depth for a single stack or 24 inches for a double. A stack 10 inches in depth is sufficient for both journals and books and can save four inches of aisle space. A 36-inch aisle between stacks is a comfortable width and allows wheelchairs to enter and exit but not turn. Minimum stack aisle width for wheelchairs is 33 inches (10:221). A stack using 12-inch "5 feet on center", this is the dimension from the center of one double stack across the aisle to the center of the next. Such measurement reveals the depth of both the shelves and the aisle. A stack using 10-inch shelves with a 33-inch aisle is described as measuring "4 feet 5 inches on center

Carrels

Carrels should be 48 inches wide 24 inches deep to accommodate bulky materials. Using a carrel 42 inches wide to save space is acceptable. Backup space for chair and user requires three feet for comfort. Carrels for audiovisual equipment should be 30 inches deep and 60 inches wide. Aisles between the carrels and stacks should be a minimum of 36 inches.

Floor Specifications

The capacity of the floor to bear the weight of the stacks filled with heavy volumes is the most important determinant in the effective use of space in a hospital library. Floors must be able to support 150 pounds of live load per square foot. Because most hospital floors are built to support a live load of about 70 pounds per square foot, this requirement often presents a problem for hospitals and may severely restrict suitable locations for the library. A building must be able to support dead load and live load. Dead load refers to the weight of the elements in the structure, such as steel, wood, and concrete. The live load refers to the elements that can be moved around in the building, such as furnishings and people.

The ability of the floor to bear the weight of stacks can only be determined by a structural engineer. The formulas presented for space assume 3-foot aisles between stacks that require a live load capacity of 150 pounds. Compact shelving requires 300 pounds. Reinforcing the weight-bearing capacity of the floor is very costly, but it provides a more flexible use of the space. Using wider aisles between the stacks reduces the amount of weight per sq.foot, but it will increase the amount of total space needed.

Staff Work Area

Each work station should have two work surfaces 30 inches by 60 inches and 124 inches by 60 inches, spanned on one side by a counter for a typewriter or computer terminal. If there is to be a separate librarians office, it should have space for two visitors chairs and perhaps space for two visitors chairs and perhaps space for a terminal with necessary work surface and a users chair. Office shelving should be generous. Storage cabinets should be no deeper than 24 inches over work counters of the same depth.

Special space in work areas should also be designated for receiving and processing mail, for holding cartons of books or bound journals on the floor, for a large waste basket, for an exit door to the corridor, for book trucks, for a sink and a refrigerator and for a coat closet.

Comparing Estimates and Making Trade-offs

When totaling the space estimated in detail for core areas, stack area and work areas, add a 6 percent configuration loss to it. The detailed space estimate should be compared to the two other estimates already prepared.

A Library Space Programme

The space or building programme is the standard document used in planning libraries. The document can be used for the following multiple purposes:

- To assist in developing initial planning concepts
- To help in the process of analyzing space needs
- To organize all the details throughout layout, construction and moving.
- To provide an excellent reference source for all planning details.
- To provide a persuasive document for all to read and evaluate
- To determine the essential needs of the library and encourage all concerned to acknowledge them
- To form the basis on which the architect can plan a satisfying facility

The space programme document functions as an outline of space requirements as well as a planning and marketing tool throughout the entire process.

The space programme presents objective facts and figures about users, staff, services, and the collection, as well as specific estimates of space required. These elements should be related to the philosophy of the library and its environment. The programme should be well organized and succinct so that it can be read easily and quickly. If the document is more than a few pages, the highlights should be summarized on the first page. A table of contents should also be provided. The following elements may be addressed in the library space programme.

Goals and objectives These should relate to the goals of the hospital.

Setting or environment This section describes the hospital user groups, the libray programmes, the library's role in the community, cooperative arrangments with local libraries, and participation in library networks.

Present conditions This section describes space problemmes, action taken to alleviate programs, and changes in use of library servicesw. It also provides statistics to indicate incrase or decrease in use.

Changes needed This section describes what need to be done, and why, to support changes in projected increase of users and services, or changes in hospital programmes.

Consequences if changes are not implemented This section includes a description of reductions in collection size, services to be limited, or number of users who won't be seated.

Profile of potential users This section lists the number of projected users by category of job status and by level of use. The profile may analyze and list users as primary and secondary users, or as heavy, moderate, or light users. It also calculates the number of seats required for users and estimates the general space required.

Estimate of space required This section provides the general estimate of space based on a percentage of potential users, as well as a detailed estimate with capacity for users, collection furniture, and staff in each area of activity.

Location This section describes factors to be considered, such as an open square or rectangular shaped space with no interior weight-bearing walls; floor load capacity per square foot of weight (150 pounds for libraries as compared to 70 pounds for patient care areas); quick and easy access; future expansion possibilities, and protection from water damage and excess noise and odours. Also included are discussions of feasible locations and possible trade-offs.

Design Considerations

Design influences people's behaviour, and thereby, affects the use of space. Planning major alternations of space requires knowledge of how people feel about space, how much distance between people need for comfort and security, and how people react within a given space. Application of these principles contributes to the efective design of space for different activities.

Private, secure and quiet work space encourages concentration. To provide this kind of space, place individual carrels at right angles to the wall so that the user is enclosed on three sides. This offers privacy and also reduces noise.

The way people use space or behave in it is also governed by the appearance or the aesthetic of the space. This principle is easily observable in restaurants. Bright colors around the information and the study area will provide a quiet, soothing environment. A library should be functional, comfortable, and attractive. Ideally, these elements should be in balance.

Design, Furniture and Flooring for Specific Areas

Library space should be flexible and should allow for the adequate operation of primary library functions. Non-assignable space-such as rest rooms, janitors closets, stairs, or corridors-should be located outside the library space. Heating, ventilation, lighting, floor load capacity, and ceiling heights should remain consistent throughout the space. In furnishings, the librarian should avoid built-in cabinets or bookcases, decorative walls, and planters in order to maintain the greatest flexibility for future change. The ideal shape for library space is the square or rectangle. It is the most workable and space-saving. If this shape is not possible, the librarian can apply the concept of the central square to the areas of heaviest user activity, the core areas, and the place most likely to change. This makes the central square the focal point of the library where people and activities coverge. Although an architect or designer designs the floor layout, librarians should review these decisions to be sure that they are functional.

Spatial Relationships

The arrangement of areas and how they relate to each other is an important consideration in the design of the floor plan. The librarian and the designer should discuss the function of each area, the relationship of each area to other areas, and the traffic flow of users and staff from area to area.

This is essential before any floor layout for new space is planned.

Areas that are frequently used for a short period of time and are monitored by staff should be located in the central core. In libraries managed by one person, it is best to arrange the core areas in a sequence to facilitate efficiency and quicker service to users, Activities that require concentration for longer periods of time should be placed away from the busy center core area.

Entrance and Exit Areas

The layout of the library should be visible as the user steps through the door. For purposes of control, there should be only one door that serves as both the entrance and the exit. Fire exits are necessary, but they can be fitted with special locks so the doors can be opened easily in emergencies

Information and Circulation Desk

The information and circulation desk should be adjacent to the entrance for both convenience and control of library materials. The most comfortable desk for both users and staff has a counter at standing height on the users side and a desk of seating height on the staff side. The desk can be bought commercially or can be designed by the architect to fit a particular situation. Working surfaces should be covered with a synthetic, nonshining laminate for durability. Bookcases can be constructed from sections of the same steel shelving used in the stacks and can be placed behind the desk. Uniform shelving used throughtout the library provides greater flexibility for future changes.

Card Catalog

The card catalog should be located close to the information desk so that the staff can easily consult it or assist users with it. Catalog drawers should be purchased with a guarantee on construction. A flat surface on or next to the catalog should be provided for the placement of tools, such as the Mesh, journals holdings list, and scrap paper. The surface can also be used for the placement of the catalogy drawer when referring to the cards at greater length.

Reference Books and Journal Indexes

Reference books and journal indexes are usually located near the information desk on steel shelving. A flat or slightly sloped counter hug on shelving at seating height is useful for consulting current indexes or reference sources. Because indexes are consulted for a short time only, stools or typing chairs on casters make good seats for this activity.

If the volume of library use warrants a reference desk for the librarian as well as an information circulation desk, a conventional office desk can be placed at a right angle to a section of the reference shelving. This forms an adequate reference center. A computer terminal for bibliographic searching can be placed here also if electrical and telephone outlets are available. Locating reference activity in full sight of users encourages the use of these services and is more convenient for a small staff.

Journal Display

The display of current journal issues should be located in the central core or square, visible from the information desk. Steel shelving with fixed slanted display shelves is most appropriate because it allows users to recognize the issue quickly by it cover, it also displays only the most current issues. Keeping the other unbound issues on the shelves with the bound issues is less confusing and more convenient for the user.

Photocopy Area

The librarian may find it helpful to set up the photocopy area close to the information desk so that staff can assist users and quickly service the machines. Special sound absorbing divider panels can be used along with book shelves to muffle the noise. The area should be well ventilated and equipped with special electrical outlets. Other items essential to the area are counter space for collating and stapling copies, a book truck for library materials, strong

for machine paper and toner, and a very large wastebasket.

Audiovisual Area

The audiovisual equipment and software should also located near the information desk so that staff can easily help users with equipment. Special carrels with high privacy screens, earphones, and electrical outlets are essential for using portable equipment efficiently. Built in audiovisual equipment cores in these carrels are not practical. They restrict use and in time become obsolete if space is available, the librarian can set up small rooms for group use of audiovisuals.

The audiovisual area can be part of the stack area, or it can be screened off with shelving. If it is included in the stack area, software should be stored on the shelves closets to the information desk. The carrels should also be placed near the desk.

Miscellaneous Items in Core Area

The following items should be considered for the core area: a dictionary stand, a wall telephone with a small shelf, a pencil sharpener, bulletin boards, book stack wastebaskets, coat racks, a book return clocks step stools, and fire extinguishers.

Seating Facilities

The librarian will want to provide a variety of seating facilities to accommodate an assortment of library activities; quick consultation, relaxed reading, group study, and concentrated study. Although a variety of seating should be provided, about 60 percent of all seating should be in carrels for concentrated study. To facilitate study, several components should be included in carrels; a shelf, a lamp, and a writing surface with a light-colour matte finish to reflect the light.

Arrangement of carrels is important. The placement of carrels in a row at right angles to the wall, facing in the same direction, helps to maintain a quiet area free of distractions, Back-to-a shelf, a lamp, and writing surface with a light-colour matte finish to reflect the light.

Back-to-back or clover leaf arrangement is conducive to concentration. Carrels placed facing the wall are often the last to be used. This arrangement exposes the users back, reducing privacy and visual control of the space around the user.

Tables absorb space in the library and should be used sparingly. A four-chair table may only seat one or two people when the chairs are less used for belongings, or when books and papers are spread out over the entire surface of the table. Therefore, only a few tables should be provided for consultation or short-term study. Group study rooms are a wise alternative to group study at tables. They can accommodate four to six people. If the room is equipped with outlets, audiovisuals can be used. A bare white wall makes an effective projection screen.

Chairs should be sturdy enough to withstand tipping . The librarian should sit in the chair before approving a selection, chairs with arms must fit under tables and carrel surfaces often it is better to pay more for a chair that guarantees durability. Sturdiness, fit, and comfort are more important than look or design. Lounge chairs add to the comfort and look of the library. They are appropriate as long as their size is proportional to the space available. Sturdy coffee tables provide a place for newspapers or journal issues and are a practical accompaniment to lounge chairs.

Shelving

Standard steel shelving provides versatility, especially when supplementary components are added, such as slanted journal display shelves, working surfaces for carrels or index consultation, slotted shelves with dividers for audiovisual software or journal issues, and coat racks that fit the standard brackets. The base of the steel shelving stack may vary in depth from 10 inches to 24 inches; the wider base prevents tipping of a free standing stack. The 10-inch base saves aisle space. The stack ranges can be braced to provide stability. It is best to avoid built-in shelving or alcoves of counter-height shelving. Freestanding, braced, double-faced stacks are preferred. They provide a uniform, clean and simple shelf agreement for users and make an effective sound barrier for study carrels.

Staff Work Area

The best location for the work area is behind the information-circulation desk. The work area should be enclosed by sound proof walls and a door with a glass panel. A pannel is preferrable to a glass wall because the wall exposes too much activity and makes it too tempting for staff to work in the offices rather than at the information desk.

The work area should be furnished with standard office furniture. Each work station should have at least two work surfaces and special counters or tables for typewriters and computer terminals. Steel shelving sections and a counter for preparing journals for binding area necessary items. Near the workroom exit to the main books, and supplies. Floor space should also be available for holding and receiving cartons of binding. Other important items that should be included in the work room are a small sink, counter space for a coffeepot, a coat closet, and large wastebaskets.

Staff work areas and offices should be comfortable, well-organized, and well-ventilated to support effective, productive performance. Plan for generous work surfaces, storage areas, and shelving space. To be prepared for future changes, extra space should be planned for at least one additonal staff member.

Carpeting

Carpet is the best material for sound absorption. It can be cleaned cheaply, and it is easy to maintain. If possible,carpet should be placed in every area of the library, Nylon or another synthetic with a low cut or loop pile and antistatic qualities is preferable to wool, which is very expensive, Carpet should be glued to the floor without padding. This gives the carpet longer wear and allows book trucks to roll more easily. If new space is planned, it is easier and cheaper to lay the carpet first and then place the stacks over it, if new carpet is to be placed in the existing space, it is easier to cut the carpet to fit around the stacks than to remove the books and the stacks to lay the carpet.

Colour Considerations

Selecting a colour scheme is important in the design of a new library. People are affected by colour, but their reactions are diverse. The use of primary colors, for example, attracts some people and repels others. Conversely, subdued tones may be oppressive to some people and soothing to others. Therefore, it is important to create an environment comfortable for most.

Choosing colours for the most effective impact requires an expert–an arachitect, an interior designer, or furniture sales person.

When selecting colours, it is best to start with the colour of the large area first-the walls. The choice of an off-white colour for the walls is the most popular solution to the problem of various colour tastes. The next area, the carpet, should have colour variations. Tweed provides such a variation and will hide dirt or lint. The ceiling should be white or a light shade so that light can be reflected effectively. Bright splashes of color can be used on small walls or on stack ends as long as the colours are kept uniform throughout the library. A mild colour should be selected for areas of concentrated study. In areas of high activity such as the information desk, the librarian can use stronger colours.

Color selections for fabrics, paints, carpets, and wood finishes should all be matched under the light and on the surface where they are to be used.

Lighting, Power, Acoustics, Heating and Cooling Systems

Adequate lighting, heating and cooling systems, and acoustics should be properly planned. The present level for overall lighting requires a higher level of illumination, from 50 to 100 feet candles depending on the detail of the work and the duration. For concentracted tasks, desk lamps provide more flexible lighting to satisfy the variations in users' needs. These lamps are more expensive to install but save energy in the long run. It is important that lighting be well diffused and that sharp contracts be avoided.

The rapid increase in the use of microform readers, slide-tape machines, photocopy machines, and computer terminals in hospital libraries has created the need for many electrical outlets and separate telephone lines. The most flexible arrangement is to install conduits through which cables can be run to provide electrical, telephone, and communication outlets as the needs arise. This capability is particularly important if the library is to have long-range flexibility in its power system.

Tolerance for noise in a library varies. In general, intermittent noise can be masked by constant noise or "White Sound" at a level of 40 to 50 decibles. This sound is more easily tolerated than even complete silence. It provide a measure of acoustical privacy, and is often provided by the heating-ventilation-air-conditioning system (HVAC). The absorption of sound by books, soft materials, and acoustical panels should be considered, as well as user and staff traffic patterns, in reducing noise levels. Walls and ceilings can be constructed to minimize sound transmission, and carpeting can be used on the floor to provide a 50 percent quieter environment than other types of flooring.

The same HVAC system that serves the hospital proper should serve the library.

Graphics

A new or refurnished library requires new and well-designed graphics to guide users in their search for resources. Signs should be posted to identify particular areas in the library, indicate direction, provide "how to" information, and mark contents of stack sections and reference shelves.

The librarian can enlist the aid of staff to plan for signs and their locations. The admistration may suggest in house help and advice on making the signs. The librarians can also consult an architect for assistance. If signs must be made by library staff, the following suggestions should be helpful.

Establishing a Consistent Format

Consistent size and colour of signs presents a unified appearance and enables users to recognize them as location and informational aids throughout the library. All messages should be kept clear and concise. Keep the number of signs to a minimum. Too many signs clutter the library and are ineffective. The use of strong contrasting colours-light and dark or warm and cool-on an off-white or neutral background will draw attention to the signs. Maps, on the other hand, provide more information in less space and inform the user of the relative locations of the rest of the collection. Keeping the same simple typeface for all signs creates consistency.

Moving the Library

Careful planning, organizing, and effective delegation of responsibility will make the library move a success. Planning the move and executing it should be a team effort. The librarian should prepare for the move by weeding the collection, taking inventory, and then measuring the collection for total current linear feet.

Looking Ahead

Rapidly changing technology and the subsequent increases in library services can cause a carefully organized ten-year plan for space to be inadequate within five years. Automation requires more space for equipment and necessitates an increase in staff as the service grows is sophistication.

To accommodate change, new space should be evaluated within one year. As service grows, space problems can be documented and reviewed periodically for necessary solutions.

At the end of a five-year period, the space can be reevaluated again. Thus, planning for the use of space becomes a continuous process that ensures efective use of space and secures the availability of new or additional space when needed.

Service for Patients

Patients have a basic need for library services that goes beyond the information needs the experience as healthy members of their communities. They need information on how to interact with the health care system, on their specific conditions and how to deal with them, and on community resources they might use after leaving the hospital.

The patients library prvides and makes accessible adequate library materials and services to patients of all ages which will assist in their rehabilitation or adjustment to their illness and /or handicapping conditions.

These standards imply the necessity for an established patients library as a basis for service to patients. Full scale patients library programme, with staffing and budgetary support is imperative. Patients are becoming active participants in the process of the consumer movement and are asking for information about their treatment. The library can offer much in the field of health education and information for patients. Libraries can provide various levels of support for health information and patient education programmes in the hospital.

Published information on patient education has expanded rapidly over the past serval years. Continuing education for patient educators is another area in which libraries can be involved. The growing body of educational material for staff members on patient teaching is a resource that should not be overlooked. The sources of patient education materials include commercial publishers, voluntary health organisations, pharmaceutical companies, professional health organisations, and individual health care delivery programmes.

To meet patients needs for health information competently, the resources of the library must be well developed in several areas. A collection of health information materials designed for the lay person and coordinated with the hospitals programmes is of primary importance.

FURTHER READING

1. Jana Bradley: Hospital Library Managment Medical Library Association In. Chicago, 1983.
2. Jacqueline Bastille: Planning Library Facilities. In Bradley J (Ed): Hospital Library Management Medical Library Asssociation, Chicago, 1983.
3. Martin RR: Library and Health information Services for Patients. In Bradley J (Ed): Hospital Library Management Medical Library Association, Chicago, 1983.

36 Planning a District Hospital

The planning and design of a hospital is a systematic process, which involves stages moving progressively from the macro-level of epidemiological surveys of the needs and demands of populations in catchment areas to the micro-level of a specific space in a building designed for a particular function or human activity. It is a multi-disciplinary activity that requires the active participation of professionals in various roles; it also requires continual interaction between the users and the professionals who are to translate functional requirements into physical forms.

At the earliest stage, what can be called a *needs assessment team* sits around the table and establishes an overall plan of the needs, the range of services to be provided, the target population or catchment area, the financial feasibility of the project and the scale of the hospital.

The table changes composition as the briefing team moves in to prepare the key document—the design brief—which translates the requirements into functions, activities, space distribution programmes and relationships and all the other information necessary for design.

The *design team,* consisting of all the people involved in designing, the physical facilities, pools the expertise of its members to produce the instruments for implementing construction, starting from preliminary and development designs and ending in the production of technical specifications, tendering documents and detailed working drawings.

The *construction team* implements the design from the approved drawings and technical specifications within the prescribed time and cost, and produces the physical facility.

The *commissioning team* staffs the hospital, commissions and procures the equipment, furniture and supplies and prepares it for operation.

By the end of the project, a multitude of people will have sat around the table and made their contributions to the project as part of the *planning team.*

In each of the stages that comprises the planning and design process, each member of the team has a role to play:

- The *health planner* establishes the need for the hospital, its role in the community and the services it will offer.
- The *functional planner* establishes the functioning of the different departments and of the hospital as a whole.
- The *financial planner* establishes the financial feasibility of the project.

Table 36.1. : Calculation of the area required for the collection of laboratory specimens

Daily demand	In the outpatient department 60% of referred patients require examination with collection of laboratory specimens 40% bring a specimen from home. • Specimen collection work is done for 1.5 hrs in the morning for outpatients. 14 collections per hr. area performed, each patient requires approximately 1.5 specimens per examination, and each patient stay half an hour for the collection.
Example.	Population 100,000 • 1.5 per 1000 require laboratory tests, 60% of them need specimen collection. • 150 beds mean 75 patients requiring laboratory tests; 20% of these must go to the laboratory for collection of specimen. • 150 outpatients × 60% = 90 patients requiring examination with collection of specimen. • 75 inpatients × 20% = 15 patients requiring examination with collection of specimen. • Total (90 + 15) 105 patients requiring collection of specimen. • Each patient is estimated to require 1.5 specimen collections. 105 × 1.5 = 157 specimen collections. • The specimen collecting section works 1.5 hrs in the morning and performs 14 collections per hr per cubicle. $\frac{157}{14 \times 1.5} = 8$ cubicles • 20% of the cubicles should be equipped for collecting vaginal specimens and have an area of approximately 9 m^2 each, the rest can be 2 m^2 each. • Net total specimen collection area: 20% of 8 = 2 cubicles of 9 m^2 each = 18 m^2 6 cubicles of 2 m^2 each = 12 m^2 Net total cubicles 30 m^2 Work area 50% 15 m^2 Net total specimens area 45 m^2 • Additional calculation for waiting-room. • 90 patients come from outpatient department and require examination with specimen collection, 50% come acompanied = 135 persons. • 135 persons who are dealt with in 2 shifts. • 15 patients come from inpatient department and are dealt with in 2 hours. • Outside waiting room 135 persons/2 shifts = 68 persons per shift at peak operating rate. • Inside waiting space for 15 patients = 15/2 = 8 patients, generally in wheel-chairs. • Each outpatient reaquires 1.00m^2 of waiting space; 68 patients require 68 m^2 of outside waiting area. • Each inpatient requires 1.5 m^2 of waiting area; 8 pateints require 12 m^2 of inside waiting area.

- The *physical planner* establishes the relation of the hospital to the town and the community that it serves.
- The *architect and* the engineering consultants provide professional planning, design and supervision of construction.
- The *builder/contractor* produces the hospital in its physical form using materials, labor and construction equipment.
- The *procurement staff* and the personnel staff form part of the commissioning team, which prepares the hospital for operation by procuring material and recruiting staff.
- The *client/user* is the owner and final user of the hospital.

These people assume either active or consultative roles at the planning table, depending on the task at hand. Table 1 gives a simplified version of

Table 36.2. : Calculation of the space required for medical record files for the outpatient and emergency departments

Data to be considered	*Example*
Size of medical record file	30 cm × 40 cm × 1 cm
Size of shelving (no. of shelves)	Shelves must be 40 cm deep. The height of the file allows for record cases 7 shelves high
• Number of medical histories per linear metre of record case (no. of medical histories per metre × no. of shelves)	• 100 × 7 = 700
Outpatient department	
• Number of consulting rooms	• 15
• Number of consultations per day per consulting room	• 15
• Number of cosultations per year (no. of consulting rooms × no. of cpd. per cr × no. of working days)	• 15 × 30 × 300 = 135,000 (rounded up to 140,000)
• Proportion of consultations leading to a new medical history file	• 20%
• New medical history files per year	• $\frac{140{,}000 \times 20}{100} = 28{,}000$
Emergency Department	
• Case load	• 10% of outpatient department = 14,000
• Proportion of emergency cases leading to a new medical history file	• 20%
• New medical history files per year	• $\frac{14{,}000 \times 20}{100} = 2800$
Outpatient and Emergency Departments together	
• Total new files per year	• 28,000 + 2800 = 30,800
• No. of years records kept in file	• 5
• Total number of files on shelves	• 30,800 × 5 = 154,000 (rounded up to 160,000)
• Linear metres of record cases needed	• $\frac{160{,}000}{700} = 228$
• Surface needed for the medical records room	Approximately 228 m^2

the stages and their corresponding inputs and outputs and the role of working professionals at each stage. It is important to note that the engineering services should be planned jointly with the layout, so that the final result is the logical outcome that meets the needs of the actual users of the hospital, offering the best available health care services to the population commensurate with the cost.

Preparation of the Design Brief

The design brief is a key document: it is the written expression of the client's needs, as expressed in consultation with various professionals, including the architect and engineers. It is important because 'a good design is based on a good brief' and 'a good brief is rich soil in which to grow a good design.' The brief should provide the following information about the hospital and its parts of units:

1. Functional content: size and content of departments, such as number of operating theatres, number of beds in wards.
2. Philosophy of service: what the departments will and will not do.
3. Workload: what hours the hospital departments will work, the shifts, maintenance time, overtime.
4. Planning principles: policies and procedures of the hospital with regard to:

Table 36.3: Stages in planning and designing a hospital

Stage	*Task*	*Input*	*Output*	*Working team*	
				Active	*Consultative*
One	Establish demand for new hospital or for hospital expansion	Information Indicators Projections	Decision to construct renovate, expand	User/ Client Planners	
Two	Prepare design brief	Services to be delivered Functional scale of hospital Functional	Design brief Client	User/ Engineers	Arichitect/
Three	Design	Design brief Additional data from consultants	Design of hospital Working documents	Architect/ Engineers	User/ Client
Four	Construction	Design of hospital Working drawings	Hospital in physical form	Architect Builder Engineers	User/ Client
Five	Commissioning	List of staff List of furniture List of equipment List of supplies	Appointment and training of staff Procurement of furniture, equipment, sup	User/Client Procurement staff Personnel staff	

- patient movement
- staff movement
- supply delivery
- disposal of used goods
- laundry service
- food service
- domestic services.

5. Staff: number and types of staff, peak periods of work.
6. Functional relationships: between departments, between rooms within a department.
7. Environmental factors and engineering: hospital policies with regard to:
   - fire protection
   - electrical supply (mains and stand-by)
   - sterilizing and sterile supply
   - security
   - hot-and cold-water supplies
   - heating and ventilation
   - lighting
   - medical gases and vacuum
   - emergency alarm system
   - other engineering services
   - landscaping and pollution control
8. Schedule of accomodations: list of all rooms and spaces in each department, type and number of occupants, sizes and activities performed in them:
9. Financial aspects
   a. Costs: budget, or programmed amounts, to include:
      - construction (a major budget item)
      - professional services (architects, engineers)
      - construction/project management services
      - fixed equipment
      - furniture and movable equipment
      - extra-utilities, if necessary
      - professional procurement and installation of equipment
      - site investigation and development, including purchase of land
      - insurance, for the fire and other liabilities required during construction

- legal counsel
- taxes, customs duty and other statutory charges
- contingencies, for unforeseen situations.

b. Possible sources of funds:
- Central Government
- gifts, donations or grants
- money generated by hospital activities prior to construction
- money to be repaid from future hospital activities

The following is a sample format and checklist of the contents of a typical design brief for a district hospital:

1. Introduction
   a. Background, project initiative
   b. Project funding, source
   c. Philosophy of service; service development plans
   d. Organization
   e. Other.
2. Site information
   a. Physical description: bearings, boundaries, topography, surface area
   b. Land use in adjoining areas
   c. Any limitations of the site that would affect planning
   d. Maps of vicinity and landmarks or centres
   e. Existing utilities
   f. Nearest city, port, airport
   g. Rainfall and data on weather and temperatures.
3. Policies for hospital operation: concepts on a general level, with implications at specific levels, such as:
   - patient movement
   - staff movement
   - delivery of supplies
   - disposal of used goods
   - laundry services
   - food services
   - domestic services
   - security
   - engineering services
   - fire protection
   - emergency alarm system
4. Zoning: grouping of departments according to zoning principles.
5. Departmental requirements: separate consideration for each department should include:
   a. Description of functions and facilities
      - procedures, operational policies
      - schedule of accomodation
      - list of rooms
      - suggested area; critical dimensions, if any
   b. Qualitative parameters
      – location, relationship to other rooms, services and departments
      – use
        - function of or activities carried out in room
        - space requirements for activities, when critical
        - numbers of staff and/or patients using room at one time
        - wheeled traffic
        - goods or materials
        - special uses and work flow
        - occupancy or time in use
      – constraints
        - privacy
        - supervision
        - security
        - separation
        - fire protection
      – environement
        - wind direction
        - lighting, natural and artificial
        - heat, humidity, sterility
        - cold, room heating
        - sound (acceptable noise levels)
        - ventilation
      – fittings, fixtures and equipment (fixed and movable)
      – loads on serviceds
        - electrical
        - heating
        - ventilation and air-conditioning
        - hot water

c. Functional relationships and physical proximities
   - closeness matrices
   - bubble diagrams
   - activity analyses, traffic movements.
d. Flexibility and future expansion: possibility of future growth, with schedule.

6. Cost of project, other financial aspects (in terms of capital and recurring costs)
   a. financing scheme
   b. cost limitations for each aspect of the project (working budget)
   c. priorities for phasing, if necessary
   d. expected flow of funding with time

Designing from the Brief

It is at this important stage that abstract ideas are translated into concrete physical facilities. In essence, the designer gains an understanding of the activities and their sequence and pictures people performing the activities; with these in mind, the designer creates the working environment, translating invisible ideas to visible spaces formed by the process of design.

Location

One of the most effective ways of determining the location of a new facility is to use a *base map* of the district and vicinity, on which one can enter, translate and compare data, facts and information. A basic mapping exercise is the first step in locating the positions of existing facilities; a graphical analysis of data on where patients come from can be used to determine the areas of influence and service of those facilities.

Service Catchment Area

The catchment area for a health facility is determined by several factors:

- Politico-administrative boundaries are usually the strongest determinant, as they set defined area and imply an established organization which directs, manages and operates the affairs of the population within its jurisdiction. In most countries, the hierarchy of physical facilities parallels that of the politico-administrative organization, so that a particular level of facility is under the jurisdiction of an equivalent level of the politico-administratrive unit throughout the country.
- Geographic boundaries are *natural physical barriers* to population movement and can therefore, also be strong determinants *of catchment areas* . Mountain ranges and bodies of water, for instance, deter cross-movement. People may cross politico-administrative boundaries to reach a facility, however, if they are deterred by a natural barrier within their own district. Geographic boundaries are often formalized into politico-administrative boundaries as a natural consequence of the development of ethnic, cohesive or homogeneous cultures on either side.
- *Time boundaries,* although invisible, *determine catchment areas* in regions without roads and easy means of transport. Populations gravitate towards the facilities that are most easily accessible, that is, the facility they can get to in the shortest time. The factor of geography also contributes to this situation, as difficult terrain takes longer to negotiate.

Factors to be considered in locating a district hospital are as follows.

- It should be within 15-30 minute travelling time. In a district with good roads and adequate means of transport, this would mean a service zone with a radius of about 25 km.
- It should be grouped with other institutional facilities, such as religious, educational (school), tribal (cultural) and commercial (market) centres.
- It should be free from dangers of flooding; it must therefore not be sited at the lowest point of the district.
- It should be in an area free of pollution of any kind, including air, water and land pollution.

- It must be serviced by public utilities: water, sewage and storm-water disposal, electricity, gas and telephone. In areas where such utilities are not available, substitutes must be found, such as a deep wall for water, generators for electricity and radio communication for telephone.

Site Selection

In the case of either site selection or evaluation of adaptability, the following items must be considered: size, topography, drainage, soil conditions, utilities available, natural features and limitations.

The site must be large enough for all the planned functional requirements to be met and for any expansion envisioned within the coming 10 years. Recommended standards vary from 1.25 to 4 ha per 100 beds; the following minimum requirements have been proposed:

25-bed capacity – 2 ha (800 m^2 per bed)
100-bed capacity – 4 ha (400 m^2 per bed)
200-bed capacity – 7 ha (350 m^2 per bed)
300-bed capacity – 10 ha (333 m^2 per bed)

These areas are for the hospital buildings only excluding the area needed for staff housing. For smaller hospitals, single-storey construction generally results in lower building cost, less reliance on expensive mechanical services and lower running and maintenance costs. Thus, hospitals up to 150 beds should be single-storey constructions unless other parameters dictate that they be multistoried.

Topography is a determinant of the distribution of form and space. A flat terrain is the easiest and least espensive to build on. A rolling or sloping terrain is more difficult and more expensive to build on, but the solutions can be interesting and innovative; by using the natural slope of the ground, the drainage and sewage disposal systems can be designed so as to result in lower construction and maintenance costs.

The terrain must allow for easy movement of water away from the site. A high point in the community is ideal.

Whenever possible, a site should be provided with surface openings to storm-water drains, drinage channels or waterways. Storm-water run-off from roads and buildings should be piped to such openings. It is also important to check that the waterways themselves are not subject to flooding and that, in floor condtioins, water will not back up on the hospital site.

The soil conditions are a determinant of foundation schemes. Ideally, the subsoil should be such that conventional, economical structural design and foundation schemes can be used.

Water-logged areas, swamps and former ricefields should be avoided. If no other site is available, however, the following steps must be taken.

When deciding the ground floor level of the buildings, care should be taken to safeguard against temporary flooding of the building in a heavy downpour.

In areas prone to regular flooding, a raised ground floor, which allows for expected peak floods, is essential. Local engineering advice on the possibilities of drainage from a site should be obtained before proceeding with its purchase, when such advice is available (e.g., from records of the local authority or relevant government department). It may also be necessary to perform percolation tests to determine the capacity of the soil to absorb liquids; this is particularly important when sewage must be treated and effluents disposed off on the site.

The soil conditions are a determinant of foundation schemes. Ideally, the subsoil should be such that conventional, economical structural design and foundation schemes can be used.

Water-logged areas, swamps and former ricefields should be avoided. If no other site is available, however, the following steps must be taken:

- Check the bearing capacity of the soil.A sufficient number of test borings or pits must be made so that the engineer can best judge the true sub-surface conditions. The results of this investigation must be submitted in a report that contains detailed recommendations for designing the foundation.

- The bearing capacity of the soil must be confirmed at key point, preferably where major foundation elements or footings are located. Some boreholes should be dug closest to the location of the basement, if any, and to the tallest structure of the building complex, including water reservoirs and the sewage treatment plant.
- Scrap unstable top layers, if necesary, and fill with well-compacted, suitable materials, like clean coarse sand.

Electrical, water and communication lines should be available. If not, generators, deep wells, water pumps and radio communication lines must be established. Health care facilities are quite ineffective if all—whether roads, water supplies and a reliable electrical supply are not available at the site.

Natural Features

Features such as natural lakes and ponds and lush vegetation are not necessarily a disadvantage and can have great potential for enhancing the building design. Building design should respond as much as possible to the site, so that the structure is in contest with the environment: a waterway that bisects a site also generally bisects the building for; this might call for an innovative dedsign solution in which the *building straddles the waterway.*

Solutions can be numerous, involving creativity and innovation, but they should be based on two over-riding considerations: (i) that the design respects and follows the laws of nature; and (ii) that the limitations imposed by the natural features do not detract from the functional performance or cost-effectiveness of the facility.

Master Physical Development

Basic documents consist of written and gaphic description of the site and its features, including:

- the title, which describes the property, the bearings and lengths of the enclosing property lines, surrounding, adjacent properties and roads, the area of the property and its encumbrances, if any;
- the survey plan, which translates into graphic and scaled form the data contained in the title
- the topographic survey, which describes graphically the configuration of the site in terms of topographic lines and shows all the physical features, including trees, fences, buildings and drains;

Before the physical planning and design of a hospital is started, the proposed site must be surveyed and a plan made. The site plan indicates the following:

- the courses and distances of the property lines, including details of party walls and foundations adjacent to the plot lines;
- dimensions and locations of any buildings, structures, easements, right-of-way or encroachments on the site;
- established curb and building lines and curb grades of streets, alleys and sidewalks at or adjacent to the site;
- all existing utility services, including their size and characteristics; the location of all piping mains, sewers, poles, wires, hydrants, manholes, etc., upon or under the site and adjacent to the site;
- official data on which elevations are based and permanent values established on or adjacent to the site;
- information regarding the disposal of sanitary wastes and storm-water and suitability of subsoil for disposal of rainwater and sewage;
- contemplated data and description of any proposed improvements to approaches or utilities adjacent to the site;
- all trees and types of vegetation within the plot; and
- elevations on a horizontal grid system of not more than 6-m interval, indicating changes of slope, to form a basis for a countour map of 50-cm intervals.

Legal Documents

Laws are generalized acts that provide parameters, guidance, supervision, direction and control over all planning and design activities. Rules and regulations implement the provisions of the law; ordinances are local laws refined and elaborated for specific areas of application; building codes embody general policies and standards for building design and construction and the requirements of modern technology to ensure the safety and optimal use, occupancy and maintenance of buildings and other structures.

Some legal documents relevant to planning and design are:

1. *Zoning regulations* With the land-use map, this document ensures that the site selected is in the proper area for the intended use. A planner who estblishes a site in the overall context of the zoning restrictions of the locality paves the way to establishing the following aspects of the project:
   - access and accessibility of the area,
   - catchment area to be served,
   - distance of other facilities and utilities required,
   - easements and rights of way, if any, and
   - sources of materials and of local-skilled and unskilled labor

   The volumetric dimensional limits of the building in terms of site coverage and building height are also dependent on zoning regulations.

   Although such regulations constrain design, they also establish the criteria that help evolve a design that is in context with the overall plan for the community, without disturbing the local ethos and environment.
2. *Building code* The building code of a country is designed to achieve the maximum safety in building construction, to establish standard requirements for the construction of buildings that can withstand powerful earthquakes and other calamities or survive them without undue damage. It contains provisions for:
   - general building requirements,
   - site requirements,
   - permits and inspection requirements,
   - types of construction,
   - fire zoning,
   - fire-resistance requirements,
   - classification and general requirements for all buildings by use or occupancy.light and ventilation,
   - labor safety and welfare during construction,
   - sanitation,
   - general design and construction requirements,
   - electrical and mechanical regulations,
   - use of specific or special materials, such as plastics and glass,
   - design and computation for earthquakes and cyclones, and
   - protection from ionizing radiation from X-ray equipment
3. *Fire code* A fire code is intended to minimize death, injury, loss and damage to property resulting from fire through national guidelines for the prevention and management of fire, by adopting safety standards, incorporating fire safety in design and construction and making provision for protective devices in buildings and structures.
4. *Other codes* Other relevant bylaws, regulations and codes include sanitation codes, environmental protection laws and water codes; these vary in form and content from one country to another. They provide detailed provisions for design and construction. By complying with them, the planner and designer ensure that:
   - the permits and licences necessary for operating the hospital will be obtained,
   - the work is within the national standards for public health and safety.

Operational Policy

The operational policy of a hospital may be developed at both the level of the whole hospital and at the departmental level. Policies at the level of the entire hospital affect all aspects and determine the disposition of the parts of the hospital on the site. They identify groupings of activities that must therefore be zoned together. Departmental level policies affect the internal organization of particular departments within the context of the whole hospital.

A simple checklist for an operational policy is as follows:

1. ***Function***
   a. *Major functions*
      i. Aims and objectives of the services to be provided (mission statement).
      ii. Patients and types.
      iii. Types of illnesses to be treated.
      iv. Activities involved (e.g., reception and documentation, diagnosis and treatment, disposal).
   b. *Minor functions*
      - Other functions contemplated (e.g., teaching, research).
      - People involved (e.g., patients, staff, researchers, students, outside faculty members).
2. ***Scale***
   - *Workload* (e.g., daily number of in-patients treated, of in-patient meals served, of X-rays taken).
   - *Manpower and staffing* needed to meet the workload.
3. ***Organization policy***

- *Patient movement.* The manner in which patients are moved on stretchers, their own beds or wheelchairs affects decisions on circulation routes and spaces, corridor widths and door widths. It also afects decisions on types of vertical routes to be used; whether stairs, lifts or ramps.
- *Staff and staff movement.* The routes taken by the staff from the outside to their places of work, how they arrive and their distribution within the hospital bears on the size and siting of staff areas and amenities, including areas for parking, changing, resting, conference and study.
- *Supply delivery.* A hospital may adopt a centralized system for storage and delivery of supplies. In this case, corridor routes by which supplies are brought from the central store to departments must be of adequate dimensions to accommodate the delivery equipment used, such as trolleys and mechanical pullers. In hospitals that opt for decentralized systems, traffic routes are simpler but a number of sub-supply posts must be provided in different departments or units.
- *Disposal of used goods.* Used goods, especially contaminated ones, very often require design solutions that involve segregation of clean and dirty streams of traffic. Segregation may also involve use of plastic bags or sealed containers, so that clean and dirty streams can use the same corridor.
- *Laundry services.* When laundry is to be undertaken within the hospital, a complete facility must be provided; if it is to be contracted outside the hospital, laundry areas may be limited to a receiving counter for clean supplies and a temporary station for soiled linen to be collected by the outside agency. Provision for washing 'foul' linen may still be necessary.
- *Food services.* A centralized kitchen from which food is brought directly to patients will be large, and centralized food management will mean that the movement of large food trolleys must be considered in the design of the corridor system. A kitchen that is decentralized to the departments and wards will be smaller at the central point but will involve satellite kitchens for tray and plate preparation and washing and storage of utensils and equipment.
- *Domestic service* A centralized domestic service will require large storage areas for fresh linen and cleaning equipment. In a decentralized system, these areas will be smaller units in different parts of the hospital.
- *Security* The number of entrances and exits is often the concern of the security unit of the

administrative office of the hospital. The decision taken on the maximum number affects circulation and circulation routes both inside and outside the hospital building.

- *Engineering services.* The checklist for this aspect will include questions like:
  - Should hot-water lines be provided in addition to cold-waterlines. If so, in what departments?
  - Should the hospital be air-conditioned? Should the air-conditioning be centralized for the whole hospital, or should it serve only selected areas? If selected areas, which departments or units?
  - What medical gaslines should be provided? Should the lines be centralized or decentralized? At what points should the lines have outlets? Or should the provisions for gas be in the form of portable tanks on carriers with rollers?
- *Fire safety* Fire safety is not limited to the provision of fire exists and fire control; fire safety should start with the design of the building. It can be improved by good planning and recognition of the specific problems of hospitals. A minimum of two compartments should be provided per floor, with proper facilities to stop fire and smoke and fire doors of appropriate standard. The larger the continuous floor area on any storey, the more fire compartments are required; this also ensures greater opportunity for progressive evacuation. Maximum amounts of fire-resistant materials should be used in constructing the buildings, in false ceilings and in partition walls, so that they have the requisite fire-resistance and flame-spread ratings as outlined in the code.
- *Communication and call systems*

The types of wired communication should be decided on,and whether all or only some of the following are required:

- internal telephones
- external telephones
- public (coin-operated) telephones
- intercoms
- patient-nurse call buttons
- emergency alarms
- public address system
- radio and television

4. ***Administration***
   - *Administrative arrangements*
   - *Office accommodation*

Site Utilization

The hospital is a rational organization of spaces in hierarchical levels: the whole hospital consists of zones, which in turn consist of spaces. The space is the smallest architectural unit in this hierarchy: here, people (patients, staff, the public, students) and goods (supplies, equipment and records) interact. Thus, the design of the hospital must proceed in the same way—from the macro to the micro level, from the general to the specific, from the whole hospital to the space. The designer must envisage the whole hospital as the sum of all the parts. Some of the items that must be analysed at the level of the whole hospital are described below.

Plot ratio The area of the site covered by buildings can be expressed in terms of the plot ratio, using the formula

$$\text{Plot ratio} = \frac{\text{total hospital floor area}}{\text{total area of site}}$$

The total hospital floor area can be obtained from the schedule of acommodations in the architect's brief, making due allowance for additional areas required for circulation.

Examples of plot ratios and subsequent possible schemes for distributing the required areas in the hospital are as follows:

A plot ratio of 1 means that a one-storey building will cover the entire area of the site.

Since it is recommended that 50% of a site area be left open for roads, other circulation routes, parking and landscaping, a plot ratio of 1 would require a solution in which the area requirements are distributed in a two-storey building.

Similarly, a plot ratio of 2 would lead to a four-storey solution and a plot ratio of 0.5 would lead to a one-storey solution.

In the suburbs, where population densities are low and land can be obtained easily, a plot ratio of no more than 0.5 should be sought. In the centre of a town, no more than 2 should be provided.

Plot ratio, however, is a measure of desirability and is not an absolute requirement. Plot ratios of more than 2 may be justified where land is expensive and use of available properties must be maximized.

Orientation

The orientation with regard to the sun and prevailing winds must be checked. It has been found that orientating buildings along an east-west axis, giving the longer sides of the building northern and southern exposures, is the most desirable. In areas where the major climatic problem is humidity rather than heat, buildings should be sited at a slight angle, either towards the east or the west, depending on the direction of the prevailing wind.

In order to overcome severe aspects of the climate at the building site, a favourable microclimate should be provided through landscaping, lawns, paving and planting trees and shrubs as well as constructing ornamental bodies of water and creating sunny and shady areas.

Illumination and ventilation are major problems in hospitals, and these are further aggravated by modern trends to construct 'deep' buildings using steel and reinforced concrete. Good ventilation in tropical climates ideally requires long, narrow buildings; but this is not always feasible, and a compromise must be found by separating activities and orientating buildings or wings of buildings. Incorrect orientation of buildings strongly affects the consumption of energy in the finished hospital.

In areas where there are heavy rains accompanied by wind, all openings should be protected against wind-driven rain. In hot, humid areas, the external surface should reflect as much solar radiation as possible, and the walls and roof should, as far as possible, be made of lightweight material with low thermal capacity.

Slope Study

On sites with steep slopes, the best areas for building must be found. As a rule, slopes of 0-10% are desirable and easy to build on; slopes greater than these require either massive cuts or massive fill or a combination of the two.

Landscaping and Horticulture

Advances in technology often entail a risk of lowering the quality of the environment. The setting up of a modern hospital on a new site is no exception. Even a funtionally well-designed building sometimes does not fit in with the environment and does not provide the level of comfort and friently surroundings necessary for patients. The solution perhaps lies, to a large extent, in proper landscaping and horticulture arrangements, which should form part of the master plan. The physical features of the land surrounding a building-shape, contours, whether open or dotted with large trees, location of other buildings affect the prevailing wind. Wind lanes are thus formed, or useful breezes might be blocked.

The most severe aspects of the climate and the handicaps of the building site should be observed in detail, so that they can be corrected to provide, as far as possible, a favorable microclimate by landscaping, grassing, paving, planting trees and shrubs, constructing ornamental bodies of water and creating many sunny and shady areas. Dense vegetation in arid areas controls hot, dusty winds, while transpiration from leaves, increased humidity and lowers the temperature. In humid areas, bushes and trees can be planted to deflect or divert winds into the building. Similarly, waterways and water channels help to reduce temperatures, and the grassing over of large areas of ground reduces glare.

Circulation

Circulation routes in a hospital consist of external and internal routes.

External Routes

These consist of traffic lines within the site, from the access point to the entrance of the building. They are generated by various kinds of exterior traffic, including:

- patients on foot,
- patients in cars or on motorcycles,
- patients in ambulances,
- visitors on foot,
- visitors in cars or on motorcycles,
- staff on foot,
- staff in cars or on motorcycles,
- supplies delivery,
- rubbish collection,
- removal of the dead,
- special route for fire trucks.

The various types of traffic should be grouped for entry into the hospital premises according to their nature. An important consideration is that traffic moving at extremely different (e.g., a patient on foot and an ambulance) should be separated. Some hospital guidelines recommend four access points to the site, in order to segregate trffic:

- emergency: for pateints in ambulances and other vehicles for the emergency depatment;
- service: for delivering supplies and collecting rubbish;
- service: for removal of dead; and
- main: for all others.

This kind of decentralized distribution of access, however, poses security and control problems, and hospital administrators prefer fewer points of entry and exit. A design solution that takes this into consideration is to have one or a maximum of two entrances and to break the main access road into several branches in a hierarchy of roads within the site.

Internal Routes

Internal traffic streams link departments; some important guidelines are as follows:

a. *Corridor size in relation to traffic intensity* A corridor 2-3 m wide can accommodate daily traffic. A corridor 3 m wide in a major hospital can accommodate a walking traffic load of 4000 people per direction per hour, or 8000 people in both directions per hour, assuming a free-flowing walking speed in hospitals of 4 km/h. The same corridor can accommodate 20-60 journeys per hour of wheeled traffic, including supplies, bed and food trolleys.

b. *Corridor size in relation to manoeuvrability* Corridors in outpatient departments and ward blocks should not be less than 2.8 m wide. A corridor must be wide enough to accommodate two passing trolleys, one of which may have a drip attached to the patient.

c. *Vertical circulation* If site limitations and functional inter-relationships lead to a multi-storey design, the folowing guidelines should be considered:

- The *stair* is the traditional and most economical route of vertical circulation however, its use as the only means of verticle circulation is limited to four storeys for walking public and staff, beyond which it must be supplemented by mechanical equipment. The stair must also be evaluated in terms of manoeuvrability; movement of trolleys and beds requires ramps and lifts.
- The *ramp* is very convenient for wheeled traffic especially when there is no electricity supply. Since its slope must be 1:15 to1:18, however, for safety, comfort and ease of movement, it requires a great deal of space. It must also be checked for maneuvrability of beds and trolleys at any turning point.
- The *elevator* is versatile for transporting all kinds of traffic vertically. Owing to their cost. However, elevator cannot always be located at points where specific departments need them. A lift system must be designed with a clear picture of departmental distribution and must be coherent with the hierarchy of circulation routes in the hospital. The key point must be determined, at which the lifts will be grouped and from

which traffic will circulate on each floor. It is recommended that the distance of an elevator from the farthest point on a floor should be no more than 30 m.

In the absence of standards, some experience in existing multi-storey hospitals confirms the adequacy of: two lift cars large enough to accomodate one trolley bed and eight passengers or 16 passengers and travelling at 105 m/min for a 100-bed hospital; and three lift cars of the same specifications for a 200-bed hospital. Adequacy is also affected, of course, by public use. It is desirble to encourage the public to use the stairs, unless they are elderly, frail or incapacitated.

- The *escalator* is a luxury provision: it is expensive to install and it devours much space. Its use is limited to ambulant people, and it cannot be used for wheeled, large hospital equipment. Its use is not recommended for any district hospital in the foreseeable future.

Growth and Change

When preparing the master plan for the hospital, imaginative foresight be used to identify the areas in which there will probably be fast growth. Growth is inevitable and is generated mainly by:

- *Growth of the community.* A community may urbanize or may change drastically as the result of an event or a catalysing situation that requires the equivalent growth of health care services.
- *Accumulated needs and requirements.* Physical effects on the building with time. Buildings deteriorate and become obsolete and even irrelevant over the years
- *Changing standards and codes.* Regulations for health and sfety change to meet advances in construction techniques and materials. A building may be declared unsafe and unfit for human use if it is not updated, upgraded and properly maintained.
- *Changing methods in medicine.* Development of new equipment, miniaturization, computerization and other new technologies in the medical field translate into new requirements for architectural design to provide better and more modern clinical services.

Physical Growth of Hospitals

Outward Growth

This is the recommended form of expansion. Thus, those areas in which growth is most probable should adjoin an outside wall; areas that are non or slow-growing should be in the central part of the building complex. Outward growth requires that departments be placed where they can expand into open space without disturbing the operation of other parts of the hsopital and infrastructure, including the road network and sewer lines. Obviously, the greatest scope for independent expansion of separate components is available in single-storey complexes with separate buildings, each of which is extendable independently of the others.

Upward (Vertical) Grwoth

This direction of growth is the option for block forms on very limited sites. It disrupts operations, particularly on the top floor of the hospital; construction materials are difficult to transport, requiring an elaborate system of scaffoldings and hoists. Excess material, although initially expensive, must be installed ahead of time, in:

- foundations that will accommodate the future load of additional floors;
- sanitary, electrical and mechanical systems that will accommodate future requirements;
- special and sometimes costly provisions to ensure that the building remains waterproof throughout the period of extension.

Downward (Vertical) Growth

This direction of growth utilizes the basement volumes, when they are not part of the original design. This can cause enormous problems of adequate headroom and in clearing the existing system of foundations and columns. Furthermore, there are problems of water proofing and damp-proofing the new retaining walls. As windows will be limited or impossible to install, there will be problems in providing natural ventilation and light. It is always desirable to avoid this type of growth, due to technical and cost considerations.

Inward Growth

This direction of growth pushes adjoining departments out of their location to make away for a growing department. It usually occurs in concentrated types of development. This type of growth disrupts the opertion of both the growing and the adjoining departments. It requires that adjoining departments:

This direction of growth pushes adjoining depatments out of their location to make way for a growing department. It usually occurs in concentrated types of development. This type of growth disrupts the operation of both the growing and the adjoining departments. It requires that adjoining departments:

- be easy to relocate and
- have convertable spaces.

Therefore, it is not economical to relocate rooms, units or departments that have comlicated engineering services, such as operating rooms, X-ray equipment, kitchens, toilets and labortories.

Growth by Fragmentation

This is the division of a single department into several subunits in different locations. Departments and other units that can be fragmented are: administration, laboratories, storage, lockers and records. Fragmentation should be avoided, however, as it poses problems of management and control, and the hospital ultimately becomes less efficient and productive owing to duplication of necessary support services.

Increments of Growth

It is most advisable to expand not in spurts with needs but by deliberate increments, thus;

- by number of beds, but in terms of ward units with their complementary manpower and supporting services.
- by functional units, in the case of a new hospital department
- by specialist rooms and their supporting units and services

Fire Safety

Fire is the perceptible phase of burning or combustion, which is the chemical combination of oxygen in air with the carbon contained in matter. The process of combustion is affected by:

- *Oxygen:* Natural air contains 21% of this element; if it is absent or insufficient, combustion will not continue unless the material iteslf has oxygen in it.
- *Heat:* Burning starts at the necesary degree of heat. Wood requires 398°C, but if it is exposed to 204°C for 30 min, it will ignite. When the ignition point of any material is reached it will start to flame if sufficient oxygen is present.
- *Nature of substance:* Thinner materials ignite more easily than thicker ones; gases and vapour are more inflammable than solids.

Smoke is a by-product of fire that contains carbon monoxide, which is harmful to human beings. It also conveys heat and may raise the temperture of substances it touches to ignition point.

Principles of Fire Safety

- *Fire avoidance* is reduction of the possibility of acidental ignition of materials, or separation of heat sources from inflammable materials. Kitchens should not be located near rooms where combustible materials, such as X-ray films and oxygen tanks, are stored.
- *Fire growth restriction* is slowing the rate of development of a fire to gain time to take mesures for control and evacuation of people. Compartmentalizing the hospital and constructing dividing walls made of fire-resistant materials will slow the spread of fire.

- *Fire containment* is restriction of the fire at its site, using fire-resistant materials and by plugging all gaps through which it could pass, to allow effective fire-fighting.
- *Fire detection* is based on early knowledge of the occurrence of fire, which ensures early action to fight it. Smoke detectors can be installed in the ceiling at various points. Interiors of rooms that contain combustible material should be visible from outside.
- *Fire control* is extinguishing fire. Fire-fighting equipment such as fire-hoses and fire-extinguishers must be easily visible and accessible for immediate use. Fire-fighting hose-reels should be of manageable length and should be located in corridors and exit routes at intervals that will allow the entire building to be covered. A fire-extinguisher should be available with each hose-reel and at the entrances to high-risk rooms, such as laboratories. Manual fire-alarms should be located at exits and be easily visible.
- *Smoke control* is the management of the action and effects of smoke. Smoke spreads very quickly and is the greatest hazard to life in case of fire. Instead of designing ceilings with voids in suspension and vertical shafts through which fire and smoke can move, such spaces must be sealed.
- *Escape provisions* are made for movement away from fire to a place of safety. Alternative escape routes must always be provided. Escape routes must be protected by sealing them from fire and smoke or by creating positive pressure in them.

Norms for fire-resistnce in buildings are as follows:

The structural framework and building elements of all buildings more than one storey high should be made of appropriately fire-resistant combinations of materials such as steel, concrete and masonry. Load-bearing walls should be limited to exterior walls, fire-walls and vertical shafts.

Bearing walls, lift shafts, chutes and other vertical shafts, walls enclosing stairways, boiler rooms, storage rooms of 10 m^2 or more should be a 2 hour fire-resistant construction.

Beams and girders supporting masonry should be individually protected with not less than 2-hour fire-resistant construction.

Columns, girders, trusses, floor and roof constructions, including beams, should be of not less than 1.5 hour fire-resistant construction.

Non-load-bearing partitions, other than corridor partitions, should be of 1-hour fire-resistant construction.

The following flame-spreading ratings should be maintained

- Interior finish of walls, ceilings of all exits, not more than 25 storage rooms and areas of unusual fire hazard
- All other areas in the building (except that up to not more than 75-10% of the aggregate wall and ceiling area may have a finish with a rating of up to 200)
- All floor finish materials not more than 75. All lift cars and platforms should be constructed of non-combustible materials, except that fire-retardant-treated materials may be used if all the exterior surfaces of the car are covered with metal. Cars of hospital lifts should have inside dimensions that will accommodate a patient bed and attendants.

Energy Conservation

Energy conservation can be adressed on two levels: practical low-level technology and sophisticated high-level technology.

The choice of the level of technology depends on a number of factors: low-technology solutions are less financially demanding and easy to maintain; high-technology equipment ensures the precise control of environmental conditions necessary for some hospital procedures but demands a high level of maintenance and spare parts inventory. The designer also has the option of combining high- and low-level technology.

High- and low-technology responses are also found with regard to power sources. High technology plants (hydroelectric, thermal, nuclear and others) produce energy for the large-scale requirements of cities and countries, both domestic and industrial. By converting waste from human beings and animals into bio-gas, a useful source of energy is harnessed for minimal light requirements.

Utilization of Solar Energy

Some departments in a hospital, such as the laundry, kitchen and wards, need a constant supply of hot water. The hot-water supply in a hospital not only requires the consumption of large amounts of conventional energy but also frequently fails, owing to lack of proper, timely maintenance and lack of availability of spare parts.

Use of simple, solar heating devices can avoid most such prloblems and ensure a reliable supply of hot water, particularly in tropical climates, where supplementary energy is needed only during the cold season. Aided by the orientation of the building, this almost maintenance-free system can provide hospitals with hot water (up to 60°C) at very low cost.

Solar energy can, of course, also be made use of natural lighting. Windows should be as tall as possible in order to provide maximal lighting against the inner wall; the angle of incidence of light from the window to the inner working areas should be not less than 27°. Special inlets with translucent covers can be placed at various places in the roof to supply glare-free light during the day in various areas of the hospital, such as corridors, waiting halls and atria.

Building Design

The implications of building design on the capital and operating costs of facilities must be fully understood at the outset. Factors to be considered are:

- Unless the external environment is severely polluted, by smog, industrial gases or noise, windows that open are the best means of ventilating most parts of a hospital. Air-conditioning is necessary in operating theatres and in a few other areas, such as intensive care units and x-ray facilities, but not in normal nursing wars, clinics or most service departments. The deep plan form of building necessitates more widespread use of expensive air-conditioning and artificial lighting.
- Buildings that require high energy result in increased capital and operating costs, and the later usually increases with time as energy and fuel costs rise. Energy thus consumes an ever-increasing percentage of the hospital budget.
- High-energy buildings require more sophisticated equipment and more maintenance. The life expectancy of air-conditioning equipment is much shorter than that of the building, so further capital must be spent on th repair and replacement of mechanical components.
- Mechanical and electrical building service equipment requires regular preventive maintenance, and trained personnel must form part of the hospital staff or be on call to keep it operational. The functioning of the building may be severely impaired when such equipment is out of action.

Master Planning

The master plan of a hospital is the basis for present and future decisions on the layout of buildings and services, changes in needs and phasing. It indicates the phasing and grouping of individual buildings and the means of communication betwen them, the scale and location of utilities necesary at various stages, and directions and limits of probable future expansion or remodelling of the hospital. Any mistake in placing buildings, access roads, sewer systems, entry points and parking facilities on the site can restrict possibilities of growth.

The architectural and engineering aspects of the project are evolved within the master plan on the basis of:

- grouping main functions, like wards, medical services, admissions and central supplies;

- establishing appropriate access routes for easy orientation of patients and visitors, with special emphasis on disabled people; and
- providing scope for future expansion to cope with an increased number of beds, supplementary functions and medical specialization, by ensuring maximum interaction between hospital units and support services.

The master plan consists of two elements: (i) determination of circulation routes and corridor systems; and (ii) location of elements on the site in relation to one another.

Circulation routes and corridor systems must be designed so that all users can find their way around with least difficulty. The main circulation loop must be discernible as such, and the hierarchy of secondary routes that in turn break into more minor traffic paths must correspond to the hierarchy of the hospital unit they serve. Simplicity should be the target of design; this reduces the requirements for signs and improves the quality of service.

The placing of elements of departments on a site should result in an optimal inter-relationship among departments and provide room for expansion. Some principles and guidelines for the disposition of the units of a hospital are as follows:

- Departments that are most closely linked to the community should be closest to the main entrance: out-patient department, emergency, administration (especially business sections), family planning, clinic and other primary health care support.
- Departments that receive their workload from those described above should be next closest to the entrance: X-ray, laboratories, dispensary.
- In-patient departments should be in the interior zones, or wards.
- Operating theatres, the delivery department and the nursery should have (1) and (2) on one side and (3) on the other, e.g., to provide easy access from the emergency department to X-ray and operating theatres. The delivery department and nursery must be separated from the operating theatre.
- Housekeeping and domestic service areas should be grouped around a service yard: laundry, kitchen, housekeeping, maintenance, storage and motor pool.
- Staff facilities should be located on the periphery near roads and public transport: staff dormitories, quarters or housing.
- Teaching facilities, if any, should be close to both staff facilities and teaching areas and to roads and public transport: student areas, educational and training components of primary health care.
- The mortuary should be in a special service yard, with a discreet entrance; it should be away from the out-patient department, ward, block and nursery.

Building Shape

The hospital should reflect the local architecture. Every community has its own concept of form and of space and of their inter-relationship, as well as having its own feeling for scale and proportion. The hospital should reflect the rhythm of the local culture, civilization and historical heritage but at the same time be flexible enough to accommodate modern methods of health care and facilities. The hospital should not be alien to its surroundings or stand out as an exception but should fit in with local life, expressing its spirit and character. The hospital building should not be a huge, unfriendly structure but should be a human, welcoming part of the community.

Layouts suitable for tropical climatic conditions include: an open-plan layout for 'hot-humid' area; a compact layout for 'hot-dry' areas; and a compact layout for 'upland' regions.

Some of the basic shapes of hospitals, and the reasons for using them, are as follows:

The *village* form is organized like a small town, in which corridors correspond to streets and departments correspond to the different land uses of a village. This design is easy to phase, which is useful when the budget is limited. It is also easy to expand, since the design is open-ended, and a wall can simply be broken down for expansion into an open space. This form requires, however, a large site; and if sufficient room is to be provided for ultimate growth, the distances betwen departments will be great.

The *modular village* form a similar to the village concept except that the departments must fit into a predetermined form. This form is useful when repeated modules are used. It results, however, in forced planning of departments to fit within the same shape; some will fit just right, other will be 'bursting at the seams' and other will have wasted space.

The *finger* plan consists of a cetnral corridor and side corridors, which link various departments branching out in 'fingers'. It is a development of the *train corridor* form in which one must pass through one component to reach the next. Since the corridors in the finger plan have single function, this form lends itself to the provision of abundant natural ventilation and lighting.

An *open-ended finger* development plan can allow for the expansion of individual blocks at different times. It also allows for staged development, by progressive extension of the main corridor as further components are required.

The *block* is a form for sites where the ground area is limited. As the hospital is developed vertically, optimal relationships between departments may be difficult to achieve and one department may be disposed on two levels. It is also a form that is difficult lto expand later. It is appropriate for designing wards, since wards have generally similar floor plans; however, structural costs are likely to be higher than those for a similar number of wards in a single-storey construction.

In the *tower and podium* design, the fastest growing departments are located in the ground-floor podium and those that are slow-growing and departments that are typical and replicable are located in the tower. This form was developed with expansion and growth as the over riding criteria. The tower, however, relies heavily on mechanical engineering services, and the structure of the tower and the location of lifts and service ducts may severely limit the central area of the podium. The roof of the podium must be constructed of fire-resistant materials so that fire will not spread from the podium via external walls and windows to the tower block.

If the site permits it, there are definite advantages to placing the tower block next to rather than on the podium.

The *court* plan closes on itself. It has the same advantages of natural lighting and ventilation as the village and finger plans but is easier to secure and more comfortable in humid tropical areas.

The *impact* plan is a 'deep' form and its proper functioning relies heavily on engineering services. Artificial ventilation and lighting must be provided for inner areas; heat generated by people and equipment must be removed by artificial cooling. This type of plan is therefore, expensive to construct, operate and maintain.

Appropriate Technology

Locally available materials and traditional building techniques should be given priority, as they are usually cheaper and better adapted to local conditions.

In general, building materials should be economical, durable, easy to clean and to maintain, sanitary and attrractive. They should also be easy to handle on the site and to replace in case of breakage or damage.

At the inception of the project, the designer must choose:

1. The types of construction method:
   - indigenous technology
   - on-site methods,
   - prefabricated modules and components assembled on site, or
   - a combination of prefabricated components and on-site construction.
2. The level of technology: low, medium or high.

Types and levels of construction technology should suit the conditions of site, geography, slope, time constraints, availability of labor and raw materials, construction equipment and other, related factors.

FURTHER READING

1. District Hospitals: Guidelines for Development. WHO Regional Publications, Western Pacific Series No. 4, 1992.

37 Planning of Health Centers

A study of activities in health centres is a pre-requisite to planning. Similar and closely-related activities should be grouped together in one area. All areas should be located in relation to one another to allow direct communication and easy flow of patients, staff and services. The design and the structural system should allow maximum flexibility and expandability.

All activities in the health centre may be grouped into four general areas:

- Waiting area, which both in layout and size will depend on local tradition, size of the health centre and patient flow as determined by the working system of the health centre. The waiting area may consist of a single waiting area for both sexes; a double waiting area, one for each sex (in this case they may be located on both sides of clinical room); there may be an additional special waiting area for maternal and child care; and, in the case of large health centres with a great variety of services, more waiting areas may be warranted. Toilets for each sex should always be provided.
- Clinical area, which consists of examination and treatment rooms. The bigger the health centre, the more specialized fcilities (such as maternal and child care room, dental treatment room, labour room, etc.) will be needed.
- Supporting services area which consists of laboratory space, which might vary from a small counter for microscopy to a full-fledged laboratory (about 18 m^2 per 1000 tests per month); pharmacy and integrated or separate storage area for other supplies; pantry or kitchen, which may even be used for training purposes if big enough (about $20m^2$); and cleaner's room (or at least a cupboard).
- Office area for clerks, sanitarians, health visitors and others (minimum of $4m^2$ per person).

In larger health centres there may, in addition, be an area for the in-patient care of emergency cases awaiting transfer or for deliveries; in that case, there should also be at least two rooms with toilet and shower facilities, as well as a clean working area for the nursing service and an area for disposal of dirty linen, etc.

The architectural programme should only be prepared after the operational policy of the centre has been established. This operational policy will determine:

- The functions to be carried out both inside and outside the centre, which will lead to an

indication of which units (e.g., examination rooms) will be necessary;
- The expected volume of attendance and of outside activities, which will indicate the workload in each unit;
- This workload, together with the knowledge of the output of each staff member concerned, will allow the determination of the number of staff necessary and the number of elements needed in each unit (e.g., the number of examination rooms);
- The flow of patients, staff and supplies;
- The supply system, including catering and laundry arrangements.

Each functional component needs a minimum of space for operational efficiency. The following are usually considered as minimum areas for the main components:

Examination room, about 10 m^2
Treatment room, about 12 m^2
Bedrooms: with 1 bed, 10 m^2
2 beds, 7 m^2
4 beds, 6 m^2
6 beds, 6 m^2

Rooms for interviews (for family planning; health visitors; nutritionist; and social worker), 6-10 m^2.

Health centre with beds should have:

Outpatient capacity up to 100 patients per day.

Staffed by two to three nurse/midwives and one administrator.

The centre is visited periodically by a mobile health team.

Inpatients are cared for by their relatives.

Programme

a. Ambulatory care and administration
   - Waiting area
   - Office for admission and medical records.
   - Storage for demonstration materials
   - Examination room (also used for sterilization; samples will be taken in the examination room)
   - Treatment room
   - Laboratory
   - Preparation and distribution of drugs
   - Sub-waiting area for laboratory and preparation and distribution of drugs
   - Drug store
   - General store
   - Toilets and shower
   - Staff toilets.

b. Obstetrics
   - Delivery room
   - Sluice
   - Shower
   - Tiolets
   - Duty and tea kitchen.

c. Inpatients
   - Two 2-bed wards (men)
   - Two 2-bed wards (women)
   - Sluice
   - Toilets and shower (women)
   - Toilets and shower (men).

Site and Location

The location should be convenient to the people it will serve. It has been observed that services are made use of, to a large extent, by inhabitants of the village where the centre is located while those living beyond 3 km from the centre hardly benefit from it. On the other hand, in towns, the network of public transportation should be taken into account. The direction of the prevailing wind must be considered, since natural ventilation is necessary. Careful attention should be paid to the topographic configuration of the site and the nature of the subsoil should also be carefully investigated.

The site should allow future expansion of the building of at least 100 percent in building area and still retain attractive grounds, the psychological effect of which on users' welfare, public goodwill and staff morale cannot be overestimated. The site should be properly planted with trees, grass and flowers to promote a cheerful and relaxing attitude of mind.

Building Materials

Local materials and traditional building techniques should generally have priority as they are cheaper and generally better adapted to local conditions and habits.

Recent research has helped in exploiting to the utmost basic local materials for low-cost building. For example, soil, sand and cement, in a ratio of 5:5:1 by volume, mixed with wear and cast into blocks (called landcrete blocks) on site either by hand or by machine in the same way as concrete blocks are cast, has provied to be a solid builing material with relatively high-bearing capacity. Walls may be whitewashed for sun reflection. Sun-dried brick may be used in combined techniques with cement plaster on both sides. The plaster is held to the walls by a mesh of fine wire-netting or by a layer of reeds. Baked brick or stone are most suitable when they are available. Floors may be made of plain concrete or landcrete mixture; in some areas of the building, for example, in clinical rooms, utility rooms and toilets, the mixture has to be covered with tiles. Roofing is a more difficult problem. Concrete hollow tiles and precast concrete units are used; brick vaults have also been successfully tried.

In general, building materials should be economical, durable, easy to clean and to maintain, sanitary and with good appearance. They should also be easy to handle on site, without the need to be carried mechanically to be put in place.

The use of local building material is advantageous with regard to maintenance, as local skill is likely to be found for necessary repairs. If the health centre is built with local materials and is well kept it will serve as a standing example to the people of how to utilize properly the available materials in order to have better homes and good living conditions.

Equipment should be simple, robust, unsophisticated, easy to handle and service.

Climate

In a hot climate—as is the case in most areas of the developing countries–the long axis of the building should be in the east-west direction. Cross-ventilation should be provided for every room that is permanently used. It has two main advantges: it produces a cooling effect; and, in hot, humid regions, it decreases the humidity through air circulation.

Fully enclosed areas must be avoided. Regarding internal ventilation, different means could be applied. A wind-catch catches the wind where it is strong, clean and cool. The wind-catch consists of a chimney-like air passage with a large opening high-up facing the prevailing wind. Set inside it is a sloping metal tray filled with charcoal that can be wetted by a tap; the air flows over this baffle and is thus cooled before entering the room. The wind-catch device can lower the indoor temperature by 10°C.

In order to improve climatic conditions, solar heat gain may be reduced by whitewashing the walls to reflect sunlight, extended roof construction to provide a shadow or by using double roofs and double external walls to allow air circulation through the outside shell of the building.

In regions with cool nights and a high day temperature, the external walls have to be built thick and from materials capable of storing the solar heat during the day and of postponing the transmission of heat until the night hours.

Climatic conditions are improved considerably in pavilion-type buildings with an inner court. If the court is shaded by trees, there will be a reduction in temperature, and there will also be cross ventilation due to the differences in temperature inside and outside the building.

The health centre should reflect the local character of architecture. Architecture and ornaments carry the rhythm of a given culture, civilization and historical heritage. The architect should understand

and fully appreciate local architecture. He should follow in his design and planning basic local characteristics of buildings.

FURTHER READING

1. Abou Zeid Rageh: Health Centres: Function, Planning and Architecture in Approaches to Planning and Design of Health Care facilities in Developing Area. Kleczkowski and Pibouleau (Eds): World Health Organisation, Geneva, 1976.
2. Jan Delru: Rationalisation of Planning and Construction of Medical Care Facilities in Developing Countries; in Approaches to Planning and Design of Health Care facilities in Developing Countries. Kleczkowski and Pibouleau (Eds): World Health Organization, Geneva, 1976.

38 Hospital Engineering Services

During the late twentieth century, technological innovation has presented almost every facet of our lives. This is especially true in the field of medicine and the delivery of health-care services. In this evolutionary process, has emerged as a centre of excellence providing a technologically sophiscated health-care delivery system. The role of engineering to assist health care professionals in the planning, design, construction and effective utilization and management of the vast array of medical devices and technologies presently available cannot be overemphasized.

Todays engineers are responsible for activities including:

- Architecture/Design
- Civil works (construction)
- Electrical works
- Mechanical works
- Advances in electronics (Telecommunication)
- Management of high technology and devices and systems (equipment, spare parts surgery, computers, medical imaging) clinical engineering.
- Facilities operations (includes heating, ventilation, and airconditioning) electric supply and distribution, central gas supply and vacuum systems, and other physical plant equipment.
- Landscape
- Environmental protection (management of biomedical waste, noise, utilities natural gas, water, etc.)
- Preventive maintenance
- Risk management
- Provision of a potable water supply and an adequate sewage disposal system are of primary importance in a hospital for the obvious reasons, both to contribute to the well-being of patients and to reduce the risks of infections and propagation of diseses, like dysentery, gastroenteritis and other water-borne diseases.
- In some developing countries, where modern amenities like an efficient water works and distribution system and a centralized sewerage system are not available, hospital planners and designers must use flexibility and ingenuity to find other solutions.

Water Supply

Water for use in hospital must be:

- free of pathogenic organisms and imitating and poisonous substances
- clear, colorless, odorless and tasteless;
- not too hard for domestic and industrial use;

- free from iron and other corrosive substances; and
- at a low, agreeable temperature

Ideally, all these requirements would be met; however, there is no such water source. Even in developed countries, water must be treated by adding chlorine to the distributing reservoir or water mains.

A complete waterworks consists of:

- *Collecting system*. This consists of the intake, where the water is drawn from the source of supply; the receiving reservoirs; the conduit through which it flows; and the pumping machinery to raise the water from one level to another until it reaches the purifying system.
- *Purifying system*. This consists of the distributing reservoirs, in which the filtered water is received, and the network of pipes that convey the water to the point of consumption. Facilities to store a 36-hour supply should be provided for a hospital.

In a simple gravity system, the force of gravity moves the water from the source to the point of consumtion. The pressure required in the system for ordinary use is 3.5 kg/cm^2; for fire protection without the aid of fire engines, however, the pressure requires is 7.0 kg/cm^2.

When there is no existing waterworks in the area, planners and designers must look for the nearest body of water, such as a spring or flowing river. In the absence of a spring or river, a deep well powered by a rotary submersible pump may be dug. Experience indicates that water extracted at a depth of 25 m is generally potable. Deeper wells yield water of better quality, but more powerful pumps and more piping are needed. An elevated water tank can be used to store the collected water. Whether the water source is a spring, a river or a well, a pipe conveyance and distribution system supported by a force pump can be used.

The minimum water requirement where water supply is a problem, is 50 litres per person per day. Normally, however, the value is 115 litres per person per day. A district hospital with about 100 patients and 200 personnel, or a total of 300 people, will need at least 34 500 litres of water per day. An additional volume of about 30 litres per person per day should be added to this basic volume in the computations for sprinkling lawns and as a standby for fire protection.

Sewerage and Sewage Disposal

Sewage is the liquid and soft solid waste of a community, and sewerage is the system by which it is removed. The sewerage system is thus the totality of the conduits, pumping stations, treatment plants and other works necessary to collect, purify and dispose of the sewage.

Normally, sewage is subjected to some preliminary treatment, such as screening, to separate the solid from the liquid waste, which is then passed through a sedimentation tank to remove minute suspended matter. The effluent from the process is then discharged into a body of water, on natural land, on prepared land, or on specially constructed filter beds of sand and gravel.

a. *Choice of disposal system*

Raw sewage contains both organic and inorganic matter. In order to determine the most efective and least expensive method of sewage disposal, the raw sewage must be analyzed for its chemical, biological and physical properties. In planning and designing a hospital, the following information must be available.

- a complete analysis of sewage at a similar institution,
- an estimate of the volume of sewage that will be produced daily,
- how it will be disposed of and
- what type of system will be used.

It should be noted that provision of on-site laundry facilities substantially increases the daily volume of sewage.

The primary aim of a disposal system is to eliminate or neutralize pathogenic bacteria that may be present in the sewage which cause cholera, diarrhoea, dysentery and typhoid fever.

It should also prevent the creation of nuisance resulting from the process of putrefaction.

At a project site where there is no existing centralized sewerge system, one of two methods of treatment of raw sewage can be used;

- In septic tanks, in which raw sewage flowing in is detained for a period of time to allow anaerobic bacteria to act on it, help in its decomposition and render it relatively inoffensive. The treated sewage is disposed of by percolation in the ground, using either a cesspool or a trench field. The suitability of the ground for this purpose must first be established by percolation tests.
- Lagooning, in which the sewage is exposed to the sun in lagoons, which could be simple ponds or ponds equipped with mechanical aerators, depending on the condition and quantity of the sewage to be treated.

More technologically advanced solutions are available, which include mechanical screening followed by sedimentation, aeration and fermentation. Such facilities require electrical energy and trained and skilled manpower to operate them; they are not recommended for small hospitals located in rural areas of developing countries.

Factors to be considered in determining the method of disposal to be adopted are cost, available area and availability of coagulants. Strong fermenting agents (microbes and enzymes) are also available that can be used to neutralize or control pathogenic bacteria.

b. *Effluent disposal and utilization*

The effluents from sewage treatment units can be discharged into lakes, streams, rivers, oceans or on the land. Sewage effluent constitutes a valuable source for recharging groundwater; however, the points of discharge must be well arranged and the quantities limited, so that there is no threat to the quality of the groundwater. Partially-purified sewage effluent can be used for fish culture and farming without further dilution, depending on local soil and hydrographic conditions. When it is used to irrigate fields, much less sewage effluent needs to be used than with fresh water, because the effluents have a higher concentration of suspended matter.

Solid Waste Disposal

A hospital produces not only liquid wastes but also a lot of garbage from the kitchens and contaminated materials from the wards, operating department and laboratory. The quantity of waste produced ranges from 2-5 kgs/bed per day. This must not be disposed of in open-air dumps but must be incinerated. The capacity of the incinerator depends on the anticipated load, and it may be run on fossil fuels or electricity. The incinerator building should be located downwind from other elements of the hospital complex. Other methods of biomedical waste management include shredding, pyrolysis, microwave, autoclave treatment, etc.

Mechanical Engineering

The significance of the combined mechanical-electrical components of a hospital can be deduced from the fact that the cost of installing the equipment is normally about one-third of the total cost of the building. The operation and maintenance costs are also more than the combined expenses for all other parts of the building. Furthermore, their expected life may be only one-half or even one-third that of the buildings.

The primary objective of the designer of the system, therefore, is to bring down the initial cost and evolve a design that has a reasonable maintenance cost. This can be done by providing the simplest mechanical devices possible while using high-quality materials; thus,the number of repairs will be reduced as will costs for labor, fuel and power. It will also ensure that the maintenances within the capability of local resources. The design should also include adequate protection of the health and safety of staff, public and pateints.

The following is a checklist of the components to be considered in the mechanical design of a hospital. Engineering consultants should be brought in at a very early stage of the design process; consultation should also take place with the necesary government authorities.

General Provisions

- General description of installations
- Fuel
- Proposed fuel with justification
- Estimated monthly and maximum daily fuel consumption
- Storage of fuel, when applicable
- Primary source of energy
- Type of heating, temperatures and pressures
- Preliminary load and breakdown of main components
- Provision for future expansion
- Number and capacity of boilers or heat exchangers
- Description of boiler and auxiliaries, control and stand-by
- Schematic diagram
- Sketch of major operational features and maintenance access.

Primary Distribution System

- General description

Domestic Heating

- Internal design criteria
- External design criteria, frequency of use
- Infiltration rate assumed
- Heating media, temperature, pressures
- Preliminary heat load, allowance for future expansion
- Scheme of circuitry
- Types of heat emitters in different areas
- Type of control operation
- Piping materials, types of pump
  - Area to be heated for each type of heating (m^2)
  - Means of absorbing thermal expansion of pipes
  - Feed and expansion provisions.

Domestic Hot Water

- Means of heating
- Design criteria, storage, maximum demand with time
- Preliminary storage and heat-up capacity
- Size of generators, allowance for future expansion
- Type of piping
- Type and capacity of cold feed system.

Steam Services

Other than for heat or hot water

- Locations (e.g., kitchen, laundry, central sterile supply department)
- Required pressure
- Criteria for load calculations
- Preliminary heat load
- Allowance for extension.

Ventilation and Air-conditioning Systems

- Description of systems (central or split type)
- Types of fan
- Areas served by each system
- Typical circuitry schemes
- Internal design criteria
- External design conditions
- Design criteria for assessing air volumes:
  - supply air temperatures;
  - ventilation to remove heat, moisture, odours, fumes;
  - minimum rates of air change per hour;
  - fresh air and recirculation requirements
- Number and capacity of fans and air-handling plants
- Sound levels
- Control operation and energy conservation
- Filter types and efficiencies
- Type of cooling and heat rejection system

- Type of humidification
- Design criteria for cooling equipment:
  - ambient conditions for cooling towers, etc. (including frequency if these are exceeded)
  - chilled water temperature
  - condenser water temperatures
- Preliminary cooling load
- Allownce for expansion
- Numbers and capacity of cooling and heat rejection plants
- Air-conditioned area (m^2)
- Ratio of design cooling load: air-conditioned area (W/m^2).

Medical Gas Services

When piped

- Gases used (e.g., vacuum, compressed air, oxygen)
- General description of system
- Allowance for extension
- Types and capacities of compressors and vaccuum pumps
- Proportion of stand-by plant used.

Fire Protection System

- Type of system, coverage and classification
- Location of control and indicator panels
- Manual call points, general locations of alerting devices, type and sequence of operation
- Details of water supply for fire-fighting
- Dry/wet riser system.

Special Service Systems

- Description and justification of any other service.

Instrumentation, Alarms, Monitors and Controls

- General description of scope and philosophy
- Type of equipment proposed.

Heating, Ventilation and Air-conditioning

Maintaining a pleasant temperature, about 22°C, is the design target for heating and air-conditioning systems in cold and warm countries. Higher or lower temperatures may be attained in specific areas through independent units to suit individual requirements.

Heating and air-conditioning and ventilation systems are related both in physical installation and in their function in the hospital departments. Air-conditioning differs from ventilation in that the temperature and humidity of the air are controlled in the former. it is expensive to provide, operate and maintain. However, it should be installed only in areas where it is essential, such as in operating theatres. Wherever possible, therefore, hospital design should minimize or eliminate the need for air-conditioning and mechanical ventilation by providing occupied spaces with adequate windows, cross-ventilated where possible, and by using internal areas for specific purposes, such as operating theatres, darkrooms and storerooms. Careful attention to sitting and design to take advantage of any cooling breezes and the use of trees to shade the building can help in optimizing natural conditions.

The ventilation of a hospital is dictated by health, comfort and safety standards. In areas where excessive heat or moisture is generated, or where objectionable odors, dust or toxic gases are present in the atmosphere, a fresh air supply and exhaust system must be provided. Electric fans can be used to augment the system as and where necessary.

Ventilation associated with kitchen, laundry and refrigeration equipment must be designed by qualified engineers in coordination with the users. Special care must be taken in designing extraction systems over cooking installations to avoid any fire hazard due to build-up of fat in exhaust ducts. Filters to trap fat carried in the exhaust fumes should be accessible and should be cleaned regularly.

Technical Requirements

Heating, ventilating and air-conditioning systems should meet the following guidelines:

a. They should provide the temperatures shown in Table 38.1 and a relative humidity of 50-60%.

Table 38.1: Temperatures to be provided in a district hospital

Area	*Temperature (°C)*
Operating theatre	21-25
Delivery room	21-25
Recovery room	24
Nursery	24-26
Intensive care	24-26

b. All air supply and air exaust systems must be operated mechanically. Fans serving exhaust systems should be located at the discharge end of the system. Minimal acceptable ventilation rates in the major areas should be as shown in Table 38.2.

c. The ventilation system should be designed and balanced to provide the pressure relationships shown in Table 38.2.

d. The ventilation systems serving sensitive areas, like operating theatres, delivery rooms, nurseries and sterile rooms, must be equipped with at least two filter beds. The exhaust from all laboratory hoods in which infections or radioactive materials are handled must have filters with 99% efficiency.

e. All filter frames must be durable and provide an air-tight fit with the enclosing ducts. All joints between segments and the enclosing ducts should be gasketed or sealed to provide a positive seal against air leakage.

f. Ducts that penetrate structures to protect against X-ray radiation should not impair its effectiveness. Ducts that pass through fire walls must be provided with automatic fire doors on both sides of the wall.

g. Duct linings, coverings, vapour barriers and the adhesives used for applying them must have

Table 38.2: Conditions for ventilation in different areas of a district hospital.

Area	*Pressure in relation to other areas*[a]	*Minimum total no. of air chagnes*	*Recirculated within*
Operating theatre	+	12	No
Emergency operating room	+	12	No
Delivery room	+	12	No
Nursery	+	12	No
Recovery room	0	6	No
Intensive care	+	6	No
Ward room	0	2	Optional
Patient area corridor	0	4	Optional
Isolation room	0	6	No
Treatment room	0	6	No
X-ray (fluoroscopy) room	–	6	No
X-ray (treatment) room	0	6	Optional
Physical therapy rom	–	6	Optional
Sterilizing room	–	10	No
Laboratory general	–	6	Optional
Laboratory, media transfer	+	4	No
Anesthesia storage room	0	8	No

[a] +, positigve; -, negative; 0, equal

a flame-spread classification of not more than 25 and a smoke-developed rating of not more than 50. Acoustic lining materials should not be used inside duct systems serving sensitive areas, such as operating theatres, nurseries and isolation rooms.

h. Cold-air ducts should be insulated wherever necessary to maintain the efficiency of the system and to minimize condensation.
i. Duct systems serving hoods should be made of corrosion-resistant materials.

ELECTRIC AND ELECTRONIC ENGINEERING

Power is supplied to hospitals in most countries by public or private utility companies. In either case, the hospital must have a back-up gasoline or diesel-driven generator for use in the case of breakdown, at least for emergency, delivery and operating rooms, selected corridors and exits, and stairs. In addition, battery or automatic generators may be used.

Components in the Electrical Design

The following is a checklist of those electrical components that should be considered in designing a district hospital. Engineering consultants should be brought in at a very early stage of the designing process. Consultation should also take place with the local electricity supply company and with any necesary government authorities regarding the mode and system of supplying high and low-tension electricity to the hospital.

- Electricity supply
- Point of mains supply
- Maximum capacity
- Supply and incoming voltage
- Tariffs and metering
- Agreements on existing installation (maximum capacity, assessed connected loads and measured maximum site demand, cable types, protection methods and discrimination).
- General description of new system (with load estimates for both essential and non-essential supplies).

Local Distribution

- General description of sub-main and sub-circuit system (routes, board locations and area of coverage)
- Cable types and sub-main load estimates
- Installation and wriring methods
- Protection methods and discrimination.

Earthing

Method adopted for each continuity and electrode system.

Sub-stations

- Type and accessibility
- Transformer and switch-gear ratings and type
- Capacity for increased load, provision for expansion.

Stand-by Plant

- Type and ratings
- Capacity for increased load
- Controls and alarms
- Sensory circuits and starting
- Fuel type and stored quantity
- Provisions for maitnenance, including access.

Distribution Boards

- General description
- Sub-main or sub-circuit protection
- Fault rating
- Capacity for increased load
- Services supplied (assessed loads and area covered).

Special Safety and Earthing

- Area, location and classifications.
- Medical procedures carried out and equipment used
- Type of protection chosen, with justification.

General Power

- Known major equipment, with assessed load (e.g. kitchen and laundry equipment, autoclaves, mechanical services plant, medical equipment)
- Typical location and numbers of plug sockets, including number per circuit
- Hazardous areas and provisions proposed.

Interior Lighting

- Area classifications
- Illumination levels
- Anti-glare design
- Types of fittings (surface, suspended, concealed)
- Lump type and color
- System data; mounting height, hours in use, reflectance
- Estimated connected load and load per circuit
- Connections to essential services with estimated loads.

Exterior Lighting

- Areas served and purpose
- Type of fitting
- Control and wiring method, including routes.

Lightning Protection

- Need
- Design criteria
- Description of proposed design
- Communications
- Justification for each type of area
- Type of system
- Areas served
- Wiring method

Other features and safety considerations, like call systems, intercommunication systems, fire alarm systems and other special installations may be included as required in the design and computations for the total electric power requirements.

Emergency Electrical Services

The hospital should have a reliable alternative source of power, in addition the normal electrical service, for emergency lighting, for operatin of essential equipment and for the safety of its occupants. The alternative source should be from:

- a generator, when the normal service is supplied from one or more central transmission lines, or
- an emergency generating set or a central transmission line, when the normal supply is generated on the premises.

The emergency generating set, including the prime mover, should be located on the premises, away from the operating department and the ward block. It should be reserved exclusively for supplying electricity in an emergency. The recommended circuits to which power should be provided are:

Lighting

- all exits, including exit signs, stairways and corridors
- surgical, obstetrical and emergency-room operating lights
- nursery, laboratory, recovery-room, intensive care unit, nursing station, labor-room and pharmacy
- generator set location, electrical switch-gear location and boiler-room
- one or two lifts, if needed for emergency
- telephone operator's-room
- computer room, when available

Guidelines for hospital illumination are shown in Table 38.3.

Equipment

- Nurses' call system
- Alarm system, including fire alarm
- Fire pump and pump for central suction system
- Blood bank refrigerator
- Sewerage or sump lift pump, if installed

Table 38.3: Guidelines for lilghting in a hospital

Area	*Recommended minimum lux*	*Area*	*Recommended minimum lux*
Autoclave room	150 -300	Laundry, general	300
Bathroom	100 -150	Laundry, mending, local	500
Blood bank	200	Library	300
Body store (mortuary)	100	Lift hall	200
Clean utility room	150	Maternity department	400
Conference room	300	Mortuary, post-mortem room	300
Consultation room	300	Mortuary, viewing room	150
Corridor, general	150 -300	Night-lighting, maternity, pediatric	
Cubicle, general	100 -150	(nurses)	100
Cubicle, treatment	300	Operating theatre, general	400
Darkroom	50	Operation theatre, operation	10,000
Delivery room	400	Operating theatre, cavity (local)	50,000
Diagnostic X-ray, couch	20-100	Pantry	100
Diagnostic X-ray, work place	300	Pharmacy	300
Dining room, general	50	Plaster room, operating theatre	400
Dining room, tables	200	Reading lights	150
Dirty utility room	150	Reception area	300
Dispensary, out-patient	300	Records, medical	150 -300
Doctor's office	300	Recovery room	300 -400
Enquiry desk, reception	500	Scrub-up, operating theatre	300
Entrance canopy	300	Shower	100-150
Entrance hall	200	Sluice sink	200
Gymnasium (physiotherapy)	300	Special baby care unit (local)	1000
Nurse's station, day	300	Staff room	100-200
Nurse's station, night	30 -100	Stores, general	100
Interview room	300	Toilets	100 -150
Kitchen	300	Workshop	300 -500
Laboratory, pathology, benches	300	X-ray room, couch	20 -100
Laboratory, pathology, local	500	X-ray room, work place	300

- Equipment necessary for maintaining telephone service
- Equipment in operating, recovery, intensive care and delivery rooms
- One electrical sterilizer, if installed.

Heating, Cooling and Ventilation System

- Operating, delivery, labor, recovery, intensive care unit, nurseries and patient rooms

The capacity of the emergency generating set should be 50-60% of the normal electrical load of the hospital, to maintain the minimum level of services.

The emergency electrical system should be so controlled that, after interruption of the normal electric power supply, the generator has brought full voltage and frequency within 10 seconds to all the emergency lighting and equipment listed above. Lights powered by storage batteries can be provided to augment the emergency lighting during the period of transfer switching, immediately following the interruption of normal service; however, these should not be used to substitute for the generator set. A typical diagram of an incoming electricity supply and of how the generator is relayed is given in Figure 38.1.

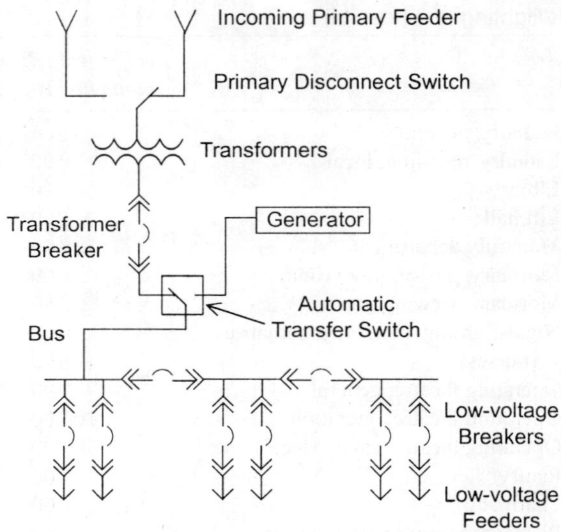

Fig. 38.1: Modified selective system of electrical distribution, including generator

PLANNING AND PROGRAMMING CONSTRUCTION

Once the basic planning and preparation of the master plan are finished, a plan should be made for the construction of the hospital. It should proceed as follows:

- plans, specifications and cost estimates;
- tender documents;
- selection of contractor and award of work;
- construction activities;
- project management and control; and
- handing over for commissioning.

Tendering

Documents for the preparation of bids by contractors for the civil, structural, architectural, electrical and other work for the hospital buildings and services should be drawn up. These documents must contain the following information:

- general conditions of contract;
- technical specifications
- tender drawings; and
- bill of quantities.

General Conditions of Contract

This should consist of:

- cover or title sheet
- index
- instructions to bidders
- bidding form
- form of agreement
- performance bond and bidding bond forms
- description of the site
- standard labor regulations and other statutory provisions applicable in the country
- right of access to the work by the owner
- details of liability insurance for bodily injury and property damage
- special conditions of contract, if any
- other relevant details, including taxes and duty.

Technical Specifications

These should supplement the drawings to describe fully the types, sizes, capacities, workmanship, finishes and other characteristics of all materials and equipment, including the codes of practices and standards, both national and international, to be followed with regard to materials, workmanship and tolerance.

Tender Drawings

These should include (i) a survey drawing and the soil investigation report; and (ii) preliminary sketches of plans, as follows:

a. Architectural and structural
   - Plans of foundations and basement, floors and roof, showing space assignment, sizes and outlines of major fixed and movable equipment;
   - All elevations and typical sections showing various finished floor levels;
   - Plot plan, showing road, paving and sidewalks; and
   - Indicative details of reinforcement of foundations, beams and columns, floor slabs and special structures, if any;

b. Mechanical and sanitary
   - Single-line diagram of all exernal and internal sewer lines and water lines, indicating diameter of pipes and location and invert level of manholes, etc;
   - Location and size of all soil, waste and vent stacks with connections to house drains and equipment; single-line layout of all ducts and piping systems, including fixture connections;
   - Diagram of riser and wet drains in the case of multistorey constructions;
   - Layout of boilers and major associated equipment, including central heating, cooling and the air-conditioning and ventilation system;
   - Air-conditioning and ventilation system, with equipment, water and refrigerant piping, ducts and exhaust ventilating duct openings;
   - Details of pumps and layout of lifts, including other handling systems;
   - Location and layout of various services in the laboratories and elsewhere, including gas tanks.

c. Electrical and asociated services
   - Plans showing space assignments, sizes and outline of fixed equipment, like transformers, main switch and switchboards;
   - Electricity entry, with switches and feeders to the public service feeders;
   - Emergency electrical system, with details of supply, feeders and circuits;
   - Fire alarm system, telephone layout and all other electrically operated systems and equipment, showing service entry, switchboards, annunciators and wiring diagrams.

Bill of Quantities

The reliability of the cost estimate of any building depends upon the accuracy of the information available at the time the estimate is made. 'Preliminary' and 'approximate' cost estimates are prepared at the briefing and planning stages,on the basis of approximate floor areas, the cost indices of previous projects and the prevailing market rates for similar projects.

When bidding for a multidisciplinary project like a hospital, contractors should know not only the technical specifications but also the approximate quantitites of each item of work (such as excavation, blockwork and shuttering), so that they can price them by considering the labor, raw materials, equipment taxes and their margin for overhead expenses and profit. Quantity surveyors estimate the quantity of each type of work, with a variation of about $\pm$ 10%, in the form of bills of quantities. If this document is prepared carefully, both the client and the bidder obtain a reasonably accurate aides of the cost of construction.

Project Management

The planning and construction of a hospital must be coordinated and monitored if they are to be carried out effectively and delays are to be avoided. A high level of discipline and good record-keeping are essential, because of the numbers of people involved at various stages, the lengthy duration and their intermittent involvement. It is therefore desirable that someone-preferably a member of the planning team with previous experience in managing planning and construction—act as a *project manager.*

The project manager is responsible for coordinating and expediting the whole process, organizing and motivating all groups, forescasting and programming their activities and monitoring and controlling their performance. The project manager is involved continuously in the project and is committed to its successful completion. It is the job of the project manager to ensure that all team members perform their tasks both on time and within the budget. He or she must obtain from them regularly updated information on all activities, both at the site and on the shop floor, so that corrective action can be taken, either to the budget and financial approvals or to the project. Above all, the project manager must see that everything is properly recorded.

The project manager must ensure that all relevant information for operating and maintaining the facility is handed over to the client. Drawing of all structures and services as they have actually been constructed must be prepared and handed over to the client for future reference.

The most important element in project management is a realistic time schedule. A basic schedule should be worked out at the early stages of the planning process, and this should serve as a framework for all activities. As the lapse of time between the decision to build and the actual taking over of a completed district hospital is very seldom less than 3-4 years, a time schedule should be prepared during the briefing stage, which should indicate the major stages and also provides for such activities as tendering, major construction activities, planning and procurement of medical equipment furniture.

Once the client has approved the start of the project, the project manager must prepare a time schedule for each of the major aspects of construction and must set a larger date for completion of the project. This schedule should indicate how construction of different elements will proceed; at what stages the working drawings and detailed technical specifications will be made available to the contractor by the architects and engineering consultants; when materials will be procured; and when plant and medical equipment will be commissioned and installed. As the choice of construction method and building materials significantly effects the schedule, it should be considered in detail at this time.

Figures 38.2a and b shows a typical time schedule for the major steps in setting up a district hospital, from the time the project is approved to when it is commissioned. This simple bar chart shows the start and finish of specific activities. It shows how they are linked, how long each will take, where they overlap, where they parallel one another, or whether there is a lag between them. Any delay are almost always followed by an increase in the cost of the project. This aspect can be monitored and controled by critical path analysis or project evaluation and review.

Critical Path Analysis

The nature of a multidisciplinary project like the building of a hospital means that complex, time-consuming, interdependent sequences of events are encountered. These can be organized by critical path analysis, which involves a diagramatic representation of the project as a network of activities. The major consecutive activities are defined as 'the critical path'. Any delay in one of the activities on the critical path will delay the overall schedule for completion of the project.

The process of network planning thus involves four steps:

- breakdown of project activities
- listing of activities
- constraints and sequential relationships of activities
- network diagramming.

It is a logical representation of all the activities, with definite points of start and finish. Once the network diagram has been completed; the duration of each activity is determined on the basis of site location, climatic conditions, availability of raw materials, quality of available labor, method of construction, height of construction, safety regulation and all other relevant factors.

The project manager should also actively control the final cost and not merely passively register payments. The client's acceptance of the budget provides the basis for economic control over the final cost (cost control), payment of contracts and variation orders (payment control) and availability and use of funds (control of cash flow).

Payments to the contractor for work done and services rendered are usually made on a fixed-price basis, either:

- as a schedule of prices, giving unit prices for the items listed in the bill of quantities (item rate contract), or as a

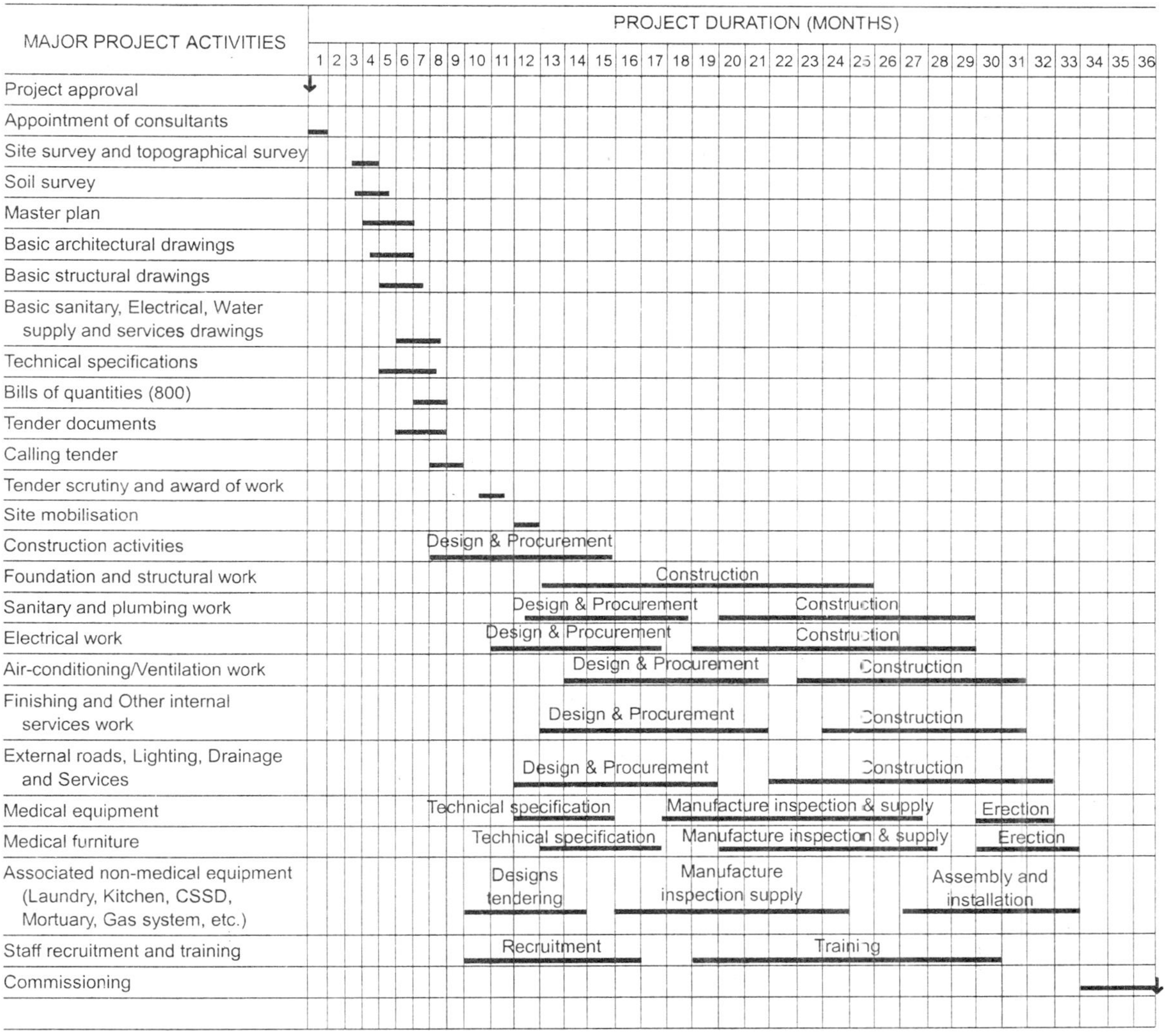

Fig. 38.2a: Project implementation scheme for a typical district hospital

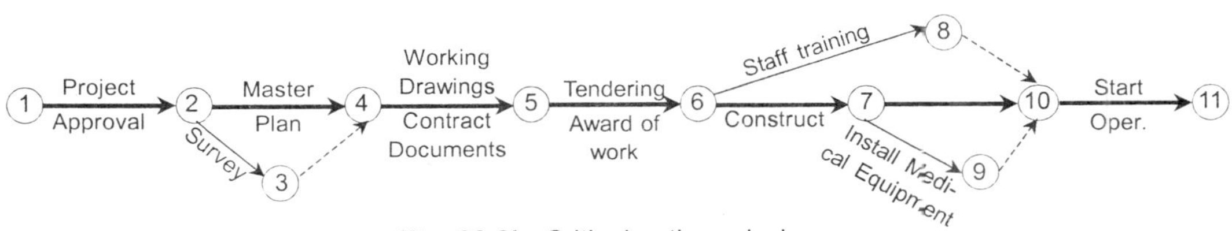

Fig. 38.2b: Critical path analysis

- lump sum for the complete work, as defined by the drawings and technical specifications (lump sum contract).

The first arrangement is the most common, in which the total price is determined by the actual quantities, measured on the site and multiplied by the unit price quoted in the contract. This is a reasonably fair and straightforward method, which works quite well for present-day construction systems.

In times of high inflation, it is the usual practice in the case of projects with a construction time exceeding one year to pay the contractor some form of compensation for rising prices, if agreed in the contract.

In current international practice, the construction agency usually gets 90% of the payment for work completed each month, and the client holds the remainder as 'retention money' until the end of the 'defects liability period', usually one year after handing over, during which time the contractor is responsible for remedying any defects in materials or workmanship in the buildings.

The final payment to the contractor is based on the final certificates of the project manager, including a final account.

Management of Medical Equipment

A system must be developed for managing medical equipment in order to use health resources effectively and efficiently. A cycle of systematic management is shown in Figure 38.3.

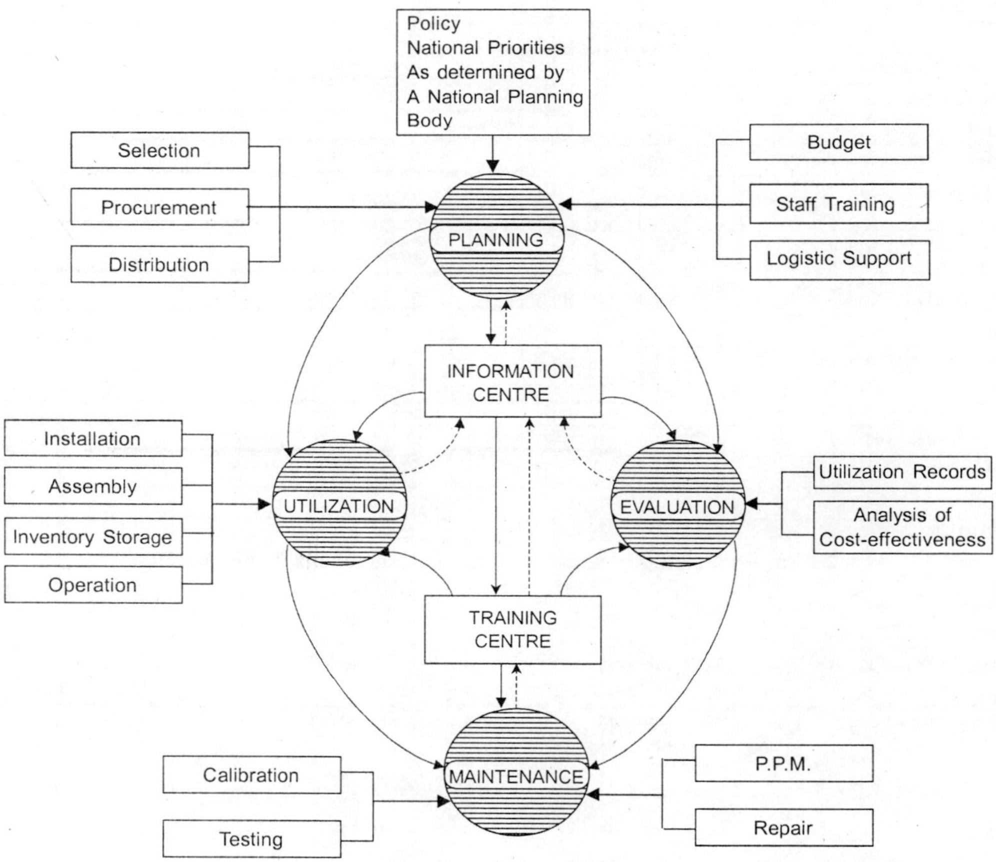

Fig. 38.3: Cycle of management of hospital equipment

Planning

Planning for the provision of medical equipment must involve the following considerations:

- the population targeted by the health service,
- their health needs,
- the health service functions required to meet those needs,
- the health care equipment required to perform- those functions and
- the available resources.

A planning group should be organized to make decisions on selection and procurement of medical equipment, on the basis of the following considerations:

The equipment must be carefully selected to ensure that it:

- gives the best value for money, weighing lifetime cost against purchase price;
- can be maintained continuously during its expected lifetime, in terms of its upkeep, repair and spare parts (a budget for maintenance contracts, spare stocks and information transfer must be provided); and
- comes from reliable, reputable and experienced manufacturers.

The financial resources available must be allocated equitably for:

- initial purchase and installation, including foreign exchange, and
- running costs.

Arrangements for maintenance should be considered at the time of procurement and should be applied systematically throughout the lifetime of the equipment. Maintenance arrangements can be made either under contract with the manufacturer or in-house by the health care technical service

Staff should be adeqauately and properly trained before being allowed to use equipment.

Utilization

The important spects of equipment use are as follows:

1. The utilization rate of equipment in current use must be increased through adequate manpower and logistic support.
2. The period of delivery, installation and assembly of equipment must be shortened.
3. Documentation about the use and maintenance of the equipment must be obtained for management purposes.
4. Inventory and storage methods must be improved and the operational procedures regulated.

Evaluation

Indices can be used to evaluate the utilization of medical equipment.

These include:

$$\text{Annual rate of operation of utility} = \frac{\text{No. of annual visits} \times \text{average operational time}}{\text{per visit/annual actual operational time}} \times 100$$

$$\text{Annual rate of effective time} = \frac{\text{No. of annual visits} \times \text{average operational time}}{\text{possible operational time per visit/annual}} \times 100$$

$$\text{Positive rate} = \text{Positive visits/total visitis} \times 100$$

$$\text{Demand for equipment} = \text{Use rate per person per year} \times \text{population/rate of effective use time of equipment possible operational quantity}$$

Cost-effectiveness and cost-benefit analysis may likewise be used in evaluating the effectiveness and efficiency of the use of medical equipment. The potential years of life saved, survival rate and quality of life are some of the indicators in cost-effectiveness analysis. Cost-benefit analysis evaluates all outcomes in economic terms.

Team Approach

A multidisciplinary approach involving team work or collective decisions must be used in ordering new equipment.

A technical committee should exist in each hospital, chaired by the hospital administrator, which reviews the equipment situation and plans for future needs. The considerations of this committee should include:

- policy for health needs,
- planning development,
- inventory,
- specification and procurement,
- budgeting,
- training of users and servicing staff,
- spare parts and
- logistic support.

When selecting equipment, the members of the technical committee should ascertain the specific health needs that must be served. The members can then proceed, taking the following factors into consideration:

- Type (not model or make) of equipment required should be identified, and general specifications should be drawn up to meet the requirements of the medical use to which it is to be put.
- All equipment needs should be identified and costed, including any training of users and servicing staff, physical facilities and auxiliary supplies, such as water,electricity, air-conditioning, protection and safety precautions.
- Technical support from the local agent must be sought and availability of spare parts ascertained.
- All technical information on operation, service, installation and spare parts must be secured before payment is made.
- Funds must be available for purchase and use of the equipment.
- In evaluating tenders, quotations must be compared and evaluated, not only in terms of price and delivery time, but also in terms of availability and quality of back-up support, spare parts and technical staff.

Human Resources Development

Both service personnel and users must be trained on the equipment in their charge if it is to be used and serviced properly, so that its useful lifespan will be prolonged and the quality of the output of the equipment will be maintained.

At the district level, training should be in the form of courses; these are augmented by training courses offered at the national level. Training must supersede the arrival of the equipment in the hospital, so that qualified staff are available when the equipment is installed.

Planned Preventive Maintenance

Planned preventive maintenance is regular, repetitive work done to keep equipment in good working order and to optimize its efficiency and accuracy. This activity involves regular,routine cleaning, lubricating, testing, calibrating and adjusting, checking for wear and tear and eventually replacing components to avoid breakdown.

Productive preventive maintenance refers to the proper selection of equipment to be made on what to include, to reduce costs; inexpensive units that are not necessarily included in the planned preventive maintenance programme can be replaced or repaired when they break down. The over-riding consideration is cost-effectiveness.

An important aspect of planned preventive maintenance is the participation and commitment of *the user*. Preventive maintenance should start with users, and the bulk of the work should be their responsibility. The task must be performed daily, with joint activities involving the user and a technician engineer at the end of the week. Highly technical repairs, which are the engineer's responsibility, may be scheduled every six months.

In order to establish an effective, efficient planned preventive maintenance system, a registry filing system is needed. The manufacturer's manual for preventive maintenance of the equipment can be supplemented by computer packages in setting up such a system; if a computer is not available, a manual file can be set up. The planned preventive maintenance administrative system requires the following.

Equipment Inventory

All equipment in the hospital that is in the care of the service workshop should be recorded on cards. All relevant information about the equipment must be entered,including its location,records of repair and maintance and the manufacturer.

A reference number is given and written on a printed paper label which is attached to each item. This number is recorded in a ledger of equipment with full identifying details.

Definition of Maintenance Task

The work that must be done to maintain each item of equipment in safe and reliable operating condition must be defined; this is known as the maintenance task. These tasks can be established by consulting the manufacturers' literature and product information.

Establishing Intervals

The frequency of the task must be decided. A heavily used item must be cleaned and checked more frequently than one which is used less often; however, minimum standards must be set. The frequency suggested in the manufacturer's manual can be used as a guide, but the actual usage should determine the maintenance procedure required.

Personnel

Individuals who are qualified and available to do preventive maintenance must be identified. Once the personnel have been listed, specific responsibilities should be assigned, perhaps in the form of a works order, giving clear instructions for the task. Each person should have a clear knowledge of his or her responsibilities. Job assignments must correspond to the training, experience and aptitude of the individual.

Reminder System

Maintenance of instruments and equipment is a continuous process: once the equipment has been inventoried, the programme must continue. It may be necessary to develop a reminder system, so that appropriate personnel are notified when certain tasks are to be performed. Whether a card index system or a computer programme is used, the date that each item of equipment is scheduled for its next preventive maintenance should be recorded. The administrator should look up in advance the jobs that need to be done and draw up a monthly or weekly schedule for the staff.

Special Test Equipment

People responsible for equipment management and maintenance should have at their disposal a range of test equipment to check the correct functioning of medical equipment as well as its compliance with the basic electrical safety standards. A wide range of tests can be undertaken, to measure different values for insulation resistance, earth continuity and leakage current in different situations, under both normal and single-fault conditions.

For the practical assessment of whether different types of medical equipment are working effectively, a number of specific analysers, calibrators and simulators are available. These allow technicians to check the function of ventilators and to calibrate blood pressure monitors, pressure transducers, electrocardiographs and the full range of monitoring equipment used in the intensive care unit. Analyzers are available for checking the effectiveness of defibrillators, electro-surgical instruments and ultrasonic phototherapy equipment. A special-purpose analyser has been developed to assess infusion devices; this had hitherto been difficult because of their very low flow rates.

Most common items of test equipment are listed below:

- *Multimeters*: Simple robust, digital multimeter with clamp-on attachment to measure high current in X-ray equipment;
- *Milliampere meter:* To measure millamperes in X-ray equipment;

- *Line resistance meter:* Low-value meter for the power requirements of X-ray equipment (mainly for generator and control units);
- *Electrocardiograph simulator:* Lead II output simulator to check the performance of the electrocardiograph;
- *Spectrophotometer standards:* To check wavelength calibrations; preferably filter standard instead of solutions, for ease of use and transportation;
- *pH meter standards:* Buffer solutions to check the accuracy of readings;
- *Oscilloscope:* Standard 50-MHz model, dual trace, for testing, fault finding and calibration;
- *DC power supplies:* Electronic power supplies, approximately 25 V DC variable and 5-V and 10-V loutputs for testing equipment;
- *Signal generator:* 0-10 MHz, since, square and sawtooth waveform generators for calibration and testing;
- *X-ray phantoms:* Various phantoms, such as hand, step wedge and grating, to test for picture quality;
- *Defbrillator tester:* To measure output (in joules).

Technical Library

A full technical library should be available. Installation and recommended spare parts manuals, annotated with the number of the corresponding equipment, should be kept together with electronic and component data books and appropriate technical books.

Surveillance

After the programme has been set up, periodic surveillance must be carried out to ensure that records are legible and that all entries are being made.

Patient Safety

It is the responsibility of those involved in equipment management to see that both stff and patients are protected from the potential hazards that exist in the hospital environment. These hazards arise from the use and presence of:

- radiation,
- electricity and
- biological materials.

The use of increasingly complex electrically-powered medical equipment in hospitals has brought about the need for a clearly defined policy to avoid the occurrence of accidental injuries to both staff and patients.

Since even a very low current, measured in milli-or even microampares, could be hazardous. Precautions must be taken to ensure proper grounding of equipment and of conductive objects that are within the reach of the patient and attending medical staff. The electrical grounding should be maintained, and periodic checks must be made to ensure that power cords are not frayed, plugs are not damaged and there is no leakage of current within the ratings specified by the manufacturers or the national standards. Medical staff should be trained to understand the need for electrical safety and some of the prlobles that can arise, so taht they can take an active role in minimizing the potential hazards and report those that occur.

Mains-powered units must have a good earth. A three-pin plug must be used on the appliance lead,which must be directly compatible with the socket outlets in the hospital. Adaptors, extension blocks and extension leads should *not* be used, since these provide an opportunity for the earth wire to be disconnected, which seriously compromises basic electrical safety.

FURTHER READING

1. Bronzino JD. Management of Medical Technology: A Primer for Clinical Engineers, Butterworth-Heinemann, Boston, 1992.
2. District Hospitals : Guidelines for Development. WHO Regional Publications, Western Pacific Series No. 4. 1992.

39 Fire Safety in Health Care Facility

A prerequisite for protecting any organization is an understanding of its structure and environment. The application of security safety principles in the hospital setting is unlike applications in any other setting. The principles and the environment must mesh as harmoniously as possible to contribute to the delivery of patient care. The protection of any facility requires the identification and assessment of organizational vulnerabilities. Although healthcare facilities have the same basic protection needs, the degree of vulnerability varies from one facility to another. Fires in medical care facilities contribute to a high loss of life and property. Fire prevention is the everyday activity that eliminates hazards and prepares people and things to react properly should a fire actually occur. Fire preventions start with the construction of the building. (Fire control pertains to the basic organizational reaction to an actual fire).

Design construction and operation of the need for evacuating occupants from the building. Protection should be provided by:

- Appropriate building design, constructions, and use of compartments (separation into fire area).
- Plans for discovering and putting out fires

Fire prevention plans adequate training of the staff on how to isolate the fire to move occupant to safety.

Construction Requirements

- Stories are counted from the primary discharge story to the highest habitable floor. At least 50 percent of the primary level must be level with or above ground.
- Multistorey buildings must be of non-combustible materials with a minimum 2 hours fire-resistive rating.
- The goal is to provide fire safety through containing the fire to room of its origin, thereby reducing the need to evacuate the building.
- Occupant load calculations for determining exit requirements must be calculated by projecting at least one person per 120 sq.ft. of floor area in sleeping areas and at least one person per 240 sq.ft in inpatient healthcare treatment areas, and/or the actual expected count of persons.
- Doors opening to the outside must have panic hardward that releases when pressure is applied from the directions of exit level.

For interior stairs, a minimum clearnance of 44 inches is required. Riser height maximum is 7 inches (minimum 4 inches). Tread depth must be a minimum of 11 inches At least ft 8 inches. of headroom must be provided. Height between landings can be no more than 12 ft. Handrails are required on each side of new stairs and ramps, and must continue the full length of the stairway. Handrails must be not less than 30 inches or higher than 34 inches above the tread. Handrails must have a clearance of at least 1½ inches from the wall, be capable of withstanding a load of 200 lb. Each set of stairs must have other doorways complying with standards relating to other doorways. A smoker proof tower is a stair enclosed designed to limit the penetration of heat, smoke, and fire gases from a fire in any part of a building.

A horizontal exit is a protected way of moving from one area to another in the same building or in an adjoining building on aproximately the same level. Single doors are permitted as a horizontal exit if they open in only one direction and are 44 inches wide or more. Horizontal exits must be 8 ft (or wider) corridors. The openings to these corridors must be protected by two swing doors, each atleast 44 inches wide. On each side of horizontal exit, there must be a total of atleast 30 sq.ft. of floor space per patient (when the square footage of corridors, treatment rooms, patient rooms, etc. is calculated).

Ramps are of special interest when ramps are used as exits, they must be wide enough to accommodate 30 persons per exit (22 persons per stair exit unit is required). Hospitals must use class A ramps in all instances. Exit capacity for a class A 44 in wide ramp is normally one ramp per 100 persons. One ramp per 30 persons using ramps and one exit per 22 persons using stairs is required in health care facilities. When used as an exit, a ramp must be separated from other parts of the facility by a 1-hour fire-resistance rating for facilities three stories or less, and by a 2-hr. fire resistance rating if four or more stories high. Openings must be protected with self-closing firedoors. Ramps must have slip-resistant surfaces. Landings must be level. All floors and fire section must be equipped with at least one exit, consisting of a door leading directly outside the buildings, an interior or exterior stair, a smoke proof tower, and a ramp or an exit passageway. Each floor or a fire section of a facility must have at least two exits that are located remotely from each other. A door to the outside, or to an outside stair, smokeproof tower, ramp, or interior stair must be provided in each fire section.

Means of access must be provided for every 30 persons in the case of horizontal travel, and for every 22 persons when the means of egress is stairs. Exit accesses must be at least 8 ft wide and free of obstructions.

Travel distance must be a maximum of 100 feet between any room door used as an exit access and the exit itself and no more than 150 feet between any point in a room and the exit. Every required exit (ramp/stair) must load directly outside at grade. The means of egress must be illuminated, and the illuminations must be continuous. Emergnecy lighting must be provided. When an electric generator with its own source of power is used, the changeover must be accomplished within 10 seconds. Provisions must be made for emergency lighting that is automatically available. To assure that emergency generators remain in readiness, they must be inspected weekly and run atleast 30 min. per month under load.

Access to exits must either be clear or be marked by easily sen signs. Exit doors and smoke barrier doors ideally should be kept shut at all times.

To maintain floor to floor separations of multistorey facility, 2 hr fire-resistive enclosures are required around vertical openings, which must be of fire-resistive construction and 1-hr fire resistive enclosures in all other buildings.

Hazardous areas must be protected by fire barriers with a fire resistance rating of 1 hr or a complete automatic extinguishment system. Hazardous areas include mechanical equipment room, the laundry, kitchen, employee locker areas, etc.

Each building must have a manually-operated fire alarm system that is electrically monitored. The fire alarm system must be arranged to notify all building occupants when any alarm stations is activated. Smoke detectors must be located no farther apart than 30 ft and not more than 15 ft from any wall. The automatic smoke detection system must both be connected electrically. New healthcare facilities must have an automatic sprinkler system. Each facility must provide portable fire extinguishers. Hand fire extinguishers are required on every floor and in every hazardous area. The travel distance to any extingusher may be not more than 75ft. Every extinguisher must be in operating condition at all times.

Every corridor must have partitions separating them from other areas. These partitions must be continuous from the floor under the health area to that of the floor above.

Corridor doors, may have wired and fixed glass upto 1,296 sq.in. in area, provided they are mounted in a steel or other suitable frame. Doors that protect corridor openings must be substantial (1 3/4 thick and of solid wood).

Smoke barriers are required as:

- Two or more compartments are required in any story housing more than 50 occupants or used by any inpatients for sleeping, and
- Smoke compartments must be limited to a maximum of 150 ft. in length. A fire resistance rating of at least 1 hr. is required for smoke barriers.
- At least 30 sq.ft per patient of usable building space must be provided on each side of a smoke barrier.
- Each patients room must have a window or a door to the outside to permit access to fresh air and/or to vent the fire to the outside. Sills must be no higher than 36 inches from the floor.

Fire Safety Programming

Basic elements of fire safety programming are:

- Prevention
- Detection
- Containment
- Evacuation, and
- Extinguishment.

Fire Preventions

Prevention encompasses the activities of the fire safety programme that occur before an actual fire, including the detection and correction of the hazards, fire control planning, employee and occupant education, design and specifications, equipment tests, drills, and fire department liaison. Facility inspections are conducted by organizational personnel. If they are conducted properly, a continuous, everyday fire inspection programme is accomplished.

Security personnel on their rounds should note and correct hazards everyday. Security staff should be particularly alert for people smoking in prohibited areas. They should also correct and report doors left open that should be closed, obstructions to fire escapes or exit doors, careless use of oxygen cylinders, and other safety violations.

Detection

Actomatic early warning detections systems are common place because fire codes generally require this equipment for hospitals.

Fire detectors require sensing units that measure the presence or change in the products of fire: flame, heat, smoke, and gases, when a standard is exceeded, the sensor is activated. When the detector senses an abnormal condition, it transmits a signal to an annunciator. The signal may also activate fire extinguishing equipment and air-handling machinery, send elevators to pre-determined locations, and release magnetic hold-open devices on doors. These functions support human response and human corrective actions.

Containment

The objective is to contain fire in the area of origin. When this is not possible, the goal is to provide successive levels of defense or areas of refuge from the fire. The five basic areas of fire containment are referred to as the unit concept. The units are : the room, the compartment, the floor, the building, and the exits, all of which have a distinct function in the fire protection system. The functions of units 1 (the room) is to provide the first barrier against the passage of smoke. The more effectively a room can be sealed, the better job it will do in containing fires. The second level of defense is the compartment. The intention is to provide two areas of refuge on every horizontal plane of the hospital. The compartment is created by smoke-and fire-resistant partitions. The function of third unit (the floor) is to prevent the spread of fire and smoke from one floor to another. For the building (unit four) to remain structurally intact for a period of time, it should maintain structural components that offer minimum contribution to any fuel load, and it should be able to withstand the effects of the fire from another structure with which it shares a common wall.

At least two exits (unit five) must be provided on each floor. Two separate means of exit should be visible from any location in the corridor.

Evacuation

Evacuation can be whole or partial, and it will follow either a vertical or horizontal flow. The typical evacuation is partial, and its route is horizontal rather than vertical. The first objective is to move patients to a safe compartment on the same floor.

Wheel chairs and carts are useful and often necessary for evacuation. Blankets can also be used.

Elevators should receive special considerations in the fire evacuation plan. Any hosptial of more than seven stories is considered a high-rise. This height is the limit of most fire department ladders. A vertical evacuation plan is mandatory for high-rise buildings. One or more elevators in a wing removed from the fire area may be used to transport patients to another floor much more quickly than when patients are carried down a stairwell. Generally, the use of elevators during fire is prohibited because of their inherent dangers in a fire.

Extinguishment

The suppression of fire is achieved either manually or by automatic extinguishing systems. The automatic water sprinkler system is the most common of the automatic suppression devices. The water sprinkler system also acts as an alarm device (these systems are installed with water flow sensors that report when water is flowing in the pipes). The sprinkler is generally activated by a holding link that melts at a given temperature. Sprinkler systems are mostly wet type rather than dry systems. Other piped extinguishing systems include: steam, water spray from carbon dioxide, dry chemical and halon agents.

The standpipe and hose systems are used to provide quick and convenient water streams. The hand held extinguishers are primarily two and one half gallon, stored pressure water extinguishers, carbon dioxide extinguishers, multipurpose extinguishers and halon extinguishers. The type at any given location is predicted on the primary type of hazard involved.

Detection and Extinguishment System

To help reduce detection time, methods of detecting smoke, heat, and fire, etc., have been developed. In addition, systems that can suppress and extinguish a fire (either manually or automatically) can be installed to reduce the amount of time before human activity would or could begin to a fire.

Detection System

Fire detection systems consist of:
- the detector portion, and
- the control /indicating portion.

Detector portion Detectors do sensing (detecting) heat, smoke, flame, gas or anything else that indicates a fire or explosion is in the making.

Detectors are also built into sprinkler heads of sprinkler systems. When the air around these sprinkler heads reaches a particular temperature, pre-set sensors snap, melt, or break, thus allowing water to flow out.

Control (indicating) portion Once a detector senses an environment in excess of a present level eg., a set density of smoke, a set temperature, a specific rate of rise in temperature, the condition has to be translated into a form (e.g. a light on a panel, a loud whistle), etc. that people can recognise in order to take appropriate action. This notification (only) is the way some systems function; others automatically cause something in addition to occur.

Fire Extinguishment System

There are two types:

- Water, and
- Chemical.

Water Systems

- Sprinkler type and
- Standpipe type.

Sprinkler systems consist of a source of water (municipal or stored), piping throughout a building, and precisely spaced sprinklers attached to these pipes near the ceiling of each area. The sprinklers have a thermal sensing part (detector) that snaps, melts, or breaks at some pre-set temperature, thereby allowing water in the pipe to discharge.

In standpipe system also there is need for a source of water and for piping to be connected to the water source throughout the building. However, instead of sprinkler heads, houses are connected to the pipes (called standpipes) at strategic points throughout a building.

Many water-type extinguishment systems require the use of pump to increase and /or maintain an adequate water pressure in the system, both initially and after the system has activated. There are equations for calculating this pressure. Today fire pumps are essential for all high-rise buildings as they are the only way to have water reach upper floors with suffcient pressure to have an effect on a fire. Fire pumps also raise the pressure in many other facilities where the water pressure from a tank or municipal supply is not adequate.

Chemical Extinguishment Systems

Various types available are:

- Carbon dioxide,
- Halon 1301, and
- Dry chemical.

Each extinguishes a fire using a different principle smothering, saturation and oxygen elimination.

Fire Protection for Fixed, Building-Wide Systems

Within a hospital there are services (systems) that encompass or connect all or major portions of the structure. Some systems such as heating, cooling, lighting, detecting, communicating, extinguishing, and collecting can be found in other types of occupied structures as well, others, however, (e.g. piped medical gas systems) are unique to health care facilities. Guidelines have been developed for the hazard. These guidelines cover the system itself, and/or the facility as a result of the systems presence, e.g., fire safety criteria during construction or installation, or criteria on the type of separation from other activities during operation.

These systems/services are grouped into following categories:

- Fire protection for environmental air building service systems (e.g heating, cooling, exhausting),
- Fire protection for electrical building service systems (e.g, electrical wiring, emergency power);
- Fire protection for specific building service systems (e.g, refuse and laundry chutes, piped gas and vacuum system).

Environmental Air Building Service Systems

Controlling the temperature (and, in many instances today, the humidity) within a building is a normal part of operating the building. The elements involved in such a system are either highly combustible (i.e., the fuels needed to generate heat) or critical in controlling smoke spread in an emergency (i.e., the forcing of air throughout the facility by a forced air system).

Fuels

Two sources of energy that are often used by healthcare facility and present a fire and explosion hazard are oil and gas. Safeguards for the handling of oil have to be developed and observed. Similarly, safeguards in the handling of gas (gas piping system) desings, materials, components, installations, inspection, testing, and purging need consideration.

Heaters

Devices used to heat a building (either by heating water or air) require different fire protections, considerations, depending on their size and the fuel utilized. Minimum requirements for safety to life and property from fire in the installation of storage tanks, accessories (piping, pumps, valves), and the oil burner itself and also criteria on the installation of central heating boilers and furnaces, direct makeup air heaters, duct furnaces; floor furnaces, etc. need to be included in the system.

Air Movers

Movement of air in buildings, (for heating/cooling), also present the possibility of moving smoke or facilitating the spread or fire in the event of a fire. There should be provisions for restricting smoke, heat, and fire spread through a duct sytem in a building; for maintaining building integrity when a duct system is used and for permitting a duct system to be used for smoke control in an emergency.

Electric Building Service System

Electricity is a conveyor of energy. It provides the "means" to do lot of things in our modern technology age. Uncontrolled, electricity can quickly heat a material so that it will burn or even explode.

Safeguarding the use of electricity include:

i. *Installation* Criteria on wiring, design, methods, material, installation and on associated electric equipment.

ii. *Emergency electrical power* Continuous electrical power in hospital is essential in the treatment of patients today.

Criteria on the power generator system needed to supply electrical power in the event the normal supply fails, how such a system is to be connected to the normal distribution system and what circuits, outlets, the system or functions are to be connected to the system, need to be followed.

Specific Building Service System

These systems are:

Piped gas system Hosptials use extensive amount of both flamable and non-flamable gases. The advantages of a piped system, for medical gases are continuous supply of gas available at any time, a lower operating cost, and a lower operating pressure (50 psi in cylinders). The disadvantages are the initial cost of installing pipes and the fire and explosion hazards of gases being circulated in pipes throughout the facility. The criteria on the in stallation and test of systems for piping gases throughout a facility (requirements for central supply system, monitors and alarms for the system, piping and valves criteria, installation and testing) need to followed.

Piped Vacuum Systems

vacuum pump to provide suctioning capability at various points throughout a facility (in lieu of individual suction machines). Some hazards exist with the use of these systems. Guidelines regarding minimum sizing, alarms, installation, maintenance, and testing of piped-vacuum systems need special consideration.

Chutes

The installation of chutes in a building is accomplished to reduce the build-up of waste, dirty linen, etc. in patient areas and do eliminate the need for personnel to go around and collect it. However, these installations pose fire hazards in that they cut through smoke barriers, thereby providing a means for fire, and smoke to spread if precautions are not taken. While eliminating a build-up of combustibles in one area, they create a build-up of combustibles in another area. Precautions have been developed (construction criteria, the chute terminal room, automatic fire suppression systems, protection for openings through which chutes penetrate, and storage rooms).

Elevators

Elevators also cut through smoke barriers. In addition to the fire problem these systems create, elevators add the "human load" factor. Criteria have been developed with regard to elevators, dumb waitors, and vertical conveyors.

Fans

Removal of certain type of dusts, air, and vapour that are flamable or combustible present several fire and explosion hazards. The include:

- the substance being removed,
- the system removing the substance, and,
- the building in which the system is installed. Criteria have been developed for such systems (system design, controls, fans, and fire extinguishment features).

Fixed Localized Systems

A multitude of activities (cooking, storing,disposal, computer operations, etc.) take place in hospitals. Other unique activities are X-rays, treatment clinics, surgical procedure, etc. As a result, fixed localized systems of fire protection for these activities have been devised.

Fire safety and storage involve the combustibility and flammability of the substance being stored; the amount being stored; The type of construction or enclosure for the substance being stored; and the type of supervision or monitoring of the storage area. Criteria for general storage, rock storage, historical type data storage, flammable liquids storage, medical gas storage , nuclear material storage and identification of hazardous material being stored, have to be fulfilled.

On-going Activities

Several locations of on-going activities including those presenting electric shock hazards,that need more attention than others are:

- Inhalation anesthetizing locations (hospitals)
- Patient-care areas of hospitals,
- Hyperbaric and hypobaric facilities
- Laboratories, and
- Non-medical areas.

Because of the critical nature of activities performed in anesthetizing locations, either localized systems are installed to provide levels of safety above that in other patient care areas, or there are more stringent requirements for any localized systems provided in these areas. Electric wiring, isolated power systems and line isolation monitors, conductive flooring piped gas and piped vacuum need special consideration.

Carrying out procedures under either compressed atmosphere or non-atmosphere is accomplished in hyperbaric and hypobaric chambers. These facilities present fire hazards because of increased oxygen content that occurs with them or within the air being supplied to persons in them. Standards on housing and fabrication, ventilation, illumination, fire protection and electric systems should be followed.

Kitchen areas present very distinct fire hazard because of the fuels used and the heat generated. Criteria for vapour removal, fire extinguishment, air movement and gas cooking equipment be followed.

The collection of combustible materials for removal purpose present a fire hazard because of the unknown condition of the material so collected. Precautions need to be taken regarding fire.

Emergency Communication Systems

Notifying occupants in a building of an emergency is an obvious necessity. The method must be effective and dependable, and it must be almost instinctively associated with an emergency requiring occupants to move or possibly be moved. Through a singal or a verbal statement, conveyance of the emergency must be clear. Standards exist for installation, maintenance and use of emergency voice/alarm communication systems. Speaker, recorded messages and/or live messages; audible and visual indicating applicances (bells, horns, chimes, strobes, etc) are optional.

Safe Practices

Operational fire protection includes safe practices that should be observed at all levels in order to help assure:

- A fire safe working environment for patients and staff, and
- Safe egressing should it be necessary during an emergency.

Norms and standards for activities in high risk areas (for safe practices) have been developed.

Inhalation anesthetizing locations of hospitals

1. Administration and maintenance
   - all anesthetizing locations
   - flammable anesthetizing locations.
2. Testing of line isolation monitors.
3. Testing of conductive floors
   - flammable anesthetizing locations.
4. Use of conductive footwear (flammable anaesthetizing locations only).
5. Anesthetic testing (flammable anesthetizing locations).
6. Use of gas cylinders (high pressure).
7. Use of anesthetic apparatus.
8 Use of electrical appliances.

Patient care areas of hospital

- Electric safety programme
- Testing of electrical grounding system
- Testing of electrical receptacles
- Testing of ground fault circuit interrupters
- Patientcare-related electrical appliances
- Use of oxygen (safe practices when respiratory therapy is administered-eliminating source of ignition, handling cylinders, use of electrical equipment rules on smoking and sparking toys, etc.)

Laboratories Criteria on safe practices exit regarding

- Maintenace and inspection
- Hazard assessment
- Orientations and training
- Flammable liquids (transfer, handling, disposal)
- Gases.

Following Areas Also Need Consideration

- Identifying hazardous areas through the posting of a standardized sign
- Hazardous chemical reactions
- Hazardous properties of flammable liquids, gases and volatile solids.

Employee Reaction

Proper employee reaction to fire is one of the fundamental factors in saving lives and property. Fire safety is a race against time, and the action taken within the finest few minutes can make the difference between a minor fire threat and a tragic disaster.

Employees must act instinctively when fire breaks out:

S	: *Save*	Patients or people if in immediate danger
A	: *Alarm*	Sound the alarm/Activate the alarm
V	: *Vents*	Close doors and windows to keep the fire contained
E	: *Evacuate & Extinguish*	Use evacuation routes and first aid fire extinguishers
R	: *Rescue*—those in danger	
C	: *Contain*—the smoke and fire	

Fire Safety Training

An employee could be the one who discovers the fire or is the first to arrive at the scene of an alarm.

There is need for continuous in-service training and new employee training classes. Fire safety training may require relearning as well as learning. Organizations have unique characteristics that require special fire planning.

Security Consideration

The role of security personnel in a fire situation is part of the overall facility fire plan. The basic responsibilities include:

- Ensuring that responding fire department personnel gain access to the hospital complex, building, and interval areas. This may require unlocking gates/doors, holding elevators, turning on lights, and even escorting fire personel to the fire area.
- Controlling traffic,
- Assisting with evacuation process if necessary
- Assisting emergency personnel throughout the emergency
- Securing the area after the conclusion of the incident.
- Preparing documentation of the fire incident.

Looking Ahead

All healthcare facilities must have a plan for the protection of all person on their premises and for their evacuation from the building in case of fire. Written copies of this plan must be available to all supervisory personnel. All employees must be periodically trained and informed of their duties in implementing the plan.

All beds must be easily movable, should evacuation be necessary. Emphasis should be placed on moving patients who are in the room of fire origin and others who are directly exposed to the fire, and on maintaining in their rooms the patients who are not immediately threatened during the fire. Fire exit drills must include actual transmission of a fire alarm signal along with a simulation of a fire condition. Quarterly drills on all shifts are required. All personnel including administrative staff, maintenance personnel and interns must be trained, as well as the nurses on duty each shift. A minimum of 12 drills must be held each year. All employees must be instructed in life safety procedures and use of devices.

FURTHER READING

1. Amin Tabish: Fire Safety in Health care facilites. *JAHA*. **9(2)**: 55-62, 1997.
2. Nicholas JE: Guide to Hospital Security. Grover Publishing Co. Ltd. England, 1983.
3. White DC: Fire Safety in Hospitals. World Hospitals. IHF, London **3**: 172-73, 1978.

40 Morgue/Mortuary

In evitable part of doctor's duty is not only caring for the living but also in helping to arrange for the disposal of those of his patients who die. The procedure of the disposal of dead is not only medico-social problem but also has a psychological aspect attached to it, which makes it very complex and delicate task. The effect of death and the look of the dead body is a great demoralizing factor for others. It, thus, becomes essential that suitable provision is made where the dead body can be transported to a place of final disposal.

Bodies are kept in refrigerated body store and examined in the post-mortem room. They usually remain in the mortuary for a very limited time. The period is longer if complicated investigations have to be carried out or of the next-of-kin are difficult to trace.

The number of refrigerated places needed in the body store will depend upon the number of deaths per day, with some allowance for week-end accidents, epidemics and the possibility of major accidents. As a general rule, four monetary places for each hundred beds is satisfactory excluding any provision in the isolation section.

The bodies are brought to the morgue on stretchers and left on stretchers in the cold room until the autopsy is performed. Then the stretcher is wheeled into the autopsy room and the body slid off the stretcher onto the autopsy table.

A depth of about 5.4 m for the body store is usually satisfactory. A body on a loose tray or stretcher may require about 3m in the cold chamber. Space is needed in front of the cold chambers for the withdrawal of trays. Clean shrouds, drapes, towels and other linen; also toilet articles that may be required in the viewing room should be available. Additional space should be considered for decomposed bodies or for those being stored for forensic purposes at 6.5°C.

The refrigerating plant should be immediately adjacent to the cold chamber. The main electrical intake and switch board may be sited here. Access for maintenance and servicing should be arranged externally so that it is necessary to enter the department. When the initial temperature of the chamber, before loading, is 5.5°C the temperature of the chambers and contents should be reduced to 3.5°C in 10 hours from loading with bodies at a temperature of 37°C. Thermostatic control will be required for each chamber. Facilities should be provided to enable the chambers not in us to be switched off. A bay of at least 6 m2 is required for the mortuary trolleys.

The post-mortem or autopsy room should be either adjacent to the morbid anatomy section of the pathology department or have direct vertical communication with it. At autopsy the organs are removed from the body and dissected. Sometimes for morphologic, micro-biological and chemical examinations are removed. Frequently photography is used as a means of recording the gross findings.

The dead body, whether previously infected or not, may a source of infection. When a post-mortem examination is being made the infection risk increases by contaminated aerosols released through squeezing sponges, sawing bones and cutting tissues. The room should have two or more post-mortem or autopsy tables. Up to 400 beds require 2 tables, each additional 200 beds another table. A two-tabled room needs about 40 m2 . About 15 m2 of space will be needed for each additional table.

There should be sufficient room for physicians, medical students and nurses to observe the autopsy. The tables of porcelain, fireclay, or stainless steel. Stainless steel is favored. A loose hardwood or cork dissecting board or platform will normally be wanted on each table as well as a rinsing sink incorporated at the foot. It is important to have a water hose as well as a saline wash readily available because water will hemolyze red cells and cause staining and discoloration of specimens.

Individual water hoses should be supplied with water from a thermostatically controlled mixing valve. Water suction pumps should not be used. Floor service ducts should be avoided. A cool spotlight should be available for use, for example, in removing the brain.

A dissection worktop will be needed for selective dissecting and the cleansing and weighting of organs. The surface of the working should be impermeable material, preferably of stainless steel.

Two large sinks with hot and cold water should be adjacent to the worktop. A flushing sluice and a wash basin are needed.

There should be a writing top, a wall mounted X-ray viewing box and a telephone facility. A smaller sterilizer should be available. A wall cupboard should be provided for saline and other solutions. Instruments and equipment store should hold the preserve stock of necessary items.

Post-mortem room must be kept clean. Impermeable and easily washable floor and wall surfaces are required, and a hose point should be available. A sluice room of about 8m2 in size should open directly off the autopsy room. A sink and a fire clay slab will be required for washing and disinfecting of instruments and bowls.

Space will be required for the soiled linen trolley, a small instrument sterilizer, and specimens. Changing rooms are required for the clinical staff and pathologists. A clean utility room for gowns, aprons, gloves etc, is needed. Each changing room should have one WC, one lavatory basin and a shower cubical. A small dirty utility room is required for soiled linen.

An office of about 12 m2 is required for the pathologist. One room for attendants is also required. A cleaner's room is required for storing the cleaning material.

In the post mortem room, lighting should ensure adequate illumination of post mortem tables and dissecting benches. Lighting in the viewing room should receive special consideration. The reasonable illumination levels are: in the post-mortem room 300 lux, at the post-mortem tables 1500 to 2000 lux, in the body store 200 lux.

41 Housing Facilities

For its smooth functioning and optimal utilisation of personnel, hospitals should provide housing facilities (within the campus) to a majority of resident doctors, nurses and technicians. There should be provision for accommodating some specialists/ faculty members.

Resident Doctors

The intern is a recent medical school graduate who spends one year full time in the hospital, assigned successively to the major services, medicine, surgery, obstetrics, pediatrics, and psychiatry. He is given professional responsibilities but works under the supervision of an attending physician and the resident in each service. He is usually assigned the day shift but may have some night duty.

The resident is a doctor who has completed his internship and elects to spend three years more in training for one of the specialities. His assignment in the hospital is thus limited to that speciality; i.e. he does not rotate among the services as does the intern. In the course of his training, he performs all the functions of the attending specialist but is still under that doctor's general supervision. The resident on duty provides continuous medical attention in the absence of the attending physician and assists him when he is at the hospital. In his later years of residency he may assume full responsibility for some patients, depending upon the character of practice in the hospital. Upon completion of his resident trraining and after passing examinations given by the specialty qualifying board, he becomes certified to practice in his specialty.

To qualify for offering internships, a hospital must have at least 150 beds with 5000 admissions annually and meet certain other qualifications regarding medical staff and methods of care. The qualifications for giving residency training are similar and usually include an intern training program and a faculty in the specialties involved.

Because resident doctors are on 24 hours a day duty, housing becomes necessary during night services. Full-time housing is less common a requirement because it is rare to find a resident doctor or intern who is not already married. For the matter, many medical students marry before graduation. Hence the housing problem within the hospital divides into two parts, first, the need for a few single rooms for the permanent occupancy of the unmarried residents and interns, and second, several rooms for those residents and interns who live outside the hospital but are on duty for the night. In planning, it is suggested that the functional program estimate the number of interns and residents and that full-time dwelling rooms be provided by the hospital for 50 per cent of the residents. In addition, the actual number of single rooms for night use as described should be calculated from the schedule of night assignment of these personnel.

A minimum program for the sleeping rooms calls for single rooms with a lavatory in each, plus central toilets and showers. If possible, a shared toilet and shower or a private one should be provided. The permanent dwelling rooms may be double, though private rooms are preferable. Some lounge or recreation space for these men should be included on the floor, plus central storage, as in a dormitory, for personal belongings. There need be no physical separation of dwelling and night rooms if both are located in the hospital building, but for reasons of construction cost and personal preference, many hospitals now plan for night quarters only to be within the hospital and all other housing in separate buildings.

Nurses and Technologists

Schools today range from one year of practical nurse training to the four-year bachelor's degree college course and, in some cases, graduate work. Most common are the schools which accept high school graduates or otherwise qualified applicants for the three year course and award the certificate of registered nurse upon graduation. There may be the option of taking another year for the college degree.

Whatever the educational pattern, it is customary to house all undergraduate student nurses in dormitories or cottages near the hospital and under its control. The program of a school of nursing deserves careful study. The idea in dormitory housing is for each nursing student to have a single room with a least a lavatory in the room and, if funds permit, a private or connecting bath. If not, central toilets and shower will serve. Double rooms are also common and are more economical of space, and there is something to be said for having young women of college age room together for sociability and exchange of eductional experience. The chief disadvantage lies in that occasional assignments to night duty may be expected, and the girls so assigned needs to sleep during the day when her room-mate may not. In spite of this circumstance, most nurses' residences do provide for two girls per room, and some hospitals simply refrain from assigning students to the night shift.

The problems of housing student technicians or others in the paramedical schools such as physical therapy, occupational therapy, X-ray, pharmacy, laboratory, and dental hygiene are little different from those for student nurses except that night shift assignments are rare. The number of students in these courses is not great, and they are usually housed in the student nurses' residence.

In all such housing the effort should be made to provide attractive quarters with a minimum of the impersonal feeling so often attached to institutional dormitories. Sometimes this is achieved through the use of color, fabrics, and furnishings, sometimes through an informal plan, even in separate cottages; more often it is not achieved. Recreational facilities are essential, plus laundary and pressing rooms and some central storage. Dining may be in the hospital or in dormitory. Student dormitory standards generally apply.

Medical Staff

Non-teaching hospital is expected only rarely to provide housing for its medical staff, though occasionally circumstances such as a remote location and a full-time staff call for it. At the other extreme, some large hospitals in metropolitan centres affiliated with a medical school may provide staff housing in addition housing for residents and interns.

Table 41.1: Functional program: housing. The program should also describe the general character of dormitory housing, whether single or double rooms, toilet facilities and other spaces, and give the number and size of various apartments which are to be planned

	100 beds	*200 beds*	*300 beds*	*400 beds*	*500 beds*
House staff	–	–	17	37	56
Night rooms in hospital	–	–	6	10	14
Dormitory rooms in or near hospital	–	–	6	12	19
Apartments elsewhere	–	–	6	12	19
Student nurses; dormitory rooms	–	–	–	10	20
Graduate nurses	30	60	90	115	140
Dormitory rooms	–	–	20	30	40
Apartments	–	–	20	30	40
Other professional staff, female	10	20	28	35	42
Apartments	–	–	5	7	9
Housing for medical staff	*Determined by local market*				
Dwelling for administrator	*Determined by hospital policy*				

Hospital Personnel

Hospitals generally should provide housing for employees, particularly those who fall under emergency category and whose services are required in different shifts.

Visitors and Relatives

There is a growing demand for transient hotel rooms for hospital visitors. This is especially true where patients come from some distance. In such cases, the hotel bed may take care of the relative or companion of the patient and even of the patient himself if he is ambulant. Although it cannot be said that the hospital has a definite obligation to provide such transient housing, it would be a great boon to have it available. Only analysis of local experience will show how much may be desirable and whether it will be self-supporting.

As with all buildings, there should be provision for adequate automobile parking in connection with housing.

The Future

As hospital care embraces more and more special categories of patients, from the acutely ill in intensive care division to the longterm or convalescent patient, the question arises whether the future may not see all housing considered as part of hospital accommodations. It would not take much to extend the spectrum to include ambulant patients and visitors in hotel rooms.

FURTHER READING

1. E Todd Wheeler: Hospital Design and Function, McGraw-Hill 1964.

RESEARCH FACILITIES

Animals are needed for diagnostic and research purposes. Diagnostic laboratories in support of the animal facilities may include capability for microbiology, hematology, blood and urine chemistries and preparation of histologic slides, both normal and pathologic.

Commonly used animals kept for stock do not require very special and very closely controlled conditions. Where breeding is concerned, the requirements may be more stringent. Highest requirements are adapted when germ-free animals are involved.

Whenever possible animal quarters should occupy the ground floor of a building to keep the labor required to handle incoming animals, their feed, bedding, cages and refuse to a minimum.

Animals' quarters should be easily identified. They should be designed with the animal' physical comfort as a primary consideration.

The environmental requirements of animal accommodations vary accoridng to the species of animals and the purpose for which they are kept.

They must be dry and easy to clean. Most of the animal attendance should be carried out from the outside. Excreta ought to be collected without disturbing the animals. Paper inserts could be used.

Good housekeeping procedures are of prime importance for limiting or preventing the exposure of personnel and experimental animals to hazardous conditions.

Animal rooms should not be overcrowded. Particular stock rooms are heavily utilized and there is a considerable heat gain from the animals. In a plastic enclosure the temperature may be 4 to 4°C higher than in the surrounding room.

Animal caging arrangements must be examined for the possibility that the cross infection between animal species will occur. This depends upon agent, animal and experimentation.

In the US, following cage spaces have been recommended:

Species	*Weight*	*Floor area cm^2/animal*	*Free height in cm*
Mouse	Upto 10 g	39	13
	10 to 15 g	52	13
	16 to 25 g	77	13
	Over 25 g	97	13
Rat	Upto 100 g	110	18
	101 to 200 g	148	18
	201 to 300 g	187	18
	Over 300 g	258	18
Hamster	Upto 60 g	65	15
	61 to 80 g	84	15
	81 to 100 g	103	15
	Over 100 g	123	15
Guinea pig	Upto 250 g	277	18
	251 to 350 g	374	18
	Over 350 g	652	18
Rabbit	Upto 2 kg	1400	36
	2 to 4 kg	2800	36
	Over 4 kg	3700	36
Cat	Upto 4 kg	2800	61
	Over 4 kg	3700	61

Germ-free animals are kept either in stainless or other heat-resistant containers of plastic or nylon which can be sterilized in an autoclave or in plastic containers which are not heat resistant and are sterilized by ethylene oxide.

Door should be about 1.15 wide and 2.15 high, and the corridors 2.2 m wide to allow easy passage.

There should be easy access to washbasins in each room. The faucet should be of screw-type to attach a hose when needed.

The floors should be nonslip, wear resistant, smooth and resistant to solvents, acids, and chemical substances present in animal urine.

Terazzo, cupric oxychloride cement, smooth hard-surfaced concrete, neoprene terazzo, hardened rubber-base aggregates and some synthetic products have proved satisfactory. mA cpmtomipis waterproof membrane may be needed. In some animal rooms squared-off fully vitriefied ceramic tiles may be used.

Large animals rooms should have floor drains fitted with hair traps and washdown facilities. The drainpipes should not be less than 10 cm in diameter.

There should be curved junctions between floor, walls and ceilings. Recesses and crackis should be avoided. Durable, waterproof, fire-resistant, seamless materials are most desirable. Paints and glazes should, in addition to being highly resistant to chemical solvents, cleaning agents, and scrubbing, also be highly resistant to high pressure sprays.

Windows are not necessary in a facility for acute animal experiments. They should be omitted where there is a risk for solar heat gian. In many cases cooling will be necessary to avoid the occurence of temperatures, which can give rise to sickness and death amongst the stock as well as uncomfortable conditions for the attendants and technicians.

Lighting should be uniformly diffused throughout the animal area.

Independent control of temperature in each room, in some cases in each enclosure, should be provided. Ideally, a system should permit individual adjustments within ± 1°C for any temperature within a range of 18° to 29° and the relative humidity should be maintained through the year within a range of 30 to 70 per cent according to the needs of the species being maintained.

The needs of some apecies are:

Mice 12°C[1], rates 21° to 23°C and 50 to 60 per cent relative humidity, hamsters max 23°C, guinea pigs min 16°C and 40 to 60 per cent humidity, rabbits 16° to 20°C and 40 to 60 per cent humidity, and cats about 20°C.

About 15 to 20 changes of air per hour have been required. Recirculation of air is not advisable.

In order to control cross-infections, the rooms should be arranged—as far as possible—on a clearn-soiled cycle with no retrograde traffic.

Emergency power for light and ventilation in the event of a power failure is necessary.

A room with diagnostic X-ray machine, fluoroscope and film developer should be provided as well as an operation unit with movable animal operation table when large animals are involved.

There should be facilities for feed and bedding supplies. Refrigerated storage is needed for perishable items such as fresh vegetables and meat. Food storage areas should be physically separate from refuse area.

Before re-use cages are decontaminated, disinfected, or sterilized, the equipment used to house infected animals should be steam-sterilized. Provision should be made for a separate room for cage-washing and sterilization.

Cage cleaning is commonly carried out by a washing machine, utilizing 83°C water under pressure to remove the fouling. Tunnel washers which can be loaded on the soiled side and which extend through a wall into a clean storage room have been recommended.

The process of cleaning and sterilizing release heat and vapour. A good standard of ventilation is necessary in the cage washing room.

After examination and autopsy, dead animals are held in the refrigerator until incinerated.

A freezer will be needed for storage of dead animals injected with radioactive isotopes and their bedding untill the radioactivity has decayed to a safe level before the animals can be autopsied and disposed of.

Waste Disposal

Animal waste comprises primarily bedding and carcasses. Local incineration is necesary, also for dead animals.

The incinerator may also handle combustible trash. Its size and design depends on the local building codes, the largest expected cadaver, and the amount of plastics to be burned.

To avoid nuisance, attention must be paid to the location of incinerators, to the prevention of undue heat transmission to surrounding areas, to the provision of a satisfactory combustion air supply and to the location of the fuel outlet.

A special corridor may openly be recommended to permit the removal of unprotected contaminated material for disinfection or disposal.

FURTHER READING

1. Ervin Putsep: The Modern Hospital: International Planning Practices. Lloyd-Luke Ltd. London 1979.

42 Landscaping

Landscape provides a picture frame and an apt setting for the building by highlighting its scale, its color scheme, by focussing the eye on important views and by screening out the negative views of the structure. It is very rightly said by the eminent architect Le-Corbusier, "The material of design and planning are the sun, the space, the vegetation, steel and concrete, in that precise order and subordination".

In hospital planning, adhering to the basic principles of environmental planning is very important. Hospital is a place where the sick come to get diagnostic and treatment facilities. In human beings any sickness causes sadness, pain, mental anguish and an overall depression. A creful landscaped environment can be of immense therapeutic value as it evoks interest and cheerfulness and brings one closer to nature.

The important principle of environmental planning is the site-structure relationship. Most of the time if the planner is sensitive the site itself offers the ideal kind of structure. Here standardization of buildings design cannot be a solution because each site with its inherent characteristics warrants for its own unique solution which will fit well into that particular environment. Sites will have their own assets and liabilities and in good planning with its vast infrastructure requirement. For example, on an undulating site the main building with wards can be placed on high points which command good views and good orientation and service areas like laundry, kitchen or depressing sights like the animal house or mortuary can be placed in the hollows whereby screening these effectively from the view. Similarly such variations in the levels can be used to create separate access routes by segregating traffic channels and entries to various departments like OPD, the maternity wards, the radiology department and the dental centre, etc.

A carefully planned landscape can create an environment which by way of visual enjoyment can exude a pleasantness which may work wonder in improving the mental outlook of a patient. Well thought of internal courtyards with shrubbery, fountains, small rock gardens will result in creating passive recreation areas as pools of stillness in the usual hustle and bustle of a hospital. Lawns opening out with carefully planned walks through clumps of shrubbery, sitting areas under thick groves of trees, small water bodies sculptures near the wards can invite people to walk out and be with nature. Similarly the out-patient zones should have highly landscape areas around them to take up the spillover of outpatient at peak hours.

The indoor environment of a hospital can present a very gloomy picture if not handled with a sensitive mind. The large open areas apart from being well, it should have a pleasant color scheme and lively interiors- as most of the time the aim is to usually uplift the spirits of the people confined in the hospital who are going through lot of pain and ill health. Here, lot of interest can be created by drawing the eye towards detail provided by variations in color scheme, sculpture, murals, indoor plants, interesting sitting out enclosures, etc. For patient who can walk around the immediate outdoors should be well landscaped with walkways and sitting out furniture.

The plant material here must be given due emphasis as it is one of the major components of landscape design. As he is to water, so is a man instinctively drawn to trees and the inviting volumes, they embrace and define. The attributes of the trees are so manifold that in the conceiving of any site volume, we first, consider its construction in relation to the existing trees. If we cannot use trees as a spatial frame, we usually draw upon the inexhaustible palette of plant material that range from the wildly free to the stiffly architectonic in their native or manicured forms.

Trees can be used as vertical elements in creating enclosures and are important in control of wind, breeze, sunlight, shadow, temperature and sound. The wind may be diverted, checked and to a large extent eliminated. It is also possible to allow it to move through desired channels with the help of trees. Sunlight may be blocked, filtered, diffused or admitted in its full glory, healing life giving force. Trees are the ideal material for helping in visual control.

Visual control is also one of the basic principles of an act of landscaping. All things seen from a space are visual ingredients of the space. Not only the extent and nature of the enclosures but the extent and nature of its revealment must be in keeping with the space thus formed. For anything that can be seen from a space is usually in the space and must be taken into account. Often objects far removed may be intorduced into the space by opening to enframing or focussing in the object. A far-off mountin peak, the dome of the monument of the hubbub of a harbor may for its therapeutic value be brought into the convalescent spaces of a hospital.

The landscape design shall also encompass the designing of open or shelters parking bays near all the major departments of the hsopital. The ugly black and roots of the low service blocks when seen from the top floor in a multistorey hospital can be turned into useful and pleasing roof gardens, if careful thought is given at the very beginning stages of planning.

43 Parking

A prevailing problem of site relates to its development for estimate the need, second to establish categroies of use and physical standards of development, and third to formulate operating policies which can be carried out effectively in the parking spaces planned.

The functional program should include a listing of the separate categories of parking to be provided, usually for medical staff, other hospital personnel, and the public, and of the number of parking spaces for each category. If there are to be restricted lots, the method of control should be indicated. Local building codes quite generally specify the quantity of stalls to be provided, and usage calls for a total for all categories ranging from one to two stalls per hospital bed. The literature on this subject documents the problem fairly well and gives standards for land use. A good rule of thumb is to use no more than one-third of the total site for parking and to figure no more than 140 cars per acre, which includes aisles but no access drivers. Key- or card-operated semaphore gates have become fairly common for control of restricted lots.

The analysis starts with estimating the need.

a. *Medical staff* Calculate peak attendance, and allow one space for each attending doctor.

b. *Hospital personnel* Allow one space for each two on the day shift.

c. *Visitor* Allow one space for each four hospital beds. The total of A, B, and C comes to one to two spaces per bed.

d. *Outpatient services* Allow four to six spaces for each doctor's suite (doctor, nurse, and two to four for patients). In large clinics allow one space for each two patient visits during the peak afternoon or morning.

e. *School of nursing* Allow one space for each full-time faculty member, plus one space for each two-day shift personnel, plus one space for each six students.

f. *Standards of planning*
   i. Use no more than one-third of total site for parking.
   ii. For each car in double line, figure 300 sqft. This will include aisles but no access roads or green strips.

The greatest pleasure in life is achieving what people say you cannot...

Part Three
Hospital Administration

44 Hospital Acquired Infection

Infections acquired as a result of a hospital stay are called nosocomial infections (the word nosocomial is derived from the Greek word for hospital; the term also includes infections acquired in nursing homes and other health-related facilities). The Centers for Disease Control (USA) estimates that from 5 to 15% of all hospital patients acquire some type of nosocomial infection. It is estimated that about 20,000 people die of nosocomial infections each year.

Noscomial infections result from the interaction of several factors: (1) microorganisms in the hospital environment., (2) the compromised (or weakened) status of the host, and (3) the chain of transmission in the hospital.

Micro-organisms in the Hospital

Although every effort is made to disinfect and check the growth of microorganisms in the hospital, the hospital environment is a major reservoir for a variety of pathogens. One reason is that the normal flora from the human body are opportunists and present a particularly strong danger to hospital patients. In fact, most of the bacteria live in healthy people, but are pathogenic only for individuals whose defenses have been weakened by illness or therapy.

In the past, most nosocomial infections were caused by gram-positive microbes. At one time, gram positive *Staphylococcus aureus* was the primary cause of nosocomial infections. Although antibiotic-resistant strains of that organism are still singnificant factors, the major causes today are gram-negative bacteria, such as *E. coli* and *Pseudomonas aeruginosa* has the ability to cause opportunistic skin infections, especially in surgical and burn patients.

In addition to the threat of opportunists in the hospital, some micro-organisms become resistant to antimicrobial drugs. For example, *P aeruginosa* and other gram-negative bacteria tend to be difficult to control with antibiotics because of their R factors, which carry genes that determine resistance to antibiotics. As the R factors recombine, new and multiple resistance factors are produced. These strains become part of the flora of patients and hospital personnel and become progressively more resistant to antibiotic therapy. In this way, people become part of the reservoir (and chain of trnsmission) for antibiotic-resistant strains of bacteria. Usually, if the host's resistance is high, the new strains are not much of a problem. But if disease, surgery, or trauma has weakened the host's defenses, secondary infections may be difficult to treat.

Compromised Host

A compromised host is one whose resistnce to infection is impaired by disease, therapy, or burns. Three principal conditions can compromise the host: (1) broken skin or mucous membranes, (2) a suppresed immune system, and (3) impaired cell activity.

As long as the skin and mucous membranes remain intact, they provide formidable physical barriers against most pathogens. Burns, surgical wounds, trauma (such as accidental wounds), injections, invasive diagnostic procedures, intravenous therapy, and urinary catheters (used to drain urine) can all break the first line of defense and make an individual more susceptible to disease in hospitals. Burn patients are especially susceptible to nosocomial infections because their skin is no longer an effective barrier to micro-organisms. A burn patient can have tissue damage caused by heat, electricity, radiation, or chemicals, all of which destroy proteins and cells in affected tissues.

The risk of infection is also related to invasive procedures, such as administering anesthesia, which may alter respiration and contribute to pneumonia, and tracheotomy, in which an incision is made into the trachea to assist breathing.

In healthy individuals, while blood cells called T lymphocytes provide resistance to disease by killing pathogenes directly, mobilizing phagocytes, and secreting chemicals that kill pathogens. Drugs, radiation therapy, steroid therapy, burns, diabetes, leukemia, kidney disease, and malnutrition can all adversely affect the actions of T lymphocytes and compromise the host.

A final factor that may compromise host defenses is impairment of the development or activities of white blood cells called B lymphocytes, which develop into antibody-producing cells. Antibodies provide immunity by such actions as neutralizing toxins, helping to lyse pathogens. Conditions that alter the actions of B lymphocytes include malnutrition and cirrhosis of the liver.

A summary of the principal kinds of nosocomial infections is presented in Table 44.1.

Table 44.1: The principal kinds of nosocomial infections

Infection	*Comment*
Urinary tract infection	Most common, usually accounting ting for about 50% of all nosocomial infections. Typically related to urinary catheterization.
Surgical wound infection	Ranks second in incidence (about 25%). It is estimated that from 5% to 12% of all surgical patients develop postoperative infections; the percentge can reach 30% for certain surgeries, such as colon surgery and amputations.
Lower respiratory infection	Nosocomial pneumonias rank third in incidence (about 12%) and have high mortality rates. Most of these pneumonias are related to respiratory devices that aid breathing or administer medications.
Bacteremia	Bacteremias account for about 6% of hospital infections. Intravenous catheterization is implicated in nosocomial infections of the blood stream, particularly infections caused by bacteria and fungi.
Cutaneous infection	Among the least common of all nosocomial infections. However, newborns have a high rate of susceptibility to skin and eye infections.

Chain of Transmission

Given the variety of pathogens (and potential pathogens) in the hospital and the compromised state of the host, routes of transmission are a constant concern. The principal routes of transmission of nosocomial infections are direct contact transmission from hospital staff to patient and from patient to patient, and indirect contact transmission through fomites and the hospital's ventilation system (airborne transmission).

Because hospital personnel are often in direct contact with patients, they can often transmit disease. For example, a physician or nurse may transmit her or his flora to a patient when changing a dressing, or a kitchen worker who carries *Salmonella* can infect a food supply.

Certain areas of a hospital are reserved for specialized care. These include the burn, hemodialysis, recovery, intensive care, and oncology units. Unfortunately, these same units also group patients together and provide environments for the epidemic spread of nosocomial infections from patient to patient.

Many diagnostic and therapeutic hospital procedures provide a fomite route of transmission. The urinary catheter used to drain urine from the bladder is a fomite in many nosocomial infections. Intravenous catheters, which pass into a vein through the skin to provide fluids, nutrients, or medication, can lalso transmit nosocomial infections. Respiratory aids can introduce contaminated fluids into the lungs. Needles may introduce pathogens into muscle or blood, and surgical dressings can become infected and promote disease.

Control of Nosocomial Infections

It is important to reduce the number of pathogens to which patients are exposed by using aseptic techniques, handling contaminated materials carefuly, insisting on frequent and conscientious handwashing, educating personnel with basic infection control measures and using isolation rooms and wards. Tubs used to bathe patients should be disinfected between uses so that bacteria from the previous patient will not contaminate the next one. Respirators and humdifiers provide both a suitable growth environment for some bacteria and a method of airborne transmission. These sources of nosocomial infections must be kept scrupulously clean and disinfected, and malarials used for bandages and intubation (insertion of tubes into organs, such as the trachea) should be sterilized prior to use. Packaging used to maintain sterility should be removed aseptically. Physicians can help improve patients' resistance to infection by prescribing antibiotics only when necesary, avoiding invasive procedures if possible, and minimizing the use of immunosuppressive drugs.

Accredited hospitals should have an infection control committee. Most hospitals at least have an infection control nurse or epidemiologist (an individual who studies disease in populations). The role of these personnel is to identify problem sources, such as antibiotic-resistant strains of bacteria and improper sterilization techniques. The infection control officer should make periodic examinations of equipment to determine the amount of microbial contamination. Samples should be taken from tubing, catheters, respirator reservoirs, and other equipment.

Patterns of Disease

A definite sequence of events usually occurs during infection and disease. There must be a reservoir of infection as a source of pathogens for an infectious disease to occur. Next, there must be transmission of the pathogen either by direct contact, indirect contact, or vectors to a susceptible.

Hospital Environment

Hospital environments become contaminated with dust, soil, chemical residues, debris, etc. as well as with organic matter and potentially infectious organisms. A safe environment is achieved by removing or destroying contamination and thereby preventing microorganisms or other contaminants reaching a susceptible site in sufficient quantities to intiate infection or any other harmful response term 'decontamination' which is used to describe this process consists of cleaning, disinfection and sterilization

Micro-organisms and the Environment

The man, the microbes and the environment are intricately intertwined: the microbes wil be present in any environment occupied by man. It is neither practical nor desirble to produce microbe-free surroundings, especially in areas of concentrated gatherings. It is however, desirable to 'minimize the number of organisms present and to favor those least likely to cause human infection, and to make it hostile to those most likely to be harmful'. The number and type of microbes present will depend on:

- the number of people in the environment
- the amount of activity
- the amount of moisture present
- the presence of material capable of supporting microbial growth
- the rate at which organisms suspended in the air are removed.

The cleaning of hospitals has two functions:

1. Non-microbiological
    - to improve or restore appearance
    - to maintain function
    - to prevent deterioration
2. Microbiological
    - to reduce the number of microbes present
    - to remove substances which will support their growth or interfere with subsequent disinfection or sterilization.

Microbiological Contamination of Hospital Environment

The organisms most commonly found in a dry environment, free from substances likely to support microbial growth, are coagulase-negative staphylococci, though to originate from patients' skin. Organisms causing nosocomial infections in patients have, however, been frequently recovered from patient surroundings.

The ability of some organisms to survive in the environment for long periods has been established: enteropathogenic strains of infecting the patient can also contaminate the wider environment of the patient, the contamination of the environment by both urine and faecal organisms may be widespread.

Hospital environmental cleaning is evidence-based and 'a cost efective method of infection control'. Furthermore, clean care establishment inspire confidence in patients and their relatives as well as in staff.

Routine Cleaning

Much of the routine cleaning process centres around maintaining the appearance of the place by removing debris and dirt. This can be adequately achieved by cleaning with household detergent and water. It is more difficult to produce an environment that is microbe-free. Organisms in the environment reach a plateau in which rates of deposition and death are in an equilibrium: cleaning will only temporarily change the numbers prsent. This suggests a constant presence of microbes in the environment. however, if not cleaned regularly, there will be a build-up of substances likely to support the growth of microbes. The hospital environment needs to be clean enough not to cause concern to patients and it should be microbiologically safe.

Cleaning Schedules

The frequency and method of cleaning is unlikely to have a major effect on the number of patients who become infected. Yet cleaning schedules should continue to remain an integral part of hospital practice because there is no guarantee that infection rates would not rise if standards are allowed to drop.

The limited resources, both financial as well as (domestic) manpower, demand that the frequency of cleaning should take note of possible risks of infection likely to be associated with each area/ room or specific item of equipment. The cleaning schedule can thus be prioritized as high, medium or low as suggested here.

High priority Daily cleaning plus regular checks and further cleaning as required. Examples include:

- beds, bedisde lockers and tables, patient chairs
- lavatories, baths and showers-including floors
- commodes-sluice rooms-including floors
- treatment rooms-including floors
- ward kitchens including floors
- patient area ward floors (dust-attracting mops)
- wet mopping as necessary

Medium priority Once or bi-weekly cleaning. Examples include:
- bed and curtain frames
- other floor areas in a ward area.

Low priority 1-, 2. or 3-monthly cleaning. Examples include:
- high dusting
- floor polishing
- office cleaning

Additional cleaning is necessary during outbreaks The cleaning schedule required flexibility to incorporate the changing circumstances of a clinical situtiion. The domestic supervisors and assistants require basic training and understanding of the what, why and how of cleaning hospitals.

Cleaning Materials and Methods

- Cleaning with household detergent and warm water remains by far the best and most effective and most commonly accepted method of removing both the contamination and microbes.
- Dry dust mopping is effective and removes the need for wet mops and buckets of water.
- The use of disinfectant solutions is justified in some instances, for example spillage of body fluids, where the environmental contamination may contribute to the indirect transmission of pathogenic micro-organisms.

Color-coded Cloths

Most establishments operate a system of color coding to ensure that cloths used for cleaning a sluice area are not used for bedside tables and lockers or in the ward kitchen.

Points to Remember

- The cleaning materials can easily become contaminated and will increase the microbial count rather than reduce it. Detergent and other cleaning fluids can heavily be contaminated with Gram-negative bacilli: Gram-positive cocci will be replaced by Gram-negative bacilli. Steps to prevent contamination of cleaning materials include:
- A through rinsing of the cleaning cloths under running hot water and then allowing them to dry (discarding cloths after each use is costly).
- Empty detergent containers should be discarded and not refilled.
- If 'spray-cleaning is practized, the spray bottle should be emptied and the bottle and nozzle washed and rinsed thoroughly and allowed to dry between use.
- Floor mops have been found to be heavily contaminated with Gram-negative bacilli.
- Used fluids and wet equipment encourage the growth of Gram-negtive bacilli. Used fluids, including water used with mops, should be discarded immediately after use and bucket and mop rinsed thoroughly under running warm water. Invert the bucket and stand the mop upright to facilitate drying. Floor mops may be sent to laundry but if this is not possible, can be disinfected using chlorine-releasing agents.
- Disinfectants are readily inactivated by organic material. The organic material should be removed with a detergent-based solution before applying disinfectants.
- Spillages of human secretions and excretions are likely to be contaminated with human pathogens and to support growth of more sensitive organisms, spillages should be cleaned promptly.

Disinfection and Sterilization

Disinfection is described as 'a process used to reduce the number of viable micro-organisms but which may not necessarily inactivate some microbial agents, such as certain viruses and bacterial spores. Disinfection may not advice the same reduction in microbial contamination level as sterilization.

Sterilization is described as a process used to render an object free from viable micro-organisms including viruses and spores.

Sterilization is required where small numbers of residual organisms on an item may be sufficient to cause disease, where exceptionally virulent organisms are suspected, or where surviving organisms may be expected to multiply on an item and reach an infective dose before its use.

For the purpose of rendering an item safe for patient use it should be clean, disinfected or sterilized. The process used depends on the risk of infection involved in the use of the item.

High-risk Items

These are items which come in close contact with a break in the skin or mucous membrane or which are introduced into sterile body areas. Surgical instruments, cardiac or urinary catheters, implants, needles, etc., are included in the 'high-risk' category. High-risk items must be sterilized

Sterilization can be achieved by:

- high temperature moist
- high temperature dry heat sterilization
- low temperature steam and formaldehyde-sterilization
- ethylene oxide sterilization
- gamma irradiation.

Moist Heat Sterilization

A temperature higher than that of boiling water is achieved by steam under pressure:

- steam under pressure • 32 lb per square inch
- temperature • 134-138°C
- time of exposure • 3 minutes

Type of Autoclave

Pourous load steam sterilizer is suitable for wrapped goods. The sterilizing cycle incorporates vacuum-assisted air removal before introduction of steam. The steam, therefore, can penetrate the good through wrapped material.

Downward displacement sterilizer is suitable for unwrapped goods. The air is removed by displacement with steam rather than by vacuum. A complete removal of air is not possible and hence the steam may not penetrate trapped air in wrapped goods.

Fluid-cycle steam sterilizer-fluid in sealed containers. Temperature/time:

- 121-124°C for 15 minutes, or
- 115°C for 30 minutes.

Low temperature steam and formaldehyde (LTSF)—for heat-sensitive instruments. Temperature/time: 73°C for 3 hours.

Hot Air Sterilization

Hot air sterilization is used for instruments which may be damaged by steam, e.g. non-stainless metals, hollow needles, glass syringes. It is also used for non-aqueous liquids, oils and powders.

Temperature/time:

- 160°C for 2 hours
- 170°C for 1 hour
- 180°C for 30 minutes

Ethylene Oxide Sterilization

This is used for heat-sensitive equipment, both wrapped and unwrapped. Temperature/time: 20-60°C for times ranging from 2 to 24 hours.

Management of Clinical Waste

Any waste generated in health care settings is called as clinical waste. The duties of employers should be identified regarding hazardous substances at work to which employees and other may be exposed: clinical waste falls within the scope of these regulations.

The Policy

The following items are suggested for an effective policy on the management of clinical waste:

- identification of categories of clinical waste
- specification of containers/enclosures to be used

- storage
- transport
- handling before disposal
- training needs (for staff at all levels)
- personal protection
- accidents and incidents (reporting, investigation and follow-up)
- spillages
- final disposal

Those in the process of developing a local policy are referred to the guidance documents. The discussion here is limited to issues which may be part of the teaching requirement for the infection control nurse.

Table 44.2: Assessment of patient care items

Category	*Treatment*	*Method*	*Items*
High risk			
In contact with a break in the skin or mucous membrane or introduced into a sterile body areas (if sterilization is not practical high level disinfection may be adequate)	Cleaning and sterilization	*Heat-tolerant:* Autoclave Hot air oven *Heat-sensitive:* Single use Ethylene oxicde Low-temperature steam and formaldehyde Sporicidal disinfectants, e.g. glutaraldehyde	Surgical instruments, laparoscopes, arthoscopes, cardiac catheters, implants, infusions, injections, needles syringes, swabs, surgical dressings, sutures.
Intermediate risk			
In contact with intact mucous membranes, body fluids, or contaminated with particularly virulent or readily transmissible organisms, or if the item is to be used on highly susceptible patients or sites	Cleaning and disinfection (or sterilization)	All the above and *Heat-tolerant:* Boiling Pasteurization Low-temperature steam washer/disinfectors *Heat-sensitive:* Disinfectants, e.g. glutaraldehyde chlorine-releasing agents, alcohol, clear soluble phenolics	Respiratory and anethetic equipment, GI endoscopes, thermometers, vaginal speculae, fluid spillage, dirty instruments prior to reprocessing, bedpans.
Low risk			
In contact with normal and intact skin	Cleaning usually adequate, disinfection if known infection risk	Manual cleaning with detergent Automated cleaning/disinfection Disinfectants	Trolley tops, operating table, wash-bowls, lavatory seats, baths washbasins, bedding, patient supports
Minimal risk			
Remote, not in direct contact with patients or immediate surroundings. Unlikely to be contaminated with a signifciant number of pathogens or be transferred to a susceptible site	Cleaning alone	Manual or automated clean-, ing damp dusting, wet mopping dust-attractant mops, vaccum cleaners	Floors, walls, furniture, ceilings, drains.

Categories of Clinical Waste

Clinical waste is categorized according to the level of risk to staff. There are five categories of waste each requiring its own control measure:

Group A

All human tissue, including blood (whether infected or not), animal carcasses and tissue from veterinary centres, hospitals or laboratories, and all related swabs and dressings.

Waste materials, where asessment indicates a risk to staff handling them, for example from infectious disease cases.

Soiled surgical dressings, swabs and other soiled waste from treatment areas.

Group B

Discarded syringe needles, cartridges, broken glass and any other contaminated disposable sharp instruments or items.

Group C

Microbiological cultures and potentially infected waste from pathology departments (laboratory and post-mortem rooms) and other clinical and research laboratories.

Group D

Certain pharmaceutical products and chemical wastes

Group E

Items used to dispose of urine, faeces and other body secretions or excretions assessed as not falling within Group A. This includes used disposable bedpans or bedpan liners, incontinence pads, stoma bags or urine containers.

The guidance suggests that the level of risk of Group E items may be difficult to assess but they may be offensive and should, therefore, be treated as clinical waste.

All staff members handle clinical waste although levels of risks will vary according to the category of waste. They require instruction and training about identifying specific categories of clinical waste.

Methods of Disposal

Incineration The incineration is the preferred method of disposal for all clinical waste. If this is not practical, the waste in Groups A and B must be incinerated. The incineration may be carried out on site or in a licensed and authorized incinerator

Disinfection Alternatives to incineration include disinfection of Group A and B waste. The waste treated in this manner will be rendered non-hazardous for disposal to landfill or to municipal incinerators or the process will reduce the risk of infection in handling and transport.

Recent advances in the management of biomedical waste include:
- Shredding
- Pyrolysis
- Microwave
- Autoclave
- Needle/syringe destroyer

Landfill is an option for the wastes from the remaining groups. The suitablility of the waste for landfill will depend on the level of risk and is offensive nature. The landfill sites have to be licensed to accept clinical waste.

Disposal into the sewer Small amounts of body fluids or tissue and wastes listed in Group E may be macerated and then discharged into the sewer. This requires approval from the sewerage undertaker or sewerage authority.

Segregation of waste A wastes, regardless of the method of disposal, should be segregated into color-coded containers. The color coding system in Table 44.3 has been recommended.

The supply of appropriate containers and sacks remains the responsibility of the supplies department

Table 44.3: Colour-coded system for segregation of waste

Colour of bag/container	*Type of waste*
Yellow	Clinical waste for incineration only
Yellow with black stripes	Clinical waste which is suitable for landfill disposal
Light blue or transparent	Waste for autoclaving or with light blue lettering equivalent treatment before ultimate disposal
Black	Normal household waste

with advice from and consultation with the local infection control personnel and estates department.

The labelling of the containers or sacks is a matter for local discussion. Some establishments prefer labelling so that the source can be identified in case of spillage or injury from an item protruding from the sack.

Staff members at all levels should receive some instructions on identification, segregation and personal protection. The importance of thorough handwashing and dry after contact with waste, whatever the category, should be emphasized.

Community Disposal

The clinical waste generated in general practice and dental surgeries, health centres and nursing homes is subject to the same regulations as in hospitals. The waste from patients' own homes remains a subject of ongoing dialogue. Many local authorities arrange a separate collection for clinical/infected waste if prior arrangements are made: yellow bags with black stripes are recommended for this method of disposal. This waste may be sent for incineration or landfill at designated, approved and licenced sites.

Management of Used Linen

Used linen may be processed on site or in a commercial laundry. Local laundering facilities are often encountered in many community elderly care units and some specialist wards usually for patients' own clothes. The soiling of clothing is as, if not more, likely to these establishments as in a ward and staff need to remain vigilant to adequate processing of clothes and their own protection when handling contaminated.

Safety points when handling waste and linen

- Use the appropriate color-coded bag.
- Do not fill bags more than two-third full.
- Check whether labelling of bags is indicated
- Bags should be securely fastened to prevent spillage.
- Prevent contamination of staff or other items or linen by using a water-soluble bags as a liner if seepage (body fluids or blood) is likely.

Infected Linen

All infected linen receives the same disinfection process as used linen. The Scottish guidance for hepatitis and AIDS viruses recommends a washing temperature of 93°C for not less than 10 minutes. The inner bag is transferred into a designated washer without being opened, followed by the outer bag. Infected linen should not be processed in a batch continuous washing machine in case of a blockage.

Heat-labile Linen

This is washed at a low temperature, i.e. 40°C, and dried at 60°C. The disinfection may be achieved by adding sodium hypochlorite to the penultimate rinse but is restricted by the presence of soiling, deterents and alkali in the wash. Hypochlorite is not suitable for fabrics treated for fire retardance.

The survival of multi-resistant enterococci, especially vancomycin-resistant *Enterococcus foecium* has been reported. The organism is said to be widespread in the environment and has been associated with a number of outbreaks. It is also possible that the organisms may persist in the washing machines and continue to contaminate the linen allowing their re-introduction into the original ward or other hospitals.

A minimum temperature of 93°C for hepatitis B is recommended. The heat inactivation at the temperatures suggested combined with the considerable dilution factors stage should render the linen safe to handle on completion of the wash cycle.

Domestic Linen

Most linen can be washed adequately in domestic washing mahcines. Special arrangements may be required for contaminated linen from people with infections. Community staff should liaise with infection control and hospital laundry personnel organization or establishment's estates department should ensure that locally-purchased washing machines have the specified programming ability to meet the disinfection standards.

Cagtegories of Used Linen

Used (Soiled)

This category includes all used linen, irrespective of state, but on occasion contaminated by body fluid or blood.

Infected

This is linen from patients with or suspected of suffering from enteric fever, and other salmonella infections, dysentery (*Shigella* spp.), hepatitis A, hepatitis B, hepatitis C and carriers, open pulmonary tuberculosis, HIV infection, notifiable diseases and other infections in Hazard Group 3. Hazard Group 3 refers to an organism that may cause severe human disease and present a serious hazard to laboratory workers. It may present a risk of spread to the community but there is usually effective prophylaxis or treatment available.

Heat-labile

Fabrics likely to be damaged by both the normal heat disinfection process and high temperature are included in this category. These need to be washed at low temperature (40°C). Chemicals such as sodium hypochlorite 150 p.m.m. available chlorine may be added to the penultimate rinse provided no soiling, detergents and alkali are present and where there is no likelihood of chemicals damaging the fabric.

Transport of Used Linen

Used (soiled and fouled) linen is placed into a polythene or nylon/polyester bag, which is usually white. Use of a water-soluble bag as a liner is recommended if seepage of body fluids or blood is likely.

Infected Linen

This is placed immediately, without sorting, into a water-soluble bag or bag with a water-soluble stitched seam of membrane. The sealed bag is then placed into a color-coded, usually red, nylon or polyester bag.

Heat-labile Linen

This is placed in a locally agreed colour-coded bag.

Disinfection of Used Linen

Used (Soiled and Fouled) Linen

This receives two wash cycles: a sluice wash is followed by a second disinfection cycle in which the load temperature, i.e. the temperature of the wash water in contact with the load, is maintained at 65°C for 10 minutes or at 71°C for 3 minutes.

Disposal of Urine, Faeces and Other Body Fluids

The main outlet for urine and faeces is a machine which sluices, washes and disinfects the urinal or the pan. The machine is connected to the sewage discharge system of the building. Alternatively, a disposable container, either a urinal or a bedpan sheet, is disposed of into a macerating machine which converts the container and the content into a pulp which is subsequently discharged as above. The washer/disinfector should indicate a minimum of 80°C for a 3-minute contact time or 83°C for 1 minute in order to ensure a safe container. The macerators have been associated with aerosol contamination of the surrounding area and should be checked. In fact much of the machinery within health care settings is governed by a code of planned maintenance programme, which the estates departments have a responsibility to fulfil.

The Sluice

There are occasions when it is necesary to release the content of a suction bottle into the sluice. There may be risk of splashes to the face or eyes. Extreme care is needed during this procedure. Eye protection may be desirable. Any contamination of the face and eyes should be rinsed off using copious amounts of water and the incident should be reported and recorded.

The Engineer's Responsibility

One other area of responsibility for engineers in relation to infection control is the prevention of Legionnaires' disease. The *Legionella* species are encountered in natural environments such as lakes, rivers and mud, and in man-made water systems such as piped water and air-conditioning systems. Water-cooled air-conditioning systems and industrial evaportive cooling towers, where large bacterial loads can build up with extensive aerosol formation, have been associated without breaks in hotels and hospitals. Planned prevention is said to be the most important defence against the disease.

Apart from regular draining and cleaning of water storage tanks, the recommendations include the storage and circulation of hot water at a minimum of 60°C. There are hazards associated with this high water temperature, especially in areas where the elderly, the mentally ill and children are nursed. The temperature of the water at the tap should be 45-50°C.

The hot water at the tap often discourages staff room washing hands appropriately or adequately: only mixer taps should be installed in clinical area.

Collection of Specimens

The value of laboratory investigation depends on the nature of the specimen. Medical staff initiate the collection of specimens but the main responsibility for obtaining samples for laboratory investigation lies with the staff involved indirect 'hands-on' care. Staff involved in collecting samples should receive training in the correct procedure.

Infectious Process

The infectious process is defined as an infection resulting 'from an encounter with a potentially pathogenic agent with a susceptible human host in conjunction with a suitable portal of entry'. The agent may already be residing on the human body (endogenous) or be from a source outside the host (exogenous). The outcome of this exposure may be a disease. Apart from the serious disease—causing microbes, people and micro-organisms coexist in harmoney most of the time. It is only when the equilibrium between the two is disrupted that micro-organisms penetrate the body's defence mechanisms and cause infection. The development of a disease thus depends both on the host and on the agent. Microorganisms which cause infection have the capacity to enter the human body and to spread throughout the tissues; they are also virulent enough to produce a disease in a susceptible host. The agents that possess these attributes are termed microorganisms of clinical signficiance.

The formula for an infectious outcome is described as:

$$\text{Risk of infection} = \frac{\text{dose + time + virulence (of microorganism)}}{\text{host susceptibility}}$$

The dose of some organisms required to cause an infection may be relatively low compared with the infective doses of other organisms.

The length of time for which an individual is exposed to the pathogen can be a contributory factor.

The virulence, i.e. the capacity of the organism to produce a disease, plays a major role in the infectious process since this capability varies with each agent.

It is the vulnerability of the human host which determines whether the above factors combine to produce an infection.

In infectious diseases the final outcome can depend as much, if not more, on the susceptibility of the person as on factors relating to the microorganism itself number of factors which increase the host susceptibility include:

- An underlying disease such as diabetes, and blood and respiratory disorders
- The therapy for disease, e.g. chemotherapy used to suppress the bone marrow in paptients with leukemia, lymphoma and those undergoing bone marrow or organ transplant
- The use of steroids and cancer-cell-suppressing (cytotoxic) drugs may result in interference with the host defences and in depression of immunity; medications such as steroids are known to increase the risk of infection
- Treatments and procedures carried out whilst in hospital, especially invasive techniques such as surgery, urinary catheterization and intravenous therapy.

Thus, infection risks are identified as host related (intrinsic), or as a result of prescribed therapeutic treatment procedures related to medical and nursing care (extrinsic).

Some of these components are considered here.

Extremes of Age

Extremes of age are defined as children aged 1 year and under, and people aged 65 years and over:

The newborn, normal-weight infant relies on maternal antibodies for protection against infection for a period of 3-6 months until its immune system is fully developed. Premature delivery and low birth weight add significantly to the infants susceptibility.

Elderly people suffer changes in their cell-mediated and humoral immunity which can lead to poor healing ability as well as poor cough reflex and poor circulation. Poor nutrition may be a common feature in the elder people. They often suffer from chronic illnesses which are associated with infection and are often on immunosuppressive drugs.

Studies have shown not only an increase in wound infection rate with advancing age but that age influences infection rate independently of other factors.

Surgical Wounds

Infection rates in clean operations are likely to become the best measure of effectiveness of an infection control programme in surgery. If surgical wound infections are to become a benchmark for successful infection control practice then nurses need to be involved in the effectiveness debate by making a positive and 'informed' contribution. Furthermore, infections in surgical patients are not limited to wounds; other body systems are equally vulnerable. The assessment of patients and appraisal of the outcome need to encompass each and every variable.

Infection Prevention

Patients admitted to elderly care wards can be highly vulnerable to infection owing to advanced age and many underlying conditions. Many patients may be admitted with lower respiratory tract infections or exacerbation of their airway diseases which can predispose them to superimposed chest infections. Many patients may develop antibiotic-associated complications which require careful infection control measures.

Immunosuppressed patients are often nursed in a single room of a medical ward. Immunocompromised patients are vulnerable to infections from opportunist organisms, i.e. organisms which rarely cause problems in an immunocompetent person. Thus, they may be vulnerable to their own endogenous organisms.

Cesarean Section

The wound infection rate following cesarean section has been placed at betwen 1 and 9 percent. Obesity, socio-economic status, length of operation, skill of operator, use of drains, previous post cesarean section infection and type of incession (horizontal versus vertical) have been described as risk factors for the development of postoperative wound infections after cesarean sections.

Women undergoing a cesarean section are catheterized prior to surgery. The procedure may vary from the catheter, inserted immediately prior to surgery, being either left to drain on a sterile pad and removed at the end of surgery, or removed immediately after emptying the bladder before surgery.

Pediatric Patients

Pediatric wards are often a mixture of non-immune and infected children. Infections of children include childhood diseases such as varicella, mumps, pertussis, measles, rubella, etc. Viral and bacterial gastrointestinal infections and other viral infections such as respiratory syncytial virus, hepatitis A and herpes are all frequently encountered amongst pediatric patients.

Intensive Care

The severity of the illness, the extensive nature of drug and invasive therapy and the frequent manipulation of the body and the devices make patients in intensive care units, whether adult, neonate or pediatric, highly susceptible to nosocomial infections.

Environmental Hygiene

Equipment such as play-pens, highchairs and scales are shared betsween children. These can easily become contaminated. Only washable equipment should be purchased and a regular cleaning schedule should operate.

Trauma Patients

Traumatized patients are at an increased risk of infection because:

- The first line of defence, skin or mucosal surfaces, is bypassed, allowing contamination a direct entry point.
- The devitalized and ischemic injured tissue becomes colonized with microbes which gain access to vulnerable sites via surgial drains, intravenous lines, urinary catheters and endotracheal tubes.
- Multiple trauma patients invariably require intensive care; these patients quickly become colonized with nosocomial pathogens.
- Trauma ill patients may require tracheostomy, are immobilized,develop bed sores and require constant manipulation of invasive devices

The steps described for invasive devices and hygiene precautions should be applied when caring for traumatized patients.

The universal precautions will protect staff members from transmission of organisms, especially blood-borne viruses.

Isolation Nursing

Specific precautions are required to prevent transmission of infectious agents from patient to patient, from patients to staff members and from health-care workers to patients. It may necessiate separating the infected or the vulnerable patient from other patients and from health-care workers using barrier clothing such as plastic aprons, disposable gloves, masks, etc.

The purpose of barrier clothing can be described as being two fold:

- The barrier prevents the infective agent from attaching to the skin or uniform thereby making the carer a means of transmission to other patients
- The barrier effectively blocks off the protal of entry into the carer.

Isolation measures are instituted to:

1. curtail the spread and microorganisms from an infected patient to susceptible individuals (source isolation)
2. prevent severely immunocompromised patients from becoming infected (protective isolation).

Source Isolation

The concept of containing infection at source was first defined by Florence Nightingale in 1863. Fever nursing, as it was called, related to the importance of contact transmission via body substances as opposed to environmental transmission. This notion of transmission via body substances has become the modern cornerstone for source isolation.

Source-specific precautions based on routes of infection include:

Category specific identifies a number of instances requiring physical separation of infected patients. The categories are based on a system that groups diseases which require similar isolation precautions. These are preset on color-coded cards which are displayed outside the room or at the foot of the patient's bed.

Disease specific considers each disease separately and allows for individualized precautions required to prevent transmission of specific organism.

Protective Isolation

Infection is a major cause of death in patients whose immune system is compromised either by a disease or its treatment or by thermal injury.

They are vulnerable to infection from:

- their own 'endogenous' micro-organisms
- opportunistic micro-organisms
- a much smaller dose of microorganisms.

It is not always possible to control the patient's own body flora but certain measures can be employed to eliminate or minimize the risk from exogenous organisms. Some health care establishments have purpose-built positive-pressure facilities with high efficiency particulate (HEPA) filters to care for such patients and practise a strict dress and equipment code. In many general district hospitals a side room attached to a general ward has to suffice. In these circumstances the hand hygiene of staff before contact with the patient and patient care equipment remains critical.

Outbreaks of Infection

Whatever the size of the outbreak the same steps are always followed. These include:

- Confirmation: depending upon the disease, an outbreak can consist of one case (e.g. rabies or botulism) or two or more patients presenting with the same symptoms are required.
- Identification of cases and characteristics: detailed histories need to be taken of all patients who are ill so that a decision can be made as to whether they should be included in the outbreak or not. Sometimes this is supported by laboratory findings but this is not always possible and clinical diagnosis is accepted.
- Verification: it is necessary that a patient's diagnosis is verified and matches that of the outbreak under investigation, e.g. the patient's symptoms and clinical history should match that of food poisoning. This is where laboratory testing of specimens and food samples helps in the investigation.
- Formulating a hypothesis: after gathering the information the outbreak group will decide on a hypothesis about the source and spread of the outbreak; this is usually a 'best guess."
- Control measures: once the hypothesis is made then precautions can be implemented to stop further spread of the infection. Until it has been decided what it is that is most likely to be causing the outbreak. It is not possible to state the preventive measures that staff should implement. However, sometimes control measures have to be started before all the facts have been ascertained.
- Final report: once the outbreak has been declared to be ended a report by the outbreak group

should be written and presented to the chief executive. It should include what caused the outbreak, control measures and their effectiveness, the number of patients affected, and finally and recommendations made to ensure that it does not occur again in the future.

Summary

Infections encountered in hospitals may be community acquired or develop after admission. The patients 'vulnerability to infection may stem from their own underlying diseases and conditions, known as intrinsic risk factors, from treatments prescribed or from care practices, known as extrinsic risk factors.

The nature of severity of the illness determines the type of treatment required, the level of physical handling the patients receive and where they are admitted. A number of practices are common to all patient-care areas irrespective of speciality, practices which are designed to manage risks and protect patients and staff. Health care workers will be in a position to manage risks and provide "informed care" if they understand the factors which contribute to both intrinsic and extrinsic risks.

FURTHER READING

1. Hoston R, Parker L, Glenister: Informed Infection Control Practice. Churchill Livingstone, New York, 1997.

45 Management: A Conceptual and Experiential Approach

Management in healthcare deals with the processes of management and leadership in healthcare practice. Management is defined as working with and through individuals and groups and other resources to accomplish organisational goals. Managers are responsible for organisational goals while leaders may only be responsible for one segment of the overall goals.

The basic premise of management is that managers set goals that represent some level of growth for a particular group in a particular environment.

The process of management is relevant to all people who seek to influence the behavior of others. The management contains four inter-related elements: Planning, organising, motivating and controlling. Technical, human and conceptual skills are required in order to carry out this process. Different levels of management require lesser or greater amounts of technical and conceptual skills; human skills are constant in all levels of management.

Tasks of a Professional Manager

The primary concern of any manager is the organisation with which he works. He is responsible for performance. Performance implies action, and action necessitates taking specific steps and doing certain tasks which a manager is expected to do to produce results.

The manager must constantly monitor the progress and activities of the organisation that it is moving in the desired direction.

Ensuring survival of the organisation is a critical task of the manager. The manager has also to actively seek growth.

Factors affecting the survival and growth include:

- Internal factors (largely controllable)
  - choice of technology
  - efficiency of employees
  - competence of managerial staff
  - organisation's image
  - financial resources.
- External factors (little or no control)
  - government policy
  - laws and regulations
  - changing customer tastes
  - attitudes and values, and
  - increasing competition.

A manager has to perform and produce results in the most efficient manner possible. Every manager has to anticipate and prepare for the increasing competition.

To plan and manage for innovation as an ongoing task, the first thing the manager must do is to maintain close contact with customer. As a manager one should keep a close watch on the technology improvements taking place and try to find a customer-oriented application for it.

Another task of any manager is building human organisation. Surround yourself with the best people you can find, delegate authority and do not interfere. A manager with a competent team has already won half the battle.

It is important to retain talent and inculcate sense of loyalty. Recognising, appreciating, and nurturing subordinate's talents will bring you rewards in terms of improved results and loyalty.

The only way a manager can be acknowledged as a leader is by continually demonstrating his leadership abilities. An effective leader must have vision, who can think and plan ahead and also have persuation to carry along all the people.

The manager has to maintain balance betwen creativity and conformity. Developing a new idea, concept or product can be very creative, challenging and exciting. To translate this idea into a reality requires detailed planning and organising of finance, marketing, administration, etc. Creativity is needed in all the functional aspects of managing.

A manager has to continuously enhance his knowleddge and skills. Training programmes aim to provide or improve knowledge and skills, which can help the manager improve his performance on the job.

Every manager has to perform the important task of a change agent. The social, political, economic, technical and cultural environment in which the organization operates is always changing. The ideal way of introducing change is that you, as a manager, simply sow the idea of the proposed change in the minds of a few people, and then let the idea grow and build till the people themselves come round to asking for the change.

The information superhighway (internet, multimedia, networking, e-mail, e-commerce, etc.) has totally changed the way managers make decisions. Managers today have access to more updated, relevant, timely and accurate information which can improve the quality of decision-making. All this helps lessen the degree of risk by reducing the level of uncertainty.

The best way to avoid public criticism and political opposition is to help all activities above board and legal. The manager should feed correct information to the media and political authorities to ensure that they view his/her organzation in the right perspective.

Improvement in information technology is resulting in an increasing trend towards democratisation of society. Exposed to better quality of life and a better lifestyle, people from the lower economic segments, aspire to the same kind of life style. The manager must understand the aspiration of workers and try to fulfil them. Giving more autonomy, responsibility, money, status and enhancing the worker's sense of self-esteem through participation in management decisions can channelize his talent or potential resentment towards more productive ends.

An organisation fulfils a need/needs of the society. It exists within the society and has a two-way interaction with it. It seeks resources (financial, human, material, etc.) from the soceity and processes them to produce services/goods for consumption by the society. In course of this interaction the manager has to deal with various segments of soceity. In fulfilling the needs of the society and interacting with various society segments, an organization creates impacts. The manager has to maintain relations with various segments of society.

Given the wide range of diverse tasks which a manager is called upon to perform, it is essential that the manager be a thinker, a doer and a people-oriented person—all rolled into one. To be effective the manager must recognize his/her strong dimension and look for an opening where his/her strength can best be utilized.

An organization is a social institution. Its very existence is dependent upon its harmonious relationships with various segments of the society.

This harmonious relationship emanates from the organization's positive responsiveness to the various segments and is closely associated with the tasks a manager is expected to perform. The process of evolving this mutual relationship betwen organization and various interestd groups begins by acknowledging the existence of the responsibilities of a manager. The responsibilities are towards customers (patients), shareholders, employees, suppliers, distributors, competitors, union, government and society.

An organisation, which wants to maintain a positive image in the society must assume and discharge with utmost sincerity in its social responsibility. Today every organisation is expected to make its contribution towards a better quality of life for the entire society.

MANAGEMENT THEORY

Management science develops a theory base from many disciplines, such as business, psychology, sociology, and anthropology. Because organizations are complex and varied, theorist's views of what succesful management is and what it should be have changed repeatedly in the last 100 years.

Scientific Management (1900-1930)

Frederick W Taylor, the "father of scientific management", postulated that if workers could be taught the "one best way to accomplish a task", productivity would increase. The four overriding principles of scientific management follow:

1. By using time and motion studies and the expertise of experienced workers, work could be scientifically designed to promote greatest efficiency of time and energy.
2. A scientific personnel system must be established so workers can be hired, trained and promoted based on their technical competence and abilities and limitations would be identified so the worker could be best matched to the most appropriate job.
3. Workers should be able to view how they "fit" into the organization and how they contribute to overall organizational productivity. This provides common goals and a sharing of the organizational mission.
4. The relationship between managers and workers should be cooperative and interdependent, and the work should be shared equally.

Max Weber, a well known German Sociologist developed similar ideas and expanded on Taylor's concepts. Weber saw the need for legalized, formal authority and consistent rules and regulations for personnel in different positions; he thus proposed bureaucracy as an organizational design.

Management Functions

Henry Fayol (1925) first identified the management functions of planning, organization, command, coordination, and control. Luther Gulic (1937) expanded on Fayol's management functions in his introduction of the "seven activities of management"–planning, organising, staffing, directing, coordinating, reporting, and budgeting–as denoted by the mneomonic POSDCORB. Eventually, theorists began to refer to these functions as the mangement process.

- Planning encompasses determining philosophy, goals, objectives, policies, procedures, and rules; carrying out long- and short-range projections; determining a fiscal course of action; and managing planned change.
- Organizing includes establishing the structure to carry out plans, determining the most appropriate type of patient care delivery, and grouping activities to meet unit goals. Other functions involve working within the structure of the organization and understanding and using power and authority appropriately.
- Staffing function consists of recruiting, interviewing, hiring, and orienting staff. Scheduling, staff development and often employee socialization also are included as staffing functions.

- Directing sometimes includes several staffing functions. However, this phase's functions usually entail human resource management responsibilities, such as motivating, managing conflict, delegating, communicating, and facilitating collaboration.
- Controlling functions include performance appraisals, fiscal accountability, quality control, legal and ethical control, and professional and collegial control.

Human Relations Management

Mary Parker Follet (1926) suggested participative decision-making (participative management) espousing her belief that managers should have authority with, rather than over, employee.

The human relations are also attempted to correct what was perceived as the major shortcoming of the bureaucratic system—a failure to include the "human element".

Studies done at the Hawthrone Works of the Western Electric Company near Chicago between 1927 and 1932 played a major role in this shifting focus. The studies, conducted by Elton Mayo and his Harward asociates, began as an attempt to look at the relationship between lift illumination in the factory and productivity.

Mayo and clolleagues discovered that when management paid special attention to workers, productivity was likely to increase, regardless of the environmental working conditions. This "Hawthrone effect" indicated that people respond to the fact that they are being studied, attempting to increase whatever behavior they feel will continue to warrant the attention. Mayo (1953) also found that informal work groups and a socially informal work environment were factors in determining productivity, and Mayo recommended more employee participation in decision-making.

Douglas McGregor (1960) reinforced these ideas by theorizing that managerial attitudes about employees (and hence, how managers treat those employees) can be directly correlated with employees satisfaction. He labelled this theory X and theory Y. Theory X managers believe that their employees are basically lazy, need constant supervision and direction, and are indifferent to organisational needs. Theory Y managers belive that their workers enjoy their work, are self-motivated, and are willing to work hard to meet personal and organizational goals.

Chris Argyris (1964) supported McGregor and Mayo by saying that managerial domination causes workers to become discouraged and passive. He believed that if self-esteem and independence needs are not met, employees will become discouraged and troublesome or may leave the organization. Argyris stressed the need for flexibility within the organization and employee participation in decision-making.

It was not until the late 1960s that researchers began to understand how complex and intertwined management and leadership are.

The Leadership Theory

The scientific study of leadership began in the 20th century. Early workers focussed broad conceptulaization of leadership, such as the traits or behaviors of the leader. Contemporary research focusses more on leadership as a process of influencing others within an organizational culture and the interactive relationship of the leder and follower.

Leadership is process of empowering beliefs and teaching others to tap their full capabilities by shifting the beliefs that have been limiting them.

The leadership roles include:

- Decision maker
- Critical thinker
- Buffer
- Advocate
- Visionary
- Forecaster
- Influencer
- Creative problem solver
- Change agent
- Diplomat
- Teacher
- Communicator
- Evaluator
- Facilitator
- Risk taker
- Mentor
- Energiser
- Coach
- Counselor
- Role model

The Greatman Theory/Trait Theory

The Greatman theory asserts that some people are born to lead, whereas others are born to be led. Trait theory assumes that some people have certain characteristics or personality traits that make them better leaders than others.

Behavioral Theories

Lewin (1951) and White and Lippit (1960) isolated common leadership styles—authoritarian, democratic and laissez-faire.

The authoritarian leader is characterized by the following behavior:

- strong control is maintined over the work group
- others are motivated by coercion
- others are directed with commands
- communication flows downward
- decision-making does not involve others
- emphasis is on difference in status
- criticism is positive

Authoritarian leadership results is well-defined group—actions that are usually predictable, reducing frustration and giving members a feeling of security. Productivity is usually high, but creativity, self-motivation, and autonomy are reduced. Authoritarian leadership is useful in crisis situations.

The democratic leader exhibits the following behavior:

- less control is maintained
- economic and ego awards are used to motivate
- others are directed through suggestions and guidance
- communication flows-up and down
- decision making involves others
- emphasis is on "we" rather than "I", and "you"

This type of leadership is particularly effective when cooperation and coordination between groups are necessary. However, democratic leadership is less efficient quantitatively than authoritative leadership.

The laisez-faire leader is characterized by:

- Is permissive with little or no control
- Motivates by support when requested by the group or individuals
- Uses upward and downward communication between members of the group
- Places emphasis on the group
- Does not criticise.

Because it is nondisected leadership, the laissez-faire style can be frustrating, group apathy and disinterest can occur. This type of leadership is appropriate when problems are poorly defined and brainstorming is needed to generate alternative solutions.

A person's leadership style has a great deal of influence on the climate and outcome of the work group.

Situational and Contingency Theories

The idea that leadership style should vary according to the situation or the employees involved was first suggested by Many Parker Follet (1926). Her "law of situation", which said that the situation should determine the directives given after allowing everyone to know the problem, was contingency leadership in its humble origins.

Fiedler's (1967) contingency approach reinforced these finding, suggesting that no one, leadership style is ideal for every situation. The interrelationship between the group's leaders and its members were most influenced by the manager's ability to be a good leaders.

Blake and Mouton's (1964) grid showed various combinations of concern or focus that managers had for or on productivity, tasks, people, and relationships. In each of these areas, the leader may rank high or low, resulting in numerous combinations of leadership behaviors.

Hersey and Blanchard (1977) also developed a situational approach to leadership. Their tridimensional leadership effectiveness model predicts which leadership style is most appropriate in each situation based on the level of the follower's maturity. As people mature, leadership style becomes less task-focused.

Tannenbaum and Schmidt (1958) built on the work of Lewin and White, suggesting that managers need varying mixtures of, autocratic and democratic leadership behavior. The primary determinanants of ledership style should include the nature of the situation, the skills of the manager and the abilities of the group members.

Contemporary Theories

Interactional Leadership Theory

The basic premise of interactional leadership theory is that leadership behavior is generally determined by the relationship between the leader's personality and the specific situation. Ouchi (1981) was among the first researchers to introduce interactional leadership theory in his application of Japanese—style management to corporate America. Theory Z, the term Ouchi used for this type of management, is an expansion of McGregor's theory Y and supports democratic leadership. Characteristics of theory Z include concensus decision-making, fitting employees to their jobs, job security, slower promotions, examining the long-term consequences of management decision-making, quality circles, guarantee of life-time employment, establishment of strong bonds of responsibility between superiors and subordinates, and a holistic concern for the workers.

Schein (1970) was the first to propose a model of humans as complex beings whose working environment was an open system to which they responded. Schein's model, based on systems theory, has the following assumptions:

- People are very complex and highly variable. They have multiple motives for doing things.
- People's motives do not stay constant but change over time.
- Goals can differ in various situations
- A person's performance and productivity are affected by the nature of task and by his/her ability, experience, and motivation.
- No single leadership strategy is effective in every situation.

To be successful, the leader must diagnose the situation and select appropriate stratagies from a large repertoire of skills. Hollander (1978) saw leadership as a dynamic two-way process. According to him, leadership effectiveness, requires the ability to use the problem-solving process; maintain group effectiveness, communicate well; demonstrate leader fairness, competence, dependability, and creativity; and develop group identification.

Nelson and Burns (1984) suggested that organizations and their leaders have four development levels and that these levels influence productivity and worker satisfaction.

- Reactive (focuses on the past)
- Responsive (leader moulds subordinates)
- Proactive (leader and followers become more future-oriented)
- HIgh performance teams, maximum productivity, and worker satisfaction are apparent.

Brandt's (1994) interactive leadership model suggests that leaders develop a work environment that fosters autonomy and creativity through valuing and empowering followers. This type of leadership affords the leader greater freedom while simultaneously adding to the burdens of leadership. The leader's responsibilities increase because priorities cannot be limited to the organisation's goals, and authority confers not only on power, but also responsibility and obligation.

Wolf, Boland, and Ankerman (1994) also emphasized an interactive leadership model in their creation of a "collaborative practice matrix"—this matrix highlights the framework for the development and ongoing support of relationships between and among professionals working together. The 'social architecture' of the work group is emphasized. Managers must learn to work synergistically with others.

Transformational Leadership

Burns (1978) suggests that both leaders and followers have the ability to raise each other to higher levels of motivation and mortality. Identifying this concept as transformational leadership, Burns maintained that there are two types of leaders in management. The traditional manager, concerned with the day-to-day operations, are termed as transactional leader; the manager, on the other hand, who is committed, has a vision, and is able to empower others with this vision was termed transformational leader.

Stout-Shaffer and Larrabee (1992) argue that the essence of transformational leadership is vision—the ability to see what is needed and to give the direction necessary to accomplish it.

Transformational leadership is an interactive relationship, based on trust, that positively impacts both the leader and the follower. The purposes of the leader and follower become focused, creating unity, wholeness and collective purpose. The high-performaing transformational leader demonstrates a strong commitment to the profession and the organization and is willing to tackle obstacles using group learning. Transformational qualities must be coupled with the more traditional transactional qualities of the day-to-day managerial role. Both sets of charcteristics need to be present in the same person in varying degrees. The organization and the environment play a critical role in the development and support of the transformational and transactional leadership skills of its employees. The reltionship must be symbiotic.

Integrating leadership and management skills:

Leadership and management skills should be integragted as they are learned. This union can best occur by:

- Using experiential learning exercises
- Demonstrating tghe leadership complement in all management functions, and
- Using a scientific approach to problem solving

Integrating leadership skills with the ability to carry out management functions is necessary if an individual is to become an effective leader/manager.

Decision-Making

Decision-making is a complex, cognitive process often defined as chosing a particular course of action. Decision-making is usually triggered by a problem but is often handled in a manner that does not eliminate the problem. Harrison (1981) has delineated the folowing steps in the managerial decision-making process.

- Set objectives
- Search for alternatives
- Evaluation alternatives
- Choose
- Implement
- Follow up and control

The professional decision-maker is self-aware, courageous, sensitive, energetic, and creative. Decision-making is an important task that relies heavily on critical thinking.

Problem Solving

Problem solving is part of decision-making. A systematic process that focuses on analyzing a difficult situation, problem solving always includes a decision-making step.

The traditional problem-solving process has following steps:

- Identify the problem
- Gather data to analyze the causes and consequences of the problem
- Explore alternative solutions
- Evaluate the alternatives
- Select the appropriate solution
- Implement the solution
- Evaluate the results

Although an effective model, its weakness lies in the amount of time needed for proper implementation.

Process and structure are beneficial to the process of decision-making and force people to be specific about options and to separate probabilities from values. A structured approach to problem solving and decision-making increases critical reasoning and is the best way to learn how to make quality decisions because it eliminates trial and error and focuses the learning on proven process.

Critical Thinking

Critical thinking is related to evaluation and has a broader scope than decision-making and problem solving. Components of critical thinking include, reasoning and creative analysis. It involves higher-order reasoning and evaluation, and has both a coagnitive and affective component insight, intuition, empathy and the willingness to take action are additional components of critical thinking.

Problem solving and decision-making must be of high quality. The following elements are considered crucial:

- Clearly defined objective
- Careful date gathering
- Generate many alternatives
- Think logically
- Choose and act decisively.

The professional approach to problem solving begins with a fixed goal and ends with an evaluation process. The successful decision maker understands the significance that each person's values, life experience, preferences, and way of thinking have on selected alternatives. The critical thinker is aware of areas of vulnerability that hinder successful decision maker.

Management Decision Making

Decision-making is a manager's most important task and is present in every phase of management process. A manager's overall effectiveness is directly related to the effectiveness of their decision-making.

The potential for autonomous decision-making and creativity within an organisation has limitations because those who advance and remain are those typically who have values and beliefs similar to that of the organization. Therefore, a balance must be found between the limitations of choice posed by the power structure within the organization and totally independent decision making that could lead to an organizational chaos.

The two major considerations in organizational decision-making are how power affects decision-making and the assumption that the management decision-making needs only to be "satisfying".

The act of making and evaluating decisions increases the expertize of the decision maker. The effective manager is aware of the need for sensitivity in decision making. Using appropriate decision-making style is a leadership role. Skill in using decision technology is a management function.

Management science has produced many tools and techniques for analyzing management problems and decision-making. These models can be very useful for a novice manager.

Planning

Planning is defined as deciding in advance what to do; who is to do it; and how, when, and where it is to be done. Therefore, planning involves choice: a necessity to choose from among alternatives.

The planning phase of the management is critical and precedes all other functions. Without adequate planning, the management process fails. Planning is a proactive function required of all managers so that personal and organizational needs and objectives can be met.

Adequate planning encourages the best use of resources. Identifying short- and long-term goals requires leadership skills, such as vision and creativity. Planning requires flexibility and energy. Plans should be specific, simple, and realistic. Because a plan is a guide for action in reaching, goal, it must allow for adjustment as unexpected events occur.

Good plans have a time for evaluation built into them so there can be a mid-course correction if unexpected events occur.

Most organisations use many types of plans that form a hierarchy from global to specific. The planning hierarchy in most healthcare organizations includes the elements of mission statement, philosophy, goals, objectives, policies, procedures and rules.

The mission statement identifies the reason an organization exists. The philosophy flows from the purpose or mission statement and delineates the set of values and beliefs that guides all organizational actions.

Management functions include determining, implementing, and evaluating the unit philosophy and an examination of values by managers.

A goal is defined as the desired result towards which effort is directed. A goal is the aim of the philosophy.

Objectives are similar to goals because they motivate people to a specific and are explicit, mesurable, observable or retrievable and obtainable. Objectives, however are more specific and measurble than goals in that they identify how and when the goal is to be accomplished.

Policies are plans reduced to statements or instructions that direct an organization in its decision-making.

Rules and regulations are plans that define specific action or nonaction. Rules are generally included in policy and procedure statements and desirable situations that allow only one choice of action.

All planning must include an evaluation step. Philosophies, goals, objectives, policies, procedures, and the need for rules changes with time and require periodic revaluation and prioritization.

All planning in the hierarchy must flow from, and be congruent with, planning done at higher levels in the hierarchy.

Benefits of effective planning include timely accomplishment of higher quality work and the best possible use of capital and human resources. Because planning is essential, managers must be able to overcome barriers that impede that planning. The organization can be more effective if movement within it is directed at specified goals and objectives.

Strategic Planning

Planning has several dimensions. Two of these dimensions are time-span and complexity or comprehensiveness. Generally, complex organizational plans that involve a long period (usually 3-10 years) are referred to as long-range or strategic plans. Strategic planning is a long-term plan that examines an organization's purpose, mission, philosophy and goals in the context of its external environment. Strategic planning forecasts the future success of an organization by matching and aligning all its copabilities with its external opportunities.

Strategic planning requires managerial expertise in healthcare economics, human resource management, political and legislative issues affecting healthcare and planning theory. It also requires the ledership skills of being sensitive to the environment, being able to appriase accurately the social and political climate, and being willing to take risks.

Healthcare facilities are particularly vulnerble to external social, economic, and political forces; strategic planning, then must address how these forces may change. It is important, therefore, that strategic plans be flexible, permitting change as external forces assert their impact on health care facilities. The realities emerging in today's rapidly changing healthcare system must be incorporated in planning for healthcare organization's future.

Because the paradigm shifts and trends impacting healthcare are constantly changing and because by the time a trend is recognized, it may already be too late to proactively plan for such a change, managers are encouraged to take a broader approach to what information they must gather in the planning process.

PLANNED CHANGE

Planned change is, change that results from a well-thought-out and deliberate effort to make something happen. Planned change is the deliberate application of knowledge and skills by a leader to bring about a change.

The three major drivers of change in contemporary healthcare are growing population, technology, and information availability.

Planned change occurs because of an intended effort by a change agent to deliberately move the system. A change agent is the person responsible for moving others who are affected by the change through its stages. Changes are implemented slowly after consultation with others.

In planned change, the manager is often the change agent.

There are three phases through which the change agent must proceed before a planned change agent must proceed before a planned change becomes part of the system. These stages include unfreezing, movement, and refreezing.

In the unfreezing stage, the change agent unfreezes forces that maintain the status quo. Thus, people become discontented and aware of a need to change. Before any change can occur, people must belive the change is needed. In movement, the change agent identifies, plans, and implements appropriate strategies, ensuring that driving forces exceed restraining forces. During the refreezing phase, the change agent assists in stabilizing the system change so it becomes integrated into the status aquo.

Three commonly used strategies for effecting change in others include:

- rational
- normative
- power
- empirical strategies
- reductive strategies
- coercive strategies

Rational-empirical strategies suggest change will result from giving information by using current data to support the change. Normative—reductive strategies use the group to socialize and influence others for change. Power-coercive strategies use rewards or force to change behavior.

Organisations are preserved by change and constant renewal. Without change, the organisation may stagnate and die.

Organisations progress through developmental stages—birth, youth, maturity, and aging. As organisations age, structure increases to provide greater control and coordination. The young organization is characterised by high energy, movement and virtually constant change and adaptation. Aged organizations have "established turf boundaries", function in an orderly and predictable fashion, and are rule and regulation focused, change is limited.

Both management and leadership skills are necessary in planned change. The change agent fulfills a management function when identifying situations wehre change is necesary and appropriate and when assessing the driving and restraining forces affecting the plan for change. The leader is the role model in planned change, is open and receptive to change and view change as a challenge and an opportunity for growth.

Stern (194) suggests 10 positive attitudes that should be adopted by leader/manager regarding change:

- problems exist to be overcome
- success involves the habit of changing habits
- Action cures fear
- The best way to escape a problem is to solve it
- Life changes occur only when beliefs change
- Look for opportunity not guarantees
- Worry is negative and results from inaction
- Discovery consists of looking at the same thing as everyone else and thinking something different
- Effective people are not problem oriented, they are opportunity-oriented
- You cannot operate on yesterdays standards and expect to be succesful today.

Managers must believe that they can make a difference. They should view change as a challenge and the chance or opportunity to do something new and innovative.

Operational Planning

Short-term (operational) planning focuses on achieving specific tasks. These plans involve a period of 1 hour to 3 years.

Time is a finite and valuable resource. If managers are to direct employees effectively and maximize other resources, they must first be able to find the time to do so. Learning to use time wisely requires both leadership skills and management fucntions.

Time management can be reduced to three cyclic steps:

- allow time for planning and establish priorities
- complete the highest priority task and whenever possible, finish one task before beginning another, and
- reprioritize based on remaining tasks and new information that may have been received.

Setting abide time at the beginning of each day to plan the day allows the manager to spend appropriate time on high priority tasks.

Using a time inventory is one way to gain insight into how and when a person is most productive.

FISCAL PLANNING

Fiscal Planning is a learned skill that improves with practice.

Scarce resources and soaring healthcare costs have strained all healthcare delivery systems. There has never been a time when healthcare organizations needed to operate more efficiently or be aware of more cost containment. Cost containment refers to effective and efficient delivery of services while generating needed removes for contianued organisational productivity. Cost containment is the responsibility of every healthcare provider, and the viability of most healthcare organizations today depends on their ability to use their financial resources wisely.

An essential feature of fiscal planing is responsibility accounting, which means that each of an organizations revenues, expenses, assets and liabilities is someone's responsibility. The person with the most direct control on any of these financial elements should be held accountable for them.

Financial planning reflects the philosophy, goals, and objectives of the organization. Fiscal planning must be proactive, flexible, and clearly stated in measurable terms; include short- and long-term planning, and involve as many people as feasible in the budgetary process. This all needs vision, creativity, and a thorough knowledge of political, social and economic forces that shape healthcare budgets.

A budget is a plan that uses numerical data to predict the activities of an organization over a period of time. The desired outcome of budgeting is maximal use of resources to meet organizational needs. The budget's value is directly related to its accuracy.

Expenses are classified as fixed or variable and either controllable or noncontrollable. Fixed expenses do not vary with volume, whereas variable expenses do. Controllable expenses can be varied by the manager. Non-controllable expenses cannot be varied.

Three types of expenditures are of primary importance: the personnel, operating, and capital budgets. The largest expenditure is on human resource because healthcare is labour-intensive. Most staffing is based on a predetermined standard that varies with each unit, department, organization, or service.

The operating budget reflects expenses that flex up or down in a predetermined manner to reflect variation in volume or services provided.

Capital budgets plan for the purchase of building or major equipment. This includes equipment that has a long life, is not used daily, and is more expensive than operating supplies.

A budgeting cycle that is set for 12 months is a fiscal year budget. Managers must rejustify their progrmme or needs every budgeting cycle in zero-based budgeting. Using a "decision package" to set funding priorities is a key feature of zero bazed budegeting.

Incremental budgeting uses current-year expenses and multiplies them by a certain figure, usually the inflation rate or consumer price index, to arrive at the budget for the coming year.

Steps in the budgetry process include:

- assess what need to be covered in the budget
- develop a plan
- implementation (ongoing monitoring and analysis)
- evaluation (review periodically and modify as needed throughout the fiscal year)

Critical pathways are one method of planning, assessing, implementing, and evaluating the cost-effectiveness of patient care. Critical pathways are predetermined courses of progress that patient should be making after admission for a specific diagnosis or after a specific surgery. Although critical pathways can be used as a tool for monitoring quality of care, they can also be used as a fiscal planning tool. Once the cost of a pathway is known, analysing the cost-effectiveness of the pathway as well as the associated cost variance is possible. With this clinical and cost variance data, decisions on changing the pathway can be made with both clinical and financial outcome projections. The advantage of critical pathways is that they do provide some means of standardizing medical care for patients with similar diagnosis.

Healthcare Reimbursement

With the advent of reimbursement for healthcare (in the USA), providers were forced to submit budgets and costs to payers that more accurately reflected their actual costs to provide these services.

The advent of Diagnostic-Related Groups (DRGs) in the early 1980s added to the need for monitoring cost containment. DRGs were predetermined payment schedules that reflected historical costs for treatment of specific patient conditions.

With DRGs, hospitals join the prospective payment system (PPS), whereby they receive a specified amount for each medicare patient's admission, regrdless of the actual cost of care. As a result of the PPS and the need to contain costs, the length of stay for most hospital admissions has decreased greatly.

The Managed Care

Managed care is a system that attempts to integrate efficiency of care with payment for the care. It is an attempt to intervene in the delivery of medical services to eliminate unnecessary and inappropriate services, without reducing quality, thereby reducing the cost of providing medical treatment. A managed-care model integrates both the financing and delivery of care. This move to integrated health plans, in which doctors, hospitals, and insurers join forces to manage care, was cornerstone of the "managed competition" approach to healthcare reform into the USA.

Key principles of managed care include the use of primary care physicians as "gatekeepers" to the healthcare system, a strong focus on prevention, a decreased emphasis on inpatient hospital care, the use of clinical practice guidelines for providers, selective contracting whereby providers agree to lower reimbursement levels in exchange for patient population contracts, utilization review, the use of formularies to manage pharmacy care, and continuous quality improvement.

Another frequent hallmark of managed care is capitation, whereby providers receive a fixed monthly payment, regardless of what services are used by that patient during the month. If the cost of caring for a specific person is less than the capitated amount, the provider profits. If the cost is greater than the capitated amount, the provider suffers a loss. The goal then for the capitatal providers is to see that patients receive the essential services to stay healthy or to keep from becoming ill, but to eliminate unnecessary use of healthcare services. This reimbursement strategy is believed to lead to undertreatment of patients.

One of the most common types of managed care organisations is the health maintenance organisation (HMO). HMOs provide healthcare in an organized system to subscribing members in a geographical area with a predetermined set of basic and preventive supplemented health maintenance and treatment services for a fixed prepaid charge.

There are four primary types of HMOs:

- Staff
- Independent Practice Association (APA)
- Group, and
- Network

In staff HMOs, physician providers are salaried by the HMO and under direct control of the HMO.

In IPA HMOs, the HMO contracts with a group of physicians through an intermediary to provide services for members of the HMO. In a Group HMO contracts with multiple independent physician group practices.

The types of plans available within HMOs typically vary according to the degree of provider choice available to enrollees. Two such plans include point-of-service (POS) and exclusive provider organisation (EPO) options. In POS plans, the patient has the option, at the time of service, to select a provider outside the network, but pays a higher premium as well as the copayment for the flexibility to do so. In the EPO option enrollees must seek care from the designated HMO provider or pay all of the cost out of pocket.

Another common type of managed care organisations is the preferred provider organisation (PPO). PPOs render services on a fee-for-service basis but provide financial incentives to consumers (they pay less) when the preferred provider is used. Providers are motivated to become part of a PPO because it ensures them on adequate population of clients.

Proponents of managed care argue that prepaid healthcare plans, such as those offered by HMOs, decrease healthcare costs between 10% and 40%, provide broader benefit for patients than under the traditional fee-for-service model, appropriately shift care from inpatient to outpatient settings, result in higher physician productivity and have high enrollee satisfaction levels.

Managers must be aware of their budgetary responsibilities and be accountable to the organization for maintaining a cost-effective environment. Managers must be skillful in the monitoring aspects of budget control.

Organizational Structure

In the organising phase, relationships are defined, procedures outlined, equipment readied, and tasks assigned. Organising also involves establishing a formal structure that provides the best possible coordination or use of resources to accomplish objectives.

An organization is formed when the number of workers is large enough to require a supervisor. Organizations are necessary because they accomplish more work than could be done by individual effort.

Organizational structure refers to the way in which a group is formed, its lines of communication, and its means for channeling authority and making decisions. Each organization has a formal and an informal organizational structure. The formal structure is generally highly planned and published, whereas the not formal structure is not implanned and often concealed.

Formal structure, through departmentalization and work division, provides a framework for defining managerial authority, responsibility, and accountability. Roles and functions are defined and systematically arranged, different people have differing roles, and rank and hierarchy are eivdent.

Informal structure is generally social in nature with blurred or shifting lines of authority and accountability.

Organizational Theory

Max Weber is known as the father of organizational theory. Weber postulated the concept of bureacracy. A bureaucracy is characterized by a clear chain of command, rules and regulations, specialization of work, division of labor, and impersonatlity of relationships.

Weber also is credited with development of the organizatgional chart to depict an organization's structure. It can help identify roles and their expectations. The organization chart defines formal relationships within the institution. Formal relationships, lines of communication, and authority are depicted on a chart by unbroken lines. These line positions can be shown by either horizontal or vertical unbroken lines. Horizontal unbroken lines represent communication between people with similar spheres of responsibility and power but different functions. Vertical unbroken lines between positions denote the official chain of command, the formal paths of communication and authority.

Dotted or broken lines on the organization chart represent staff positions. Because the positions are advisory, a staff member provides information and assistance to the manager but has limited organizational authority. Staff positions enable a manager to handle more activities and interactions than would otherwise be possible. Advisory (staff) positions do not have inherent legitimate authority.

Unity of command is indicated by the vertical solid line between the people. This concept is best described as one person/one boss. Each person has one manager to whom they report and to whom they are responsible. The scalar chain can be flat (in decentralized organizations) or tall (in centralized organizations). A lack of unity of command results in some conflict and lost productivity.

Span of control also can be determined from the organization chart. The number of people reporting to any manager represents that manager's span of control and determines the number of interactions expected of him or her.

Level of Management

In large organizations, several levels of managers often exist. Top-level managers look at the organisation as a whole, coordinating external and internal influences, and generally make decisions with few guidelines or structures. Their responsibilities include dtetermining the organizational philosophy, setting policy, and creating goals and priorities for resource allocation. Top-level managers have a greater need for conceptual and leadership skills.

Middle-level managers coordinate the efforts of the lower levels of hierarchy and are the channel between lower- and top-level managers. They carry on day-to-day operations but are still involved in some long-term planning and in establishing unit policies. They need greater human skills.

First level managers are concerned with their specific units work flow. They deal with immediate problems in the unit's daily operations, with organizational needs, and with personal needs of the employee. First level managers need greater technical skills.

The decision-making hierarchy, or pyramid, is often referred to as a scalar chain. In organizations with centralized decision-making, decisions are made by a few managers at the top of the hierarchy. Thus, more centralized the decision-making, longer the scalar chain.

Decentralized decision-making diffuses decision making throughout the organization and allows problems to be solved by the lowest practical managerial level. The larger the organization, the greater need to decentralise decision making. With decentralized organizations, the hierarchy of decision making is said to be flat, with a very short scalar chain.

One of the limitations of the organization chart is that, although it defines authority, it does'nt define responsibility and accountability. Authority is the official power to act and direct the work of others. Responsibility is related to job assignment and must be accompanied by enough authority to accomplish the assigned task. Accountability is the moral responsibility that acompanies a position.

Organizational culture is the total of an organization's beliefs, history, taboos, formal and informal relationships, and communication patterns. There is no one "best" way to structure an organization. One must always consider such variables as the size of the organization, the capability of its human resources, and the commitment level of its workers. The sturcture should be clearly defined so that employees know where they belong and where to go for assistance.

The integrated manager takes responsibility for ensuring that subordinates also understand the overall organisational structure and the structure at the unit level.

Leadership requires that problems are pursued through appropriate channels, that upward communication is encouraged, and that unit structure is periodically evaluated to determine if it can be redesigned to enable more lower-level decision making. The effective manager recognises difficulties inherent in advisory positions and uses leadership skills to support staff in these positions. This is accomplished by granting sufficient authority to enable advisory staff to carry out the functions of their role.

It is important for the manager to be knowledgeable about the organization's culture. He/She understands the organization and recognises what can be moulded or shaped and what is constant. Thus, the interaction between the manager and the organization is dynamic.

Shared governance refers to an organizational design that empowers staff by making them an integral part of patient care decision making and providing acountability and responsibility in their work.

Organizational structure is effective when the design is clearly communicated. Communication is facilitated, decisions are made at the lowest possible level, informal groups are encourged, and future leaders are developed.

Empowering Subordinates

The empowerment of staff is a hallmark of transformational leadership. Empowerment means to enable, develop, or allow. It is an interactive process that develops, builds, and increases power through coopertion, sharing, and working together. Empowerment occurs when leaders communicate their vision, employees are given the opportunity to make the most of their talents, and learning, creativity and explorations are encourged.

Managers empower subordinates when they delegate assignments to provide learning opportunities and allow employees to share in the satisfaction derived from achievement.

The key to establishing and keeping authority and power in an organization is for the manager to be able to accomplish four separate tasks:

- A small authority-power gap must be maintained;
- Subordinates should be empowered whenever possible;
- Authority should be used in such a manner that subordinates view that happens in the organization as necessary and,
- When needed, political strategies must be used to maintain power and authority.

Following stragtegies are suggested for enhancing power:

- expand personal resources
- present powerful picture to others
- hard work
- determine the powerful in the organization
- learn the language and symbols of the organization
- increase professional skills and knowledge
- maintain a broad vision
- use experts and seek counsel
- be flexible
- develop visibility and a voice in the organization, and
- empower others

A manager's ability to gain and wisely use power is critical to his/her success.

Organizing Patient Care

For organizing functions to be productive and facilitate meeting organisation needs, the manager must know the organisation and its members well. Leadership roles include:

- Periodically evaluate the effectiveness of the organizational structure for the delivery of patient care
- Determines if adequate resources and support exist before making any change in the organisation of patient care
- Examines the human element in work redesign
- Inspires the work group towards a team effort
- Organizes work activities to attain organizational goals
- Uses a patient care delivery system that maximises resources, people, material, and time
- Uses scientific research to support changes

The five primary means of organizing nursing care for patient are:

- Total patient care
- Functional nursing
- Team and modular nursing
- Primary nursing, and
- Case management.

Total patient care, utilizing the case method of assignment, is the oldest form of patient care organization and is still widely used today.

Functional nursing organization requires the completion of speciific tasks by different nursing personnel.

Team or modular nursing organization uses a leader who coordinates team members in the care of a group of patients.

Primary care nursing is organized so the patient is at the centre of the structure. One nurse has 24-hour responsibililty for the nursing care plan.

Case management is similar to primary nursing and derived from managed care. The case manager in managed care focuses on coordinating, planning and evaluating care; case management is used most frequently in complex patient care situations, using critical paths and case MAPs.

Differentiated nursing practice delineates different roles for nurses based on their skill, knowledge, educational level, and motivation.

The care MAP (multidisciplinary action plan) is a combination of critical path and a nursing care plan except times when nursing interventions should occur are indicated.

Organizing is an improtant management function. The work must be organized so organizational goals are sustained. Activities must be grouped so resources, people, materials, and time are used fully.

The manager groups activities to facilitate communication. Integrating leadership roles and management functions ensure that the type of patient care delivery model selected will provide quality care and staff satisfaction and that change in the mode of delivery will not be attempted without adequate resources, appropriate justification, and attention to how it will affect group cohesiveness.

STAFFING

Hospitals are labor intensive organizations. This large work force comprises of highly skilled, competent professionals. Ensuring the adequacy of skilled staff to accomplish organizational goals is an important management function.

Staffing responsibilities begin with planning because the philosophy and fiscal resources of the organisation influence the mix and the numbers of staff.

The first step in the staffing process is to determine the type and number of personnel needed. It is important to predict future staffing needs and proactively plan to meet those needs.

Successfully recruiting an adequate workforce depends on many variables, including financial resources, the organization's reputation, competitive salaries, etc.

Effective recruiting methods include advertisement, career days, and literature.

Managers share the responsibility for recruitment. Managers must be skilled in planning, conducting and controlling interviews.

Selection of the staff should be based on the requirements necesary for the job; these criteria should be developed before beginning the selection process.

Indoctrination consists of induction, orientation, and socialization of employees.

Productivity is directly related to the quality of an organization's personnel. Active recruitment allows institutions to bring in the most qualified personnel for a position. After those applicants have been recruited, managers using specified criteria have a critical responsibility to see that the best applicant is hired.

After determining present and future staffing needs and recruiting, interviewing, selecting, and placing personnel, the manager must see that the staff is appropriately socialized and trained in order to build a cohesive and effective team.

The socialization of people into roles occurs with all roles and is a normal sociological process. Two methods used to socialize others are social interaction and education.

Socialization is a complex process directed at the acquisition of appropriate attitudes, cognition, emotions, values, motivations, skills, knowledge, and social patterns necessary to cope with the social and professional environment. The manager supports employees during difficult role transitions. Mentoring and role remodelling are encouraged, and role expectations are clarified.

A well-planned and implemented indoctrination programme is a wise investment of organizational resources.

The manager recognizes the ultimate responsibility for staff development and uses appropriate teaching theories to assist with teaching and training staff.

The manager must ascertain that adequate numbers and an appropriate mix of personnel are available to meet daily unit needs and organizational goals.

Scheduling policies and staffing patterns are directly related to the management phases of planning and organising.

The manager must plan for adequate staffing to meet patient care needs. Efforts must be made to avoid overstaffing and understaffing as patient census and acuity fluctuate.

Fair and uniform staffing and scheduling policies and procedure must be written and communicated to all staff. Continued efforts should be made to use innovative and creative methods of staffing and scheduling. Flexitime is a concept modern organizations use to allow employees to have varying hours of starting and leaving times. Self scheduling allows employees the opportunity and the responsibility to make their own work schedules.

The effective manager knows that establishing trust helps build the team spirit needed to deal with temporary staff shortages. The manager also looks for innovative methods to overcome staffing difficulties.

Directing

In planning and organizing, managers attempt to establish an environment that is conducive to getting work done. In directing (coordinating), the manager sets those plans into action. Creating a motivating climate is critical element in meeting employee and organisational goals.

Because human beings have constant needs and wants, the person is always motivated to some extent. All human beings are motivated differently, however, because they have different needs and desires.

Managers cannot intrinsicly motivate people because motivation comes from within the person. The humanistic manager can, however, create an environment in which the development of human potential can be maximized.

Maslow stated that people are motivated to satisfy certain needs ranging from basic survival to complex psychological needs and that people seek a higher need ony when the lower needs have been predominantly met.

Hertzberg maintained that motrivators or job satisfiers, are present in the work itself and encourge people to want to work and to do that work well. Hygiene or maintenance factors keep the worker firm being dissatisfied or demotivated but do not act as true motivators for the workers.

Vroom's expectancy model say that people's expectations about their environment or a certain event will infleunce their behavior.

McGregor shows the improtance of a manager's assumptions about workers on the intrinsic motivation of the worker. These assumptions are labeled theory X and theory Y influence worker motivation.

Positive reinforcement is one of the most powerful motivators the manager can use.

The success of a motivational strategy is measured by the increased productivity and benefit to the organization and by the growth in the person, which motivates him/her to accomplish again.

Besides being a role model for staff, managers must try to mentor future managers and encourage monitoring relationships between subordinates. Identifying employee goals and fostering their attainment allow the manager to motivate employees to reach personal and organizational goals.

Organizational Communication

Organizational communication is a mangement function; it must be systematic, have continuity, and be fully integrated into the organizational structure, encouraging an exchange of views and ideas.

Communication forms the core of management activities and cuts across all phases of the management process.

Basic elements common to communication include the sender, receiver, message, mode, and climate of the interaction.

Communication is large organizations in particularly difficult due to their complexity and size.

Communication channels used by the manager in the organization may be upward, downward, horizontal, diagonal, or through the grapevine.

The clarity of the message is significantly affected by the mode of communication used. In general, the more direct the communication, the greater the probity of clear communication. The more people involved in filtering the communication, the greater the chance of distortion.

Written communication is used most often in large organizations.

Effective managers are congruent in their verbal and non-verbal communication, so followers are clear about the messages they receive.

Rapidly flourishing communication technologies have great potential to increase the efficiency and effectiveness or organizational communication. However, well-developed leadership and management skills are needed to ensure that such technological advances are used safety and appropriately.

Communication is critical to successful management. A manager has the formal authority and responsibility to communicate with many people in the organization.

Delegation

Delegation can be defined as getting work done through others or as directing the performance of one or more people to accomplish organizational goals.

Everyone needs to feel that he/she makes a difference to the success of the organisation. The difference may be small, but when they are empowered, people feel that what they do has meaning and significance.

Delegation is a major skill that must be learned. Delegation is not an option for the manager—it is a necessity.

Delegation should be used for assigning routine tasks and tasks for which the manager does not have time. It also is appropriate as a tool for problem solving and compatibility building in subordinates.

In delegation, managers must clearly communicate what they want done, including the purpose for doing so. Managers must delegate the authority and the responsibility necessary to complete the task.

The right to delegate and the ability to provide formal rewards for successful completion of delegated tasks reflect the legitimate authority inherent in the management role. Delegation provides a means of icnreasing unit productivity. It is also a management tool for subordiante acomplishment and enrichment.

Delegation requires high-level managerial and leadership skills.

Managing Conflict

Conflict is defined as the internal or external discord that results from diferences in ideas, values, or feeling between two or more people.

There are three primary categories of conflict: intrapersonal, interpersonal, and intergroup. Intrapersonal conflict occurs within the person. It involves an internal struggle to clarify contradictory values or wants.

Interpersonal conflict happens between two or more people with differing values, goals, and beliefs.

Intergroup conflict occurs between two or more groups of people, departments, or organizations.

The conflict proces has five stages:

- Latent conflict
- Perceived conflict
- Felt conflict
- Manifest conflict
- Conflict aftermath

The optimal goal in resolving conflict is creating a win-win solution for all involved. An effective manager recognizes which conflict management or resolution strategy is most appropriate for each situation.

Common conflict resolution stragtegies include:

- Compromising
- Competing (forcing)
- Cooperating—accommodating—smoothing
- Avoiding
- Collaborating

Managing conflict efectively requires an understanding of its origin. Some of the most common sources of organizational conflict are communication problems, organizational structure, and individual behavior within the organization. Diversity in gender, culture, and age also have the potential to create conflict in an organization.

Following strategies can be used to deal effectively with conflict:

- Urging confrontation (urge the subordinates to attempt to handle their own problems)
- Third party consultation
- Behavior change
- Responsibility charting
- Structure change
- Soothing one party

Negotiations may be competitive or collaborative, but collaborative negotiations generally has a more, poisitive outcome. A major goal of effective negotiation is to make the other party, feel satisfied with the outcome. The focus in negotiation should be to create a win-win situation.

Consensus is always an appropriate goal in resolving conflicts and in negotiation. Consensus means that negotiating parties are able to reach an agreement that all parties can support, or at least not oppose, even through it does not represent everyone's priorities.

The manager who creates a stable environment that minimizes the antecedent conditions for conflict has more time and energy to focus on meeting organizational and human resource needs.

Because knowledge is power,the more informed a negotiator, the greater his/her bargaining power.

Collective Bargaining

Two constraints that may affect the directing aspects of management are collective bargaining and legislation concerning employment practices. Managers must be able to see collective bargaining and employment legislation following perspectives:

- The organization
- The worker
- Societal
- Personal

Collective bargaining is defined as activities occuring between organized labor and management that concern employee relations. Such activities include negotiations of formal labor agreements and day-to-day interactions between unions and management.

Unionization and legal constraints will be seen less burdensome if managers remember that both primarily protect the rights of patients and employees. If managers perform their jobs well and work for organizations that desire to"do the right thing" by accepting their social responsibility, they need not fear unionization and legal constraints.

An effective manager always seeks to do what is just when making decisions that deal with unions. She/he maintins required staffing and ensures a safe working environment. Rights of the organization and employee are protected as the manager uses personnel policies in a non-discriminatory and consistent manner. The emphasis is on flexibility and accommodation of employment legislation and union contracts.

Controlling

During the controlloing phase of management process, standards are set, performance is measured, and action is taken to correct discrepencies between standards and actual performance.

Organisations need some control over productivity, innovation, and quality outcomes. Controlling should be viewed as a way to learn and grow, both personally and professionally.

Examples of management controlling functions include the periodic evaluation of unit philosophy, mission, goals, and objectives; the measurement of individual and group performance against pre-established standards; the monitoring of expenses and use of supplies; and the auditing of patient goals and outcomes.

Quality control, a specific type of controlling, refers to activities that evaluate, monitor, or regulate services rendered to patients.

Effective quality control requires managers to have skill in both leadership and management.

Measuring quantitative data is often fairly simple. Qualitative data are, however, more elusive, and their measurement is more difficult. Accurate assessment of qualitative data requires managers to consistently use a specific and systematic process:

- The criterion or standard is determined
- Information is collected to determine if the standard has been met
- Educational or corrective action is taken if the criterion has not been met.

The first stage is the establishment of control criteria or standards. A standard is a predetermined baseline condition or level of excellence that constitutes a model to be followed and practiced. Each organization must set standards and objectives to guide invididual practitioners in performing safe and effective care.

Clinical practice guidelines provide diagnosis-based, step-by-step interventions to doctors and nurses to follow in an effort to promote high quality care and yet control resource utilization and costs.

Benchmarking is the process of measuring products, practices and services against best performing organization.

An audit is a systematic and official examination of a record, process, or account to evaluate performance.

Structure audits monitor the structure or setting in which patient care occurs (e.g., the finances, medical records, nursing service structure, environmental structure, etc.).

Process audits are used to measure the process of care or how the care was carried out.

Outcome audits determine what results, if any, follow from specific medical or nursing interventions for patients.

Total quality management is based on the premise that the patient is the focal element on which production and service depend. Quality is built into the service or product, rather than assuming that inspection of and removal of errors lead to quality.

Quality control provides managers the opportunity to evaluate organizational performance from a systematic, scientific, and objective view point. To do so, managers must determine what standards will be used to measure quality care on their units and then develop and implement quality control progrmmes that measure quality care on their units and then develop and implement quality control programmes that measure results against those standards. All managers are responsible for monitoring the quality patient care.

Inspiring subordinates to establish and achieve high standards of care, vision, risk taking and accountability will help achieving excellence in providing care. An effective manager seeks to achieve a balance between quality and cost containment that does not violate professional obligations to patients and employees.

Performance Appraisal

To determine how well employees carry out their duties, performance appraisal is used. It is a sensitive and important part of the management process, requiring much skill. When accurate and appropriate appraisal assessments are performed, the otucome can be very positive.

In performance appraisal, actual perfromance is evaluated, not intent. Performance appraisals let employees know the level of their job performance as well as any expectations the organization may have of them.

The effectivensss of a performance appraisal system is only as good as the tools used to create those assessments. Some of the appraisal tools commonly used in healthcare organizations include:

- That rating scales (method of rating a person against a set standard)
- Job dimension scales (rating scale is constructed for each job classification)
- Behaviorly anchoring rating scales (behavioral expectation scales)
- Checklists (the weighted scale, the forced checklist, the simple checklist)
- Essays (the free form revised (decribes employees strengths and areas where improvement is needed).
- Self-appraisals
- Management by objectives (MBO) (an excellent tool for determining individual employee progress)
- Peer review

Performance appraisal is a major responsibility in the controlling function of management.

Discipline

Discipline is a positive and necessary tool in promoting subordinate growth. The optimal goal in constructive discipline is assisting employees to behave in a manner that allows than to be self-directed in meeting organisational goals. To ensure fairnesss, rules should include the components of forewarning, immediate application, consistency and impartiality.

Problem employees are those employees who exhibit chronic disruptive rule breaking or behavior requiring disciplinary interventions.

Except for most serious dereliction, discipline should be administered in progressive steps, which include verbal admonishment, written admonishment, suspension, and termination.

In performance deficiency coaching, the manager actively brings areas of unacceptable behavior or performance to the attention of the employee and works with him/her to establish a short-term plan to correct deficiencies.

The grievance procedure is essentially a statement of wrong doing or a procedure to follow when one believes that a wrong has been committed. All employees should have the right to grieve disciplinary action that they believe has been arbitrary or unfair in some way.

The presence of a union generally entails more procedural, legalistic safeguards for administering discipline and a well-defined grievance process for employee who believe they have been disciplined unfairly.

When discipline is constructive, fair, and consistent, it provides the structure needed for high unit morale and productivity. When discipline is destructive, vindictive, and inconsistent, unit morale and productivity plummet. The skills of the manager plays a key role in determining the climate for discipline and how discipline is administered at the unit level.

Management functions are more controlling because they involve the enforcement of established rules, policies and procedures. Although good managerial practice greatly reduces the need for discipline, some employees still need external direction and discipline to accomplish organisational objectives. Discipline allows the violating employee and all the employees to understand clearly the expectations of the organization and the penalty for failing to meet those expectations.

The effective manager is able to balance the need for employee growth and organizational structure.

Ethical Decision Making

In an era of markedly limited physical,human, and financial resources, nearly all decision-making by managers involves some ethical component. Much of the difficulty people have in making ethical decisions can be attributed to lack of formal education in problem solving and decision making. Many systematic approaches to ethical prloblem solving are appropriate for the manager. These approaches include the use of theoretical problem solving and decision-making models, ethical frameworks, and ethical principles.

The quality of ethical problem solving should be evaluated in terms of the process used to make the decision. If a structured approach to problem solving is used, data gathering is adequate, and multiple alternatives are analyzed then, regardless of the outcome, the manager should feel comfortable that the best possible decision was made at that time with the infromation and resource available.

Four of the most commonly used ethical frameworks for decision making include utilitarianism, duty-based reasoning, right-based reasoning, and intuitionism. These frameworks assist the people involved in the problem solving to clarify their values and beliefs.

Principles of ethical reasoning explore and define what beliefs or values form the basis for our decision making. These principles include autonomy, beneficence, non-maleficence, paternalism, utility, justice, truth telling, deception, promise keeping, and confidentiality.

Ethical issues are inherent in through but at all aspects of the management process. Professional codes of ethics are a guide to the highest standards of ethical practice for doctors and nurses.

Managers by virtue of their many roles, must be advocates for their patients, subordinates, and the profession. Advocacy is helping others to grow and self-actualise and is a leadership role.

The effective manager recognizes that ethical issues pervade every aspect of leadership and management. The manager should make the best possible decision at that time with the information and resources available The manager should become an expert at using systematic approaches to problem-solving or decision-making. Leadership roles focus on the human element involved in ethical decision-making.

NEW PARADIGM OF HEALTHCARE MANAGEMENT

There must be a shared belief that the hospital exists to care for sick and injured people. All other activities, whatever they may be, are secondary to this and each and every management process must have the patient at its heart.

The driving force in the hospital must be multidisciplinary clinical teams, assisted and supported by management financial and personnel expertise. The service of the organization is delivered by doctors, nurses, technicians, etc. They hold the intimate knowledge of patient needs and it is vital that this unique knowledge is harnessed in the effective management of the service. To do this, clinicians must be helped and genuinely supported by administrative staff.

The design of the clinical services must be geared to the needs of the patient rather than those of the staff.

In the ideal scenario, decisions are taken on the basis of hard fact and expert knowledge by all stakeholders, rather than on the basis of politics or convenience. There is the ideal of decisions at every level of the organization being taken in the light of a clinical perspective.

It takes considerable skill and a thorough understanding of the principles of change management to bring about major organizational change effectively and with the minimum of pain.

The creative and innovative manager will find the management role extremely stimulating, enjoyable and, above all interesting.

The new paradigm of health care management requires planning of healthcare delivery which takes account of the needs of the patients in terms of quality care by doctors, nurses and paramedical staff who are all experienced in dealing with both the patient's clinical condition and with the type of care required at that moment in time. They must be involved in the planning process.

The overall goal must be to improve services for patients. The appropriate strategic objectives and criteria by which improvements in healthcare delivery will be judged should be identified and agreed, by consensus whereever possible. These criteria should include:

- Appropriate and effective quality of care;
- Good access to facilities;
- Well-integrated care (working across organizational boundaries);
- Efficient care delivery;
- Care delivery that is economical in its use of resources;
- What is required to provide good teaching facilities;
- What is good use of skills, in particular allowing service availability and quality to be maintained by creating a setting and way of working that is attractive to potential recruits in the future.

Right-sizing and Redundancy

The process of tailoring the work force to the needs of the organization has become an important aspect of management. Redundancy should be a part of an overall approach to achieving the best fit of work force to organization. If redundancy does eventually become necessary, it should be approched positively, decisively and in a constructive way.

Redundancy occurs when the employer ceases to carry on the business for which the employee was employed or ceases to carry on the business in the place where the employee was employed. It also occurs when a requirement for a parituclar kind of work either ceases or diminishes or a requirement for a particular kind of work in a particular place either ceases or diminishes.

Organizational change involving displacement and possible redundancy should be anticipated, at least to the extent of the production and maintenance of a clear procedure for dealing with the human resource issues. The approach should, as far as posible, be agreed with the staff through whatever local machinery exists for this purpose.

Measures to avoid redundancy include:

- Elimination of uneconomic working practices wherever this is practiceable.
- Natural wastage, which will include restrictions on recruitmenf in affected and related stff groups/disciplies. This could involve the use of temporary contarcts if a service has to be maintained for an interim period.
- Positive commitment to retraining and redeployment of staff
- Identifcation in forward planning of any possible future redundancy situations, with an immediate action plan designed to minimize the effect on permanent staff.

An employee offered a new post to avoid redundancy should be provided with full details of the alternative employment.

It is also important to have rules about the way in which vacancies are filled by redeployed staff and to ensure that these are consistently applied.

Right-sizing is a process of change management. As such, individuals will perceive it to be threatening to their status, power base, economic and social needs, and to their general well-being. Managers affecting the change should have a clear view of what he/she wants to do and keep his/her eye on the objective throughout, set out the new arrangements and identify those jobs no longer required, involve staff at an early stage, and draw up aprocedure to facilitate the changes (agree this with the staff) and apply it consistently.

Achieving organizational change and right-sizing in an efficient and fair way can be achieved by following some of the basic approaches set out above.

Outsourcing

Outsourcing is the flexible route to success. Offering greater flexibility and efficient utilization of resources, it is fast becoming an integral part of increasing productivity and providing excellent quality service to patients.

Pressures to cut costs while delivering better quality service has forced everyone to look at workplace structuring—and the health service is no exception. One of the key facets of this change has been a reassessment of the way human resources are organised and deployed. With labour as the most expensive commodity, a more flexible staffing strategy means increased productivity with reduced costs. More and more organizations are now turning to outsourcing as a solution to shift in demands.

Contracting out enables an organization to respond to and plan for changes in work patterns with the advantage of being able to predict the unpredictable in terms of cost and productivity. A professional and responsible contractor can held to firm cost estimates against agreed specifications, with a direct and positive impact on budgeting and cost control. By using staff as and when required, and paying on the basis of skills rather than length of service, running overheads can significantly be reduced.

In the health service, outsourcing staff ready to work from the moment they arrive not only maximises productivity but ensure the quality of the service can be delivered at a continuously high level of excellence.

Using contract workers to fill either specialist roles or those peripheral to the main business, frees up permanent employees and enables them to put their skills to better use, so helping them to achieve greater motivation and job satisfaction as well as productivity.

To gain maximum benefit from outsourcing it is critical to find the right source who can demonstrate a successful track records with your organization and who have recognized quality accreditation.

Business Process Re-engineering

Achieving more from less is an increasing preoccupation for hospitals. The rapidly changing environment in which hospitals operate creates the simultaneous need to improve both quality and efficiency.

Business process re-engineering is defined as the fundamental rethinking and radical redesign of business process to achieve dramatic improvements in critical, contemporary measures of performance such as cost, quality, service and speed. Process may be described as a set of logically-related tasks formed to achieve an outcome valued by customers. Process in healthcare may include outpatient, inpatient and emergency care.

In hosptials, responsibility is generally allocated by functional contribution to a process. Patients travel through hospitals metamorphically (and sometimes physically) horizontally, and yet hospital management structures are organized vertically.

It is not posible to create excellence across hospital services without fundamental redesign of core healthcare processes.

The hospital administration must be commited to initiate, sustain and achieve successful bsiness re-engineering progammes. Strong visible and invisible support of the hospitals' powerful groups is essential.

Hospital staff must understand why the organization is to go forward with a re-engineering programme. A well-communiated strategic vision provides the context within which large-scale organisational change can take place.

Communication with interest groups is essential for a business process re-engineering pragramme and to sustain organizational tolerance and understanding once it has commenced.

Focus on something of value to internal and external stakeholders: time and quality are both excellent targets. Cost reduction dissociated from quality improvement will discourage staff participation and without strong staff support, such programmes will fail.

Re-engineering teams should comprise the hospital's "brightest and best". The team members must be credible and influential people within the hospital. They must display a wide range of skills and aptitudes as they work in a highly ambiguous, intense and stressful environment to develop creative process solutions.

Line managers must be closely involved in the redesign and early testing of healthcare processes. They are critical to any successful implementation so their ownership of new processes is essential.

Re-designing work creates different jobs and requires different reward systems. New reward systems facilitate and encourage changes, which occur too slowly, compared to the speed of process redesign and implementation, can result in faltering organizational performance.

Excellent programme management smooths the sequence of process reesign, prototyping and piloting, human resource management, netgotiations with trade unions, outsourcing arrangements and overarching communications. Meticulous planning includes scanning the environment to anticipate obstacles and taking appropriate action.

Re-engineering health care processes requires a sophisticated benefits tracking system to ensure that all targetted benefits are achieved. Clinical and managerial leadership's reinforcement of the importance of achieving benefits is essential.

Business process re-engineering is a mechanism for radical change that breathes life into the excellent ideas which normally lie dormant within a hospital. To be successful, such programmes must harness the energy, creativity and ambition to improve patient care that bonds together those working in healthcare.

Risk Managment

The primary aim of risk management is to be proactive in the reduction of risks to the lowest level reasonably practicable. Managers should undertake formal risk assessment of the workplace. To do this you must identify hazards and assess the risk involved.

- A hazard is something with the potential to cause harm.
- A risk is the likelihood of the hazard occuring.

Essential risk management responsibility is usually develoved to the line manager but identification of risks may come from several sources. These may include:

- Questionnaire
- Analysis of accident figures
- Analysis of sickness figures
- Observation by staff with specialist skills
- Review of policies already in place
- Formalized risk assessment.

Organizing control measures will help make your risk management strategy change your organization into a proactive health and safety culture. The control measures should include policy and safe system of work.

A written health and safety policy is not only a legal requirement but can also bring many benefits. The policy should be written by a multi-disciplinary team including specialist advisers such as manual handling adviser, radiation emission control officer, fire prevention officer, etc. The policy should include:

- Resources available for implementation.
- State clear responsibilities for implementing the policy.
- State who is responsible for specific areas of health and safety.
- Provide clear understanding that employee cooperation is essential.

Resources should be targeted at areas of greatest benefit, the following to the considered as a minimum:

- Management of health and safety
- Food safety and hygiene
- Fire
- Lifting and handling
- Infection control
- Waste management
- Electricity

- Substances hazardous to health
- Display screen equipment
- Radiation
- Noise
- Pressure systems
- Asbestos
- Legionella
- Flammable and explosive substances
- Personal protective equipment
- Workplace health, safety and welfare
- Work equipment
- Construction design and management

In addition to these, the need also to be well understood policies in four areas which can be considered to be the tools of health and safety management:

- Training
- Health and safety audit
- Risk assessment
- Incident reporting.

The underpinning principle behind health and safety policy is risk assessment. This is the process of identifying hazards, evaluating the risks associated with them, and selecting appropriate solutions.

A policy that is thoroughly thought and has the backing and firm commitment of the organization should lead to a proactive health and safety culture which will eventually be reflected in a better quality of patient care.

Empolyers have a particular duty for the provsion and maintenance of safe systems of work so far as is reasonably practicable. A safe system of work is needed when a hazard cannot be eliminated and an element of risk remains. A safe system of work is one resulting from a formalized and a systematic examination of a task to identify hazards and their risks. It provides recommendations to ensure that safe methods are implemented to eliminate hazards or eliminate or reduce the risks involved. Safe system of work include:

- Task assessment
- Hazard identification
- Define safe methods
- Implement
- Monitor

The system should be applied to all tasks in all areas of work and to all personnel.

Health and safety training should be provided for employees:
When recruited into the employer's undertaking

- before being exposed to new or increased risks because of
  - introduction of new equipment;
  - introduction of new technology;
  - introduction of new work system;
- repeated periodically when appropriate;
- adapted to any new risks;
- occur during normal working hours

It is advisable to maintain detailed records. Who is responsible for maintaining these records should be clearly identified. These should record:

- what training was provided;
- when provided;
- the course contents;
- who was the instructor;
- verification of the employee's attendance and his/her statement conforming he/she feels competent to meet the required performance as trained.

Monitoring provides the information to enable you to review activities and decide how to improve performance.

Identifying hazards and their associated risk will help indicate the extent of risks which your organization is taking. Organizing control measures helps change your organization into a proactive health and safety culture. Monitoring and auditing ensures that your organization is achieving the right results.

Quality Improvement

The development of consumersim and rising public expectations have led to a desire for increasing amounts of information to be made available. There has been a demand for the adoption of measurement-based approaches to quality assurance.

Measuring performance in non-clinical areas is relatively straightforward. However, in the clinical arena, meaningful data are hard to find and difficult to interpret.

A holistic view of quality is one that emphasizes the results of addressing trends and improvements over time. The most valuable contribution of quality data will be to help providers to determine the correct cost and quality trade-offs in the provision of care.

If an organization is committed to pursuing continuous quality improvement, it should be able to handle performance indicators.

An organization that performs well will have done so because of a great deal of hard work by staff from every discipline and every level of that organization.

Striving for quality should be part of everyone's daily busienss. Three diamensions of quality are encompasses by the strategy; the patient's perspective, the professional perspective and the managerial perspective. Achieving a balance between these three dimensions is crucial to the delivery of high-quality care. The basic principles of this strategy include:

- Building on what is there;
- Making sense of quality;
- Developmental approach (continuous incremental improvement)
- Clearly defined responsibilities;
- Integration (in daily life and managerial agenda).

Helped by an effective organizational structure and manager support at speciality level, a range of performance mesurement systems have to be developed. Combined with knowledge of problem-solving techniques and skills in change management, services should be able to effectively address areas of concern.

Health service should be underpinned by a strong ethical framework, an ethic which might be expressed as:

- Preservation of the autonomy of the individual (democratic consent)
- Bring no harm (non-maleficence)
- Justice (explaining the basis on which personnel health need/due is calculated).

Audit should be directed at quality of care. It should include setting of standards, compare performance with these to lead to beneficial change. Audit is a tool, which can be used to examine any aspect of healthcare.

We need to continually to stress the ethical value of audit, to recognise that those healthcare workers who have primary responsibility for individual patients are confronted with very difficult decisions.

So emphasizing the ethical basis for audit is essential if we wish to get the commitment of professionals, which is necesary to the efective implementation of audit.

Control to making the audit to work is the engagement and commitment of all health professionals. It needs:

- Conceptual change • clinical audit
- Organizational change • centre stage
- Implementation • good management

We need to change our perception of audit and strengthen the organizational framework within which it is developed.

Productivity

Productivity has become a central issue in health services management over the last ten years. Staffing is the major cost in the health care delivery, averaging 50-70 percent of total budget allocated to health. In a service that is constantly pressed to keep up with demand it should be a key role of management to ensure that staffing is achieving optimum value for money. Improving productivity offers more opportunity to release existing resources than any other single factor in healthcare organization.

A systematic approach to workforce planning, ensuring that it is an integral part of the business planning process operating within the management and service delivery strcuture of the provider is required to measure and assess productivity.

Workforce planning should operate at unit level (clinical directorate) and should also allow for cooperate management to set an overall framework which reflects the organization's priorities and takes account of the cost, volume and quality parameters. The process has six major stages:

- Setting objectives
- Setting out the current profile
- Developing a supply-based forecast
- Developing measures of productivity
- Demand modelling and target setting
- Setting strategic targets

Quality and unit labor cost can go hand in hand. Indeed it should be a fundamental objective that each time a process and/or staffing profile is reviewed with a view to achieving greater productivity, a quality gain is also achieved.

Facilities Management

First impressions tend to stick. Negative first impressions will perhaps damage patient confidence. Good experience will help the caring process and make the job of other colleagues down the line easier and more effective.

Facilities management is a key element in the delivery of healthcare pursuing the idea of 'putting people first'. The benefits of facilities management are improved quality, reduced costs and better use of resources.

Facilities management (FM) is the process by which an organization delivers and sustains agreed support service levels within a quality environment to provide full value in use to meet strategic objectives.

Considering the hospital as a 'hotel' for healthcare, FM makes significant contributions to patient care and therapy. If a patient is admitted to a bed, why should he/she not feel as though he/she is in a hotel. This hotel service starts with the initial contact made between the hospital and the patient. The areas that can be considered under FM include:

- Linen (Laundry)
- The food and beverages (catering)
- Sanitation
- Reception
- Grounds and gardens
- Foyer
- Parking
- Entrance

To provide a continually improving quality and commercially-oriented cost-effective service to ptients, a number of initiatives are required like CQI/TQM, ISO 9002, benchmarking, etc.

There is a need for staff at every level in the organization to have assistance to realize their potential and perform to the best of their ability in their chosen jobs.

Positive performance management will involve:

- Clarifying the role
- Setting goals
- Planning personal development
- Reviewing regularly and annually.

Each manager should prepare an action plan for implementation. The staff should only be paid their full allowance when all elements of the agreement (quality, productivity and attendance) are met.

FM should make a major impact on improved patient care and the patients should say that our hospitals are like a five-star hotel.

FURTHER READING

1. Argyris C: Integrating the individual and the organisation. New York: John Wiley and Son. 1964.
2. Blake RR: The managerial grid. Houston: Fulf Publishing. 1964.
3. Burns JM: leadership, New York; Harper & Row 1978.
4. Drucker PF: Managing for the future: The 1990s and beyond. New York: Truman Talley/Dutton. 1992.
5. Fayol H: General and Industrial management. London: Pitman & Sons. 1925.
6. Hersey P, Blanchard K: Management of Organisational behaviour: Utilising human resources. Englewood Cliffs, NJ: prenltice Hall, 1977.
7. Mayo E: The human problem of an industrialised civiliation. New York: Mcmillan, 1953.
8. Marquis BL, Huston CJ: Leadership Roles and Management Function in Nursing: Theory and Application. Philadelphia: Lippincott. Willisms & Wilikins, 2000.

9. McGragor D: The human side of enterprise. New York: McGraw Hill. 1960.
10. Ouchi WG, Theory Z: How American business can meet the Japanese challenge. Reading MA: Addison Wesley, 1981.
11. Schein EH: Organisational Psychology. Englewood Cliffs, NJ: Prentice-Hall, 1970.
12. Skinne BF: Science and human behaviour. New York: Free Press, 1953.
13. Taylor FW: The principles of scientific management. New York: Harper & Row, 1911.
14. Vroom VH, Jago AG: The new leadership. Engle wood Cliffs, NJ: Prentice-Hal, 1988.

46 Staffing Pattern

Human Resource Management

An organization is nothing without human resources. Since every hospital is made up to people, acquiring their services, developing their skills, motivating them to high levels of performance, and ensuring that they continue to maintain their commitments to the organization are essential to achieving organizational objectives. Getting and keeping good people is critical to the success of every organization.

Those organizations that are able to acquire, develop, stimulate, and keep outstanding workers will be both effective and efficient. Survival of an organization requires managers and workers coordinating their efforts towards an ultimate end. Human resource management is a process of acquisition, development, motivation and maintenance of people.

For a 500-bed hospital following staff is required. This should serve as a guideline rather than a rule.

ADMINISTRATION

Hospital Director

Medical Director should be whole time preferably with post graduate qualification in hospital administration and requisite experience. He should be assisted by one whole time Deputy Medical Superintendent and two Assistant Medical Superintendents preferrably qualified in hospital administration.

Specialities

The following speciality services should be provided:

- Internal Medicine
- General Surgery
- Obstetrics and Gynecology including Family Welfare
- Pediatrics including neonatology
- Orthopedics
- Physical medicine and rehabilitation
- Otorhinolaryngology
- Ophthalmology
- Burns and Plastic surgery
- Dermatology and Venerlogoy
- Dental Surgery
- Psychiatry
- Anesthesia and critical care medicine
- Radiology and Imaging
- Laboratory services
- Blood transfusion services

- Toxicology and forensic medicine
- Community medicine and Public health.

Distribution of Beds

Speciality	*No.of beds*	*%*
Emergency medicine	75	35
General surgery	100	
Obs and Gyne including Family Welfare	75	25
Pediatrics including neonatology	75	
Orthopedics	50	10
Otohinolaryngology	25	5
Ophthalmology	25	5
Psychiatry including de-addiction	25	5
Burn and plastic surgery	12	2½
Dental surgery	12	2½
Demotology and venerology	12	2½
Critical Care medicine (ICU)	12	2½

Staffing Pattern in Deployment of Various Categories of Staff

Medical Staff

Director/Hospital Administrator 1
Medical Superintendent should be whole time having a defined post-graduate qualification in Hospital Administration and adequate experience.

Dy. Medical Director/
Dy. Hospital Administrator 1
To assist Medical Director in all administrative matters. Should be having post-graduate qualification in hospital administration and requisite experience.

Asstt. Medical Director/
Asstt. Hospital Administrator 2
One as Dy. Medical Supdt. (OPD and Emergency) and one as Dy. Medical Supdt. (Indoor and Service areas).

Senior Specialists 16
One each for different speciality services viz. General Medicine, General Surgery, Obs. and Gynae., Pediatrics, Orthopedics, Otorhinolaryngology, Ophthalmology, Burns and Plastic Surgery, Psychiatry, Anesthesia, Radiology, Pathology, Forensic Medicine and Community Medicine. The above posts are felt essential for a 500-beded hospital as this hospital is envisaged to provide specialized services.

Junior Specialists 40
Two for Emergency Service, four for General Medicine, Four for General Surgery, Four for Obs. and Gynae. including FW, Three for pediatrics including neonatology, Three for Orthopedics, One each for Burn and Plastic Surgery, Otorhinolaryngology, Ophthalmology, Dermatology, Dental Surgery and Psychiatry, Five for anesthesia, Three for Pathology (one each Patho, Micro and Bio), Three for Radiodiagnosis and one each for Community Medicine and Blood Bank. These posts are more in number because in a 500-bedded speciality hospital, round-the-clock coverage on call) by Junior Specialists is a must.

General Duty Medical Officer 65
Ten for Emergency Services, eight for General Medicine, ten for General Surgery, ten for Obs. and Gynae, eight for Pediatrics and eight for Orthopedics, two each for Otorhinolaryngology, Ophthalmology and Psychiatry, one each for Burn Plastic Surgery, Dental Surgery and Dermatology, and two for Blood Bank.

Nursing Staff

Chief Nursing Officer/Nursing Superintendent 1
One post is considered essential for over all administration of the nursing staff.

Dy. Nursing Officer 1
To assist Nursing Superintendent.

Asstt. Nursing Officer 4
One each for Office Administration, Emergency Services, Operation Theater and indoors including labour room).

Nursing Supervisors 25
One for OPD, three for Emergency Deptt., two for OT, three for Labor Room and one each for indoor wards or Nursing Units.

Staff Nurses 200
Twelve for Emergency Deptt., twelve for Major OT., two for Minor OT., ten for Labor Room, two for Blood Bank, two for Obs. and Gynae. OPD and one hundred and sixty for indoors.

Para Medical and Others

Public Health Worker 1
Health Educator 3
Health staff is required for health education which is an essential service to be rendered to patients attending the OPD.

Medical Social Worker 1
Medical Social Guide 8
To guide people and to help them at psychoemotional evel.

Psysiotherapist 2
Occupational Therapist 1
Vocational Guide 1
For rehabilitation, physiotherapy, occupational therapy and vocational guidance.

Medical Record Officer 1
Medical Record Tech. 3
Medical Record Clerk/Receptionist 16
For Medical Record Department.

Chief Dietician 1
For overall supervision of kitchen.

Dietician 1
Junior Dietician 4
To assist dietician in management of kitchen.

Steward 4

Head Cook 2

Cook 12

Cook Aide/Helper 12

X-ray technician 1
For overall supervision

Sr. Radiographer 2

Jr. Radiographer 10
Of these, four for round-the-clock emergency department coverage and rest for Radiology Department.

Dark Room Assistant 5
Four round-the-clock ccuerage of Radiology Deptt. and Emergency.

Lab. Technician 5
One in Pathology, Two in Hematology, One in Microbiology and One in Biochemistry.

Lab. Assistant 10
To assist Lab. Technicians.

Blood Bank Technician 4

Blood Bank Asstt. 8

CSSD Supervisor 1

CSSD Technician 2

CSSD Asstt. Gr. I and II 8

Boiler Attendant 2

Laundry Supervisor 1

Laundry Technician 1

Laundry Operator 20

Laundry Orderly 10

Laundry Tailor 1

OT Technician 2
For main operation theatre.

OT Assistant 10
For round the clock duty.

Plaster Room Technician 4

Dresser 8
For OPD Minor OT and emergeycy.

Chief Pharmacist 1
For overall supervision.

Junior Pharmacist 6
For main operation theatre.

ECG Technician 6
For round-the-clock duty.

Audiometry Assistant 2
For Otorhinolaryngology.

Refractionist 2
For Ophthalmology.

Orthopist 1
For Ophthalmology.

Dental Hygienist 3
For Dental section.

Dental Mechanic 1
For Dental section.

Mortuary Technician 1
For overall supervision.

Mortuary Attendant 5
For round the clock duty.

General Administrative Staff

Administrative Officer 1
One for overall officer administration.

Accounts Officer 1
One for all financial matters including accounts.

Public Relation Officer 1

Office Superintendent 4
One each for different sections viz. general, establishment, budget and accounts.

Jr. Accounts Officer/Accountant 2
To assist Accounts Officer.

Cashier 2
For disbursing/receiving cash.

Head Clerk/UDC 10

Stenographer 10

Jr. Assistants 30
Besides working Office Administration, also required for some other area, like Dietetics, Laundry, CSSD, Pharmacy, Hawaldar Office, etc.

Despatch Clerk 2

Messenger/Peon 10
For working in various offices.

Material Management Officer 1
Overall supervision and control and central stores.

Asstt. Material Management Officer 2
To assist Stores Officer.

Stores Assistants 4
One each for Medical, Surgical, General and Stationery stores.

Stores Attendants/Helper 8

Ancillary Staff

Sanitary Superintendent 1
Supervision and control and housekeeping and class IV staff.

Sanitary Supervisor 6
For found the clock duty.

Sweepers 125
Half of these are required for indoors and rest for OPD, Service Areas and Office Administration.

Nursing Aides 100
Nursing orderlies 25
Half of these are required for indoors and rest for OPD, Service Areas and Office Administration.

Fire and Security

Security cum Fire Officer 1
Responsible for overall general and fire safety arrangements.

Asstt. Security Officer 1
To Assist Security Officer.

Security Supervisor 5
For round the clock duty.

Security Guards 60
For round-the-clock security and safety of whole hospital complex.

Engineering Services

Executive Engineer 1
Responsible for overall control of emergency services.

Asstt. Engineer (Civil) 2

Asstt. Engineer (Elect.) 2

Asstt. Engineer (A/C) 1

Asstt. Engineer (Horticulture) 1

Asstt. Engineer (Workshop and Electronic) 1

Electricien 8
For round the clock duty.

Carpenter 1

Plumbers 2

Builders 1

A/C Operator 4

Lift Attendant 12

Gardener 12

Sewage Cleaner 4

Khalasi 6

Workshop Supervisor 1

Workshop Mechanic 2

Blacksmith 1

Glass Blower 1

Painter 1

Transport cum Ambulance Services

Transport Officer 1

Asstt. Transport Officer 1

Drivers 12

Cleaners 6

Telecommunication

Telephbone Supervisor 1

Telephone Mechanic 1

Telephone Operator 10

Paging Room asstt. 6

Class 'D' Employees

Ward Boy/Orderlies 1
Per 10 beds + 30% leave reserve.

Sweepers 1
Per 10 beds + 30% leave reserve.

GENERAL GUIDELINES

Medical Staff

a. For all departments having direct responsibility for patient care:
   - Sr. Specialist 1
   - Jr. Specialist 2
   - House officers 4 per 30 to 40 bed unit

   In addition
   - House Officer 1 per 10 bed
   - Jr. Specialist 1 per 30 to 40 bed

b. For departments not directly related with patient care/para-clinical deptts.
   - Sr. Specialist 1
   - Jr. Specialist 1 per 100-150 beds module.

Staffing Pattern for 100-Beded Hospital

1. *Administration:* Medical Director should be whole time.
2. *Specialities:* The following speciality services should be provided:
   General Medicine, General Surgery, Obs. and Gynae. including Family Welfare, Pediatrics including Neonatology, Orthopedics including Physiotherapy, Otorhinolryngology, Ophthalmology, Dental Surgery, Psychiatry, Anesthesia, Radiology including Ultrasound, Pahthology including Blood Bank Services, Community Medicine and Public Health.

Department	Addending					Consulting					Residents					Interns					Fellows		Totals				
	100	200	300	400	500	100	200	300	400	500	100	200	300	400	500	100	200	300	400	500	400	500	100	200	300	400	500
Medicine	6	12	16	25	30	10	20	30	35	40	—	—	4	8	12	—	—	—	—	—	—	3	16	32	50	68	85
Internal	5	8	11	17	21	8	16	25	26	30	—	—	4	8	12	—	—	—	—	—	—	—	13	24	40	51	63
Cardiology	1	3	3	4	4	2	4	4	6	6	—	—	—	—	—	—	—	—	—	—	—	2	3	7	7	10	12
Dermatology	—	1	2	3	3	—	—	1	1	2	—	—	—	—	—	—	—	—	—	—	—	—	—	1	3	4	5
Allergy	—	—	—	—	1	—	—	—	—	—	—	—	—	—	—	—	—	—	—	—	—	—	—	—	—	—	1
Neurology	—	—	—	1	1	—	—	—	2	2	—	—	—	—	—	—	—	—	—	—	—	1	—	—	—	3	4
Surgery	10	18	22	30	34	4	12	16	20	24	—	—	3	6	10	—	—	—	—	—	—	1	14	30	41	56	69
General	10	16	15	18	18	4	10	8	6	5	—	—	3	6	10	—	—	—	—	—	—	—	14	26	26	30	33
Orthopedic	—	1	4	5	6	—	2	4	3	4	—	—	—	—	—	—	—	—	—	—	—	—	—	3	8	8	10
Neuro	—	—	—	1	1	—	—	—	1	2	—	—	—	—	—	—	—	—	—	—	—	1	—	—	—	2	4
Thoracic	—	—	—	1	2	—	—	—	1	1	—	—	—	—	—	—	—	—	—	—	—	—	—	—	—	2	3
Urology	—	1	2	3	4	—	—	2	4	6	—	—	—	—	—	—	—	—	—	—	—	—	—	1	4	7	10
Eye	—	—	—	1	1	—	—	—	2	2	—	—	—	—	—	—	—	—	—	—	—	—	—	—	—	3	3
ENT	—	—	1	1	1	—	—	2	3	3	—	—	—	—	—	—	—	—	—	—	—	—	—	—	3	4	4
Oral	—	—	—	—	1	—	—	—	—	1	—	—	—	—	—	—	—	—	—	—	—	—	—	—	—	—	2
Obstetrics	4	6	8	14	16	—	4	10	18	24	—	—	1	4	6	—	—	—	—	—	—	1	4	10	19	36	47
Obs.	4	6	8	13	14	—	4	10	16	21	—	—	1	4	6	—	—	—	—	—	—	1	4	10	19	33	42
Gynae.	—	—	—	1	2	—	—	—	2	3	—	—	—	—	—	—	—	—	—	—	—	—	—	—	—	3	5
Pediatrics	—	2	4	5	8	—	4	6	10	12	—	—	—	2	2	—	—	—	—	—	—	—	—	6	10	17	22
Psychiatry	—	—	3	4	5	—	—	2	5	10	—	—	1	2	3	—	—	—	—	—	—	1	—	—	6	11	19
Public health	—	—	—	—	1	—	—	—	—	1	—	—	—	—	1	—	—	—	—	—	—	1	—	—	—	—	4
Pathology	½	1	2	2	3	—	—	1	1	2	—	—	1	2	2	—	—	—	—	—	1	2	½	1	4	6	9
Radiology	½	1	2	2	3	—	—	1	1	2	—	—	1	3	3	—	—	—	—	—	—	—	½	1	4	6	8
Physical medicine	—	—	—	1	1	—	—	—	—	—	—	—	—	—	1	—	—	—	—	—	—	—	—	—	—	1	2
Anesthesiology	—	—	1	1	2	—	—	—	—	1	—	—	—	—	1	—	—	—	—	—	—	—	—	—	—	—	2
Interns	—	—	—	—	(Rotate among the services)						—	—	—	—	—	—	—	6	10	15	—	—	—	—	6	10	15
Total	21	40	58	84	103	14	40	66	90	116	—	—	11	27	41	—	—	6	10	15	1	9	35	80	141	212	284

Fig. 46.1: Estimate of minimum medical staff, hospitals, 100 to 500 beds

Department	100 beds				200 beds				300 beds				400 beds				500 beds			
	Day	Ev.	Nt.	Tot.	Day	Ev.	Nt.	Tot.	Day	Ev.	Nt.	Tot.	Day	Ev.	Nt.	Tot.	Day	Ev.	Nt.	Tot.
Nursing services	40	19	8	67	71	38	19	128	103	60	34	197	119	73	37	229	155	97	51	303
Patient care	20	14	8	42	41	30	18	89	64	47	29	140	73	54	32	159	103	76	46	225
Medical & surgical	14	10	6	30	28	20	12	60	28	20	12	60	35	25	15	75	42	30	18	90
OB	6	4	2	12	8	6	3	17	10	8	4	22	12	10	4	26	20	16	7	43
Pediatrics	—	—	—	—	5	4	3	12	7	5	3	15	7	5	3	15	14	10	6	30
Psychiatry	—	—	—	—	—	—	—	—	5	4	2	11	5	4	2	11	6	5	3	14
Others	—	—	—	—	—	—	—	—	14	10	8	32	14	10	8	32	21	15	12	48
Operating suite	14	2	—	16	21	3	—	24	28	8	—	36	32	11	—	43	36	12	—	48
Delivery suite	5	3	—	8	6	4	—	10	7	4	4	15	10	6	4	20	10	6	4	20
Emergency	1	—	—	1	3	1	1	5	4	1	1	6	4	2	1	7	6	3	1	10
Adjuncts	13	1	—	14	25	2	—	27	43	5	—	48	66	5	—	71	82	10	—	92
Laboratory	4	1	—	5	9	1	—	10	13	2	—	15	20	2	—	22	26	4	—	30
Radiology	4	—	—	4	10	—	—	10	13	2	—	15	20	2	—	22	22	4	—	26
Diagnosis	4	—	—	4	9	—	—	9	12	2	—	14	18	2	—	20	20	4	—	24
Therapy	—	—	—	—	1	—	—	1	1	—	—	1	2	—	—	2	2	—	—	2
Physical Medicine	3	—	—	3	4	—	—	4	10	—	—	10	15	—	—	15	20	—	—	18
Physical therapy	3	—	—	3	4	—	—	4	8	—	—	8	12	—	—	12	2	—	—	14
Occu. therapy	—	—	—	—	—	—	—	—	2	—	—	2	3	—	—	3	18	—	—	4
Pharmacy	2	—	—	2	2	1	—	3	3	1	—	4	5	1	—	6	14	2	—	8
Medical social service	—	—	—	—	—	—	—	—	2	—	—	2	3	—	—	3	4	—	—	4
Medical illustration	—	—	—	—	—	—	—	—	2	—	—	2	3	—	—	3	6	—	—	6
Service department	47	12	3	62	74	22	8	104	109	33	10	152	131	57	14	202	167	76	18	261
Dietary	10	7	—	17	16	12	3	31	24	18	4	46	32	24	5	61	42	30	5	77
Housekeeping	7	3	1	11	14	6	1	21	22	10	1	33	27	16	2	45	34	21	3	58
Laundry	5	—	—	5	8	—	—	8	12	—	—	12	17	—	—	17	22	—	—	22
CSS	10	—	—	10	18	—	—	18	22	—	—	22	20	10	—	30	25	15	—	40
CGS	5	—	—	5	6	—	—	6	8	—	—	8	9	—	—	9	12	—	—	12
Building maintenance and operation	10	2	2	14	12	4	4	20	21	5	5	31	26	7	7	40	32	10	10	52
Administration	30	1	1	32	38	4	4	46	48	4	4	56	64	5	5	74	87	5	6	98
Offices	16	1	1	18	19	3	3	25	22	3	3	28	26	4	4	34	28	4	4	36
Medical records	4	—	—	4	4	1	1	6	6	1	1	8	8	1	1	10	9	1	2	12
Auxiliary	10	—	—	10	15	—	—	15	20	—	—	20	30	—	—	30	50	—	—	50
Total hospital	130	33	12	175	208	66	31	305	303	102	48	453	380	140	56	576	491	188	75	754
Employees per bed	—	—	—	175	—	—	—	157	—	—	—	151	—	—	—	144	—	—	—	151
Ambulatory patient facilities	8	—	—	8	12	—	—	12	20	—	—	20	30	—	—	30	40	—	—	40

Fig. 46.2: Estimate of hospital service staff. Departmental figures may vary + 100 or – 50 percent. Shifts are 7.00 A.M., 3.00 P.M. and 11.00 P.M.

3. Distribution of beds:

Speciality	*No. of beds*
General medicine	25
General surgery	15
Obs. and Gyne. including FW	15
Pediatrics including Neonatology	15
Orthopedics	10
Others (including Otorhinolarynlogy) Ophthalmology, Dental and Psychiatry)	20

4. Staffing pattern–Deployment of various categories of staff.

FURTHER READING

1. Amin Tabish: Towards Professionalisation of Hospital Administration. Management in Medicine, England **12(2)**: 1998.
2. Bureau of Indian Standards Basic requirements for Hospital Planning Part I and Part II) 1995.
3. Bajaj Committee Report-Ministry of Health and Family Welfare, Govt. of India, 1983.
4. National Institute of Health and Family Welfare-Guide to staffing pattern for hospitals-Technical Report No. 5.
5. Study Group on Hospitals and Health Care (Haldipur Committee)-Ministry of Health and Family Welfare, Govt. of India, 1978.
6. Shakti Gupta: Hospital Staffing Norms Journal of Academy of Hospital Administration, Vol 1 No. 1 and 2, 1989.

47 Waste Management and Ecohealth

Environment in which we live is an ecosystem or an integration of physical and social relations. In adopting ecosystem health practices, it is necessary that environmental hazards are equated with a population, in terms of local environmental conditions as a reference. This will mean that reconstructing an ecosystem will be in complete consonance with the majority of the people's needs

Environmental concerns have long been the subject of international interest. Global concerns have acquired a new urgency. Over the past 20 years the content and the quality of the discourse on the environment have been completely transformed. By its sheer volume, the authoritative scientific evidence available on environmental problems commands the attention of the government and the public alike.

Hospital wastes have always been considered as potentially hazardous in view of the inherent potential for dissemination of infection. By hospital wastes, it means specially the bio-medical waste generated in different departments of the hospital. Hospitals generate on average, between 1 and 2 kg of waste per bed per day. It is estimated that about 85 per cent of the waste generated is non-hazardous, about 10 per cent is infectious wastes and 5 per cent non-infectious but hazardous waste. Disinfecting right at source and disposal by incineration (which completely destroy micro-organisms of all types), has been the timetested and most widely advocated method for safe management of hospital waste. General hygiene is a pre-requisite for good waste management. The rising trends of Hepatitis-B Virus and HIV/AIDS infection has led to an increasing awareness about the risk associated with this lackadaisical practice and the need to evolve and implement strategies for safe and sustainable methods of disposal of waste material generated. Careful management of wastes from the point of generation to safe disposal is of paramount importance. Waste survey (an important component of the waste management scheme) helps in evaluating both the type and quantity of waste generated in a hospital.

Hospitals in countries with inadequate disposal facilities may dump contaminated hospital waste on open rubbish tips. This presents a great risk to the people particularly the rag-pickers. All hospital waste should be disposed of, so that it presents no risk of injury/contamination.

Types of hospital waste include clinical waste (soiled dressings, body fluids, IV needles and syringes, drainage bags, pathology waste, blood products, amputated limbs), laboratory waste (high risk category), non-clinical waste (paper and plastics), kitchen waste, radioactive waste).

Segregation at source and safe storage is the key to whole waste management process because it is at this stage that wastes are segregated into different schemes. By segregation, a hospital can reduce total treatment cost, reduce the impact of this waste on the community, and reduce the chances of infecting healthcare workers. Treatment is mainly required to disinfect or decontaminate by chemical disinfection of waste right at source. After this treatment, the residue can be handled safely, transported, stored and disposed. Infectious waste needs to be destroyed by the recommended methods of like autoclaving and microwaving. Major portion of the sharps are the needles, which can be cut by a needle cutter and contained in a bleaching powder solution or autoclaved or/and shredded or be destroyed by a needle destroyer.

A simple color-coding system should be used to separate waste so that the different components can be treated safely. To ensure the smooth operation of a color-coding policy different colored containers should be provided throughout the hospital so that the waste can be separated at source. Wards should be provided with two separate color-coded containers–one for clinical and one for non-clinical waste. All waste from operating theaters should be defined as clinical waste. Office waste (usually paper) is defined as non-clinical waste. All waste leaving the pathology department should be defined as clinical waste and must be rendered safe before disposal. Waste from pathology should be autoclaved prior to incineration. A separate color should be used in each kitchen work area. Color coded plastic bags (minimum gauge 225 μm for high risk waste and 100 μm for low risk waste) should be used. The destination of the bags will depend on the color coding. The color coded bags in the wards should be emptied when they are two-thirds full. They should be tied securely to the neck and labeled clearly. The bags should be carried by the neck and taken to a predesignated area for collection. The collection staff should ensure that the waste is segregated properly according to colour-coding and sent to the appropriate destination. The bag should be stored in vermin and vandal-proof cages ready for transportation to their destination. The color coded bags should be handled only after they have been secured. Porters should wear protective clothing (heavy duty gauntlets or gloves and overalls) when transferring the bags. Under no circumstances should any member of staff put their hands into any waste container. After compaction, non-clinical waste can be disposed of at a land-fill site. Clinical waste requires incineration or, failing this, must be covered with lime and buried. Where incineration facilities are not available, clinical waste can be treated with lime and buried in the hospital grounds. Liming is the cheapest and most effective means of getting rid of clinical waste in areas where incineration facilities are not available. Chemical disinfection is cost-effective and does not require large investments. Some of the disinfectants include Sodium Hypochlorite (0.5%), Bleach (10 grams of bleach in 1 litre water), Savlon 1 per cent and Glutaraldehyde 2 per cent. Non-clinical waste should be removed by the local authority or an independent contractor and disposed of independently or at the municipal dump. No clinical waste, needles or syringes should be sent to the municipal dump–the hospital must not be responsible for increasing the risk of disease. There is a very real risk of acquiring blood-borne disease from sharps contaminated with blood products. All sharps, including fine-bore needles, must be single-use only (never recycled). All sharps containers must be leak-proof and puncture-proof and carry a *biological hazard* sign.

The disposable material should be given high priority by ensuring its destruction and eliminating reuse. Shredding is a technique that causes a reduction in the volume of the waste (up to 90%) besides preventing its reuse. Waste sharps and Solid wastes generated from disposable items other than tubing catheters and i.v. sets can be subjected to shredding. It should be ensured that waste is disinfected by chemicals/micro waving/autoclaving before shredding.,

The biodegradable waste is comparatively easy to handle. It should be disposed after its biodegradation which can be accomplished by bio-digestion (using bacteria or earth worms or by Pit composting). After complete decomposition it can be used as biofertilizer.

Chemical hazardous wastes (solvents, chemotherapy waste, pathogenic chemicals, radioactive waste and waste anesthetic gases) may be segregated and properly managed. Minimization of the waste, careful segregation and safe disposal of that waste, which cannot be recycled, is important.

During incineration the chlorinated polyvinylchloride emits chlorinated dioxins and related compounds, which are toxic substances having deleterious effects in very low doses as these gases are constantly present in the environment. Thus it is advisable to use non-chlorinated bags. An improved method of incineration-*pyrolysis*-is now available in which extremely high temperature, burning process under low oxygen conditions is employed. This system reduces emission limits of gases, which pollute the environment.

Radioactive Waste

Radioactive wastes are clearly defined. Methods of their management are established. These wastes are disposed as per guidelines of Atomic Energy Regulatory Board/BARC. Adequate installations must be provided to deal safely with radioactive wastes in liquid or solid form. A storage tank for radioactive waste is an advantage when isotopes with short half-life are used. Radioactive waste from telecurie and brachycurie treatment is in the kilocurie or 100 millicurie range with a half life of about five years. These preparations, as well as cobalt 60, are regarded as no longer usable after a few years. These wastes are not bulky but are highly active and need to be fully screened at all stages. Waste from nuclear medicine and other applications are bulky but with a half-life of less than 14 days can be treated as inactive waste after 24 half life periods. After this period the radioactivity is surveyed by dosimeters. Once it is found that the radioactivity limits are below the maximum permissible limits it is diluted and disposed in the normal channels under strict supervision. The gross quantity of radioactive material released into the sewage system by any hospital should not exceed 37 GBq/year. Iodine 125, with a half life of 60 days, needs special storage. Maximum activity of iodine-131 that can be discharged into sewage system should not exceed 100 mico curie per day, and average monthly concentration in the effluent at the discharge point should not exceed 0.6 micro curie per liter. Solid radioactive wastes like syringes, cotton, glassware, gloves, etc. are stored in well-protected Hot Lab which is properly shielded by lead blocks and allowed to decay for more than 10 half lives. After surveying its radioactivity limit (less than 135 mill curie/ cu mm of solid waste) it is incinerated.

Liquid Waste

A survey by the WHO indicates that three of every four humans alive today do not have enough water to drink or, if water is available, the supplies are contaminated. Water is unfit to drink when it contains human sewage, animal waste, or other pollutants. However, the situation can be reversed through the proper management of water resources. Water purification procedures prevent pathogenic microorganisms from reaching the body, while sewage treatment process removes pathogens from body waste products. After water has been used, it becomes sewage. Sewage includes all the water from a household that is used for washing, as well as toilet wastes.

Hospital generates liquid waste, which is either infectious or chemical in nature. To avoid the exposure to general public, it is necessary that the waste be properly treated. The liquid pathological waste should be treated with a chemical disinfectant. The solution should then be treated with a reagent to neutralize it. This can be flushed into the sewer system.

Sewage Treatment

Systems for the treatment of human waste range from the primitive outhouse, which is nothing more than a hole in the ground, to the sophisticated sewage treatment facilities. All operate under the same basic principle: water is separated from the waste, and the solid matter is broken down by micro-organisms to simple compounds for return to the soil and water.

The usual first step in sewage treatment is called *primary treatment*. In this process, incoming sewage receives preliminary treatment–large floating materials are screened out, the sewage is allowed to flow through settling chambers so that sand and similarly gritty material can be removed, skimmers remove floating oil and grease, and floating debris is shredded on ground. After this step, the sewage passes through sedimentation tanks, where solid matter settles out. Sewage solids collecting on the bottom are called sludge. The sludge is removed on either a continuous or intermittent basis or the effluent (the liquid flowing out) then undergoes secondary treatment. Primary treatment removes approximately 25 per cent to 35 per cent of the biochemical oxygen demand (BOD) of the sewage. BOD is a measure of the biologically degradable organic matter in water. BOD is determined by the amount of oxygen required by bacteria to metabolize the organic matter. The classic method of measurement is to use special bottles with air-tight stoppers. Each bottle is first filled with the test water or dilutions of the test water. The water is initially aerated to provide a relatively high level of dissolved oxygen and is seeded with bacteria if necessary. The filled bottles are then incubated in the dark for five days at 20 degree C, and the decrease in dissolved oxygen is determined by a chemical or electronic testing method. The more oxygen that is used up as the bacteria degrade the organic matter in the sample, the greater the BOD–which is usually expressed in milligrams of oxygen per liter of water. The amount of oxygen that normally can be dissolved in water is only about 10 mg/litre. Typical BOD value of waste water may be 20 times this amount. If this waste water enters a lake, e.g., bacteria in the lake begin to consume the organic matter responsible for the high BOD, rapidly depleting the oxygen in the lake water.

Secondary treatment, which is primarily biological, is designed to remove most of dissolved organic matter (the greater part of BOD remaining in the sewage after primary treatment) and reduce the BOD. In this process, the sewage undergoes strong aeration to encourage the growth of aerobic bacteria and other micro-organisms that oxidize the dissolved organic matter to carbon dioxide and water. Two commonly-used methods are *sludge system* and *trickling filters*.

Primary sludge accumulates in primary sedimentation tanks; sludge also accumulates in activated sludge and in trickling filter secondary treatments. For further treatment, these sludges are *often* pumped to *anaerobic sludge digesters*. The process of sludge digestion is carried out in large tanks, from which oxygen is almost completely excluded. However, considerable amounts of undigested sludge still remain. To reduce its volume, the sludge is pumped to shallow drying beds or filters. It is then carried away for disposal. It can be used for landfill or as a soil conditioner, or it can be incinerated.

Some communities have developed tertiary treatment plants to tackle biologically degradable organic matter (remaining after primary and secondary treatment) particularly when the effluent is discharged into recreational lakes. The effluent from secondary treatment plants contains some residual BOD. It also contains about 50 per cent of the original nitrogen and 70 per cent of the original phosphorus. Tertiary treatment is designed to remove essentially all the BOD, nitrogen, and phosphorus. Tertiary treatment depends less on biological treatment than on physical and chemical treatments. Some systems encourage denitrifying bacteria to form volatile nitrogen gas. Nitrogen gas is converted to ammonia and evaporates into the air in stripping towers. Finally, chlorine is added to the purified water to kill or inhibit any remaining micro-organisms and to oxidize any remaining odor producing substances.

Tertiary treatment provides water that is suitable for drinking, but the process is extremely costly. Secondary treatment is less costly, but water that has undergone only secondary treatment contains many nutrients that pollutes water. Even now, waste water with coliform counts below 2.2/100 ml is being used to irrigate food crops.

The effluent generated from the hospital should conform to the prescribed limits: pH 605-9, suspended solids 100mg/l, oil and grease 10mg/l, BOD 30 mg/l, COD 250mg/l, Bio-assay test 90 per cent survival of fish after 96 hours in 100 per cent effluent.

Biological Analysis of Water

Among the most frequently used indicator organisms are the coliform bacteria. Coliform bacteria are normally found in the intestinal tracts of humans. They are able to survive for extensive periods of time in the environment. Escherichia coli is the most important indicator organism within this group.

The *membrane filter technique* is a popular laboratory test in water microbiology. Another method for testing water is the *standard plate count technique*. A third test is a statistical evaluation called *the most possible number*.

The three basic steps in the preparation of water for drinking include: sedimentation to remove bulky objects; filtration to eliminate the vast majority of microorganisms; and chlorination to destroy the last remnants of microbial life.

Ecohealth

Because our health conditions are an integral part of our environment, we cannot always assume that ill-health is manifested by disease. Rather, ill-health is usually a condition of weakness or stress, and regardless of the symptoms, there is an accompanying loss of 'balance' owing to the change in the environment. It is essential to diagnose and reverse the weakness process before serious consequences follow.

If health planning is to include certain environmental hazards, it cannot continually reduce 'environment' to the physical condition of a particular disease. Given the accelerated pace of industrialization, environmental hazards should be adequately addressed at the planning stage. A technology mission should be constituted to reduce environmental health hazards in areas with high ecostress.

Ministry of Environment and Forests has notified the rules for the Management and Handling of Bio-medical waste, 1998. According to this Act the state government shall establish a prescribed authority with such members as may specified for granting authorization and implementing these rules. The Advisory Committee was constituted by the state government that comprises experts in the field of Healthcare, Veterinary sciences, Municipality and Environment management, State Pollution Control Board and NGO.

There are strong economic and social reasons for aggressively protecting the environment by creating incentives to reduce and manage such spillovers/environmental problems. Effective responses to these problems are vital to the struggle for sustainable development.

Green Productivity

If development is to be sustainable, there is a need to moe beyond pollution prevention and ensure that both productivity improvement and environmental protection are achieved simultaneously.

Green productivity is a strategy for enhancing productivity and environmental performance for over-all socioeconomic development. It is the application of appropriate productivity and environmental management tools, techniques, technologies to reduce the environmental impact of organization's activities, goods and services. It is a strategy of integrating environmental and social considerations with business and other activities.It is applicable to all sectors including service establishments, schools, as well as the community. The objective is to attain higher level of productivity for serving the needs of society and to protect and enhance the quality of environemnt. Green productivity will definitely have a role to play in productivity and qualityoriented industry and service organizations. It can help organizations reduce their expenditure on environmental protection through means like source reduction, waste minimization, pllution prevention and cleaner production. Organizations can thus achieve productivity improvement and at the same time protect the environment that will enable sustainable development. It leads to gains in profitability through improvements in productivity and environmental performance. Sustainability is thus the vision or the driving force. Sustainable development refers to development that meets the needs of the present generation without compromising the ability of the future generation to met their needs. This also means the use of services and products that meet basic needs of human beings and improve quality of life. The entire life cycle of these products and services must be based on minimizing use of natural resources and toxic substances, and resulting emissions, in order not to compromise the ability of future generations to meet their needs.

For any development strategy to be sustainable, it needs to focus on quality, profitability and environment—triple focus of Green Productivity. Natural resources are conserved thereby reducing environmental degradation. Reducing the amount of material and energy use to make or supply services or goods can directly cut the costs thereby ensuring profitability. The savings may come from lower production and waste management costs or may take the form of avoiding the cost of potential enviornmental liabilities.

Distinguishing characteristics of Green Productivity include environmental compliance, productivity improvement, integrated people-based approach, and information driven improvement. The *kaizen* approach of continuous quality improvement forms the basis. The concept of CQI is achieved by adopting the tenets of the PDCA (Plan, Do, Check and Act) cycle. This cycle is aimed at insuring productivity improvement programmes.

Any changes that have to be made to benefit society have to therefore be made at the market place. This means that the development strategy like Green Productivity must aim at changing consumption by pushing products and services so that societal economics is not compromised with and at the same time the natural environment on which society depends is not degraded.

Ecological principles of accountability, polluter pays and the precautionary principles bring in the element of responsibility and place the onus for environmental restroation on the polluter. Precautionary principle advocates a cautious, proactive and anticipatory approach. It is applicable in situation when the impact of an event is long-term and difficult to reverse. Pollution prevention, cleaner production and source reduction are all based on this precautionary principle of environmental protection.

A systematic implementation framework must be adopted by organizations to translate the guiding principles of Green Productivity (GP) into practice. This framework integrates the use of the GP methodology, the GP tools and the GP techniques harmoniously according to the guiding principles of GP.

48 Telemedicine

Technology available today suggest futuristic possibilities of modes of treatment. Computer-assisted imaging techniques providing morphological and functional information on the individual organism have gained a great acceptance for diagnosis and surgical planning.

The aim of increased technical support should be to achieve:

- Higher precision, accuracy and efficiency
- Shorter time of intervention and anesthesia with less blood loss
- Reduction of stress and strain for the patient as well as for the operating team
- Quality standardization on an expert level even for a broad clinical application, and

The possibility of developing new less invasive operative strategies using new support systems (image guided extracorporeal shockwack Lithotripsy is a well established example for the potentials of computer assisted therapy including robot technology).

Telemedicine—providing health care at a distance—has emerged as an important means of important in areas where the full range of clinician services are unavailable.

There is worldwide need to improve to delivery of health care in both qualitative and quantitative terms, particularly respecting its cost-effectiveness. This is especially true for health care delivery in remote areas, interaction between health care professionals at differing sites, and interaction between health professionals who remain at their work site while interacting with patients at their home.

Applications of Telemedicine

Examples of successful applications of telemedicine include.

Transmission of radiological pictures and microscopic pathology slides prepared by medical technical staff in remote primary hospitals to radiologists and pathologists in specialist centers for interpretation has substantially enhanced the delivery of healthcare in the USA, the UK, Sweden, Russia, Greece, and Norway.

Surgery

Robots have been used successfully in operating theaters for neurosurgery, Orthopedic surgery, urological surgery and ENT surgery. Robot surgery has been shown to have advantages over an intervention with regard to spacial accuracy, reliability and precision. It is possible to use multisensory inputs from a remote operating theatre to create the perception that the operator is physically present and thus allow the remote surgeon to regain natural hand-eye co-ordination and receive tactile feedback.

Other applications include Home care (ECG monitors for home use to monitor patients with cardiac disorders), Dermatology (Skin rash Video camera consultations by General practitioners in remote surgery settings with dermatologist in Urban specialist centres), Primary care (General practitioner consultation with specialists), and District nursing (transportable video camera brought to patients homes have allowed remote medical consultations).

Telemedicine can reach and extent to almost any aspect of the practice of medicines. Because of its interactive nature, it can provide the means for integrating intellectual and other resources and ensuring continuous education at all level within a healthcare system.

Telemedical conferencing also offers great advantage for pre-and postgraduate training. Larger audiences can be created for and inter-institutional collaboration in creating such courses expands the creative and financial basis for producing and delivering courses of the highest quality.

The implementation of telemedicine involves both professional and legal matters. Telemedical procedures need to be introduced in an ordered fashion. Academic departmets are being formed with the aim of developing and evaluating telemedical procedures while taking professional, psychological, communicational, sociological and economic aspects into consideration.

The Benefits the Technology Offers

Telemedicine is a simple concept that provides a wide range of cost-effective solutions for healthcare providers for local, regional and global applications. Real-time patient management and diagnostics can be provided for any location, no matter how remote. Global networking can be accessed providing, remote and distributed point of care evaluation by expert clinicians. The successful application of telemedicine in areas like healthcare infrastructure, realtime monitoring, image diagnostics, telecardiology, tele-emergency services, telefetal monitoring, clinical studies. Although simply said, telemedicine must be expertly executed if the real benefits are to be realised.

Computer-Assisted Medical Interventions

Computer-assisted imaging techniques providing morphological and functional information on the individual organism have gained great acceptance for diagnosis and surgical planning.

The possibility of developing new less invasive operative strategies using new support systems like Image guided Extracorporal Shockwave Lithotripsy (ESWL) is a well-established example of computer-assisted therapy including robot technology).

A surgeon who has to define an optimal strategy of a surgical intervention uses various kinds of information such as pre or intraoperative X-ray projections, CT, NMR, US Video endoscopy, anatomical models and computer-assisted therapy research is to support the matching of the total information represention, slices, sections, surfaces and other signals. Surgeons can be supported by computer-based planning system providing three-dimensional reconstruction and analysis of multimodal information.

Recent developments in the area of computer assisted surgery offer different technological solutions to translate the high geometric accuracy of the properative imaging and planning into a precise intraoperative execution.

Once the spatial relation between the computer-based model and the operating site is known, the translation of geometrical information is possible in both directions.

Different systems including passive navigation systems as well as active robot systems have already been introdued into clinical application.

Robot could potentially provide a precise computer-based active link to the image space and the preoperative planning.

FURTHER READING

1. K Radennacher, G Brandt, G Rau: Robot and computer-assisted medical interventions. New World Health IHF. London 51-4, 1997.
2. Putsep E: Modern Hospital—International planning practices. Lloyd-Luke, London, 1979.

49 Appendices

Appendix–1

CONSTITUTION OF THE COMMUNITY HOSPITAL

Name

The name of the hospital shall be ____________________ Community Hospital.

Purpose

The purpose for which the hospital exists is to provide the comprehensive health care to the community without discrimination as to ethnic origin, party of religion, and to provide training for health personnel.

Controlling Bodies

A. The Hospital Management Board, subject to
B. The ________________ (a higher body) _________ representing the ___________ Community.

Hospital Management Board

A. *The Board* shall consist of fifteen members:
   - 5 from the—community appointed by —(of people having some understanding and concern for health matters, and broadly representative of all sides of the community-men and women, church and mosque, traditional rulers and business leaders)
   - 3 from the—College of Medicine appointed by—(only relevant if cooperation with university)
   - 2 from—Local Government, appointed by the Chairman
   - 2 from the State Government appointed by the State Health Management Board
   - 3 hospital officers, the Medical Superintendent, the Matron and Hospital Secretary

B. *Officers of the Board* these shall consist of a Chairman and a Secretary
   1. The Chairman shall be appointed by the traditional leader in Council from among the five community representatives he appoints to the Board
   2. The Secretary–Shall be elected triennially from among the members of the Board. He shall keep the minutes of Board Meetings, conduct Board correspondence, and in consultation with the Chairman, issue the notices calling meetings of the Board; and do all such things as the necessary for the better execution of his office.

C. *General Meetings* the Board shall meet every six months at—Notices, with copies of the agenda prepared in consultation with the Medical Superintendent and Chairmen shall be sent by the Secretary to all members not less than twenty-one days before the date for which the meeting was called.

Emergency Meeting of the board may be called at the request of the Chairman and Secretary, or at the written request of five members of the Board. Notice of Emergency meeting with the business to be considered, shall be delivered by hand to all members not less than five days before the date for which the meeting is called. Decisions taken shall be subject to approval at the next General Meeting.

D. *Quorum* six members shall form a quorum at a General Meeting for the purpose of transacting business.

E. *Functions*
1. Control and define the general policy of the hospital.
2. Accept and adopt the Annual Statement of Accounts, and the Budget.
3. Appoint the Auditors
4. Receive the Annual Report from the Medical Superintendent
5. Appoint the Hospital Officers–the Medical Superintendent, the Matron and the Hospital Secretary.
6. Approve the appointment of Senior Staff and confirm their dismssal.
7. Appoint the Executive Committee consisting the Chairman, the three Hospital Officer, and two others to hear, and to act on urgent matters between the Board meetings.

On Establishment, the Executive shall:
- determine the fixed establishment, and review as necessary
- consider rates of pay and conditions of service, and make recommendations to the Board
- appoint senior staff, subject top confirmation by the Board, and del with all other staff matters.

On Finance, the Executive shall:
- authorise the opening of bank accounts in the name of the Hospital
- examine the Annual Statement of Accounts and Budget, and Auditor's Report, and make recommendations to the Board
- examine tenders for capital works approved by the Board, and award contracts.

8. Appoint other such committees as may be necessary for the good management of the Hospital, and determine the terms of reference.
9. Have power to recommend amendments to this Constition. These shall be tabled at the Meeting, but no voted on till the next. A three-fourths majority of the members present and voting shall be necessary to confirm the amendment.

Bye-Laws

1. The Officers of the Hospital shall have the following responsibilities:

a. *Medical Director/Hospital Administrator* He shall be person with registrable medical qualifications, and appropriate experience. He shall be the Executive Head of the Hospital, and shall see to its efficient and satisfactory administration. He shall, however, delegate the duties specified which fall within other departments.
- He shall be the recognised correspondent for the hospital on all official matters.
- He shall be responsible for the admission, proper treatment and discharge of all patients.
- He shall make recommendations to the Executive and/or board for all matters to do with Senior Staff, other than those of the nursing service.
- He shall appoint or dismiss any employee.
- He shall commence, carry on or defend all actions and proceedings concerning the Hospital.

b. *Nursing Superintendent* The Matron shall be a persons with registrable nursing and midwifere qualification. In consultation with the Hospital Administrator shall be responsible for the satisfactory administration of the Nursing Services in the Hospital.
- She shall be the recognised correspondent with official bodies on matters concerning the Nursing Service.
- She shall in consultation with the Medical Superintendent, make recommendations to the Executive and/or the Board for all matters to do with qualified staff of the Nursing Services.
- She shall be responsible for the discipline and care of the nurses, and all auxillary staff attached to the Nursing Service, including maids and cleaners.
- She shall be responsible for the general cleanliness of the hospital, and for the care of linen and nursing supplies.

c. *Hospital Secretary* He shall be a person with a training in administration (or accounting), and suitable experience.

- He shall be in consultation with the Medical Superintendent, be responsible for the general and financial administration of the Hospital, and will see that proper accounts of the hospital money are maintained.
- He will be responsible for the ordering of supplies, other than drugs ordered by the Pharmacy section.
- The maintenance staff shall be responsible to him for the maintenance and repair of the buildings, equipment and vehicles, and for the general up keep of the hospital and grounds.
- He shall in consultation with the Medical Superintendent, appoint junior clearical and labour staff, and in consultation with the appropriate head of the section, junior technical staff.
- He shall conduct such correspondences as the Medical Superintendent may assign him.

2. *Voting* Subject to the exception noted below:
   - each member of the Board shall have one vote.
   - the Chairman shall exercise his vote with the other members' voting.
   - in case of a tie vote the motion is lost.
   - there shall be no voting by proxy.

   Exception

   The Hospital Officers on the Board shall not vote on any matter concerning appointment or dismissal of Hospital Officer. When the status, salary and allowines or personal conduct, of a Hospital Officer comes up for discussion, the Officer shall privileged to make a statement concerning the matter, and the shall withdraw.
3. *Quorum* Unless otherwise stated then not less than half the members of any commodities or subcommittees in the Hospital shall from a quorum for the purpose of transcting business.
4. *Absentee members* If a member of the Board fails to attend three consecutive meetings without reasonable excuse, a replacement shall be called for.
5. *Right of approval* Any member of the Senior Staff shall have the right of appeal to the Hospital Management Board against any decision of the Hospital Officers taking against them Junior staff shall be right of appeal to the Executive.

Appendix–2

GENERAL EVALUATION AND CHECKLIST FOR ANY EXISTING BUILDING

This checklist is applicable to any building, either a health care facility or a building being converted to a health care facility.

Basic Structure Type ______

Materials

Concrete ______

Steel (fireproffed) ______

Wood ______

Exterior Finish ______

Roof construction ______

Window Type(s) ______

Special Features ______

______

Basic Size and Shape ______

Height ______

No. of stories:

Above grade ______

Below grade ______

Zoning

Frontyard setback ______

Rearyard setback ______

Left side yardback ______

Right side yard setback ______

Utilities

Water, domestic ______

Water, fire ______

Building connection ______

Sewer, sanitary ______

Electric ______

Gas ______

Telephone ______

Television ______

Alams ______

Parking

Normal (patients, staff visitors) ______

Handicapped ______

Emergency ______

Lighting ______

Accesss ______

Description of Terrain (trees, shrubs, grade) ______

______

______

Interior Egrees (describe how)

Corridor ______

Exit doors ______

Ramps ______

Stairs ______

Rating or Fire-resistance Level of Exits ______

______

______

Handicapped: conditions of Exit and Access ______

______

______

Fire Alarms

Audible

Parking ______

Normal (patients, staff visitors) ____________

Handicapped ____________

Emergency ____________

Lighting ____________

Access ____________

Visual

Smoke Alarms ____________

Heat Detectors ____________

Tied to fire alarm system? ____________

Sprinkles ____________

Standpipes ____________

Pull Stations ____________

Within 5 feet of exits? ____________

Roof Access (for fire department) ____________

Fire Fighting Equipment ____________

____

Interior Partitions (describe for each area)

Corridors ____________

Rooms ____________

Public Facilities ____________

Stairs ____________

Shafts ____________

Note: Include floor, walls, base, dado and ceilings

Heating, Ventilating, and Air Conditioning System(s) [Describe, indicating existence of fire and smoke dampers]

____

Plumbing (Describe, including gas) ____________

____

Electric (describe) ____________

____

Emergency Generator(s) [describe, including size and capacity] ____________

____

Emergency Lighting (describe)

On generator(s) ____________

On battery (ies) ____________

Low-voltage System(s): Intercom, Music, Paging, Closed-circuit Television, Radio (Describe) ____________

____

Basic Service Company (name, teletphone number, contact

____

Goods Receiving Area

Doors: height ____________

Door Size ____________

Turnaround for large trucks ____________

Parking for sales people ____________

Separate road access and exit ____________

____

Fuel receiving ______

Trash removal ______

Laundry ______

Food ______

Medical goods ______

Gas (Propane, oxygen, etc.) ______

General goods ______

Storage space ______

Offices ______

Incrating ans sorting ______

Workshops

Carpentry ______

HVAC ______

Plumbing ______

Electric ______

Engineering

Offices (including toilets, showers, and lockers) ______

______

Mechanical spaces ______

______

General Condition of Existing Building(s): [describe, indicating any deterioration, such as leaky roof, cracked concrete, trim rot, extreme interior wear particularly floor, doors, walls), or remedial work needed, such as on brick pointing, windows, door weather stripping] ______

______

______

______

______

______

Appendix–3

FIRE SAFETY IN HOSPITALS

	Meetings the requirements		*Not applicable*
	Yes	*No*	
I. **Facility Fire Protection**			
A. Location of building			
1. Adjacent buildings' hazard levels (state building codes)			
2. Fire exposure			
B. Area around building			
1. Bulk storage of flammable gases			
2. Bulk storage of flammable liquids			
3. Bulk storage non-flammable (oxidizing) gases			
4. Bulk of non-flammable (oxidizing) liquids			
5. External water supplies (tanks) for fire protection			
6. Hydrants			
7. Incinerators/compactors			
8. Fire lanes			
9. Parking gases			
C. Structural protection			
1. Chimneys, fireplaces, etc.			
2. Flame spread of finish materials			
3. Floor-ceilling assemblies			
4. General construction protection (building codes)			
5. Laboratories in health care facilities (HPC)			
6. Lightning protection			
7. Rooftop heliport			
8. Separation of mixed occupancies			
9. Solid-fuel-burning appliances			
10. Walls			
11. Windows and doors			

D. Life safety considerations
   1. Building services
   2. Construction features
   3. Exit access/exists/exists discharge
   4. Fire protection
   5. General health care requirements)
   6. Handicapped provision (each state, either in the building code or separate iegislation)
   7. High-risk consideration
   8. Laboratories in HCF
   9. Operating features

E. Detection/Extinguishment system
   1. Detection systems
   2. Extinguishment system

F. Other fire protection equipment
   1. Fire pumps
   2. Houses

G. Fixed building-wide service system
   1. Fuels for heating system
      Bases
      Liquids
   2. Heaters
      Gas
      Oil
   3. Air movement/restrictions (fire and smoke dampers)
   4. Electrical Service Normal
   5. Specific building services
      Chutes (waste, linen, etc.)
      Elevation/escalators
      Fans
      Piped gas systems (flammable)
      Piped gas systems (non-flammable)
      Piped gas systems (labs, HCF)
      Piped gas systems (non-HCF labs)
      Piped vacuum systems (med-surg)

H. Fixed, loccalized system
   1. Storage areas
      Flammable liquids

Gases	______	______	______
General	______	______	______
Historical data	______	______	______
Identifying hazard level	______	______	______
Nuclear material	______	______	______
Rack	______	______	______
2. For anesthetizing locations	______	______	______
3. For other patient care areas	______	______	______
4. For laboratories in HCF	______	______	______
5. For compactors	______	______	______
6. For computer areas	______	______	______
7. For kitchens	______	______	______
8. For hyperbarbaric facilities	______	______	______

II. **Operation Fire Protection**

A. Systems and their maintenance

1. Automatic fire detectors	______	______	______
2. Emergency electric power systems	______	______	______
3. Normal electric power systems (patient care areas)	______	______	______
4. Other extinghishing systems	______	______	______
5. Piped gas systems	______	______	______
6. Piped vacuum systems (med-surg)	______	______	______
7. Signal systems (for detector)	______	______	______
8. Sprinkler systems	______	______	______

B. Other fire protection equipment

1. Fire houses	______	______	______
2. Fire pumps	______	______	______
3. Portable fire extinguishers	______	______	______
C. Employees safety-electrical	______	______	______
D. Response to disasters (internal and external)	______	______	______

Index

G

H